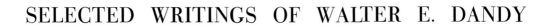

SELECTED WRITINGS OF WALTER E. DANDY

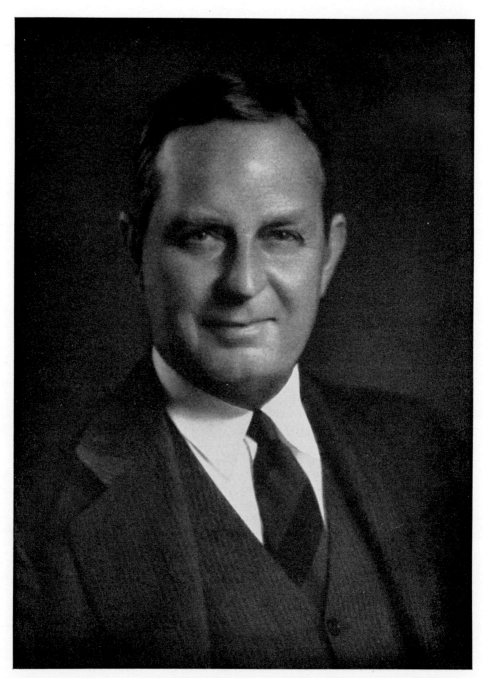

WALTER E. DANDY

Selected

Writings

of

WALTER E. DANDY

Compiled

by

Charles E.
Troland, M. D.

and

Frank J.
Otenasek, M. D.

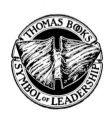

CHARLES C THOMAS · PUBLISHER
Springfield · Illinois · USA

CHARLES C THOMAS · PUBLISHER

BANNERSTONE HOUSE

301-327 East Lawrence Avenue, Springfield, Illinois, U.S.A.

Published simultaneously in the British Commonwealth of Nations by

BLACKWELL SCIENTIFIC PUBLICATIONS, LTD., OXFORD, ENGLAND

Published simultaneously in Canada by

THE RYERSON PRESS, TORONTO

Library of Congress Catalog Card Number: 57-5607

Printed in the United States of America

CONTENTS

Chapter   *Page*

1. The Blood Supply of the Pituitary Body 3
2. The Nerve Supply to the Pituitary Body 9
3. An Experimental and Clinical Study of Internal Hydrocephalus 14
4. Extirpation of the Pineal Body 18
5. Internal Hydrocephalus 25
6. Ventriculography Following the Injection of Air into the Cerebral Ventricles .. 39
7. Extirpation of the Choroid Plexus of the Lateral Ventricles in
    Communicating Hydrocephalus 45
8. Rontgenography of the Brain after the Injection of Air into the Spinal Canal .. 55
9. Localization or Elimination of Cerebral Tumors by Ventriculography 61
10. The Diagnosis and Treatment of Hydrocephalus Resulting from Strictures
    of the Aqueduct of Sylvius 73
11. The Diagnosis and Treatment of Hydrocephalus Due to Occlusions of the
    Foramina of Magendie and Luschka 89
12. The Cause of So-called Idiopathic Hydrocephalus 101
13. An Operation for the Removal of Pineal Tumors 117
14. Prechiasmal Intracranial Tumors of the Optic Nerves 124
15. An Operation for the Total Extirpation of Tumors in the Cerebello-pontine
    Angle. A Preliminary Report 138
16. A Method for the Localization of Brain Tumors in Comatose Patients 139
17. The Diagnosis and Localization of Spinal Cord Tumors 155
18. Studies in Experimental Epilepsy 179
19. Section of the Sensory Root of the Trigeminal Nerve at the Pons 188
20. Studies on Experimental Hypophysectomy 190
21. An Operation for the Total Removal of Cerebellopontile (Acoustic) Tumors .. 198
22. Intracranial Tumors and Abscesses Causing Communicating Hydrocephalus ... 219
23. Pneumocephalus (Intracranial Pneumatocele of Aerocele) 226
24. Abscesses and Inflammatory Tumors in the Spinal Epidural Space (So-called
    Pachymeningitis Externa) 246
25. A Sign and Symptom of Spinal Cord Tumors 260
26. Treatment of Chronic Abscess of the Brain by Tapping 265
27. Glossopharyngeal Neuralgia (Tic Douloureux) 267
28. Removal of Right Cerebral Hemisphere for Certain Tumors with Hemiplegia .. 277
29. Meniere's Disease 281
30. Arteriovenous Aneurysm of the Brain 301
31. Venous Abnormalities and Angiomas of the Brain 333
32. An Operation for the Cure of Tic Douloureux 378
33. Where is Cerebrospinal Fluid Absorbed? 409

CONTENTS

Chapter   *Page*

34. Operative Relief from Pain in Lesions of the Mouth, Tongue and Throat 412
35. An Operative Treatment for Certain Cases of Meningocele (or Encephalocele) into the Orbit 416
36. Loose Cartilage from Intervertebral Disk Simulating Tumor of the Spinal Cord 420
37. An Operation for the Treatment of Spasmodic Torticollis 428
38. Changes in Our Conceptions of Localization of Certain Functions in the Brain 437
39. The Course of the Nerve Fibers Transmitting Sensation of Taste 438
40. Congenital Cerebral Cysts of the Cavum Septi Pellucidi (Fifth Ventricle) and Cavum Vergae (Sixth Ventricle) 467
41. Effects of Total Removal of Left Temporal Lobe in a Right-handed Person: Localization of Areas of Brain Concerned with Speech 480
42. Physiological Studies Following Extirpation of the Right Cerebral Hemisphere in Man 484
43. Treatment of Meniere's Disease by Section of Only the Vestibular Portion of the Acoustic Nerve 497
44. Benign Encapsulated Tumors in the Lateral Ventricles of the Brain: Diagnosis and Treatment 500
45. Cerebral (Ventricular) Hydrodynamic Test for Thrombosis of the Lateral Sinus 503
46. The Effect of Hemisection of the Cochlear Branch of the Human Auditory Nerve. Preliminary Report 509
47. Removal of Cerebellopontile (Acoustic) Tumors Through a Unilateral Approach 512
48. The Treatment of So-called Pseudo-Meniere's Disease 516
49. The Treatment of Carotid Cavernous Arteriovenous Aneurysms 521
50. The Treatment of Bilateral Meniere's Disease and Pseudo-Meniere's Disease ... 523
51. Polyuria and Polydipsia (Diabetes Insipidus) and Glycosuria Resulting from Animal Experiments on the Hypophysis and its Environs 526
52. Operative Experience in Cases of Pineal Tumor 533
53. Etiological and Clinical Types of So-called Nerve Deafness 547
54. Intracranial Pressure Without Brain Tumor 549
55. Studies on Experimental Hypophysectomy in Dogs 568
56. Intracranial Aneurysm of the Internal Carotid Artery 581
57. The Operative Treatment of Communicating Hydrocephalus 584
58. Subdural Hematoma 590
59. The Treatment of Internal Carotid Aneurysms Within the Cavernous Sinus and the Cranial Chamber 613
60. Papilledema Without Intracranial Pressure (Optic Neuritis) 628
61. The Central Connections of the Vestivular Pathways 634

Chapter   *Page*

62. Intracranial Aneurysms 639

63. Section of the Human Hypophysial Stalk 641

64. Removal of Longitudinal Sinus Involved in Tumors 646

65. Results Following the Transcranial Operative Attack on Orbital Tumors 653

66. On the Pathology of Carotid-Cavernous Aneurysms (Pulsating Exophthalmos) 667

67. The Surgical Treatment of Intracranial Aneurysms of the Internal Carotid Artery 682

68. Serious Complications of Ruptured Intervertebral Disks 685

69. Aneurysm of the Anterior Cerebral Artery 692

70. Intracranial Arterial Aneurysms in the Carotid Canal 694

71. Results Following Ligation of the Internal Carotid Artery 706

72. Newer Aspects of Ruptured Intervertebral Disks 715

73. Pathogenesis of Intermittent Exophthalmos 718

74. Treatment of Rhinorrhea and Otorrhea 729

75. Diagnosis and Treatment of Strictures of the Aqueduct of Sylvius (Causing Hydrocephalus) 740

76. Arteriovenous Aneurysms of the Scalp and Face 750

77. Results Following Bands and Ligatures on the Human Internal Carotid Artery 767

78. The Location of the Conscious Center in the Brain—The Corpus Striatum 776

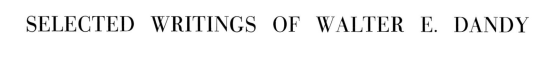

SELECTED WRITINGS OF WALTER E. DANDY

This volume is dedicated to the memory of Doctor Walter E. Dandy, a pioneer and most gifted neurosurgeon. The funds for its publication have been donated by his immediate family, some of his residents and friends.

I

THE BLOOD SUPPLY OF THE PITUITARY BODY*

WALTER E. DANDY, M.D. AND EMIL GOETSCH

INTRODUCTION

Studies made in the Hunterian Laboratory[1] by Reford, Crowe, Homans, Goetsch and Cushing, based upon a series of over two hundred canine and feline hypophysectomies, have supported Paulesco's view that a fragment of the pars anterior is essential to the maintenance of life, a total hypophysectomy being invariably fatal in the course of a few days, the length of survival depending somewhat upon the age of the animal. During the course of these investigations it was found that the gland could be separated from its dural pocket and left dangling by the stalk alone without destroying its vitality. Division or ligation of the stalk, on the other hand, often led to profound histological alterations, evidently due to an anaemic necrosis confined largely to the centre of the anterior lobe. It had been suggested by Paulesco that stalk separation is equivalent to a total hypophysectomy, presumably as a result of such necrosis; and the experiences in this laboratory tended at first to confirm this view. Later observations, however, have shown that although stalk separation will often lead to a certain degree of central necrosis of the pars anterior, total isolation of the gland, not only from the infundibulum but from its dural attachments as well, is necessary before the procedure becomes equivalent to a total removal; and even in this case fragments of the structure, thus isolated, may under favorable circumstances become revascularized in part, the operation therefore being comparable to a total homo-transplantation of the gland into the tissues elsewhere.

More complete information in regard to the sources of the glandular blood supply has become essential to a better understanding of these operative experiences, and at the suggestion of Dr. Cushing these studies have been made with this end in view.

The present paper deals with the mammalian circulation as observed in the dog — the animal employed for most of the experimental studies. It is presumable that the findings apply as well to man, but we have had no suitable opportunity for a proper injection of the human gland.

PRIOR DESCRIPTION OF THE CIRCULATION

The first mention in the literature of the pituitary circulation is an incidental reference by Duret ('72) in his classical work upon the blood supply of the brain in general. He refers to a small bilateral branch which passes from the posterior communicating artery to the infundibular wall. Heubner, two years later, made a similar reference.

From the time of these casual comments, although it was generally appreciated that the anterior lobe was a very vascular organ and contained peculiar sinusoidal spaces, the subject has been given little attention, until Herring's recent excellent and concise description of the internal circulation of the cat's hypophysis.[2] Herring was the first to show that the anterior and posterior lobes possess independent blood supplies, the former coming down through the stalk, the latter entering the posterior lobe from behind. No comment was made, however, on the origin of these vessels. Substantially

*Reprinted from *The American Journal of Anatomy*, *11:* 2, January, 1911.

the same results were obtained a few years ago by Dr. G. J. Heuer in unpublished studies carried on independently in this laboratory.

Our observations, as will be seen, entirely confirm the views of Herring upon the general plan of the gland's internal ciculation, but especial emphasis is placed upon the grosser circulation, in view of its experimental and surgical importance.

MATERIAL AND METHODS

Immediately after death the animals were injected headward through both common carotid arteries, during which process the principal veins of the neck were ligated or a tourniquet applied to obstruct the venous return of the injection mass. Of the numerous colored masses, we have derived the best results from a 10 per cent gelatin mass with carmine or vermillion for the veins and capillaries, and Prussian blue or ultramarine for the arteries. Satisfactory injections may be obtained by following a primary carmine injection by one of Prussian blue, a double injection being obtained — the veins red and the arteries blue — since the larger granules of the blue mass are unable to pass through the capillaries.

Carmine gelatin, although the best general injection mass, is a very capricious substance, requiring careful preparation, for if too alkaline it diffuses through the vessel wall, or if too acid it precipitates. We are indebted to Dr. M. J. Burrows of the Rockefeller Institute for the benefit of his experience in the rather elaborate preparation of this mass.

To secure an injection of the venous supply alone, Prussian blue was injected headwards into the internal jugular vein, there being no valves in the canine jugular to prevent the reversed stream from reaching the intracranial veins and venous sinuses. After the gelatin had been hardened by cooling, a block of tissue containing the hypophysis and its meningeal envelopes intact was carefully removed, preserved in glycerine or creosote, and either studied by the aid of the binocular after clearing, or fixed and sectioned for microscopical study.

GENERAL CONSIDERATION OF THE CIRCULATION

The blood supply of the hypophysis is so abundant as to seem, were it actually an unimportant gland, more than commensurate with its functional needs and the possibility of harm from vascular disturbances.

Situated in the centre of the circle of Willis, it receives the first installments of blood to the brain, its numerous vessels converging from all parts of the circle like spokes to the hub of a wheel, while the venous outflow is equally abundant and the vessels similarly disposed.

There are three fairly independent circulations to the subdivisions of the gland in correspondence with their structural independence: (1) The supply to the anterior and intermediate lobes: (2) to the posterior lobe; and (3) to a structure which has been discovered during the course of these investigations and which we shall designate the "parahypophysis."

Vessels of the Anterior Lobe

The anterior lobe receives its blood supply from numerous small arteries which converge toward the stalk of the hypophysis. The great majority of these vessels arise from the anterior half of the circle of Willis. Thus the anterior communicating artery, which is usually small in the dog, sends off from eight to ten small branches in its course across the optic chiasm; and each posterior communicating artery sends off from three to five more. Futhermore, a pair of vessels on each side is given off by internal carotid artery, immediately before its trifurcation into the anterior, the middle cerebral and the posterior communicating arteries. Thus, all told, from eighteen to twenty or even more separate small vessels, barely visible to the unaided eye, converge directly toward the infundibular stalk. In addition other vessels from the posterior half of the circle of Willis stream in a fine network over the corpora mamillaria and converge toward the posterior surface of the infundibulum. Upon reaching the stalk these vessels immediately subdivide into capillaries which empty into the dilated channels of the anterior lobe. These channels are lined merely by a single layer of endothelial cells which lie directly in contact with the anterior lobe cells. The sinusoidal spaces are so numerous and so large as to make the anterior lobe one of the most vascular structures of the body, comprising as they do a large part of the volume of the gland. Inasmuch as the anterior lobe contains no arteries or veins, arterial injections, owing to the large size of the granules, tend to stop at the capillaries of the stalk of the hypophysis.

The injected hypophysis, viewed in the gross by the aid of the binocular, shows numerous parallel longitudinal channels uniformly distributed throughout the gland and varying slightly in size. These are evidently the main channels, from which smaller ones are redistributed, although histologically all have the same single endothelial lining. There is, however, no very great difference in their size, although in specimens injected under a relatively high pressure it is often possible to see vary large spaces, out of proportion to the surrounding channels, owing to the irregular disposition of the injection mass.

The venous return from the anterior lobe is very similar in arrangement to the arterial inflow. These channels reform into capillaries and, very soon, into numerous small veins in the stalk, from which the collecting vessels radiate to the basilar circle of veins which overlies but has an arrangement very similar to the arterial circle of Willis. There are six or seven of these relatively large collecting trunks, which pass laterally and singly into the basilar veins lying deep under the temporal lobe, and thence upward around the crura cerebri to discharge into the venae magnae Galeni. There is also a network of venules which emerge from the posterior part of the stalk and pass over the Corpora mam-

illaria, ending in several veins that empty into a transverse connection between the basilar veins which forms the posterior arc of the Willisian venous circle.

Vessels of the Pars Intermedia

Certain portions of the pars intermedia are also very vascular — much more vascular than the posterior lobe, though less so than the anterior. It derives its circulation from three sources. The thicker, tongue-like portion near the stalk, which is more or less merged with the upper part of the anterior lobe, receives its blood from the vessels of the stalk and from others which cross from the brain substance immediately adjacent. The thin epithelial investment of the pars nervosa, on the other hand, is entirely devoid of vessels, as Herring states. The abundant capillary network, which intervenes between these two histologically different structures constituting the posterior lobe, does not penetrate into the layers of the investing cells. The capillaries of the vascularized tongue of pars intermedia, however, are in immediate contact with the base of the cells and follow their villous formations. From these capillary beds of pars nervosa there are two possible ways of escape for the blood — upward into the veins of the stalk and base of the brain, and backward into the veins of the pars nervosa and thence into the circular sinus by the vascular system which remains to be described.

Vessels of the Posterior Lobe

The posterior lobe is the least vascular of the anatomical subdivisions of the hypophysis. This is very easily recognized in the fresh uninjected specimen, the anterior lobe appearing a pinkish-yellow color in marked contrast to the glistening and whiter posterior lobe. Injected specimens naturally bring out this contrast much more strikingly.

The circulation of the posterior lobe enters the gland at the posterior pole of the pars nervosa and is entirely independent of the systems heretofore described.

Each internal carotid shortly after it enters the cranial chamber and turns forward in the carotid groove, gives off a small branch; these two vessels unite in front of the posterior clinoid process to form the single median trunk which enters the hypophyseal posterior lobe at the point where a small area of firm dural attachment is appreciable in the usual dissection to liberate the gland. It is well to bear in mind that these branches of the carotid lie between the two layers of dura forming the circular sinus, and therefore really in a sense lie in this sinus, just as the internal carotid itself lies in the lateral sinus.

The artery enters the posterior lobe near its centre dividing immediately into numerous large branches which stream outward toward the periphery. There is, however, no marked difference in the inherent vascularity of any part of the posterior lobe until the capillary bed is reached at the extreme periphery under the epithelial investment.

The veins collect the blood and pass to the point of dural attachment in much the same arrangement as the arteries. A single large central vein enters the circular sinus at this point (cf. fig. 3, m. v.) immediately above the entrance of the artery, the two being closely adjacent. In addition, there are other smaller veins which empty independently into the sinus.

Collateral Circulation

Although the anterior and posterior lobes have independent blood supplies, the question arises as to the possible vascular communication between structures so intimately related. Is the collateral circulation sufficient to preserve the glandular function in case of occlusion of the blood supply to one or another of the anatomical subdivisions of the gland? Is separation of the vessels of the stalk equivalent to a transplantation of the anterior lobe? There is doubtless some collateral circulation between the anterior and posterior lobes through the pars intermedia as mentioned above — namely, at the relatively narrow area of pars intermedia above the cleft, which elsewhere prevents contiguity of pars anterior and pars posterior. Histologically we should judge that this would be sufficient, especially in view of the small fragment of anterior lobe which apparently will suffice for the preservation of life.

Naturally the final test of the practical efficiency of this collateral must be determined by experimental operative methods. Paulesco records cases of stalk separation which caused consequent degeneration of the anterior lobe cells. One must, however, be certain that this small collateral area of pars intermedia has not also been destroyed by the operative manipulations, thereby preventing the possibility of preservation by collateral.

In a few operations on dogs by one of us (Goetsch), in which the blood supply through the stalk was interrupted by the placement of a silver wire "clip" (equivalent to the ligation of the stalk), no evidences of physiological deficiency or histological degeneration of anterior lobe cells were observed.

In one of Dr. Cushing's hypophyseal operations for acromegaly by a transphenoidal route it was intended merely to remove the floor of the sella turcia and to freely incise the dural pocket enclosing the greatly enlarged gland, in the hope of thus relieving the neighborhood symptoms. A fragment of the exposed anterior lobe was removed for examination, and during the necessary manipulations the gland was broken from its stalk and there was a gush of cerebrospinal fluid, much as in an experimental canine hypophysectomy when the gland is detached from its infundibular connections. The patient died in forty-eight hours with symptoms comparable to those seen in animals after a total hypophysectomy; and post-mortem hostological studies showed an anemic necrosis involving practically the entire pars anterior, whereas the pars nervosa and its epithelial covering (pars intermedia) remained normal in appearance, its individual and isolated blood supply having been remote from possible operative injury.

The Circulation of the "Parahypophysis"

As has been stated in discussing methods, after the injections were made a block of tissue containing the gland within its intact meningeal envelopes was removed and cleared in glycerine. On examining the base of the cleared specimen with the binocular dissecting microscope, a minute button-like structure was seen lying below the mid-point of the gland and between the two layers of the dura which originally lined the base of the sella turcia. This structure had been previously observed in a number of the serial longitudinal sections which had been made as a routine after all of the experimental hypophysectomies. No especial importance had been attached to it and it naturally had escaped histological observation in all of the cases in which the dura had not been removed and sectioned together with the gland. It is an epithelial body and appears to be an organ which is invariably present and one which may have some physiological significance. It contains under normal conditions none of the typical anterior lobe (eosinophilic) cells. A minute median pit in which the body rests is usually discernable in the centre of the sella turcia after the removal of its lining dura.

This epithelial body has a separate circulation distinct from the others which have been described. The arterial supply seems to be of two-fold origin. A minute artery enters the gland posteriorly, and by reconstruction of two specimens its origin can be traced by a relatively long intradural course to each posterior lobe artery, the two uniting into a single trunk before reaching the parahypophysis. Moreover the small intradural branch from each internal carotid artery gives an additional bilateral arterial supply. A single small vein apparently passes into the bone at the situation of the above mentioned pit, though it is probable that there may also be a connection in the dura with the network of venous channels, which are somewhat radially arranged around the parahypophysis. This structure therefore should retain its circulation intact in procedures similar to the experimental hypophysectomies in which the gland is removed by an operation conducted from under the temporal lobe. It would be the first to suffer in all operations such as those which have been employed in man in which the gland is approached from below through the sphenoidal cells.

SUMMARY

The anterior lobe receives its blood supply from about eighteen or twenty small arteries which converge toward the stalk from the various components of the circle of Willis. These vessels immediately break up into numerous large sinusoidal channels, in apposition with the cells and lined only by endothelium. Hence, there are no veins or arteries proper in the anterior lobe. The venous supply is very similar in arrangement to the arterial system; the veins passing from the stalk to a venous circle immediately overlying the circle of Willis and draining into the vanae magnae Galeni.

The pars intermedia derives its supply from the vessels of the stalk, from the posterior lobe. A collateral therefore exists at this point between the anterior and posterior lobes, probably sufficient to preserve the function of at least the adjoining portion of either lobe if its individual supply is cut off.

The posterior lobe receives its arterial supply from a small artery found by the union of a symmetrical branch from each internal carotid. One large vein and other small ones enter the circular sinus immediately above the artery.

The "parahypophysis" has an individual blood supply of two-fold origin; a posterior vessel from the union of two branches from the posterior lobe arteries and a bilateral branch from the internal carotid arteries.

In concluding, it is a pleasure to express our gratitude to Dr. Harvey Cushing for his suggestions during the course of the work.

REFERENCES

[1] 1. Is the pituary gland essential to the maintenance of life? *The Johns Hopkins Hosp. Bull.*, 1909, 20, no. 217.

2. The hypophysis cerebri: clinical aspects of hyperpituitarism and of hypopituitarism. *J. A. M. A.*, 53: 249, 1909.

3. Effects of hypophyseal transplantation following total hypophysectomy in the canine. *Quart. J. Exper. Physiol.*, 2: 389, 1909.

4. The functions of the pituitary body. *Am. J. Med. Sc.*, 1910.

5. Experimental hypophysectomy. *The Johns Hopkins Hosp. Bull.*, 21: 127, 1910.

6. Concerning the secretion of the infundibular lobe of the pituitary body and its presence in the cerebrospinal fluid. *Am. J. Physiol.*, 27: 60, 1910.

[2] Herring, P. T. The histological appearances of the mammalian pituitary body. *Quarterly J. Exper. Physiol.*, i: 154, 1908. In this article Herring gives an excellent photograph (Fig. 16, p. 154) of the injected feline hypophysis, which shows unusually well the relatively greater vascularity of the anterior lobe. This condition is rarely and with difficulty brought out by a simple arterial injection, which usually shows little more than in our Figure 4.

II

THE NERVE SUPPLY TO THE PITUITARY BODY*

It is but natural that neglect of an organ itself should yield a proportional lack of interest in its more detailed structure and even more so, in its less important adjuncts —the blood and nerve supply. Such has been true of the pituitary body.

The recent tremendous stimulus produced by Paulesco's[1] sudden transformation of the hypophysis from a structure of vestigial curiosity to a vitally essential organ, has borne its fruit in the rapid accumulation of co-working histological,[2] experimental[3 4 5 6] and clinical[7 8] observations. Though still very meager our information is now sufficient to have established a hypophyseal clinical entity, amenable in many cases to medical and surgical treatment.

Forming as it does a link in the chain of internal secreting glands, the hypophysis, essentially of hormone action, must be regulated as other glands in this system, by an autonomic nervous mechanism.

Recent studies from the Hunterian Laboratory[5] by Goetsch, Cushing and Jacobson gave evidences of hypophyseal influence over carbohydrate metabolism. It has been shown that sugar tolerance is dependent upon the functional activity of the posterior lobe of the pituitary body. It was later shown by Dandy and Fitz Simmons (observations unpublished) that a piqure of the hypophyseal region in rabbits produced a heavy glycosuria, therefore giving results similar to a piqure of the so-called Bernard's sugar center in the floor of the fourth ventricle. These results have been amplified by Weed, Cushing and Jacobson.[6]

The combination of glandular or hormone activity and the results of mechanical stimuli (presumably of nervous origin) has suggested the possibility of a neurohypophyseal sugar center.

The rational interpretation of this and other physiological data has been handicapped by the uncertainty and meager evidence of the regulatory autonomic nervous mechanism. Accordingly at the suggestion of Dr. Cushing under whose direction the experimental hypophyseal investigations have been conducted, the determination of the source and distribution of the nerve supply was undertaken.

Lying as does the hypophysis in such close proximity to the carotid arteries with their abundant superimposed plexus of sympathetic nerve fibers, it is but natural to assume that this is the source of the hypophyseal nerve supply. Indeed evidence of this is found in the infrequent passing reference to a nerve filament which could be traced from this plexus to the hypophysis.

EARLY REFERENCE TO THE NERVE SUPPLY

Probably the earliest reference to a hypophyseal nerve supply is the casual mention by Bourgery ('45) that he observed sympathetic nerve fibers passing to the pituitary body. Further substantiation is subsequently given in similar casual mention by Fontona, Cloquet, Bock, Ribbes,[9] and possibly others.

In his Anatomie des Menschen ('79) Henle[9] devotes a paragraph to the hypophyseal nerve supply and supplements this description by a drawing of the carotid sympathetic system, which includes a cluster of two or three twigs running from each plexus to the pituitary body. This is the most extensive description of the hypophyseal nerve supply extant. He casts doubt upon the previous discovery of nerve fibers

---

*Reprinted from *The American Journal of Anatomy*, *15:* 3 November, 1913.

to this gland and concludes that on account of the inherent difficulties they have mistaken fibrous filaments of connective tissue for nerve filaments, saying, "Ohne Zweifel beruhen diese und manche ältere Angaben auf Verwechselung fibroser Balkchen mit Nervenfasern, doch zeigte mir das Mikroskop in dem Netzformigen zwischen Carotis und Hypophyse ausgespannten Gewebe feine Nervenfaserbundelchen dieselben, von denen Luschka sagt, dass sie zwei bis drei jederseits, in den vorderen Lappen der Hypophyse sich einsenken." It is based upon this paragraph and drawing by Henle that an occasional brief mention of hypophyseal nerve supply is found in the more detailed and comprehensive anatomies, the majority, however, passing over the matter in silence.

The internal distribution of the hypophyseal nerves was studied by Berkley ('94) [10] in a series of Golgi stained sections. He observed numerous varicose nerve filaments in the interior of the gland, the lobus anterior and pars intermedia in particular, but some also in the posterior lobe. The external connections of the nerves were not studied. On account of his inability to observe nerve cells in the gland, he presumed they were of extraneous origin and thought they probably come from the sympathetic system.

MATERIAL AND METHODS

The purpose of this paper is to consider only the relatively grosser aspects, i.e., the origin, course and distribution of the hypophyseal nerve supply. The histological distribution and relation of the ultimate filaments to the gland cells have not been considered. It is analogous in character to a recent publication[11] dealing with the blood supply of this organ.

The difficulties of deductions and the impossibility of an accurate conception of the nerve supply based upon gross human dissection have been shown (Henle) [9] by the supposedly erroneous observations of early investigators in mistaking connective tissue trabeculae for the very delicate nerve

filaments, which are almost beyond the range of naked vision. These observations are based upon the canine and feline gland, the animals used in the experimental investigations in the Hunterian Laboratory. The anatomical environment of the pituitary body in these forms is such that the difficulties of a tightly enclosed, deeply imbedded and adherent gland encountered in man and the ape are obviated. The hypophysis dangles from the brain and is readily removed with the brain after liberation of its single point of dural attachment posteriorly, so that the entering nerves may be studied in their true relations, without tearing or distortion.

We have used almost exclusively the specific methylene blue intra vitam method of staining the nerves. For the details of this technique we are greatly indebted to the excellent contribution by J. Gordon Wilson.[12] Three essentials are necessary for the successful use of this stain: the exsanguination of the tissues must be thorough in order to get a sharply defined picture of the nerves, since the combination of the methylene blue with blood presents a diffuse, indistinct picture with poorly stained nerves; the nerves must be superficial or covered only by a thin layer of tissue; the air must come in contact with the nerves, otherwise no differentiation takes place.

During the final stages of bleeding the anaesthetized animal from the femoral arteries, a one-twentieth per cent isotonic solution of methylene blue "nach Ehrlich" at body temperature was injected into both carotid arteries and continued until the injecting fluid emanated perfectly clear from the femorals. A tourniquet was then applied around the neck below the point of injection under a pressure sufficiently low to insure filling of the cephalic vessels without danger of diffusion or rupture.

On account of the capricious character of this stain, litters of very young puppies or kittens were injected at the same sitting, so that the defects of some might be supplemented by better staining of others. The total nerve supply then is a summation of results, a reconstruction as it were.

After a few minutes to allow penetration of the stain, the skull was opened and a block of tissue, including the hypophysis with its vessels and nerves in their normal relations, was removed from the base of the brain. The hypophysis was gently retracted so as to allow full exposure of one side to the air. The nerves then assume their differential blue. These specimens were immediately studied under the binocular microscope. The study of fixed specimens with post mortem staining was far less satisfactory, because of the collapse of blood vessels, with which the nerves are intimately associated, the more stiffened picture, and the deficient maintenance of the blue in the nerve fibers.

NERVES TO THE ANTERIOR LOBE

The key to the nerve supply of the pituitary body is the arterial supply to this organ. In a recent publication from this laboratory, it was shown[11] that the anterior lobe received an extensive blood supply from a large number of minute vessels, most of which, even when injected, were beyond the range of naked vision. These vessels radiate from the Willisian circle to the hypophyseal stalk like spokes to the hub of a wheel. The majority of these branches are from the anterior and posterior communicating arteries. The network of sympathetic nerves comprising the carotid plexus is continuous along the three main branches which result from its trifurcation. The distribution, however, is very uneven. A few fibers continue along the anterior and middle cerebral arteries for a short distance but the great majority are found on the two communicating arteries which supply the hypophysis; the posterior communicating artery is particularly well supplied. From these extensions of the carotid plexus numerous filaments are given off and pass along the blood vessels to the stalk of the hypophysis, from which they delve into the substance of the anterior lobe and are lost to view. Some arterial branches have as many as three or even four small filaments, the majority, however, only one or two. The course of the fibers is fairly direct and very few branches are given off. These filaments frequently entwine the vessels but no minute plexuses or anastomoses are visible after leaving the plexus on the main trunks. No nerves have been observed on the external surface of the anterior lobe. All nerves going to the hypophysis are in contact with the sheaths of minute blood vessels. On reaching the stalk it is of course impossible to trace this relation further. Their distribution in the gland has not been observed.

NERVES OF THE PARS INTERMEDIA

Only by dissection of the hypophysis can the nerve supply of the pars intermedia be traced. By gently separating and retracting the posterior lobe from the clasping mitten-like anterior lobe, it is often possible to trace a single nerve fiber with its branches passing down the stalk and spreading out over the pars intermedia which envelops the posterior lobe.

NERVES OF THE POSTERIOR LOBE

It has been shown that the posterior lobe is supplied by a median artery which is formed by the confluence of two branches, one from each carotid artery immediately after its entrance into the cavernous sinus. In the canine this vessel enters the posterior lobe at the only point of dural attachment. Vital nerve staining is somewhat more difficult in this region on account of the relatively thicker dural covering which excludes the action of the air and necessitates a delicate dissection of this vessel. For a long time we were unable to find any trace of a nerve entering the posterior lobe. Several branches were always visible at the origin of the vessels from the carotid but the fibers were lost in the dura before the posterior lobe was reached.

However, it was finally possible to demonstrate nerve fibers actually entering the posterior lobe along the artery. Certainly the disparity between the nerve supply to the posterior and anterior lobes is most striking—in the anterior lobe almost superabundant, in the posterior lobe very few. This contrast may in some measure be due to the difficulties mentioned above; we are however disinclined to lay much emphasis on them.

A most striking color contrast is demonstrated upon removing the hypophysis after vital staining. The anterior lobe is a yellowish white, the posterior a deep indigo blue, possibly due to the (autogenic?) nervous character of the posterior lobe. The blue is of a hemogeneous character, no nerve fibers being differentiable under the higher magnifications of the binocular microscope. The intensity of the blue is even much more marked than that of the adjacent, deeply staining oculomotor nerve.

NERVES OF THE PARAHYPOPHYSIS

This little 'nubbin' resting in a small depression in the floor of the sella, usually enclosed in dura, is present in over 80 per cent of canines, and is evidently a remnant of the embryonic Rathke's pouch. In some adults it may be traced to the pars intermedia; it varies greatly in size and histological character. It has an individual blood supply, a small artery given off by each posterior lobe artery. Frequently it has been possible to trace a nerve some distance along this vessel toward this "body" but never have we been able to observe a definite nerve connection.

OTHER BRANCHES OF THE CAROTID PLEXUS

During observations on the hypophyseal nerve supply naturally the distribution of the sympathetic filaments were noted in the immediate vicinity. The dura of the sella region is exceptionally well supplied with filaments from the carotid plexus. Several branches run from the carotid plexus direct

to the oculomotor nerve. A couple of twigs were also observed entering the optic nerve; these branches were from the nerves in the adventitia of the anterior cerebral artery. There is thus afforded a direct nervous autonomic path between the optic and oculomotor nerves and between these and the sympathetic trunk.

SUMMARY

The nerve supply to the pituitary body is from the carotid plexus of the sympathetic system. Numerous branches radiate to the stalk along the hypophyseal vessels and are immediately lost to view in the substance of the anterior lobe.

The posterior lobe nerve supply is very scant, in marked contrast to the extensive innervation of the anterior lobe.

The pars intermedia receives its nerves from the stalk.

There is connection between the carotid sympathetic system and the oculomotor and optic nerves.

The absolute differentiation between secretory and vasomotor nerves is of course a matter of much dispute and is impossible. The impression, however, from the character and course of the nerve fibers their greatly increased number in the region of the hypophysis, and their disappearance at a distance from the hypophysis, the differences between the supply of the anterior and posterior lobes, the connections established with the other cranial nerves, leads us to regard them as secretory, in contradistinction to vasomotor, the existence of which in the cranial chamber has not been observed.

It is a pleasure to express my gratitude to Dr. Harvey Cushing for his suggestions during the progress of this problem.

REFERENCES

[1]Paulesco, N. C.: *L'hypophyse du cerveau*. Paris, Vigot Freres, 1908.

[2]Herring, P. T.: The histological appearance of the mammalian pituitary body. *Quart. J. Exper. Physiol.*, 1: 121–159, 1908.

[3]Howell, W. H.: The physiological effects of extracts of hypophysis cerebri and infundibular

body. *J. Exper. Med., 3:* 245–258, 1898.

[4]Reford, L. L. and Cushing, H.: Is the pituitary gland essential to the maintenance of life? *Johns Hopkins Hosp. Bull., 20:* 105–107, 1909.

[5]Goetsch, E., Cushing, H. and Jacobson, C.: Carbohydrate tolerance and the posterior lobe of the hypophysis cerebri. *Johns Hopkins Hosp. Bull., 22:* 165–190, 1911.

[6]Weed, L. H., Cushing, H. and Jacobson, C.: Further studies on the role of the hypophysis in the metabolism of carbohydrates. The automatic control of the pituitary gland. *Johns Hopkins Hosp. Bull., 24:* 33, 1913.

[7]Marie, P.: Sur deux cas d'acromegalie; hypertrophie singuliere non congenitale des extremites superieures, inferieures et cephalique. *Rev. de Med., vi:* 297–333, 1886.

[8]Cushing, Harvey: *The Pituitary Body and its Disorders.* Philadelphia, 1912.

[9]Henle: *Anatomie des Menschen,* 3, 1879.

[10]Berkeley, Henry, J.: The finer anatomy of the infundibular region of the cerebrum including the pituitary gland. *Brain, 17:* 575, 1894.

[11]Dandy, Walter E. and Goetsch, Emil: The blood supply of the pituitary body. *Am. J. Anat., 9:* 137, 1911.

[12]Wilson, J. Gordon: Intravitam staining with methylene blue. *Anat. Rec., 4:* 267, 1910.

III

AN EXPERIMENTAL AND CLINICAL STUDY OF INTERNAL HYDROCEPHALUS*

Walter E. Dandy Kenneth D. Blackfan, M.D.

Numerous methods have been suggested for the treatment of internal hydrocephalus, none of which have been productive of satisfactory results. So long as the etiology of this condition remains obscure, the treatment must necessarily be only symptomatic. In the hope of clarifying its etiology and thus affording a rational working basis for its relief, we have undertaken this investigation.

The present communication, which is presented as a preliminary report, includes observations on dogs after the production of experimental hydrocephalus, together with observations on patients suffering from the disease. We have also considered the manner and the place of formation and of absorption of the normal cerebrospinal fluid and the relation of these factors in the production of this pathologic condition.

HYDROCEPHALUS EXPERIMENTALLY PRODUCED

From a survey of the literature we have been unable to find any record of hydrocephalus having been produced experimentally. In our experiments an obstruction has been placed in the aqueduct of Sylvius, and thus the only way of exit for the cerebrospinal fluid from the third and the lateral ventricles has been occluded. An internal hydrocephalus has invariably resulted. The following is the procedure:

A bilateral suboccipital decompression is made through an occipital midline inci-

sion. After exposure of the cerebellum it is retracted upward, and the foramen of Magendie carefully enlarged by incising the membrane joining the cerebellum and medulla. A piece of cotton in a small gelatin capsule, placed on the end of a graduated carrier, is inserted through this enlarged foramen of Magendie and gently passed along the floor of the fourth ventricle into the aqueduct of Sylvius, where it is deposited by withdrawal of the carrier. The symptoms which are observed following the operation are principally lethargy and vomiting (general pressure symptoms) dating from the time of operation. When carefully performed there are no irritative or destructive symptoms from the operation. This hydrocephalus therefore is due to a purely mechanical obstruction in the aqueduct, as there is no interference with the veins of Galen.

Since the venous obstruction is considered a possible cause of hydrocephalus, a series of experiments was conducted in which the vein of Galen and the straight sinus were ligated. In none of these cases did hydrocephalus result.

ABSORPTION OF THE CEREBROSPINAL FLUID

There are many theories concerning the place and manner of the absorption of cerebrospinal fluid. In the study of absorption in the experimental and clinical work we have used almost exclusively phenolsulphonephthalein. This inert colored solution, first introduced into practical medicine as a renal test by Rowntree and Geraghty, has since been shown to be an accurate index of fluid absorption when the

*Reprinted from *The Journal of the American Medical Association, LXI:* 2216 and 2217, Dec. 20, 1913.

renal function is normal. It is very stable, is excreted in the urine with great rapidity, is easily detected in minute traces and is readily adapted to accurate quantitative estimation.[1]

Since an internal hydrocephalus can be experimentally produced by occluding the aqueduct of Sylvius, it is evident that absorption of fluid from the ventricles is less rapid than its production. In the studies of the absorption from the ventricles of patients with an internal hydrocephalus due to obstruction in the aqueduct, after an introduction of phenolsulphonephthalein in the lateral ventricles, there is excreted in the urine from 0.25 to 1 per cent. during a period of two hours; but when it is injected into the subarachnoid space of the same patient there is an excretion of from 35 to 60 per cent. in the urine in the same period of time. This demonstrates that the absorption of cerebrospinal fluid takes place almost entirely in the subarachnoid space.

It is evident that the fluid must be absorbed either into the blood or lymph-vessels. When phenolsulphonephthalein or other inert colored solutions are injected into the subarachnoid space, they appear in the lymph of the thoracic and right lymphatic ducts only after an interval of from thirty to fifty minutes, and only a faint trace is present even after two hours, whereas, they appear in the blood in three minutes and in the urine in six minutes and, as mentioned above, from 35 to 60 per cent. is excreted in the urine at the end of two hours. These facts indicate that the cerebrospinal fluid passes directly into the blood and that the lymph-vessels are not concerned in its absorption. There are three principal views regarding the manner in which the cerebrospinal fluid passes into the blood: (1) by means of stomata arranged along the venous sinuses; (2) through the pacchionian granulations, and (3) by a general process of osmosis.

When a suspension of fine granules is injected into the subarachnoid space the granules do not pass into the blood except in very minute quantities and after a long interval of time. Consequently the assumption of special openings (stomata) from the subarachnoid space into the venous sinuses seems unlikely. This applies to granules injected into the subarachnoid space under normal conditions of pressure. If pressure is used, especially on young tissues, foreign materials can easily be forced into the veins. In adult animals this requires a very high pressure. It should be noted that stomata were formerly believed to exist in the peritoneum to explain the absorption from this cavity, but this has been shown not to be the case.

That the pacchionian granulations do not play any special role in absorption can, we think, also be shown. These granulations are absent in many species of animals, are always variable in number and size and develop principally in adult life. After fine granules are injected into the subarachnoid space, local collections are deposited along the sinuses—especially the superior longitudinal sinus—in the interstices of the fibrous meshwork which forms the walls of the sinuses. These deposits are in all essentials similar to those in the pacchionian granulations. There is always a layer of dura and arachnoid separating these masses of granules from the blood in the veins. This is a much greater mechanical barrier to absorption than is present in the exposed capillaries of the pia-arachnoid.

After the injection of phenolsulphonephthalein into the spinal subarachnoid space (the communication with the cerebral subarachnoid space being closed), there is found to be a quantitative absorption proportionately as great as from the entire subarachnoid space. This shows that the absorption from the spinal subarachnoid space is similar to that from the cerebral. It is obvious, therefore, that cerebrospinal fluid is absorbed by a diffuse process from the entire subarachnoid space and is not restricted to any special locality, as, for instance, the region of the venous sinuses or the pacchionian granulations.

From the foregoing observations, absorption from the subarachnoid space appears to be very similar to that from the pleural and peritoneal cavities, though it is somewhat less rapid.

FORMATION OF THE CEREBROSPINAL FLUID

It has long been known that there is an active formation of cerebrospinal fluid as evidenced by the rapidity with which the fluid reforms after it has been withdrawn either by lumbar or ventricular puncture. The endowment of the chorioid plexus with an elaborate blood-supply indicates that it is a structure with a special function. Since the work of Faivre (1854) and Luschka (1855) showing the secretory character of the cells, the chorioid plexuses have been regarded as glands, from which at least part of the cerebrospinal fluid is formed. The discovery of secretory granules by *intra-vitam* staining by Francini, and also by Bibergeil and Levaditi, leaves but little doubt as to the secretory nature of this function.

We have shown that practically no absorption takes place in the ventricles, at least under the pressure from an abnormal accumulation of fluid. Since this is true and since hydrocephalus results from an experimental block in the aqueduct of Sylvius, it is evident that the fluid forms in the ventricles. These facts demonstrate an irreciprocal permeability of the fluid-forming structures, and emphasizes the secretory rather than the mechanical formation of the cerebrospinal fluid.

OBSERVATIONS ON PATIENTS WITH HYDROCEPHALUS

In these cases we have applied the phenolsulphonephthalein test in order to determine the amount of absorption from the ventricles, the amount of absorption from the subarachnoid spaces and whether or not there was free communication between the ventricles and the subarachnoid spaces. Subsequently the results of these tests have been compared with the pathologic findings. Phenolsulphonephthalein, as has been said before, is perfectly harmless, and when used for injection into the ventricles or subarachnoid spaces produces no reaction.

From observations made on patients without hydrocephalus it has been possible to establish a normal standard for the excretion of phthalein after its injection into one or the other of these cavities. In all cases the kidney function has been shown to be normal. When injected into the ventricles phenolsulphonephthalein normally appears in the urine in from ten to twelve minutes, and after two hours from 12 to 20 per cent. is excreted. After its injection into the subarachnoid space, it appears in the urine in from six to eight minutes, and from 35 to 60 per cent. is excreted in two hours.

When phenolsulphonephthalein is injected into the ventricles, it appears in the lumbar spinal fluid within two or three minutes. In hydrocephalus this becomes a most important test, for it enables one to determine accurately the patency or obstruction of the channels of exit from the ventricles to the subarachnoid space. Furthermore, fluid passes upward into the ventricles after the injection of phenolsulphonephthalein into the lumbar subarachnoid space.

By comparing the results of these tests with those obtained in hydrocephalus, we are enabled to establish two types of this disease. In the first type, after the injection of phenolsulphonephthalein into the ventricles, the time of its appearance in the urine is greatly delayed (from twenty to forty-five minutes) and the quantity excreted in two hours is practically negligible (from 0.25 to 1 per cent.). The excretion of phenolsulphonephthalein in this group after its injection into the subarachnoid space, however, is practically normal (time of appearance from six to eight minutes, quantity excreted in two hours from 35 to 60 per cent.). Furthermore, after the injection of phenolsulphonephthalein into the ventricles, it has not, in the cases observed, appeared in the spinal fluid. In this group, we have found at necropsy an obstruction to the passage of cerebrospinal fluid from the ventricles to the subarachnoid space. In two cases there was a congenital closure of the aqueduct of Sylvius, a third showed old adhesions obliterating the basal foramina of Magendie and Luschka, and in the fourth these foramina were closed by a thick tuberculous exudate which completely covered the base of the brain.

In the second type the excretion of phenolsulphonephthalein after its injection into the subarachnoid space is greatly diminished (from 8 to 15 per cent.), and the appearance time delayed (from twenty to thirty minutes). The amount excreted after its injection into the ventricles likewise is greatly diminished, undoubtedly due to the low subarachnoid absorption. In contradistinction to the first type the communication between the ventricles and the subarachnoid space is open. This is shown by the prompt (from two to three minutes) appearance in the spinal fluid of phenolsulphonephthalein after its injection into the ventricles. We have had the opportunity of examining two patients of this type, but as yet have made no pathologic observations. In both there has been an antecedent history of meningitis, one of which was due to the meningococcus.

These two types of hydrocephalus may be readily differentiated by determining the patency or occlusion of the channels of exit from the ventricles. In Type 1 these channels are obstructed and hydrocephalus results because there is no absorption from the ventricles. In Type 2 the channels are patent and hydrocephalus is due to the diminished absorption from the subarachnoid space.

It is a pleasure to express our gratitude to Professors Halsted, Howland and Cushing for suggestions during the course of the work, and for the opportunity of carrying out these investigations.

REFERENCE

[1] It should be emphasized, however, that ordinary solutions of phenolsulphonephthalein are made up in alkali, which is sufficient to militate against its use in the central nervous system. To overcome this defect we use a neutral solution specially prepared for us by Hynson, Wescott & Co.

IV

EXTIRPATION OF THE PINEAL BODY*

The pineal body until recently has been regarded merely as a very curious vestigial inheritance, serving in the chain of evolution as a reminder of a far distant functioning pineal or central eye. There seems to have been nothing in its macro- or microscopic appearance sufficiently noteworthy to stimulate the especial interest of either anatomists of physiologists. Its inaccessible location has, perhaps, deterred experimenters from undertaking investigations of apparently so little promise.

Tumors of the pineal had not infrequently been reported by pathologists, but there was nothing which seemed significant correlative in the pathological findings and the clinical signs and symptoms. The marvelous story of the thyroid, parathyroids, hypophysis, and adrenals is, no doubt, largely responsible for the recent endeavors to promote the pineal to a position of like importance among the endocrine glands.

In 1898 Heubner[1] presented a case of markedly precocious sexual and less pronouncedly precocious somatic development. The patient was a boy of four and one-half years with pubic hair 1 cm. long, penis and testicles as large as the normal at puberty. The mammae were conspicuous. The body development was equal to that of a boy of eight or nine. He was abnormally fat. A diagnosis of tumor of the hypophysis was made. The following year this case was reported by Oestreich and Slawyk,[2] who found at autopsy a teratoma of the pineal. Almost simultaneously Ogle[3] reported a very similar case, a boy of six years with precocious sexual development. The precocity was principally evidenced by an enlarged penis and the presence of pubic

hair. The testicles were about normal in size. In this instance also a teratoma of the pineal was found post mortem.

Marburg,[4] in 1907, collected from the literature about forty cases of pineal tumor and added a case of his own. Marburg's patient presented no precocity either sexual or somatic; he was merely too fat. Marburg endeavored to establish a pineal clinical entity, and ventured even to pronounce upon the degree, in a given case, of the activity of this gland. He classified all pineal glandular symptoms under the three heads, hypopinealism, hyperpinealism, and apinealism. Hypertrophy of the genitals and precocity were found in hypopinealism, adiposity in hyperpinealism, and cachexia in apinealism.

According to this conception, the pineal and pituitary would seem to have antagonistic activities. Hyperthrophy of the pineal is expected to produce an adiposity indistinguishable from Frohlich's dystrophia adiposogenitalis of hypopituitarism. Atrophy of the pineal would be accompanied by genital and somatic hypertrophy and precocity, whereas acromegaly results from hyperplasia of the pituitary gland. Cachexia is described with both apinealism and apituitarism.

It was Marburg's view that the pineal, normally functioning only during the early years of life, inhibited genital and somatic growth and sexual characteristics, and that its partial destruction by tumors with the resultant hypopinealism permitted, uncontrolled, the development of these features. Consequently, tumors in older youths and adults would not cause sexual abnormalities, because the pineal in them had ceased to function. This view is in accord with the anatomical evidences of its involution after the early years of life.

---

*Reprinted from the *Journal of Experimental Medicine*, XXII: 2, 1915.

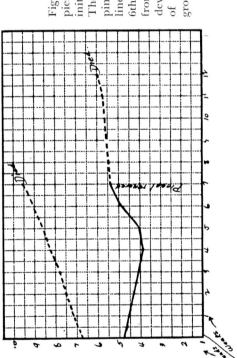

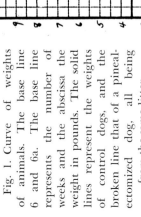

Fig. 1. Curve of weights of animals. The base line 6 and 6a. The base line represents the number of weeks and the abscissa the weight in pounds. The solid lines represent the weights of control dogs, and the broken line that of a pineal-ectomized dog, all being from the same litter.

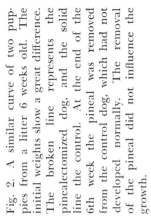

Fig. 2. A similar curve of two puppies from a litter 6 weeks old. The initial weights show a great difference. The broken line represents the pinealectomized dog, and the solid line the control. At the end of the 6th week the pineal was removed from the control dog, which had not developed normally. The removal of the pineal did not influence the growth.

It must be emphasized that at the time of Marburg's publication there had been absolutely no significant experimental investigations on the pineal and that his classification is based solely on clinicopathological observations; also that of about forty cases of tumor of the pineal gland only in the two above mentioned instances was there any sexual, somatic, or mental precocity. In several cases varying degrees of adiposity had been noted. It is also worthy of note in passing that in both cases of sexual precocity the tumor was a teratoma.

Since Marburg's publication many cases of pineal tumor have been added, the total now being about sixty cases. Von Frankl-Hoch-wart's[5] case, also a teratoma of the pineal, in a boy of five and one-half years, rather large for his age, showed sexual hypertrophy and precocity two months before death. The patient developed a deep voice and the genital hair was equal to that of a boy of fifteen. There was also mental precocity. Raymond and Claude[6] added a case which presented increasing adiposity, and somatic development but without sexual changes. With the exception of a rather frequent adiposity the other cases have shown but little to indicate glandular influences.

Experimental work has since been added but with contradictory results. In general, attempts have been made to reproduce so called hyperpinealism by feeding pineal extract and apinealism or hypopinealism by extirpation of the pineal. In feeding experiments by McCord[7] on guinea pigs, chickens, and dogs, an increase in weight together with earlier sexual maturity and sexual characteristics resulted. Dana and Berkeley[8] fed pineal extract of young bullocks and calves to guinea pigs, rabbits, and kittens, and noted a 25 per cent increase in weight over the controls. Later fifty children were injected with pineal extract, but they grew in height and weight less rapidly than the controls, though a distinctly greater mental improvement was observed. These observers think there is no doubt that injections of pineal will clear low grades of mental deficiency. These claims are quite similar to those of McCord, who noted mental precocity in his pineal-fed puppies.

Attempts have been made to remove the pineal by Exner and Boese,[9] Foa,[10] and Sarteschi.[11] The results of these investigations add even more confusion. Exner and Boese found absolutely no changes following complete or partial removal of the pineal. Sarteschi found adiposity, greater somatic and genital development, and sexual precocity in young dogs. Following extirpation of the pineal of chickens, Foa observed a premature development of the primary and secondary sexual characters.

Briefly, therefore, adiposity may result by feeding pineal extract (McCord, Dana, and Berkeley) or by complete or partial removal of the pineal (Sarteschi). Sexual and somatic precocity may result from feeding pineal extracts (McCord, Dana, and Berkeley), or from partial or complete removal of the pineal body (Foa, Sarteschi), or nothing may result from its partial or complete destruction (Exner and Boese). Such is the paradoxical experimental support for Marburg's hypothesis of pineal function.[12]

The foregoing is presented as a purely objective, concise summary of our present knowledge of the pineal. A detailed consideration of the clinical and experimental observations will be given in a subsequent communication. The purpose of this paper is to report briefly the results of pinealectomy in a series of young puppies and to describe the method which has been evolved for extirpation of the pineal body.

EXPERIMENTAL REMOVAL OF THE PINEAL

In the higher mammals the pineal is so deeply situated, so minute, and so intimately associated with important and easily injured structures that its removal by operation has been regarded as impractical. It is covered by the splenium of the corpus callosum and by the vena Galena magna. It lies between the anterior corpora quadrigemina, and consequently is just above the aqueduct of Sylvius. It is situated almost exactly in the center of the brain. Its removal necessitates opening the third ventricle, the posterior wall of which it forms a part. The greatest of the dangers encountered in the removal of the pineal is hemorrhage, and especially hemorrhage into the ventricles. The greatest difficulty is the definite recognition of the gland.

Foa has successfully excised pineals from chickens, but with the exception of Sarteschi's work, the removal of the pineal in higher mammals has not been successful. Exner and Boese attempted its removal in dogs but soon yielded to the more expedient but objectionable method of cauterization. By these investigators the cautery was inserted blindly through a trephine opening in the skull. This procedure was accompanied by a very high mortality. From a series of ninety-five animals, death resulted from the operation in seventy-five. The principal cause of death was hemorrhage. This is not surprising, since a successful introduction of the cautery must almost necessarily perforate the vena Galena magna. Sarteschi's operative results were almost equally disastrous. Of fifteen dogs operated upon only three survived. He ascribes the mortality to hemorrhage, trauma, and anesthesia. He ligates both carotid arteries as a preliminary procedure, divides the superior longitudinal sinus, and arrives at the pineal by separating the cerebral hemispheres and elevating the splenium. The destruction of both carotid arteries and the superior longitudinal sinus seriously complicates the interpretation of results. Destruction of the great vein of Galen may also be an important complication. Into this vein passes practically all the blood from the interior of the brain. The collateral venous supply for the vein is so inadequate that its occlusion results in an internal hydrocephalus. The amount of cerebral destruction incident to the above mentioned procedure of Sarteschi is also significant.

EVOLUTION OF THE OPERATION UPON THE PINEAL BODY

In a series of experiments on internal hydrocephalus by the author[13] three years ago, the vein of Galen was occluded by the application of a silver clip, and in the development of this procedure a field of operation very close to the pineal was made accessible, and thus the possibility of removal of this structure was suggested.

By elaboration of the method of approach, an operation was devised which is free from the objections inherent to operations which entail cerebral destruction, vascular injury, or the endangering of the vitality of other cerebral structures. The results which might be noted could be attributed only to the uncomplicated loss of the pineal body. The operation to be described was successfully performed on young puppies from ten days to three weeks old under ether anesthesia plus a preliminary, relatively high dose of morphia. Despite the long duration of the operation, which usually required two and one-half to three and sometimes four hours, the animals recovered very quickly, and on the following day were almost as active and playful as the controls.

An opening about 2 cm. in length was made in the vault of the skull, extending posteriorly to the inion and mesially to the midsagittal line. The dura was opened to and reflected over the superior longitudinal sinus. The occipital lobe was then carefully retracted and following the ligation of a small vein, which bridges the space between the brain and the falx cerebri, the tip of the tentorium cerebelli (osseum) was quickly exposed and the terminus of the vena Galena magna brought into view. Then a very tedious and painstaking liberation of this vein was begun. By alternately freeing the vein with careful blunt dissection and controlling the hemorrhage with pledgets of cotton, the inferior surface of the vein was liberated and the corpora quadrigemina exposed. The vein was then carefully elevated in order to work beneath it, and the median groove between the corpora quadrigemina was slowly followed anteriorly until the pineal body was reached. The pineal was then caught in a small biting forceps and removed. From a series of twelve dogs, of varying ages, not one survived the operation longer than one to two hours. Invariably the postmortem examination disclosed the ventricles full of blood, which was presumably the cause of death. The bleeding from the numerous venous and arterial radicles in the enveloping pia always resulted at the time of removal of the gland. Extirpation of the pineal necessitated opening the third ventricle because of the incorporation of this structure in its posterior wall.

Two years later the same plan of attack was again tried, but the pineal was dissected out more thoroughly before removal in order to minimize the hemorrhage when the ventricle was opened. Another addition to the technique of the operation and one which has proved of the greatest importance was to open the third ventricle at a point over the pineal body before attempting its removal. This not only permitted more room by release of the fluid, but, more important still, it collapsed the cerebral ventricles so that if hemorrhage should occur it would not be into the open ventricles and thus cause distention of the brain and possibly rupture of the cortex.

With these modifications this operative procedure became successful. The small amount of bleeding which resulted was sponged away with pledgets of cotton and was always under control.

The operation as performed was, however, very unsatisfactory because of its great difficulty and the length of time required for its accomplishment. The most patient and assiduous care in the control of hemorrhage by wet and dry cotton pressure had to be exercised. It was necessary to hold the head quite motionless during this long and tedious procedure. With practice the pineal could usually be recognized because of its constant and dominant position at the junction of the median quadrigeminal groove and the third ven-

tricle. However, very frequently, despite the greatest caution, the pineal would become covered with blood clot and unrecognizable and, perhaps, occasionally would be sponged away. When this was believed to have occurred an area of tissue from this accurately located position was removed and examined microscopically. In all such cases a second piece of tissue was excised in order to insure complete removal of the gland. This, too, was studied with the microscope. In many instances the pineal area was further treated by an electric cautery needle. At times even with the greatest care, death resulted from bleeding into the ventricles. Successful complete extirpation resulted in only about 25 per cent of the cases operated upon in this manner.

NEW METHOD OF PINEALECTOMY

The foregoing method was very capricious. To be of practical value the pineal body must be more easily reached and removed with greater certainty and less mortality. Consequently a new and simple method of attack has been evolved. Though more delicate and requiring more painstaking care, it can be done almost as easily as a canine hypophysectomy. The new operation can be done in less than one hour. It differs from the preceding operation in that the pineal is reached from in front through the third ventricle rather than from behind. In this way the extensive bleeding consequent to liberation of the vein of Galen is obviated, sidetracked as it were, and the operation can be performed almost bloodlessly. This is accomplished by dividing the splenium of the corpus callosum in the midline for a distance of about 2 cm. from its posterior terminus. This exposes the transparent roof of the third ventricle which is distended by the contained cerebrospinal fluid. A large anemic area is visible in the midline of the roof of the ventricle, between the two small veins of Galen. This is perforated and the opening enlarged backward to the origin of the vena Galena magna by releasing the blades of the forceps. The entire third ventricle is thus brought in full view and the pineal body is readily seen under the origin of this vein, in the median quadrigeminal groove. The pineal body can easily be grasped in the jaws of the cupped biting forceps and completely removed.

Practically no bleeding occurs during the exposure of the gland. A little bleeding follows its removal but this can easily be controlled by a minute tampon of cotton. With collapsed ventricles the bleeding is outward through the wound and is therefore not to be feared. Not infrequently the aqueduct of Sylvius may be filled with blood. This has never caused any mortality because, before closure, the mould of clotted blood may be readily extracted, the aqueduct of Sylvius being in full view. To insure complete excision a second piece of tissue was invariably removed from the pineal region. With this method of operating there has been, as I have said, practically no mortality. It is, however, quite easy to become disoriented, even when following carefully the procedure which I am advocating. If bleeding and laceration of tissue are avoided, as they can be, and the midline is adhered to, there is little danger of losing one's bearings.

In every case a histological examination is made of all the tissue obtained at the operation and, after death, of the immediate region from which the pineal was removed.

RESULTS FOLLOWING PINEALECTOMY

Our operations for extirpation of the pineal have been mainly upon young puppies, from ten to three weeks old. Of these one is living fifteen months after the operation; one died of distemper one year after operation; several survived the pinealectomy three to eight months. It is exceedingly difficult to raise puppies in the confined quarters of our laboratory. We were, however, unable to note any difference in the resistance of the operated and the control animals to the usual diseases.

When litters of puppies could be obtained, one or more of the animals were kept as controls. Little importance, however, should be attached to such comparisons because of the great variations found in members of the same family. The pineal was also removed in several adult male and female dogs, and three of these are living longer than four months after the operation.

SOMATIC DEVELOPMENT, ADIPOSITY, AND MENTALITY

Careful observations have been made of the growth of the pinealectomized animals. Skiagraphs have been taken at various periods, but there has been no evidence of either superior or inferior somatic development or adiposity (Figs. 1 and 2), save perhaps in a single instance. In this animal there was a slight increase in weight for a brief period about one year after the operation; this is disappearing, so that now it is scarcely noticeable. It might be attributed to overfeeding. There is nothing in the behavior of the pinealectomized animals to suggest mental precocity.

SEXUAL PRECOCITY

We have observed nothing to support the view that the pineal gland inhibits the sexual functions and that its removal is followed by excessive sexual development. Two bitches have lived for one year following the removal of the pineal; both were in heat ten months after the operation, or when about one year old. In neither animal has pregnancy resulted, and in neither was any abnormality observed in the generative organs.

The pinealectomized young male puppies observed for periods of from three to eight months, contrasted with members of the same litter, have given no evidence of sexual precocity or retardation.

GROSS AND MICROSCOPIC STUDY OF THE GLANDS OF INTERNAL SECRETION

Examination has been made of the various ductless glands which were obtained at autopsy. In none was a definite macro- or micro-scopic change observed. The tissues examined include the thymus, parathyroids, thyroid, hypophysis, adrenals, pancreas, liver, spleen, lymph glands, testes, ovaries, and mammary glands.

SUMMARY AND CONCLUSIONS

1. Following the removal of the pineal I have observed no sexual precocity or indolence, no adiposity or emaciation, no somatic or mental precocity or retardation.

2. Our experiments seem to have yielded nothing to sustain the view that the pineal gland has an active endocrine function of importance either in the very young or adult dogs.

3. The pineal is apparently not essential to life and seems to have no influence upon the animal's well being.

It is a pleasure to express my gratitude to Professor Halsted for his interest and suggestions during the course of this investigation.

REFERENCES

[1]Heubner, *Allg. med. Centr.–Ztg., lxviii:* 89, 1899.

[2]Oesterich, R., and Slawyk, Riesenwuchs und Zirbeldrusen-Geschwulst. *Virchows Arch. f. path. Anat., clvii:* 475, 1899.

[3]Ogle, C., (1.): Sarcoma of the Pineal Body, with Diffused Melanotic Sarcoma of the Surface of Cerebrum. (2.) Tumor of Pineal Body in a Boy. *Tr. Path. Soc. London, 1:* 6, 1898.

[4]Marburg, O.: Zur Kenntnis der normalen und pathologischen Histologie der Zirbeldruse; die Adipositas cerebralis, *Arb. neurol. Inst. Univ. Wien, xvii:* 217, 1908; Die Adipositas cerebralis. Ein Beitrag zur Pathologie der Zirbeldruse. *Wein. med Wchnschr., lviii:* 2617, 1908.

[5]von Frankl-Hochwart, L.: Uber Diagnose der Zirbeldrusentumoren. *Deutsche Ztschr. Nervenh.,* 1909, *xxxvii:* 455, 1909.

[6]Raymond, F., and Claude, H.: Les tumeurs de la glande pineale chez l'enfant. *Bull. l'Acad. med. Paris, lxiii:* 265, series 3, 1910.

[7]McCord, C. P.: The Pineal Gland in Relation to Somatic, Sexual and Mental Development. *J. A. M. A., lxiii:* 232, 1914.

[8]Berkeley, W. N., Dana, C. L., Goddard, H. H. and Cornell, W. S.: The Functions of the Pineal Gland, with Report of Feeding Experiments. *M. Rec., lxxxiii:* 835, 1913. Dana and Berkeley, The Functions of the Pineal Gland. *Month. Cycl. Pract. Med., xxviii:* 78, 1914.

[9]Exner, A., and Boese, J.: Ueber experimentelle Exstirpation der Glandula pinealis. *Deutsche Ztschr. f. Chir., cvii:* 182, 1910. Uber experimental Exstirpation der Glandula pinealis. *Neurol. Centralbl., xxix:* 754, 1910.

[10]Foa, C.: Ipertrofia dei testicoli e della cresta dopo l'asportazione della ghiandola pineale nel gallo. *Pathologica, iv:* 445, 1911–12.

[11]Sarteschi, U., La sindrome epifisaria "macrogenitosomia precoce" attenuta sperimentalmente nei mammiferi. *Pathologica, v:* 707, 1913.

[12]It should also be noted that Pellizzi (Pellizzi, G. B., La sindrome "macrogenitosomia precoce." *Neurol., Centralbl., xxx:* 870, 1911, in 1910, presented two cases of somatic and sexual precocity without substantiation of the diagnosis, as cases of "la sindrome epifisaria macrogenitosomia precoce." In the absence of anatomical proof and the rarity of a correct clinical diagnosis of pineal tumor, this evidence can not be accepted. It was in Pellizzi's laboratory that the experimental work of Sarteschi was conducted.

[13]Dandy, W. E., and Blackfan, K. D.: Internal Hydrocephalus, an Experimental, Clinical and Pathological Study. *J. A. M. A. lxi:* 2216, 1913. Internal Hydrocephalus, eine experimentelle, klinische und pathologische Untersuchung. *Beitr. klin. Chir., xciii:* 392, 1914; An Experimental and Clinical Study of Internal Hydrocephalus. *Am. J. Dis. Child., viii:* 406, 1914.

V

INTERNAL HYDROCEPHALUS*

SECOND PAPER†

WALTER E. DANDY AND KENNETH D. BLACKFAN

In a recent communication a series of cases of internal hydrocephalus was presented and subdivided into two apparently distinct anatomic varieties — obstructive hydrocephalus and communicating hydrocephalus. These two groups were sharply differentiated by an anatomic difference, demonstrated by the introduction of a neutral solution of phenolsulphonephthalein into the cerebral ventricles and almost immediately testing for its presence in the spinal fluid. In the obstructive type, this solution introduced into the ventricles failed to appear in the spinal fluid; in the communicating type it appeared promptly in the spinal fluid.

Clinically, the two varieties appeared identical, and it was only by this test that hydrocephalus could be subdivided. The growth of the head seemed about equally rapid, the etiology was equally obscure, and either variety might be congenital or acquired.

By an estimation of the amount of phenolsulphonephthalein excreted by the kidneys following the intraventricular and intraspinal introduction, a quantitative absorption of cerebrospinal fluid could be estimated in each type of hydrocephalus and a second very important physiologic difference was demonstrated. In the obstructive type of hydrocephalus the absorption, which is restricted to the cerebral ventricles, is practically nil — less than 1 per cent, as contrasted with a normal of 12 to 20 per cent (Fig. 2). In the communicating type, the absorption is 2 to 5 per cent, as contrasted with the same normal (Fig. 1). The similarity of the two groups is that in both there is a tremendous diminution in the absorption of cerebrospinal fluid. This is the reason hydrocephalus develops in both the obstructive and communicating types of hydrocephalus; that is, diminished absorption of cerebrospinal fluid with an unaffected production.

It was also shown by a series of experiments that cerebrospinal fluid is produced in the ventricles and is absorbed in the subarachnoid space, and that the blood vessels of the entire spinal and cranial subarachnoid space participate in the absorption. It was further shown that in the obstructive type of hydrocephalus, the absorption of cerebrospinal fluid from the spinal subarachnoid space was normal. Hydrocephalus then resulted because a mechanical obstruction prevented the cerebrospinal fluid from leaving the ventricles of the brain, where there is no absorption, to the subarachnoid space, where the absorption may be normal.

In the communicating type of hydrocephalus there was a great diminution in the absorption of cerebrospinal fluid from the subarachnoid space. Although the cerebrospinal fluid passed freely from the ventricles, hydrocephalus resulted because an adequate absorption did not occur from the subarachnoid space.

*Reprinted from *The American Journal of Diseases of Children*, xiv: 424–443, Dec. 1917.

†First Paper: Dandy, W. E., and Blackfan, K. D.: Internal Hydrocephalus. An Experimental, Clinical and Pathological Study. *A. J. D. C.*, *8:* 406, 1914. Also, *Beitr. z. klin. Chir.*, *93:* 392, 1914. A preliminary report appeared in *J. A. M. A.*, *61:* 2216, 1913.

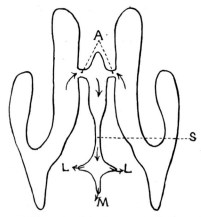

Fig. 1. Diagram of the cerebral ventricular system, showing the intracerebral course of the cerebrospinal fluid. The three arrows at the base (L, L, and M) show the only three points of exit from the entire ventricular system. A block at A would produce a unilateral hydrocephalus involving only one ventricle; a block at S would produce an internal hydrocephalus involving both lateral ventricles; and to obtain a complete obstruction at the base, the two foramina of Luschka and the foramen of Magendie (L, L, and M) would have to be occluded.

A-foramen of Monroe; S-aqueduct of Sylvius; L, L-foramina of Luschka; M-foramen of Magendie.

From a physiologic standpoint, therefore, both varieties of hydrocephalus result from the same cause — a diminished absorption. Although there is an anatomic difference in the patency or closure of the foramina of exit from the ventricles, the absorption is only slightly greater where the foramina are open.

In the previous communication a series of cases of obstructive hydrocephalus was shown in which the pathologic findings verified the clinical evidence of an existing obstruction to the outflow of cerebrospinal fluid from the ventricles. Since then, numerous other cases have been studied, in all of which an obstruction was invariably found when the phenolsulphonephthalein test indicated such an obstruction during life. It is needless to present these cases in detail, as they merely confirm the previous observations, differing only in the

details of the character and location of the obstruction. The accompanying tabulation of these cases (Table II) gives in condensed form all the fundamental facts concerning the added group of cases of hydrocephalus with obstruction.

Although a small series of cases of communicating hydrocephalus was studied by the foregoing mentioned methods and presented in the earlier paper, we were unable to obtain any pathologic examinations to explain the clinical findings, and final conclusions on the etiology of this form of hydrocephalus were necessarily deferred, although the conclusions suggested from the tests strikingly anticipated the subsequent pathologic findings. It is largely the purpose of this communication to fill this pathologic deficiency and give the findings at necropsy of four cases of communicating hydrocephalus and to present the pathologic findings which result in the production of this so-called idiopathic disease. All the cases studied are from the services of Professor Halsted and Professor

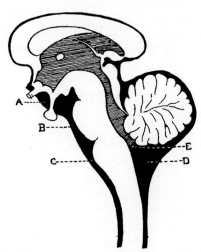

Fig. 2. Diagram representing the midsagittal view of the brain stem, showing the ventricular system (in cross lines) and the subarachnoid system (in black). The communication between the two systems is at E (foramen of Magendie). The foramina of Luschka are not shown.

A-cisterna interpedicularis; B-cisterna pontis; C, D-cisterna cerebellomedullaris (cisterna magna).

TABLE I

CASES OF COMMUNICATING HYDROCEPHALUS STUDIED WITH PHENOLSULPHONEPHTHALEIN TEST

Cases	Age	Absorption After Ventricular Injection		Absorption After Subarachnoid (Spinal) Injection		Communication, Ventricles and Subarachnoid Space; Appearance in Spinal Canal; Ventricular Injection, Min.	History	Postmortem Findings
		Time of Appearance, Minutes	Two-Hour Absorption, Per Cent	Time of Appearance, Minutes	Two-Hour Absorption, Per Cent			
1. R. G.	18 months	30	2.0	..	11.0	1	Definite history of meningitis at 7 months hydrocephalus followed immediately	Living
2. M. R.	11 mos. (during meningitis) (during hydrocephalus) 9 months later 3 years later	13-15 20	6.5 0.5	.. 8 8	14.0-9.5 15.0 60.0	7 2	Meningitis followed by hydrocephalus, which healed spontaneously	Living (spontaneous recovery)
3. H. N.	8 months	25 25	4.4 4.0	.. ..	10.0 10.0	20 13	Hydrocephalus noted 6 weeks after birth; acute illness 3 days after birth; meningitis (?)	Living
4. J. C.	16 months	30	4.0	..	....	1	....	None
5. W. F.	6 months	..	4.5	..	16.0	3	Congenital.........	Living
6. W. F.	4 months	..	3.0	..	....	2	Convulsion and fever three days after birth	Living
7. E. W.	3 months	..	3.0	..	8.5	1	Meningitis (meningococcus)	None
8. P. G.	8 months	..	5.0	..	10.0	Less than 7 min.	....	None
9. F. C.	4 months	..	2.0	..	....	7	Meningocele.........	Adhesions at base
10. H. B.	4 months	..	..	..	....	5	Meningocele.........	Adhesions at base
11. F. W.	6 months	16 25	2.0 1.0	12 ..	10.0 ..	Slight in less than 4½ hours, None in an observation several weeks later	Meningocele large head at birth	Adhesions at base

Howland, and it is due to their privileges and continued interest that this contribution is made possible.

I. COMMUNICATING INTERNAL HYDROCEPHALUS

(a) *Demonstration of the Communication.* Eleven cases of communicating hydrocephalus have been studied. In each of these the communication has been demonstrated by the phenolsulphonephthalein test. This is the only absolute method of differentiation of the two types of hydrocephalus. One can often tell from the amount of fluid obtained by lumbar puncture whether a communication exists, but more frequently this is misleading. If only 3 or 4 cc. are obtainable on more than one occasion, it is fairly safe to assume that the obstruction is complete and exists at the foramina of Luschka and Magendie, because all the fluid formed from the choroid plexus is retained in the ventricles. On the other hand, if an obstruction exists at the aqueduct of Sylvius, a large amount of fluid can be obtained by lumbar puncture because the choroid plexus of the fourth ventricle, including the flocculi, is still producing fluid which passes freely into the subarachnoid space. It must be remembered that even in the highest grades of hydrocephalus it is impossible to withdraw more than a certain amount of fluid by needle, either from the ventricle or the subarachnoid space, because a balance between intracranial and extracranial pressure is reached before the ventricles are emptied, and air cannot enter the needle to displace more fluid. False interpretations can be avoided and the existence of communication or obstruction determined with accuracy by the phenolsulphonephthalein test. It should be emphasized again that the ordinary solution of phenolsulphonephthalein is strongly alkaline and produces a marked reaction. A neutral solution which can be used with a minimum degree of danger has been prepared for us by Hynson, Wescott & Dunning. The solution should be freshly prepared.

Phenolsulphonephthalein appears in the spinal fluid in one to three minutes after its introduction into the ventricles where hydrocephalus does not exist. Almost the same obtains in communicating hydrocephalus, although the time in many cases is five to seven minutes, and in one instance was twenty minutes. This increased period was reduced to thirteen minutes by the upright position.

The increased amount of cerebrospinal fluid present in hydrocephalus seems to cause no appreciable delay in the transmission of the dye from the ventricles to the spinal canal. Why the delay should be so much greater in the single instance is not entirely clear, although adhesions along the spinal cord suggest a possible explanation. In cases which adhesions are present at the base of the brain, the same condition frequently exists along the entire spinal canal, and it is natural to assume that these may delay the descent of the dye.

One patient showed a trace of phenolsulphonephthalein when a lumbar puncture was made four and a half hours after the ventricular introduction, although it was absent one-half hour after its introduction. Several weeks later a similar test was performed and there was a complete obstruction. We must assume a very trivial communication to have existed in this case, and later to have been closed over. At necropsy very dense adhesions totally occluded the foramina of exit from the fourth ventricle. No doubt this cordon of adhesions was becoming progressively tighter and the first phenolsulphonephthalein test caught the condition in the terminal stages of the transition from a communicating hydrocephalus to an obstructive hydrocephalus.

(b) *Quantitative Absorption in Communicating Internal Hydrocephalus.* There is very little to add to our previous report on the quantitative absorption of cerebrospinal fluid except the confirmation of additional material. The variation of the amount of absorption is within narrow limits; the average is 3 to 4 per cent during a two-hour period, the highest 5 per cent, and the lowest 0.5 per cent. The absorption following introduction into the normal ventricle is 12 to 20 per cent. When introduced into the spinal canal the variation is also small. The average two-hour absorption is 10 per cent, the highest 16 per cent, the lowest 7 per cent, the normal 35 to 60 per cent. The time of first appearance in the urine is also greatly delayed following either intraventricular or intraspinal injection.

One interesting case has been under observation for four years. The child was first seen with an acute epidemic cerebrospinal meningitis, and the absorption tests showed a moderate delay and diminution in absorption following the ventricular test. The ventricles were shown to communicate with the subarachnoid space. A few weeks later, after the subsidence of the acute meningitis, the child was again brought to the hospital apparently becoming blind and having an enlarged head, with a bulging tense anterior fontanel. Large amounts of cerebrospinal fluid were obtainable both from the ventricles and the subarachnoid space. The condition was obviously internal hydrocephalus, which was shown to be of the communicating variety. The absorption from the ventricles (0.5 per cent) and subarachnoid space (14 and 9.5 per cent on two occasions) was characteristically low. Phenolsulphonephthalein appeared in the spinal canal two minutes after its introduction into the ventricles. The condition seemed hopeless, and the parents were so instructed. Much to our surprise, four years later the patient again appeared, with a fractured skull, but the hydrocephalus had apparently cleared, and the child on discharge appeared entirely normal. Tests at this time showed 50 per cent, or a normal phenolsulphonephthalein output from the subarachnoid space. The roentgenogram of the skull was negative.

(c) *Pathological Findings in Communicating Internal Hydrocephalus.* A pathologic examination has been obtained in four cases of communicating hydrocephalus. Three of these have been studied in the above series and the fourth is a specimen which has been in the pathologic museum for several years. Because of the similarity of the findings in all cases, the results will be grouped and individual mention made only of accessory details.

Each of the four cases presented exactly the same pathologic condition — a barrier of very dense adhesions at the base of the brain. In each case the foramen of Magendie and one foramen of Luschka were sealed by adhesions and the other foramen of Luschka was patent to a certain degree, and through this single channel the fluid escaped from the fourth ventricle and therefore from the ventricular system. The adhesions completely encircled the brain anterior to the patent foramen of Luschka; and the basal cisternae — cisternae magna, cisterna pontomedularis, and cisterna interpeduncularis — were completely obliterated by these adhesions. The adhesions in each instance were most dense in the region of the medulla and cerebellum and became less pronounced in the chiasmal region. Minor adhesions were scattered over the surface of the brain. In one case the adhesions were present over the base, with additional dense adhesions completely binding the tentorium to the posterior surface of each occipital lobe, the superior surface of both cerebellar lobes, and completely encircled the midbrain as it passed through the opening in the tentorium cerebelli. In each instance an apparently complete encircling mass of adhesions sealed off the base of the brain so that the cerebrospinal fluid could not pass forward to the cerebral subarachnoid space, but only downward into the spinal canal. The obliteration of the various basilar cisternae, which are the centers from which cerebrospinal fluid is distributed over the cerebral subarachnoid space, may in itself be sufficient to eliminate the cerebral subarachnoid space from absorption, even without the encircling adhesions.

No doubt in many cases both foramina

of Luschka may be obliterated, with a patent foramen of Magendie, or vice versa. In any case, the communication between the ventricles and subarachnoid space, though limited to one foramen at the base, is ample, being at least larger than the aqueduct of Sylvius. After passing from the ventricles, however, the absorption is limited to the *spinal* subarachnoid space and a minimal area of the subarachnoid space around the cerebellum.

The phenolsulphonephthalein tests show a reduction in absorption from the subarachnoid space to about one-fourth or one-fifth of the normal. This roughly corresponds to the diminution of the subarachnoid absorbing area due to the elimination of the cerebral subarachnoid space by adhesions.

In each instance the adhesions between the brain and the dura were dense, necessitating their incision to prevent tearing the cortex during the removal of the brain. Special emphasis should be placed on the necessity of demonstrating the adhesions during the progress of the postmortem examination, for after they have been separated their demonstration becomes difficult. This is especially true when, the adhesions are thin and toward the periphe-

TABLE II

CASES OF INTERNAL HYDROCEPHALUS WITH OBSTRUCTION,—

Cases	Age	Absorption After Ventricular Introduction		Absorption After Spinal Introduction		Communication Ventricle and Subarachnoid Space: Time of Appearance
		Time of Appearance, Minutes	Two-Hour Absorption, Per Cent	Time of Appearance, Minutes	Two-Hour Absorption, Per Cent	
1. P. G.	7 months	45	0.75	6	62	None in 45 min.
2. A. H.	6 months	40	1.0	..	..	None in 2 hours
3. N. P.	6 weeks	45	1.0	..	..	None in 20 min.
4. N. M.	2 years	40	0.50	6	35	None in 2 days
		35	0.50			
5. M. R.	13 months	40	0.50	8	25	None in 1½ hrs.
		20	0.9			
6. F. W.	6 months	16	2.0	12	10	Trace in less than 4½ hrs.
		25	1.0			None in 2d observation in 3 hours
7. M. N.	5 months	30	1.5	..	35	None in 30 min. Faint trace in 14 hours
8. R. C.	2 months	..	1.2	..	30	None in 2 hours
9. R. S.	6 weeks	..	2.0	..	..	None in 2 hours
10. L. S.	19 months	..	1.5	..	56	None in 2 hours
11. J. S.	8 months	..	0.5	..	35	None in 2 hours
12. J. B.	3 months	..	0.5	..	..	None in 40 min.
13. A. C.	16 months	..	0.5	..	..	None in 1 hour
14. J. M.	2½ years	..	2.0	..	..	None in 1 hour
15. J. F.	5 years	..	0.5	..	45	None in 1 hour
					41	

ry of their distribution. One not infrequently sees a large area of adhesions over the cerebral cortex which causes no internal hydrocephalus. This is probably due to the fact that the base is the distributing center for all the fluid that covers the brain, and the closure of the cisternae prevents the distribution, whereas a large cortical area can easily be compensated for by the normal excess of the absorbing area.

The presence of adhesions is responsible for the fact that fluid accumulates in the brain and not outside the brain, or, in other words, that an internal and not an external hydrocephalus results. This is because the brain is tightly bound to the dura, and more important, because the fluid-containing and fluid-absorbing subarachnoid space is obliterated over most of the brain, and especially at the distributing center in the cisternae.

The truth of the following paragraph from our former paper has been substantiated by the results of the pathologic examinations:

We have had no pathologic examination on patients with hydrocephalus of the communicating type. It is very likely that the diminished absorption from the subarachnoid space is due to adhesions

—STUDIED WITH THE PHENOLSULPHONEPHTHALEIN TEST

Duration of Excretion		History	Postmortem Findings
Ventricle	*Spinal Canal*		
3% excreted in 12 hours; three days later, concentration of phenolsulphonephthalein in the urine was diminished	Less than 12 hours	Tuberculous meningitis; meningocele since birth	Exudate over base of brain occluding the foramina of exit
. . . .	. . . .	Congenital; myelomeningocele also present	Occlusion of aqueduct of Sylvius
. . . .	. . . .	Congenital	Total absence of aqueduct of Sylvius
11 days; 6.1% first 24 hours: 7.5% second 24 hours 5.7% third 24 hours	21 hours	Congenital	Died at age of 5 years. Double obstruction: one at aqueduct, the other at foramina of Magendie and Luschka
7 days	. . . .	Meningitis at 4 months; previously normal	Absence of foramina of Luschka and Magendie. Fourth ventricle a large cyst. Marked thickening of piaarachnoid
. . . .	48 hours	Congenital; syringomyelocele; no history of meningitis	Chronic inflammatory process: adhesions at base occluding foramina of exit
. . . .	. . . .	Congenital	Living
. . . .	. . . .	Congenital	Obstruction at foramina of Magendie and Luschka; enormous fourth ventricle, like a huge cyst
. . . .	. . . .	Congenital	No necropsy
. . . .	. . . .	Meningitis lasting one month when 1 year old	Living
. . . .	. . . .	Meningitis congenital. .	Very dense adhesions at base of brain disclosed at operation; child still living
. . . .	. . . .	Congenital	No necropsy
. . . .	. . . .	Acute meningitis.	Thick exudate of acute meningitis at base of brain
. . . .	. . . .	Acute meningitis.	Living
. . . .	. . . .	Tumor.	Glioma in midbrain occluding aqueduct of Sylvius

which diminish the size of the subarachnoid space. Adhesions anterior to the foramina of Luschka, by causing obliteration of the cisterna magna, would prevent the passage of fluid into the general cerebral subarachnoid space as effectually as if the aqueduct of Sylvius were obliterated. The two groups would then be essentially similar, differing only in the fact that the spinal subarachnoid space participated in absorption in the communicating type.... How much alteration in the meninges alone, without adhesions, interferes with absorption, cannot be stated. It seems to us probable that the major part if not all of the disturbance is due to the limitation of the subarachnoid space.

II. OBSTRUCTIVE INTERNAL HYDROCEPHALUS

A series of fifteen cases of obstructive internal hydrocephalus has been studied, in each of which the obstruction has been clinically demonstrated by the phenolsulphonephthalein test. In addition to these, numerous other cases have been observed in which tumors have caused the hydrocephalus, but they have not been included. Several other cases have been seen at necropsy, but are also not included because they were not previously observed clinically. In ten of these fifteen cases the obstruction has been verified by a postmortem examination. One was due to an acute tuberculous meningitis which sealed the foramina of Luschka and Magendie. Another case was an acute cerebrospinal meningitis in which the base was covered by exudate. Four cases had complete occlusion of the aqueduct of Sylvius, three of which showed histologic epithelial remnants of this structure, and the fourth was due to a solitary tubercule in the midbrain which had grown into and totally occluded the aqueduct of Sylvius. One of these cases with iter obstruction had a second obstruction by adhesions, completely closing both foramina of Luschka and the foramen of Magendie. This child (N. M. 4) lived five years and was under observation most of that time, and despite an enormous hydrocephalus, did not lose all evidences of intelligence. At necropsy there was in addition to the hydrocephalus a congenital urethral obstruction and a double hydronephrosis. The brain presented a great dilatation of the third and lateral ventricles anterior to an iter obstruction, and a dilatation of the fourth ventricle, anterior to the closure of the basal foramina of exit. Adhesions between the cerebellum and dura no doubt restricted the dilatation of the fourth ventricle and mechanically prevented its enlargement into a great cyst. It was impossible to have suspected the presence of the second or iter obstruction. The obstruction at the base was certain because of the very scant amount of cerebrospinal fluid (2 to 4 cc.) obtainable at successive lumbar punctures.

(*a*) *Demonstration of the Obstruction.* In each of these fifteen cases, phenolsulphonephthalein failed to appear in the spinal fluid following its introduction into the lateral ventricle. In one instance (F. W. 6) a trace was present, appearing at some time in the interval between one-half and four and a half hours. Several months later the obstruction had become complete and phenolsulphonephthalein did not appear in the spinal canal. There was a corresponding reduction in the absorption from 2 to 1 per cent, and a corresponding increase in the appearance time. The significance of these observations will be mentioned later, in considering the interrelationship of the two types of hydrocephalus. In each of the fifteen cases the output of cerebrospinal fluid was under 2 per cent as compared to the normal of 15 to 20 per cent, and readily explains the cause of the hydrocephalus. The spinal absorption in several cases was entirely normal; in several it was quite low, 10 to 30 per cent, as compared to the normal of 35 to 60 per cent. In these cases the amount of absorption is really immaterial in the production of the hydrocephalus, because the fluid never reaches the meninges. Its importance, however, is in the prognosis following operative intervention, for with

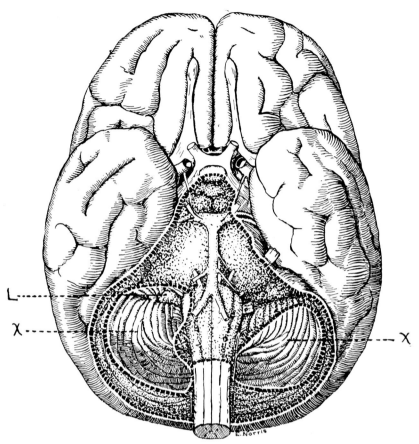

Fig. 3. Diagram of the base of the brain, showing in diagram form, roughly, the distribution of the adhesions over the base of the brain responsible for the communicating type of internal hydrocephalus.

X, X represent areas on the cerebellar hemispheres which are relatively free from adhesions. L represents the foramen of Luschka, which is patent only on this side. The opposite side is completely obliterated by adhesions. The adhesions extend along the tentorium on both the superior and inferior surfaces.

a low spinal absorption (10 to 30 per cent) the release of the obstruction would then transfer an obstructive hydrocephalus to a communicating hydrocephalus, and only modify but not cure the disease. It would only make its development less rapid.

The total time for elimination of the dye after ventricular introduction was studied in only a few cases, in each of which the excretion was carried over a period of several days; in one case eleven days on two different occasions. The excretion following spinal introduction varied from normal to two days, an index of which time is given by the two-hour output in the urine.

COMPARISON OF THE TWO TYPES OF HYDROCEPHALUS

Both types of hydrocephalus are due to a diminution in the absorption of cerebrospinal fluid. Both are obstructive, differing only in the location of the obstruction. In the so-called obstructive variety, the obstruction is within the ventricular system. In the so-called communicating hydrocephalus, the obstruction is in the subarachnoid space. In communicating hydrocephalus the obstruction is probably always the result of adhesions, which, of course, means that an inflammatory process has existed before birth if the hydro-

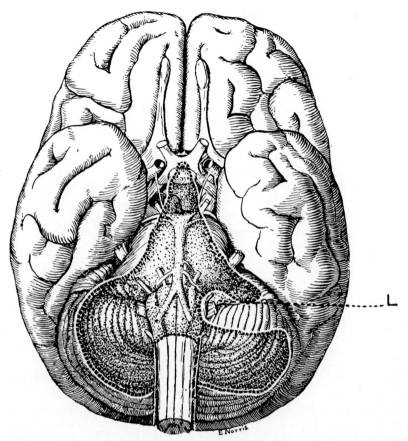

L - - - - - -

Fig. 4. A diagram of the base of the brain showing roughly the extent of the adhesions at the base.

L is the patent foramen of Luschka, on one side only. The other foramen of Luschka and the foramen of Magendie are completely obliterated by adhesions. In this case the adhesions did not involve the tentorium, but only the base of the brain.

cephalus is congenital, or it may develop at any time after birth. Such an inflammation of the meninges may seal the three foramina of exit from the fourth ventricle and produce an obstructive hydrocephalus, or it may leave one, two, or all the foramina patent and seal off the cisternae, producing the communicating type of hydrocephalus; or it is possible to do both; that is, the foramina may all be closed and the meninges sealed anterior to the foramina. This, of course, would produce the obstructive hydrocephalus, and the meningeal obliteration, though of no consequence (because the fluid does not reach the meninges), could be demonstrated clinically only

by tests as a greatly reduced absorption from the subarachnoid space. Case F. W. 6 is such an instance of a combination of the two types. At first there was a minute and greatly delayed communication. The process was undoubtedly progressive, as later the obstruction became total and the absorption following ventricular introduction correspondingly diminished. In all of our cases of communicating hydrocephalus the foramen of Magendie has been closed, together with one foramen of Luschka. A gradual reduction in the size of the remaining foramen of Luschka would change the communicating hydrocephalus to obstructive hydrocephalus, as in the foregoing case, whereas clinically the transition would scarcely be noticed. It is, of course, of the greatest importance to determine whether the absorption from the subarachnoid space is normal or approximately so before attempting any operative procedure designed to relieve the obstruction. As mentioned previously, the transference from an obstructive to a communicating hydrocephalus would add but little to the patient's welfare.

MENINGOCELE AND INTERNAL HYDROCEPHALUS

The frequent association of a meningocele with internal hydrocephalus has long been known, and quite frequently an internal hydrocephalus has been observed to develop following the removal of a meningocele. This seems to us most probably due to the removal of the absorbing area of the meningocele, which was just sufficient (or nearly so) to maintain the balance between the production and absorption of cerebrospinal fluid. With its removal the production of fluid becomes sufficiently greater than absorption to cause increased dilatation of the ventricles.

In eleven patients with communicating hydrocephalus, three had a meningocele; and in fifteen cases of obstructive hydrocephalus, a meningocele was present in three. The formation of a meningocele in conjunction with a communicating hydrocephalus, arising in early intra-uterine life, seems explainable by the pressure which causes the cerebrospinal fluid to take the path of least resistance, usually in the lumbar region, which is the last part of the spinal canal to be bridged over. The presumption is natural that a meningocele signifies an increased pressure of cerebrospinal fluid in the spinal canal, or a communicating hydrocephalus. But that this is not necessarily true is shown by its existence in three cases of obstructive hydrocephalus. In one, however, the hydrocephalus was originally of the communicating variety, and when first seen by us was in the last stages of the transition to a total

obstruction. The other case was a myelocystocele, the cerebrospinal fluid having no communication with the sac, which was now blind, and even the original communication with the central canal of the spinal cord was closed in several places. The relationship of the meningocele to the obstructive hydrocephalus in the remaining case could not be ascertained because of the absence of a pathologic examination.

In all cases with a meningocele which have recently come under our observation, careful studies have been made of the amount of absorption from the spinal canal in addition to other evidence of internal hydrocephalus. Only in those cases in which a normal absorption is present from the spinal canal have we removed the meningocele, and in these cases have observed no subsequent secondary effects on the brain. The phenolsulphonephthalein output from the spinal canal we regard as a thoroughly reliable index of the function of the meninges, and know of no other way in which a safe decision can be made in the operative treatment of a meningocele.

THE RELATION OF MENINGITIS AND OTHER FACTORS TO INTERNAL HYDROCEPHALUS

It is our opinion, based on the clinical studies and pathologic findings, that the great majority of cases of hydrocephalus result from meningitis. A hydrocephalus of short duration may occur during the meningitis, due to the tubercle bacillus, the pneumococcus, and doubtless other organisms. Chronic hydrocephalus is to be expected only following a meningococcus meningitis. That a very mild form of what was probably meningococcus meningitis has been the cause of a number of our cases seems evident from some of the history, but the illness has been so slight and recovery so prompt that the mother has looked on it as a "cold," "stomach trouble," or some illness incident to teething, and it is only by careful questioning that the illness is recalled. Yet after these mild

TABLE III
SUMMARY OF ETIOLOGIC FACTORS IN CASES OF INTERNAL HYDROCEPHALUS

Hydro-cephalus	Meningitis			Con-genital Malfor-mation; Not Inflam-matory	Tumor	Uncertain Whether Congenital or Inflamma-tory Process; Foramina at Base Oc-cluded	No Proof of Char-acter of Lesion Because no Exam-ination
	Clinical Alone	Necropsy or Opera-tion Alone	By His-tory and Operation or Necropsy				
Obstruc-tive	2	2	3	3	1	1	3
		46.6%		(20%)	(6.6%)	(6.6%)	(20%)
Communi-cating	4	3	..	..	.	..	4
		63.6%					(37.4%)

Excluding those cases in which no evidence is obtainable because of absence of examination by operation or necropsy:

1. The percentage of meningitis cases in obstructive hydrocephalus is 58.3 per cent.

2. The percentage of meningitis cases in communicating hydrocephalus is 100 per cent.

3. The percentage of meningitis cases in both obstruvtive and communicating hydrocephalus is 80 per cent.

4. The percentage of congenital malformation causing hydrocephalus (in all cases) is 15.8 per cent; and excluding communicating hydrocephalus, is 25 per cent.

symptoms hydrocephalus may result.

At necropsy adhesions are found which have the usual basal distribution of other types of meningitis, and these adhesions are the cause of the internal hydrocephalus. At necropsy exactly the same findings are obtained in cases which have an internal hydrocephalus at birth; that is, adhesions over the same general distribution, affording proof of the existence of an intra-uterine inflammatory process. What organism is responsible for these lesions is entirely unknown. So is also the organism that causes intra-uterine lesions of other serous membranes. In no instance have we been able to elicit any illness of the mother occurring during gestation which could account for the meningitis in the child.

An analysis of the accompanying table (Table III) shows the high percentage of cases in which meningitis is the basis for the hydrocephalus. The figures are intended only to give the results from a small group of cases and may no doubt be greatly altered with increasing numbers. Both types of hydrocephalus are caused by

this process, as heretofore mentioned. It is really difficult to understand how the communicating hydrocephalus can be caused by any other process than a meningitis, because of the rather diffuse area necessary to be invaded to produce these results. In this series of eleven cases of communicating hydrocephalus, four gave a definite history of meningitis, but from these no anatomic examinations were possible; three others gave no history of meningitis, but the condition was evidently congenital, because each had had a lumbar meningocele and at necropsy each of these gave all the evidences of an old extensive basilar meningitis. Of the four remaining cases in this group, three were evidently of congenital origin, the enlargement of the head being noticed very shortly after birth, and the fourth was noticed when the child was three months old and may also have been congenital, no illness having been noticed between the time of birth and the enlargement of the head. As an anatomic examination was not made in any of these four cases, the etiology remains entirely obscure.

Two cases of obstructive hydrocephalus (M. R. 4 and R. C. 8) present an almost indistinguishable anatomic picture. In each patient the foramen of Magendie and both foramina of Luschka were entirely absent, and the posterior fossa was filled with a cyst, resulting from a dilated fourth ventricle. The other ventricles were proportionately dilated. In one of these cases the child was perfectly normal until four months old, when a typical mild meningitis developed. The hydrocephalus followed immediately. At necropsy only a few minor adhesions were found. Had not the history been definite, the condition could easily have been regarded as congenital and the foramina at the base as congenitally absent, but the condition was unquestionably due to the meningitis, few traces of which remained. The other case with a similar anatomic picture was of congenital origin and the foramina were likewise closed. Whether an intra-uterine inflammatory process caused the condition similar to the extra-uterine meningitis of the other case, or whether the foramina were congenitally absent, could not be decided.

Congenital obliteration of the aqueduct has been adequately presented in the previous paper. Recently, Schlapp and Gere[1] presented additional cases of the same character.

One tumor has been included in this series. Tumors, of course, with rare exceptions, produce only the obstructive type of hydrocephalus. In infancy they are extremely rare and it is only in early childhood that this becomes an important factor to consider. As age increases hydrocephalus becomes more the result of tumor and relatively less the result of meningitis, on account of the increasing frequency of tumors.

SPONTANEOUS CURE OF INTERNAL HYDROCEPHALUS

Spontaneous recovery is not infrequent in internal hydrocephalus. This is evident from the cases seen from time to time of arrested growth of the abnormally large head. We have at least three cases under observation in which the diagnosis is clear, and in which there has been no change in the size of the head of the patient for years. Another child was studied through an attack of meningitis into the stage of hydrocephalus. After being lost sight of for three years, she returned apparently entirely cured. Many patients with meningitis recover without an internal hydrocephalus, and no doubt many cases of hydrocephalus follow meningitis and sooner or later recover.

Spontaneous recovery naturally depends on the cause of the disease. A spontaneous cure in a case of hydrocephalus with a congenital or other obstruction at the aqueduct seems entirely impossible, but it is not difficult to imagine recovery following the gradual disappearance of adhesions. This is especially true when one realizes how adhesions may disappear. The reverse may also be true and adhesions in the meninges as elsewhere may be progressive and increase the hydrocephalus. It is also possible to imagine a sudden rupture of the thin wall of a large fourth ventricle cyst, producing a new foramen of exit to the subarachnoid space. It is not improbable that the majority of cases having a meningocele but no hydrocephalus, represent a regressive stage or cure of an old intra-uterine hydrocephalus. Otherwise it is difficult to understand the formation of many meningoceles.

SUMMARY AND CONCLUSIONS

1. Twenty-six cases of internal hydrocephalus have been studied, fifteen of the obstructive and eleven of the communicating variety.

2. These cases have been studied with intraventricular and intra-spinal injections of phenolsulphonephthalein.

3. Postmortem examinations have demonstrated an obstruction in every case in which an obstruction has been shown clinically by this test. The obstruction may be a congenital malformation or inflammatory process or tumor, and occur at any

part of the ventricular system, but usually at the aqueduct of Sylvius or the foramina of Luschka and Magendie.

4. In all cases of obstructive hydrocephalus there is practically no absorption from the ventricles, and frequently (although not neecssarily) a normal absorption from the subarachnoid space. Hydrocephalus results because the fluid is mechanically prevented from passing from the ventricles, where the fluid forms, to the subarachnoid space, where it is normally absorbed, and where only it can be absorbed.

5. Communicating hydrocephalus is caused by a barrier of adhesions at the base of the brain which mechanically prevents the cerebrospinal fluid from reaching the cerebral subarachnoid space, where the greatest part of absorption normally takes place. The various cisternae or centers for the distribution of cerebrospinal fluid are more or less obliterated by adhesions.

6. Absorption of cerebrospinal fluid is a general process, from the entire subarachnoid space, and communicating hydrocephalus results because only a fraction of this area can be utilized for absorption.

7. These pathologic findings harmonize with the clinical phenolsulphonephthalein tests, which show a greatly diminished absorption from the subarachnoid space.

8. Obstructive and communicating hydrocephalus are, therefore, essentially the same, and in reality all are due to obstruction. In the obstructive variety the obstruction is in the ventricular system; in the communicating variety the obstruction is in the subarachnoid space.

9. Obstructive hydrocephalus may, by operation or spontaneously, change to communicating hydrocephalus, or the reverse may occur spontaneously. Careful studies with the phenolsulphonephthalein test will indicate these possibilities.

10. Meningitis is by far the greatest etiologic factor in both types of hydrocephalus and probably always causes the communicating variety. This may be either prenatal or postnatal. The meningitis may be of a very mild grade and easily overlooked.

11. There is a definite relationship between a meningocele and internal hydrocephalus; both usually probably result from the same cause. The removal of a meningocele may aggravate a fairly well balanced or even arrested case of internal hydrocephalus. This probably results from a diminution of the absorbing area.

12. Spontaneous recovery of internal hydrocephalus sometimes occurs.

13. We feel that the surgical treatment of internal hydrocephalus has now a definite anatomic basis and hopeful prospects. The operative results of a series of cases will appear in a subsequent communication.

REFERENCE

[1]Schlapp, M. G., and Gere, B.: Occlusion of the Aqueduct of Sylvius in Relation to Internal Hydrocephalus. *Am. J. D. C., 13:* 461, 1917.

VI

VENTRICULOGRAPHY FOLLOWING THE INJECTION OF AIR INTO THE CEREBRAL VENTRICLES*

The value of rontgenography in the diagnosis and localization of intracranial tumors is mainly restricted to the cases in which the neoplasm has affected the skull. In an analysis of the x-ray findings in one hundred cases of brain tumor from Doctor Halsted's Clinic, Heuer and I[1] have shown that in only 6 per cent of the cases did the tumor cast a shadow, and in these it was only the calcified areas that were differentiated by the x-rays from the normal cerebral tissues.

In those instances (9 per cent of our cases) in which tumor has encroached upon the sphenoid, ethmoid or frontal sinus, the invading portion casts a shadow in the rontgenogram. Such shadows are due to the displacement of the normally contained air by tissues which are less pervious to the x-ray. This group of shadows is of minor practical importance because the growth can be recognized by the destruction of the walls or bony septa of the sinuses.

Since the x-rays penetrate normal brain tissues, blood, cerebrospinal fluid and non-calcified tumor tissue almost equally, any changes in the brain produced by altered proportions of these components will not materially alter the rontgenogram.

Although skull changes are shown by the x-ray in 45 per cent of our cases and are frequently pathognomonic, on the whole they represent late stages of the disease. As intracranial tumors come to be diagnosed and localized earlier, the value of the x-ray will be correspondingly diminished.

For some time I have considered the possibility of filling the cerebral ventricles

with a medium that will produce a shadow in the radiogram. If this could be done, an accurate outline of the cerebral ventricles could be photographed with x-rays, and since most neoplasms either directly or indirectly modify the size or shape of the ventricles, we should then possess an early and accurate aid to the localization of intracranial affections. In addition to its radiographic properties, any substance injected into the ventricles must satisfy two very rigid exactions: (1) It must be absolutely non-irritating and non-toxic; and (2) it must be readily absorbed and excreted.

The various solutions and suspensions used in pyelography — thorium, potassium, iodide, collargol, argyrol, bismuth subnitrate and subcarbonate, all in various concentrations — were injected into the ventricles of dogs, but always with fatal results, owing to the injurious effects on the brain. Marked oedema, serosonguineous exudate, and petechial hemorrhages resulted. The severe reactions that are sometimes encountered after the intraspinous injection of most therapeutic remedies indicate the dangers even from carefully prepared solutions. A slight acidity or alkalinity may result even in death. It seems unlikely that any solution of radiographic value will be found which is sufficiently harmless to justify its injection into the central nervous system. Suspensions are precluded because they are not absorbed.

Ventriculography, therefore, seems possible only by substitution of gas for cerebrospinal fluid. It is largely due to the frequent comment by Doctor Halsted on the remarkable power of intestinal gases "to perforate bone" that my attention was drawn to its practical possibilities in the

*Reprinted from *The Annals of Surgery,* July, 1918.

brain. Striking gas shadows are present in all abdominal and thoracic radiograms. The stomach and intestines are often outlined by the contained air, even more sharply than when filled with bismuth. A small collection of gas in the intestines often obliterates the kidney outlines. A perforation of the intestines may be diagnosed by the shadow of the air that has accumulated under the diaphragm. Gas gangrene may be diagnosed by the air blebs (of B. welchii) in the tissues. Pneumothorax is sharply outlined because the normal lung tissues are eliminated. The paranasal sinuses and mastoid air cells show up in a thick skull by virtue of the air, and pathological conditions of the sinuses are evident because inflammatory or tumor tissue replaces the air. From these and many other normal and pathological clinical demonstrations of the radiographic properties of air it is but a step to the injection of gas into the cerebral ventricles — pneumoventriculography.

Methods. Several gases are inert and readily absorbable, and in these respects satisfy the requirements for injection into the cerebrospinal system. Although it is possible other gases give even better results, we have used only air in the injections here described. The merits of other gases are now being studied.

In order to obtain a skiagram of the lateral cerebral ventricles filled with air, it is necessary to remove at least more cerebrospinal fluid than the contents of one ventricle and to replace this fluid with an equal quantity of air. Before closure of the fontanelles, one can readily make a ventricular puncture through the interosseus defect. After union of the sutures, it is necessary to make a small opening in the bone.

Air and water in a ventricle behave exactly as they would in a closed flask. Following any change in position the fluid gravitates to the most dependent part and the air rises to the top. Owing to the free communication between the third, the right and the left lateral ventricles through the foramina of Monro, fluid and air will readily pass from one ventricle to the other. Because of the curves in the ventricular system, however, it is obvious that in any given position, only part of the ventricular fluid can gravitate to the point of the needle, so that this amount only can be aspirated. If desired, fluid can be removed from the remaining recesses by tilting the head, just as one manipulates a curved tube to replace the fluid with air. Theoretically, it should be possible to remove nearly all the ventricular fluid by suitable manipulations of the head, but for practical purposes enough fluid can be obtained from one correct position. Visualization of the ventricular system will best indicate the most appropriate location for ventricular puncture and the proper position of the head. It will then be seen that the most fluid can be obtained from a puncture in the anterior part of either lateral ventricle (Fig. 2). The head should be placed with the face down and partially rotated so that the ventricle to be aspirated is beneath and the needle enters at the most dependent point possible. This position permits the maximal drainage of fluid from the opposite lateral and the third ventricles. Aspiration through a puncture in the posterior or descending horn permits a fairly complete removal of the fluid from one ventricle and from that portion of the other lateral ventricle which is anterior to the foramen of Monro. In the aspiration of fluid from the posterior horn of the lateral ventricle, the patient must lie with the face directed upward and backward and the head rotated from 30 to 40 degrees toward the side of the needle.

The exchange of air for cerebrospinal fluid must be made accurately. If the air injected is greater in volume than the fluid withdrawn, acute pressure symptoms will result. To attain accuracy we have used a Record syringe with a two-way valve attachment (Fig 1). A small amount of fluid (20 cc.) is aspirated and an equal quantity of air injected. This is repeated until all the fluid has been removed. By aspirating and injecting in small quantities, injury to the brain from negative pressure is prevented. Not knowing the size of the ventricles beforehand, we have no way of estimating the amount of air necessary to fill one ventricle. For this reason we have preferred the removal of all the fluid that can be readily obtained. This has been found to be but little greater than the contents of one ventricle.

Needless to say, owing to the lighter weight of air, the ventriculogram represents the ventricle farthest from the x-ray plate. To insure the best results the sagittal plane of the head should be parallel with the plate. Valuable assistance can also be obtained from anteroposterior x-rays. The head should then be placed so that the sagittal plane is vertical, preferably with the occiput resting on the plate. With the latter precaution a more even distribution of air on the two sides is obtained and the ventriculogram represents the anterior portions of both lateral ventricles. For special points in diagnosis additional anteroposterior views may be taken of the posterior and descending horns of the ventricle by placing the forehead on the plate.

Results Following Injection. We have injected air into the cerebral ventricles at least twenty times. In some instances the injection has been repeated. The amount of air injected has varied from 40 to 300 cc., the larger quantities in cases of internal hydrocephalus. Only once has there been any reaction, and in this case the injection (300 cc.) was made forty-eight hours after the first stage of an operation for cerebellar tumor. The reaction was

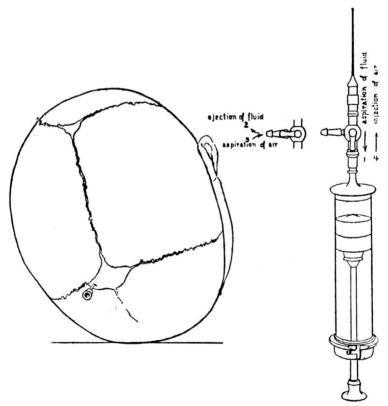

Fig. 1. Showing oblique position of head for aspiration of fluid and injection of air. The forehead is resting on plate. Note point of entrance of the needle into anterior fontanelle on dependent side. Figure on right shows record syringe and two-way valve attachment used for this purpose.

characterized by a rise of temperature, nausea, vomiting, and increased headache, all of which quickly relieved after release of the air by a ventricular puncture. Ten days later, a large cerebellar tumor was removed, the patient making an uneventful recovery. All of the injections have been made in children varying from six months to twelve years of age. Invariably the lateral ventricle has been sharply outlined in the radiogram. In two instances the third ventricle and the foramen of Monro were visible. In none, however, have we observed the fourth ventricle or the aqueduct of Sylvius. The practical value from the pneumoventriculography is expected principally from the shadows of the lateral ventricles.

Day by day the air shadow diminishes and eventually disappears. In a case of internal hydrocephalus it required two weeks. Possibly in more normal cases the time may be less, as air in other body tissues vanishes much more rapidly. In all probability absorption of air injected into the ventricles takes place by the same channels as in the case of the ventricular cerebrospinal fluid. In a previous communication[2] it has been shown that cerebrospinal fluid is almost entirely absorbed

from the subarachnoid space; that only a very slight absorption takes place from the ventricles. Phenolsulphonephthalein in a closed ventricular system disappears in from ten to twelve days, whereas it is absorbed in from ten to twelve hours when the ventricles communicate with the subarachnoid space, where the absorption of cerebrospinal fluid normally takes place.

Air introduced into the ventricles acts in no way differently from the air included at every intracranial operation. Following tumor extirpation especially, the resulting defect fills with air which, unless displacd by salt solution, is shut in when the dura and scalp are sutured. For a few days pending its absorption from tumor defects the patient may be conscious of the movement of the air when the head is turned, but its presence is without any other effects.

The Value of Ventriculography. Even in the few cases here reported ventriculography has proven of great practical value. For the first time we have a means of diagnosing internal hydrocephalus in the early stages. Internal hydrocephalus is one of the most insidious diseases of the brain and is rarely diagnosed before a considerable amount of cortical destruction has resulted. This is true of adults as well as of

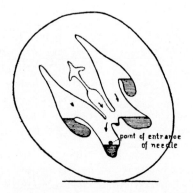 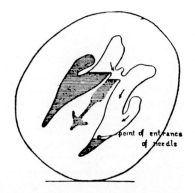

Fig. 2. Diagrams showing relative amounts of cerebrospinal fluid that can be removed from a single ventricular puncture; (1) when forehead is down (a) and (2) when occiput is down (b). Shaded area represents the fluid which remains in the ventricular system after the greatest possible quantity has been removed. Unshaded area represents maximum quantity of air which can be injected to replace the fluid withdrawn. It is evident that more fluid can be removed when the puncture is made anterionly and the forehead is dependent.

children. With exact visualization of the ventricles the findings are pathognomonic. Not only the existence of hydrocephalus but its degree and the amount of brain destruction are at once evident from the ventriculogram.

In one case (in an infant six months old) an internal hydrocephalus was suspected from a bulging fontanelle, but the ventriculogram showed no enlargement of the ventricles. Another child (three years old) remained drowsy for several days after apparent recovery from an attack of epidemic cerebrospinal meningitis. The spinal fluid was clear and contained no organisms. The ventricular fluid was turbid and organisms were present; the ventriculogram demonstrated a greatly enlarged ventricle. The diagnosis of obstructive internal hydrocephalus, clinically unsuspected, was made with absolute certainty from the ventriculogram.

In two other children measurements of the head were normal but hydrocephalus was suspected because of abnormally large fontanelles. In each case the ventriculogram demonstrated ventricles which nearly filled the cranial chamber.

One of the most interesting diagnoses, made possible only through the ventriculogram, was in a colored child eight months old. The head was definitely larger than normal, indicating the probability of an internal hydrocephalus. Over the anterior fontanelle, but slightly to one side, was a protruding tumor suggesting a meningocele, and this diagnosis had been made. Air injected into the lateral ventricle passed directly into the tumor. In the lateral ventriculogram the tumor was seen to arise from the greatly distended ventricle by a narrow neck. An anteroposterior ventriculogram showed this communication to be unilateral. The diagnosis of a ruptured cortex with a (false) ventricular hernia was established, and subsequently verified at necropsy.

In another case a large cerebellar tumor was removed from a boy twelve years old. The large head, the marked convolutional atrophy of the skull, blindness, and the location of the tumor, made the diagnosis of internal hydrocephalus certain, but only the ventriculogram gave an accurate estimation of its advanced degree and the amount of brain destruction.

Without a ventriculogram the diagnosis of internal hydrocephalus in children is frequently guess-work; with the ventriculogram the diagnosis is absolute.

We have as yet not obtained a normal ventriculogram. In one of these cases the ventricle was small but not known to be normal. It is possible that one of the earliest signs of internal hydrocephalus may be alteration in the shape of the ventricle due to the pressure effects on parts of the wall which are least resistant. The obliteration of the angle between body and posterior horn suggests this probability, but ventriculograms of the intervening stages and the normal are lacking.

We have not yet applied ventriculography to adults, but expect to do so in all cases in which the diagnosis is obscure. In a boy of twelve years the ventriculogram was even sharper than in younger children. In adults we should expect the ventriculogram to be at least as sharp or possibly even more so because of the greater contrast between the density of air and bone. Several possibilities are anticipated from ventriculograms in adults: (1) The enlarged ventricles in internal hydrocephalus should be absolutely defined. (2) Tumors in either cerebral hemisphere may dislocate or compress the ventricle and in this way localize the neoplasm. (3) Tumors growing into the ventricles may show a corresponding defect in the ventricular shadow. (4) A unilateral hydrocephalus may be demonstrable if the air cannot be made to enter the opposite ventricle.

CONCLUSIONS

1. The outlines of the lateral cerebral ventricles can be sharply outlined by the x-ray if air is substituted for cerebrospinal fluid.

2. The injection of air into the ventricles has had no deleterious effects in twenty cases.

3. Ventriculography has already proved of great practical value in the diagnosis and

localization of many intracranial conditions. It is invaluable in internal hydrocephalus.

Note.—*Explanation of Figures.*—Two pictures are shown in each figure number. The upper one is the untouched photographic reproduction of the x-ray plate; the lower is the same photograph retouched by Miss Norris in order to overcome photographic loss of detail, and especially to emphasize the lines and special points which would otherwise be lost to the reader.

REFERENCES

[1]Rontgenography in the Localization of Brain Tumor, Based Upon a Series of One Hundred Consecutive Cases. *Johns Hopkins Hosp. Bull.,* xxvii: 311, 1916. Also: A Report of Seventy Cases of Brain Tumor. *Johns Hopkins Hosp. Bull.,* xxvii: 224, 1916.

[2]Dandy and Blackfan: *Am. J. Dis. Child., viii:* 406, 1914; *xiv:* 24, 1917. Also *J. A. M. A., lxi:* 2216, 1913.

VII

EXTIRPATION OF THE CHOROID PLEXUS OF THE LATERAL VENTRICLES IN COMMUNICATING HYDROCEPHALUS*

No form of treatment, either medical or surgical, has yet a valid claim to the cure of a single case of hydrocephalus, except in those cases caused by tumor and relieved by tumor extirpation. But hydrocephalus is a curable disease. This is demonstrated by the not infrequent cases which have been cured spontaneously, though usually at a time when cerebral destruction has left the patient a hopeless imbecile. The reason for nature's successes is that the cause has been either circumvented or overcome. The reason for medical or surgical failures is that the cause has not been recognized. All forms of therapy have been entirely empirical. They have been directed toward the effect rather than the cause. They have lacked not only the etiology and pathology of the disease but even a knowledge of the circulation of cerebrospinal fluid before pathological changes have occurred.

Hydrocephalus should no longer be classified as an idiopathic disease. Its pathology and, in large part, its etiology are definitely established.[1] With the cause recognized, a rational form of therapy is indicated. I make this statement principally upon the results of our own investigations, which have been conducted in the past five years. These studies include the paths for the circulation of cerebrospinal fluid, the place and manner of formation and absorption of cerebrospinal fluid, the experimental production of hydrocephalus, the pathogenesis of many cases of hydrocephalus studied clinically by the phenolsulphonephthalein test, and the pathology

of the various so-called types of hydrocephalus by post-mortem examination. The present communication is directed to the treatment based upon these observations.

A knowledge of the type of hydrocephalus is an absolute prerequisite to its treatment. The timeworn symptomatic classifications are incoordinate and confusing. The classification on the following page is presented, based upon the etiology and pathology of the disease:

The vast majority of cases of hydrocephalus are included in one of the two groups: (1) Communicating hydrocephalus; (2) obstructive hydrocephalus. The other types are rare. It will be noted that no separate subdivision has been made into internal and external hydrocephalus. It is a question whether external hydrocephalus ever really exists as a primary condition. It seems to be a secondary transformation of a primary internal hydrocephalus. This metamorphosis is probably due to a local or general atrophy of the cerebrum permitting escape to the exterior by these artificial channels. Because of the rarity of this condition, however, our facts are not sufficient to make a positive stand in this statement. It is conceivable, though not proven, that it may also result from a transfer of cerebrospinal fluid from the subarachnoid space to the subdural space in communicating hydrocephalus. The exact status of so-called external hydrocephalus is still in doubt. With this rare exception, nearly all hydrocephalus is internal; that is, the accumulation of cerebrospinal fluid is in the ventricles. It is internal for the very good reason that cerebrospinal fluid forms in the ventricles and cannot reach the exterior (obstruc-

*Reprinted from *The Annals of Surgery*, December, 1918.

45

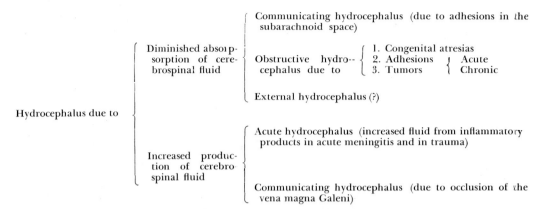

Hydrocephalus due to

- Diminished absorption of cerebrospinal fluid
  - Communicating hydrocephalus (due to adhesions in the subarachnoid space)
  - Obstructive hydrocephalus due to
    1. Congenital atresias
    2. Adhesions — Acute
    3. Tumors — Chronic
  - External hydrocephalus (?)
- Increased production of cerebrospinal fluid
  - Acute hydrocephalus (increased fluid from inflammatory products in acute meningitis and in trauma)
  - Communicating hydrocephalus (due to occlusion of the vena magna Galeni)

tive hydrocephalus) ; or at most it reaches only a small fraction of the external absorbing surface — the posterior cranial fossa and spinal canal (communicating hydrocephalus). In either case the fluid dams back at its source. If cerebrospinal fluid could reach the subarachnoid space over the entire exterior of the brain, it would be absorbed and hydrocephalus could not exist.

Another rare type of hydrocephalus is that due to thrombosis of the vena magna Galeni. Owing to insufficient collateral venous circulation, hydrocephalus then results from an increased production of cerebrospinal fluid by venous stasis, just as ascites often follows stenosis of the inferior vena cava. I have produced this type experimentally, but have seen no instance clinically. Only a few cases have been reported in the literature.

In acute meningitis of inflammatory origin there is undoubtedly an increased production of fluid from the products of the inflammation. It is questionable whether an increase of fluid by exudation should be classified with true hydrocephalus. It is probably external as much if not more than internal, because the infection has a general but principally external distribution. It subsides with the decline of the infection and is not of practical import in considering the treatment of hydrocephalus. An increase of fluid also follows trauma to the brain in fractures of the skull. It is probably of vascular origin, and usually subsides rapidly.

Fundamentally the two main types of hydrocephalus — obstructive and communicating — are similar. Both are due to an obstruction in the cerebrospinal fluid circulatory system. In our series of cases in children the relative frequency is nearly the same. In the former the obstruction is in the ventricles and in the latter in the subarachnoid space. The only reason for subdividing hydrocephalus into groups is that the anatomical differences in the two types necessitate an entirely different operative procedure for the treatment of each.

In this paper only the treatment of the communicating type of hydrocephalus will be considered. A form of treatment for hydrocephalus with obstruction will be presented in a later communication. For a proper understanding of the basis for the operation herein proposed, a brief explanation of the underlying etiology and pathology is necessary.

The Etiology and Pathology of Hydrocephalus with Communication. It is the communicating type of hydrocephalus which has caused all hydrocephalus to be considered idiopathic. Though numerous explanations have been proposed, no pathologic findings have been presented until recently. All the ventricles communicate with each other and with the subarachnoid space, and post-mortem examinations of the brain have heretofore revealed nothing to the naked eye. The reason for the negative findings has been an inadequate knowledge (1) of the post-mortem appearance of the normal subarachnoid space and the pia arachnoid membranes; (2) of the alterations produced by pathological changes; (3) of the relation of the subarachnoid space to the absorption of cerebrospinal fluid; and (4) the anatomy and physiology of the cerebrospinal fluid circulatory system.

The only satisfactory time to observe changes in the meninges is when the brain is being removed. Adhesions of an extensive nature will then be seen and divided, but later will show very little in the preserved specimen. In cases of communicating hydrocephalus the meninges will be opaque and thickened, the normal filmy pia arachnoid will be replaced by a firm, fibrous, adherent membrane. This will be especially noted in the cisternae at the base of the brain. The adhesions are often so dense as to tear the brain during their liberation. It is the distribution or location of these adhesions, not their extent, which determines the production of hydrocephalus (Fig. 1). Adhesions encircling the midbrain where it passes through the incisura tentorii, will destroy all communication between the posterior and middle cranial fossae and thereby eliminate the entire subarachnoid space over both cerebral hemispheres from participation in the absorption of cerebrospinal fluid. Hydrocephalus will invariably result from such a process. Adhesions which close the cisternae at the base of the brain will also produce hydrocephalus just as effectively.

The extraventricular cerebrospinal circulatory system may be compared to the trunk and branches of a tree — the cisternae representing the trunk, the subarachnoid spaces over the cerebral hemispheres the branches. Obliteration of the cisternae by adhesions is equivalent to transection of the trunk of a tree. All distal communication will be destroyed and hydrocephalus will follow. Large areas of adhesions may be present over the cerebral hemispheres with only local effects and with no effect upon the general cerebrospi-

nal fluid circulation. This is analogous to the absence of a relationship between the destruction of branches and the life of a tree. The absorbing function of these local areas is easily compensated by the subarachnoid space over the remainder of the brain.

In each of our cases these adhesions have also obliterated either one or two of the three foramina (Luschka and Magendie) by which the ventricles and the subarachnoid space normally communicate (Fig. 1). One foramen remaining patent will maintain an adequate transfer of cerebrospinal fluid. Should the adhesions close all three foramina at the base instead of only one or two, an obstructive hydrocephalus would result. In short, communicating hydrocephalus is due not to a reduction in the avenues of communication between the ventricles and the subarachnoid space but to a blocking of the primary trunks of the subarachnoid space, thus preventing cerebrospinal fluid from passing to the branches. The distribution of cerebrospinal fluid is thereby limited to that small part of the subarachnoid space in the posterior cranial fossa and the spinal canal. It does not include any of the subarachnoid space over either cerebral hemisphere, which is by far the most important area for absorption.

Cerebrospinal fluid is absorbed from the entire subarachnoid space. Adhesions obstructing the main stem of the subarachnoid space therefore limit the absorbing area to a fraction of the normal, and the diminished absorption results in accumulation of cerebrospinal fluid—hydrocephalus.

We have spoken of adhesions almost exclusively as the cause of communicating hydrocephalus. It is conceivable that certain tumors filling or compressing the cisternae may produce similar results. We have as yet no proof of this possibility. All of the cases observed by Dr. Blackfan and myself have had a meningitis, which has been both prenatal and postnatal. There is frequently a definite history of meningitis preceding the development of hydrocephalus, but this cannot always be obtained.

Studies with the phenosulphonephthalein test enabled us to predict ante mortem the pathologic findings. By the dye it was possible to measure the amount of absorption from any region by the quantitative excretion in the urine. It was found that normally practically no absorption occurs from the entire ventricular system (less than 1 per cent. in two hours). All the cerebrospinal fluid is absorbed from the subarachnoid space; 40 to 60 per cent. being excreted in a two-hour interval, which has been adopted as an arbitrary standard of time. In a large series of cases of communicating hydrocephalus the absorption from the subarachnoid space was found almost invariably to be only 8 to 10 per cent., or about one-fifth of the normal.

In view of the fact that experiments on animals have demonstrated that absorption of cerebrospinal fluid is from the entire subarachnoid space, the lowered absorption in communicating hydrocephalus must mean a reduction in the extent of the absorbing area and at a fairly constant location. The localization of the adhesions blocking the cisternae or surrounding the mesencephalon harmonized the physiological and clinical tests and the pathological findings. The frequent history of an antecedent meningitis is additional confirmatory evidence, should such be necessary. The experimental production of this type of hydrocephalus by duplicating nature's pathologic processes, leaves no doubt of the etiological and pathological basis of communicating hydrocephalus. This experimental proof will shortly appear, together with that of the other types of hydrocephalus.

In operations upon the brain of cases of communicating hydrocephalus, one is impressed by the absence of fluid in the sulci. The sulci are practically obliterated, and only vascular lines separate the convolutions. If hydrocephalus were due to occlusion of such fanciful structures as stomata into the venous sinuses or the Pacchionian bodies, as has been proposed, one

should expect distended subarachnoid spaces up to the points of obstruction. The absence of extracerebral cerebrospinal fluid proves the non-existence of any such mechanism, and indicates the lack of communication of the part of the subarachnoid space with the fluid-containing spaces; in other words, an obstruction must exist at some place nearer the origin of the cerebrospinal fluid.

The Diagnosis of Hydrocephalus with Communication. Clinically, the two types of internal hydrocephalus are identical. Neither by the history nor the physical examination can they be differentiated. Frequently, the communicating type can be diagnosed by the large quantity of cerebrospinal fluid which can be obtained by lumbar puncture, but there is such great variability in the amounts of fluid obtained in both types of hydrocephalus that the results are frequently of little value. The differentiation between the two types of hydrocephalus can be simply, harmlessly and absolutely made by the phenolsulphonephthalein test.

One cubic centimetre of neutral phenolsulphthalein[2] is introduced into either lateral ventricle; a lumbar puncture is done one-half hour later. If communication exists, the dye will by that time have appeared in the spinal fluid. If an obstruction exists in the ventricular system, the spinal fluid will remain colorless. This test is the only way in which guess-work can be eliminated.

Previous Treatment of Communicating Hydrocephalus. Because of the great number of operations suggested, tried, and found failures, their consideration individually would require too much space and yield little of practical value. With rare exceptions, no attempt has been made to differentiate the two types of hydrocephalus. The usual treatments have been directed toward a disposition of the fluid, (1) either by transferring the fluid to the exterior of the brain, to the scalp, the retroperitoneal space, the peritoneal cavity, or some other space; or (2) by making a communication with some part of the venous system, either directly or by a vascular transplant; (3) in addition to periodically repeated lumbar and ventricular puncture, attempts have been made to establish a more or less continuous drainage to the exterior, always, of course, with death from secondary infection. Other attempts have been made to reduce the formation of cerebrospinal fluid by ligating one or both carotid arteries, by injection of irritants into the ventricles, compression of the head, etc.

All attempts to drain into body spaces are futile because the tissues wall off the fluid and soon cease to absorb it. Moreover, the openings into the spaces remain patent only temporarily. Puncture of the corpus callosum might at first sight appear to be an ideal procedure, but it is practically identical with punctures elsewhere. Fluid side-tracked by an opening of the corpus callosum or of other parts of the brain does not pass into the subarachnoid space, but into the avascular subdural space, where absorption is little if any greater than in the ventricles or in the scalp. Moreover, the openings in the corpus callosum or elsewhere closes in the course of a few weeks. Fluid can reach the *subarachnoid spaces* over the brain only through the normally designated distributing channels — the cisternae. Permanent communication between the ventricles and the cisternae can be maintained only through the fourth ventricle and by means of the foramina of Luschka and Magendie, or, in their absence, by openings artificially produced in this region.

The fate of vascular communications is similar. The opening into the veins, sinus or transplant functions but briefly. Such openings can hardly be expected to function properly, because they should handle in a few minutes all the fluid which is produced in several hours, and would be functionless the remainder of the time. Normal absorption of cerebrospinal fluid takes place slowly, by a process of osmosis through membranes and not into prepared openings or stomata.

Scientific Basis for Operative Treatment. The logical treatment of any disease is the removal of the cause. In communicating hydrocephalus the treatment of the cause, that is, the removal or liberation of adhesions, is precluded by present surgical limitations. The area of adhesions is too extensive, too diffuse, and in a location inaccessible for operative interference. The ideal treatment would be restoration of the cisternae through these adhesions, and even if reconstruction were possible reformation of the adhesions must always remain a possibility.

In view of these deterring factors, treatment of the cause must for the present at least be deferred. From the results of experiments on animals a new and scientific form of treatment is suggested, by which it is hoped to circumvent the cause. This treatment aims to restore the balance between fluid production and fluid absorption by reducing the production of cerebrospinal fluid to a level where it can be absorbed. By experiments on animals, the results of which will appear shortly, the following facts have been established:

(1) If the foramen of Monro is occluded, a unilateral hydrocephalus results;

(2) But if the entire choroid plexus of this ventricle is removed at the time the foramen of Monro is occluded, this ventricle will be obliterated;

(3) Therefore, cerebrospinal fluid forms from the choroid plexus, and not from the ependyma.

(4) Following total occlusion of the aqueduct of Sylvius the development of hydrocephalus is greatly retarded by the extirpation of the choroid plexus of both lateral ventricles. In this experiment the cerebrospinal fluid, which is produced proximal to the obstruction, can be derived only from the choroid plexus of the third ventricle.

The conclusion from these experiments is if all the choroid plexuses of the four ventricles could be removed, the formation of cerebrospinal fluid would cease and hydrocephalus could not result or if present its development would cease. To cure obstructive hydrocephalus by removal of the choroid plexus, it would be necessary to remove all of the choroid plexuses because there is no absorption in the ventricles; but in communicating hydrocephalus, there is about one-fifth of the normal absorption. It would not therefore be necessary to remove the entire amount of choroid plexus but to reduce its volume until the amount remaining would not produce cerebrospinal fluid faster than it could be absorbed. In other words, it would be necessary to remove roughly four-fifths of the total amount of choroid plexus to reduce the fluid formation to the 8 to 10 per cent absorption (one-fifth of the normal) which occurs in communicating hydrocephalus.

It is not feasible to remove the choroid plexus from the third ventricle and very difficult to extirpate flocculi in the fourth ventricle. Roughly the choroid plexuses of the combined third and fourth ventricles is about one-fifth the total amount in all the ventricles. The plexus is in the two lateral ventricles therefore comprise about four-fifths of the total. It is relatively easy to remove the choroid plexus from both lateral ventricles. A bilateral extirpation from the lateral ventricles should, therefore, according to our present conceptions, reduce the formation of cerebrospinal fluid to a point where it can be absorbed by the restricted patent area of the subarachnoid space.

The problem, however, is not purely one of mathematics. Casually, one would expect that the removal of 75 per cent of the productive structure would reduce the formation to meet absorption which is 20 to 25 per cent of the normal, but it should do even more, for in hydrocephalus fluid is formed at a greatly reduced rate because of the changed intracranial pressure from fluid accumulation. It has been demonstrated that the formation of cerebrospinal fluid is to a large extent at least mechanical. This can easily be demonstrated by inducing venous congestion by compression of the veins of the neck. We know that fluid forms at a greatly lessened rate in hydrocephalus due to the increased intracranial pressure, because if it formed at the normal rate (which we know) the head would grow at a tremendous speed. Although nature can modify the rate of fluid production she is unable to reduce its formation to the level at which it can be absorbed. The removal of the choroid plexus from both lateral ventricles should be more than is necessary, but it seems preferable to remove too much with no consequent danger, than to run the risk of an insufficient removal, in which event a progressive destruction of the brain will inevitably result. Hydrocephalus even when developing at the slowest rate causes a rapid atrophy of the brain. It is of course obvious that if more than the necessary amount of choroid plexus is removed, extra- and intravascular pressure differences will produce sufficient fluid to maintain the necessary amount of fluid to fill the ventricles.

The Operation.[3] The steps in the removal of the choroid plexus are clearly shown in the accompanying drawings by Miss Norris. A small circular bone flap is made over the parietal eminence. The wound is made well posterior to the Rolondic area and in a salient part of the occipital lobe. After ligating numerous vessels on the cortex by circumvection, the cortex is bloodlessly incised and this incision carried into the ventricle. From the exposure which is over the junction of the body and descending horn of the lateral ventricle, the entire extent of the ventricle can be brought into view. The opening in the brain is maintained by an open nasal dilator, or when the ventricle is very large the brain wall must be elevated by a spatula which is inserted into the ventricle. It is necessary to remove all the cerebrospinal fluid in the ventricle to get a view of the choroid plexus; the brownish-red flocculent choroid plexus can then be easily followed from the foramen of Monro to the tip of the descending horn.

The choroid plexus is picked up in

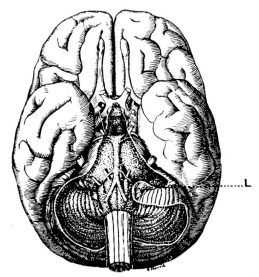

- - - - - - L

Fig. 1. Diagram to show the distribution of adhesions over the base of the brain in a case of communicating hydrocephalus. All the cisternae are obliterated. Communication between the ventricles and subarachnoid is restricted to one foramen of Luschka (L). The other foramen of Luschka and the foramen of Magendie are sealed by the adhesions. Ablation of the cisternae prevents cerebrospinal fluid reaching the cerebral subarachnoid space.

forceps at the foramen of Monro, and the vessels ligated by a silver clip. A pledget of moist cotton is inserted into the foramen of Monro to prevent blood gravitating into the third ventricle. The plexus is then transected and gently stripped backward from its narrow attachment to the floor of the body of the ventricle. When the glomus is reached the stripping from the body of the ventricle is stopped and the choroid plexus picked up at the tip of the descending horn. This part of the choroid plexus is also stripped backward to the glomus; the remaining attachment of the glomus is then liberated and the entire choroid plexus removed in toto. Bleeding from the denuded area of velum interpositum is slight and easily controlled by moist saline cotton pledgets. Special care must be taken to leave no bleeding points.

The collapse of the brain following evacuation of the ventricular fluid causes a remarkable infolding of the cerebral walls, the extent depending of course upon the size of the ventricle and thickness of the cortex. In advanced cases a tremendous cavity results, which is filled before closure with salt solution to restore the collapsed cerebral wall as nearly as possible to its natural convexity.

A remarkable exposure is obtained during the operation in the ventricle. One can see the third and opposite lateral ventricle and the septum lucidum which is frequently perforated in many places owing to pressure atrophy.

The opening in the cortex is closed with a series of interrupted fine silk sutures which are held by the delicate pia arachnoid membrane. The dura and scalp are carefully closed also with silk, special care being taken to prevent any subsequent leak of cerebrospinal fluid.

Result. I have extirpated the choroid plexus in four cases of hydrocephalus from Professor Halsted's Clinic. All of these have survived the operation, although three died two to four weeks after the operation. One patient has survived a bilateral choroid plexectomy ten months, and shows no evidence that the disease is advancing. During and following the operation the reaction seems to vary directly with the grade of the disease. If the ventricle is small the operation will be well tolerated even by a very young baby. When the ventricles are large and the cortex is greatly thinned and marked enlargement of the head has resulted, a very severe reaction occurs during the operation and the convalescence is very slow. In the highest grades of hydrocephalus death will follow almost immediately upon release of the fluid, or a very severe reaction will result at once and death will quickly follow. In the advanced cases we can hold out very little encouragement from operative procedures of any kind which will necessitate release of fluid and consequent collapse of the brain. There is, however, little object in attempting a cure of the disease in this advanced stage because the child would be left a hopeless imbecile. In the three cases of this series which subsequently died the hydrocephalus was of the extreme grade. In each of these there was an immediate operative collapse, beginning with pallor of the face and body, rapid feeble pulse which quickly becomes imperceptible, cold clammy perspiration, rapid, shallow and irregular respirations — in other words, typical shock. These changes invariably begin with evacuation of the ventricular fluid, and are undoubtedly due to differences of pressure which affect all the blood-vessels and directly or indirectly the centres in the medulla. Following escape of the fluid the thin brain walls collapse like a wet cloth. In addition to the differences in intra- and extravascular pressures, the mechanical kinking of the large vascular trunks by angulation of the infolding brain must have a pronounced effect upon the circulation.

In each instance there was a gradual recovery, and death came from two to four

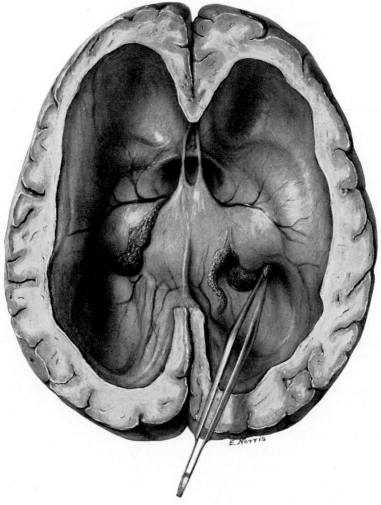

Fig. 2. Coronal section through hydrocephalic brain, showing method of stripping choroid plexus from its attachment to the floor of the ventricle. The right plexus has been stripped from the foramen of Monro to the end of the glomus and at the tip descending horn is shown grasped by the forceps in the process of being stripped to the glomus. The entire plexus is then lifted from its bed.

weeks later. In two cases death was no doubt due to gradually progressive acute intracranial pressure which we now would be able to recognize and probably alleviate. In a third case the cause of death is still uncertain, though undoubtedly a result of the operation. The temperature rose to 108° four hours after operation; remained around 102° to 106° for two weeks. Though conscious, the ability to swallow was lost and not regained. At autopsy no cause for death could be observed.

In the fourth case, which is still living and well and with no evidence of progress of the disease, no post-operative effects were observed, despite the fact that within three weeks of birth three operations were performed, one for the removal of a large myelomeningocele and two for the bilateral extirpation of the choroid plexus. Feeding was uninterrupted; the temperature at no time rose over 100°, and the rising curve of body weight was not even temporarily affected.

This case was kindly referred to me by Dr. J. Whitridge Williams, who made a most unusual diagnosis of hydrocephalus immediately following the child's delivery in his clinic. The head was not enlarged but the fontanelles were wider and a trifle fuller than normal. The myelomeningocele also suggested the possibility of hydrocephalus. A ventriculogram[4] showed a well developed hydrocephalus with complete obliteration of the posterior horn of the lateral ventricle. In no other way could this very early tentative diagnosis have been substantiated.

Unfortunately in this case our diagnosis of communicating hydrocephalus has been to a large extent conjectural. The large myelomeningocele filling the lumbar region precluded successful lumbar puncture, so that we were unable to determine by the phenolsulphonephthalein test whether communication was present, or indirectly by quantitative absorption whether the hydrocephalus was of the communicating type.

The absorption of phenolsulphonephtha-lein following injection into the ventricle was 2 per cent, which is a little higher than in obstructive hydrocephalus and about what obtains in communicating hydrocephalus. This is not considered conclusive by any means, as the difference between the ventricular absorption in the two types of hydrocephalus is not great enough to be a decisive test. The meningocele is by no means evidence in favor of a communicating and against an obstructive hydrocephalus.

Wherever possible both choroid plexuses should certainly be removed. This requires two operations, the length of time intervening depending upon the reaction following the first operation. Only one of our cases has had a bilateral extirpation. It is doubtful whether the removal of the choroid plexus of one ventricle would produce more than a retardation of the disease, which, of course, would be of no ultimate benefit.

Even though one case is apparently well ten months after a bilateral extirpation, no conclusions are justifiable on the basis of a single case or in such a short period of time. The operation is presented without claims of cure, but because of its apparently sound scientific foundation it is hoped and expected that cures will result.

CONCLUSIONS

1. Any treatment of hydrocephalus must be based upon the etiology and pathology of this disease.

2. Communicating hydrocephalus is caused by an obstruction in the subarachnoid space causing diminished absorption of cerebrospinal fluid.

3. This obstruction is probably nearly always due to adhesions following meningitis.

4. These adhesions close the cisternae through which all cerebrospinal fluid is distributed to the subarachnoid space over the cerebral hemispheres.

5. Absorption is reduced to one-fourth or one-fifth of the normal, roughly corresponding to the volume of subarachnoid

space which contains cerebrospinal fluid.

6. It is at present impossible to reestablish the cisternae by surgical means.

7. By experiments it has been demonstrated that cerebrospinal fluid forms from the choroid plexus.

8. An operation is presented for the cure of this type of hydrocephalus by removal of the choroid plexus of both lateral ventricles. This removes, roughly, four-fifths of the total amount of fluid-forming structures. It is hoped the cerebrospinal fluid which forms from the choroid plexus can be absorbed in the small amount of subarachnoid space which remains in the third and fourth ventricles.

9. Choroid plexectomy is of value only in communicating hydrocephalus. Any treatment therefore presupposes an accurate diagnosis of the type of hydrocephalus. This is best made by the phenolsulphonephthalein test.

10. The operation has been performed on four cases. One case is alive and apparently well ten months after the operation.

11. Sufficient time has not elapsed to speculate on the practical results of the operation.

12. The operation can be safely performed in moderately advanced cases of hydrocephalus.

REFERENCES

[1]Dandy, W. E., and Blackfan, K. D.: Internal Hydrocephalus. An Experimental, Clinical and Pathological Study. *J. A. M. A., lxi:* 216, 1913; *Am. J. Dis. Child., viii:* 406, 1914; *Beitr. z. klin. Chir., xciii:* 392, 1914. Internal Hydrocephalus, Second Paper. *Am. J. Dis. Child, xiv:* 424, 1917.

[2]This solution has been specially prepared by Mr. H. A. B. Dunning, of Hynson, Westcott & Dunning. A serious reaction will follow the use of the ordinary phenolsulphonephthalein solution used for kidney studies.

[3]I am greatly indebted to Professor Halsted for many suggestions in the development of this operative procedure, as well as in the experimental work upon which the operation is founded.

[4]Dandy, W. E.: Ventriculography Following the Injection of Air Into the Cerebral Ventricles. *A. S.,* July, 1918.

VIII

RONTGENOGRAPHY OF THE BRAIN AFTER THE INJECTION OF AIR INTO THE SPINAL CANAL*

(From the Department of Surgery, The Johns Hopkins Hospital and University)

As was shown in a recent publication,[1] one or more of the cerebral ventricles can be sharply outlined in a rontgenogram if the ventricular fluid be withdrawn and replaced by an equal quantity of air. In the course of this work it was soon noted that in many cases some of the air had passed out of the ventricular system and could be seen in filaments on the surface of the brain, that is, in the sulci. In order to reach the sulci from the point of injection in a lateral ventricle, the air must have followed the normal pathways by which cerebrospinal fluid circulates. It must have passed through the foramen of Monro into the third ventricles, thence into the fourth ventricles, through the aqueduct of Sylvius, and then, having left the ventricular system, it must have entered the cisterna magna by way of the foramen of Magendie and the paired foramina of Luschka. Finally, from the cisterna magna it must have passed along the various cisternae under the base of the brain and then by numerous branches have reached the termination of the subarachnoid space — the sulci. Not infrequently, the entire subarachnoid space was graphically defined by the air shadows.

These observations at once gave promise of new possibilities in intracranial diagnostic study. Many lesions of the brain affect part of the subarachnoid space directly or indirectly. In hydrocephalus of the communicating type, adhesions at the base of the brain obliterate the cisternae and the cerebrospinal fluid cannot reach the sulci over the cerebral hemispheres; a local area of subarachnoid space may be obliterated by a tumor situated on or near the surface of the brain; a defect in the brain due to atrophy must necessarily be filled with cerebrospinal fluid, which may maintain communication with the subarachnoid space. These, and no doubt many other conditions, should be demonstrable by the absence or by the presence of air over the cerebral hemispheres.

After the injection of air into a cerebral ventricle a certain amount will soon appear on the external surface of the brain if the head is carefully manipulated so that the air is guided to the small aqueduct of Sylvius and the fourth ventricle. But the time of escape of air from the ventricles and of its appearance in the cerebral sulci are variable. The more completely the ventricles are filled with air the greater the probability that it will appear externally; and the more dilated the iter and the foramina of Luschka and Magendie (as in hydrocephalus) the more readily will air appear externally. Nevertheless, it was evident that at best the amount of air that will reach the cerebral sulci must vary greatly, according to the conditions existing in each individual case.

The problem therefore before us was: How can we in every case be sure of obtaining a complete injection of the subarachnoid space? The solution lies in the direct injection of air into the spinal canal. By this method the influence of the ventricular system is entirely eliminated; the air passes directly into the cisterna magna and thence into the ultimate ramifications of the subarachnoid space.

The technic is essentially similar to that described elsewhere for intraventricular in-

---

*Reprinted from *Annals of Surgery*, October, 1919.

jections. A small quantity of spinal fluid is withdrawn and an equal amount of air injected into the spinal canal. This process of substitution is repeated until the fluid ceases to appear on aspiration. There is no need to sterilize the air, because it is always free from pathogenic organisms.

Undoubtedly this procedure is not devoid of danger. Medullary distress, even fatal results, might well follow from increased intracranial pressure if the amount of air injected were even slightly in excess of the fluid withdrawn. The danger would certainly appear to be much greater in intraspinous than in intraventricular injections, because in the latter direct pressure on the medulla in large measure is inhibited by the tentorium cerebri. In my own cases no bad effects have followed and the results have led me to believe that with proper care and judgment the procedure is entirely harmless. I have always left the open needle in the spinal canal for two or three minutes after the injection has been finished, thus rendering the intraspinous pressure directly under control. If the needle is left open, the intraspinous becomes equal to the atmospheric pressure, which is less than the normal intraspinous pressure. This reduced pressure is an additional safeguard against any possible development of a "reactive" intracranial pressure.

The position of the body is all-important in intraspinous injections—in fact, in all air injections, because the air rises as the fluid gravitates. The head must be at least twenty degrees higher than the needle. With each injection the air will then rush to the brain and a new supply of fluid will fall to the point of the needle. No doubt the sitting posture would be more satisfactory, because it would allow a more complete and uniform injection of the subarachnoid spaces over both cerebral hemispheres. In the recumbent position, which I have used exclusively, mainly for the comfort of the patient, it is possible that the injection may be more complete over the surface of the higher hemisphere than over the lower hemisphere, and that on turning the patient from one side to the other (in order to take both right and left lateral views of the head) important changes in the distribution of the air may be induced by the effects of gravity. In the sitting posture, rotation of the head would not alter the position of the air in the spaces, because gravity would not be brought into play, and a more accurate photograph of the "air mantel" on each hemisphere would be obtained. If, however, the intracranial subarachnoid space is thoroughly injected, there should be but little change due to gravity and the recumbent posture should prove practically as effective as the sitting posture. Additional experience will probably indicate the position of choice.

I have injected air intraspinously into eight patients — four children and four adults — from Professor Halsted's service, without any bad effect. The amount of air has varied from 20 to 120 cc. In one patient a mild headache followed but disappeared in three hours; vomiting but no headache occurred in another case; in the others no complaints were made. In reality, the effects should be much the same as those following the usual lumbar puncture.

One difficulty in the injection procedure should be mentioned. The aspiration must be gentle because the needle may plug at times, presumably with fibres of the cauda equina. If the suction is very gentle this may be obviated. In no case was there pain from injury to the nerves.

It must always be remembered that spinal punctures are very dangerous in all patients with intracrannial tumors. A spinal puncture should never be made (if a tumor is present) unless the intracranial pressure has been previously relieved by a ventricular puncture or by some other procedure.

What becomes of the air? Air disappears from the subarachnoid space quite rapidly. It is absorbed as from other tissue spaces and undoubtedly passes directly into the blood. Usually no air is demonstrable in the rontgenogram twenty-four hours after the injection. Absorption from the subarachnoid space is many times faster than from the ventricles.

Practically all cerebrospinal fluid is absorbed from the subarachnoid space; very little from the ventricles, and the absorption of ventricular fluid occurs only after it has passed into the subarachnoid space.[2] When air is injected into a lateral ventricle, its rate of absorption seems to depend upon the freedom of access to the subarachnoid space. If the ventricles are normal the air will disappear in the course of a few days. If an internal hydrocephalus is present, the absorption time is greatly increased because an obstruction prevents the air from reaching the subarachnoid space. In cases of ventricular dilatation it may require two to three weeks for the air to disappear. The rate of absorption of air from the ventricles and the subarachnoid space appears to be relatively the same as that for the absorption of fluids from these cavities, although the absolute time required is greater for the absorption of air.

Rontgenography of the Normal Subarachnoid Space. If the spinal and intracranial subarachnoid spaces are normal, the air which has been injected intraspinously will fill all the intracranial spaces. The cisterna magna shows as an air-filled space of varying size, anterior to the squamous part of the occipital bone. The cisterna chiasmatica, which is the anterior terminus of the cisternae, usually shows quite distinctly, and from it several branches may be seen passing upward into the cerebral sulci. The intensity of the shadow of the cisternae under the medulla, pons, and midbrain is greatly modified by the dense bone at the base of the skull, notably the petrous part of both temporal bones. The continuity of the shadow of all the cisternae can, however, nearly always be traced if the x-ray is good and the injection has been complete. The sulci appear as a network of lines over all the surfaces of the cerebral hemispheres. In general appearance the injected sulci suggest very closely

the shadows of the vessels in the diploe, although the arrangement is different. In the earlier ventriculograms, in which only a few sulci contained air, the shadows were erroneously looked upon as markings of the diploetic veins. Sulci have not been observed around the cerebellum, but frequently an envelope of air can be seen completely surrounding it. This envelope of cerebellar air is continuous with the cisterna magna. In one plate in which the upper part of the spinal canal was included, the spinal subarachnoid space was full of air, and in this column of air the shadow of the spinal cord was very distinct.

The cerebellum frequently appears as an island. Since the tentorium cerebelli is in apposition with part of the pericerebellar subarachnoid space, the shadow of this space marks the under surface of the tentorium. In cases in which the lateral ventricles are enormously dilated, a ventriculogram will delimit the upper margin of the tentorium. By combining the upper and lower shadows in such a case, the outlines of the tentorium are quite sharply seen. Mention of this is made merely to show how sharply the x-rays will differentiate tissues in a medium of air.

Localization of Intracranial Lesions by Intraspinous Injections of Air.[3] The cisternae may be regarded as the vital part of the subarachnoid space. Inasmuch as they form the trunk of the subarachnoid tree, all cerebrospinal fluid must traverse them in order to reach the cerebral sulci. The sulci are important because in them practically all cerebrospinal fluid is absorbed. Any obstruction in the cisternae, therefore, leads to hydrocephalus because of a diminished absorption of cerebrospinal fluid. Hence it becomes of the utmost importance to determine whether the cisternae are patent or whether they have been obliterated. Intraspinous air will always reach the sulci if the cisternae are patent; and conversely, if the air does not reach the sulci, the cisternae must be obstructed at some point. Furthermore, with a good x-ray one can see just where the obstruction is situated.

In this series of eight cases, the location of the lesion has been accurately determined in three. In the remaining five, the subarachnoid space was normal. In the three patients in whom the lesion was located by means of intraspinous air, other methods had entirely failed. The findings in these cases will be briefly stated.

In a case of hydrocephalus, 110 cc. of air were injected intraspinously. It filled the cisterna magna, extended along the cisterna medullaris and was stopped at the point of obstruction in the cisterna pontis. This obstruction, due to adhesions from meningitis, had prevented the air reaching the sulci and thereby caused hydrocephalus. Necropsies have shown that communicating hydrocephalus is usually caused by adhesions in the cisternae.[4] I have since produced this disease in animals by occluding the cisterna with a perimesencephalic band of gauze.[5]

The injection of air gave still further information. Although it could not reach the cerebral subarachnoid space, which is normally the path of least resistance, it passed through the basal foramina of Luschka and Magendie, the fourth ventricle, the aqueduct of Sylvius, the third ventricle, the foramen of Monro, and partially filled a lateral ventricle. The fact that the air passed into the ventricle showed that the hydrocephalus was of the communicating type. It should be noted that air has not been observed to enter the ventricle except in hydrocephalus. Normally, the cerebellum is in such close apposition to the floor of the fourth ventricle that, despite the absence of valves, the retrograde flow of air into the fourth ventricle is prevented. It is conceivable that the precise localization of the obstruction by the air method may render operative relief for the obstruction possible.[6]

Our second case presents an even more interesting pathology. The patient was a child three years of age. She had passed through an attack of acute cerebrospinal meningitis, but instead of complete recovery, lethargy and vomiting had ensued. Internal hydrocephalus was suspected by Doctor Blackfan, and confirmed by ventriculogram. A month later a second ventriculogram showed a measurable increase in the size of the lateral ventricle, but the rate of growth was markedly less than in the typical form of this disease. The air passed freely along the cisternae and into the sulci over a very restricted area of the cerebral cortex, not more than one-fourth of all the sulci showing the injection. Nor could it be determined whether the injected area was bilateral or unilateral. Exactly the same rontgenographic findings were present in the two x-rays taken a month apart; in fact, the same convolutions could be traced in both. The sulci could be followed into the cisterna chiasmatica.

These data supply a new conception of the pathology of hydrocephalus. The inflammatory process has sealed off all the main branches which radiate from the cisternae, with the exception of one or possibly more which supply the anterior fourth of the cerebral cortex on one or possibly both sides. Absorption of cerebospinal fluid from this restricted area has been sufficient to retard to a great extent, though not to prevent, the development of hydrocephalus. Should more branches from the cisternae subsequently open, it is quite probable that, owing to the increased absorption which would follow, the accumulation of fluid will be entirely arrested. Such a development could easily explain many spontaneous cures in hydrocephalus. It is very doubtful if these pathological changes in the brain would be detected at necropsy.

A third case was in a boy of nineteen, who was suffering from intracranial pressure. An internal hydrocephalus was discovered. But what had caused the hydrocephalus? From his symptoms a tentative diagnosis of a cerebellar tumor was made, and since the signs and symptoms pointed to both sides equally, a vermis tumor seemed most likely. After a thorough cerebellar exploration

I was unable to find any trace of the tumor. The foramen of Magendie was normal. Three weeks after this operation, the phenolsulphonephthalein test showed that a complete obstruction was present at some point between the third ventricle and the foramen of Magendie. Air (120 c.c.), injected intraspinously, was stopped in the anterior end of the cisterna pontis; none reached the cerebral sulci. These findings could admit of only one interpretation—the pressure of a tumor in the region of the aqueduct of Sylvius, which had occluded it and the cisterna pontis. At operation a tumor as large as a hickory nut was found in the midbrain, and partially removed after bisection of the vermis of the cerebellum. The iter had been completely obliterated by the tumor.

Another interesting radiographic finding in the case was the enormous amount of fluid which had collected at the base of the brain after the first operation. We have frequently noticed after cerebellar operations in which a tumor was not found that such an accumulation of fluid followed, but the explanation had never been clear. The x-ray picture seems to indicate that the closure of the cisternae causes the fluid to accumulate, or, in other words, bring about a localized hydrocephalus; the fluid forms in the fourth ventricle (the iter being closed). Another point of interest in this rontgenogram is the sharp outline of the spinal cord.

A fourth case was that of a boy of eighteen. Hydrocephalus of a year's standing had followed an acute illness which had been diagnosed as measles. At operation the hydrocephalus was found to be due to closure of the foramina of Luschka and Magendie by dense adhesions. I made a new foramen of Magendie and wanted to be sure that it was functioning before allowing the patient to go home. Six weeks after the operation, air injected into the ventricles passed through the new foramen of Magendie and filled the cisterna magna and many of the cerebral sulci. We now could feel certain not only that the foramen of Magendie was patent, but also that all the subarachnoid space was receiving cerebrospinal fluid for absorption. The boy has since resumed his studies in college.

It also seems probable that we shall be able to localize spinal cord tumors by means of intraspinous injections of air. In one of our cases, the spinal cord and the surrounding air-filled space are sharply outlined. Should the spinal canal be obliterated, either by a tumor or possibly by an inflammatory process, it is conceivable that the air shadow will extend up to the level of the lesion. Its intensity will naturally be greatly reduced by the great density of the spine, and particularly of the bodies of the vertebrae. A lateral view of the spine, by eliminating the maximum amount of bone, will probably give the best results. If the spinal canal is not obliterated by the tumor, the injected air will pass freely into the intracranial subarachnoid space, none being left in the spinal canal. This happened in one of our cases in which a spinal cord tumor was suspected. The passage of air into the brain was difficult to explain at the time of the injection, as the symptoms had been present for four years and a tumor of such duration would certainly have blocked the spinal canal. At operation a chronic transverse myelitis was found. Instead of an enlargement of the spinal cord, there was a constriction, which readily explained the failure of air to stop at the suspected zone.

As yet we have not had an opportunity of studying the radiographic findings in tumors of the cerebral hemispheres. It is conceivable that local effects may be noted in the sulci, or possibly even the direct or indirect effects of pressure on the cisternae may be discovered.

The practical value of intraspinous injections has been thoroughly established by the results in the few cases here reported. As a matter of fact, we shall often be able to localize a tumor from either a ventriculogram or from an x-ray of the subarachnoid space alone, an analysis of the signs and symptoms of the individual case enabling us to determine which should be tried first. From the data obtainable from the combination of intraventricular and intraspinous injections it is difficult to see how intracranial tumors can escape localization.

CONCLUSIONS

1. By substituting air for cerebrospinal fluid through a lumbar puncture, all parts of the subarachnoid space can be clearly seen in a rontgenogram.

2. Not infrequently, an air shadow will completely surround the cerebellum, showing clearly its size and shape.

3. The spinal cord can be seen surrounded by a column of air.

4. The cisternae appear as large collections of air at the base of the brain; the cerebral sulci as a network of tortuous filaments of air.

5. After an intraspinous injection, provided that the subarachnoid space is intact, the air will always fill the cerebral sulci.

6. But if the cisternae are blocked at any point by a tumor or adhesions, the air will not be able to reach the cerebral sulci.

7. The exact position of the obstruction in the cisternae can often be seen in the radiogram. In one of our cases of communicating hydrocephalus, the obstruction was in the cisterna pontis. In a second case of communicating hydrocephalus the cisternae were patent but all except one or two of the main branches were occluded. In a third case a tumor was located in the midbrain solely by means of the radiogram.

8. In a case of hydrocephalus, air passed from the spinal canal into the lateral ventricle, demonstrating the patency (and dilatation) of the foramina of Magendie and Luschka, the aqueduct of Sylvius, and the foramen of Monro. The hydrocephalus was, therefore, of the communicating type.

9. A case of hydrocephalus was cured by constructing a new foramen of Magendie. Six weeks later, air injected into the ventricles passed through the new foramen, showing that it was still functioning. The air also filled the cerebral sulci, an indication that the entire arachnoid space was patent.

REFERENCES

[1]Dandy, W. E.: Ventriculography Following the Injection of Air Into the Cerebral Ventricles. *A. S.*, July, 1918. Fluoroscopy of the Cerebral Ventricles. *The Johns Hopkins Hosp. Bull.*, February, 1919.

[2]Dandy, W. E., and Blackfan, K. D.: Internal Hydrocephalus. *Am. J. Dis. Child.*, *viii:* 406, 1914. Second paper: *Am. J. Dis. Child.*, *xiv:* 424, 1917. Also: *J. A. M. A. lxi:* 2216, 1913.

[3]The rontgenographic detail in these plates we owe to the skill of Miss Mary Stuart Smith, in the x-ray service of Doctor Baetjer.

[4]Dandy, W. E., and Blackfan, K. D.: Internal Hydrocephalus (second paper). *Am. J. Dis. Child.*, *xiv:* 424, 1917.

[5]Dandy, W. E.: Experimental Hydrocephalus. To appear in *Annals of Surgery*.

[6]In the December number of the *Annals of Surgery*, 1918, I presented a form of treatment for communicating hydrocephalus. If it should be possible, in a certain number of cases, to restore the channel of the cisternae, this treatment would be superior to a bilateral choroid plexectomy.

IX

LOCALIZATION OR ELIMINATION OF CEREBRAL TUMORS BY VENTRICULOGRAPHY*

It seems incredible that a brain tumor as large as one's fist can exist in either cerebral hemisphere and still escape localization by expert neurologists and neurologic surgeons. Yet nearly all cerebral tumors eventually attain this size, and a very high percentage of them can neither be accurately localized before operation nor be found by an exploration of the brain.

In a recent analysis of a series of seventy cases with neoplasms of the brain, Dr. Heuer and I[1] have shown that of forty-five cases which were presumably located in the cerebral hemispheres, twenty, or 44.4 per cent, escaped detection at operation; and at the time of that publication we considered this a high record in verifying the location of cerebral tumors. This percentage is not strictly correct, for several of the cases were submitted to more than one operation before the tumor was disclosed. On the other hand, in many cases which seemed to present definite signs of localization, the tumor could not be found because it was situated too deeply in the brain.

A more careful analysis of these figures disclosed to an even greater extent the limitations of the neurological signs which are helpful in localizing brain tumors. Nearly all of the tumors which could be localized with certainty were in one of three locations,[2] in each of which the signs are pathognomonic: (1) hypophyseal or third-ventricle tumors gave the characteristic disturbances of the optic tracts and destruction of the sella turcia; (2) precentral or postcentral lesions were evident by the contralateral motor or sensory disturbances; and

(3) neoplasms affecting the motor or sensory centers produced the typical deficiencies of speech. The remaining cases which were localized exclusively by other methods, such as changes in the eye-grounds, disturbances of the other cranial nerves, etc., really comprised a very small group.

There is only one satisfactory form of treatment for brain tumors, i.e., complete operative extirpation of the tumor. It is not conceivable that neoplasms of the brain ever disappear spontaneously or are cured or even benefited by any form of medical therapy. Nor, in our experience, has radium or the x-ray produced even temporary beneficial results. All attempts at medical treatment only cause delay which is disastrous to the individual; just as in the growth of malignant neoplasms of the breast, there is a time in the development of the tumor when its removal is possible and relatively easy and a complete cure will result. This opportunity is now too frequently lost in tumors of the brain because the diagnosis is made too late and because time is lost in misdirected and useless therapy. The treatment of intracranial tumors is now passing through the incipient and least fruitful stages, and is roughly where the treatment of breast tumors was twenty-five years ago, or where the treatment of appendicitis was thirty years ago. In both of these conditions the treatment has gradually become exclusively surgical and every effort has been directed toward an early diagnosis. The results of these efforts are now so thoroughly recognized that for all delay in treatment the physician in charge is held responsible.

When intracranial tumors are recognized and localized early, extirpation will be relatively simple and the permanent results

*Reprinted from *Surgery, Gynecology and Obstetrics,* April 1920, pp. 329–342.

will be vastly greater than those of today. The character and position of many tumors will, of course, preclude the perfect results which obtain in the operative treatment of appendicitis today, but they will undoubtedly surpass the operative results in early malignant lesions of the breast. Gliomata arising very deeply in the brain or in vital parts of the brain must still be looked upon as hopeless, but the vast silent areas harbor most of the incipient brain tumors, and from these regions tumors can be removed with impunity. There are even important areas which, with proper caution and due respect, no longer challenge us with *noli me tangere,* and from which tumors can be extirpated without permanent disability. At the present time, the operative procedures are greatly in advance of the methods of diagnosis, and in competent hands are fairly adequate. Small *enucleable* brain tumors can be removed with very little danger, and even large enucleable tumors can be removed with but a slight mortality, though the haemorrhages in these cases require an operator of large experience. Small *infiltrating* tumors can be removed with the contiguous brain tissues with but little danger, but there is little chance of removing a large infiltrating tumor without a recurrence. Other things being equal the results, immediate and remote, are directly proportional to the stage of growth of the tumor.

Only as a last resort should an exploratory craniotomy or a decompression be done. A subtemporal decompression, though the simplest major cranial operative procedure, is often not only a useless operation to the patient but is frequently accompanied by a pronounced injurious effect. As a routine procedure it is questionable whether it does more good than harm. In all cases of hydrocephalus no relief can possibly result, for the cause of the hydrocephalus nearly always being in the brain stem, is unaffected and the ventricular dilatation continues to increase as rapidly as the extra space afforded by the bony defect will permit. This of course causes greater brain destruction. In advanced cases the result is not infrequently fatal, particularly so when the larger procedure of a combined exploration and decompression is performed. To perform a decompression or an exploration, an internal hydrocephalus should always be excluded. If a hydrocephalus is present a cerebellar exploration is usually, though not invariably, indicated. But here again the question of diagnosis is all important. It is frequently just as difficult to tell whether a lesion is in the cerebral or cerebellar hemispheres as it is to define its exact location.

At best a decompression is only palliative treatment and by the delay between the time at which a decompression is made for a so-called unlocalizable tumor and the later operation for its removal, after self-localization, the patient's chances of a complete cure have dwindled tremendously. The crux of the whole matter is that no brain tumor can be cured without operative removal; and that the earlier the diagnosis and localization is made the better the chances of a cure. The future outlook in the treatment of brain tumors is dependent almost entirely upon early recognition and localization of the tumor.

In a recent publication by the author, a new method—ventriculography or pneumoventriculography—was introduced, by which it was hoped that intracranial localization would be greatly assisted. At that time the procedure had been tried in only a few cases, but the results were such as to indicate alluring probabilities. I now hope to show the efficiency of this method in *cerebral* lesions and where all other means at our command have failed to localize the growth. I venture the prediction that by an intelligent use of this method[1] in the hands of competent neurological surgeons but few cerebral tumors will escape localization. During the past two years I have completely removed over twenty brain tumors in Professor Halsted's service. Many more have been partially removed or treated by palliative procedures. Many of the tumors treated partially, and therefore unsatisfactorily, could have been completely removed had they been received earlier. The time will come when it will be just as reprehensible for a physician to delay the proper treatment in a case of brain tumor as it is now to await developments in a case of acute appendicitis. When one considers the terrible train of events which must inevitably follow the development of a brain tumor—blindness, headache, paralysis, aphasia, etc.—the burden of the delay must fall heavily upon those who are responsible for the failure correctly to diagnose the lesion or at least for the neglect in sending the patient to a competent neurologist or neurological surgeon.

PROCEDURE FOR LOCALIZATION OF THE TUMOR BY VENTRICULOGRAPHY

Each lateral ventricle occupies a large area in the interior of its corresponding cerebral hemisphere. It is evident that a tumor of any size situated in either cerebral hemisphere will modify the shape, size, and position of the corresponding lateral ventricle. Quite frequently the lateral ventricle in the opposite hemisphere will be dislocated and its size also will be greatly modified. These changes in the ventricles, both homolateral and contralateral, yield many opportunities for locating brain tumors by ventriculography. Fortunately following the injection of air into one lateral ventricle, it is possible to obtain a roentgenogram of each lateral ventricle separately, and thus determine alterations produced by a tumor in either cerebral hemisphere. Owing to the angles of the ventricular system, it is possible to fill only one lateral ventricle with air when the head is in a given position. After a roentgenogram has been taken, the head must be carefully turned in such a manner that the air can pass the various ventricular angles and the interventricular foramina (of Monro) and the third ventricle, and thus reach the opposite lateral ventricle. After a lateral view of each ventricle has

been photographed, the head should again be carefully turned in order to direct the air into the anterior horns of both lateral ventricles; the occiput will then be on the plate and the roentgenogram will give the size, shape, and position of the anterior part of both lateral ventricles. Then by placing the forehead on the plate, the size and position of the body, and of the posterior and descending horns, can be demonstrated. It would seem that most tumors must give some manifestations of their presence in one of these views, and the findings must therefore absolutely indicate the position of the tumor.

To introduce air into the ventricles of an adult, it is of course necessary to make an opening in the skull. This can be done either under local or general anaesthesia, the choice largely depending upon the patient. Personally, I prefer local anaesthesia with a responsive patient. The procedure need be but slightly painful and after transferring the patient to the x-ray room his co-operation eliminates respiratory movements and allows a much better exposure; moreover a considerable period of anaesthesia is avoided during the time necessary to dress the wound and transfer the patient to the x-ray room.

A ventriculogram will in many cases at once tell whether the tumor is cerebral or cerebellar. In the latter cases an internal hydrocephalus will be evident by the symmetrically enlarged lateral ventricles.

In some cases it will be found that the size of the ventricle has been so reduced that it is impossible to withdraw sufficient fluid to make the injection of air a safe procedure. It is then best to make a ventricular puncture on the opposite side and inject air into this ventricle, though occasionally both ventricles are too small. Not infrequently we can localize a tumor merely by the difference in size of the two lateral ventricles as determined by the ventricular puncture or often by the abnormal position at which either ventricle may be reached. In a general way a very small ventricle is presumptive though of course not absolute evidence of a cerebral as against a cerebellar tumor or a tumor of the brain stem; when there is a difference in the size of the two lateral ventricles the tumor is usually on the side of the smallest ventricle. Even a bilateral ventricular puncture, which is only occasionally necessary, is a small procedure compared to an exploratory craniotomy or even to a decompression, and the results obtained in localization of the growth not infrequently make the puncture far more valuable than an exploratory craniotomy. In infants and very young children, a puncture can be made through an open fontanelle or through sutures which have been separated by the abnormal pressure.

During the past six months I have used ventriculography in over seventy-five cases from Professor Halsted's clinic. The majority of these cases had hydrocephalus; in many cases ventricular dilatation was suspected and the injection of air made the diagnosis certain. In many others the injection was made in order to determine whether the disease was progressive or stationary, in other words, as a means to determine whether or not operative treatment should be instituted. These cases will not be considered here but will appear in a subsequent paper. I shall describe here only the instances of tumors in the cerebral hemispheres or for very strong reasons suspected of being located there, and only those in which the ventriculogram has been the *sole* means of diagnosis. In many cases the localization of the growth has been easily determined by signs and symptoms and in such instances there is at present no purpose in instituting ventriculography, though I feel that eventually this method may be important in differentiating the type of tumor and determining the kind of operative treatment which is necessary. This possibility is strongly suggested by two of the cases which will be described, but such a decisive stand in treatment, which in many cases might eliminate exploration of the tumor, will only be determined by an extensive experience in the

interpretation of the x-ray findings in a large series of brain tumors.

Five cases are described here, each representing entirely different findings and showing the range of usefulness of this procedure when tumors of the cerebral hemisphere are suspected. Ventriculography will be seen to exclude a cerebral tumor when the lesion is situated elsewhere; precisely to locate the tumor when it exists in either cerebral hemisphere. In two of these cases there was no localizing sign by which the location of the tumors was even suspected. In both, the ventriculograms showed the precise location of the growth. In one case the tumor was entirely removed and the patient is now well; he had previously submitted to two exploratory craniotomies but the tumor could not be found. In the second case a decompression had been done; after localization of the tumor by a ventriculogram, a very large infiltrating glioma was found at operation but could not be removed. The patient was spared further useless operations by the ventriculographic localization of the tumor. In a third case the signs were differently interpreted; a large localized bulging in the right temple seemed to indicate an underlying tumor. There was a complete sensory and motor paralysis of the trigeminal nerve which could have resulted from pressure on the gasserian ganglion; or the paralysis might have been due to involvement of the trigeminal root in the posterior cranial fossa. The ventriculogram conclusively determined the location. In a fourth case, an exploratory craniotomy in a case of focal epilepsy disclosed a greatly dilated ventricle—apparently hydrocephalus; subsequently the ventricles were injected with air and the ventricular dilatation was found to be unilateral—a very rare condition. A fifth case can hardly be included as a result following ventriculography for air could not be injected, but the attempt at the procedure was responsible for locating the tumor. The ventricle was found by a ventricular puncture to be markedly dislocated to the left, but it was so small that only a few drops of fluid could be obtained from the needle. Under such conditions it is not safe to inject air. The dislocated position of the ventricle could only be caused by a tumor in the opposite side of the brain. The extremely small size of the ventricle must be due to the intracranial pressure produced by the tumor. The neoplasm was found in the right prefrontal region and completely removed.

LOCALIZATION OF A TUMOR IN THE OCCIPITAL LOBE, BY VENTRICULOGRAPHY

The difficulties and ofttimes the impossibilities of correctly localizing a brain tumor by the older methods and the simplicity of making the diagnosis by ventriculography will be seen in the observations which follow.

A sallow young man of 23, consulted me for disturbances caused by a tumor of the brain. The diagnosis of a cerebellar tumor had been made by one of America's foremost neurological surgeons and a cerebellar operation performed by him one year previously; the tumor was not found and consequently no relief was obtained. A year later he complained of constant headaches, with severe periodic exacerbations, and particularly of a progressive loss of vision. That the patient had a brain tumor was evident at a glance. A huge cerebellar hernia had followed the first operation and at once indicated a high degree of intracranial pressure. There was a bilateral choked disc measuring 6 diopters in each eye. But the position of the tumor was obscure. The only real objective finding was a complete deafness on the right side; bone conduction as well as air conduction was entirely absent. There was a suggestive Romberg; at times a slight fine nystagmus, and a suggestive bilateral ataxia of the fingers. The patient insisted that the deafness followed the operation. He was sure of this because he had been in the telephone business and had used both ears equally well, moreover the deafness was noticed

immediately after recovery from the cerebellar operation. The subjective symptoms were equally confusing and at that time could not be correlated into the results of a single intracranial lesion. His illness dated back 4 years, at which time severe attacks of bifrontal headaches and vomiting occurred periodically and steadily progressed in frequency and severity. Sixteen months ago diplopia appeared and after lasting for 2 weeks, disappeared and never returned. One month later the left half of the face became anaesthetic over night. He claims the left side of the face was paralyzed also. (He says he could not close the left eyelid and the left corner of his mouth drooped.) The sensory change was quite typically confined to the trigeminal area, ending sharply at the midline. The sensory (and motor) changes of the face last about two weeks. The left side of the face is still subjectively slightly numb, but there is no objective sensory or motor difference between the two sides. There was a sudden exacerbation of the headaches at the time of onset of these facial disturbances and vision then began steadily to diminish first in the left eye, later in the right. It is worthy of note that neither arm nor leg were affected at this time or subsequently. Two months after the onset of these symptoms, the previously mentioned cerebellar operation was performed. Four months later the patient had a convulsion and remained comatose for 4 days. No localizing signs were noticed by anyone during the convulsion. The patient insists that following this period of coma the large occipital hernia which resulted from the operation almost disappeared and later gradually resumed its natural fullness and hardness. There had been a slight disturbance of gait with a tendency to stagger; but it was inconstant and the patient thought it no more than his general weakness could easily explain. No staggering had been observed by his friends. The visual fields showed great restriction of vision in both eyes. There was only slight vision for color in the left eye and this seemed to show a nasal hemianopsia; this was not considered significant because it was the terminal phase of color vision and the field of vision in the right eye showed no such form. A slight grade of convolutional atrophy was present in the skull, indicating that an intracranial pressure existed.

The problem then was how much reliance to place upon the patient's subjective sensations, which seemed paradoxical. It was difficult to see how a complete deafness could result on the right side from the operation as he had claimed. It was impossible to put much confidence in his assertion that the left side of the face was paralyzed (facial nerve). He might easily have thought his face was paralyzed because of anaesthesia; or as happens most frequently the facial paralysis, if present, may have been on the opposite side. As is well known patients and even physicians often mistake the side of facial paralysis. If the *left* trigeminal nerve (V) had been paralyzed, obviously the *right* auditory nerve (VIII) could not be destroyed by the same lesion. The patient could not by any possibility mistake the side which had been anaesthetic (cranial nerve V). If the facial nerve paralysis had been present and had been on the left side it seemed conceivable that a lesion in the left cerebellopontile angle could explain the anaesthesia and facial paralysis, but it would be necessary to disregard entirely the right auditory paralysis (nerve VIII) which he claimed had followed the operation. On the other hand if the auditory paralysis (nerve VIII) had resulted from the tumor and not from the operation a cerebellopontile tumor could explain it and also a possible right facial palsy (VII) but not the anaesthesia of the left side of the face (V). In either case it seemed most probable that the tumor was located in either cerebellopontile angle or possibly in a lobe of the cerebellum. To support this was the transient nystagmus, suggestive Romberg and ataxia, and possibly a slight staggering gait. Transitory hemianaesthesia of the face and facial paralysis are not uncommon in angle tumors. The absence of sensory or motor weakness of the arm and leg seemed to indicate that any facial paralysis must be a peripheral involvement of the facial nerve (VII) rather than involvement of the facial area of the pyramidal tract.

As a result of these deductions I was led again to explore the cerebellar region. It seemed either that the tumor might have been overlooked by the previous operator or that a tumor lying deeply in the cerebellum might by this time have grown nearer the surface. All these presumptions and analyses proved false. A thorough exploration of the cerebellar region and both cerebellopontile recesses revealed no evidence of a tumor. The foramen of Magendie was normal. The large hernia was mainly due to an enormous collection of cerebrospinal fluid, which of course would inevitably reform. Though greatly disappointed at the negative outcome of two big operations, the patient still hoped for a diagnosis which we saw little hope of attaining. A ray of hope appeared in ventriculography, but its value at that time had not been tried. The procedure was mentioned as a possibility to the patient; its uncertainties and possible dangers were emphasized. He eagerly grasped the opportunity.

Seventy-five cubic centimeters of cerebrospinal fluid were removed from the right ventricle and an equal amount of air substituted. Roentgenograms of both right and left lateral ventricles were taken, first in profile and then in an anteroposterior view. The shape of the right lateral ventricle is normal although it may be slightly enlarged. (The normal variations in size of the lateral ventricles have not yet been accurately determined.) The size of the left lateral ventricle was the same as the right but it suddenly ended near the middle of the body of the ventricle. The anterior horn and the anterior portion of the body of the left ventricle were almost exactly like the corresponding parts of the right ventricle, but no air reached the posterior end of the body, the posterior horn or the descending horn of the left ventricle. These portions of the ventricle therefore threw no shadows and were absent in the roentgenogram. The air shadow terminated at a sharp curved line, with concavity directed forward. These findings could admit of but one interpretation—the tumor had completely occluded the body of the ventricle and had prevented the air reaching the posterior and descending horn. The tumor must, therefore, be situated in the left occipital lobe. The anteroposterior ventriculogram showed the left ventricle pushed toward the right and partially occupying the right half of the cranial chamber. The right ventricle is also dislocated farther to the right than its normal position. The anteroposterior ventriculogram alone would have shown the tumor to be in the left cerebral hemisphere, but the lateral view of the left ventricle disclosed the exact location of the tumor.

As a subsequent operation a craniotomy was performed directly over the tumor in the left occipital lobe. An area of tumor about 1 by 1 centimeter reached the surface of the brain. After circumvection of the blood vessels, the cortex over the tumor was divided and the tumor readily shelled out of its bed. It was perfectly encapsulated except at one point; here the tumor arose from the ependyma in the upper outer wall of the descending horn, near its junction with the posterior horn. It was, of course, necessary to open the ventricle widely and thoroughly resect the wall of the ventricle from which the tumor arose. The glomus of the choroid plexus had attached itself to the tumor. It was stripped away and left intact. The ventricle was apparently completely occluded by the intruding growth. The descending horn of the ventricle was definitely enlarged (localized hydrocephalus); the body of the ventricle was well over to the right of the midline exactly as the anteroposterior ventriculogram had indicated. The entire tumor with the wall of the ventricle was removed. It is now two years since the operation and the patient is perfectly well

and at work. There has also been a marked restoration of vision.

In the light of the operative findings, it is now evident that the patient's history was largely correct, but I am still uncertain about the facial paralysis. The auditory nerve paralysis (nerve VIII) undoubtedly resulted in some way from his first operation. The sudden but transient attack of severe headache, vomiting, left trigeminal anaesthesia (nerve V) was due to a sudden occlusion of the ventricle by the ingrowing tumor. A left facial paralysis (nerve VII) could not by any chance have occurred. A right facial paralysis is conceivable from pressure of the localized hydrocephalus, on the face center of the pyramidal tract, but this hardly seems probable. He probably mistook the anaesthesia for motor paralysis. The block in the ventricle had produced an acute hydrocephalus localized to the descending horn of the ventricle (because the ventricle is situated distal to the obstruction). This sudden localized hydrocephalus compressed the gasserian ganglion or the three branches of the ganglion, producing the left trigeminal anaesthesia. The tumor was situated too far posteriorly to have produced *direct* pressure on the gasserian ganglion. A channel in the ventricle subsequently opened and the sensory and possibly motor paralyses were relieved to a great extent. The enlargement of the descending horn is now understood, for there is only one outlet for the cerebrospinal fluid in the descending horn and that is into the body of the ventricle.

DIFFERENTIAL DIAGNOSIS BETWEEN A TUMOR IN THE TEMPORAL FOSSA AND CEREBELLOPONTILE ANGLE

The above localization of a cerebral tumor when a cerebellar neoplasm is suspected, has a counterpart in the following diagnosis of a cerebellar tumor when a temporal lobe tumor is suspected. At least there are very valid reasons for the differences of opinion in the diagnosis.

A girl of thirteen suffered from headaches most of her life, but during the past three years they had become gradually more violent. There were numerous spells of projectile vomiting. Since childhood a large swelling in the right temple had caused a marked facial disfigurement. Diplopia had been present at times. Only recently signs of cerebellar involvement had appeared. There was a definite Romberg with tendency to fall to the right; staggering gait with tendency to waver toward the right; a slight but definite ataxia of the right hand; a slight diminution in hearing on the right; adiadochocinesia, and nystagmus. All these were outspoken objective evidences that the cerebellum was involved. There was a bilateral choked disc which measured six diopters in each eye. But the outstanding features of the case were the large boss in the right temporal region, a complete sensory and motor paralysis of the fifth nerve and a right facial paralysis which was also nearly complete. The boss and the anaesthesia had been present for several years. The masseter and temporal muscles were completely atrophied on the right side there being no muscular response whatever; the anaesthesia over the entire trigeminal area was complete. Taste was lost on the anterior two-thirds of the tongue. The right corneal reflex was absent. There was no hemianopsia, but a general restriction of the visual fields and of the visual acuity. Hearing was present but less acute on the right. There were two possible locations for the growth and plausible reasons for each diagnosis. During the previous three years she had been to two very prominent surgeons, each of whom had wished to remove the tumor mass from the temporal region. They thought the growth was a bony tumor which had originated there, and in its later growth had projected into the cerebellar fossa, producing the cerebellar signs of comparatively recent onset. There were three very good reasons for this diagnosis. First, the large local protuberance had all the appearance of a tumor; second, the complete paralysis

of the trigeminal nerve and its long duration before the more recent involvement of the other cranial nerves particularly the facial nerve (VII), and the auditory nerve (VIII) which arise very close to the fifth nerve. The complete fifth nerve palsy (V) could easily be explained by direct pressure of the presumed tumor of the middle cranial fossa on the gasserian ganglion, especially since the trigeminal paralysis had been present for years and was complete. The x-ray showed increased density in the right parietal region; this was definite but not sufficiently pronounced to be a primary tumor of the bone; if a tumor at all it could only be an underlying soft tumor of the brain. On the other hand the assumption of tumor in the region of the gasserian ganglion or elsewhere in the middle cranial fossa, rendered the explanation of the cerebellar signs difficult. Only an extension of the tumor through the tentorium cerebelli into the posterior cranial fossa could produce the cerebellar signs. Such an extension of a tumor may indeed occur but it is quite exceptional. On the other hand in the origin of the tumor was in the region of the cerebellum, how could one explain the large unilateral boss in the temporal fossa? It could only be said that occasionally in hydrocephalus, there is a localized bulging in the temporal fossa, but I have never seen one so prominent. Such an explanation of course presupposed a hydrocephalus which was not known to exist and it further assumed that the hydrocephalus dated back to early childhood when the skull was very plastic. The head was possibly slightly larger than normal. The swelling had been present as long as the parents could remember, but they thought it was still growing although very slowly. Paralysis of the temporal and masseter muscles accentuated the prominence of the swelling but could not explain it as relative rather than actual.

The solution of the confusion in the diagnosis lay in the presence or absence of an internal hydrocephalus. If an internal hydrocephalus was not present the boss in the temporal region would probably be due to a tumor in that locality and the right lateral ventricle would probably show signs of dislocation or compression from the tumor. On the other hand if a hydrocephalus was present it could not have resulted from a tumor in the temporal fossa but the tumor must have been situated in the posterior cranial fossa. Except in rare instances, only tumors in the brain stem or cerebellum can produce a symmetrical bilateral internal hydrocephalus.

The entire operative procedure for relief of such a case was dependent upon the ventriculogram. The ventricles were found by ventriculography to be greatly and equally dilated. Unfortunately the patient was in the terminal phase of pressure when she arrived and her condition did not warrant a cerebellar operation. A subtemporal decompression would have accomplished nothing beneficial but would no doubt have ended fatally. At necropsy the tumor was found in the cerebellar region as indicated by the internal hydrocephalus shown in the ventriculogram. It was an invasive glioma probably of congenital origin. No doubt the tumor had remained comparatively dormant for years and then resumed a sudden activity.

In both this case and the preceding one the tumor could not be located by the usual methods. In the first case two operations were performed in the wrong location because of misleading signs and symptoms. In the second, two surgeons wished to operate on the temporal region and were prevented only by the patient's hesitancy to undergo the operations. I thought the tumor to be in the cerebellar region but the diagnosis could not be certain; others regarded the tumor as in the middle cranial fossa instead of in the posterior cranial fossa. Although a very high grade of hydrocephalus existed, only the ventriculogram could prove it. In both cases the ventriculogram alone was decisive.

LOCALIZATION OF AN INOPERABLE SUBCORTICAL CEREBRAL TUMOR

Another instance of a brain tumor clinically unlocalizable, but clarified by the ventriculogram, was in a man aged thirty-seven.

His symptoms were almost fulminating —headache and vomiting of only three months' duration. A bilateral choked disc of four diopters was the only possible objective finding. A subtemporal decompression had been performed by Dr. Heuer but the tumor grew so rapidly that the decompression had ceased to be of value in less than a month. A right ventricular puncture was then made under local anaesthesia Because of the extreme intracranial tension which was indicated by a very tight decompression I was afraid of acute pressure symptoms and injected less than 30 cubic centimeters of air which was sufficient to fill only the descending horn of this ventricle, but the size of the left ventricle was so reduced that the injected air was ample to fill it entirely. The ventriculogram therefore indicated a normal right ventricle and a left ventricle greatly and fairly uniformly reduced in size. The various horns of this ventricle were about equally affected. The anterior horn, however, was pushed backward and downward by the tumor. Later a left craniotomy was performed and the tumor was found to be a very extensive infiltrating glioma but coming to the surface in the frontal region. The surface compression of the convolutions suggested an extensive subcortical involvement of the frontal and temporal lobes. The tumor was too large to attempt removal, but an extra large decompression was performed to further alleviate his symptoms.

UNILATERAL HYDROCEPHALUS DEMONSTRATED BY VENTRICULOGRAPHY

During a recent craniotomy for Jacksonian epilepsy in a child of six years I was surprised to find what seemed to be a large cyst in the right post-Rolandic region.

On incision this cyst proved to be a huge lateral ventricle. The posterior horn and the descending horn had lost their normal configuration because of the tremendous distention. There had been no reason to suspect an internal hydrocephalus; the eye-grounds were normal; the roentgenogram of the head showed no signs of intracranial pressure. There was a distinct abnormality of the surface of the brain. Extensive obliteration of both the cerebral arteries and veins in the parietal and occipital-lobe had left a pale white, soft cortex posterior to the Rolandic fissure. Numerous tiny new arteries passed through the meninges, apparently a recent and new development to replace those which had been destroyed.

For months prior to the operation and since the onset of the Jacksonian epilepsy, the patient had had a high irregular fever, a marked tachycardia and at times had been comatose. Apparently there has been an extensive vascular thrombosis at this time.

After convalescence from the operation, permission was obtained from the parents, to inject air into the ventricles for ventriculographic observations. The results of these studies are graphically shown in the accompanying ventriculograms. The hydrocephalus is unilateral, a most unusual condition. The left ventricle was of normal shape, its size somewhat larger than normal though I have not had a sufficient number of normal ventricles to tell how large the normal variations may be. The right ventricle was a tremendous cyst but the enlargement is principally posteriorly, where the vascular affection was most pronounced. In the strict sense this cannot be a true hydrocephalus, for there is, at least now, no increased intracranial pressure. The unilateral dilated ventricle is undoubtedly due to softening of the cerebral walls from the vascular disturbance. The softened area atrophied from the pressure in the ventricles. In a true unilateral hydrocephalus the foramen of Monro must necessarily be occluded. At a subsequent

operation I removed the choroid plexus from the dilated ventricle and occluded the foramen of Monro by a transplant of fascia as I have done on animals, following Professor Halsted's suggestion. There was immediate cessation in the attacks but this phase of the story will be considered in a subsequent paper.

The condition in this case could not have been known, even after the operation, without a ventriculogram. In fact a ventricular puncture and a roentgenogram would have given the same information without the exploratory craniotomy, and the patient might have been spared the first operation.

LOCATION OF A CEREBRAL TUMOR BY VENTRICULAR PUNCTURE WHEN THE VENTRICLE IS TOO SMALL TO PERMIT THE INJECTION OF AIR

In some cases of brain tumor, possibly due to a very rapid growth of the tumor, the size of the ventricle on the side of the tumor and at times even of the contralateral ventricle is so reduced that only a few drops of fluid can be obtained by a ventricular puncture. In these cases enough fluid cannot be aspirated safely to permit the injection of the air for the purpose of obtaining a ventriculogram. If air should be injected under such conditions, an acute rise of intracranial pressure might follow, possibly with disastrous results. But in these cases there is usually a definite dislocation of the ventricle; this is frequently great enough to cause difficulty in locating the ventricles by a puncture. But when the ventricle is found, its position may explain the location of the tumor.

A young woman of twenty-four was suffering from a rapidly growing intracranial tumor. The signs and symptoms gave absolutely no clue to the location of the growth. Pursuant to our newer conception of the importance of an early localization of the growth, I made a right ventricular puncture and found the ventricle dislocated toward the left side, but only three or four drops of fluid escaped from the needle. Since air could not be injected under these circumstances without risk, a ventricular puncture was at once made on the left side but the left ventricle was no larger and despite the high grade of intracranial pressure (6 diopters swelling in each optic disc) only a few drops of fluid escaped and no more could be aspirated. This ventricle also was dislocated markedly to the left. It was evident that the tumor must be in the right cerebral hemisphere and that it had pushed both lateral ventricles toward the left; however, the exact localization of the tumor on the right side could not be made in any way. In view of these findings a right exploratory craniotomy was performed and a large extracortical circumscribed tumor completely removed from the right frontal lobe. The patient recently left the hospital perfectly well.

CONCLUSIONS

1. Ventriculography is invaluable in the localization of obscure brain tumors. So-called unlocalizable tumors comprise at present over half of the total number.

2. Practically all brain tumors either directly or indirectly affect some part of the ventricular system.

3. Hydrocephalus is easily demonstrable by ventriculography and when present usually though not always restricts the location of the tumor to the posterior cranial fossa—that is, the brain stem or the cerebellum.

4. Local changes in the size, shape, and position of one or both ventricles as shown by the ventriculogram will accurately localize most obscure tumors of either cerebral hemisphere.

5. Every effort should be made to localize the tumors before resorting to any operative procedure.

6. The usual subtemporal decompression is useless and dangerous when a hydrocephalus is present, that is when the tumor is in the brain stem or cerebellum.

7. A suboccipital decompression (cerebellar operation) is extremely dangerous when the lesion is in the cerebral hemispheres.

8. To differentiate between cerebral and cerebellar lesions is frequently one of the most difficult tasks in intracranial localization. Ventriculography at once separates these two groups and indicates the operation of choice.

9. The only cure for brain tumor is extirpation. The results in terms of complete cures of brain tumors will be in proportion to the early localizations which are made. A decompression is a purely palliative procedure and should be adopted only when the tumor cannot be located. Ventriculography permits of an early and accurate localization of the growth when all other methods fail.

10. It is possible to get a separate profile ventriculogram of the whole of each lateral ventricle. Any change in size or contour is easily demonstrated. Antero-posterior views will show the same points in cross section but they are chiefly useful in showing any lateral dislocation of the ventricles.

11. The results in localization of five types of cases of brain tumor are shown with ventriculograms. In all but one of these, the ventriculogram was the only means by which a positive localization could be made. One tumor occluded a lateral ventricle and dislocated both lateral ventricles. Another tumor altered the size and shape of one lateral ventricle. In a third case a cerebral tumor, though suspected, was eliminated by the hydrocephalus. In a fourth case a unilateral hydrocephalus was demonstrated.

12. Occasionally the size of both ventricles is so reduced that air cannot be safely injected. In one case the dislocated position of both ventricles, which were greatly reduced in size, made the localization possible.

13. Ventriculography is also useful in *precisely* localizing the growth. This permits of an exploration *directly over the tumor* and greatly simplifies the operative procedures.

14. Many useless and harmful operations will be spared the patient by a judicious use of ventriculography.

15. Doubtless the type of tumor will often be indicated by the ventriculogram. Such knowledge will be useful in prognosis and in determining whether radical or palliative operative treatment should be instituted. These determinations will result from accumulated experience in the interpretation of the ventriculograms together with the correlative operative findings presented in a large series of cases.

16. With experience and care in the use of ventriculography, I believe few tumors will escape accurate localization.

REFERENCES

[1]Heuer, G. J., and Dandy, W. E. A report of seventy cases of brain tumor. *Bull., Johns Hopkins Hosp., xxvi:* 224, 1916.

[2]These statments, of course, have reference only to lesions of the cerebral hemisphere and do not include tumors of the brain stem or the cerebellum. This paper is intended to consider only the localization of tumors which are supposed to be situated in the cerebral hemispheres.

[3]Dandy, W. E. Ventriculography following the injection of air into the celebral ventricles. *Ann. Surg., lxviii:* 5–11; fluoroscopy of the cerebral ventricles. *Johns Hopkins Hosp. Bull., xxx:* 29–33, roentgenography of the brain after injection of air into the spinal canal. *Ann. Surg.,* October, 1919.

X

THE DIAGNOSIS AND TREATMENT OF HYDROCEPHALUS RESULTING FROM STRICTURES OF THE AQUEDUCT OF SYLVIUS*

The purpose of this paper is to describe a type of hydrocephalus which occurs most frequently in infants, to give its pathology both gross and microscopical, to present the methods of diagnosis, and particularly to suggest a new form of treatment for this condition. To separate hydrocephalus into types is becoming increasingly difficult and, as our knowledge of this disease, but recently regarded as idiopathic, becomes better established, we are concerned less with subdividing it into groups and more with isolating the character and the exact location of the lesion which is causing the condition. Indeed, as the anatomy of the cerebrospinal spaces and the circulation of the cerebrospinal fluid become more clearly understood, hydrocephalus begins to appear as a single disease with varied anatomical manifestations, which are dependent upon the location of the underlying cause.

Hydrocephalus is always secondary to a primary cause and it should now be possible in every instance to locate the primary lesion, though its discovery, while at times simple, is usually sufficiently difficult to exhaust all the newer methods at our command. Moreover, in the chronic form of the disease (which is practically always referred to), there is but slight hope of spontaneous cure; there is no hope whatever from any medicinal therapy; the only hope lies in surgically correcting the cause of the disease, which is almost always an obstruction in the cerebrospinal spaces. The maximum results of surgical treatment, when this becomes proficient, and it is rapidly becoming so, will always be dependent on an early and accurate diagnosis.

The cases which comprise the particular group referred to in this paper are due to stenosis of the aqueduct of Sylvius. The vast majority of these cases begins in the prenatal period. The disease develops rapidly both during the prenatal and the postnatal life, though the manifestations may not be clearly evident for some time after birth. In 1914, I reported with Dr. Blackfan a series of eighteen cases of hydrocephalus, and in 1917 a series of twenty-five cases,[1] in which complete studies on the absorption of cerebrospinal fluid were made during life. Tests were devised to differentiate the types of hydrocephalus and other tests to obtain an index of the functions of the ventricles and the cerebrospinal spaces. The subdivision of most cases of hydrocephalus into two main classes, communicating and obstructive, still holds. In reality, nearly all cases of hydrocephalus are due to an obstruction, but in the so-called obstructive group the obstruction is in some part of the ventricular system. In the so-called communicating group, the ventricles are in communication with the subarachnoid space and the obstruction, usually adhesions, lies in the various parts of the subarachnoid space. The differentiation into these two great groups is clinically possible and easy of accomplishment by using a colored dye test. If, after injection of the dye into a lateral ventricle, it quickly appears in the spinal canal (lumbar puncture), there is a communication between the ventricles and the subarachnoid space, and this type of hydrocephalus is known as "communicating." The absence of the dye in the spinal fluid denotes an obstruction at some point in the ventricular system; this type is called "obstructive."

*Reprinted from *Surgery, Gynecology & Obstetrics,* October, 1920, pp. 340–358.

Obviously, this differentiation is of the utmost importance in determining the type of surgical treatment which is necessary.

From the later series of twenty-five cases, necropsy was obtained in eleven; of this number, four were caused by obliteration of the aqueduct of Sylvius. Doubtless, several more had a similar lesion, but the absolute proof from necropsy was lacking.

Fourteen of the total number of cases in the series were shown by the dye test to be of the obstructive type and the remaining eleven to be of the communicating type. An analysis of the fourteen cases of the obstructive type shows the relative incidence of those cases in which the obstruction was at the aqueduct of Sylvius. Necropsy was obtained in eight of these fourteen cases, and in half of them (four cases) the aqueduct was occluded and, of course, this obstruction was the etiological factor in each instance, for the aqueduct cannot be occluded without hydrocephalus resulting. Two of these eight cases were under observation during an attack of acute meningitis, and hydrocephalus was observed to follow this illness. In one case the meningitis was tuberculous, and in the other it was of influenzal origin. Six cases remain of this obstructive group (of the eight cases in which a postmortem examination was obtained), in which the hydrocephalus was of congenital origin: four of these had an obstruction at the aqueduct of Sylvius and two at the base of the brain (occluding the foramina of Magendie and Luschka by adhesions). This percentage (66 per cent) should, I think, express about a fair relative incidence of obstructions at the aqueduct of Sylvius in all cases of *congenital hydrocephalus* of the *obstructive* type. In other words, congenital occlusions at the aqueduct of Sylvius are probably at least twice as frequent as those at the foramina of Magendie and Luschka.

Since the publication of the above series, I have had twenty-five additional cases of hydrocephalus; ten were of the communicating and fifteen of the obstructive type. Postmortem examinations were obtained in five of the ten cases of communicating hydrocephalus and, as in the previous series, the disease was caused by an inflammatory process which sealed the branches of the subarachnoid space, usually the cisternae. Necropsies were obtained in five of the fifteen cases of obstructive hydrocephalus, and in each the obstruction was located at the aqueduct of Sylvius. In three additional recent cases of hydrocephalus which have been treated by operation, total occlusion at the aqueduct has been found in each instance. Undoubtedly, the same cause would be present in many of the remaining seven cases had a postmortem examination been made. In this series of twenty-five cases, 50 per cent of the autopsies and operations showed the aqueduct of Sylvius to be occluded (exactly the same percentage as in the other series). Stenosis of the aqueduct is, therefore, the causative lesion in about one-half of all cases of hydrocephalus occurring congenitally.

CASES OF STENOSIS OF THE AQUEDUCT OF SYLVIUS COLLECTED FROM THE LITERATURE

Magendie[1] described an occlusion of the aqueduct of Sylvius in 1842; a marked dilatation of the lateral ventricles was also mentioned and discussed as having a probable relationship to the stricture, but this view was finally dismissed and the ventricular dilatation was regarded as incidental rather than causative.

Prior to Magendie's epoch-making publication, in which mention of the stricture of the iter was a mere incident, rational pathological descriptions were scarcely possible, for the normal was not known. Not until then was it known that the cavities in and around the brain contained fluid; Magendie discovered the foramen of Magendie, but even this opening is disputed to the present day. The foramina of Luschka were described several years later. Strictures of such a minute and apparently unimportant channel as the aqueduct of Sylvius could hardly have elicited any serious comment.

Oppenheim [2] (1900) discovered a unique abnormality of the aqueduct at the necropsy of a patient who had suffered from a malady which had been diagnosed as myasthenia gravis during life. A thin bridge of tissue longitudinally bisected the iter; in addition, numerous tiny nodules composed of lymphocytes protruded into the lumen of the aqueduct. The bisecting bridge had a very thin fibrous tissue center and was completely covered on either side by ependyma. There was no dilatation of the third or lateral ventricles, and in all probability the abnormality produced no injurious primary or secondary effects.

Bourneville and Noir [1] (1900) described a total occlusion of the iter, but, curiously, they placed no importance on the absence of this channel. Even tremendous enlargement of the third and both lateral ventricles of this case, contrasted to the normal small fourth ventricle, produced no impression on these authors who had the etiology of hydrocephalus in their hands but utterly failed to grasp it. They conclude, "Nothing whatever distinguishes this autopsy from that on any other case of hydrocephalus. Nevertheless we note the complete obliteration of the aqueduct of Sylvius which is not ordinarily present." Even at this recent date, the cause of hydrocephalus was not recognized! The most careful and painstaking postmortem examinations frequently revealed the correct pathological lesions, but they were dismissed because they conflicted with current whimsical theories. Even the great Monro, nearly a century and a half ago, found several pathological specimens with mechanical obstructions in the ventricular system but, in his endeavor to prove the ventricles to be independent of any communication with the exterior of the brain, discarded these findings as insignificant.

Touche [2] records a most remarkable case of hydrocephalus which began with a series of convulsions when patient was four years of age. There was nothing in the history to indicate that the acute illness was or was not an inflammation, but the head began to enlarge shortly after this illness, prior to which the child had been perfectly normal. The patient lived to be twenty nine years old, at which time there was almost complete paralysis of both arms and legs, almost total lack of intelligence, and pronounced limitations of the extra-ocular movements. At autopsy, the third and both lateral ventricles were enormously dilated, the iter was completely occluded, and the fourth ventricle was not enlarged. Touche was the first among the references I have found who attributed the hydrocephalus to the obliteration of the aqueduct, though he does not discuss this relationship. No microscopic study of the mesencephalon was made.

Spiller [3] (1902) reported two cases, each with a cicatricial stenosis of an interventricular passage, one at the foramen of Monro, the other at the aqueduct of Sylvius which is not ordinarily the stricture microscopically and describes an hypertrophy of glia enclosing numerous minute rests of the epithelial lining of the aqueduct. The stenosis of the foramen of Monro (followed by unilateral hydrocephalus) was also due to a cicatrix. He thought both occlusions to be of inflammatory origin, possibly tuberculous, and to be the cause of the hydrocephalus in each.

In an admirable article, Guthrie [1] (1910) reported studies in hydrocephalus from a large series of postmortem examinations of patients who died of meningitis or its sequelae. His views on the relationship of meningitis to the production of hydrocephalus were most sane and on the whole far in advance of contemporary articles on hydrocephalus. He emphasizes a relationship of diseases which is certainly correct and all-important, but one which is even now poorly recognized. Eight cases of complete occlusion of the iter were included in his report; in six, the occlusion was undoubtedly inflammatory and occurred during the progress of the meningitis. In two cases of hydrocephalus (which alone of his series are included in this report of cases collected from the litera-

TABLE OF CASES OF STRICTURE OF THE AQUEDUCT OF SYLVIUS COLLECTED FROM THE LITERATURE

	Author	Age of Patient	Time of Onset of Symptoms	Antecedent or Other Illness Etiological Factors	Signs and Symptoms	Gross Pathology	Microscopic Pathology	General Statement
1	Oppenheim	Adult			Treated as bulbar paralysis	Bridge across aqueduct	Hypertrophy of glia Numerous small nodules	No symptoms of intracranial pressure because obstruction slight, if any
2	Bourneville and Noir	9 years	At 6 months or before	Mother had smallpox – premature delivery	Epilepsy Spasticity Sexual precocity	No trace of aqueduct		Child always weak. No intelligence. Somatic development not unusual. Marked sexual precocity Lays no emphasis on occlusion of aqueduct
3	Touche	29 years	At 4 years	Convulsions for 2 months	Large head. Absence of mentality. Bilateral paralysis almost complete. Partial opthalmoplegia	Aqueduct occluded completely. Third and both lateral ventricles large. Fourth normal size	None	Patient lived 25 years after hydrocephalus was evident
4	Spiller	19	Doubtful		Difficulty in walking Staggering dizziness	Aqueduct closed third and lateral ventricles. Fourth normal	Tiny opening microscopically Neuroglia increased Ependymal cells in groups	Headaches since childhood
5	Guthrie					No trace of aqueduct		Fourth ventricle small
6	Guthrie					No trace of aqueduct		Fourth ventricle also dilated No evidence of meningitis at necropsy
7	Dandy and Blackfan	6 months	Noticed at birth	None	Large head, circumference 40 centimeters Arms and legs spastic	Total occlusion of aqueduct. Small pouch at third ventricle	Microscopic remnants of aqueduct Hypertrophy of glia	Myelomeningocele also present Third and both lateral ventricles large
8	Dandy and Blackfan	6 weeks	Large head at birth	None	Large head, circumference 50 centimeters Convulsions began second week. Extra-ocular palsies, nystagmus	Cerebral hemispheres almost completely destroyed. Aqueduct completely occluded	No microscopic remnants of aqueduct. Increased production of glia	Very advanced. Total occlusion must have existed early in intra-uterine life. Fourth ventricle mere slit. Third and both lateral ventricles extremely large

	Author	Age	Head history	Trauma	Clinical findings	Obstruction	Glia	Remarks
9	Dandy and Blackfan	5 years	Head large at birth. Abnormal at 4½ months. Never able to hold up head	None	Head 54 centimeters grew to 72 centimeters. Strabismus. Spasticity of arms and legs. Wassermann negative	Double obstruction (1) Aqueduct Sylvius (2) Foramina of Luschka and Magendie		Patient was observed 5 years. Some development of speech and slight intelligence despite progress of disease. Hydronephrosis (bilateral) due to a congenital obstruction of the urethra
10	Schlapp and Gere	3½ years at death	Head large at birth	Fall when 2¾ years old. Unconscious several minutes vomiting. Headaches, epilepsy and irritability began 6 weeks later	Unsteady gait, irritability, headache, convulsions. No extra-ocular palsies. Choked disc. No ataxia. No Romberg. Slight nystagmus. Head 62 centimeters	Complete occlusion of aqueduct. Tiny cysts	Increase of glia. Cellular changes in wall of ventricles, probably inflammatory	The large head at birth suggests a congenital origin through the trauma may be important either for originating the stricture or for causing a partial one to become complete
11	Schlapp and Gere	5½ months	Head large 1 month. Normal at birth	Instrumental delivery	Convulsions. Head 63 centimeters. Limbs spastic. Knee kicks active	Complete closure of aqueduct. Upper part of aqueduct greatly dilated. Brain membrane thick	Increase in glia	
12	Schlapp and Gere	2½ years	Head large at birth, gradually increased	None mentioned	Head 67 centimeters. Never able to move arms or legs. Probably blind or deaf	Cortex ½ centimeter. Ventricles large. Aqueduct entirely closed	Hypertrophy of glia	
13	Schlapp and Gere	6 months	Large since birth		One eye turned out since birth. Blind. Bilateral ankleclonus and Babinski	Head 19½ centimeters. Tumor of fourth ventricle	Hypertrophy of glia with cyst formation entire length of aqueduct	
14	Schlapp and Gere	15 months				Head 67 centimeters. Several small gliomata occlude aqueduct completely		
15	Schlapp and Gere					Little brain tissue left	Cellular reaction around aqueduct which is closed	Evidence of syphilis

	Author	Age of Patient	Time of Onset of Symptoms	Antecedent or Other Illness Etiological Factors	Signs and Symptoms	Gross Pathology	Microscopic Pathology	General Statement
16	Schlapp and Gere	Birth	Before birth			Aqueduct closed	Increase of glia small slit open microscopically	
17	Dandy	2 months	1½ months	None	Head 40.5 centimeters	Tiny opening of a q u e d u c t remains	Increase of glia	Talipes equinovarus. Spina bifida. Myelomeningocele Obstruction of the aqueduct is not quite complete
18	Dandy	4 months	Head large at birth	Easy labor	Head 68 centimeters Slight strabismus Child died of pneumonia No operation	Thin band across aqueduct	None made	This band could undoubtedly have been treated at operation, probably permanently
19	Dandy	3 months	1½ months	Easy labor Head noticed to be large at age of 6 weeks	Head 50.5 centimeters	Total occlusion of aqueduct	None made	Tube was passed over aqueduct; because the cerebellum was not split, the view was obscured. Death followed operation
20	Dandy	3 months	Head large at birth		Head 48.75 centimeters One month later was 53.75 centimeters	Total occlusion of aqueduct	None made	Death followed incision of ventricle

ture), there was neither a history nor any postmortem evidence of meningitis, but the aqueduct of Sylvius was totally occluded in each. The possible relationship of meningitis to the formation of these strictures, as implied by Guthrie, will be discussed later.

Schlapp and Gere[2] (1911) presented a series of four cases, each having complete occlusion of the iter; later (1917) the number was increased to seven.[2a] All of these cases were carefully studied microscopically.

PATHOLOGY OF STRICTURES OF THE AQUEDUCT

All of these cases, including the three entered by Blackfan and myself,[3] have essentially the same microscopic pathology which was described by Spiller. In each instance, only epithelial remnants of the lining ependyma remain, and an hypertrophy of the glial tissue replaces the defect. In one of our cases, not a trace of epithelium could be found in any of the sections, but the other two which were so examined had microscopic tubular remains of ependyma; but no possible channel could be reconstructed from the third to the fourth ventricle through this connective tissue.

In the gross, the region of the occluded iter differs but little from the surrounding mesencephalic tissue. There is usually no increased density noticeable to the touch and one gets the impression of a normal mesencephalon minus the aqueduct. In one of our cases, however, the region of the aqueduct appeared fairly sharply circumscribed, almost like a tumor; it was much harder and more fibrous but microscopically the picture was similar to that of the others.

In four of our seven cases, the entire length of the aqueduct was occluded. In one, the stricture was not quite complete, though phenolsulphonephthalein did not appear in the spinal fluid within a half hour after it had been injected into the lateral ventricle, as it normally should when the aqueduct is patent. In one case, the

stricture was a very thin diaphragm which transmitted light and should easily have been amenable to treatment. In another case, there were two obstructions in the ventricular system, one at the iter, the second at the base of the brain. The fourth ventricle, which intervened between the strictures, was markedly dilated as should be expected from failure of its fluid to escape into the cisterna magna. The stricture at the aqueduct was only about 3 millimeters in length. Apparently one of Guthrie's cases, also, had two such obstructions and at the same locations, for the fourth ventricle was enlarged, a finding which could not occur unless both foramina of Luschka together with the foramen of Magendie were closed. In two of the cases described by Schlapp and Gere, only the posterior end of the aqueduct was occluded, the anterior part being dilated up to the point of the stricture. This was also true in one of our specimens.

It is hardly necessary to note that in every case in which the aqueduct of Sylvius is occluded, the third and both lateral ventricles are dilated, the degree varying with the time which has lapsed after the stricture has formed. The size of the fourth ventricle is not increased except in those rare cases in which the foramina of Luschka and Magendie are also occluded; it is usually, though not invariably, smaller than normal because of the superimposed pressure of the hydrocephalic ventricles, although this pressure is greatly reduced by the comparatively inelastic tentorium cerebelli which holds the heavy cerebral hemispheres. The reason the third and both lateral ventricles dilate is because the closure of the aqueduct of Sylvius removes the only avenue by which the cerebrospinal fluid can escape from these ventricles. And, since there is only a trivial amount of absorption through the walls of the ventricles and a constant formation of fluid within the ventricles from the choroid plexus, the ventricles must continue to enlarge. To compensate for this enlargement, the brain is steadily destroyed. In most of the cases included in this series and reported by various authors the ventricles had reached extreme dilatation and the amount of cerebral cortex which remained was small. In two of our cases, there was only a film of brain remaining and this was attached to the leptomeneninges; and in many areas of considerable size the brain tissue was entirely absent.

By the newer methods, it is now possible to determine the presence of hydrocephalus in the earlier stages of its development. It is no longer necessary to await progressive enlargement of the head with the great destruction of brain tissue. In one of our cases, the hydrocephalus was suspected at birth on account of the presence of a myelomeningocele and of an unusually large anterior fontanelle.

The presence of a meningocele should always be looked upon as a suspicious sign that hydrocephalus may be an accompanying condition which may be far more serious than the meningocele. The cause of the frequent association of hydrocephalus and meningocele is as yet not entirely clear, but the importance and frequency of the relationship cannot be overestimated.

THE CAUSE OF STRICTURE OF THE AQUEDUCT

During early embryonic development, the aqueduct of Sylvius shows no differentiation from the remainder of the neural tube. Everywhere the entire neural canal, including the aqueduct of Sylvius, therefore, must necessarily have been patent and lined by epithelium. It is easy to understand how the foramina of Luschka and Magendie may be impermeable, simply because they have failed to develop, because they are secondary openings from a primary closed neural tube; but no such hypothesis is tenable in explaining stenosis of the aqueduct of Sylvius. Since, therefore, the aqueduct of Sylvius is primarily an open tube, its closure must be secondary and never due to agenesis. The presence of microscopic epithelial remains and occasionally of a minute patent channel, evi-

dent at times even macroscopically, serve as supporting evidence that the iter has been in existence but has been subsequently occluded by some abnormal process.

The aqueduct is the weakest and at the same time the most important link in the ventricular system. Its lumen should normally be open for the passage of cerebrospinal fluid which is constantly but very slowly being poured through it. The hypertrophy of glia cannot be regarded as a tumor because it has not the cellular element of a tumor; moreover, it does not proliferate beyond the immediate region of the iter.

Glia behaves essentially as does connective tissue. Its growth must be secondary and not primary. It would be difficult to imagine a primary rampant growth of connective tissue beyond the confines of a normal epithelial lining. It would appear more probable that a primary destruction of the epithelial lining of the aqueduct had resulted and the natural attempt of nature to heal the breach by glial tissue had resulted in the stenosis of the iter at the affected zone. Such an hypothesis, and of course more it cannot be, is supported by the method of formation of stenoses elsewhere in the body, either by trauma plus infection, or even by infection alone. The closure of only a portion of the aqueduct in many cases supports the view that an epithelial defect is primary, for a primary connective-tissue growth would hardly be so restricted.

We know that intracranial intra-uterine inflammations do exist, because adhesions are so frequently found over the surface of the brain. We have no information by which it is possible to decide whether these inflammatory changes are the result of bacteria or merely toxins, but this differentiation is irrelevant. There is every reason why the aqueduct of Sylvius should be most susceptible to any such intra-uterine inflammatory changes. Its relatively great length, together with its tiny caliber, makes it a place of least resistance both to trauma and in inflammatory changes or to both;

and it is easily conceivable that only a relatively slight injury to the aqueduct, either by trauma or by toxins, would be necessary to produce sufficient destruction of the epithelium to result in a stricture—which could scarcely be reparable by any method of nature.

In this connection, there are several findings in the above series of cases which are important. Oppenheim's case was characterized by a number of small nodules which protruded into the lumen and which were made up of clusters of lymphocytes. Similar lymphocytic changes, which have been interpreted as inflammatory by the authors, were described by Schlapp and Gere in two of their cases. In all of our cases, and doubtless most of the others which are recorded here, the process is too old to record any cellular inflammatory reaction, had such changes been present at the time of onset of the lesion. It is not necessary to relegate all possible inflammatory changes to the overcrowded and underreasoned syphilitic category, for there must be many types of mild inflammatory changes of which we know very little at the present time. Guthrie's observations bear the greatest weight in this connection. He found in postmortem examinations of a series of patients who had died of meningitis, 8 instances in which total occlusion of the aqueduct had resulted from the inflammations. In all of his cases, the meningitis was postnatal. Undoubtedly, the aqueduct is much more resistant to injury after birth and becomes progressively more so; this statement is made upon the relative infrequency of stenosis of the aqueduct with increasing age. If, therefore, inflammations can occlude the aqueduct so frequently after birth, a relatively trivial infection or irritant would doubtless produce the same disastrous results in the tender period of intra-uterine life.

ANALYSIS OF THE CLINICAL MANIFESTATIONS IN THIS SERIES

A large head of varying size is the only constant feature of these cases and, obviously, the large head is a manifestation of all types of hydrocephalus and not of obstructions of the aqueduct in particular. The size of the head is only very roughly proportional to the size of the lateral ventricles. At birth the head may be only slightly enlarged or, as usually happens, may attract no attention whatever and still the ventricles may be several times the normal size. Any appreciable enlargement of the head means a very great enlargement of the ventricles and a corresponding amount of destruction of brain tissue. The size of the head is, therefore, only a very rough index of the condition of the contents of the cranial chamber; the small head is a very poor index, if any at all; the large head is a very good index. After the first few years of life, the size of the head changes but slightly despite great enlargement of the ventricles, because the united bones preclude much separation. We have made several diagnoses of early hydrocephalus soon after birth by carefully examining the anterior fontanelle for enlargement, fullness, and alteration of shape. Not infrequently the anterior and posterior fontanelles are continuous, owing to separation of the interparietal suture. The anterior fontanelle will also usually project farther forward than normal and farther lateralward by separation of the interfrontal and frontoparietal sutures respectively.

It is quite remarkable how a limited amount of intelligence may continue to develop in young children in spite of the rapid progressive destruction of the brain. Even with an enormous head, measuring 60 to 70 centimeters in circumference, the child may learn to speak distinctly though, of course, with a greatly restricted vocabulary. A considerable amount of destruction of the brain may be tolerated in the early stages of hydrocephalus without any or with only moderate mental inferiority; this holds true only so far, after which the mental changes progress rapidly and, of course, are irreparable.

Many hydrocephalic children have a downward displacement of the eyes due to depression of the roof of the orbit. Owing to this displacement, the sclera shows above the iris and the iris is partially covered below. Quite frequently there is also a considerable limitation of the various extra-ocular movements. This is usually symmetrical, though one set of muscles may be more involved in one eye than the other. I believe these palsies are due, not to implication of the quadrigeminal bodies as could be readily inferred from the close proximity of these bodies to the iter, but rather to the pressure of the bulging, distended third ventricle which presses upon the third, fourth, and sixth nerves directly. Were the affection in the quadrigeminal bodies or in the nuclei of the third nerves which are located in the mesencephalon, the extra-ocular palsies would be complete rather than partial.

Convulsions are not uncommonly present, though probably the majority of patients are not so afflicted, or have only an occasional attack; the attacks are general and may be both petit mal and grand mal. Their explanation is still obscure because of our meager knowledge of the underlying cause. Spasticity of the arms and legs is also frequent, doubtless from pressure of the intraventricular fluid on the thinning pyramidal tract. Eventually, this destruction leads to complete paralysis of the arms and legs.

Blindness is not infrequent, even when the head can enlarge quite readily. The optic nerves are directly compressed by the distended third ventricle which thus produces the loss of vision. Ankle clonus, Babinski and Oppenheim reflexes are present with varying frequency. The reflexes are usually exaggerated, in keeping with the degree of spasticity. One might expect to find a choked disc constantly, but most cases have a primary atrophy instead; the explanation for this fact is that the third ventricle acts as a tumor and presses on the optic chiasm directly, thus occluding the space in the sheath of the nerves.

But all of these signs and symptoms are not present in every case or even type of hydrocephalus. They are the manifestations of hydrocephalus, and have no direct bearing upon the primary lesion in the aqueduct of Sylvius or elsewhere. Moreover, there is no sign or symptom which is characteristic of a stricture of the aqueduct of Sylvius as such. A tumor in the midbrain blocking the aqueduct of Sylvius has signs which are pathognomonic, but only because the contiguous nuclei or the quadrigeminal bodies are involved. Were the hypertrophied glia a progressive lesion, it would likewise involve these contiguous structures and produce the same signs but, being restricted, only the signs of pressure are usually present.

CASE WITH TWO OBSTRUCTIONS, ONE AT THE AQUEDUCT OF SYLVIUS, THE OTHER AT THE FORAMINA OF LUSCHKA AND MAGENDIE

This patient was five years old at the time of his death. He had been under observation from time to time for four and one-half years, during which time the size of his head steadily increased. The patient was the third of five children, the others being hearty and well. There is no history of tuberculosis or syphilis in the family. The birth was at full time and the delivery not abnormal though more difficult than the others. When one month old, the patient had two "inward spasms"; the head was thrown back and the eyes rolled up; these spells were apparently convulsions and never reappeared. There has never been a history of meningitis. When three months old, it was definitely agreed that his head was abnormally large. Before this time, however, the neighbors had commented on the "large round head." When four and one-half years old, he had "screaming spells" almost daily, but these were not associated with convulsions or vomiting. At this time, the family physician made the diagnosis of water on the brain. Feeding was uneventful and he thrived and his body grew normally. He was never able to hold up his head, to sit up or to walk. When a year old, it was noticed that his left arm was weaker than the right. The fontanelles remained open and wide. When nine months old, the anterior fontanelle measured 11 centimeters transversely and 9 centimeters anteroposteriorly. The posterior fontanelle was closed. Two years later (two and one-half years old) the fontanelle measured 10 by 9.75 centimeters. The head measurements at various intervals are as follows:

When 6½ months old, 52.5 centimeters.

When 9 months old, 54.0 centimeters.

When 13 months old, 56.0 centimeters.

When 14 months old, 57.0 centimeters.

When 15 months old, 57.8 centimeters (puncture of corpus callosum done 1 month ago.)

When 23 months old, 62.0 centimeters.

When 29 montns old, 64.0 centimeters.

When 33 months old, 65.0 centimeters.

When 60 months old, 68.0 centimeters (at time of death).

This happens to be the first case of hydrocephalus in which the absorption from the ventricles and the subarachnoid space was tested by the phenolsulphonephthalein test. It was found that the dye appeared in the urine 55 minutes after injection into tne ventricle and in two hours following the appearance time only 0.5 per cent was excreted by the kidneys which were shown to have a normal function. Spinal punctures, repeatedly made, yielded only 2 to 3 cubic centimeters of clear fluid, containing none of the phenolsulphonephthalein, thereby demonstrating the absence of communication between the ventricles and the subarachnoid space. When phthalein was injected into the ventricles, a normal absorption, 35 per cent in two hours, was obtained. The cause of the hydrocephalus is evident from these studies. An obstruction was indicated and, because of the very small amount of fluid obtained at lumbar puncture,

the obstruction was thought to be at the foramina of Luscnka and Magendie. These observations were made before the institution ot surgical treatment was advisable.

A puncture of the corpus callosum was made when the child was fourteen months old, but no beneficial results were obtained. The child died when five years old of bilateral pyonephrosis which was caused by a congenital urethral stricture. The foramina of Magendie and Luschka were occluded but the surprising finding was the second obstruction at the aqueduct of Sylvius. The third ventricle and particularly the lateral ventricles were tremendously distended. The fourth ventricle was moderately distended.

Had the obstruction been solely at the aqueduct of Sylvius, the size of the fourth ventricle would not have been increased and, conversely with an obstruction at the aqueduct, the fourth ventricle could dilate only when the foramina of Luschka and Magendie are obstructed.

CASE OF PARTIAL BUT NEARLY TOTAL OCCLUSION OF THE AQUEDUCT OF SYLVIUS

Patient was first seen when six weeks old. It was apparent at that time from the large fontanelle that hydrocephalus was present though the size of the head was normal, and no abnormality of the head had been suspected by the parents. In two weeks, the circumference of the head increased 3 centimeters and then measured 39 centimeters. A meningocele had been partially excised two days after birth, and the patient was brought to me to complete the excision of the meningocele. The wound had healed and no nerve palsies had followed. The sagittal suture was open, uniting the anterior and posterior fontanelles.

A ventriculogram shows a large lateral ventricle, at least four times the normal size, leaving a greatly reduced cortex. On spinal puncture, only 5 cubic centimeters of fluid were obtained and indigo-carmine, which had been injected into the lateral ventricle, did not appear in the spinal fluid in 35 minutes. Unfortunately, a puncture was not made 1 hour after the injection, for a trace of fluid might have been present at that time. This inference is made because at autopsy the aqueduct was reduced to a channel of filiform size. It was really still a partial obstruction though nearly complete, and sufficiently complete to cause the high grade hydrocephalus. The foramina of Luschka and Magendie were patent and of normal size. The third and both lateral ventricles were greatly dilated, the fourth ventricle was very small. Undoubtedly, this is a progressive lesion and shortly the lumen would have been completely closed as in the other cases.

DIAGNOSIS OF A STRICTURE OF THE AQUEDUCT OF SYLVIUS

An occlusion of the aqueduct of Sylvius can now be accurately localized. It is first necessary to prove the existence of hydrocephalus; second, to find whether it is of the obstructive or of the communicating type; and finally, if obstructive, to locate the obstruction. Unfortunately, hydro-

cephalus is now usually diagnosed only in the late or relatively late stages of the disease by the characteristic enlargement of the head; at this stage, the diagnosis is just as easily made by the parent as by the physician. Moreover, when any considerable enlargement of the head is present, the destruction of the brain is so great that the pratical value of the diagnosis is relatively slight, for any effective treatment would leave the patient mentally deficient.

In the early stages of hydrocephalus in children, and in all cases after union of the sutures, the diagnosis of hydrocephalus is extremely difficult. But the important time to make a diagnosis is at the beginning of the disease, before the large head has made the diagnosis unquestioned. It is not with in the scope of this paper to deal with this most important phase of hydrocephalus — the early diagnosis — but it should always be eagerly borne in mind and when suspected, the patient should be referred to a competent authority to ascertain definitely whether or not this condition is present. This diagnosis can now be made with absolute certainty and the degree of the ventricular dilatation determined with ab-

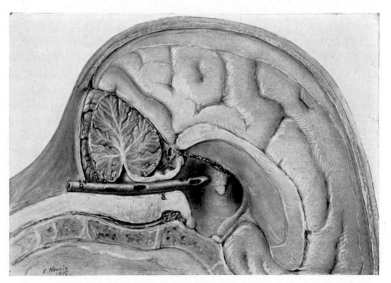

Fig. 1. Sagittal view of brain showing tube in position in the aqueduct of Sylvius. Openings are made in that part of the tube which lies in the third and fourth ventricles. The tube is firmly anchored to the dura with a silk suture at b. The tube is buried complete when the occipital muscles and the skin are closed.

solute accuracy by ventriculography, and when moderately advanced, not infrequently the condition can be recognized by an x-ray without ventriculography. Without these methods, the determination of the presence or absence of hydrocephalus in the early stages is entirely guesswork, that is until the tell-tale growth of the head has taken place. Careful weekly measurement of the head should always be made until any suspicion of hydrocephalus is allayed or verified. When the diagnosis of hydrocephalus is made, the proper treatment, which depends entirely upon the type of hydrocephalus, should be instituted without delay.

When the diagnosis of hydrocephalus has been made, a simple and safe procedure will determine whether the ventricles communicate with the subarachnoid space and thus determine into which of the two great groups — obstructive hydrocephalus or communicating hydrocephalus — the particular case belongs. One cubic centimeter of indigo-carmine (or of a carefully neutralized solution of phenolsulphonephthalein, though I have ceased to use this in the ventricles because of an occasional reaction) should be injected into a lateral ventricle and thirty minutes later a lumbar puncture made. If the ventricles communicate with the subarachnoid space, the color will have appeared in quantity in the spinal fluid by this time or very shortly thereafter. The hydrocephalus would, therefore, be of the communicating type and one could be certain that there was *no obstruction* in any part of the ventricular system. For the purposes of this paper it would exclude any occlusion of the aqueduct of Sylvius.

On the other hand, if the dye does not appear in the spinal fluid in this allotted period of time, one could know just as positively that an obstruction existed at some part of the ventricular system; it might be at the foramen of Monro — a rare possibility — or more probably either (1) at the aqueduct of Sylvius or (2) at the basal foramina of Magendie and Luschka

(all three must be occluded to produce hydrocephalus). In cases of congenital hydrocephalus, as indicated by statistics given at the beginning of the paper, the chances are about two to one that the obstruction is at the aqueduct of Sylvius, and about one to two that the foramina of Magendie and Luschka are occluded. There are some rarer exceptions to these interpretations which need not be considered here.

The precise location of the site of the obstruction can be accomplished only by ventriculography.[10] If the obstruction is at the aqueduct of Slyvius, the shadow of the third and particularly of the lateral ventricles will be shown to be greatly dilated, *but no air will be present in the fourth ventricle. If air is in the fourth ventricle, the obstruction cannot be at the aqueduct of Sylvius.* Further differentiation of the types of hydrocephalus by air injections will be considered in greater detail in a paper which will appear shortly. The absence of a shadow of the fourth ventricle must not be taken, as conclusive evidence of an occlusion at the iter unless one is confident of a perfect and complete injection, that is one which has almost completely filled both lateral ventricles and in which the head has been properly manipulated in order to permit the air to pass into and remain in the fourth ventricle.

AN OPERATIVE TREATMENT FOR STRICTURES OF THE AQUEDUCT OF SYLVIUS

The difficulties encountered in treating lesions of the aqueduct of Sylvius would appear almost insuperable, but I have been encouraged to the possibilities of a direct attack upon the mesencephalon even in infants by the increasing number of cases in which the aqueduct has been exposed during the extirpation of cerebellar tumors. At least twenty-five times during the past year it has been possible to watch the cerebrospinal fluid pour through the aqueduct (often enlarged by the hydrocephalus which follows tumors) into the fourth ventricle. On two occasions, a pineal tumor has been exposed and in several instances the exposure of tumors of the anterior part of the vermis or the removal of huge tumors of the cerebellum left this structure in full view. In animals long tedious operations for removal of the pineal body were borne with impunity even when the puppy operated was only three or four days old.

In dogs I have found that an obstruction could be placed in the aqueduct and produce hydrocephalus;[11] later, it could be removed and the hydrocephalus cured. Moreover, an accumulated past experience with the surgical treatment of hydrocephalus would seem to indicate strongly that the treatment of hydrocephalus must be directed toward an attack on the cause of the disease. All efforts at circumventing the cause, such as a puncture of the corpus callosum, or puncture of the wall of a lateral ventricle, are doomed to failure because of anatomical and physiological facors which must be recognized but which have been disregarded or not known in the empirical treatments instituted heretofore. It seems impossible to produce an opening in the third ventricle which will drain the cerebrospinal fluid into an absorbing area except by way of the normal route into the fourth ventricle. It is necessary that cerebrospinal fluid pass into the cisternae before it can be distributed into the finer radicles of the subarachnoid space, for it is only there that an adequate absorption of the fluid is possible. The fluid can only reach the cisterna magna by way of the fourth ventricle through the foramina of Luschka and Magendie, and the fourth ventricle can only be reached through the aqueduct of Sylvius. Following a puncture of the corpus callosum, the cerebrospinal fluid passes into the subdural space in which absorption is no greater than in the ventricle from which the fluid escaped. Moreover, the opening in the roof of the ventricle remains patent for a brief period only. All small openings through any considerable thickness of brain tissue must

cicatrize unless lined by epithelium and, pending closure of the opening, the fluid which escapes becomes encysted unless it is poured into an absorbing area.

In an attempt to treat the cause directly, I propose a method of reconstructing the obliterated aqueduct of Sylvius. In probably the majority of cases which are collected here, the entire aqueduct is obliterated by a very dense fibrous scar. It is hardly to be expected that any new channel as long as the iter can be permanently maintained after reconstruction, when the entire aqueduct is involved. But in those cases where only a small portion of the aqueduct is occluded, and ideally perhaps where the aqueduct is crossed by a thin diaphragm, or where the obstruction is only partial, a restoration of the iter should appear to be a hopeful possibility.

The operation has been performed twice, on children one year and five years of age. There was very little reaction to the operation in either case. The older child died seven weeks later of pneumonia; the younger child is still living. There is, of course, no way that the operator can tell beforehand the longitudinal extent of the obstruction in the iter. It is thus necessary to subject all, in whom the intellectual indications are favorable, to the operation, without which there is not the slightest chance of improvement.

Should there be any doubt as to the site of the obstruction, the absolute decision can be made at the operation without delay or difficulty. After eliminating a foramen of Monro obstruction, by proving communication between the two lateral ventricles, there are only two other possible locations for the occlusion — the foramina of Magendie and Luschka, and the aqueduct of Sylvius. Fortunately, the same incision is made for the treatment of either lesion. Patency or occlusion of the foramen of Magendie can readily be determined by an operator of experience. The patency or occlusion of the foramina of Luschka is of less importance, for one foramen is adequate to permit egress of all the cerebrospinal fluid. If the foramen of Magendie is patent, the occlusion, by elimination, must be at the aqueduct of Sylvius. On the other hand, two cases of double stricture in this series, one at the aqueduct, the other at the foramen of Magendie, emphasize the danger of assuming that the aqueduct is patent after the occlusion of the foramen of Magendie has been relieved. The indigo-carmine test will precisely determine this point.

The steps in the operation are shown in the accompanying drawing (Fig. 1). After a bilateral exposure of the cerebellum, the vermis is elevated with a small spatula, exposing a normal foramen of Magendie and fourth ventricle. Into this a fine catheter is gently passed forward until it is met by the obstruction at the aqueduct of Sylvius. To get a satisfactory exposure it is necessary to divide the lower half of the vermis in the mid-line and carry this incision through the roof of the fourth ventricle. A nasal dilator introduced into this defect permits a good exposure of the funnel-like anterior terminus of the fourth ventricle and the entrance to the aqueduct of Sylvius. A small sound entering this orifice meets the obstruction and is carefully forced through it into the third ventricle. Fluid at once freely escapes through the opening which again establishes communication between the third and fourth ventricles. Larger sounds are then passed to increase the size of the lumen. A small rubber catheter is pushed into the newly made channel (Fig. 1) and left in position for a period of two to three weeks after the operation. The tube is perforated in numerous places to prevent closure of the lumen by fibrin. The walls of that part of the tube which lies in the aqueduct are smooth and are without perforations. The anterior part of the tube projects into the third ventricle, the posterior part is in the fourth ventricle and lies on the pons and medulla. It is anchored with a silk ligature to the dura at the foramen magnum. The end of the tube is cut off at this point and the lumen closed by a

ligature. The excess tube which traverses the entire length of the fourth ventricle is necessary to preclude the possibility of the tube becoming dislocated and lost. The nuchal muscles are carefully closed over the wound, giving a good protection of tissues over the large foreign body which is quite deeply buried and is free from skin infections during its abode in the brain.

Such a big foreign body is necessarily accompanied by a reaction of considerable severity which ultimately necessitates its removal at a second operation. I have endeavored to leave the tube in place as long as possible, hoping for epithelization of the iter, and thereby preservation of lumen after the tube has been removed. In one case which died, the tube was left in place 2 weeks, and in the second case it remained 3 weeks. The reaction of the patient to the tube is evident as a general lethargy, loss of appetite, vomiting, loss of weight, temperature elevation, and a full and tight anterior fontanelle, in other words, the manifestations of general intracranial pressure. Signs of pressure quickly disappear after the tube is removed.

It will doubtless seem a radical procedure to hemisect or even partially hemisect the vermis of the cerebellum. I have three patients who are perfectly well after complete removal of the vermis and part of both lobes of the cerebellum, the operations being necessary to remove large tumors. They have no effects of this complete section. In ten other cases, partial section of the vermis has been necessary and has been devoid of any apparent ill effects. Certainly, it is necessary to see every step in remaking the aqueduct. Inferiorly, the pyramidal tract and the nuclei of the third nerve are so near and, above, the vein of Galen is in such intimate contact that a false passage will obviously have serious results. Moreover, an attempt to pass a sound blindly by palpation could scarcely be successful.

In the surviving patient in which the tube was inserted into the aqueduct there are no disturbances. It is now over a year since the operation. His movements are entirely without ataxia. He can hold up his head and walk with no sign of staggering gait or loss of equilibrium. He is talking both English and Norwegian quite freely but it is too soon to predict the final outcome.

SUMMARY AND CONCLUSIONS

1. Cicatricial stenosis of the aqueduct of Sylvius is the most frequent lesion in congenital hydrocephalus (about 50 per cent), and is found in a large percentage of cases of hydrocephalus occurring in infancy and early childhood. It may occur (though rarely) in adult life.

2. Hydrocephalus *always* follows occlusion of the aqueduct. The third and both lateral ventricles progressively dilate. The fourth ventricle, being posterior to the obstruction, does not enlarge.

3. In the gross, the occluded aqueduct appears to be replaced by a fibrous tissue which microscopically is neuroglia. Microscopic remnants of the aqueduct are usually but not invariably found.

4. The stenosis may occupy the entire length of the aqueduct, or varying parts; it may be only a thin even transparent membrane. Again, the stricture may be only partial.

5. Strictures of the aqueduct of Sylvius can be diagnosed and accurately localized. The indigo-carmine test will indicate that an obstruction is present; ventriculography will be the means of precisely locating the obstruction.

6. Spontaneous relief is not possible. Surgical attempts to drain the fluid from the third ventricle to the exterior of the brain have all proved futile. The openings invariably close and the fluid cannot absorb in the subdural space.

7. A surgical procedure is suggested which is directed toward the cause. A new aqueduct of Sylvius is constructed; a tube is left in place for two to three weeks. It is hoped the epithelium will regenerate and establish a new canal.

8. This operation has been performed on two cases, both recovering from the operation. One patient died of pneumonia several weeks later, the second seems well one year after the operation.

REFERENCES

[1]Dandy, W. E., and Blackfan, K. D.: Internad hydrocephalus, an experimental, clinical, and pathological study. *Am. J. Dis. Child.,* viii: 406, 1914. *Beitr z. klin. Chir.,* xciii: 392, 1914. *Am. J. Dis. Child.,* xiv: 424, 1917 (second paper).

[2]Magendie, F.: *Recherches physiologiques et cliniques sur le lequide cephalo-rachidien ou cerebrospinal.* Paris, 1842.

[3]Oppenheimer: *Monatschr. f. Psychiat. u. Neurol., Berl.,* March, 1900, p. 177.

[4]Bourneville and Noir: *Le Progres med.,* July 14, 1900, p. 17.

[5]Touche: Bull. et mem. Soc. med. d. hop., Paris, xix: 141, 1902.

[6]Spiller: *Am. J. M. Sc., cxxiv:* 24, 1902.

[7]Guthrie, L. S.: *Practitioner, lxxxv:* 47, 1910.

[8]Schlapp and Gere: *Am. J. Dis. Child., xiii:* 461, 1917. *Proc. New York Path. Soc.,* 1911, p. 64.

[8a]An additional case is not included here because the obstruction at the aqueduct was due to a tumor. The symptoms, incidence and treatment of such lesions are entirely different and will be considered subsequently.

[9]Dandy and Blackfan. *Loc. cit.*

[10]Dandy, W. E.: Ventriculography following the injection of air into the cerebral ventricles. *Ann. Surg,* July, 1918; Fluoroscopy of the cerebral ventricles. *Bull. Johns Hopkins Hosp.,* February, 1919; Roentgenography of the brain after the injection of air into the spinal canal. *Ann. Surg.,* October, 1919; Localization or elimination of cerebral tumors by ventriculography. *Surg., Gynec. & Obst.,* 329, 1920.

[11]Dandy, W. E.: Experimental hydrocephalus. *Ann. Surg.,* August, 1919.

XI

THE DIAGNOSIS AND TREATMENT OF HYDROCEPHALUS DUE TO OCCLUSIONS OF THE FORAMINA OF MAGENDIE AND LUSCHKA*

Every case of hydrocephalus has a specific cause which can and should be located by clinical tests during life. In a great many instances this cause is easy of correction by operation with a resultant cure of the disease. I realize that this is a very sweeping statement concerning a disease which has been considered idiopathic and for which no treatment has been successful. The purpose of this paper is to describe a group of cases of hydrocephalus caused by closure of the foramina of Luschka and Magendie, to show the pathology by postmortem specimens, to describe the means by which it can be diagnosed clinicaly, and particularly to describe an operative procedure which will produce its cure. In previous papers, [1] I have described the pathology, methods of diagnosis, and operative procedures for the treatment of other types of hydrocephalus. In this type of hydrocephalus, the treatment is ideal in that the cause can be attacked directly and with every prospect of permanency. It is one of the most common of the types of congenital hydrocephalus, being surpassed in frequency probably only by the group of cases with an obstruction at the aqueduct of Sylvius. To be effective, the treatment must be applied in the early stages of the disease.

A clear conception of the anatomy of the cerebrospinal spaces, within and without the brain, is an absolute prerequisite to the introduction of a successful method of treatment. It must be appreciated that the normal equilibrium of cerebrospinal fluid is absolutely dependent upon communication between the ventricles of the brain and the subarachnoid spaces. In the ventricles, cerebrofluid is produced; in the subarachnoid space, it is absorbed. The balance between the formation and the absorption of cerebrospinal fluid is maintained solely by three openings which connect the fourth ventricle with the cesterna magna. These openings are the paired foramina of Luschka and the median foramen of Magendie. These openings are neither myths nor artefacts. Although they are now incorporated in the modern text books of anatomy, there is a very uncertain attitude toward their acceptance by many authorities, both anatomical and surgical, and their demonstration is usually even more indefinite. By many, they are looked upon as "functional" rather than anatomical openings. There can be no reason for this hesitancy in their acceptance and no basis for a controversy as to their exact nature. They are just as definite and as precisely outlined as the foramen of Monro or the aqueduct of Sylvius. Nor is this an academic discussion. It is one of the greatest practical import, for surely no neurological surgeon can be competent to make a differential diagnosis of lesions of the cerebellar region, and far less to perform cerebellar operations, who has not a perfect understanding of the importance of the foramen of Magendie and who does not know the foramen when he sees it and who does not expose it at every cerebellar operation in which the exploration has not disclosed the lesion. To those who do not question the existence of the foramen of Magendie, these statements, doubtless, seem superfluous, but constantly the ques-

*Reprinted from *Surgery, Gynecology & Obstetrics*, February, 1921, pp. 112-124.

tion is asked by men of authority: Is the foramen of Magendie a real opening, or is it not an artefact produced by dissection of the delicate membranes? The answers to this query are many and admit of no equivocation.

An anatomical dissection after death shows the three foramina, through each of which a probe can easily be passed without injury to any membranes. The foramen of Magendie is exposed at most cerebellar operations and through it the floor of the fourth ventricle is always evident. The three openings can easily be demonstrated at a postmortem examination (without any dissection) by cutting the mid-brain transversely and injecting (without pressure) into the aqueduct of Sylvius a colored solution; the color will pass from the fourth ventricle to the exterior through the foramina of Luschka and Magendie, but through no other openings.

ARE THE FORAMINA OF LUSCHKA AND MAGENDIE NECESSARY?

The whole problem of hydrocephalus hinges on this question. As early as 1790, the renowned anatomist, Monro, the discoverer of the foramen of Monro, denied any communication between the ventricles and the subarachnoid space. A curious defect in his argument was that, in a case of hydrocephalus, there were no openings and the ventricular system was intact. So it was in his case, for he missed the cause of the hydrocephalus—the closure of the foramina at the base. Magendie described the foramen which bears his name, in 1825. It seems incredible that, at this late date, a large part of his epoch-making contribution should have been devoted to proving that the cerebrospinal system contained fluid and not air or vapor. His foramen of Magendie was received with skepticism and open hostility. Renault, 1829, found the foramen of Magendie absent in the horse and dog, and his observations were even confirmed by Magendie, though the latter still thought his foramen important in man. Magendie's explanation of the

function of the foramen was not impressive and was incorrect in the light of our present knowledge. He assumed the cerebrospinal fluid to form in the pia and thought it passed upward through his new foramen into the ventricles of the brain. And when he found a case of hydrocephalus (1842) in which the foramen of Magendie was closed, a satisfactory explanation was not forthcoming, though he still thought in some way the closure of the foramen to be the cause of the disease, as it undoubtedly was. Monro had the cause of hydrocephalus before him, but missed it because of his eagerness to prove a theory. Magendie maintained confidence in his anatomical findings, in spite of the conflict with his theories, and should receive credit for the first case of hydrocephalus in which the described pathological findings were the cause of the disease.

Krause (1843) and Todd (1847) described the foramen of Magendie as an artefact produced either by pressure or tearing of the tissues. Virchow (1854) very strongly disclaimed the existence of a foramen of Magendie or any other open communication between the ventricles and the subarachnoid space. With Virchow's strong opposition it is but natural that Magendie's foramen should by that time have been thoroughly discredited. But another discovery of the greatest importance appeared in the same year as Virchow's publication, and gradually the prevailing but erroneous views have been transformed. Luschka discovered a foramen on each side of the fourth ventricle at the point of emergence of the flocculus from the fourth ventricle. He also confirmed Magendie's discovery of a mesial foramen, thus making three foramina which established communication between the ventricles and the subarachnoid space (the cisterna magna). The foramina of Luschka were found to be constantly present in man and all mammals. The absence of the foramen of Magendie in the horse and dog is immaterial because the two foramina of Luschka are ample to assume its function. Nature has made in man the foramen of Magendie as an additional safeguard against possible closure of the fourth ventricle; this is in marked contrast to the absence of such safeguards in case of closure of the aqueduct of Sylvius. Key and Retzius (1875) and Retzius (1896) confirmed the presence of the foramina of Luschka in examinations of many brains. They found the foramen of Magendie absent in two of one hundred cases examined and the foramina of Luschka closed in three instances. No mention is made whether the three foramina were absent in the same brains, nor of the incidence of hydrocephalus in the brains examined. Cannieu (1898), however, made similar examinations and looked upon all the openings as artefacts and considered the ventricles a closed system and everywhere lined by epithelium. Testut and Schmorl, also, shared this view.

In recent communications[1,2] I have shown the absolute necessity of communication between the ventricles and the subarachnoid space. I have shown by experiments on animals that cerebrospinal fluid is formed from the choroid plexus which are located in each of the four ventricles, and that in no part of the entire ventricular system is there any appreciable absorption. It is for these reasons that the foramina of Luschka and Magendie are necessary. They permit the fluid to pass to the absorbing area of the brain—the subarachnoid space. The normal ventricular pathway for cerebrospinal fluid is from each lateral ventricle through its foramen of Monro into the third ventricle, thence through the aqueduct of Sylvius into the fourth ventricle and from there into the cisterna magna through the foramina of Magendie and Luschka. There are no other openings which allow communication betwen the ventricles and the subarachnoid space; all other openings which have been described are artefacts; nor has it been possible to establish artificial openings in other parts of the brain to replace these openings when they become closed, except by the operation which will

be proposed; here alone, the anatomical conditions are such as to favor the restoration of these openings.

From another viewpoint, the foramina of Luschka and Magendie can be shown to be indispensable. Closure of these three foramina in the same brain will, without exception, result in hydrocephalus. This we have shown experimentally by producing hydrocephalus in dogs; and clinically it has been observed in a number of patients, in many of whom postmortem examinations have been made.

It is entirely possible, in fact it frequently happens, that one or even two of the three foramina at the base may be occluded and the remaining opening is adequate to allow the ventricular fluid to pass from the ventricles into the subarachnoid space. On the other hand, it does not mean that if one, or even all, of these foramina are open, hydrocephalus may not result. In the communicating type of hydrocephalus precisely this condition is present, but the hydrocephalus is due to an entirely different cause — the obliteration of the cisternae or their branches. The inflammatory process which seals the cisternae or their branches usually obliterates one or two of the three foramina, though not infrequently all three openings are closed, in which case the hydrocephalus becomes obstructive.

THE PATHOLOGY OF OCCLUSIONS OF THE FORAMINA OF MAGENDIE AND LUSCHKA

There are, apparently, two types of occlusions of the foramina of Luschka and Magendie: One which occurs congenitally and is well advanced at birth, the second which occurs at all ages. The latter always follows some form of meningitis; the former may or may not be the result of an intrauterine inflammation.

In the cases which are apparently of congenital origin, the characteristic large head of hydrocephalus is usually noticed about the second or third month, though, of course, the brain is largely destroyed by this time, showing that the disease has existed for a long time, — undoubtedly far back into intra-uterine life. I have seen four of these cases at postmortem examination; in all, the time of recognition of the hydrocephalus was approximately the same and, therefore, doubtless the disease arose at about the same period of foetal life. In each of these cases, the aqueduct of Sylvius was treble its normal size, the fourth ventricle greatly enlarged, though there was great difference in the actual size of the fourth ventricle and the shape and size of the cerebellum. In two cases, the vermis was absent (Fig. 1), the two lateral lobes of the cerebellum were small nubbins, laterally placed in the angles of the posterior cranial fossae and connected by a broad expanse of a rather thin, transparent membrane which, in the absence of the vermis, was now the roof of the fourth ventricle. This membrane was fastened tightly to the lateral margins of the medulla and pons and everywhere the fourth ventricle was hermetically sealed, giving it the appearance of a huge cyst. This cyst was not adherent to the dura and there were no signs of any pre-existing inflammatory process in the posterior cranial fossa. The third and fourth cases differed from this description only in degree; in each the vermis was present, the fourth ventricle was a large cyst everywhere covered by cerebellum and hermetically sealed. One lateral pouch (lateral recess) was very transparent and extremely thin, but everywhere intact; this pouch was really a secondary bulging cyst which had protruded through a ring of denser tissue which corresponded with foramen of Luschka. In these cases no traces of a pre-existing meningitis were seen.

Recently, in all postmortem examinations of cases of hydrocephalus, we have injected a colored solution into the spinal canal to observe its distribution in the subarachnoid space and in the ventricles. In two of these cases (with occlusion of the basal foramina) the solution surrounded the entire brain but did not enter the large dilated fourth ventricle, proving conclusively that the obstruction was complete and the fourth ventricle, therefore, devoid of all communication with the subarachnoid space. One can pass a probe into the regions in which the foramina are normally present and one meets a bulging but closed pouch instead of the usual normal opening. Again, colored solutions injected into the fourth ventricle fail to reach the exterior as in the normal brain. If one holds the specimen before a light and looks through the enlarged aqueduct of Sylvius into the fourth ventricle, the transparent membrane can be beautifully seen surrounding the margins of the medulla and pons and stretching upward across a space about 1 centimeter wide before attaching itself to the inferior margin of the cerebellum. If the brain is carefully removed, the arachnoid membrane, which forms the outer layer of the cisterna magna, can be dissected from the base of the brain, exposing the cystic membrane which forms the sides of the fourth ventricle and is entirely distinct from the pia-arachnoid. The presence of this delicate arachnoid tissue, not adherent or only slightly adherent to the contiguous brain tissue, may be looked upon as evidence against an old inflammatory process, at least of a severe grade.

We know that the foramina of Magendie and Luschka are secondary openings in a primary, closed, ventricular system. Blake [1] and Heuser [2] have shown these foramina to develop in the pig embryo by a gradual thinning of the wall of the ventricle. Owing to the early period of onset of the hydrocephalus *in utero,* and to the absence of adhesions, I am led to believe that this type of hydrocephalus results from the failure of these foramina to develop, rather than from a secondary closure after their developments. On the other hand, the same picture may result from a very mild inflammatory process which has sealed these foramina and has left few, if any, additional traces such as adhesions in its wake. It is not impossible that some very mild type of inflammation may seal these openings,

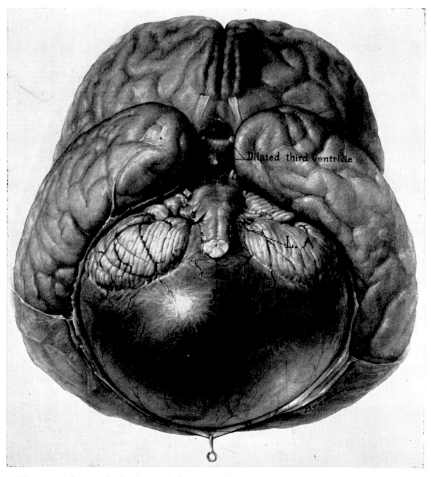

Fig. 1. Advanced hydrocephalus resulting from complete closure of the foramina of Magendie and Luschka. All the ventricles are dilated up to the point of obstruction. Owing to the absence of adhesions, to the absence of the vermis of the cerebellum, together with presence of hyrodcephalus at birth, we have looked upon the occlusion of these foramina to have been due to their failure to develop rather than to a secondary closure. 1, Where foramen of Luschka should be; it is closed. m, Where foramen of Magendie should be; it is closed.

though such an explanation certainly seems less probable.

There is a second group of these occlusions of the basal foramina, which occurs in infants, in which an old inflammatory process is everywhere manifest. We have seen three cases of this kind at necropsy and one at operation. The base of the brain is then sealed to the dura, over areas of considerable extent; the meninges are thickened and tough, and the contiguous brain itself is usually thickened and rigid. The cisterna magna and the other cisternae are usually obliterated by adhesions. The foramina of Luschka and Magendie are occluded either completely or almost completely. The floor of the fourth ventricle also shows marked evidences of the inflammation, rugae of scar tissue are present, and the size of the medulla and pons is increased by the inflammatory tissue. Two of these cases have followed a definite meningitis. In the third case, hydrocephalus was undoubtedly present at birth; the delivery was difficult and the head was unusually large; a lumbar myelomeningocele was also present. In this latter case, doubtless, an inflammation had been present early in intra-uterine life. This is evident by the presence of the meningocele and by the high grade of hydrocephalus which was manifest soon after birth. In a fourth case, a dorsal meningocele was present at birth and hydrocephalus was observed two months after birth. A dense scar covered the foramen of Magendie and the contiguous region. The cerebellum was firmly bound to the medulla and pons, there being no bulging fourth ventricle between. A large cerebellar hernia projected into the spinal canal. The pia-arachnoid was adherent to the dura over most of the area exposed at operation. Undoubtedly, an intra-uterine inflammatory process had produced both the hydrocephalus and the meningocele. In all of the cases with marked evidences of an old inflammatory process, there is a striking difference from those of the non-inflammatory type. Following the inflammatory process, the cerebellum is usually, but not always, firmly bound to the border of the medulla and pons, thus effectually preventing the fourth ventricle from bulging as a cyst between these structures, as occurs in the noninflammatory type. The difference between a total and a partial occlusion of the foramina of Luschka and Magendie is one which is readily made at necropsy and just as easily by a clinical test, and is all-important in the matter of treatment of the individual case.

A group of two adult cases completes the pathological picture of occlusions at the basal foramina. The pathology of these cases was seen at operation and not at necropsy. At operation, the foramina of Luschka can be seen directly only with difficulty, but the examination of the foramen of Magendie gives all the necessary information. If the foramen of Magendie is patent, hydrocephalus will not result even should both foramina of Luschka be closed. On the other hand, if the foramen of Magendie is closed, hydrocephalus will result only if both foramina of Luschka are also occluded. *But, given a dilated fourth ventricle and a closed foramen of Magendie, the closure of this foramen is always the cause of the hydrocephalus.* On the other hand, given a normal fourth ventricle and a closed foramen of Magendie, the closure would not be significant. The latter stipulation, however, is only of theoretical value for there would be no symptom requiring operation.

In one of the two adult cases, a dense scar at the foramen of Magendie was the only evidence of a pre-existing inflammation, but this evidence was indisputable. In this young man, who was nineteen years old, the pathological features differed from those of the congenital type of occlusion of these foramina only in the presence of this scar; the cystic fourth ventricle bulged on each side between the cerebellum and medulla which were separated by the pressure of the accumulated fluid. The scarred foramen of Magendie was sufficiently extensive and rigid to retain the cerebellum in the posterior cranial chamber and prevent the protrusion of the lobes through the foramen magnum into the spinal canal (cerebellar hernia). In the second adult case, the fourth ventricle was of tremendous size and both lobes of the cerebellum had herniated far into the spinal canal. The foramen of Magendie was tightly sealed by adhesions which, however, were not present over the lobes of the cerebellum. The cerebellum and medulla were also tightly adherent, thus effectually preventing the fourth ventricle from bulging between these structures. The operative findings of these two cases were almost exactly like that of the infant in whom an intra-uterine inflammation had closed the foramina of Luschka and Magendie.

To sum up the pathology of these nine cases, the fundamental features were always similar. The foramina of Luschka and Magendie were closed. The absence or presence of the vermis, the position of the cerebellar lobes, the presence or absence of the bulging fourth ventricle between the inferior surface of the cerebellum and the medulla, the presence or absence of a cerebellar hernia into the spinal canal were all dependent upon local differences in type or extent of the causative lesion and, doubtless, also upon the time at which the lesion developed. In four cases, the cause of hydrocephalus is presumed to be a failure of the foramina of Magendie and Luschka to develop, though a mild intra-uterine inflammation can not be excluded. In two cases, a definite inflammatory process in infancy caused the condition, and in a third case, a definite intra-uterine inflammation had been the cause. Two adult cases were caused by a mild meningitis which, clinically, was not recognized as such but the pathological findings needed no clinical confirmation.

THE DIAGNOSIS OF OCCLUSIONS OF THE FORAMINA OF LUSCHKA AND MAGENDIE

Since occlusions of the foramina of Luschka and Magendie occur at varying periods of life, I shall divide the consideration of the clinical manifestations and the differential diagnosis into the period of infancy and of later life. Seven of our cases occurred in infancy and two in adult life. In infancy, the clinical picture is that of hydrocephalus; in adult life, the clinical picture is hard to differentiate from that of a cerebellar tumor. Infants, of course, give none of the cerebellar signs such as ataxia, adiadokokinesia, nystagmus, Romberg, and disturbances of gait; the signs are purely those of increased pressure of the intraventricular fluid and this is shown solely by enlargement of the head and separation of the sutures. At this early age, an enlargement of the head is almost pathognomonic of hydrocephalus. But, as hydrocephalus is a symptom and not a cause, there is nothing about the enlargement of the head which

denotes the location of the cause, i. e., the obstruction.

There is no clinical picture which is distinctive of any particular type of hydrocephalus, at least none is recognized as yet. It is only by the tests which have been recently introduced that we are able to determine the location of the obstruction which causes the hydrocephalus. In a recent publication,[1] we have shown how lesions of the aqueduct of Sylvius may be localized. The localization of occlusions of the foramina of Magendie and Luschka is made by the same methods. It is first necessary to determine that hydrocephalus is not of the communicating type but is due to an obstruction in the ventricular system. This is done by the indigocarmine test; in obstructive hydrocephalus, the color does not appear in the spinal canal after its injection into a lateral ventricle. There are two locations at which the obstruction can exist: (1) the aqueduct of Sylvius or (2) the foramina of Luschka and Magendie (an obstruction at the foramen of Monro must also be thought of, but its incidence is rare). One can, at times, get a fair indication of the position of the obstruction by the amount of cerebrospinal fluid which can be obtained by lumbar puncture but, at best, such deductions are most capricious. In occlusions of the aqueduct of Sylvius, several cubic centimeters of fluid may be obtained by a simple tapping and by aspiration, whereas in occlusions of the foramina of Magendie and Luschka, usually only a few drops will be obtained and little, if any, more can be aspirated. The reason for this difference is that, in lesion of the basal foramina, the foramen magnum is well plugged by a cerebellar hernia or by the dilated ventricle without a hernia. But this differentiation is not always so simple, for at times only a small amount of fluid is obtained when the obstruction is at the aqueduct of Sylvius, owing to the foraminal herniation of the cerebellum. An absolute determination of the precise location of the obstruction can be made only by the use of ventriculography. Following a complete removal of the ventricular fluid and the substitution of air, the latter will reach the point of the obstruction but can not pass beyond. If the aqueduct of Sylvius is obstructed, the third ventricle will be clearly shown but no air will reach the fourth ventricle. If, in hydrocephalus, the fourth ventricle and aqueduct of Sylvius are filled with air, both will be enlarged and the boundaries of each will be sharply defined. Such findings will eliminate an obstruction at the aqueduct of Sylvius and place the obstruction at the foramina of Luschka and Magendie, provided, of course, an obstructive hydrocephalus has been demonstrated by the indigocarmine or phenolsulphone-phthalein tests. In obstructions at the foramina of Luschka and Magendie, the air will not fill the cisterna magna, whereas in communicating hydrocephalus, the cisterna magna will not only contain air but will usually be considerably enlarged.

The clinical diagnosis of a postinflammatory occlusion of the foramina of Luschka and Magendie in adult life is more difficult. This is true mainly because the diagnosis of *hydrocephalus* is more difficult and when the diagnosis of hydrocephalus is finally made, the chances are that the obstruction is due to a tumor, particularly when there has been no antecedent history of meningitis. In infants, intracranial tumors need scarcely be considered, so that the diagnosis of hydrocephalus, which is made with relative facility, presupposes an inflammatory condition or one of the congenital defects, both of which lesions are not frequent at that age.

I had never heard of an inflammatory occlusion of the foramina of Luschka and Magendie in adult life, so that the first case came as a surprise, the preoperative diagnosis of a cerebellar tumor having been made. The second case was, likewise, diagnosed a cerebellar tumor because of unilateral localizing signs and symptoms. In neither case, therefore, can we claim credit for making the clinical diagnosis. I have since seen a case which, on examination, gave almost the identical findings which were present in the second case; the diagnosis of an inflammatory occlusion of the foramina of Luschka and Magendie was considered but a cerebello-pontine tumor was found. I know of no way that an absolute diagnosis of this type of lesion can be made as yet; but it is always possible to diagnose the hydrocephalus, after which the operator must be prepared to find the lesion which is causing the obstruction and thereby producing the hydrocephalus.

The first patient with this inflammation was eighteen years old. He complained of general headache and loss of vision, and, at times, a staggering gait. Eight months before admission to the Johns Hopkins Hospital, the patient was seized with sudden severe headaches in the forehead and suboccipital region. These persisted, though with varying intensity. Seven months ago and one month after the onset of his illness, a sudden severe headache was quickly followed by twitching of his limbs and his right leg became paralyzed and without feeling. This paralysis lasted only a few hours and never recurred, though a similar attack a month later was accompanied by the loss of power in the right arm; this was also transient. A staggering gait was present at times, principally during exacerbations of headaches. Soon an impairment of vision was noticed in the left eye and shortly afterward in the right eye. There had been a rapid loss of sight in both eyes until there was little vision remaining in either eye, the left being definitely worse than the right. There is complete loss of color vision and great reduction in the fields of vision; (he could not read the large headlines of a newspaper). Diplopia had been present at times. Nausea and vomiting were present only on one occasion. There was a bilateral choked disc which measured six diopters in each eye. The neurological examination was strikingly negative except for a slight, even questionable, Romberg. There was no ataxia, no nystagmus, no adiadoko-kinesia, no extraocular palsy and the gait was entirely normal during several examinations. There was no difference in the reflexes on the two sides. Aside from the uncertain Romberg, there was only one localizing sign which could be made out objectively and that was a convolutional atrophy of the skull. This roentgenographic finding is almost pathognomonic of hydrocephalus and, therefore, referred the lesion to the posterior cranial fossa. At operation, the hydrocephalus was found to be due to a dense scar at the foramen of Magendie.

After operation we inquired into the past history very closely for an illness which could have been responsible for the production of this scar. There was never an illness which at all resembled meningitis, but the mother regarded his present illness as a sequel to an attack of "measles" which antedated his present cranial symptoms by four months. She had even volunteered this when the history was taken before the operation but his recovery from the attack seemed complete and there was a four months' interval of practically normal health. This illness was probably measles; there was an epidemic; a rash, photophobia, and fever were present; he was confined to bed five or six days. There had been no headaches, cervical rigidity or pains in the legs or back during the illness.

The second case was a man of thirty-six who had wondered about from physician to physician looking for relief from terrific headaches and dizziness. Two, not only futile but injurious operations, had been performed by well meaning but thoroughly incompetent surgeons. His illness dated back four years when, without warning, he suddenly fell unconscious. Previous to this time he had had only occasional headaches but since then the pain never remitted. Nearly every morning and frequently during the day, vomiting accompanied the headaches and the patient was soon too weak to continue his work. Although he never fell, there was always a feeling as though he would "topple forward on his head." After these symptoms had persisted for a year there was a sudden and unexplained cessation of all symptoms for nearly a year. Then the headaches, dizziness, and vomiting again returned as before but with even greater violence.

Vertigo was increased by any change of position or by lying on the back. The headache was then always present and was both frontal and suboccipital.

Bilateral decompressions, previously performed, were bulging knots. The following positive neurological signs were obtained: (1) Nystagmus in all directions; (2) slight weakness of the left external rectus muscle (sixth nerve); (3) jaw deviates to left (fifth nerve); (4) hyperaesthesia in pain, touch, and temperature, on left diminution of left corneal reflex (left fifth nerve); (5) Romberg positive, but patient tends to fall in every direction; (6) complete nerve deafness (left eighth nerve) but patient says he has been deaf in this ear since childhood; (7) slight ataxia in left hand; (8) convolutional atrophy of the skull and destruction of the posterior clinoid process (x-ray); (9) bilateral choked disc; (10) slight left fascial weakness (seventh nerve).

The diagnosis of hydrocephalus was clear, but the unilateral weakness of the left face and loss of sensation in the left trigeminal area, loss of the left corneal reflex, weakness of the muscles supplied by the left trigeminal nerve led me to the diagnosis of a left cerebellar tumor and possibly one in the left cerebellopontine angle. A completely occluded foramen of Magendie and a greatly dilated fourth ventricle made the diagnosis at operation. Doubtless, the unilateral signs and symptoms were due to the pressure of fluid in the left lateral recess of the fourth ventricle.

After carefully examining the clinical findings in these two adult cases, I am forced to the conclusion that without a history of an antecedent meningitis, there could be little certainty in making a diagnosis of occlusion of the foramina of Luschka and Magendie before operation. Of probably the greatest significance is the absence or the relatively slight intensity of the usual signs which are present in cerebellar lesions, such as ataxia, nystagmus, staggering gait and Romberg. In the second case, the complete cessation of all symptoms for a year is suggestive of such a lesion rather than a neoplasm.

The diagnosis of hydrocephalus can frequently be made in the later stages from the roentgenogram but in the early or moderately advanced stages of the disease the diagnosis can only be made by ventriculography. The methods of arriving at the diagnosis are essentially the same in infants and in adults. The diagnosis of hydrocephalus is all-important. The precise localization of the cause of the hydrocephalus before operation is not indispensable, for the same operative approach is necessary for obstructions at the foramina of Luschka and Magendie or the aqueduct of Sylvius. But if a hydrocephalus is proved, it is absolutely required of the surgeon that this obstruction be found at operation and of the findings there can be no equivocation.

Several years ago, I described with Dr. Blackfan occlusion of the foramina of Luschka and Magendie in an infant with hydrocephalus, but, so far as I am aware, this case and those which I have described here are the only instances of this lesion in the literature. I am confident none has been found at operation.

THE TREATMENT OF OCCLUSIONS OF THE FORAMINA OF LUSCHKA AND MAGENDIE

It is obvious that the only satisfactory treatment of any form of hydrocephalus is the treatment of the cause. In occlusions of the foramina of Luschka and Magendie, the entire ventricular system is devoid of any communication with the subarachnoid space and to cure the hydrocephalus it is necessary to make one opening between the fourth ventricle and the cisterna magna to assume the function of the three which are blocked. But before operating it is necessary to know whether the ultimate radicles of the subarchnoid space are open and whether there is a normal absorption of fluid from the subarachnoid space. Following meningitis, particularly in children, the cisternae are blocked as well as the foramina of Luschka and Magendie, so that the reconstruction

of a new foramen of Magendie would lead to no beneficial results because the ventricular fluid would have access to only the restricted area of the subarachnoid space posterior to tentorium cerebelli. The subarachnoid space should be tested in one of two ways, first by the intraspinous phenolsulphonephthalein test and second by an intraspinous injection of air. If over 30 per cent of the phenolsulphonephthalein is absorbed in two hours, a cure can be expected if the cause is corrected. Intraspinous injections of air will give the same information. The air will reach all the parts of the subarachnoid space which are open. If, therefore, the cerebral sulci show in the roentgenogram, there is a graphic demonstration that the absorbing spaces are open to the reception of fluid if its escape from the ventricles is made possible. The absence of air in the cerebral sulci denotes a closure of the cisternae and precludes an operative cure of the hydrocephalus. Such a finding would be accompanied by a low phenolsulphonephthalein output, usually less than 10 per cent in 2 hours.

PRODUCTION OF A NEW FORAMEN OF MAGENDIE AT OPERATION

The usual bilateral exposure of the cerebellum is made exactly as is done for the extirpation of cerebellar tumors. The operator will quickly learn to recognize the normal foramen of Magendie at a glance and to know whether it is open or closed. I rarely expose the cerebellum without seeing the foramen of Magendie, either because it is necessary to look for it or because after the removal of a tumor from this region, it is usually brought directly into view. It will probably occur to the reader to ask why it is not necessary to expose and determine the patency of the foramina of Luschka. The exposure of these openings is possible but much more difficult and not important. It is necessary to have but one of the three foramina patent and, if the foramen of

Magendie is open, it is not necessary to search further. If the foramen of Magendie is occluded the size of the fourth ventricle will indicate the condition of the foramina of Luschka.

I have operated upon three cases in which a total occlusion of the foramen of Magendie has been found. The findings in each were quite different. In an infant of three months, the vermis was entirely absent and the lateral lobes of the cerebellum pushed lateralward into the outer angles of the fossa was filled with the tremendously dilated fourth ventricle covered only by a membrane. The hydrocephalus was extreme, so that puncture of the ventricle quickly resulted in death. The lesion disclosed at operation in the boy of 19 was sharply localized to the foramen of Magendie and the immediately contiguous region to either side. A very dense scar bound the cerebellum and medulla and, because of its rigidity, precluded a herniation of the lateral lobes into the spinal canal. To either side of the scar, the tissues were normal. A thin, bluish wall bulged between the cerebellum and medulla and, because of its thinness, offered an ideal situation for the construction of a new foramen. The absence of any signs of an old inflammatory process in this region seemed to preclude a closure of the newly made foramen, especially in view of the steady flow of cerebrospinal fluid through it into the cisterna magna. In the second case, the procedure was different, the medulla was closely applied to the cerebellum preventing the fourth ventricle bulging between these strictures as in the preceding case. It was, therefore, impossible to reconstruct a new foramen of Magendie in the space between the medulla and cerebellum, as in the other case, with any prospect of maintaining a permanent opening. The scar at the foramen of Magendie was much more localized and was confined almost to the normal limits of the foramen of Magendie. A large bilateral cerebellar hernia into the spinal canal made the ex-

posure of the scarred foramen of Magendie difficult. To construct a new foramen, it was necessary to excise the entire scar at the foramen of Magendie. The recurrence of the scar in this case remains a possibility; in the preceding case, recurrence seems impossible.

POSTOPERATIVE COURSE AFTER CONSTRUCTION OF A NEW FORAMEN OF MAGENDIE

Each of the adult cases left the hospital a month after operation, apparently perfectly well. The boy of 19 has since resumed his studies at college. Every symptom has been completely relieved. His vision has greatly improved, both in range and acuity. Color vision, which before operation was entirely gone, has returned. Unfortunately, the older case has been lost track of, so that his ultimate condition can not be reported.

In one of these cases, we have demonstrated by ventriculography not only that the new foramen of Magendie is patent and functioning but that the hydrocephalus has been cured. Six weeks after leaving the hospital, the patient returned for observation and air was injected into a lateral ventricle in order to test the new foramen. The roentgenogram showed the tremendous enlargement of the lateral ventricles; the third ventricle, the aqueduct of Sylvius and the fourth ventricle are sharply outlined. The air has passed through the new foramen of Magendie—which is marked by the silver clips which were placed over a divided blood vessel at operation—into the cesterna magna. The air is even seen to fill the cerebral sulci, showing that the most remote branches of the subarachnoid space receive fluid from the ventricles and that, therefore, the hydrocephalus has been cured.

CONCLUSIONS

1. Blocking of the foramina of Luschka and Magendie invariably produces hydrocephalus. Patency of one of the three foramina prevents the development of hydro-

cephalus, provided the subarachnoid space is normal.

2. A group of cases is presented with occlusion of these foramina and with a hydrocephalus resulting therefrom.

3. Undoubtedly, the disease, occurring in adult life, follows an inflammatory process which may or may not have been clinically evident. Probably, failure of the foramina to develop accounts for the hydrocephalus in many cases which are recognized soon after birth; in other infants an intra-uterine or postnatal inflammation is the cause.

4. Although the general results of the occlusion are the same in every case, there are marked local anatomical differences due to the extent of the inflammatory process and the time of its development.

5. There are no clinical features which permit one to make an absolute diagnosis of occlusion of the foramina of Magendie and Luschka. In every instance, both in adults and infants, the diagnosis of hydrocephalus is possible; the exact site and the character of the obstruction causing the hydrocephalus can be determined by ventriculography and by the phenolsulphonephthalein test.

6. The lesion can always be found at operation.

7. An operative treatment is presented. Two adult cases have apparently been cured by this procedure, which attacks the cause directly.

REFERENCES

[1]Dandy, W. E.: Extirpation of the choroid plexus of the lateral ventricles in communicating hydrocephalus. *Ann. Surg.*, December, 1918. The diagnosis and treatment of hydrocephalus following strictures of the aqueduct of Sylvius. *Surg., Gynec. & Obst., xxxi:* 340, 1920.

[2]Dandy, W. E. and Blackfan, K. D.: Internal hydrocephalus. *Am. J. Dis. Child, viii:* 405, 1914; *xiv:* 424, 1917. *J. A. M. A., lxi:* 2216, 1913; *Beitr. z. klin. chir., xciii:* 392, 1914.

[3]Dandy, W. E.: Experimental hydrocephalus. *Ann. Surg.*, August, 1919.

[4]Blake, J. A.: The roof and lateral recesses of the fourth ventricle. *J. Comp. Neurol., x:* 1920.

[5]Heuser, C. H.: Cerebral ventricles in the pig. *Am. J. Anat. xv:* 213.

[6]*Surg., Gynec. & Obst., xxxi:* 340, 1920.

XII

THE CAUSE OF SO-CALLED IDIOPATHIC HYDROCEPHALUS *

Until recently all cases of hydrocephalus were considered idiopathic. We think it is now fair to assume that those cases in which an obstruction in the ventricular system can be demonstrated may be liberated from this *terra incognita* and may now be classified according to an established pathology; for there can no longer be any doubt concerning the cause of obstructive hydrocephalus. Any lesion which occludes the ventricular system will always produce stasis of fluid and dilatation of the ventricles proximal to the obstruction and will not change the size of the ventricles distal to it. There can be no exception to this rule. The proof of this causative relationship has been amply provided in recent necropsy material[1] and in the experimental production of the disease at will.[1,3,4,5]

The purpose of this paper is to present proof — which I believe is just as positive — of the cause of the remaining big group of this disease — *communicating hydrocephalus, i. e.,* of that type of hydrocephalus in which all the ventricles are in communication with the subarachnoid space. In the course of intensive studies on the absorption of cerebrospinal fluid in hydrocephalus it was found that in the communicating type the absorption from the subarachnoid space was greatly reduced. A reduction in the amount of the absorbing spaces which are reached by the cerebrospinal fluid was suspected as the cause and a hypothetical pathology suggested along this line of reasoning.[1] Later, four cases of communicating hydrocephalus were studied at necropsy and in each adhesions were found which obliterated the cisternae; hence it was assumed that, by preventing

the cerebrospinal fluid from reaching the great absorbing spaces over the cerebral hemispheres, these adhesions had caused the hydrocephalus.[2] We realized, however, the necessity of a more graphic demonstration of the lesion and of proof of its effects before these findings could be accepted beyond question.

There are two ways in which an obstruction of the cisternae can be clearly shown — one after death, the other in the living patient. (1) If a colored suspension is carefully injected into the spinal canal before making an autopsy[3] the color will reach but cannot pass an obstruction in the cisternae. (2) If air is injected into the spinal canal of a living patient, the roentgenogram will show the air extending up to but not beyond the point of obstruction in the cisternae.[6,7] Unless these tests are positive, an obstruction in the cisternae or elsewhere cannot be presumed to exist nor considered to be the cause of communicating hydrocephalus. If properly applied, either test will prove conclusively that an obstruction either is or is not present.

A third and equally important proof must be forthcoming before the cause of communicating hydrocephalus can be regarded as solved: it must be shown that a lesion similar to the one described in these cases of communicating hydrocephalus and similarly situated will cause hydrocephalus when experimentally produced in animals.

COMMUNICATING HYDROCEPHALUS EXPERIMENTALLY PRODUCED

In the studies presented here, all of these exactions have been met. First I have produced communicating hydrocephalus in

*Reprinted from *The Johns Hopkins Hospital Bulletin*, Vol. XXXII, No. 361, March, 1921.

dogs by making a barrier of adhesions in the mesencephalic cisternae.[3] Shortly before necropsy on these animals a suspension of India ink was substituted for an equal amount of cerebrospinal fluid which had been aspirated from the cisterna magna through a puncture of the occipito-atlantal membrane. When India ink is introduced into the spinal canal of an animal whose cerebrospinal spaces are intact, the color will find its way within two hours to every point of the subarachnoid space over both cerebral hemispheres. But in the experimental animal with the perimesencephalic band of adhesions, the passage of the ink is abruptly terminated by the obstructing band and none of the color reaches the surface of either cerebral hemisphere (Figs. 2 & 3); furthermore, as a result of the hydrocephalus which has developed, the foramina of Luschka and Magendie have become so dilated that a retrograde flow of ink is freely permitted into all the cerebral ventricles (Fig. 2). The entrance of ink into the furthermost recesses of the ventricles (which normally occurs only at times) shows that the color has had every opportunity to reach the cerebral sulci, but is precluded from doing so by the obstruction.

DEMONSTRATION OF OBSTRUCTION IN THE SUBARACHNOID SPACE AT POST-MORTEM EXAMINATION

Knowing from the experiments that an obstruction in the cisterna produces communicating hydrocephalus, it then remains to prove that all or at least many cases of this disease have this as the causative lesion. The graphic color method should be applied to all human necropsy material in which hydrocephalus is suspected or known to be present. It is important that pressure be avoided in introducing these colored solutions, for delicate adhesions, though sufficient to cause an obstruction during life, may be easily ruptured and in this way artificial results may be obtained. In animals, the color can be introduced without

pressure during life and the normal circulation will convey the fluid to all the spaces which are patent. In necropsy material the results, though less perfect, will be satisfactory if the color is introduced by gravity for 15 or 20 minutes.

Despite studies in a large series of cases of hydrocephalus, we have had but one opportunity of applying this method at a post-mortem examination in a case of hydrocephalus with communication. In this instance the results were just as striking as in the experimental cases which have been described; the color filled the cisternae, even the cisterna interpeduncularis, covered the cerebellar subarachnoid spaces, but failed to reach any of the sulci over either cerebral hemisphere. On the other hand, the ink passed freely into every part of the cerebral ventricles, deeply staining their walls, for both foramina of Luschka and the foramen of Magendie were widely open. No gross adhesions could be seen either in the vicinity of these openings or even along the cisternae; nevertheless, the cerebral sulci could not be reached by the colored solution, because the branches issuing from the cisternae were sealed. The character of the pathological lesion will be discussed later; the test demonstrates that an obstruction exists in the cisternae and with the additional support of the experimental evidence no doubt can exist that this obstruction is the cause of the hydrocephalus.

WHY SHOULD AN OBSTRUCTION IN THE CISTERNAE CAUSE HYDROCEPHALUS?

Doubtless obstructions, similar to those which we are about to describe in communicating hydrocephalus, have been present in all necropsies of this disease. The adhesions may not be striking, and at times could be missed entirely, if one did not look for them. Indeed in some cases the lesion may be due to defective formation of the cerebrospinal spaces in the early embryo. These pathological findings become significant and all-important only when the anatomy of the cerebrospinal spaces and the manner and place of the formation and the absorption of cerebrospinal fluid are fully understood.

Cerebrospinal fluid circulates in a mesothelial-lined vascular system which is just as definite as the vascular systems for blood, lymph or bile. A clear conception of the gross plan of this vascular system can be obtained from the accompanying diagram by Max Brodel (Fig. 4). The cavities in the interior of the brain (the ventricular system) are concerned only with the *production* of cerebrospinal fluid; the spaces on the exterior of the brain (the subarachnoid spaces) are normally concerned only with the *absorption* of cerebrospinal fluid. The balance between the production and absorption of fluid is maintained by three closely grouped communicating openings — the foramina of Luschka and that of Magendie. Only through these openings can fluid escape from the entire ventricular system; consequently, closure of these openings always produces a stasis of fluid — hydrocephalus — in all the ventricles. But in communicating hydrocephalus, these conduits are open, either entirely or in part, depending upon the extent and position of the pathological lesion. This type of hydrocephalus is caused by interference with the absorption of the cerebrospinal fluid in the subarachnoid spaces. The real absorbing area of the subarachnoid space is the great network of subarachnoid spaces over the cerebral hemispheres — the cerebral sulci. Here the cerebrospinal fluid is distributed over a very extensive surface of blood capillaries of the pia and passes directly through the capillary walls into the blood by osmosis. Numerous large branches convey the fluid to these spaces from the cisterna chiasmatis and the cisterna interpeduncularis, which together serve as a distributing center for all the cerebrospinal fluid which is destined to reach the cerebral hemisphere. Since all the ventricular fluid, on leaving the ventricles, first reaches the cisterna magna (by way of the foramina of Luschka

and Magendie), a relatively long passageway under the medulla, pons, and midbrain must be traversed before this fluid can reach the cisterna interpeduncularis and the cisterna chiasmatis, whence it can be distributed to the cerebral sulci by the major branches, as described (Fig. 4). The finer anatomy and histology of these spaces have been well described by Weed.[8,9]

By experimental methods, which have been mentioned in earlier publications, it has been shown that from three-fourths to four-fifths of the cerebrospinal fluid is absorbed from the subarachnoid spaces of the brain, and the remaining one-quarter or one-fifth in the spinal subarachnoid space. It is doubtful if any absorption occurs in the cisternae, these channels probably serving only as large conduits to carry the fluid to the surface of the brain, much as the ureters carry the urinary secretion to the bladder. An obstruction in the cisternae under the medulla, pons or mesencephalon (that is, at any point between the foramina of Luschka and the cisterna interpeduncularis) will produce a stasis of fluid up to the point of obstruction and cause hydrocephalus just as effectively as would a block at the aqueduct of Sylvius or at the foramina of Luschka and Magendie. It will be remembered that through the membranous tentorium cerebelli which separates the posterior and middle cranial cavities there is but one opening, and this is only a little larger than the brain stem (mesencephalon) which passes through it. It is evident that when adhesions close the incisura tentorii and obliterate the mesencephalic cisterna, collateral channels for the distribution of cerebrospinal fluid have no possible way to develop.

INTRA VITAM METHOD OF DEMONSTRATING AN OBSTRUCTION IN THE SUBARACHNOID SPACE

The value of intraspinous injections of air will be apparent when it is realized that every part of the subarachnoid space can be reproduced[6] in the roentgenogram, just as every part of the ventricular system can be reproduced by an *intraventricular* injection of air.[7] At times, the ventricles also can be injected from the spinal puncture and, again, the subarachnoid space may be partially or wholly injected by way of the ventricular puncture. The patient is placed in the recumbent position, with the head exactly horizontal and higher than the body. This position must be carefully maintained until the skiagram has been taken. In the normal adult, about 30 to 60 cc. of fluid can be obtained by lumbar puncture and an equal quantity of air, which is substituted, will fill all parts of the subarachnoid space. The cerebral sulci are shown as a network of lines over the brain. The presence or absence of these air-filled sulci is the crucial observation of all intraspinous injections. Normally, the sulci will always be filled. When they can be seen over the entire cerebral hemisphere, it is evident that every part of the subarachnoid space is patent. Intact subarachnoid spaces may be interpreted to mean that hydrocephalus, if present, cannot be of the communicating type; if, therefore, hydrocephalus is present (with air-filled sulci) an obstruction must be located in the ventricular system. On the other hand, the absence of air in the cerebral sulci means that an obstruction exists in some part of the subarachnoid space; it also indicates that hydrocephalus must exist because the cerebrospinal fluid (air) cannot reach the absorbing spaces of the cerebral hemispheres; the hydrocephalus with such pneumographic findings would be of the communicating type or possibly of an obstructive type, which, if corrected, would only be transformed into a communicating type.[6,7]

When intact, the cisternal conduit can often be seen throughout the entire course, even through the dense petrous portion of the temporal bone; the major branches can frequently be seen passing directly from the cisterna chiasmatis and the cisterna interpeduncularis to the cerebral sulci; and when an obstruction exists at any point

along the cisternae, it is located definitely by the furthermost point of the air shadow. The cisterna magna is usually clearly outlined. A marked variation has been found in its size; to a certain extent, I believe its size depends upon effects of adhesions, which are so frequently present; for if the cerebellar lobes are firmly bound to the dura in the neighborhood of the foramen magnum, it is clear that the size of the cisterna magna will be reduced and that its enlargement which would otherwise naturally occur with hydrocephalus will be impossible. In obstructive hydrocephalus the size of the cisterna magna is usually reduced by the backward pressure of the superimposed dilated ventricles, the contents of which have no avenue of escape into the cisternae.

LOCATION OF OCCLUSIONS IN THE SUBARACHNOID SPACE

Obviously an obstruction can exist at any part of the subarachnoid tree and the results, in terms of hydrocephalus, will be dependent upon the location of the obstruction. The obstruction may be in the trunk of the tree (the cisternae); it may occlude all the main branches which carry fluid from the cisternae to the cerebral sulci; it may occlude some, but not all, of these branches; or finally, more or less extensive local areas of the subarachnoid space may be obliterated. An obliteration of the cisternae or of all the distributing branches will prevent any cerebrospinal fluid from reaching any of the cerebral sulci; occlusion of some but not all the branches of the cisternae may or may not produce hydrocephalus according to the number of cerebral sulci which continue to receive fluid through the branches which remain intact; or a low grade of hydrocephalus may develop because part of the fluid will be handled by the patent sulci. Extensive local areas of the cerebral subarachnoid space may be destroyed without the occurrence of any hydrocephalus, because the normal subarachnoid spaces are far in excess of the normal requirement for absorption; this is demonstrated by the results of every cranial operation, following which adhesions obliterate extensive areas of subarachnoid spaces with no effect upon the balance of cerebrospinal fluid.

OBSTRUCTION IN THE CISTERNAE

The most frequent location for an obstruction in communicating hydrocephalus is in the cisternae. This was first observed in the four cases which were carefully studied at necropsy and will be seen in the results which are to follow in the patients who have been studied by cerebral pneumography. One must not infer from this statement that adhesions only in the cisternae exist in these cases, but merely that these are the adhesions which are directly responsible for the production of the hydrocephalus. As a matter of fact, there are frequently more or less extensive adhesions along the entire base of the brain, particularly over both cerebellar lobes, and even over the cerebral hemispheres. Frequently one or two of the three basal foramina (Luschka and Magendie) may be sealed by these adhesions and at times the lumen of the third opening may be implicated. When all three openings are occluded, obstructive hydrocephalus results; when one or more foramina are patent, the hydrocephalus is of the communicating type.

Certainly the vast majority of all cases of communicating hydrocephalus follow meningitis and, being a post-meningitic process, the obstruction of the cisternae is in keeping with the basilar involvement of most forms of meningitis. It is also worthy of note that the great majority of these cases occur in infants and young children in whom meningitis is so prevalent and in whom the delicate meninges are more susceptible to permanent injury. At times the meningitic process may be of prenatal origin. This is shown by the frequent occurrence of this type of hydrocephalus at birth and by the presence of the basilar adhesions as the etiological factor; also by the coexistence of a meningo-

cele which is doubtless caused by the same general process.

In more than half of our cases of communicating hydrocephalus the disease has definitely arisen at some time after birth, usually following an illness which has been variously diagnosed, but which a careful history will prove to have been meningitis. Again, the hydrocephalus has almost certainly followed an acute illness, perhaps even very mild, but which on the most careful inquiry has yielded none of the signs or symptoms of meningitis. In these cases adhesions have been found, either at necropsy or at operation, denoting that this illness must have been meningitis. At other times, though quite rarely, it is even possible to find at the base of the brain and elsewhere adhesions which could have been caused only by a pre-existing meningitis, although no illness may have been observed by the parents. These facts show the importance of a careful history of all patients suffering from intracranial pressure; they show that characteristic full-blown signs and symptoms of meningitis are not always present; and that the post-meningitic adhesions are not necessarily in proportion to the severity of the attack of meningitis. The situation, not the extent, of the pre-meningitic adhesions determines the onset and severity of the resulting hydrocephalus.

Communicating hydrocephalus can, of course, result from obstruction of the cisternae by tumors of the pons and mid-brain and even by tumors situated in the middle cranial fossa; instances of these relationships have been reported in previous papers.[6,10] The effects on the circulation of the cerebrospinal fluid are exactly the same whether the occlusion of the subarachnoid space is caused by tumor or by adhesions; but because of differences in treatment, the consideration of occlusions by neoplasms will not be considered here.

In seven out of ten patients with communicating hydrocephalus studied by cerebral pneumography, the obstruction has been located in the pontine or mesencephalic cisterna. In each of these, the column of air ended abruptly under the pons or mid-brain and no air reached the cerebral sulci; in each, the air passed freely into the lateral ventricles, demonstrating the free communication between the ventricles and the spinal subarachnoid space; in each, the cisterna magna was also seen, but its size varied greatly. In one instance it was scarcely visible, doubtless because adhesions between the cerebellum and the adjacent dura had obliterated this usually large chamber of fluid. In other instances the cisterna magna was greatly enlarged — even to the same degree as the fourth ventricle. The pontine and mesencephalic cisternae showed some variation in size.

Several times, when performing cerebellar operations on patients with hydrocephalus, I have been impressed with the fact that the cisterna magna, which usually covers nearly one-half of the posterior surface of both cerebellar lobes, was very small and at times were scarcely recognizable. Invariably in these cases the cerebellum was tightly bound to the dura by adhesions. These operative findings, together with the necropsy observations, explain the cause of the pneumographic variation in the size of the cisternae.

It has doubtless, occurred to many, as to ourselves, to ask why hydrocephalus should be *internal* when the fluid can pass from the ventricles to the exterior. The fact that the cerebrospinal fluid forms in the ventricles and that the fluid is dammed back to its source only partially answers this question. The full answer is now clear. When an obstruction exists in the mesencephalic or pontine cisternae, the extraventricular distribution of cerebrospinal fluid is restricted to the subarachnoid spaces in the posterior cranial fossa, and usually these spaces are reduced to less than normal size by the post-inflammatory process. The cisterna magna will be proportionately as large as the fourth ventricle when its enlargement is not precluded by adhesions; in other words the accumulation of cerebrospinal fluid and the dilatation of the

fluid-containing spaces will occur up to the obstruction (the causative lesion) and the size of the various collections of fluid in these spaces will be dependent on the resistance offered.

OCCLUSION OF ALL THE MAIN BRANCHES OF THE CISTERNA INTERPEDUNCULARIS AND THE CISTERNA CHIASMATIS

In two of our cases the occlusion was not in the cisternae but in the large branches which radiate from the cisternae interpeduncularis and chiasmatica and which carry the cerebrospinal fluid to all the surfaces of the cerebral hemispheres. Although the anatomical features of the two cases differed greatly, fundamentally they were similar in that the cisternae were patent but all the branches were sealed. In each case the clinical diagnosis of communicating hydrocephalus was established by the phenolsulphonephthalein test. In each the site of the obstruction was determined by cerebral pneumography. In one case the findings were verified by necropsy and the intraspinal color test; and in the other by operation and the clinical tests. There was nothing unusual in the history of either case, the disease having been noticed soon after birth and having progressed with the usual rapidity until a tremendously large head had resulted. In one a partial fluid balance eventually had been established, as frequently happens, and at the age of four the fontanelles had slowly closed. The other child was only eight months old and the rate of growth of the head had not diminished.

After the injection of air into the younger child, the roentgenogram showed the air to have stopped in the cisterna immediately behind the sella turcica, *i. e.,* at the cisterna interpeduncularis. Only a small amount of air had been injected into the spine, and this passed freely into the lateral ventricles, but not a trace could be found in the cerebral sulci. which normally should fill with greater ease than the ventricles. The cisterna magna and the cisternae under the brain-stem were small. At necropsy the spinal cord was injected with India ink. The distribution of this color was exactly that of the air as shown by the roentgenogram. The ink did not extend beyond the cisternae although it reached the region of the optic chiasm. On the other hand, all the recesses of the cerebral ventricles, as well as the entire subarachnoid space surrounding the cerebellum, were filled with the black suspension, showing that the ink had had ample opportunity to reach the cerebral sulci, but had been prevented from doing so by an obstruction. No adhesions were evident during removal of the brain, nor could any be found later on careful inspection of the brain. In all of our other cases of communicating hydrocephalus, adhesions had been found at necropsy and one or two of the basal foramina (Luschka and Magendie) had been included in these adhesions and their closure had resulted. But in this case the foramina of Luschka and that of Magendie were open and larger than normal. In the accompanying photograph, a wire has been inserted into the three foramina to show their position and condition. The patency or closure of each of these foramina can always be demonstrated easily and absolutely if the probe is passed from the fourth ventricle outward along the lateral recess. The personal equation cannot enter into the determination.

But in the absence of any demonstrable adhesions, and in the presence of an intact cisternal conduit, why do not the cerebral sulci fill? We know that they cannot fill, because both the air before death and the ink after death have been unable to reach them, and by the two tests, either of which should be absolute, an obstructing lesion has been located in identically the same position. There can be only one explanation for the failure of fluid to reach the cerebral sulci, namely, the absence of the main branches which carry the fluid from the cisternae to the cerebral hemispheres. These branches may be absent either because they have been obliterated by adhe-

sions following meningitis or they may have failed to develop. The absence of adhesion leads me to suspect the latter to be the cause, though the proof is lacking. Weed[8] has shown the cerebrospinal spaces to be a secondary splitting of the peri-encephalic mesenchyme and their development to follow closely upon the opening of the basal foramina, which result from a gradual thinning of the walls of the fourth ventricle; prior to this time the ventricular system is closed. At times these foramina fail to develop[11] and hydrocephalus results, and doubtless the same agenesis, perhaps easier to understand, may account for the failure either of the cisternae or of its branches to develop.

It is worthy of note that in this case the cisterna is small, whereas it should be larger owing to the accumulated fluid up to the obstruction. The absence of this expected enlargement must indicate a rigid wall, which might be of inflammatory origin or it might be the congenital impediment which prevented the further development of the cisternae in foetal life.

In the second case the pathological features at first glance will appear to show little in common with the preceding case. The pathology was disclosed by operation and not by necropsy, but as there was ample opportunity to observe the entire surface of the brain, excepting most of that in the posterior cranial fossa, a post-mortem examination would be of little additional value. Air was injected into a lateral ventricle and not into the spinal canal. As mentioned above, the phenolsulphonephthalein test showed a communicating hydrocephalus. At two operations both hemispheres were explored, and over neither was cerebrospinal fluid found in the cerebral sulci. A huge cyst filled the base of the cranial chamber and extending upward pushed the brain away from the floor of the skull. The cyst extended from one side of the skull to the other, and on each side it was continuous with the cisternae chiasmatica and interpeduncularis. In fact, on each side it was a direct extension of these cisternae. Moreover, when the cyst was opened (on either side) the brain-stem could be seen as far as the pons, owing to the tremendous size of the cisternae under the mid-brain and pons; and doubtless the medullary cisterna was of corresponding size. The chemical analysis of this vast accumulation of fluid showed it to be the same as the cerebrospinal fluid in the lateral ventricles. Furthermore, the phenolsulphonephthalein test demonstrated communication between the ventricles and these extra-cerebral cysts, but only after half an hour. In other words, the communication was by a devious path and was not direct. The absence of air in the cysts after ventricular injection also eliminates any direct communication, and finally, at operation there was seen to be no direct communication.[12]

We are dealing, therefore, with a case of communicating hydrocephalus in which the obstruction is at the branches which pass from the cisterna interpeduncularis and the c. chiasmatis to the surfaces of the cerebral hemispheres (there being no fluid in the cerebral sulci). The walls of the cisternae, gradually yielding to the pressure of the accumulating fluid, allow the formation of the huge cysts instead of the usually restricted cisterna under the brain. No adhesions of note were found at either operation, so that the assumption of a meningitis would be without a history of this affection and without any anatomical evidence of its existence. The most plausible explanation of the cause of this condition is the congenital failure of the large branches of the cisternae to develop. In the preceding case it is possible that the cisternae may have been obliterated rather than that the branches have failed to develop; in this case the cisternae are well open, in fact they are greatly distended; under the midbrain the cisterna is as large as one's index finger.

An external hydrocephalus differs from the above picture only in that the fluid is distributed over the hemispheres instead of being confined to a localized cyst of more restricted size. In fact, in this case the hydrocephalus was transformed into an external hydrocephalus merely by opening the cyst, but the fluid, passing over the arachnoid membrane instead of under it, poured into the subdural space instead of the subarachnoid space, where there was only a slight absorption. The pathology of this case really forms a connecting link which explains the relationship between external hydrocephalus and internal hydrocephalus; this relationship and the general subject of external hydrocephalus will be considered in detail in a forth-coming publication.

OBSTRUCTION OF SOME BUT NOT ALL THE MAIN BRANCHES OF THE CISTERNAE

In the accompanying ventriculogram evidence of a very early hydrocephalus will be seen. It developed in a three-year-old child under observation in the service of Professor Howland. She was first treated for a typical illness of acute meningococcus meningitis, from which there was an apparent recovery, though very shortly lethargy and vomiting ensued. Six weeks after the onset of the attack of acute meningitis and two weeks after apparent recovery,[13] hydrocephalus was first suspected. At this time, the cell count in the cerebrospinal fluid was ten. The sutures of the skull were separated; a suggestive cracked-pot sound was obtained. There was no choked disc and no other sign of intracranial pressure. Without the ventriculogram the diagnosis of hydrocephalus could never have been substantiated. With the absolute verification it is probably the earliest recorded case of hydrocephalus. The ventriculogram was different from that of any previous case which has come under my observation. Air passed from the ventricles and finally reached the cerebral sulci but only in a very restricted segment over the frontal lobe. Such a finding might have been assumed to be due to an imperfect injection of air, but one month later another ventriculogram was made and precisely the same segment of subarachnoid space and exactly the same sulci were injected. In this interval of thirty days between the two ventriculograms, the lateral ventricle had increased in size, though the rate of growth was considerably less than in the usual development of hydrocephalus. The phenolsulphonephthalein output from the spinal canal rose from 13 per cent to 22 per cent; the latter percentage was found at the time the first ventriculogram was made; unfortunately, no test was made when the second ventriculogram was obtained. It is evident, from the phenolsulphonephthalein test, that a partial compensation has occurred, for, with 22 per cent absorption (normal 35-50 per cent), the hydrocephalus could not be full-blown. The ventriculogram was also interpreted to mean that the filling of part of the subarachnoid spaces denoted that a greater amount of cerebrospinal fluid (12 per cent more by the phenolsulphonephthalein test) than in the usual quantitative absorption in communicating hydrocephalus with an obstruction in the cisterna was being absorbed in this restricted area and that a partial compensation had developed, as it should have done.

The branches of the cisternae can be traced directly from the cisterna chiasmatis to the cerebral sulci of the frontal region. Numerous perpendicular air shadows are clearly shown just above the cisterna interpeduncularis and rising vertically from it but ending blindly. These shadows, I believe, represent the branches of the cisternae which are obstructed and which should supply the remainder of the cerebral hemispheres with fluid. The air extends in these branches up to the point of the obstruction in each individual branch.

This patient has been seen at intervals for the past two years and has recovered completely. We have proof from the pneumographic records not only of the existence of a hydrocephalus, which could not have been diagnosed otherwise, of its unusual rate of development, and of its spontaneous cure, but, more important, we have the findings in the transition stages

and, we think, the reason for the compensation and eventual cessation of development of the hydrocephalus. Whether at one time *all* the cisternal branches were occluded and *some* subsequently opened, producing a partially compensating hydrocephalus; whether additional spaces were reestablished after our studies were made and permitted the condition to change from a partially compensating hydrocephalus to a complete cure, we have not the pneumographic evidence to prove or disprove.

I do not believe that it is possible for a hydrocephalus to occur, if all or even many of the cerebral sulci can be shown to fill with air or if the phenolsulphonephthalein output after a spinal injection measures 35 per cent in two hours. From a large series of cases of hydrocephalus, there has been no exception to disprove this statement. We are, however, not yet sufficiently familiar with the roentgenographic pictures of the cerebral sulci to make many positive claims as to prognosis in these unusual types of hydrocephalus.

SUMMARY AND CONCLUSIONS

(1) The cerebrospinal fluid circulates in a closed vascular system. This is just as well defined as the vascular system for blood, lymph, bile or urine.

(2) The ventricular system, in which fluid is produced but not absorbed, is lined with a high cubical and columnar epithelium; the subarachnoid space, in which the cerebrospinal fluid is absorbed, is lined with low mesothelial cells. Nearly all the cerebrospinal fluid is absorbed in the cerebral sulci.

(3) Collateral circulation is almost precluded either in the ventricles or in the cisternae. An obstruction in these spaces, therefore, results in a hydrocephalus, just as closure of a ureter results in a hydronephrosis. If the obstruction is situated in any part of the ventricles (usually the aqueduct of Sylvius or the foramina of Luschka and Magendie) the hydrocephalus is of the obstructive type; if it is situated

in the cisternae (or in the main branches of the cisternae) it is of the communicating type.

(4) That the cause of communicating hydrocephalus (the remnant of so-called idiopathic hydrocephalus) is an obstruction in the cisternae is conclusively demonstrated in three ways. (a) Experimentally communicating hydrocephlaus can be produced by blocking the mesencephalic cisterna. (b) The obstruction can be graphically demonstrated in the experimental animal or at necropsy in the human by injecting a suspension of India ink into the spinal canal; the color stops abruptly at the obstruction. (c) In all living patients the obstruction can be clearly shown by cerebral pneumography after air has been injected into the spinal canal; the air also stops at the obstruction, and can be sharply outlined in the roentgenogram.

(5) The obstruction in the subarachnoid space is most frequently located in the mesencephalic or pontine cisterna.

(6) However, the obstruction need not necessarily be in the cisternae; it may be in the large branches which carry the fluid from the cisternae chiasmatica and interpeduncularis to the cerebral sulci. Any number of these branches may be occluded. If all the main branches are obstructed, the hydrocephalus will be the same as if the occlusion were in the cisterna. If some of the branches remain unobstructed, the degree of hydrocephalus will be modified proportionately; a complete cure may even result because of the absorption which takes place in the remaining patent areas of the subarachnoid space.

(7) Adhesions, which follow meningitis and occlude the cisternae, cause the vast majority of cases of communicating hydrocephalus. They also cause many cases of obstructive hydrocephalus, by blocking the foramina of Luschka and Magendie. Adhesions give infallible proof of a preexisting meningitis. A history of meningitis may be easy, difficult or impossible to obtain. The post-meningitic occlusions have no relation to the severity of the attack and the number of adhesions but rather to the location of the adhesions

(8) In two cases the hydrocephalus appeared to be due to a congenital failure of the cisternae or of its branches to develop. Tumors in the pons, medulla, or mid-brain also produce partial or complete obstruction of the subarachnoid space and therefore cause communicating hydrocephalus.

(9) Pneumographic records are shown demonstrating the existence of a very early stage of communicating hydrocephalus, the cause of the hydrocephalus, the reason for its unusually tardy development, and for its spontaneous arrest.

REFERENCES

[1]Dandy, W. E., and Blackfan, K. D.: Internal Hydrocephalus—an Experimental, Clinical and Pathological Study. *J. A. M. A.*, lxi: 2216, 1913; *Am. J. Dis. Child.*, viii: 406, 1914.

[2]Dandy, W. E.: Experimental Hydrocephalus. *Ann. Surg.*, August, 1919, p. 129.

[3]Weed, L. H.: *The Experimental Production of an Internal Hydrocephalus.* Publication 272, Carnegie Institute of Washington, p. 425.

[4]Thomas, W. T.: Experimental Hydrocephalus. *J. Exper. Med.*, xix: 106, 1914.

[5]Dandy, W. E., and Blackfan, K. D.: Internal Hydrocephalus. Second paper. *Am. J. Dis. Child.*, xiv: 424, 1917.

[6]Dandy, W. E.: Roentgenography of the brain after the injection of air into the spinal canal. *Ann. Surg.*, October, 1919, p. 397.

[7]Dandy, W. E.: Ventriculography following the injection of air into the cerebral ventricles. *Ann. Surg.*, July, 1918, p. 5.

[8]Weed, L. H.: An Anatomical Consideration of the Cerebrospinal Fluid. *Anat. Rec.*, xii: 461, 1917.

[9]Weed, L. H. Cells of the Arachnoid. *Bull. Johns Hopkins Hosp.*, xxxi: 343, 1920.

[10]Dandy, W. E.: Localization or Elimination of Cerebral Tumors by Ventriculography. *Surg. Gynec. & Obst.*, April, 1920, p. 329.

[11]Dandy, W. E.: The Diagnosis and Treatment of Hydrocephalus resulting from the closure of the foramina of Luschka and Magendie. *Surg., Gynec. and Obst.*, February, 1921.

[13]A pneumoccus panophthalmitis also developed, necessitating removal of the eye, from which the meningococcus was grown in pure culture.

[14]A description of the remarkable anatomical changes in this case would only add confusion if presented here. They are therefore omitted and will appear in a subsequent publication dealing with other phases of hydrocephalus. My purpose

here is to correlate all the anatomical variations of communicating hydrocephalus into a single disease with a fundamentally similar pathology and etiology.

DESCRIPTION OF PLATES

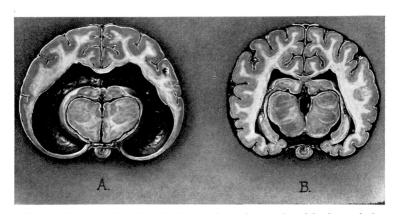

Fig. 1. Section of a dog's brain to show the grade of hydrocephalus which resulted from the perimensecephalic band of adhesions. On the right is a section of a normal brain as a control. The hydrocephalus is of three months' development.

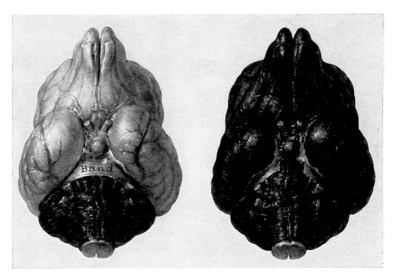

Fig. 2. Drawings by Max Brodel to give a graphic demonstration of the reason for the development of communicating hydrocephalus after the formation of the perimesecephalic adhesions. India ink had been substituted for cerebrospinal fluid in the spinal canal two hours before the animal was sacrificed. On the right is a control animal in which the same quantity of ink was injected at a similar time before death. In each case the ink has had the distribution which the cerebrospinal fluid would have. In the normal (right), the ink has thoroughly and evenly covered every part of the brain's surface because all of the cerebrospinal spaces receive the cerebrospinal fluid. In the experimental animal the ink has stopped sharply at the perimesencephalic band. None of the ink has been able to reach the cerebral hemispheres, although the cerebellum has been as well

covered as the normal. In Fig 7 it will be seen that in the normal brain the ink has not entered the lateral ventricles, whereas in the experimental animal the ventricles have filled with ink. Since the ventricles fill with ink, there can be no question that the injection is inadequate, for the ventricles are farther forward than the obstructing band.

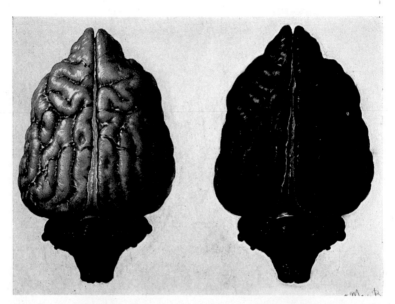

Fig. 3. Dorsal view of the same brains (as Figs. 1, 2) to show the distribution of the ink on this surface. It will be seen that the ink has not extended beyond the tentorium (owing to the perimesencephalic band), whereas in the normal the entire brain is covered. Hydrocephalus results from this band because the trunk of the subarachnoid tree is occluded and cerebrospinal fluid cannot reach the spaces over the cerebral hemispheres where most of the cerebrospinal fluid absorbs.

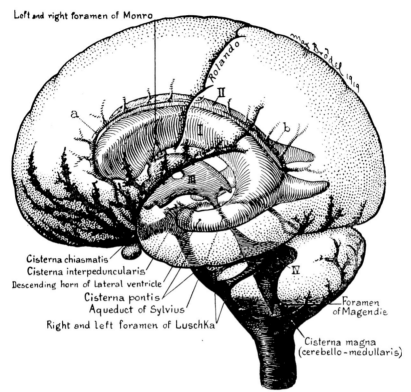

Fig. 4. Drawing by M. Brodel to show the general plan of the vascular system for cerebrospinal fluid. Fluid forms in the cerebral ventricles and is absorbed in the subarachnoid space. The paired foramina of Luschka and the median foramen of Magendie are the only openings by which the ventricular fluid can leave the ventricles and reach the subarachnoid space. Obstructions at these openings and the aqueduct of Sylvius or at the foramen of Monro produce hydrocephalus involving the ventricles anterior to the obstruction. Obstructions in the subarachnoid space are just as effective in producing hydrocephalus. The sites of these obstructions and their effects will be shown in the succeeding diagrams.

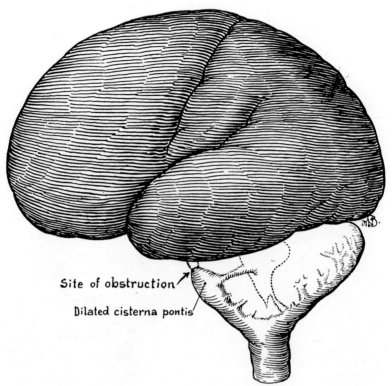

Fig. 5. Diagram to show the disturbance in the circulation of cerebrospinal fluid following an obstruction at the mesencephalic or
pontine cisterna. The black area represents the absorbing spaces,
which cannot be reached by the cerebrospinal fluid owing to the
obstruction. Hydrocephalus results because this vast area (where
three-quarters to four fifths of the cerebrospinal fluid is normally
absorbed) can no longer perform its function. The mesencephalic
and pontine cisternae are the usual sites for post-meningitic obstructions in communicating hydrocephalus.

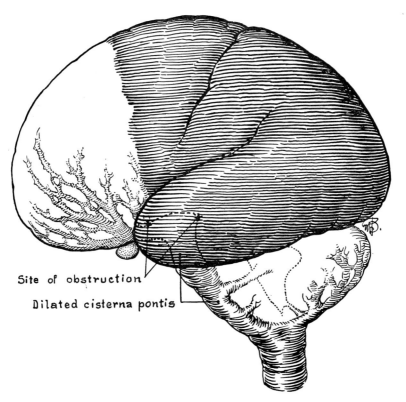

Fig. 6. Diagram showing the effect on the cerebrospinal fluid circulation when some, but not all, of the branches from the cisternae interpeduncularis and chiasmatica are occluded. The black area represents the subarachnoid space which does not receive cerebrospinal fluid. In the clear zone the circulation is intact.

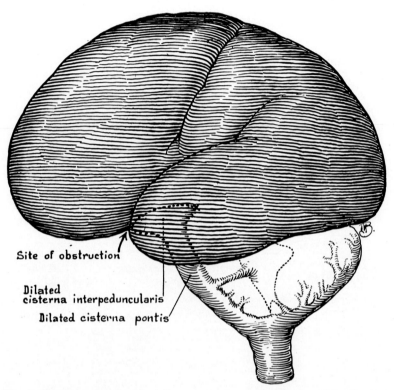

Site of obstruction

Dilated
cisterna interpeduncularis

Dilated cisterna pontis

Fig. 7. Diagram showing the effect upon the cerebral subarachnoid space when all the main branches, which carry the fluid from the cisternae interpeducularis and chiasmatica, are occluded. Exactly the same absorbing area is eliminated and the hydrocephalus which results in identically the same. In our cases of this type absence of these branches was regarded as probably due to a congenitally defective development of these spaces.

XIII

AN OPERATION FOR THE REMOVAL OF PINEAL TUMORS *

Tumors of the pineal body have rarely been diagnosed and substantiated. The total number of authenticated pineal tumors is less than one hundred and almost all have been accidental findings at necropsy. In most instances the clinical diagnosis of a pineal neoplasm has been made upon inadequate and fallacious observations and deductions and a totally different lesion has been found at necropsy. But it is now possible to make a correct diagnosis of this lesion; at times the exact diagnosis cannot be made but the lesion can be restricted to the mesencephalon with the pineal growth the highest probability. Naturally the absence of a correct localization of this lesion has precluded any operative interference with this region, and with the advent of accurate localization, the need of a practical surgical approach for the enucleation of pineal tumors is imperative. It is the purpose of this paper to introduce such an operative procedure. The diagnosis of tumors of the pineal body will be withheld for a subsequent communication.

Several years ago I evolved an operative procedure by which it was possible to remove the pineal body in dogs.[1] The operation as finally developed could be conducted without mortality and without any noticeable after-effect upon the well-being of the animal and resulted in no apparent mental or physical change. The operation which is presented here for patients suffering with pineal tumors is very similar to this canine operation.

The operation has been performed on three patients. In the first instance a silent

cerebellar tumor had secondarily involved the region of the pineal body and the corpora quadrigemina; after exposure of the tumor, no attempt was made to remove it, because of its infiltrating character. This case, however, showed that a good exposure of this region is possible. On two subsequent occasions, tumors of the pineal body have been completely removed. In one case an encapsulated tubercle of the pineal body was extirpated, the patient recovering only to die 8 months later, presumably of the effects of other tubercles of the brain, although as he was then at home no necropsy was obtained. After the removal of the tubercle, however, the signs by which his lesion was located quickly disappeared. The gross appearance of this growth at the time of operation suggested an endothelioma and it was only subsequently that the microscope revealed its true nature to be a tubercle. It was hard, nodular, and perfectly encapsulated; it measured 5 centimeters by 4 centimeters. The results of this case demonstrated not only the feasibility of the removal of tumors of the pineal body but also the absence (in this case at least) of any injurious mental or physical effects due to the operation.

The extirpation of the second pineal tumor was very much more difficult. The tumor was much larger and since the vena Galena magna and both small veins of Galen passed directly through the tumor and could not be dissected from it, the removal of practically all of these veins was a prerequisite to enucleation of the tumor. This tumor weighed 26 grams. It was very hard, fairly nodular, and perfectly encapsulated. It required a painstaking dissection to free the growth from the extensive

*Reprinted from *Surgery, Gynecology and Obstetrics,* August, 1921, pages 113-119.

117

vascular attachments, but it was finally readily lifted from its bed without any bleeding. The patient lived forty-eight hours, dying presumably of the shock due to the magnitude of the operation. His vitality was doubtless impaired by a cerebellar operation which was performed ten days previously and at which the tumor was found; but it was entirely inaccessible for removal by this approach. One can, of course, only wonder whether there might have been a different outcome had his full strength been retained. One must also consider whether the complete removal of all the main trunks of the intracranial venous system — the large vein of Galen and both small veins of Galen — would be compatible with life. I know of no previous instance in which these veins have been removed or even ligated. In dogs I have ligated the vena Galena magna without effect when the ligation is distally placed but when proximally placed a mild grade of hydrocephalus has resulted. In this case, however, at least 7 centimeters of this vascular trunk on either side were removed. Whether the collateral venous system in the human brain could be developed to compensate for this tremendous loss can only be surmised; it does seem doubtful, but there was no alternative to the removal of these veins with the tumor.

THE TREATMENT OF PINEAL TUMORS

Tumors of the pineal body can be helped by only one form of therapy, i.e., operative removal. Any treatment which is less than this can have no possible value. The symptoms which bring the patient to the physician are invariably those of intracranial pressure due to an internal hydrocephalus which is caused by occlusion of the aqueduct of Sylvius directly over which the tumor is situated. Other signs of local character follow the direct pressure of the tumor upon the corpora quadrigemina and upon the structures in the mesencephalon. There can be no relief of the hydrocephalus except by removal of the obstructing lesion.

No palliative benefits can possibly accrue from a decompression or from the too oft performed puncture of the corpus callosum. A decompression removes an area of bone which is nature's only protection against the tremendous intraventricular pressure and local cerebral injury must follow at the operative area and without any possible compensatory benefit to the afflicted individual. A callosal puncture admits of no relief because the fluid released absorbs with no greater rapidity in the subdural space, into which it passes, than in its former habitat in the ventricle; moreover, the opening remains patent only for a brief period, closing as all non-epithelialized cerebral wounds must do owing to the reparative processes of the neuroglia.

The operation, therefore, which I am about to propose is designed to remove the tumor directly. The accompany drawing and diagram by Mr. Broedel clearly show the various stages in the operation. The approach to the tumor is made possible by a very large parieto-occipital bone flap (Fig. 1), the mesial margin of which extends to the superior longitudinal sinus. The exposure of this sinus is frequently a relatively bloody procedure because of the venous lakes, which are usually both large

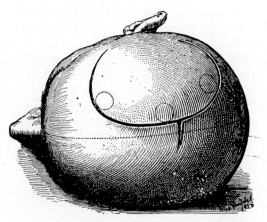

Fig. 1. The skin incision and the openings for the bone flap are outlined permitting a thorough exposure of the posterior two-thirds of the cerebral hemisphere. The incision extends almost to the mid-line and is made large enough to permit exposure of the posterior two-thirds of the cerebral hemisphere.

and numerous and the control of haemorr-hage must be quick and effective. If the bone flap does not extend to the mid-line a secondary defect must be rongeured away from the mesial margin of bone until the sinus is reached. The dura is then opened and reflected over the inferior longitudinal sinus. In doing so, the cerebral veins which bridge the subdural space between the brain and the logitudinal sinus are gradu-ally elevated, doubly ligated with fine silk ligatures, and divided. The number of these veins in the necessary field of opera-tion varies from one to six or even more. It is well if possible to avoid ligature of the Rolandic vein for a transient hemiple-gia will follow. Usually, however, it is necessary to ligate all the veins posterior to the Rolandic vein. It is hardly necessary to add that for this reason and because of possible speech disturbances, the cranio-tomy should be performed on the right side; and because tumors of the pineal body are always in a strictly central posi-tion, exposure of the growth is equally easy on either side. In the case in which

the tubercle was removed, the tumor was approached from the left side because a de-forming operation had been previously performed on the right. No speech distur-bances followed in this case, although there was a weakness of the right side for several days.

After division of the cerebral veins the entire half of the cerebral hemisphere can be retracted and the falx exposed. The inferior longitudinal sinus is quickly pass-ed and the corpus callosum brought into view as the brain is still further retracted (Fig. 2). This part of the operation is bloodless and is quickly and easily accom-plished. Until now there is no evidence of an underlying tumor. The posterior half of the corpus callosum is then care-fully incised in the mid-line (Fig. 3) for a distance of 3 or 4 centimeters and the hemi-spheres still further retracted. The tumor will then be brought into full view. Under the fornix of the corpus callosum the vena Galena magna will always be brought into full view at its entrance into the sinus rectus (Fig. 4). In one of the cases here

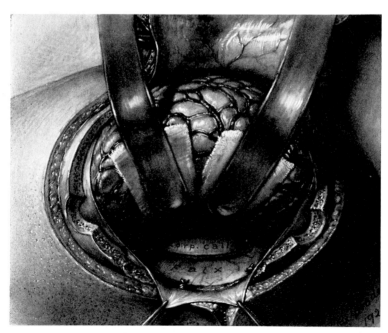

Fig. 2. The cerebral hemisphere is retracted exposing the corpus callosum and the falx. Note the ligated stumps of the cerebral veins as they enter the superior longitudinal sinus.

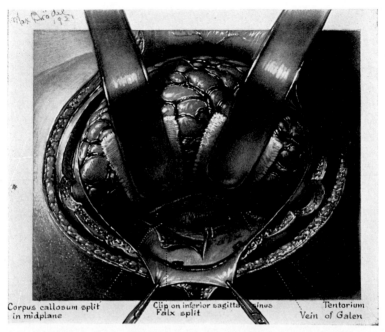

Fig. 3. The corpus callosum has been divided longitudinally exposing the tumor of the pineal body and the entire length of the vena
Galena magna and the terminus of each small vein of Galen. Note
the divided falx and inferior longitudinal sinus.

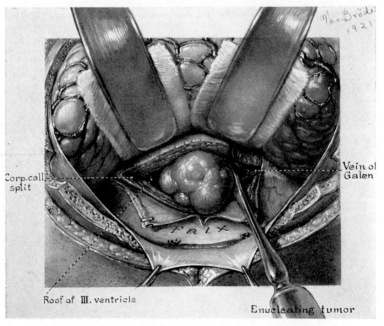

Fig. 4. Demonstrates the enucleation of the encapsulated pineal tumor. This particular growth was a tubercle of the pineal.

reported, the tumor lay anterior to the large vein of Galen and between it and the corpus callosum. In the other case about one-half centimeter of the great vein of Galen was free between the upper margin of the tumor and the beginning of the sinus rectus, an amount sufficient to permit double ligation and division of the vein between the ligatures. In the first case the tumor tubercle stripped readily from the vein (Fig. 4), and no bleeding resulted from the dissection. After the tumor was extirpated the great vein of Galen was seen as a tortuous trunk which when straightened would probably measure 4 centimeters in length; the third ventricle was not opened during the enucleation of the tumor. The bed from which the tumor was removed was the roof of the third ventricle and its appearance was exactly like the photographs seen in text books showing the small vein of Galen on either side of the mid-line running a straight longitudinal course of probably 5 centimeters before they were again lost in the substance of the brain (Fig. 5).

In the second case the tumor was so large that an adequate exposure was obtained only by dividing the falx cerebri (and with it, of course, the inferior longitudinal sinus). It was then possible to retract the brain to both sides. Each small vein of Galen was carefully dissected where it crossed from the tumor to the brain and divided between silk ligatures. Several small tributaries of these veins were separately tied and divided as they emerged from the tumor. No dissection was made blindly; the tumor (Fig. 6) was gradually enucleated with ease. During the removal of this tumor the third ventricle was opened and the tumor extended so deeply that the operator's finger reached the posterior clinoid process of the sella turcica. It will

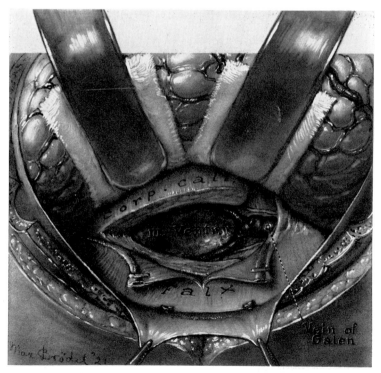

Fig. 5. After removal of the tumor the roof of the third ventricle in this case remained intact and the large vein and the two small veins of Galen are brought into view. The large vein is quote tortous; the two small veins unduly separated by the growth between them.

be evident from the ability to tie ligatures at this great depth (Fig. 8, frontispiece) and from the deep dissection of tumor which lay immediately over posterior clinoid process that operative exposure is probably sufficient. A great deal of this room is afforded by the release of fluid from the lateral ventricle by a puncture early

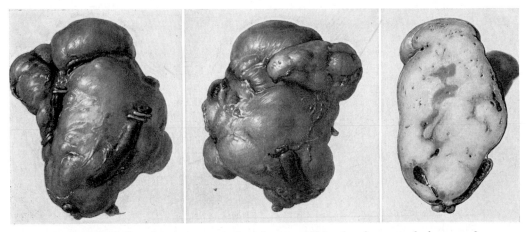

Fig. 6. Drawings of the pineal tumor, reduced one-twelfth, showing actual shape and appearance on section. Note the veins of Galen clinging to the tumor.

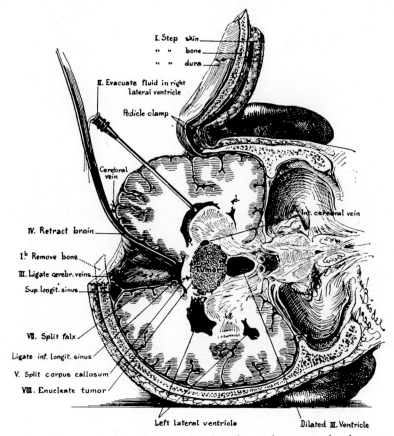

Fig. 7. Diagram by Mr. Broedel showing the various steps in the operation. The labeling adequately tells the operative story.

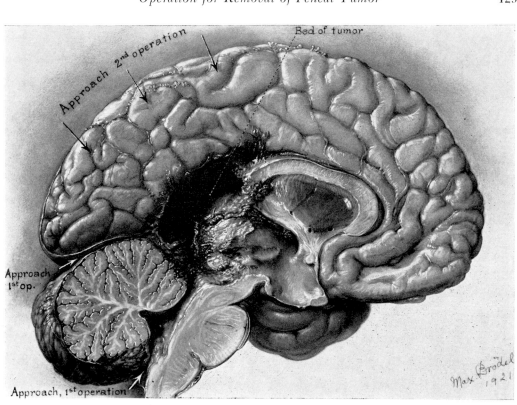

Fig. 8. Drawing of mid-sagittal view of brain from which a pineal tumor was removed. The bed from which the tumor was removed shows its location and relative size. The tumor was exposed first by following up the fourth ventricle. It was then exposed by an approach over the cerebellum and under the tentorium but the removal was seen to be possible only by operative precedure just described.

in the operation. The hydrocephalus while so destructive of brain tissue has its compensating benefits in the amount of fluid which can be released thus allowing the reduced bulk of brain to be easily retracted from the operative field. Were it not for the release of fluid not only would the exposure of the tumor be very difficult but the necessary retraction of the brain would be very injurious to the cerebral hemisphere.

REFERENCE

[1]Extirpation of the pineal body. *J. Exper. Med.,* *xxii:* 237, 1915.

XIV

PRECHIASMAL INTRACRANIAL TUMORS OF THE OPTIC NERVES *

This paper gives a general discussion of prechiasmal tumors of the optic nerve; and reports two cases with the pathologic findings, and the conclusions drawn from the author's experience. The detection of this lesion is the direct outcome of an address delivered before the Hartford (Conn.) Academy of Medicine, on the diagnosis and localization of brain tumors. Dr. F. L. Waite and Dr. E. Terry Smith, who had been attending these patients, then suggested the possibility of an intracranial tumor, from the Department of Surgery of the Johns Hopkins Hospital and University.

The two cases which form the basis of this paper are presented because I believe they represent a type of lesion which may be responsible for many cases of unexplained blindness, and because with proper treatment of the cause, the vision may be more or less completely restored. The lesion in question is an intracranial tumor involving the prechiasmal segment of the optic nerves in the neighborhood of the optic foramina. Postmortem records establish a group of cases fundamentally similar, but I have found no record of the clinical diagnosis of such a lesion and none, therefore, in which such a tumor has been treated surgically. There is a very definite and important pathologic relationship between these tumors and those of the intraorbital division of the optic nerve. This relationship, long obscured by the paucity of postmortem examinations and the proper correlation of those which have been made, now becomes of the greatest practical concern in all tumors involving the optic nerve, for not only does the eyesight but quite frequently the life of the patient depend upon a correct diagnosis and adequate surgical treatment.

The diagnosis of a prechiasmal tumor of the optic nerve is at present none too sharp and at best there is an element of uncertainty, but the early stage at which the diagnosis of these first cases has been made, encourages the hope that the history and the signs, altho few, may be sufficiently definite to lead to the recognition of the lesion with greater precision, and before the advent of those late and hopeless manifestations which indicate the spread of the tumor either into the orbital cavity or into the brain. In the two cases which are presented here, the tumors were so small and so precisely confined to the optic nerve, that the location of the growth was not betrayed by any signs of intracranial pressure or by involvement of the optic chiasm thru extension of the growth posteriorly, or by exophthalmos from its extension anteriorly. In one case, the clinical picture was that of gradual blindness, and nothing else; not even was there a suggestion, either by signs or symptoms, that an intracranial lesion was present: in the other, there were superimposed features which conformed to no recognized lesion but which, in general, indicated an intracranial disturbance. In one case, the vision returned from blindness to normal in less than two weeks after the operation; in the other, there was considerable return of sight after a partial removal of the tumor.

The presentation of a definite pathology for a group of cases of blindness of obscure origin, is particularly pertinent at this time when the literature is surfeited with articles on "optic neuritis." It is not to be inferred from this statement that I look

*Reprinted from the *American Journal of Opthalmology,* 5: 3, March, 1922.

upon optic neuritis as the false conception which has been claimed in rather heated discussion by very able authorities. The existence of this clinical entity is undoubted. It is backed by evidence too conclusive. I have had several instances in which the optic neuritis has been substantiated by pathological proof. However, as is true in all new discoveries, it is most unfortunate that such extravagant claims are made upon very hasty and fallacious observations and accompanied by no objective demonstration of pathology — opinions, on the whole, dominated by an over zealous personal equation. Eventually, of course, optic neuritis will settle down to a concrete clinical entity with a well defined pathologic basis, but until then patients innumerable are doomed to useless, dangerous, even fatal rhinologic operations, and many are sidetracked from the detection of the real cause of their ailment until the lesion has grown beyond the pale of operative assistance. As long as optic neuritis remains a diagnosis of exclusion, as it is so largely at the present time, this exclusion demands the collaboration of experts who are thoroughly competent to exclude. Intracranial tumors have too frequently been missed by over zealous enthusiasts searching for optic neuritis. Over eager neurologic surgeons, also, are by no means blameless, for too many cases of optic neuritis have been subjected to needless cranial surgery, under the impression that a brain tumor existed. But on both sides the fault lies with the individual. Our means of diagnosis, tho still far from what they should be, are nevertheless adequate to eliminate all but the exceptional cases from these errors.

The differentiation between a mechanical swelling of the optic disc — "choked disc" — and an inflammatory swelling of the disc — optic neuritis — is only too frequently impossible by ophthalmologic examination. But what information is lacking with the ophthalmoscope, can usually be compensated by a careful history and by other examinations. At times, of course, the differentiation between an optic neuritis and a brain tumor may not be easy, but it should always be possible and without risk to the patient. Speaking from the standpoint of a neurological surgeon, I can say that any brain tumor which can cause a choked disc can be accurately diagnosed and precisely localized; and conversely, it can be told with equal accuracy when a tumor is not present.[1] And, I believe, infections of the nasal sinuses can also be detected or eliminated with a high degree of accuracy without resorting to rather blind exploratory operations on the paranasal sinuses. There is, therefore, little excuse in confusing these lesions. The mistakes are made by those who are not thoroughly competent to pass upon intracranial or rhinologic conditions. The differential diagnosis between a prechiasmal tumor and an optic neuritis will be considered later.

CASES

The history and operative findings on the two tumors of intracranial portion of the optic nerve are as follows:

Case 1. Mary C., referred by Dr. F. L. Waite of Hartford, Conn., is a very bright and physically normal girl of 13. When seven years old, or six years before admission to the Johns Hopkins Hospital, she had a spell of vomiting lasting a week. There was no associated abdominal pain or other disturbance which should accompany an acute abdominal ailment; but during this period of vomiting, diplopia developed and the left eye turned distinctly outward, demonstrating the intracranial origin of the vomiting. There was no headache associated with the attack. Within a week the crossed eye had returned to normal. About this time, dimness of vision first appeared in the right eye. There was no pain or aching in the eyeball and none referred elsewhere. Little further change developed until three years ago, when, during a mild attack of influenza, another vomiting spell persisted for several days and again the right eye became crossed. The vision was then so much impaired that she had to quit school. The crossed eye gradually returned to normal. During the past three years, there have been three additional attacks of vomiting, each lasting nearly a week, and at each time *both* eyes were crossed. Coincident with the strabismus there has been drooping of the upper eyelids—apparently bilateral. Altho some improvement in the strabismus has been noted following the subsidence of the vomiting, a more or less permanent weakness of the eye muscles has persisted and varied in intensity from time to time. During the past three attacks, there has been a little aching in the eyes, but this subsided with the disappearance of the vomiting. Exophthaloms has never been noticed in either eye.

The loss of vision has been very gradu-ally progressive in both eyes, but more in the right. Dr. Waite's careful notes show that she was blind in the right eye at least three years ago—at which time she first consulted him. At that time (1918) the vision in the left eye was 20/60; failing gradually, it was 10/200 in March, 1920, and 8/200 in June, 1920, and was the same on admission to the Johns Hopkins Hospital (April, 1921). *Patient has never had a headache in her life* and, except for the loss of vision, would be "in fine shape." From the physical, neurologic and special examination, the following positive and

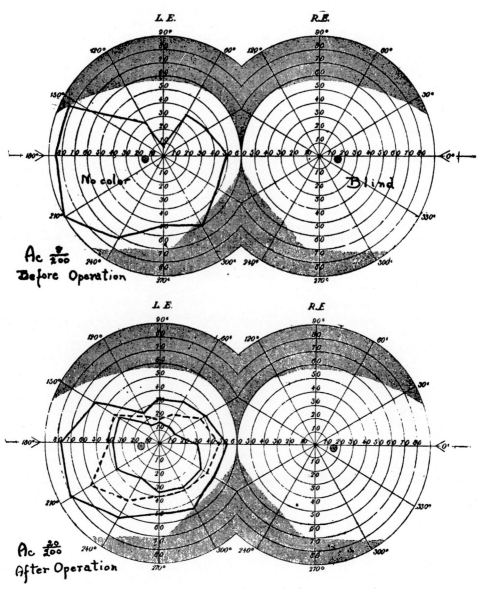

Fig. 1 Visual fields of patients before and after removal of tumor.

negative items are summarized:

1) The right eye is totally blind.

2) The visual field for form was preserved in the left eye, but was somewhat contracted; visual acuity—8/200; complete loss of color perception; no hemianopsia (Fig. 1).

3) Both optic discs have a brilliant atrophic pallor; the margins are sharply defined; the lamina cribrosa are very distinct; there is no choked disc and no change in the size or shape of the retinal vessels.

4) The right eye moves outward, inward and slightly downward, but not upward. The left eye moves laterally, slightly downward, not medially or upward. There is a slight but definite ptosis of both upper lids. Both pupils react fairly actively to light, directly and consensually.

5) There was an unusually large calcified shadow of the pineal body (roentgenogram).

6) The sella turcica is slightly but distinctly enlarged; it is rather cone shaped with the base of the cone upward.

7) The size and position of the lateral ventricles were normal (pneumoventriculography).

8) The examination of the cerebrospinal fluid was negative. The Wassermann reaction from both the blood and cerebrospinal fluid was negative.

9) The paranasal sinuses were entirely negative.

Reasoning Toward a Diagnosis

Despite the absence of headache, there was reasonable certainty in the diagnosis of an intracranial lesion, because of the transient bilateral extraocular palsies which always accompanied the spells of periodic vomiting. The fleeting character of the ocular changes indicated a lesion which varied in size. An intracranial lesion giving such variable signs is most likely a cyst or some abnormal collection of cerebrospinal fluid. The progressive blindness extending over such a long period of time seemed to indicate a tumor. But where could there be a tumor which would produce bilateral palsies of all the extraocular muscles and at the same time a bilateral loss of vision approaching blindness and at the same time without hemianopsia? The large extraordinary shadow in the pineal region was suggestive of a tumor of the pineal body, especially since a growth in this region would readily explain the bilateral changes in the eye muscles, and it could also explain the transient character of these disturbances. But a pineal tumor would cause blindness only if a hydrocephalus existed, for all pineal tumors produce symptoms of intracranial pressure only thru the secondary effects of hydrocephalus, which results from occlusion of the subjacent aqueduct of Sylvius. A choked disc and changes in the vessels of the retina would be expected, tho not necessarily demanded, of a pineal tumor which produced hydrocephalus; but a hydrocephalus was positively excluded by cerebral pneumography—the lateral ventricles being entirely normal. If there was a pineal tumor, it certainly was not causing blindness and, for the same reasons, it was not causing the ptosis, for the nuclei of the third, fourth and sixth cranial nerves could be reached only after the aqueduct of Sylvius had first been compressed.

Could all the findings be explained by a tumor elsewhere? In only one other location could a growth give bilateral ptosis and extraocular palsies at the same time, i. e., in the region of the sphenoidal fissure, thru which the third, fourth and sixth nerves pass into the orbit. But a tumor in this region must be very wide to involve these nerves on *both* sides, so large in fact that intracranial pressure would certainly have existed. Moreover, the olfactory nerves should have been affected, but they were not. Such an hypothetically located tumor also made it difficult to explain the vision which was still present, for the optic nerves necessarily would have been in the center of a very large tumor mass. Moreover, the size of the sella was only slightly greater than normal; the posterior clinoid processes were not destroyed, so that the existence of a tumor of any size in this region was almost precluded; and if a pituitary tumor should be present (almost an impossibility) why no evidences of heminaopsia?

The presence of a primary optic atrophy could not be questioned, therefore, a tumor must be located somewhere along the optic nerves, and presumably between the optic foramina and the chiasm. Any form of toxic neuritis advancing so slowly and so progressively, seemed inconceivable; moreover, the paranasal sinuses were normal.

At operation, two entirely independent tumors were found (Fig. 6), one completely surrounding each optic nerve

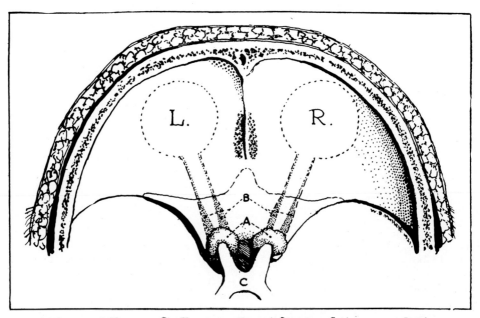

A - Exposed Tumor - B - Tumor on Dural Sheath of Nerve in Orbit,
C - Optic Chiasma

Fig 2. Diagram showing the position and size of the tumors of the optic nerve. Tumors are symmetric collar like growths surrounding each optic nerve at the optic foramen and passing forward into the orbit.

at the optic foramen. The growths were small, almost perfectly symmetric, collar like growths. They were pale grayish pink, not unlike granulation tissue; the periphery of the growth was rather fluffy, much like seaweed, but toward the nerve it became quite firm. The entire diameter of each tumor including the optic nerve was about 1.5 cm.; posteriorly it extended along the nerve about 0.75 cm. and was very loosely attached except at the point where the dura is reflected. The tumor also grew thru the optic foramen into the orbit for a distance of about 1.5 cm., but it extended only as a linear strand in the orbit and did not surround the nerve. Here also it was merely adjacent to and not adherent to the nerve. The optic foramen did not seem enlarged. The intraorbital course and extent of the tumor on the left nerve could not be followed, for the orbital roof was not opened, but the intracranial appearance of the two tumors was practically identical. The tumor on each nerve arose from the dural sheath and in its slow fibrous growth had gradually constricted and strangled the optic nerve. The growths

were not perfectly circular. Each budded externally as a small nubbin, and possibly may have abutted on the structures which passed thru the sphenoidal fissure, but this lateral extension was so tiny that such a nerve involvement was neither visible nor scarcely conceivable. The finding to which I am more inclined to attribute extraocular palsies is the big collection of fluid surrounding the tumor—undoubtedly a compensatory product which formed to protect the brain from this intrusive foreign mass. Nature has a well known method of surrounding the surface of many tumors with a bed of fluid which acts as a buffer between the neoplasm and the brain. All cerebello-pontine tumors are so covered. The principal reason for the belief that the pocket of fluid was responsible for the strabismus is that it was certainly responsible for the transient attacks which dated back several years, lasted only a few days and were always associated with vomiting. Palsies following the direct growth of the tumors would have persisted and increased and the growth was too gradual, and even in its final size too small, to have produced either the sudden transient disturbance or the permanent weakness of these muscles. The solid tumors were also far too small to produce vomiting or any signs of intracranial pressure. This collection of fluid was really an extension of the cisterna chiamatis. Another striking feature was the length of the optic nerves, a finding which one sees in all pituitary tumors when the chiasm has been lifted up and pushed backward, stretching the optic nerves as they grew; and in this particular instance the elongation of the optic nerves was possible only from the pocket of fluid, for the tumors extended less than half way between the optic foramina and the optic chiasm. After the release of this big collection of fluid, the entire sella turcica and the suprasellar region could be readily inspected without traction on the optic nerves. This inspection is not easy unless the optic nerves have been stretched and unless the cisterna chiasmatis is greatly enlarged. Doubtless, the slightly enlarged sella turcica was the result of the long continued pressure of the abnormally large cisterna chiasmatis.

The gross appearance of the tumor at once suggested the typical dural endothelioma which we see so frequently arising from the dura and pushing the brain before it. The difference was only in size. Whereas the optic nerve tumors were tiny structures, the dural endotheliomata of the brain are frequently as large as one's fist. Histologically, the tumors from both the right and left nerve were identical and were exactly like the dural endotheliomata of the brain, with the additional features of a psammoma. The body of the tumors was made up of fibrous tissue, arranged in whorls, strands and columns. The fibrous tissue could easily be mistaken for that of a spindle celled sarcoma. In the connective tissue were nests of the characteristic whorl like onion bodies— deeply red staining hyalin, lamellated crescents.

The tumor surrounding the right optic nerve was totally removed. It was necessary to strip the dura from the optic nerve, it being an integral part of the tumor. The tumor had, also, grown forward into the orbit for a distance of $1\frac{1}{2}$ cm. The removal of this part of the growth necessitated the resection of part of the superior wall of the orbit. The left nerve being so far distant from the operative field (a right sided craniotomy having been performed), only a partial removal of its tumor was possible. This removal, nevertheless, restored the vision of the left eye to 20/200 within two weeks after the operation, color fields returning also and being practically normal. Vision in the right eye, however, has not yet improved. The vision in this eye is known to have been totally absent for over three years, and this probably was of much longer duration. Whether vision so long lost can return, I am not prepared to say.

Case 2. The second patient was a normal appearing boy of eight years, referred by Dr. E. Terry Smith of Hartford, Conn. One year before admission to the hospital, his teacher noticed that his vision was not good. An immediate examition by an oculist disclosed almost complete blindness of the right eye and a marked diminution in the vision of the left. According to his father, there have been vascillations in the vision, but on the whole it has decreased, tho very slowly. When a year old, a fork's prong is said to have pierced the right eyeball. The history about this point is rather vague, and it was not certain whether the eye had been blind since that time. His father thinks, however, his eyes had been examined subsequent to that accident and nothing found abnormal. On admission to the Johns Hopkins Hospital, there was only slight vision in the right eye and a little more in the left. No definite evidence of hemianopsia. Color is not perceived in the right and only slightly in the left eye. Visual acuity is 20/200 in left eye; fingers are seen at a distance of two inches with the right eye (Fig. 3). Dr. Smith first saw this patient 4 months ago and at that time the vision in the left eye was 20/100, and practically nil in the right. Aside from a slight pallor of both optic disc, the neurologic examinations were entirely negative. The paranasal sinuses had been repeatedly examined with entirely negative results. The skiagram of the head showed nothing abnormal. The verebrospinal fluid was normal and the Wassermann reaction was negative both from the blood and cerebrospinalfluid. He had never had headache or vomiting. There were no extraocular palsies, and he has never had diplopia. In other words, aside from a very slowly developing blindness, there was no subjective or objective evidence of an intracranial affection. In view of the negative findings and solely by exclusion, I was inclined to

assume the diagnosis of optic neuritis of
some indeterminable toxic origin. The
striking resemblance to the preceding case,
however, forced the possible diagnosis of
a prechiasmal tumor and, bearing this in
mind, the patient was advised to return
home for further observation of his vision. During the succeeding two months,
three examinations were made by Dr.
Smith and in each there was a decided
reduction in vision over the preceding test.

In the right eye, he had become totally
blind; and with the left he could only
distinguish a bright light; he could no
longer count fingers. He then returned
for an exploration of the chiasmal region
by an intracranial operation.

A right craniotomy extending well forward over the frontal region was performed. The right optic nerve was normal as
far as one could judge. There was a small
circumscribed tumor about the size of a

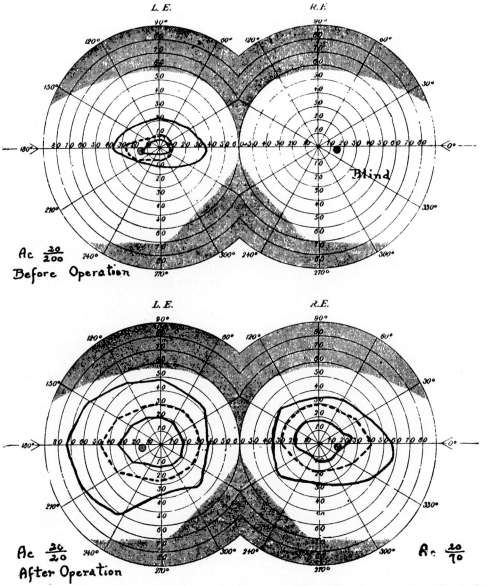

Fig. 3. Visual fields of patient before and after operation. The preoperative visual field
was taken two months before operation. At the time of the operation this remaining vision
was lost and patient was then blind in both eyes.

cherry beneath the *left* optic nerve, and by pushing it upward causing the nerve to arch sharply. A thin band of fibrous tissue over the optic foramen and the anterior clinoid process held the optic nerve tightly against the tumor and produced a distinct constriction of the nerve. A marked pallor of this nerve gave a striking contrast to the normally pink color of the right side. This band being incised, the nerve was at once released from the clutches of the tumor. The operative exposure had been made from the right side of the head because of the prior and greater visual loss on the right; the tumor was, therefore, too far distant to permit of its removal with safety. Fearing bleeding, because of its apparent vascularity and inaccessible position, I did not even dare remove a piece for diagnosis. The exact nature of the tumor could, therefore, not be determined, and as the major part of the tumor was hidden from view by the optic nerve, its point of origin could not be accurately determined. I feel, however, that it probably arose from the dural sheath at the optic foramen. The tumor did not seem to enter the optic foramen; it was not a small extension of a larger growth; the exposure at operation was adequate to determine this point with certainty; it seemed most likely an endothelioma. The incision of the band produced all the relief which could be obtained with safety; subsequently the tumor can be easily removed by an operation directed from the left side of the head.

An amazing restoration of vision (see charts) followed the simple division of the binding band over the left nerve (Fig. 3). The visual loss was, therefore, due to a physiologic block of the nerve; apparently there was little if any destruction. I have yet been unable to understand the loss of vision in the right eye since it was not directly affected by the tumor; equally puzzling is the rapid restoration of vision in this eye. It can, of course, be explained only on a sympathetic basis. The visual acuity within two weeks after the operation had returned to 20/20 in the left and 20/70 in the right. Almost a normal field of vision including color returned in each eye. A letter received from his father as this paper is being written (six months after the operation) says his vision continues to improve and he is now attending school.

PATHOLOGIC ASPECTS OF PRECHIASMAL TUMORS

The tumors which are here reported are representative of a well known tho not extensive group of endotheliomata or psammomata. They arise from the dural sheath of the optic nerve and heretofore have been described only for the intraorbital part of the nerve. This particular tumor is unusual in that it is bilateral, is perfectly symmetric and so small after at least six and probably many more years' growth. These cases are, so far as I can determine, the only reported instances of intracranial optic nerve tumors which have been diagnosed clinically and found at operation.* There is no reason to believe that intracranial optic nerve tumors should be different from those of the intraorbital part, except that within the skull the optic nerve is devoid of the dural sheath. All *intracranial* tumors of the optic nerve arising from the dura must therefore arise at the optic foramen, where the dura is reflected, and secondarily project into the cranial cavity. The three tumors here described arose at just that point.

Intraorbital optic nerve tumors have been thoroly collected and reported from time to time. Willemer[2] (1879) collected from the literature probably the first series of twenty-seven cases; Jocqs[3] (1887) found sixty-two cases; Braunschweig[4] (1893) ninety-four cases; Finlay[5] (1895) one hundred and seventeen; Byers[6] (1901) one hundred and eighteen and Hudson[7] (1912) one hundred and fifty-four cases which together with an appended list of twenty-eight cases brought the total to one hundred and eighty-two. There is little to be added to the excellent contributions of Byers and

---

*Since this paper was sent to the press, I have found a very similar case recorded from a necropsy by Schott (*Arch. f. Opth., vi:* 276). A small circumscribed tumor (5x5 m. m.) was found on each optic nerve in the region of the optic foramen. Each tumor was a pasammommoma, containing many onion like formations. Their presence was not suspected during life. The patient was fifty-five years old and blind.

of Hudson. In each the literature is well covered and all the available histologic data, usually obscured in the chaos of a changing pathology, has been carefully scrutinized in order to bring them into a harmonious grouping. While these tumors may assume various histologic appearances, they may all be run down to the usual connective tissue derivatives with protean expression. Hudson has added an abstract of each of his 182 cases. Byers has considered principally the intradural tumors of which there are 102, and has appended sixteen cases of extradural tumor. Parsons[8] (1902) collected eighteen cases of dural (extradural) tumor. Hudson has assembled the cases into three groups: (1) those arising from the connective tissue of the nerve — intradural — (he uses the term gliomatosis) (one hundred and eighteen cases) ; (2) those due to fibromatosis of the nerve sheath (six cases) ; and (3) endothelial tumors arising from the dura and analogous to endothelial tumors of the membranes of the brain; many of these tumors contain the psammoma bodies. The still simpler classification of Byers — intradural and dural tumors — subordinates all the histologic features of these growths.

From the standpoint of practical treatment, much can be learned from the clinical tables of the cases collected by Byers and Hudson, and I have drawn upon them freely. Probably the most important feature of all is the high percentage of intraorbital tumors which have also an intracranial extension of the growth. Apparently this applies about equally to the intradural and dural tumors. In most of the cases there is direct continuity between the intraorbital and intracranial parts of the tumor. The narrow optic foramen, which is usually but not necessarily enlarged from the effects of the tumor, gives the growth an irregular dumbbell appearance. In some cases, the intraorbital part of the tumor may be larger than the intracranial and the reverse may be true. In a few instances, there have been multiple discrete tumors involving each nerve or both nerves, and

occasionally even the optic chiasm is included. In a few instances the tumor has grown backward along the base of the brain as far as the pons and medulla. At other times, it has grown upward into the brain and may even have pierced the 3rd or one of the lateral ventricles. The intracranial involvement in intraorbital optic nerve tumors was emphasized by both Byers and Hudson, but at the time of their publications there seemed little that could be done to cure a patient when the tumor had passed thru the optic foramen into the interior of the skull.

The exact proportion of intraorbital tumors which grew into the cranial chamber can, of course, not be estimated with any degree of accuracy from the cases collected from the literature. The clinical diagnosis of brain tumors has been too unsatisfactory to give any accurate data, for tumors of the brain may grow to a tremendous size before they will be suspected. Many of these tumors have developed very slowly. A case reported by Byers, died of the intracranial growth ten years after the orbital tumor had been removed, and one by Pagenstecher and Steffan[9] died twenty-five years after the removal of the tumor of the orbit. Frequently, the intracranial extension of the tumor has been known by the fact that tumor tissue has been cut thru when the orbital tumor has been removed, making of course an incomplete removal of the neoplasm; but this operative report has often been lacking, and often pathognomonic symptoms of the late phases of the intracranial growth or the postmortem proof has given the inadequate information at hand. From one hundred and two cases of intradural tumor in Byers' series, at least twenty-three gave indisputable evidence of an intracranial involvement; and from Hudson's series of one hundred and eighty-two cases, seventeen additional cases have been found i. e., cases which have not been included in Byer's series. From one hundred ninety-one cases of both series (cases not duplicated) there are, therefore, forty cases (21%) in which the intracranial involvement is certain. The actual percentage is, of course, very much higher, for the ultimate results of most cases cannot be obtained, either because the patients cannot be obtained. On the other hand, Byers states that from his one hundred and twelve cases "only eight are known positively by record to have continued in a good state of health beyond five years."

An analysis of Hudson's tables, from the viewpoint of the operative findings, strikingly shows the great proportion of cases in which orbital tumors are complicated by an intracranial extension of the growth. The reports from the operators who have removed the orbital tumor show, that in at least fifty-one out of one hundred and eighteen intradural tumors the tumor removal was probably incomplete (43%); and from thirty-four dural tumors, thirteen (or 39%) were probably incompletely removed. Sixty-four of the total number of one hundred and fifty-two cases were therefore only partially removed (42%). As many cases which were not completely removed would never be so reported, the actual percentage of orbital tumors having intracranial extension would be much higher.

Even more astounding and impressive is the analysis of all the reported necropsies in the entire series of cases reported by Byers and by Hudson. Of twenty-three postmortem examinations which were obtained in cases of intraorbital optic nerve tumors, twenty-one showed an intracranial growth and in only one instance did the cranial cavity contain no tumor. Fourteen of these autopsies were obtained on patients who died of meningitis within a few days after the orbital tumor had been removed; the intracranial tumor, therefore, was present when the orbital growth was treated; three necropsies were obtained when the patient subsequently died of intracranial pressure; and in five necropsies the tumors were found in patients who died of an intercurrent disease; in two of these, the tumor of the optic nerves was an unexpected finding, tho the patients had been blind.

Apparently both dural and intradural tumors of the optic nerve give intracranial involvement in about equal proportion. From one hundred and eighteen cases of intradural tumors in Hudson's list, twenty were definitely known to have had intracranial tumors (17%), and seven of thirty-four dural tumors had tumors in the cranial cavity (20%). The actual percentage in each variety is, of course, very much higher.

The most striking clinical difference between the intradural and dural tumors within the orbit, and doubtless the same is true of those within the cranium, is the average age of onset and the rate of the tumor's growth. Again we refer to the excellent tables of Byers and Hudson, both of which are so complete in every detail. Among the intradural tumors, 62% develop the symptoms of onset in the first decade of life and 90% before the twentieth year. The dural tumors, however, are distributed fairly evenly according to decades, slightly more than half being accounted for after the 30th year of life. The dural tumors on the whole grow very much more slowly than the intradural tumors, tho exceptions to this rule occur in both varieties of tumor.

THE DIAGNOSIS OF PRECHIASMAL TUMORS

While *intraorbital* tumors of the optic nerve are early betrayed by exophthalmos, the interposed optic foramen precludes this pathognomonic clinical information in *prechiasmal* optic nerve tumors, at least until the orbit has been secondarily invaded. The pure prechiasmal tumors, such as those entered in this paper, that is tumors affecting only the intracranial part of the optic nerve, will probably give only a progressive loss of vision in one or both eyes. In the early stages of the tumor's growth, the mass is too small to produce any signs of intracranial pressure, and when these do appear, it can be fairly certain that the tumor has become very large and will almost certainly have completely blinded the patient. In each of these cases, there has been a *primary* optic atrophy, with a pale bluish white glistening disc and no changes in the size or shape of the veins or arteries in the fundus. In many of the orbital tumors, swelling of the disc (optic neuritis) has been reported. The cause of this swelling is not exactly clear, but it has been reported so frequently that it has been regarded as authentic. Whether a similar ophthalmologic picture could be obtained in prechiasmal tumors, must be left open. However, in a large series of intracranial tumors producing a primary optic atrophy from direct pressure on the visual tracts, I have never seen a choked disc until the tumor had grown large enough to have produced marked intracranial pressure. In fact, the ophthalmologic examination is often sufficient evidence to make the diagnosis of a brain tumor compressing the optic nerves directly. One must, of course, think of the probability of intraorbital pressure producing a choked disc just as does intracranial pressure. Both the orbit and cranium are closed chambers with inadequate vent for any unusual or rapidly increased pressure.

The skiagram of the head should show no abnormality in the earlier stages of growth of these tumors; there should be no discernible change in the anterior or posterior clinoid processes. There may be changes in the visual fields such as an atypical nasal or temporal hemianopsia on the affected side; this would not be unexpected, but there is no definite evidence of it in the scant examinations afforded by these cases. The differential diagnosis between some form of optic neuritis and a prechiasmal tumor lies principally in the character and rapidity of the visual loss and the character of the eye grounds. A typical optic neuritis gives a more rapid, even at times fulminating, history of visual loss, and is usually accompanied by marked changes in the eyegrounds (neuroretinitis). There are the added but variable manifestations of optic neuritis — central scotoma and enlarged blind spot. Prechiasmal tumors will produce a very gradually progressive loss of vision, the time depending, of course, on the character of the tumor and (this may not be absolute) the fundus should show the characteristics of a primary optic atrophy. There has been nothing in the history of these two cases to suggest a central scotoma. There are, of course, instances of so-called toxic neuritis, in which a known or possibly even an unknown toxin will produce blindness, and the disc will not be unlike that of the primary optic atrophy due to pressure of a tumor on the nerve. There is frequently a central scotoma or enlargement of the blind spot in these forms and also the affection is apt to be bilateral. Unless one has a very definite history of a specific toxin, the diagnosis of toxic neuritis must be one of last resort, and one solely of exclusion of all other possible factors. Intracranial tumors other than those which are of primary origin in the optic nerve, can give a similar clinical picture, and when small and implicating the optic nerve directly, there is no way of making a differential diagnosis. The indicated therapeutic measures, however, would be identical, so that this refinement of diagnosis is not essential. By far the most frequent tumor in this region is the pituitary tumor, which typically, but by no means always, produces a hemianopsia of the bitemporal type; it moreover nearly always shows in the skiagram the characteristic destruction of the sella turcica. There are extremely few pituitary tumors which have been diagnosed without one or the other and usually both of these two objective findings: (1) destruction of the landmarks of the sella turcica, (2) hemianopsia, usually bitemporal, occasionally homonymous.

The most difficult diagnosis to make or to exclude is a second intracranial lesion when an orbital tumor has been removed and apparently does not pass thru the optic foramen. The signs which such a tumor should give have already been given by the intraorbital tumor and, therefore, cannot be considered. The diagnosis of the intracranial extension of these tumors must then await one of three objective signs: (1) extension of the visual defect either to the chiasm or the opposite optic nerve, (2) roentgenologic evidence of destruction of the landmarks in the region (principally the sella turcica), (3) the advent of signs of intracranial pressure.

OPERATIVE TREATMENT OF OPTIC NERVE TUMORS

In considering the treatment of prechiasmal tumors, I of course include all tumors of the optic nerve in the prechiasmal region, whether primary in the orbit or cranium; and because of the intimate relationship between the orbital and intracranial tumors, it is necessary to consider all optic nerve tumors in a general way. Until now, the treatment of orbital tumors has been restricted to the removal of the intraorbital tumor. The future of the patient has then been left to chance. And we have seen from the ultimate results, inadequate as they are, that a very high percentage of these patients die of an intracranial tumor. One cannot do better than quote the well stated conclusion of Byers in regard to this aspect of intraorbital optic nerve tumors: "The danger is not from recurrence in the strict sense of the term, but from the continued development of the intracranial portion of the tumor which it is impossible to remove at the time of the operation." This statement was made twenty years ago. Only now has surgery developed to meet this condition.

There are, therefore, two problems to meet in the treatment of all optic nerve tumors, whether intraorbital or intracranial. First and most important, to save the life of the individual and second to save the vision which remains and, if possible, restore that which is gone. I shall merely mention here eand shortly publish elsewhere an operative procedure by which both of these objects can be attained. It is not to be inferred that all cases of optic nerve tumor can be cured. Much depends upon the stage at which the diagnosis is made and also upon the character of the tumor. If the intracranial tumor is diagnosed in the late stages there is little point in any operative procedure; the tumor would be too large and would have grown too far back along the base of the brain. Again, in very young children with a rapidly growing tumor, doubtless sarcoma, probably nothing could be done. But in the vast majority of cases, the entire intracranial tumor could be removed and with little danger to life. Fortunately, the optic nerve is more or less suspended in the cranial chamber so that its resection, if necessary, would not be difficult and if a tumor is appended to the nerve its dissection from the nerve would be comparatively simple. The operative procedure consists in turning down a large bone flap, well forward, so that the exposure of the optic tracts is not impeded by lack of room. The procedure was originally intended solely for the intracranial part of the tumor, but in one case the growth extended into the orbital cavity and the roof of the orbit was easily removed, and the intraorbital portion of the tumor enucleated at the same time. The roof of the orbit can then be replaced as in Kronlein's operation. The intracranial operation is advocated for all tumors in which an intracranial optic nerve growth is known to be present. I am not yet prepared to say how far this procedure should be adopted in intraorbital tumors of the optic nerve. It must depend upon a more careful report of the pathology of optic nerve tumors, i. e., exactly what proportion of these tumors have intracranial extension of the growth. If it is found from autopsies and reliable clinical data that most orbital tumors enter the cranium, then this intracranial operation (which combines the intraorbital also) will be found the safest procedure in the beginning, rather than to await the verdict of the operator who has done a local removal of the orbital tumor. In safe hands, the operation itself is practically without danger; it is the removal of large growths which adds the danger.

The reports in the papers of Byers, Hudson and all other authors, of the terrific mortality from meningitis following the removal of intraorbital tumors, reflects the bad treatment of these tumors in the past. There is now, of course, little excuse for any procedure which will permit meningitis. No operation should be performed thru a field which cannot be sterilized and protected. For this reason, operations thru the palpebral fissure and conjunctive cannot be too strongly condemned. A cerebrospinal fistula results when the optic nerve is severed and it is then almost impossible to prevent meningitis. Kronlein's operation seems the best and safest of the local procedures; it gives the best exposure, and the operator can work thru an aseptic field.

When a local operation has been performed for the orbital tumor and it is found that its complete removal is impossible, the intracranial operation must then be done, for unless the tumor can be completely removed, total blindness and death are inevitable. Whatever operative procedure for an intraorbital tumor we may consider best and safest at the onset, this must be adequate to assure the patient that an intracranial extension of the growth does not exist, for when following the interval after the operation the intracranial growth later becomes evident from symptoms of intracranial pressure, the chances of life are gone; the tumor is then too large. As is true in all other intracranial tumors, an early diagnosis simplifies the operative procedure, reduces its dangers and affords the patient the best chance of life and preservation of function.

SUMMARY AND CONCLUSIONS

1. Two cases of tumors of the intracranial part of the optic nerve are reported.

2. In one case there were two bilateral, symmetric tumors at the optic foramen. Each of these tumors was a psammoma, i. e., a dural tumor, usually considered a dural endothelioma. In the second case,

there was a single tumor on the left optic nerve at the optic foramen. In both cases there was bilateral loss of vision.

3. The symmetric tumors entered the orbit thru the optic foramen, the other tumor was strictly intracranial.

4. One was diagnosed clinically; the other was suspected after an earlier diagnosis of optic neuritis; both were found at operation.

5. From the case with the bilateral tumors, all of one tumor and part of the other was removed. The vision was greatly improved as a result.

6. In the second case, the tumor could not be removed because it was under the optic nerve on the side opposite the operative approach. A band of adhesions bound the tumor to the anterior clinoid process, and its incision liberated the nerve from the clutches of the tumor and complete restoration of vision resulted.

7. A very high proportion of intraorbital optic nerve tumors extend into the cranial chamber. Local operations on the orbital part of the tumors in these cases are, therefore, not only futile but give the patient a false sense of security until it is too late.

8. The only justifiable local treatment of intraorbital tumors is one which at once assures the patient that an intracranial extention either does or does not exist.

9. If either a primary intracranial tumor of the optic nerve or a secondary intracranial extension of an intraorbital tumor is present, only an intracranial operation which aims at the removal of the tumor, offers the patient any chance of the preservation of life or vision.

10. An operation is proposed, the object of which is to remove the intracranial or the combined intracranial and intraorbital tumors when both are present.

11. The differential diagnosis of prechiasmal intracranial tumors from other lesions is considered.

REFERENCES

[1]Dandy, W. E.: Localization or Elimination of Cere-

bral Tumors by Ventriculography. *Annals of Surgery,* April, 1920.

[2]Willemer, W.: Uber eigentliche d. h. sich innerhalb der aussern Schiede entwickelende Tumoren des Sehnervn. *Arch. f. Ophth., xxv:* 189, 1879.

[3]Jocqs: *Des Tumeurs du Nerf Optique.* These de Paris, 1887.

[4]Braunschweig: Die primaren Geschwulste des Sehnerven. *Arch. f. Ophth., xxxix:* 1–93, 1893.

[5]Finlay, C. E.: *Arch. Ophth.,* N. Y., *xxiv:* 224–242, 1895.

[6]Byers, W. G. M.: Primary Intradural Tumors of the Optic Nerve. *Roy. Victoria Hosp., Montreal, I:* 3–82, 1901–03.

[7]Hudson, A. C.: Primary Tumors of the Optic Nerve. *Roy. Lond. Ophth. Hosp. Rep., xviii:* 317–439, 1910-12. *Tr. Ophth. Soc. U. Kingdom, Lond., xxiii:* 116–134, 1902-03.

[8]Parsons, J. H.: Primary Extradural Tumors of the Optic Nerve.

[9]Pagenstecher and Steffan. *Arch. f. Ophth., LIV:* 300, 1902.

XV

AN OPERATION FOR THE TOTAL EXTIRPATION OF TUMORS IN THE CEREBELLO-PONTINE ANGLE. A PRELIMINARY REPORT. *

The most frequent tumor in the cerebello-pontine angle is an encapsulated endothelioma arising from the leptomeninges. Rather loosely embedded in the lateral wall of the brain-stem, it is potentially a benign tumor by virtue of its encapsulation. Its complete removal offers a permanent cure to the afflicted individual but its extirpation has been attended by a mortality so high as to render such attempts inadvisable. In fact, the complete removal of such tumors with recovery has been regarded as impossible. As a result, a partial intracapsular enucleation has been the operation which has seemed to offer most to the patient, but it is obvious that such treatment of a potentially benign lesion is most unsatisfactory to the patient, for the tumor must inevitably recur.

Five years ago, I completely removed such a growth from a patient who has since remained well. The growth was extirpated *in toto* by careful dissection around the tumor. Subsequently, two other tumors of the same type were similarly removed, but the results of such a method were too capricious and the mortality was too high.

Gradually a procedure has been evolved by which I believe these neoplasms can be successfully removed and with relative safety; the mortality should be little

*Reprinted from *The Johns Hopkins Hospital Bulletin, xxxiii:* 344, September, 1922.

higher than from a subtotal removal of the contents of the tumor. The last two patients with cerebello-pontine tumors have been treated by this procedure and are well. The last patient was a particularly bad risk because of a partial hemiplegia and hemianaesthesia and inability to swallow. She quickly recovered from the operation. In one patient, the operation was performed in two stages; in the second in one stage. The latter method is far preferable because in the interim between stages the capsule becomes friable and more difficult to handle.

The purpose of this preliminary report is to present the salient features of the operative procedure. A bilateral suboccipital exposure of the cerebellum is performed with as much exposure of the affected angle as possible. The interior of the growth is removed with a curette. Following this, the capsule is picked up with forceps and beginning at the upper and lower poles, carefully drawn away from the medulla, pons and mid-brain. The traction brings into view the several small veins and arteries crossing from the brain-stem to the tumor. These vessels are ligated individually with silver clips or fine silk ligatures and divided. Gradually, in this painstaking way, the whole tumor is delivered from its bed without bleeding, and without trauma to the brain-stem. The cranial nerves stretched by the tumor are automatically liberated as the capsule falls away from them.

XVI

A METHOD FOR THE LOCALIZATION OF BRAIN TUMORS IN COMATOSE PATIENTS *

THE DETERMINATION OF COMMUNICATION BETWEEN THE CEREBRAL VENTRICLES AND THE ESTIMATION OF THEIR POSITION AND SIZE WITHOUT THE INJECTION OF AIR (VENTRICULAR ESTIMATION)

If the character and location of all brain tumors were known or easy of determination, the treatment would be greatly simplified. If it could be demonstrated that the character or position of the tumor was such as to prevent its removal, palliative treatment would at once be instituted as the utmost resource at our command. But if both the character and position of the tumor were known to be such as to make its removal probable or even a possibility, every effort would be directed toward its extirpation, this being the only hope of a cure.

Unfortunately, however, not all of this information is as yet attainable even after all examinations have been made. In only exceptional cases, as for instance tumors of the brain-stem and of the left temporal lobe, can we know that its extirpation either is not possible or is not justifiable. Although there are often indications that tumors either do or do not lend themselves to extirpation, the evidence on this point is most unreliable and may be just as misleading one way as the other. With few exceptions, the character of the tumor is not ascertainable until the growth is actually seen and examined at operation. Because of the progressive, necessarily destructive, and fatal course of these lesions unless completely removed by operation, the patient's only hope lies in the assumption that *all* tumors are curable until proven otherwise.

*Reprinted from *Surgery, Gynecology and Obstetrics*, May 1923, pages 641-656.

Fortunately, we are now able to determine the *location* of practically all brain tumors, so that by their inspection at operation the character of the growth can at once be known and either the palliative or curative treatment instituted at that time. With very few exceptions, the kind of tumor can be accurately told by its gross appearance at operation as by a microscopical examination. Roughly estimated, not many more than 50 per cent of all brain tumors are localizable by neurological and roentgenological examinations, and it is for the localization of the other half that cerebral pneumography is of the greatest value.

We believe very firmly that no surgical treatment should be attempted until the location of the tumor is as precisely known as possible; that *primary* palliative treatment should never be done until a tumor is known not to be removable. We feel that the only treatment for brain tumors is to treat the *cause* directly; and that the tumor should be *completely* extirpated, and promptly, when possible.

There are times when this procedure may seem impractical or very difficult. Particularly is this true in those patients who are seen for the first time in the last stages of intracranial pressure, i.e., when in coma or when coma is impending. But under such circumstances, an accurate localization is far more important than when the patient's general condition is good. The correct treatment will often save the patient's life, while a misdirected operation will merely hasten the end. Cerebral pneumography[1] has been invaluable in these cases, for the patient may be so deeply unconscious that the results of the neurological examination may be negligible and the history obtained from others either inaccurate or misleading. However, in these cases the use of cerebral pneumography may, in itself, be very serious on account of the aggravations of pressure symptoms due to the effects of the air (a factor now largely under control), but still more so because of the time lost in making the examinations, and may reduce, more than it helps, the chances of a cure.

If, under these circumstances, it were possible to make a localization of the tumor without injecting air into the ventricles, the patient's chances would be considerably increased. It is the purpose of this paper to propose a quick method by which a localization can usually be made *in such emergencies*. It is not without its possibilities of error but, taking everything into consideration, it seems to offer the most to the patients in their very desperate condition. It is recommended with hesitation and only as an emergency procedure. It is possible that the procedure may be useful in a few cases where the information obtained is sufficient to eliminate a definite region of the brain, when it seems certain that the tumor can be in one of only two possible situations. At all other times when there is doubt as to the tumor's location, presuming, of course, that the patient's condition is favorable, the other precise method of cerebral pneumography should be used.

The method proposed is to *estimate the size, position, and intercommunication of the ventricles by aspiration of the fluid in the lateral ventricles (and at times from the cisterna magna)*. We have learned from necropsy material but particularly from ventriculography that practically all brain tumors which cause intracranial pressure alter the size, shape, or position of part or all of the cerebral ventricular system; and the situation of tumors is, therefore, determined by the deviations in the size,

shape, and position of the ventricles.

The position of the lateral ventricles can be determined by ventricular punctures; their size by measuring the fluid in the ventricles; and their communication with each other by injecting a dye into one ventricle and testing for the color elsewhere in the ventricular system. This information, while it leaves much still to be desired, is usually at least sufficient to tell whether either cerebral hemisphere or the cerebellum is the likely seat of the tumor.

Since the introduction of cerebral pneumography, it has been our custom to make a small perforator opening in the occipital region of *both* sides of the skull. Frequently one ventricle is collapsed or displaced by a tumor and cannot be reached by ventricular puncture, but it will be exceptional for both ventricles to be inaccessible. Usually the puncture of only one ventricle is necessary for cerebral pneumography, but since we cannot foretell which ventricle can or cannot be reached, and since at times both ventricles must be tapped, it is better to have both ventricles under control. The two openings can be made as easily and safely as one. The part of the lateral ventricle, the vestibule, is most accessible from this point. Moreover, the vestibule of the ventricle is, on the whole, less easily collapsed and dislocated than other parts of the ventricle. At times we have used bilateral punctures of the anterior horns of the ventricles but here the ventricles are smaller and consequently harder to enter. Moreover, dislocation and collapse of both anterior horns is more likely because they are closer together and, therefore, more equally affected by any pressure directed from the side. The vestibules and posterior horns are farther apart and are less equally occluded by the same pressure. Another anatomical factor which carries weight is that the anterior puncture must be nearer the midline and consequently through a field of larger veins which are nearing the longitudinal sinus. These may easily be punctured, whereas the posterior puncture is through a less vascular area. The lateral puncture into the descending horn has been used very sparingly and practically never bilaterally. At times a patient has previously had a decompression performed and an attempt may be made to enter the ventricle under these circumstances. A lateral puncture of the left side would hardly be considered because of the important speech areas which the needle must traverse. For ventricular estimations we have used the same posterior approach to the ventricles. *Punctures of both ventricles are then always necessary* (Fig. 1).

THE POSITION OF A LATERAL VENTRICLE

By experience it will be known that a normal lateral ventricle should always be entered from a given point when the ventricular needle is inserted in the proper direction and to a given depth. With practice one acquires a certain degree of confidence in this determination. If the ventricle is enlarged from hydrocephalus, it will be even more easily reached and usually at less depth. When neither ventricle can be *reached* by properly directed punctures, it is strong evidence that hydrocephalus is not present, and this will at once signify that the tumor cannot be in the cerebellum, third ventricle, or brain-stem. When the ventricle is entered, it is usually not possible to say more than that the ventricle is not dislocated. Whether the ventricle is of normal size or enlarged, can be determined only by *measuring* the fluid which it contains. If only a few drops of fluid escape from the needle, the ventricle may be considered smaller than normal, but attempts to aspirate will always make this deduction safer. Occasionally, neither ventricle can be reached in the normal position, but one or both may be entered at a distance to the right or to the left. Such a displacement, when definite and particularly when known to be the same on both sides, can be explained only by the effects of a tumor; and the tumor must be

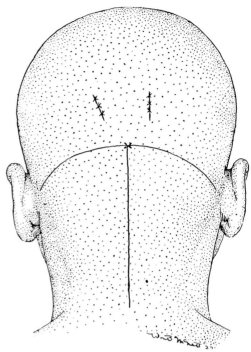

Fig. 1. To show the position for bilateral ventricular punctures. A cerebellar incision is outlined for orientation. For the puncture, either a slight oblique or ventrical incision can be made.

on the side *from* which the dislocation has occurred. If the lateral deviation of the ventricles has been shown by a *posterior* ventricular puncture, it is presumptive evidence of a tumor in the posterior half of the cerebral hemisphere, for tumors in the anterior half of the hemisphere will hardly cause such a pronounced dislocation of the vestibules of the lateral ventricles. Doubtless more and greater deviation of the anterior horns would be demonstrable by puncture of the anterior horns, but the evidence of dislocation of the ventricles from a puncture is far less important and less reliable than the computation of the size of the ventricles. In one of our cases, however, the sole information of the tumor's position was learned from the dislocation of the ventricles (Case 4). Both lateral ventricles were so small that no fluid could be aspirated but each ventricle was reached far to the right of its normal position.

SIZE OF THE LATERAL VENTRICLES

From a large series of ventriculograms it has been found that the size of the normal lateral ventricle is most variable. Indeed, to differentiate between a large normal, and a small hydrocephalic, ventricle, often requires close study. But apparently the lateral ventricles in the same patient are of equal size unless there is some lesion to cause inequality.

We have also learned that the lateral ventricle is always smaller on the side of a cerebral tumor (excluding a resultant localized hydrocephalus) than on the opposite side and usually the difference is very striking. Indeed, the ventricle on the side of a tumor is usually so small that it cannot be reached by a ventricular puncture or, if reached, only a few drops of fluid will escape. Occasionally, as in one of the cases reported here, the size of both ventricles may be tremendously reduced, but usually there is a considerable difference in their size. For this reason, if we find one lateral ventricle from which 25 cubic centimeters of fluid can easily be aspirated, and only 1 or 2 cubic centimeters can be obtained from the other ventricle, we may feel fairly confident (after excluding a block in the ventricle) that the tumor is on the side of the small ventricle. Again, if we can easily aspirate 25 cubic centimeters of fluid from a lateral ventricle, it is fairly safe (there are exceptions) to assume that a tumor does not exist in that hemisphere, for such a tumor would by this time have consumed that space in seeking room for expansion (we are now considering only patients in coma or with coma impending). And if both lateral ventricles are of equal size, it would be fairly safe to assume the presence of hydrocephalus and, therefore, that the tumor is in the cerebellum, brain-stem, or third ventricle. For practical purposes, we have come to look upon the aspiration of 25 cubic centimeters of fluid as a standard quantity upon which to draw conclusions. The aspiration of more fluid would usu-

ally require the injection of air to prevent too much negative pressure. In this connection, it should be emphasized that any conclusions drawn from the amount of fluid obtained by ventricular puncture alone, i.e., without aspirating fluid, are too capricious to be in any way reliable. The amount of fluid which spurts from a ventricular needle, except when the ventricle is very small, only indicates in a rough way the degree of intracranial pressure. From a ventricle of normal size or even smaller than normal, there will be a considerable spurt of fluid; a hydrocephalic ventricle may not give more. It is the reserve in the ventricle after the pressure relief which is important. A ventricle of normal size would exhaust its fluid in only partially relieving the intracranial pressure, and there would be no fluid in reserve for aspiration, but, from a hydrocephalic ventricle, additional fluid will still easily be obtained after the pressure has been relieved.

A small ventricle in one cerebral hemisphere will eliminate a tumor of the cerebellum, brain-stem, or third ventricle, but will not eliminate a unilateral hydrocephalus or focal hydrocephalus on the other side; and conversely, the demonstration of a hydrocephalus on one side does not prove a tumor to be in the cerebellum, brain-stem, or third ventricle. It is never safe to draw conclusions from one lateral ventricle alone; the status of both ventricles must always be determined (Fig. 1); inferences from both still leave too many possibilities of error. It is hardly necessary to add that in drawing conclusions of such character, one must be very confident of his ability to reach a normally placed ventricle; also that some extraneous factor such as a plugged needle is not causing erroneous deductions to be drawn.

COMMUNICATION BETWEEN THE VENTRICLES THE INDIGOCARMIN TEST

An additional method of ventricular estimation is most useful in further reducing the chances of error in those cases in which the tumor has caused hydrocephalus. If 1 or 2 cubic centimeters (depending on the size of the ventricle) of indigocarmin[1] is injected into a lateral ventricle, aspiration of the contralateral ventricle will easily indicate whether or not the two lateral ventricles are in free communication (Figs. 2 and 3). If the dye does not pass from one ventricle to the other, there must be a tumor in the anterior or the middle and not the posterior cranial fossa. If both ventricles are dilated and the dye passes freely to the opposite side, the tumor will be in the posterior cranial fossa. Exceptions to the latter assumption are some pineal tumors and also those long-standing cases of hydrocephalus where an artificial communication between the lateral ventricles has resulted from pressure atrophy of the septum pellucidum; these atrophic openings have assumed this function of the foramina of Monro. This dye test is also useful in deciding whether the lateral ventricles com-

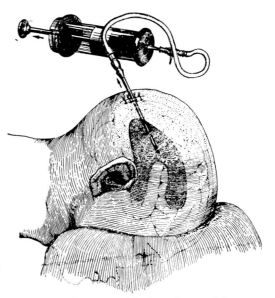

Fig. 3. Diagram, with lateral ventricles outlined indicating the approximate course of the ventricular needle.

municate with the cisterna magna or the spinal subarachnoid space. At times it may be uncertain whether the lateral ventricles are hydrocephalic or merely of large but yet normal size. Again, the ventricles may be hydrocephalic but it may not be clear whether a tumor or another condition is responsible, i.e., whether the hydrocephalus is due to an obstruction or to an increased production of fluid. If an obstruction (usually a tumor) is the cause of hydrocephalus, the dye will not appear in the cisterna magna or the lumbar subarachnoid space. If the hydrocephalus is due to an increased production of cerebrospinal fluid (cardio-vascular-renal; chronic inflammatory reaction, etc.), the dye will freely pass into the cisterna magna or the spinal subarachnoid space. This communication or obstruction can be determined by aspiration through a lumbar puncture or a cisternal puncture (Ayer's puncture) or by operative exposure of the cisterna magna. We are strongly prejudiced against lumbar punctures in all cases where intracranial tumor is suspected, because of frequent medullary injury; except where intracranial pressure is first relieved

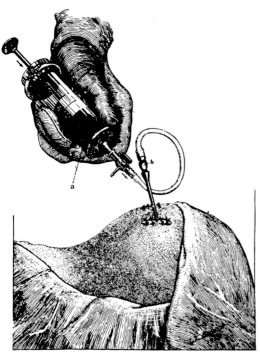

Fig. 2. To show method of ventricular puncture and aspiration of the ventricle and injection of indigocarmin (a).

by ventricular puncture, it should never be done and even then we would be most hesitant when a patient is in coma. Ayer's puncture would be at least equally dangerous for the same reason and also because the cisterna magna will always be-obliterated by tumors in the posterior fossa. In cases where there is doubt and a tumor of the posterior fossa seems a probability, it is much safer to expose the cisterna magna. If the tumor is present, the operative procedure is necessary and if not present, we have erred on the safer side and done no harm. Uncertainty of this kind must be rare but one such example recently came to our attention and will later be considered in some detail (Case 5).

The possibilities of this method developed during an exploration of the left cerebral hemisphere in a patient in deep coma from intracranial pressure.

A few hours after his arrival at the hospital, patient suddenly became unconscious. Fairly satisfactory examinations were made by Drs. Boggs and Thomas. The presence of an intracranial tumor or abscess was known because of the headaches, torpor, vomiting, and bilateral choked disc. There were, however, no positive localizing neurological findings except Jacksonian convulsions beginning in the right hand, spreading over the *right* side and eventually becoming bilateral. This history seemed sufficient to indicate a left cerebral lesion and this side of the brain was explored. In view of a history of sudden pain in the frontal region (bilateral), high fever for three weeks, swelling and closure of the *left* eye, immediately preceding patient's present illness, it was thought likely by both Drs. Thomas and Boggs that the lesion might be an abscess rather than a tumor. It should also be noted that the left pupil was much larger than the right. There had never been any localization of the headaches. He had had many convulsions while at home but in none had any focal character been observed. It was during examination in the hospital that the Jacksonian attack was seen. There was no motor or sensory inequality and the reflexes on the two sides were equal; no

Babinski or ankle clonus on either side. There was bilateral choked disc of six diopters. The x-ray examination was negative. There seemed little doubt that the lesion was on the left side. Before beginning the operation, characteristic Cheyne-Stokes respirations developed and his color was cyanotic. Feeling that, should a tumor be found, his condition would not warrant its removal, only a decompression was planned, but in such deep coma the ordinary sized decompression would have been of little value. It is our custom in such extreme coma quickly to turn down a small bone-flap on the suspected side of the tumor. The operation can be done as quickly as the usual subtemporal decompression, and it has two great advantages: (1) it allows us to obtain very valuable information of the character of the tumor, thereby giving additional possibilities of treatment, and (2) if the tumor is found to be inoperable, all or part of the bone-flap can be removed, giving a larger and more effective decompression. At times a cyst may be encountered and its simple evacuation will give far more effective relief than any form of decompression alone. Ofttimes the patient's condition is sufficiently good to permit complete extirpation of a favorable tumor even at this operation. At other times an enucleable tumor may be encountered but the patient's condition may be too poor to permit its removal at this time but at a subsequent stage. Partial or total removal of the bone-flap will serve as a decompression until a succeeding stage. Experience alone can decide whether a one-stage or two-stage operation should be done in such emergencies. The general condition of each patient must be the guide in each. Always the one-stage operation is preferable, other things being equal, but tumor extirpations are such tremendous undertakings that it is always better to err on the side of safety and, when the patient's condition is not the best, to reserve extirpation for a second stage.

According to the above plan of treatment, a small bone-flap was quickly reflected on the left. A very tense dura was exposed and incised concentrically. No anaesthetic was given at any time during the operation. The brain was allowed to protrude slowly through the dural defect and a big cerebral herniation bulged through the dural defect. No abnormality of any part of the cerebral cortex could be seen or palpated. The configuration of the lateral ventricle could easily be mapped out throughout practically its entire extent, a finding which usually denotes a large ventricle. A ventricular needle was passed into the vestibule of the ventricle and 25 cubic centimeters of fluid was aspirated. It contained 21 cells, suggesting that the lesion was probably an abscess. After release of the fluid, the outline of the ventricle was sharply shown by the indentation of the sunken cortex. The bone-flap was removed and the galea and skin quickly closed. These findings were interpreted as follows: with a ventricle so large, a tumor could not exist in this hemisphere and particularly as the enlargement was of the entire ventricle and not of a portion only. But is seemed possible from this data alone, to tell even more than merely to exclude this hemisphere as the seat of the tumor. When this ventricle was emptied there still remained intracranial pressure, i.e., there was still a big hernia of the brain through the dural opening. If the tumor were in the cerebellum or the brain-stem, there would be a bilateral hydrocephalus and after a puncture with aspiration of the fluid in this ventricle, the pressure in both cerebral hemispheres would be equally released, at least sufficiently to allow the brain to sink below the level of the dura, thus making the intracranial pressure negative instead of positive. We were, therefore, forced to conclude that a tumor mass must exist in the other (right) cerebral hemisphere; that the hydrocephalus (if such it was) must be confined to the side of operation and therefore be unilateral. The unilateral hydrocephalus must be due to closure of the third ventricle and the foramen of Monro on the operated side.

No benefit resulted from the decompression and the patient died on the following day. At necropsy an abscess of the *right* frontal lobe was found. We had operated on the *left* side because of a Jacksonian convulsion beginning in the right hand! Had his condition warranted air injection, the location of the abscess could have been easily determined. The misplaced confidence in the Jacksonian attack need not concern us here. We are merely warned that apparently positive signs are not always reliable. Had the operation been performed on the side of the lesion, allowing drainage of the abscess, a better result might conceivably have followed, even in his extreme condition.

During the past six months four other patients[1] have entered the Johns Hopkins Hospital in a comatose condition due to intracranial tumor and in whom no information leading to the location of the tumor could be elicited either from the history of friends and relatives or from the purely objective examinations of the comatose patients. In three of these patients the estimation of the ventricular capacity alone made the localization of the tumor possible. In the fourth, both lateral ventricles were so reduced that only drops of fluid could be obtained from either side, but the ventricles were so definitely dislocated toward the right that the tumor was localized to the left cerebral hemisphere. Two of these patients are now cured after total extirpation of dural endotheliomata. A third died twenty-four hours after total removal of a cerebello-pontine angle tumor and the fourth died of ventricular haemorrhage two days after extirpation of a glioma which projected into the ventricle. Three were completed in one stage, the fourth in two stages. Possibly a two-stage operation would have been wiser in the two patients who did not recover.

Case 1. *Patient comatose. Diagnosis: Brain tumor. Presumptive localization: Left cerebral hemisphere. Localization following ventricular estimation: Tumor in posterior fossa. Operative finding: Tumor right cerebello-pontine angle. Total removal; death 18 hours later.*

A sparely nourished woman, age 48, was seen in consultation in another hospital. For several hours she had been deeply unconscious following a lumbar puncture.

Over a period of four or five years she had complained of general headaches, perhaps greater over the vertex. These gradually increased in frequency and severity, and throughout the past eight weeks were almost intolerable. At times, vomiting followed the severe headaches and gave a certain amount of relief. The right eye had been blind for three weeks, and only light perception remained in the left. During the past few weeks she had complained of a weakness of the right arm and leg. A slight facial asymmetry and weakness of the right arm had been noticed by her husband. Recently she fell when the right knee gave way. There had also been pain in the right arm at times. She had never complained of deafness or any unusual feeling in her face (involvement of nerves VIII and V). She was no deeply unconscious that the examination was entirely objective; except for a bilaterally symmetrical choked disc of 6 diopters, there was no positive neurological finding, though possibly the right side of the face moved less on deep stimulation of the surpra-orbital nerve; but the difference was not sufficiently definite to be considered positive. The reflexes were equal. There was no Babinski or ankle clonus on either side. No extra-ocular palsies could be detected; she had never complained of diplopia. The spinal fluid made at the above ill-advised lumbar puncture, contained globulin and a 4+ Wassermann. The blood pressure was 168-122; pulse 120. The diagnosis of an intracranial tumor was clear, owing to the bilateral choked disc, the long history of headaches, vomiting, and gradual loss of vision. The localization of the tumor was not clear, but from the history of weakness of the entire right side, a presumptive diagnosis of a left cerebral tumor, possibly frontal, was made. She was, therefore, draped for an exploration of the left cerebrum, but since the diagnosis was only tentative and based on the history, puncture of both lateral ventricles was first made to confirm or contradict this diagnosis. Twenty cubic centimeters of fluid was easily aspirated from each lateral ventricle and more could have been withdrawn. Indigocarmin injected into the left ventricle was quickly recovered when the right was aspirated. Such large ventricles were considered proof that our presumptive diagnosis was incorrect; that a tumor could not be present in either cerebral hemisphere and, since there was free communication between the

ventricles, the neoplasm was probably in the posterior cranial fossa. The patient was then redraped for a cerebellar operation. The usual bilateral cerebellar exposure was made. A characteristic encapsulated tumor presented in the right cerebello-pontine angle (Fig. 4). Realizing that a cerebellar decompression would hardly be helpful, since the obstruction to the iter was caused by a firmly imbedded tumor which would not be affected by the removal of bone, an intracapsular enucleation was considered the only possible method of producing palliation. This was easily performed, but since her condition had remained unchanged, the removal of the capsule also seemed possible with little extra time and effort. It was, therefore, completely extirpated. There was no bleeding at any time, the individual arteries and veins being caught in silver clips. Consciousness did not return following the operation, death coming 18 hours later. In retrospect, it doubtless would have been wiser to have been content to leave the capsule in place and to complete its removal at a subsequent stage, particularly as the slightest injury to the medulla would greatly add to her danger. It is worthy of passing note that the Wassermann (4+) was of no significance and might have been very misleading.

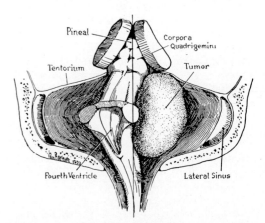

Fig. 4. Diagram of cerebello-pontine tumor located in Case 1 by ventricular estimation. The tumor has blocked the aqueduct of Sylvius causing symmetrical dilatation of the lateral ventricles; free communication between them is determined by the injection of indigocarmin into one ventricle and aspiration of the color in the other.

Case 2. *Patient comatose. Diagnosis:*
Brain tumor. Presumptive localization:
Tumor of left cerebellum or right frontal
lobe. Localization from ventricular esti-
mation: Tumor in posterior fossa. Two-
stage operation: Total removal encapsu-
lated dural endothelioma arising from
tentorium cerebelli. Recovery.

A well nourished woman of fifty-five
years was seen in Rochester, New York,
in consultation with Dr. John R. Booth.
For the past two days she had gradually
become increasingly drowsy and during
the night lapsed into coma. Although
no response to questions was obtainable,
she still moved at times. Though the wife
of a physician, she had complained so
little that he could offer nothing which
was helpful in making a localization of
her lesion. For only the past 2 months
had she complained of general headaches,
intensified by defaecation. Frequently
there was vomiting. For a few days there
had been diplopia but this had disappeared. For five weeks there had been
dizziness and an uncertain, unsteady gait
with possibly a tendency to deviate to the
left. At times she had spoken of a weakness of the left leg and arm, but nothing
suggesting ataxia or nystagmus had been
observed. A severe acute infection of the
right frontal sinus had immediately preceded her headaches, and this had been
looked upon as the cause of her present
illness. Except for a choked disc of about
seven diopters in each fundus oculi, the
examination was entirely negative. No
nystagmus could be elicited; there was no
noticeable strabismus. No difference in
the muscle tone of either arm could be
detected on quickly flexing and extending
the forearm. The reflexes were normal
and equal on the two sides. No Babinski
or ankle clonus. White blood count,
15,000; pulse, 120; temperature, 99.2°.
There was little evidence upon which to
defferentiate between a right frontal
tumor or abscess and one in the left cerebellum. The strongly emphasized frontal
infection (sinuses now clear), the leucocy-
tosis of 15,000, and the history of a weakness of the left side, were weighed against
a possible history of staggering gait and
tendency to fall to the left.

She was at once brought to Baltimore
and sent directly to the operating room.
She stood the journey surprisingly well,
there being very grave doubt that she
would reach the destination. The operation: 25 cubic centimeters of fluid was
aspirated from each lateral ventricle. It
was under great pressure. The reasoning
from these data was essentially like that
in the preceding case. Ventricles of such
size were considered incompatible with
a tumor in either cerebral hemisphere
and indicated an infratentorial tumor.
A bilateral cerebellar decompression was
made. The left lobe was so much larger
than the right that a tumor in the left
cerebellar hemisphere was unquestioned.
A cyst was excluded by a puncture of the
hemisphere. No attempt was made to
learn more about the tumor because of
her desperate condition. During the next
few days consciousness returned and her
strength quickly followed. Had we been
able to consult the patient, the differential diagnosis would not have been
difficult. The staggering gait and tendency to fall to the left had not been equivocal. She had been very dizzy for some
time and because of this had been unwilling to lie on the left side. She had not
communicated these symptoms to her
husband because of her unwillingness to
worry him.

A month later, an encapsulated dural
endothelioma weighing 40.5 grams and
arising from the inferior surface of the
tentorium (Fig. 5), was removed *in toto*.
It was completely hidden from view by
the overlying left lobe of the cerebellum
so that it was not actually seen at the
first operation. She made an uneventful
recovery.

Case 3. *Patient comatose. Diagnosis:*
Brain tumor. Localization not presumed.
Localization after ventricular estimation:
Right occipital lobe. Operation: Removal
dural endothelioma arising from superior
surface of tentorium. Recovery.

Patient is a well-nourished woman, age
fifty; referred by Dr. J. S. Horsley of
Richmond, Virginia. On arrival at the
Johns Hopkins Hospital she was unconscious and had been so for about five
hours. Only very deep stimulation of the
supra-orbital nerve brought response. Respirations were of the typical Cheyne-
Stokes type, with breathless intervals of
forty seconds; pulse slow, full, and bound-
ing, sixty per minute. Her present trouble

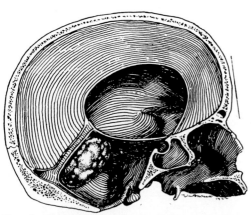

Fig. 5. Diagram to show position of dural endothelioma arising from the inferior surface of the tentorium cerebelli (Case 2). Dilatation of the lateral ventricles with free communication was determined by the ventricular estimation test. The cause of the hydrocephalus was obstruction of the aqueduct of Sylvius.

began only three months before admission, with severe headaches on the top of the head—never more localized. In the beginning the headaches would last two or three hours and recur two or three times a week. Gradually they increased in frequency and severity and for the past month they have been almost constant. There was some pain and tenderness in the back of the head and some stiffness of the neck. She became dull and slept a great deal. Nausea and vomiting began about a month after the onset of headaches and for two days during the last week she vomited almost continuously. Two weeks before admission her eyes became crossed. About this time she also saw half of things, but her physician could find no hemianopsia. Dr. Horsley and Dr. Vaughan saw her for a few hours and apparently made out a hemianopsia to the left, but, as Dr. Horsley's notes had not yet arrived, our only information about the hemianopsia was brought through the husband. We had no way of knowing how definite this finding might be.

The examination showed a paralysis of the *left* external rectus, the eye being turned strongly inward and a bilateral choked disc of six diopters. There were no differences in the reflexes on the two sides, no Babinski or ankle clonus. No

difference in the muscle tone could be detected. The one objective finding, therefore, was paralysis of the *left* external rectus muscle (nerve VI). The possible history of a hemianopsia to the left would not harmonize with palsy of the left nerve VI. but the value of implication of the sixth nerve is too capricious to be taken seriously. Here we should have been misled had it been considered a localizing sign. The suboccipital headache and cervical rigidity suggested the possibility of a cerebellar tumor, though no history of staggering gait could be elicited.

Bilateral ventricular punctures were attempted; the right ventricle could *not* be reached, the left ventricle was encountered in a position which did not appear abnormal, but only 10 cubic centimeters of fluid could be withdrawn. Again an attempt was made to reach the right ventricle, but again without success. We were safe in excluding a tumor of the posterior crainal fossa because there was no hydrocephalus. The inability to reach the right ventricle was presumptive evi-

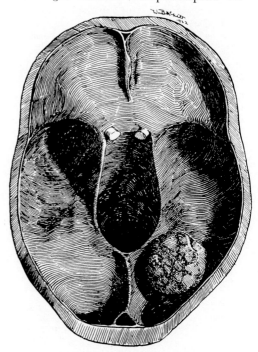

Fig. 6. Diagram to show the position of the dural endothelioma arising from the superior surface of the tentorium (Case 3). It was located by the ventricular estimation test. The tumor was completely removed; uneventful recovery.

dence of a tumor on this side, especially when taken in conjunction with a fairly normal sized ventricle on the left, and if the tumor was on the right it would more probably be located posteriorly because of the closure of the posterior horn and vestibule; this part of the ventricle would hardly have been completely occluded, or at least it would have seemed less likely, from a tumor located anteriorly in the hemisphere. A presumptive diagnosis was then made of a tumor of the occipital lobe. Operation: A bone-flap was turned down exposing the posterior two-thirds of the right cerebral hemisphere. The brain under high tension quickly herniated through the dural opening. No tumor was visible, though practically the entire outer surface of the brain could be inspected. Posteriorly, however, the brain was distinctly paler than elsewhere, the convolutions were wider and the sulci so flattened that they were practically devoid of the normal mantle of cerebrospinal fluid; all of which indicated an underlying tumor. The inferior tentorial surface of the occipital lobe was then explored and about 1 centimeter beneath the outer surface, a well-rounded edge of tumor presented. A perfectly encapsulated dural endothelioma was gradually brought into view and totally extirpated without unusual difficulty. It weighed 22 grams. Recovery uneventful.

Case 4. *Patient comatose. Diagnosis: Brain tumor. No localization presumed. Localization after ventricular estimation: Left cerebral hemisphere, probably occipital. Operation: Removal deeply situated subcortical glioma projecting into the lateral ventricle. Death two days later of intraventricular haemorrhage.*

Patient was a well-nourished woman of thirty-seven. When first seen with Dr. L. A. Krause, she was extremely restless but unresponsive. In the interval of about an hour before reaching the hospital, she became so deeply comatose that strong supra-orbital pressure brought no response. She became cyanotic and respirations were very shallow and pulse which had been 60 to 70 quickly mounted to 140. When placed in the ventral position there was some improvement, which became so great when a ventricular puncture was done as to allay immediate apprehension and allow us to proceed with the operation.

Her history and examination were easily adequate to make the diagnosis of an intracranial tumor. Although she had suffered from headaches nearly all her life, they had become much more severe four months ago and had since been practically constant. The headaches have been frontal, at the vertex and occipital regions, but never confined to one side. About four months ago blurring vision was noticed; this became so bad that she could not read the music notes (she was a music teacher). Double vision was present at times. There had been no complaint of hemianopsia. The vision in the left eye seemed worse than the right. To see objects with her left eye she would be compelled to turn her head around in this direction. (This was considered at the time as possible evidence of hemianopsia; the tumor's location, however, would have caused homonymous hemianopsia to the right instead of to the left).

Vomiting spells had been frequent, sometimes four or five attacks a day. Nausea was present most of the time and caused great distress. A month before admission she became unconscious and remained so for an hour, but is said not to have had a convulsion. Dr. Krause, who saw her for the first time only twenty-four hours before my examination, made out more active reflexes on the right, but no other changes. The reflex difference was not evident when I saw her. No Babinski and no ankle clonus were present. A bilateral choked disc of six or seven diopters was the only positive finding.

Attempts were made to tap both lateral ventricles but at first neither could be reached. The right ventricle was finally entered, probably 2.5 centimeters to the right of its proper position (as nearly as could be estimated from the deeply concealed tip of the needle), but only a few drops of fluid escaped and apparently under no increased pressure (when ventricles are so greatly reduced in size, the few drops of fluid which escape from the needle indicate a cavity too small to register intracranial pressure). The left ventricle was also reached far to the right. It was so compressed that no fluid escaped through the end of the needle; the only proof that the left ventricle had been reached was a few drops of clear fluid which escaped from the needle after its withdrawal. The diagnostic reasoning from these observations was as follows: the lesion could not be in the posterior fossa because there was no hydrocephalus; it was probably in the left cerebral hemisphere because both lateral ventricles were definitely dislocated to the right; the almost complete obliteration of the posterior part of both lateral ventricles, together with the great dislocation of this part of the ventricles, indicated that the location of the tumor was probably in the occipital region. Accordingly, the left occipital region was explored. Although no tumor was on the outer or inferior surfaces of the brain, an underlying lesion was indicated by the pallor and breadth of the convolutions and obliteration of the fluid-containing sulci. Transcortical exploration just back of the supramarginal gyrus disclosed a well-circumscribed tumor about 3 centimeters below the surface of the brain (Fig. 7). The position of the tumor would indicate a probable glioma, but it was extremely hard—almost of stony consistency—and seemed to separate readily from the brain tissue; moreover, a large, smooth nodule projected into the vestibule of the ventricle. For these reasons, the possibility of an ependymal tumor was considered. The most distant parts of the tumor became increasingly more fixed and less circum-

scribed; it was then clear that the tumor was a glioma and could not be completely removed, unless possibly after removing the main mass of tumor the outskirts could be excised later with normal brain tissue. A tumor mass weighing 105.5 grams was removed with considerable difficulty by finger enucleation leaving of course fringes of the tumor, even though invisible. The vestibule of the ventricle was opened. The bleeding was controlled after a large vein entering the vena Galena magna had been ligated. After removal of the tumor the incisura tentorii was in plain view, in fact it was here that the large bleeding vessel was "clipped." The glomus of the choroid plexus was exposed in the open ventricle. The bleeding was apparently entirely checked for some time before closure; but the possibility of a tiny ooze into an open ventricle is always the source of apprehension. Two days later she died of intraventricular haemorrhage.

POSSIBILITIES OF ERROR FROM VENTRICULAR ESTIMATION

It is well to reiterate that there are great possibilities of error in this procedure for reasons which we shall show. It is justifiable to disregard these possible mistakes only when the patient's condition is so serious as to preclude cerebral pneumography or when there is only a slight element of doubt of the location of the tumor which may be eliminated in this way. The whole procedure, of course, is dependent upon knowledge of ventricular topography, upon the confidence in one's ability precisely to reach the normal ventricle and in the interpretation in terms of intracranial pathology of the results of the punctures.

The first element of uncertainty lies in the great variation in size of the normal lateral ventricles. A lateral ventricle in one individual may be four or five times as large as in another. A big normal lateral ventricle may even be larger than a small hydrocephalic ventricle. From a small lateral ventricle 10 to 15 cubic centimeters of fluid can usually be aspirated, but from ventricles apparently equally

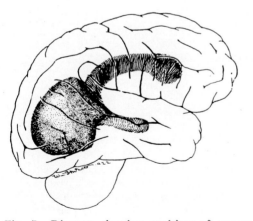

Fig. 7. Diagram showing position of tumor in occipital lobe (Case 4) located by ventricular estimation test. Tumor, which was a glioma, projected into the lateral ventricle. Patient died 2 days later of a slow bleeding into the ventricle.

normal 30 to 40 cubic centimeters may be obtained, and there are all sizes between. It is evident, therefore, that large normal ventricles may easily be mistaken for hydrocephalic ventricles, if ventricular estimation alone were depended upon for a localization of the growth. There would really be no way of making the differentiation by this method. In order to emphasize this danger, the following case in point is briefly presented. Had this patient been comatose at the time of entrance to the hospital, and if his localization had depended on ventricular estimation, doubtless a cerebellar operation would have been performed and his tumor would have been missed.

This patient was blind from intracranial pressure but had absolutely no signs of the tumor's location. The accompanying ventriculograms indicate the location of the tumor and oversize of the lateral ventricles — surely normal for this individual and not increased in any conceivable way by the tumor's pressure. Despite the great size of the tumor — 143.5 grams — a dural endothelioma — this ventricle still yielded 30 cubic centimeters of fluid, an amount which would easily indicate a hydrocephalic ventricle. The tumors was completely enucleated and an uninterrupted recovery followed.

It will be seen from these ventriculograms that the tip of the posterior horn extends so nearly to the surface of the brain that the ventricular needle would have to penetrate only about 1 centimeter of brain tissue to reach it. Such a finding could easily lead to the assumption that the ventricle was greatly dilated.

Probably an even greater element of error in the use of this method is in cases of hydrocephalus. Bilateral hydrocephalus may develop from tumors of the pituitary, third ventricle, pineal body, cerebellum and brain-stem, or more precisely from tumors which can produce an obstruction anywhere between the foramina of Monro and the foramen of Magendie, i.e., roughly about three-quarters of the longitudinal extent of the brain. From the interpreta-

tion of the findings of ventricular estimation as just described, on the law of probability the tumor would be in the posterior cranial fossa, but a very high percentage of cases with bilateral hydrocephalus are in the middle and not the posterior cranial fossa. Tumors of the pituitary, third ventricle, and some tumors of the pineal body, can be eliminated by the indigocarmin test. The elimination of these growths (of ever-inrceasing importance) reduces the chances of error to the small group of tumors of the pineal and of the contiguous part of the brain, i.e., those tumors which occlude the aqueduct of Sylvius but do not close the foramina of Monro. From a practical standpoint, however, the chance of curing or even temporarily relieving a patient in coma from bilateral hydrocephalus when the tumor lies elsewhere than in the posterior cranial fossa is slight. In the presence of a *bilateral* hydrocephalus, the two lateral ventricles communicating, there is justification, from a practical standpoint, of a cerebellar exploration. And with the dye test, practically all tumors of the posterior fossa can be found at operation.

EXCLUSION OF TUMORS BY VENTRICULAR ESTIMATION

Coma resulting from other intracranial lesions simulating tumor — chronic meningitis. At times other conditions may produce coma which is very difficult or even impossible to differentiate from that of brain tumor. This is particularly true when coma is so far advanced that there is not time for extended examination. Such a case was recently seen in consultation with Dr. Horning of York, Pennsylvania.

The patient, a large strong man of fifty-five years, had been in partial coma for forty-eight hours. He was then deeply unconscious, though deep supra-orbital pressure brought response. The respirations were characteristically of Cheyne-Stokes type. Until two weeks ago he had seemed well in every way. Bifrontal headaches beginning at that time quickly became so severe that he was forced to bed. The headaches had been practically constant and of steadily increasing intensity. When he attempted to walk his gait was like that of a drunken person and unless supported he would fall. A squint appeared about a week ago. Urinary and fecal incontinence developed with coma. A choked disc of 4 diopters completely obliterated both nerve heads. Pulse 70; temperature 99.6°; blood pressure 185-100. The urine contained a few cells and more than a trace of albumin. On two examinations previously made by Dr. Horning, a trace of albumin was found. Left cardiac dullness extended 13.5 centimeters from the midline; the heart sounds were clear. There was no oedema of the eyelids or ankles. Aside from a slight abducens palsy, the neurological examination revealed no positive findings. The reflexes were equal and normal, no Babinski or ankle clonus; no difference in the muscle tone of the two sides. There was no history of a blow on the head. There was no rigidity of the neck.

The cause of the coma was by no means clear. A cardio-vascular-renal syndrome was considered. The blood pressure of 185, trace of albumin and white cells in the urine, made a nephritic condition possible, but these findings did not seem sufficient for such profound intracranial as well as systemic changes. On the other hand, the history of headaches of only two weeks' duration before the onset of coma, is most unusual for an intracranial tumor. But all of his symptoms had been referable to the head, i.e., headache, staggering gait, and strabismus; these and a bilateral choked disc made an encephalopathy clear. A brain tumor seemed the most plausible explanation of all the facts in our possession and possibly a cerebellar tumor because of the staggering gait. But the evidence was not conclusive even that it was a tumor, largely because the history was too short and the symptoms and coma too fulminating (not impossibilities, however). Nor were we willing to make a positive localization to the cerebellum; staggering gait might be due to weakness, intensity of headache, or dizziness. Ventricular estimation tests showed both lateral ventricles large (25 cubic centimeters easily obtained) and indigocarmin easily passed from one ventricle to the other. The ventricular fluid was under pressure. If a tumor, it was therefore not in either cerebral hemisphere, but must be in the posterior fossa. If a tumor was in the posterior cranial fossa, the dye would not pass into the cisterna magna or the spinal subarachnoid space. A spinal puncture or an Ayer's puncture or exposure of the cisterna magna would determine the presence or absence of such a tumor. Because of the great danger of lumbar punctures and of Ayer punctures in intracranial tumors, we were forced for reasons of safety to a direct exposure of the cisterna.

The presence of the dye on quantity precluded a tumor and made the diagnosis of hydrocephalus of the communicating type due to some condition other than a tumor. The cisterna magna was oversize and the cerebellar tonsils were not herniated into the foramen magnum. Both of these findings made a cerebellar tumor highly improbable. Hydrocephalus of this character is probably due to an increased production of fluid rather than to an obstruction with decreased absorption. Possibly in this case it may have been due to a cardio-vascular-renal syndrome, though this is by no means yet clear. Death came thirty hours later. A complete necropsy was made by Dr. MacCallum. He reports a mild chronic inflammatory process along the base of the brain. The condition was doubtless, therefore, a chronic meningitis of unknown origin. Bacteria were not found. There was no tumor in the brain. However, we are concerned here only with the diagnosis and elimination of the tumor.

SUMMARY OF CASES

About six months ago, a left craniotomy was performed on a patient in the terminal stages of coma from intracranial pressure, presumably due to a tumor or abscess. The sole means of determining upon which side the exploration should be made was a Jacksonian convulsion beginning in the right hand. Though considered a most trustworthy localizing manifestation, it proved misleading on this occasion, for at necropsy an abscess was found in the right frontal lobe, i.e., it was homolateral to the side of the convulsion. During the operation, information was gained from the lateral ventricle which led us to the adoption of a procedure which we may call "estimation of the cerebral ventricles." Its object is to localize growths in such emergencies. The information leading to this end is derived from a determination of the capacity, location, and intercommunication of the cerebral ventricles, particularly the lateral ventricles. Since this first case, five other patients have been seen in coma from intracranial pressure. In none of them was there any information obtainable, either from the history of friends and relatives or from the restricted objective examination of the unconscious patient, which was considered of merit in determining the location of the lesion. In four of these patients the lesion was a tumor and in the fifth an acute hydrocephalus of chronic meningitis origin. In the last case, a tentative diagnosis of tumor was made but given up as a result of the "ventricular estimation" tests. Possibly an analysis of the fluid at the time might have shown an increased cell count, but unfortunately this examination was not made because the fluid was blood-stained. The Wassermann from the ventricular fluid was negative. Each of the four tumors was correctly localized by these tests and in each instance the tumor was found at operation and removed. Two of these patients succumbed on the following day and the other two, after complete removal of dural endotheliomata, recovered and are now entirely well.

SUMMARY OF REASONS FOR VENTRICULAR ESTIMATION

Three determinations are made: (1) The position of the lateral ventricles by the ventricular puncture; (2) the size of each lateral ventricle by measurement of amount of ventricular fluid aspirated from each lateral ventricle; (3) the communicability of the lateral ventricles (or other parts of the cerebrospinal system) by injecting indigocarmin into a lateral ventricle and then aspirating fluid elsewhere (de-

pending on part of the ventricular system to be tested).

If we know the actual size of each lateral ventricle, we can infer, with a certain degree of accuracy, whether a tumor can exist in either cerebral hemisphere. If one lateral ventircle is small (or collapsed) and the other larger, a tumor will probably be on the side of the small ventricle (with exceptions). If both lateral ventricles are large, a tumor will probably not be in either hemisphere but in the posterior cranial fossa (with more exceptions). The exceptions are principally instances in which hydrocephalus results from tumors in the middle or even at times the anterior cranial fossa. The indigocarmin test is principally useful in eliminating and identifying these exceptions. From its use we are usually able to say whether there is any obstruction in the ventricular system anterior to the aqueduct of Sylvius. An obstruction anterior to the aqueduct of Sylvius will (with exceptions) prevent the dye from passing from one lateral ventricle to the other. On occasions, which are probably not frequent, it is necessary to know whether an obstruction exists at or posterior to the aqueduct of Sylvius; this is almost equal to determining whether a tumor or some other condition is causing the coma. For information of this character, it is necessary to inject the dye and test for its presence in the cisterna magna (or spinal canal). It is safer to expose the cisterna magna by operation than to employ lumbar puncture. It is only when both ventricles are so nearly occluded that only a few drops of fluid can be obtained, that we are forced to rely solely upon the information from a ventricular puncture. A definite displacement of both lateral ventricles will then indicate the location of the growth. It is, of course, possible even with large tumors that there may be no dislocation, or at best it will not be sufficiently marked to draw any conclusions. I have seen such a case at necropsy: a tumor arising in the midline had grown to each side and occluded practically all of the posterior three-fourths of both lateral ventricles. This in one of the situations in which the method is defective.

SUMMARY OF ARGUMENTS FOR AND AGAINST VENTRICULAR ESTIMATION

The method is relatively simple, easily performed, relatively harmless, and requires very little time. The principal danger to life is in puncturing an intraventricular haemorrhage. Though this is always an actual danger, it is not deterrent when we consider the magnitude of the problem of saving an unconscious patient. It requires very little, and at times no extra, time, but the relief of intracranial pressure by release of fluid is more than compensatory. The greatest drawback is the possibility of an incorrect localization. Were it not for this very great element of error (described above), the procedure could be used as a substitute for cerebral pneumography. But the element of error is of such magnitude that the procedure should be used only in emergencies, where the more precise methods would add danger to an already overstrained intracranial tension. I am not so certain that in time it may not appear advisable to use it in cases of hydrocephalus, but at present this does not seem indicated. There are many instances where we could have made the correct localization of an intracranial tumor by this method and spared the patient discomfort and a certain degree of danger, but there are other tumors which would surely have been missed at operation had it alone been employed. The treatment of brain tumors is always too serious and too all-dependent on a precise localization, to run the risks of an incorrect operation based upon a mistaken diagnosis which has been made with even an element of chance or guesswork.

REFERENCES

[1] I regret that press of time has so far precluded the publication in detail of the large series of brain tumors in which the use of cerebral pneumography has been the means of localizing the growth. It is hoped that this may appear in the ensuing year.

[1] We formerly used phenolsulphonephathalein for this test but if quantitative determinations are not necessary, indigocarmin will do just as well. Apparently it is not irritating, whereas phenosulphonephthalein, even when carefully prepared, may be very decidedly so.

For some time we have injected indigocarmin into a lateral ventricle as a routine procedure in all cases where a cerebellar operation is performed for tumor. It gives a striking objective demonstration of the location of the tumor, for the dye will not appear until the obstruction has been reached and passed and, if by chance the hydrocephalus is not due to tumor, the pressure of the dye in the cisterna magna will be excellent proof.

[1] Other comatose patients afflicted with brain tumors have been operated upon during this period, but they have had signs which have indicated the location of the growth. The cases here reported are all in whom the procedure has been used since its adoption.

XVII

THE DIAGNOSIS AND LOCALIZATION OF SPINAL CORD TUMORS *

Surgery produces few results more brilliant than the restoration of function following the extirpation of spinal cord tumors. Although the only possibility of a cure to patients so afflicted is by total removal of the neoplasm, defects in the methods of diagnosis and localization have, until recently, withheld from many the fruits of operative procedures. Fortunately, these deficiencies have so far been overcome that it now seems possible not only to diagnose and accurately localize every spinal cord tumor, but also to confidently exclude tumors in the differential diagnosis. These advances make possible precise surgical treatment for tumors and they eliminate exploratory laminectomies when the lesion is not a tumor.

Until Froin's [1] discovery (1903) that a yellow heavy albumen cloud—"Xanthochromie et coagulation massive"—was a sign of spinal compression, the diagnosis and localization of spinal cord tumors was made solely upon a careful history and neurological examination. Froin's syndrome was the beginning of a series of important chemical, microscopic, hydrostatic, and hydrodynamic tests of the spinal fluid, of punctures other than the routine lumbar puncture, and finally of mechanical aids by injections of extraneous materials into the spinal canal.

Soon after Froin's discovery it was found that a very slight increase of protein in the spinal fluid, often so slight as to be demonstrable only by delicate chemical reactions, was nearly as significant as the heavier cloud of Froin's syndrome. But neither an increase in globulin nor the

presence of xanthochromie is pathognomonic of a spinal cord tumor, for both are often present in other lesions of the spinal cord and in many intracranial lesions including tumors. An increased globulin content of spinal fluid, therefore, only indicates a lesion of the central nervous system and is of no localizing importance.

Another method advanced by Pierre Marie, Foix, and Robert [2] (1913) made it possible not only to eliminate intracranial tumors, but also to localize tumors of the spinal cord within certain rather wide limits. They introduced *double* spinal punctures. Carefully examining the cerebrospinal fluid from each of these punctures, they discovered qualitative differences in the spinal fluid above and below a tumor—"l'hyperalbuminose, presque nulle dans le liquide superieur, etait au contraire considerable dans le liquide inferieur." But punctures of the spinal canal above the cauda equina carry such obvious potentialities of harm that they have never become more than locally popular. Moreover, only by chance or by repeated punctures could a tumor be localized with even a fair degree of accuracy. The introduction of the cisternal puncture in animals by Wegeforth, Ayer and Essick [3] (1919) opened up this field of study anew. Ayer [4] (1920) soon made clinical application of the cisternal puncture, and in a large series of spinal cord lesions, with and without a block of the spinal canal, used the cisternal puncture in combination with lumbar punctures. He verified and greatly amplified the findings of Marie, Foix and Robert in painstaking studies of the fluids above and below tumors. Though seemingly dang-

*Reprinted from *Annals of Surgery*, January, 1925.

erous, this brillant method has been shown by the reports of cases now in the thousands to be quite safe, at least in competent hands.

Ayer also made use of an even more important test in connection with these double punctures, namely the differences in the pressure of the spinal fluid above and below the spinal block. At the cisterna magna the pressure of the cerebrospinal fluid was always higher than at the lumbar canal when there was a complete block between these two points of puncture; but these pressures were always identical when the spinal canal was not occluded. For example, when the intracranial pressure is artificially raised by venous congestion resulting from compression of the jugular veins, the cisternal pressure (being the intracranial pressure) was instantly raised to a much higher level and as quickly subsided when the jugular compression was released. During the same test the lumbar spinal pressure would rise to an equal height if there was no intervening obstruction, but a block in the spinal canal above the lumbar puncture would prevent the transmission of the increased intracranial pressure to the lumbar puncture and its level would remain practically unchanged.

Antedating the studies of Ayer, and appearing shortly after those of Marie, Foix, Robert and Bouttier,[5] was the method of Queckenstedt[6] (1916). Using lumbar punctures alone, he first observed that the pressure in the lumbar canal rose following compression of both jugular veins when there was no obstruction in the spinal canal, but that the spinal pressure did not materially change when an obstruction existed in the canal. This test is very much simpler than the methods of Marie, Foix and Robert and of Ayer and gives as much information of practical value. By obtaining all the available data from the use of Queckenstedt's method, *i.e.,* chemical, microscopic examination of the spinal fluid, together with the hydrostatic and hydrodynamic studies, it has

been claimed that it is possible to obtain all the information necessary to diagnose or eliminate a total block of the spinal subarachnoid space. There are, however, tumors — as I shall show — with only partial closure of the spinal canal and which escape detection by Queckenstedt's test; but for the same reason they will also be missed by the other procedures mentioned.

The surgical treatment of spinal cord tumors demands both a correct diagnosis and a precise localization, but by none of the above methods can a localization be obtained. With this problem in mind, the author[7] conceived the idea of replacing some of the cerebrospinal fluid by something which would cast a shadow in the x-ray. The delicate spinal cord would not tolerate any of the rontgenologically opaque solutions which were used at that time for the diagnosis of urological lesions. Air (including other gases) then seemed to be the only solution of the problem—it was readily absorbed and had possibilities of shadow production because its density was less than the cerebrospinal fluid which it replaced, the spinal cord, and the tumor to which it was brought into juxtaposition. It was hoped that the upper level of air would define the lower level of tumors or other obstructions in the spinal canal, and that the presence of air in the cranial chamber owuld eliminate a tumor with certainty.

At that time it was shown (1) that the spinal cord could be thrown in relief by the surrounding column of air; (2) that obstructions in the cisterna pontis could be precisely located, and (3) in one case a tumor of the spinal cord was strongly suspected but eliminated by the air test —operation subsequently showing the lesion to be a constriction of the cord resulting from an old inflammation. The paucity of material at that time prevented the actual demonstration of a tumor localization for which the method was intended. Soon thereafter, Wideroe[8] (1921) and Jacobeus[9] (1921) located spinal cord

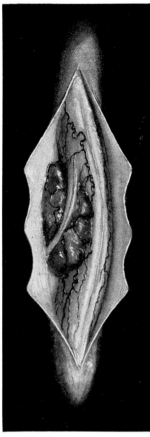

Fig. 1. Endothelioma apparently arising from the pia-arachnoid showing a nerve root running over its surface.

tumors by this method, though the shadows were rather vague and looked upon as easily susceptible of erroneous interpretation.

This communication was originally intended to present the results obtained from a series of intraspinous injections of air, but the brilliant discovery of Sicard [10] makes necessary a reconsideration of the entire subject. What seemed impossible has been accomplished. Sicard has discovered and utilized an oil (lipiodol) which holds sufficient iodine in suspension to cast a heavy shadow in the x-ray. Lipiodol can be injected into the spinal canal without pain either immediately or subsequently, and apparently without any harmful effect. The oil can be made to gravitate to the tumor's level where its rontgenographic shadow will mark the tumor's location. A detracting feature is that the oil remains indefinitely in the spinal canal, but Sicard's reports lead us to believe that this prolonged stay is not harmful.

From a careful analysis of our series of spinal cord tumors during recent years, I have attempted to estimate the relative importance of these accessory diagnostic aids; in how many cases a careful neurological examination will fail to give all the information necessary both for diagnosis and localization; and, when necessary, which tests are advisable. I have included in this survey a brief account of the tumors and the operative results.

There are 36 consecutive cases of spinal cord tumors in this series; all, with two exceptions, have been verified by operation during the past six years. The exceptions were a gumma diagnosed by clinical tests and cured by antisyphilitic therapy, and a high cervical tumor which was found at necropsy. Included under the broad designation of tumor are chronic inflammatory lesions which, by their steady growth and tumor formation, give symptoms similar to those of true neoplasms; and they demand the same treatment.

THE PATHOLOGY OF SPINAL CORD TUMORS

There is no single satisfactory method by which tumors of the spinal cord can be grouped—a story not unlike that of intracranial tumors. Although a cytological classification is on the whole the safest and would appear to be the ultimate solution for all tumors, the histological picture of neoplasms of the central nervous system is still susceptible of too many interpretations to be used exclusively as a differentiator. Particularly is this true in the differentiation of gliomata from sarcomata, and again in the separation of sarcomata from endotheliomata. Doctor Bloodgood [11] has shown how unreliable is even expert opinion on the purely his-

TABLE 1

Meningeo-mata	Extradural Neuromata	Other Benign Tumors	Inflammatory	Glioma and Sarcoma	Carcinoma
10 cases Ages: 27, 40, 40, 41, 47, 47, 56, 58, 59, 62	4 cases Ages: 25, 38, 38, 50	(1) O s t e o m a from body of vertebra @ 51 (2) Embryonal fibrous tumor arising in body of vertebra, piercing dura @ 14 (3) Shell of bone between dura and leptomeninges @ 22 (4) Angioma @ 59 (5) Angioma @ 58 (6) Angiofibroma arising in thorax @ 19	(1) Gumma @ 37 (2) Tubercle (intra-medullary) @ 30 (3) Post-inflammatory diffuse lesion @ 49 (4) Extradural tuber-culoma @ 27 (5) Extradural mass of s t a p h y l o-coccus aureus origin @ 42	9 cases Ages: 11, 11, 12, 14, 15, 29, 29, 33, 45	2 cases. Ages: 46, 54.
Total 10	4	6	5	9	2

tological interpretation of tumors of the breast. The histological diagnoses of tumors of the brain and spinal cord are equally as faulty.

I have made no attempt to clarify these defects of classification. Rather, I have avoided attempts at finer differentiation. For example, gliomata and sarcomata have been grouped together. A typical glioma is entirely different both in the gross and under the microscope from a typical sarcoma, but there are many intermediate pictures in which the personal equation largely determines into which class they belong. From a practical standpoint, they are essentially alike; neither is curable by extirpation.

Under meningeomas have been grouped tumors arising both from the dura and from the leptomeninges. There are seven of the former and three of the latter. There can be no question of the derivation of the dural tumors because of their firm outgrowth from the dura. Many of these contain numerous psammomas bodies and they are often classified under psammomas. Presumably those which have no such attachment and lie loosely imbedded in the pia-arachnoid, and seemingly do not arise from a spinal nerve, have their origin in the leptomeninges.

Although the character of many tumors is easy to determine, in others all the available information — from the operat-ing table, the gross and microscopic examinations—should be utilized before attempting interpretation. A tumor easily recognized as a dural endothelioma may, by microscopical examination alone, be reported as a sarcoma. As a matter of fact, there are few tumors which the trained surgeon cannot recognize almost as well at the operating table as under the microscope — certainly the differentiation between a malignant and benign tumor can rarely be open to question when the tumor is exposed at the operation. I believe the differentiation of gliomata and sarcomata from the gross inspection at operation, both of the tumor's character and its point of origin, is on the whole safer. Before grouping gliomata and sarcomata together, I tabulated only two of the former and seven of the latter, basing the separation on the origin of the tumor within the cord (glioma) or without the cord (sarcoma). In two of the seven cases grouped as sarcomata, the point of origin was apparently in the lumbar enlargement. At least the tumors penetrated the cord but, except for this small part, the great mass of the tumor was free in the spinal canal, tightly packing but not invading the nerve roots of the cauda equina into the sacral canal. They are well recognized by neurologists and surgeons as a fairly well defined type of slowly growing tumors with insidiously developing symptoms. Adson [12] refers to them as ependymal gliomata. Their point of origin would seem to indicate that this view is probably correct, though their gross appearance is more like sarcomata.

It will be evident that gliomata are far less frequent than the same type of tumors in the brain. This is probably due to the smaller volume, both relative and absolute, of the glia owing to the great concentration of the nerve paths in the spinal canal. Conversely, the meningeomata are relatively far more frequent in the cord than in the brain.

Aside from these two great groups of tumors, one is impressed with the great number of totally different and unusual tumors affecting the spinal cord. There are no less than eighteen different varieties of tumors in this small series of thirty-six cases. The presence of only two cases of carcinoma in our series might appear to indicate that metastases to the spine were rare. Unfortunately, they are exceedingly common, but their clinical recognition makes operation unnecessary. They are therefore, not included among our certified tumors.

The extradural neuromata (4) are all very hard, perfectly encapsulated fibrous tumors. The fibrous tissue is irregularly arranged in layers, whorls, and pallisades. Into each a sensory and also motor nerve were traced, but the structure of the nerves was soon lost in the tumor. Each tumor had a dumb-bell shape, being constricted in the intervertebral foramen and expanding mesially but extradurally in the spinal canal and externally against the pleura. It seems probable that the point of origin of these tumors is at the point of its constriction—*i.e.,* in the intervertebral canal and possibly from the ganglion. Two of our four cases were so full of giant cells as to suggest the histological diagnosis of giant-cell sarcoma.

Of unusual interest are the extrathecal inflammatory lesions, which behave like very rapidly growing tumors. One of these was tuberculous, the other apparently due to staphylococcus aureus. In each the attenuated organism had invaded the fat between the laminae and the dura. Multiple minute foci were surrounded by a dense fibrous mass which, because of its increasing size, assumed the character of a tumor and compressed the cord. The tuberculous mass followed a local trauma. Our presumptive diagnosis was a tuberculous abscess, despite the fact that there was no involvement of a vertebral body. The diagnosis of the staphylococcus mass was only suspected when the level of the tumor was marked on the skin. It was found to bisect the scar resulting from the healing of a severe carbuncle. This coincidence at once suggested that the old carbuncle, which shortly preceded the symptoms, was responsible for a secondary inflammatory mass outside the spinal canal; the high cell count (45) supported this hypothesis.

One other exceptional type of tumor, or possibly pseudotumor, was a shell of bone surrounding the posterior half of the spinal cord and cauda equina for a length of at least nine vertebrae. It lay between the dura and pia-arachnoid and, though snugly imbedded except in one short space where a nerve root tunnelled the bony formation, it was nowhere firmly attached. I have seen no reference to any such formation in the literature and have little to offer in its explanation. In a way, it suggests, on a grand scale, the pia-arachnoid plaques which one so frequently sees in explorations of the spinal cord. The two angiomata deserve special mention. Both were entirely venous and therefore without pulsation. The gross appearance was that of a mass of worm-like venous channels which entirely obscured the dorsal half of the cord from view. One was a single and sharply defined mass 8 cm. long, the other consisted of one large cluster and several smaller discrete patches joined together by a tortuous mid-dorsal vein. On removing these masses, one sees that one or more of the veins enter the substance of the cord.

In explorations of the cord, less pronounced but very definite venous masses are not infrequently encountered; presumably they cause no harm, but their detection may misdirect the operator's search away from the real lesion. I have been guilty of one such mistake, the tumor (one vertebra higher than the angioma) being found and removed a year later. Curiously, his symptoms disappeared after removal of the angioma, and reappeared several months later, and the new sensory level was two segments higher than at the former admission.

The remaining tumors of interest will be briefly considered under "Operability of Tumors."

OPERABILITY OF SPINAL CORD TUMORS

The high percentage of operable intraspinal tumors is in striking contrast to that of the intracranial chamber with which it is natural to seek a comparison. The outstanding reason for this difference is the very favorable ratio of meningeomata to gliomata. Fourteen (40 per cent) of this series of 36 tumors are encapsulated fibrous tumors: meningeomata (10) and extradural neuromata (4). All except one were totally extirpated, without mortality, and in none has there been any evidence of recurrence. The single exception was a leptomeningeal tumor on the ventral side of the first and second cervical vertebrae and just protruding into the intracranial chamber. It was an accidental finding at necropsy. The only difference of importance between tumors arising from the dura and tumors of the leptomeninges is that the former are harder, very firmly attached to the dura, and more difficult of removal. If their attachment is on the ventral or ventrolateral part of the dura, the removal becomes even a greater undertaking because the spinal cord must be gently retracted to the side to give room for extirpation. If the dural tumor is situated laterally or dorsally, it is always preferable to excise the dural attachment also and transplant in its stead a piece of fascia. When attached on the ventral aspect, the dural venous sinuses prevent excision of the dura; the operator must then be content with scraping the dura, but even after such treatment there has been no instance of recurrence. It is often best to first remove the interior of the tumor and then the capsule. This plan of attack is principally applicable in the ventral or ventrolateral tumors, or when the tumor is relatively large. The intracapsular removal gives more room and allows the collapsed tumor to fall away from the spinal cord. The most important feature of any tumor extirpation is the avoidance of injury to the spinal cord. Resection of one or even two unimportant sensory roots, and at times even a thoracic motor root when the tumor is situated ventrally, allows the cord to be drawn away so that it can be covered with a layer of moist cotton which acts as an effective buffer to traumatic insults when working on the tumor.

The tumors arising from the pia-arachnoid are just as encapsulated (Fig. 1) but, the attachment being of a filmy nature, they can be easily elevated from their bed in toto. The neuromata are even more favorable for extirpation. Being entirely extradural the spinal cord is not exposed and is protected from operative injury by the intervening dura. It is necessary to remove the pedicles and transverse processes of the contiguous vertebrae in order to thoroughly expose the tumor and permit its safe extirpation. The transparent pleura and the moving lung beneath it afford a beautiful picture after the tumor has been removed.

Unless the paralysis has endured too long, perfect restoration of function will usually follow extirpation of all of these tumors. The single exception was a patient whose limbs were firmly fixed in contraction and in whom, aside from a bilateral Babinski, no reflexes could be elicited. Sensory, motor, and sphincter functions had been totally abolished for two and a half years.

When one sees the deep depression in the spinal cord produced by one of these tumors—usually the spinal cord seems reduced to about one-half its normal cross-section—one marvels at the perfect function that returns. The conclusion can be safely drawn that despite this gross depression in the cord, the fibre tracts are still intact for some time after complete paraplegia develops. Only the transmission of impulses is blocked. Doubtless much of the reduction in size of the cord is due to loss of water and of the vascular bed—a protective compensation similar to that which has been shown to exist, but to a much greater extent, in tumors and destructive lesions in the cranial chamber.[13] The rapidity of return of function after removal of the tumor is remarkable. If paralysis has not been longer than a few weeks, movements will frequently begin in thirty-six to forty-eight hours, and the patient will be able to walk out of the hospital in less than a month. The longer the paralysis has persisted, the slower will functions return, but even after paralysis of several months' duration, complete return of function will follow, though it will be much slower. The quick recovery of motor and sensory power after removal of spinal cord tumors is apparently quite analogous to the quick return of vision after extirpation of pituitary tumors—the functions in both instances being "physiologically blocked."

In addition to the possible perfect results from this group of encapsulated tumors, there are eight other cases of diverse nature in which a perfect recovery resulted —six following extirpation of the tumor, one after antisyphilitic treatment, and one following radium. From the total of thirty-six tumors, therefore, there are 21, or 60 per cent, which could be totally extirpated or otherwise so treated that complete restoration of function will result. These statistics are identical with those of Adson.[14] In addition, there is a patient afflict-

ed with a venous angioma who improved so rapidly after its removal that he walked out of the hospital, but who has since been lost to view. While there is reason to believe he is also cured, the proof of subsequent reports is lacking. The other six benign tumors which were completely extirpated with restoration of function are: (1) A tumor in a girl of fourteen, produced a characteristic Brown-Sequard syndrome. This tumor was surely of congenital origin, for it filled the body of the sixth cervical vertebra, leaving the bony cortex intact except at the point of perforation. Piercing the bony shell posteriorly, it perforated the spinal dura laterally and flared out into an intraspinal tumor which caused her symptoms. The entire tumor, both within the spinal canal and the body of the vertebra, was shelled out intact. She has remained perfectly well three years. Histologically, the tumor is like that of a dural meningeoma. (2) A sharply defined finger-like osteoma projecting from the body of the vertebra into the anterior surface of the cord; patient *aet.* fifty-one. (3) Six years ago a remarkable shell of bone lying over the dorsal half of the cord between the dura and the pia and extending from the ninth thoracic to the first lumbar vertebrae, inclusive, was removed from a girl *aet.* twenty-two. Five years later, and after complete recovery of function, motor weakness again developed and a bony shell of exactly the same type was removed from the second to the fifth lumbar vertebrae, inclusive. Curiously, this slab of bone had five articulations, whereas the former specimen was solid, the difference doubtless being due to the effect of the fixed and movable vertebrae. (4) An extrathecal solid tubercle with well-defined limits was removed from a girl of twenty-seven, and (5) a very hard fibrous inflammatory mass containing many small subacute foci had formed extradurally in a man of forty-two, several weeks after a carbuncle had healed directly over the site of the present tumor.

In the last two cases the return of power

has been slower. A study of the differences in time necessary for function to return suggests a rule that the rapidity of functional return is inversely proportional to the rapidity of functional loss from the tumor's growth. A rapidly growing tumor strangulates the cord and injures it, whereas a slowly growing tumor gives the cord a chance to gradually adapt itself to the intruder.

The only gumma in the series was in a woman *aet.* thirty-seven, who was on the service of Professor Thomas. There was complete block of the spinal canal. The symptoms and signs were those of a Brown-Sequard hemi-lesion. Until the Wassermann of the spinal fluid was found to be positive, the lesion was considered to be a tumor. Under antisyphilitic treatment, recovery was complete and she has remained well for three years. The last tumor to be included with those completely yielding to treatment, was in a girl of nineteen. Five (5) years ago she entered the hospital because of a rapidly developing paraplegia and loss of sphincter control. The x-ray disclosed a very large intrathoracic shadow. The intraspinal growth was a prolongation of this thoracic tumor which had evaded the vertebrae and reached the spinal cord. Doctor Finney explored the thoracic tumor, found it to have expansile pulsation and to be inoperable. A needle was inserted into it and blood spurted from the lumen. A presumptive diagnosis of angiosarcoma was made; a small piece of tissue was removed for microscopic diagnosis, but unfortunately was lost. Seemingly hopeless, she was given radium treatment by Doctor Burnham, and quickly her paralysis began to clear. In a few months she had completely recovered and has remained well to the present time (five years). It is interesting to note that despite the disappearance of the spinal cord disturbance, the radium had no effect upon the size of the rontgenographic thoracic shadow. The thoracic tumor has never given her symptoms. This brilliant result from radium treatment,

however, has been exceptional. It is only fair to say that in nearly all the remaining inoperable cases radium has been tried, but without any noticeable benefit, and in two recent cases deep x-ray has been of no greater help. Possibly the vascular character of this unusual tumor was responsible for the marked susceptibility to radium, whereas tissues of the nervous system are more refractile.

The incurable spinal cord tumors, sarcomata and gliomata (9), carcinoma (2), tubercle (1), comprise thirty-three and one-third per cent of all the tumors in the series. Unfortunately, with few exceptions, there is no certain way by which the *character* of the tumor can be foretold. Xanthochromia usually indicates a glioma or sarcoma, but this is not invariably true; an inflammatory lesion and a dural edothelioma gave this color change. Ofttimes the existence of a metastatic tumor can be known by finding a primary growth, frequently but not always, in the pelvis. Many operations would be avoided if gliomata and sarcomata could be differentiated from the curable tumors, but in the absence of such positive information, exploration of the tumor is always indicated. But the operation on many incurable tumors is well worth while, for the removal of the laminae gives additional room, thereby acting as a decompression, effectively alleviating backache which is often excruciating; and at times a decompression may even permit a temporary return of some motor, sensory, or sphincter function by allowing tumors to "lift" from the spinal cord. The operative mortality in spinal cord tumors should be practically nil. There is one death in this series—from shock. This was one of the first of the series and followed removal of extensive multiple angiomata of the cord. This death would surely be avoided now. The completion of the operation in one stage, unless there are individual contra-indications, is practically always possible and preferable. In none of our cases have two stages been necessary. In children, often quite ill, it would be impossible to remove many of the extensive growths at one time, but these growths are mostly malignant or recurrent and attempted removal is not indicated; nor is it necessary to expose the entire extent of the tumor, unless to give a palliative decompression.

The operative technic needs little comment. The precise localization is all important. With this accomplished, the removal of laminae from two, or at most, three vertebrae, is adequate. Even in the cervical region this produces no noticeable weakness. I have no experience with hemilaminectomy. It is far better to remove all the laminae necessary than to hamper the exposure and removal of the tumor in the slightest degree. Ether anaesthesia has been used exclusively. Ether well administered has so few disadvantages in spinal cord surgery that, except in unusual conditions, the need of local or paravertebral anaesthesia, has never appeared—a marked contrast to many advantages of local anaesthesia in intracranial surgery. Far more important than any type of operation is the best possible exposure of the tumor, so that its removal is easy and free of danger to the cord. At times, despite scrupulous care in removing spinal cord tumors, urinary retention will develop. The treatment of this will be mentioned later.

THE CLINICAL FEATURES OF SPINAL CORD TUMORS

Probably the outstanding impression of our study of spinal cord tumors is the accuracy with which most spinal cord tumors can be diagnosed and localized, using only a careful history and neurological examination. It is exceptional when the information from these sources, backed by an experience which makes interpretations safe, is not adequate both for diagnosis and localization. Spinal cord tumors are so frequently overlooked because their frequency, both absolute and relative, is not appreciated. Given a gradually progressive bi-

lateral loss of motor power with spasticity, the burden of proof is on any diagnosis other than a spinal cord tumor. This is the most likely lesion and almost the only one offering the patient relief. If there is a sensory level in addition to the motor loss, the location of the tumor is at once precisely made. Rectal, and particularly vesical sphincter disturbances, though usually appearing much later, complete the great triad of symptoms resulting from spinal cord tumors. Other symptoms, though important, are of lesser significance.

Sensory Level. The most important of all objective determinations in spinal cord tumor suspects is the level of hypaesthesia or anaesthesia. Although usually easy to elicit, it may be very difficult, especially in tumors affecting the cauda equina. In thirty-five out of our thirty-six cases a sensory level was present, though in two of these it appeared only after a lumbar puncture. In the only case without a sensory level, the tumor was accidentally found at necropsy.

The importance of great care in the sensory examination is shown by the fact that in five of these thirty-five patients (14 per cent) a sensory level was missed by two of our examiners and picked up by the third. In each instance the sensory level was detected by testing for touch with a wisp of cotton. The finer changes in touch and pain denote a sensory level just as definitely as if there were a much greater hypaesthesia or even an anaesthesia.

Not infrequently there is a zone of one or two segments characterized by a lesser degree of hypaesthesia (occasionally there may be hyperaesthesia). This zone corresponds with the tumor's level and is doubtless due to its local effect. Although diminished sensation is usually bilateral and symmetrical at the time the patient comes to the physician for help, it may at times be unilateral.

Two patients in this series presented the Brown-Sequard syndrome, so characteristic of lateral hemi-lesions of the cord.

In each this unilateral hemianaesthesia, contralateral to the lesion, and upper segment motor paralysis with loss of muscle sense on the side of the lesion, were detected by Professor Thomas. Both were cervical tumors, one a fibroma, the other a gumma. While under observation, the signs in each case changed from those of a strictly hemi-lesion of the cord to changes indicating partial involvement of the other half also. A careful history of many patients will give a story of a hemi-lesion and almost always of a partial hemi-lesion. Not only sensation but also motor disturbances appear on one side, days, weeks, months, or even years (in one patient two years) before the other side.

A careful history of the sequence of, events will often tell in which part of the cross-section of the spinal canal the tumor is located. Initial sensory disturbances suggest a tumor on the posterior aspect of the cord. Motor symptoms preceding sensory loss, indicate a tumor situated more anteriorly; and a Brown-Sequard syndrome may be looked upon as evidence, that the tumor is located laterally. The rapid progress of the signs and symptoms from one side of the body to the other, suggests that the tumor is either on the dorsal aspect of the cord or is intramedullary.

In a strikingly high percentage of these, patients, regardless of the location of the tumor in the cord, the subjective sensory changes have begun in the toes, and gradually progressed up the foot, leg, and the abdominal walls to the permanent sensory level. Doubtless, this is due to the topographical distribution of the sensory fibres in the cord.

Only once have two operations been necessary to find a tumor after determining the sensory level. One year after a negative exploration, the tumor was found one vertebra higher and in this interim the sensory level had shifted two segments upward. Possibly the sensory level on the first admission had been inaccurately made, though even a year later the diminished sensation was so slight as to have escaped detection until very delicate tests were used. At the first operation a well-defined angioma was removed from the dorsal surface of the cord at a level corresponding to the sensory findings at that time and, curiously, both sensory and motor symptoms almost entirely disappeared.

Motor Loss; Rigidity, and Flaccidity. Other disturbances of function included in the clinical picture, though of more concern to the patient, are of secondary value in making a localization of the growth. The chief complaint of practically every patient is a gradual motor loss and associated with this are the manifestations of upper motor segment paralysis —spasticity below the lesion and involuntary muscular jerkings (convulsions). There are exceptions to this rule, however. In two of our cases there was *complete flaccid paralysis*: in one the lesion was an extradural tubercle and in the other an extradural sarcoma; in both the progress of the disease was very rapid, seven and ten days, and on admission to the hospital the loss of power, sensation, and sphincter control was complete. Such a clinical picture is analogous to that accompanying a complete traumatic transverse section of the spinal cord. A third patient also had flaccid paralysis, but this was a sarcoma involving the cauda equina; and as lesions of the cauda equina involve peripheral nerves, a flaccid paralysis is to be expected.

Involuntary jerkings of the affected extremities are a frequent source of annoyance before complete paraplegia ensues and again when motor function is returning. Frequently they are described by patients as convulsions, which they doubtless are—though, of course, being of spinal origin they are without loss of conciousness. They probably occur, but in varying intensity, in most cases, though our records are not complete on this point. In only one case is there specific mention of their absence.

Pain. Three kinds of pain result from spinal cord tumors: (1) localized pain from direct involvement of the sensory nerves by the tumor, (2) pains from pressure on the sensory tracts in the cord, (3) aching from intraspinous pressure.

Localized pain along the course of a sensory nerve — so-called root-pain — was present in at least twelve, or one-third of our cases. The pain was always severe, at times of a sharp lancinating character, much like the lightning pains of tabes, at other times a constant dull aching pain. But always the location of the pain has been unchanged and without exception it has been unilateral. Usually these pains antedate the onset of the spinal cord symptoms. In one instance the pain had existed ten years, another four, one "a number of years," and several for many weeks or months. That the pain has been due to the tumor during all these months and years, is a safe deduction, because it always refers back to the nerve involved in the tumor. It may be significant that nine curable tumors, and the other three were sarcomata. In the three latter cases the pain preceded the cord symptoms by only two months. It would appear that the duration of this localized pain might be a useful prognostic sign. In none of the intramedullary tumors (there were only three, however) was there pain of this character. It is not to be expected that intramedullary tumors should produce this type of pain, for they do not implicate the spinal nerves. The distribution of this pain in the series was: "kidney region," three cases; "lower ribs" (1); down arm (2); in axilla (1); shoulder blade (2); left groin (1). One patient was subjected to a nephrotomy operation for a presumed kidney stone because of sharp attacks of pain in this region. Whether one will eventually be justified in making a diagnosis of a spinal nerve

or spinal cord tumor solely on the history of such a constant pain, is doubtful. As yet I know of no cases which have been operated from such a diagnosis.

Pain from pressure on tracts in the spinal cord at times also antedates both recognizable sensory and motor changes. In seven of our thirty-six cases such pains have been recorded. It is interesting to note that both intramedullary tumors (gliomata) had severe pains down both legs. Usually sensory loss appears soon after the onset of these pains, but in one case a tumor at the third dorsal vertebra gave tingling pains down the right leg two years before the left leg and four years before there was any noticeable motor or sensory disturbance. It is worthy of note that the tumor was situated more to the left side of the cord, *i.e.,* contralateral to the subjective pain. Seemingly in keeping with the progress of the subjective sensory changes noted above, practically all of these pains have radiated down the legs, regardless of the location of the tumor along the spinal cord. In a tumor at the first cervical segment, there had long been sharp shooting pains down both legs. In two cases the pain radiated "to the knees," in two there was burnnig sensation down the left leg, and in another the tingling pain was for a long time restricted to the big toe of one foot. In the remaining cases there was no restriction of the pain other than "down both legs."

Girdle sensations were mentioned in ten cases, though doubtless they were present more frequently than the records indicate. This very common complaint is merely the patient's interpretation of the sudden change between the normal and the disturbed sensation, a transition which is usually so symmetrical as to make the suggestion of a band quite applicable.

The remaining type of pain is really a backache and is due to the excessive pressure within the inexpansile walls of the vertebral canal. It is exactly analogous to headache from increased intracranial pressure and, like it, is relieved by the removal of the laminae—a spinal decompression. Backache of this character was present in fourteen cases. Its intensity varies, at times it is excruciating and is the outstanding complaint. It is always made worse by movement of the spine. The patients soon learn that the sitting position gives them the greatest comfort; at times they may be unable to lie down to sleep. The effect of posture on the alleviation of this pain is so characteristic that it is sometimes possible to make a snap diagnosis of spinal cord tumor when told that the patient can only obtain relief by the sitting posture.

Vesical and Rectal Disturbances. Not the least dreaded sequelae of spinal cord tumors—sphincter changes—were present in some degree in at least twenty-five of the thirty-six cases. That vesical control, previously unaffected, was lost in two cases immediately after lumbar puncture, is sufficient warning that this procedure is by no means harmless. Usually sphincter disturbances do not appear until both motor and sensory changes are quite advanced. The character of the urinary disturbance has varied. Typically, a hesitancy in urination preceded retention, and retention passes into incontinence, but this sequence is by no means constant. Not infrequently incontinence will be transient, control again restored, and later again be lost. At times incontinence may be the first expression of this disturbance. Although vesical and rectal loss of control are usually affected about the same time, bladder disturbances often appear first and exist for some time before the rectal sphincter is affected. In one case the patient was incontinent for urine eighteen months before rectal control was disturbed. In the two rapidly developing complete paraplegias, retention developed, though in one dribbling of urine first appeared and retention followed two days later. We are still unable to feel satisfied with any treatment of retention of urine, though it is our present belief that catheterization, with scrupulous cleanliness, carried out regularly every six or eight hours, probably carries less danger of cystitis and pyelitis than a retention catheter or by allowing the bladder to overflow.

Reflex Changes. Typically, the deep reflexes below the segment affected by the tumor are exaggerated; the abdominal reflexes are absent, Babinski reflexes present, and ankle clonus positive on both sides. As tumors, however, vary in the transverse injury of the spinal cord, there are modifications of this standard picture; often there is asymmetry in the reflexes on the two sides. For example, in the cord affections with a Brown-Sequard syndrome, the reflex changes appear only on the side of the tumor, the motor tracts on the opposite side being as yet unaffected. In complete or nearly transverse lesions, of which there are seven in the series, no reflexes were obtainable or if present were very feeble. Tumors of the cauda equina affecting the distal neurone should not and do not produce increase, but rather a decrease in these reflexes. In the two cauda tumors of our series, the reflexes were abolished, the paraplegia in each being almost complete and flaccid.

Ankle clonus was noted in fifteen of our cases, but doubtless the actual number is higher. In only five cases of the series were the abdominal reflexes unaffected.

Blood Wassermann. Examination of the blood for the Wassermann reaction was taken routinely in every case and with the single exception of the gumma was reported negative.

X-ray Examinations. Routine x-ray examination of the spine in the suspected zone was helpful in only two cases. In one there was a dense shadow of a great primary intrathoracic tumor, and in the other there was destruction of the transverse processes of the sixth and seventh

TABLE II
TABLE SHOWING THE INCIDENCE OF TUMORS ACCORDING TO DECADES

Age	1-10	11-20	21-30	31-40	41-50	51-60	61-70	Total
Benign	..	1	5	3	7	5	1	22
Malignant	1	5	2	2	3	1	..	14
Total	1	6	7	5	10	6	1	36

cervical vertebrae, and in addition a calcification of the cervical extension of the tumor. In one case where the body of the vertebra was filled with a fibrous tumor, and in another where the laminae were markedly eroded, subsequent examination of the x-ray plates still failed to disclose these defects. There are probably few tumors of the body lying adjacent to bone in which the x-ray is less helpful. This is not a reflection on the x-ray, but rather upon the rarity of bony changes, and also upon the background which makes difficult the detection of even considerable destruction of bone which may occasionally develop. Even very gross changes could hardly be evident except with stereoscopic vision. The well-known destructive changes in the vertebrae due to a carcinoma are excluded from this generalization. Except in rare instances, spinal cord tumors do not reach the interior of bodies of the vertebrae.

Age of Patients Afflicted with Tumors of the Spinal Cord. The accompanying table shows the frequency of benign and malignant tumors according to decades.

A few conclusions are warranted: (1) encapsulated, curable tumors are uncommon under the age of twenty, and the overwhelming proportion are malignant, (2) that benign encapsulated, curable tumors appear in a fairly even proportion between the ages of twenty and sixty, and (3) incurable tumors, though less frequent than benign, are also fairly evenly distributed during the same period; (4) from this series of cases 70 per cent of all tumors appearing after the second decade were removable and permanently curable.

Duration of Symptoms. The accompanying table indicates that from the duration of the patient's symptoms little inference can be drawn as to the curability or incurability, encapsulation or non-encapsulation of the tumor. It has always been our impression that very rapidly growing tumors are more probably malignant, and those of long duration are more suggestive of benign growths. While this impression still holds to some extent, there are too many exceptions to look upon it as more than a very rough indicator.

LUMBAR PUNCTURE AND SPINAL FLUID EXAMINATIONS

Twenty-four (24) of the thirty-six cases (66 per cent) had lumbar puncture and spinal fluid examinations. This is a much higher percentage than is now necessary. While there are no great contra-indications to spinal puncture, we have avoided subjecting patients to unnecessary examinations which are more or less painful, and which carry certain potentialities

TABLE III
TABLE SHOWING THE DURATION OF SYMPTOMS BEFORE ADMISSION FOR OPERATION

Age	3 Months	4–6 Months	7–12 Months	1–2 Years	2–3 Years	3–4 Years	4–5 Years	5 + Years	Total
Curable	..	2	3	5	3	1	4	4	22
Incurable..............	3	3	..	3	2	2	1	1	15
Total..............	3	5	3	8	5	3	5	5	37

of harm, even though they may be transient. Surely, if there is the least doubt as to the nature of the lesion, spinal punctures are necessary. I have previously noted that in three instances a sensory level suddenly appeared after a lumbar puncture. This information in two instances, however, was obtained at the cost of a sudden startling paraplegia and urinary retention. Elsberg and Stookey [15] report an increase in the patients symptoms in ten cases from their series. Although the removal of the tumors shortly afterwards always gives complete return of all functions, these sequelae of the puncture were naturally very alarming to the patients and made us wonder if a more careful sensory examination might not have detected the sensory level and made lumbar puncture unnecessary. The cause of the occasional sudden increase in spinal cord injury following lumbar puncture is not entirely clear, but it would seem that the sudden release of cerebrospinal fluid probably forces the tumor downward owing to the unrelieved and unopposed pressure above the tumor. It will be recalled that tumors produce deep depressions in the spinal cord, and dislocation of the tumor downward probably allows it to injure the part of the spinal cord which projects under the tumor. If such an explanation is correct, it would seem impossible that similar cord injuries could occur after cisternal puncture.

From examination of the spinal fluid in twenty-four cases, the following information was obtained: Xanthochromia was present in eight as follows: a long-standing dural meningeoma (slightly yellow), an extradural inflammatory mass, a tuberculous extradural mass, a gumma, three sarcomata, one extradural and two intradural, and one glioma. Globulin was recorded sixteen times; occasionally there was a slight increase, but usually a heavy (4+) cloud was present.

The cell count was recorded sixteen times as follows: one cell (4), two cells (2), three cells (2), four cells (3), nine cells (dural meningeoma), fourteen cells (extradural sarcoma), fifteen cells (extradural tuberculoma), forty-five cells (verified) (chronic staphylococcus extradural mass), and sixty-one cells (not verified) (evtradural sarcoma).

An increase in globulin, while not invariably present, is the usual finding and is present in all types of tumors. Xanthochromia was found only once in the intra- and extra-dural encapsulated fibromata and was present in three of the four inflammatory lesions and in many of the sarcomata and in the only glioma case from which fluid was obtained. Important as is this information, it can hardly be claimed that it is necessary either for diagnosis or localization after a careful neurological examination has been made.

AIR INJECTION ROUTINE. INTERPRETATION OF RESULTS

The procedure has been described in an earlier publication. [16] A syringe with a rubber connection containing a two-way cock is attached to the lumbar puncture needle. Ten (10) cc. of fluid is aspirated from the spinal canal and an equal amount of air injected. The patient is recumbent, but at an angle of about 50° to 60°, this position being assumed to allow the air to rise quickly in the spinal subarachnoid space and, unless an obstruction exists, to pass at once into the cranial subarachnoid space. When air reaches the head, the patient immediately complains of a fairly sharp pain, first in the posterior, then the middle, and then the anterior part of the side of the head which is uppermost. Usually these successive localizations of the air's progress are noted by the patient. *So constant and characteristic is this pain that it seems to be positive evidence that there is no complete block of the spinal canal. On the other hand, if the patient does not complain of pain in the head after a spinal injection, there must be a spinal block.* The rontgenographic evidence of the presence or absence of air in the cranial chamber in a series of cases has already substantiated the above subjective results. The presence of air in the cerebral ventricles or sulci denotes the absence of a total spinal block; the absence of air indicates a total block.

Variable amounts of air are injected, depending upon the individual case. If air reaches the head at once, 10 cc. will give as much information as any greater amount. If air does not pass into the cranial chamber, it is better to inject as much air as the spinal canal will hold in order to get the maximum effect of the air shadow for rontgenographic localization of the tumor. Below a tumor which occludes the spinal canal, air does not cause pain, ache, or any injurious effect, either immediately or subsequently. The absorption of the air from the spinal canal is sufficiently rapid to prevent any trouble. We have tried various positions of the spine with reference to the x-ray plate in order best to define the air shadow. We now take only a single stereoscopic plate, the patient lying on the back and the rays passing straight through. This position gives the constant dense background of the vertebral bodies, against which the artificial air shadow is best thrown in relief. In lateral or partial lateral views, the loss of this constant background makes difficult the evaluation of the spinal air shadow against the variable air and visceral shadows of the thorax and abdomen. Curiously, air in the spinal subarachnoid space produces practically no pain comparable with that in the cerebral subarachnoid space. However, nerve root pains resulting from the irritation of the air will radiate along the course of the nerves which are fixed by the tumor. Though usually unilateral, these pains may at times be bilateral. When a tumor is present these pains have always marked its location. However, I have occasionally observed similar pains, of more fleeting character and of less constancy, when no spinal block was present. Pains of this kind are, therefore, of importance as corroborative but not absolute evidence of a tumor's location.

An additional determination of interest and of some value is the quantity of air which can be aspirated when the spinal canal is blocked. In several instances, 30 cc. have been obtained when tumors were located in the mid and lower thoracic regions where most of our tumors have been. When that part of the spinal canal below the tumor has been drained of cerebrospinal fluid, as evidenced by the reaspiration of air, the volume of this part of the spinal canal can be estimated with fair accuracy. The value of this determination is that it roughly marks the region where the air level may be sought with the x-ray.

RESULTS AIR INJECTIONS

Case I. Mrs. D. H., aged forty-nine. Two negative explorations had been performed (one and one-half and two years ago) at another hospital for a presumed spinal cord tumor. The symptoms were of four and one-half years' standing. There is now complete paralysis of all muscles of lower extremities with strong contractures. Sensation ended sharply at the tenth thoracic segment. Loss of rectal and vesical control is complete. The spinal fluid was slightly yellow (Xanthochromia), 9 cells and 4+ globulin.

Queckenstedt's Test.—Indicates no obstruction; fluid beginning at 15 centimetres quickly rose to 40 with jugular compression and fell with release of the compression.

Air Injection.—Thirty cc. of fluid was aspirated and an equal amount of air was injected. More fluid could not be obtained. *Immediately after the air was injected, pain radiated to the kidney region on the right side.* For years this had been the site of her spontaneous pain. Headache did not follow. Skiagram of the head showed no air in the cerebral sulci. *The air column was plainly defined at the eighth thoracic verte-*

bra.

A dural endothelioma was completely removed, but due to the long duration of her paralysis no function had returned one year later.

Comment.—The history alone should easily have been adequate both for the diagnosis and localization of this tumor, the negative operations notwithstanding. It is interesting that after such a long period of growth (four and one-half years) Queckenstedt's test should still fail to show a block in the spinal canal; also, that air disclosed a complete block when Queckenstedt's test indicated a patent canal. Another point of importance is that the original pain was duplicated by the air test. The fact that only 30 cc. of fluid could be obtained (after which the air was reaspirated) was additional proof of an obstruction in the spinal canal and roughly indicated its location.

Case II. Mrs. E. S., aged forty-five. Pain and rigidity of back for four years, pain intensified by movement. Paralysis has been gradually increasing for over a year. There is a faint but definite sensory level at the twelfth thoracic segment on both sides. The ankle jerks are absent; Babinski negative. The spinal fluid is yellow, contains four cells, globulin 4+.

Queckenstedt's test indicates no obstruction.

Air Injection.—Thirty-five cc. of fluid was aspirated and the same amount of air injected. There were no referred pains or sensations and no headache following the injection. More fluid was not obtainable, only air being reaspirated with further trials. As an experiment, an additional amount of air was injected under pressure. The resistance to the injection was very distinct. At first nothing was noted, but there soon appeared pain in the head, and air-filled cerebral sulci were then demonstrable in the skiagram. Additional aspirations again brought only air into the syringe, showing that the obstruction of the spinal canal was still essentially complete. After all of these tests the skiagram showed a sharp tumor level at the eleventh (11) thoracic spine.

A very extensive glioma (entirely within the spinal cord), was found at oper-

ation. Extirpation was not attempted.

Comment.—Again the history and neurological examination should have been sufficient both for diagnosis and localization. Queckenstedt's test failed to show an obstruction, which the air test both indicated and accurately defined. It is of interest that with an increase of pressure, air could be forced past the obstruction. The amount of fluid which could be obtained from the spinal canal was about the same as in the preceding case.

Case III. W. W. is a colored boy, aged six, with gradually increasing paralysis of the lower limbs (more left). Backache has been very severe. There is a bilateral very faint sensory level at the first lumbar segment. The first and second lumbar spines are tender to deep pressure. Babinski is negative on both sides; left K. K. not obtainable; right normal. The spinal fluid is distinctly yellow; globulin 4+.

Queckenstedt's Test.—The spinal fluid rose from 180 to 300 on jugular compression and instantly fell to the original level on release of pressure, indicating that there is no obstruction in the spinal canal.

Air Injection.—At the same lumbar tap, 40 cc. of air was injected. More fluid could not be obtained. Headache did not follow the injection, nor were air-filled sulci present in the skiagrams of the head. The lower surface of the tumor was sharply defined as a conical shadow at the level of the first lumbar vertebra. Moreover, along each of the spinal nerves below the level of the tumor was an oval air shadow about a centimetre long. These pouches were dilatations of the subarachnoid space at the point of emergence of the spinal nerves, and were due to the high pressure of the fluid caused by hydrocephalus of the communicating type. This finding has been unique. In addition to the spinal cord tumor, this patient had a growth in the region of the pituitary body and another along the brainstem. The latter caused hydrocephalus by obstructing the cisterna pontis. The pressure of the spinal fluid distended the arachnoid sheath of each of the nerves—as shown by the air shadows.

On careful inspection of the rontgeno-gram, a narrow column of air can be seen on the right side of the tumor, and extending laterally from it is a patent subarachnoid pouch along one spinal nerve. The obstruction to the air was complete, although fluid apparently passed freely around the tumor, doubt-less where the column of air partially encircled one side of the tumor.

It is worthy of note that three days after the above tests, a Queckenstedt test was again made. The initial pres-sure was 300 mm. water. On jugular compression, the pressure rose to 340 but did not fall with release of this pressure—*i.e.*, the spinal canal had now begun to show evidence of an obstruc-tion to fluid.

Operation.—A small fibromyxoma was removed from the lumbar enlargement and the beginning of the cauda equina.

Case IV. William B., aged fifty. A pro-gressive loss of power and sensation had been gradually developing for four months. There was a sensory level at the ninth thoracic segment. Urinary incontinence had just appeared. The abdominal reflexes were absent; no ankle clonus. The spinal fluid was entirely negative. Dorsal flexion of the big toe on both sides.

Queckenstedt's Test.—The spinal fluid rose from 90 mm. to 135 on jugular compression, but fell very slowly, event-ually reaching the same level. The slow fall of the fluid level may be regarded as suggestive of a block, though on repeated jugular compression the same quick rise of fluid occurred.

Air injection into spinal canal: Thirty cc. of air replaced an equal amount of spinal fluid; no pain in head; no air-filled cerebral sulci in the rontgenogram of the head. A rontgenographic shadow of the air is well defined at the level of the ninth thoracic vertebra.

Operation.—External dumb-bell shaped neurofibroma arising from the eighth thoracic nerve in the region of the gang-lion. The tumor projected through the intervertebral foramen and again en-larging pushed against the pleura. Total extirpation of the tumor was followed by rapid and complete restoration of motor, sensory, and vesical function.

Comment.—The story of a gradually progressive paraplegia with a sharp sen-sory level should have made additional evidence unnecessary. The air injection was made in this instance only to satisfy one who was unconvinced. Again, Queckenstedt's test failed to prove a block, which the air injection both proved and located.

Case V. Agnes E., aged twenty-seven. Patient complained of a constant severe pain in the back and along the margins of the ribs. The pain dated from a blow on the back eight weeks ago. Paralysis and anaesthesia of both legs rapidly be-gan one week ago and was now complete. The fourth thoracic spine was very ten-der to pressure. The paralyzed limbs were *flaccid*. All reflexes were absent below the sensory level (sixth thoracic segment). Spinal fluid: slight Xantho-chromia, fifteen cells, globulin 4+.

Queckenstedt's Test.—From a primary level of 115 mm. the cerebrospinal fluid rose to 145 mm. on jugular compression but failed to return when the pressure was withdrawn. There was no oscillation of the fluid with respiration.

Air Injection.—Twenty-five cc. of air was injected after withdrawing an equal amount of fluid. That the air did not reach the head was shown by the absence of headache and the absence of the air-filled cerebral sulci in the rontgenogram. A fairly sharp line of the upper limit of the column of air was located at the fourth dorsal segment. *Following the air injection, the original nerve root pains were greatly intensified.*

Operation.—A large solid extrathecal tuberculoma was removed from the dor-sal surface of the dura at the level of the third and fourth thoracic vertebrae. It was tightly wedged between the laminae and dura causing compression of the spinal cord. The extradural fat was in-corporated in the inflammatory mass. Restoration of all functions followed operation, though much more slowly than in the preceding case.

Comment.—Although a sharp sensory level was present, a myelitis had to be considered because of the rapid paraly-sis. The air test was, therefore, necessary only in diagnosis; the sensory level was adequate for localization.

Case VI. Lena D., aged twenty-three. (Reported by kindness of Professor H. M. Thomas.) Her chief complaints were: severe and presistent pain in the cervical spine and down arm; weakness of the left arm and leg; numbness of the right arm and leg. A typical Brown-Sequard syndrome was present with characteristic reflex changes. The Wassermann from the blood was positive. Spinal fluid: straw-color; four cells; globulin 4+; *positive Wassermann*. Under antisyphilitic treatment signs and symptoms disappeared.

Queckenstedt's Test. — The Cerebrospinal fluid rose from a level of 195 mm. to only 210 mm. on compression of the jugular veins, and did not return when the jugular pressure was released. These results indicate a total occlusion of the spinal canal.

Air Injection.—No air reached the cranial chamber. The air level was only fairly clear at the 5th cervical vertebra; tracheal air shadows always make superimposed artificial air shadows difficult of interpretation. Pain in both arms (the original pain) instantly followed injection of the air.

Treatment and Comment.—A presumptive diagnosis of a spinal cord tumor was made. The positive Wassermann in both blood and spinal fluid, caused the diagnosis to be shifted from a tumor to a gumma. Following antisyphilitic treatment by Doctor Thomas, she recovered completely.

Several months later she consented to a second air injection. The air at once passed into the cranial chamber and caused headache. In the rontgenogram air could be seen both in the cerebral sulci and the lateral ventricles. *With the cure of her symptoms there was therefore proof that the obstruction in the spinal canal had disappeared.*

Case VII. H. T., aged fourteen. Because of a most intense backache and pain, patient's only position of comfort was sitting upright. Her symptoms, which were of only three weeks' duration, had progressed so rapidly that she was now completely paralyzed and anaesthetic below the eighth thoracic segment. There was marked tenderness on deep pressure of the sixth thoracic spine. The paralysis

was flaccid and all reflexes below the sensory level were abolished except that there was a positive Babinski on both sides. Spinal fluid: four cells, positive globulin, no Xanthochromia.

Queckenstedt's Test.—The pressure of the cerebrospinal fluid registered 180 mm. and did not rise when the jugular veins were compressed. This indicated a complete obstruction.

Air Injection.—Only 20 cc. of fluid could be aspirated; pain along both eighth dorsal nerves followed the injection. Air did not reach the head. The lower margin of the tumor was sharply defined by the air shadow in the rontgenogram.

Comment.—Queckenstedt's test was quite positive. The air test showed a complete block and accurately localized it, though it could hardly be claimed that either test was essential either for the diagnosis or localization.

DIAGNOSIS AND LOCALIZATION OF TUMORS WHEN THE LUMBAR CANAL IS CLOSED

Case VIII. W. W., aged forty-nine. During the past seven years patient has had three attacks of very severe lumbar pain radiating down the legs. The attacks were two years apart, came without warning, persisted about three months, holding him bedfast, and then passed off without any after effects. After the last attack (two years ago) difficulty in walking began, steadily increased, and for six months he had been confined to bed. There was now bilateral spastic paralysis with little voluntary power and some loss of sensation beginning at the eighth thoracic segment. The sensory level was detected only by using wisps of cotton and finer shades of heat and cold; K. K. and Achilles reflexes hyperactive; bilateral Babinski; no ankle clonus.

Spinal Fluid.—Less than 0.5 cc. of clear fluid could be obtained; 2 cells; globulin +.

Queckenstedt's Test.—Manometric reading not possible because only drops of fluid obtainable; jugular compression did not increase the flow.

Air Injection.—No fluid could be aspirated; nor was it possible to force more than a cubic centimetre of air into the spinal canal because there was no free space. Air pressure applied to the spinal canal caused sharp pains to radiate down both legs.

Comment.—It seemed clear that some lesion had practically obliterated the spinal canal at the site of puncture (3rd lumbar vertebra). But the sensory level was at the sixth thoracic vertebra (8th segment). If both observations were correct, the lesion would extend over a length of at least nine vertebrae—hardly a probability if the lesion were a tumor. A diffuse chronic inflammatory process was disclosed from the sixth to the ninth thoracic vertebrae and, though not followed further, it surely extended into the lumbar canal. The cord was to a large extent destroyed and replaced by numerous cystic spaces lined by dense fibrous tissue. They were isolated from each other and apparently also from the subarachnoid space above. The fluid obtained from lumbar puncture was doubtless from one of these pockets. We were greatly puzzled at the time by the seemingly paradoxical findings. The chief practical inference which might have been drawn was that it was a lesion so extensive as to have permitted no benefit by operation. This would have spared a useless laminectomy. Recently another case has been under observation with almost precisely similar findings, and he was advised that operation was contra-indicated.

The pain referred down the legs when the air was forced under pressure (several times repeated), is almost surely explained by stimulation of the nerve roots which were in contact with the local cystic pocket. The other case just referred to gave excruciating pain down only one leg, but each slight pressure gave identically the same pain. Even had there been no sensory level, the evidence from the lumbar puncture and air test alone should have localized the lesion to the lumbar spinal canal.

Case IX. A boy of eighteen had suffered from dull aching pain for over four years and until recently had shown nothing objective except that he was less adept at play than other boys. There had been some scoliosis and he held the lumbar spine more or less rigidly.

Two months ago while at camp his right leg began to drag. He was a precocious youngster and a diagnosis of hysteria had been repeatedly made by the most competent medical advisors. It was only after the left leg also became affected that I saw him. His lumbar spine was very rigid and tender on deep pressure. Although sensation at first seemed unimpaired, very careful tests showed a faint but definite hypaesthesia at the twelfth thoracic segment (9th thoracic vertebra.) The following is a recapitulation of the essential reflexes: K. K. and Achilles slightly hyperactive; Babinski negative; no ankle clonus; Kernig positive both sides.

Spinal Fluid.—None could be obtained on three successive attempts.

Queckenstedt's Test.—On one occasion blood-tinged fluid rose to 140 mm., and on jugular compression climbed to 160 but did not return on release of the venous obstruction.

Air Injection.—It was impossible to inject air for there was no space. A severe backache resulted when increased pressure was applied.

Comment.—Our interpretation, which proved to be correct, was that a tumor filled the lumbar canal at the site of puncture and that the arterial blood-tinged fluid was additional evidence of this. Although the tumor (an extensive glioma or sarcoma) could not be removed, immediate relief of the backache resulted from the decompressive laminectomy. Some motor function also returned following this simple relief of pressure.

Case X. Five years ago I removed a hemi-cylindrical shell of bone lying between the dura and the pia-arachnoid and extending from the eighth to the twelfth thoracic veretebrae. Complete relief of all signs and symptoms followed. Loss of motor function with spasticity was again developing slowly and made us fear a recurrence. But there was no evident sensory impairment. There was a suggestive ankle clonus on the right, a bilateral Babinski, slightly increased reflexes, and a positive Romberg. Spinal fluid could not be obtained. Queckenstedt's test could, therefore, not be applied.

Air Injection.—No air could be pushed into the spinal canal.

Comment.—That the needle had entered the spinal was certain, for pain radiating down the legs was evidence that the needle caught the nerves of the cauda equina. It was our belief that the lumbar canal was completely filled, probably by tumor similar to the one previously removed higher up in the spinal canal. The lumbar region was exposed at operation and a hemi-cylindrical bony shell extending from the twelfth thoracic to the first sacral vertebrae was removed. The tumor, if such it may be termed, was similar to the one previously removed from the thoracic region and of which there was no sign of recurrence. The bony mass completely filled the spinal canal and prevented the escape of fluid from the lumbar puncture.

Summary.—The three tumors in the lumbar spinal canal in this series have shown only faint sensory changes in two instances and none in the third. In one case no fluid and in two only a few drops flowed from the needle, because the tumors had completely or almost completely filled the lumbar canal. But in none could fluid be aspirated and in none could air be injected. The absence of fluid and the inability to push air into the spinal canal, I believe to be important evidence of a tumor or some other type of space-obliterating lesion in this region. It is, however, recognized that localizations upon such evidence are open to the objection that the spinal puncture might be faulty. At the time of these operations, Sicard's method had not yet appeared. Had we felt any doubt as to the position of the lesion, we would have injected air into the cisterna magna and elevated the hips to allow the air to pass caudally. Since the advent of Sicard's method, any hesitancy in diagnosis or localization could better be cleared by his oil.

I have had no tumors situated caudal to the site of the lumbar puncture. It is clear that neither the diagnosis nor the localization of these tumors could be accomplished by any information from lumbar puncture or Queckenstedt's test. While it is probable that air injections might be useful for this purpose, if the injection were made into the cisterna magna and the pelvis elevated, I should now much prefer Sicard's procedure.

THE USE OF SICARD'S "LIPIODOL" IN THE DIAGNOSIS AND LOCALIZATION OF SPINAL CORD TUMORS

As previously noted, Sicard's oil contains iodine which casts a striking opaque shadow in the x-ray; the iodine is so well protected by the oil that no noticeable irritation of the cord follows its introduction into the spinal canal. When half a cubic centimetre (or less) of this oil is injected into the spinal canal, the oil normally descends to the most dependent part of the spinal canal. The injection can be made either into the lumbar canal or, much better, into the cisterna magna (Ayer's puncture). The disadvantage of a lumbar injection is that the head must be dependent, sometimes for many minutes, making a most uncomfortable position, and the best incline obtainable is far short of the vertical position. When introduced by the cisternal route — a simpler and less painful procedure than lumbar puncture—the sitting posture offers the maximum opportunity for gravitation of the oil. Another disadvantage of the lumbar injection is that the nerve roots at the lumbar enlargement sometimes catch and hold the oil, thus suggesting an obstruction when none really exists. I have seen two negative explorations of this region, both made for obstructions indicated by lipiodol, whereas had the oil been injected into the cisterna this mistake could hardly have occurred. While the oil gravitates quite readily, it is tenacious and can easily be retained if it does not get a good start or if the position is not sufficiently upright. We have also been warned by Sicard that the inclusion of air with the oil may retain the oil at the point of injection.

Since all of our cases were studied before Sicard's discovery, I am unable to include any results in tumor localization from lipiodol. However, I have used it in ten cases in which spinal block followed fracture of the spine and in cases where the diagnosis of spinal cord tumor was considered and excluded by the method. In one instance an obstruction was located at the lumbar enlargement by a lumbar injection of lipiodol, and a second at the cervical enlargement by a cisternal injection. Since multiple lesions were surely present, operation was not advised. Several times under the fluoroscope we have observed gravitation of the opaque shadow. If the patient is sitting and the injection is made into the cisterna—surely the method of choice—the oil drops very quickly to the bottom of the dural sac. With the full play of gravity there seems to be little possibility that the progress of the oil will be impeded except by a real obstruction. I have seen no harm result from the oil. Aside from a temperature reaction lasting over two weeks in one patient, I have seen no ill effect. There has been no pain either at the time of injection or subsequently.

SUMMARY AND CONCLUSIONS

There is but one treatment for spinal cord tumors—removal by operation. Sixty per cent of all spinal cord tumors can be totally removed and without chance of recurrence. The operation should be attended by no mortality.

A careful history and a painstaking neurological examination are adequate to make both a correct diagnosis and a precise localization in probably over 90 per cent of all spinal cord tumors. In the remaining 10 per cent the accessory methods—air or lipiodol injections—will make the diagnosis and localization accurately. As the precision of neurological examination diminishes, the need for air or lipiodol injections increases proportionate-

ly. Fortunately, these tests do not add any appreciable danger and very little discomfort. When there is the slightest doubt of the presence of a lesion or of its character, their advantages should be utilized. Operative procedures (laminectomies) are no longer warranted until the localization of a lesion has been positively determined.

Examination of the spinal fluid gives information which, though important, is rarely essential. The not infrequent loss of sphincter, motor, and sensory function following lumbar puncture, makes this simple procedure objectionable—even contra-indicated unless one is prepared to immediately follow up any adverse effect by extirpation of the tumor. Though the originator of the air injection method, I have always had an aversion to the use of any accessory examinations unless, of course, they gave necessary information. The dependence on mechanical methods should always be deprecated if by their employment one makes neurological examinations with less painstaking care.

Queckenstedt's test is too unreliable to be considered at all trustworthy. In only two cases was a complete closure of the canal positively shown by the failure of the spinal pressure to rise and fall following compression of the jugular veins. In three cases the results were equivocal, there being a less pronounced rise and at other times a delayed fall after an apparently normal rise. In four other cases there was no evidence of a spinal block, when the air test demonstrated a complete block. At best, the procedure is limited to diagnosis and is of no help in localization.

As between air and lipiodol injections, something is to be said for and against each method. There are really but two objections to the use of Sicard's lipiodol —(1) it remains indefinitely in the spinal canal and (2) at times may lodge where there is no tumor. The latter objection is hardly tenable, however, for when the oil is properly used the true level of the obstruction should be indicated. Should the prolonged stay of lipiodol in the spinal canal ultimately prove to be entirely harmless (as seems possible), then there should be no drawback to its use. The value of lipiodol in cases where it is indicated, overwhelms these objections which then become of minor concern. If a tumor is present it can always be located with absolute precision by lipiodol. The density of the shadow is most striking. Its employment makes the diagnosis and localization almost fool-proof. Surely the possibility of error in localization when properly employed, is less than in all other methods combined. It can almost be said that little information other than that obtained from the use of lipiodol is necessary for the localization, even the diagnosis of a tumor. And doubtless one can exclude spinal cord tumors with equal certainty when the passage of lipiodol is unobstructed. It would be difficult to imagine that a tumor which gave symptoms could be present if lipiodol passed freely from the cisterna magna to the caudal end of the spinal canal. It is in those cases where a tumor does not exist that one need consider the objection, as yet theoretical, to the prolonged stay of lipiodol in the nervous system. When a tumor is exposed at operation, the lipiodol can be removed; but when a tumor does not exist the lipiodol must remain.

It is entirely possible that lipiodol might locate a block earlier than air, for the viscosity of the oil would probably prevent, or at least retard, transit of the oil around a tumor which air could still pass. However, we have had no opportunity of making a practical application of this hypothesis. In all of our certified tumors in which air has been used, there has been a total subarachnoid block in one instance when an abnormal pressure was used; and in none of the cases in which a tumor has been excluded by the interpretation of the air injection, has a tumor since appeared. Our inference from this fact would be that except when

tumors arise within the cord, occlusion of the spinal subarachnoid space, demonstrable either by air or lipiodol, would occur soon after sensory and motor symptoms appear.

The indications for air injections are much the same as for lipiodol. The advantage of air over lipiodol is that it is quickly absorbed. The principal disadvantage is that in localizing the level of a tumor the air shadow is far less sharp. Whereas the lipiodol shadow is as striking as a bullet, the x-ray plates must often be carefully scrutinized for the air shadow. Unless the location of the tumor is known to be within a restricted part of the spinal cord (a determination which can be roughly made by measuring the volume of fluid in the spinal canal), the search for the air shadow would be very difficult. Air shadows in the cervical region are too uncertain to be reliable because of the strong superimposed shadow of tracheal air. Usually a tumor level can be clearly shown in the thoracic and lumbar canal. For tumors caudal to the site of lumbar puncture, an air shadow could define a tumor only if the pelvis was raised, but none of our tumors have been in this region. For localization of tumors which are known to be present, lipiodol is, therefore, far superior to air. Moreover, an inferior x-ray plate will make a better localization with the use of lipiodol than the best x-rays after the injection of air.

The greatest use of air is in the diagnosis or elimination of tumors; its localizing value is subsidiary. It is extremely simple, and except for a slight transient headache is without harmful effect. Air will apparently diagnose or eliminate tumors with a certainty equal to that of lipiodol, and it has the added advantage that no foreign material remains permanently in the central nervous system.

Our present attitude toward the diagnosis and localization of spinal cord tumors may be summed up as follows:

(1) A careful history and neurological examination will be sufficient both for diagnosis and localization in over 90 per cent of the cases of spinal cord tumor. The importance of a painstaking examination is shown by the fact that in five of our cases sensory changes were missed by two observers and picked up by the third, who thereby made it unnecessary to use air or lipiodol for localization. By using air or lipiodol (only when required) the diagnosis and localization can be made in the remaining 10 per cent of these cases.

2. Use *air* to *diagnose or eliminate* a tumor when the neurological examination is not adequate for this purpose.

3. Use *air* (same injection) to *localize* a tumor when it is possible.

4. Use *lipiodol* for localization when a tumor is known to be present and where other means fail. The lipiodol can then be removed at operation.

5. Lumbar puncture alone is not a procedure of merit. The limited information it yields is overbalanced by the potentialities of serious harm. If used in conjunction with air or lipiodol, the information obtained is greater than the possible injury. Any injurious effect from lumbar puncture can be corrected by immediately removing the tumor.

6. Lumbar puncture is necessary for air injections. Ayer's cisternal puncture is far superior for the lipiodol test.

7. The importance of a dry lumbar puncture tap is indicated in three cases, but there is danger of error in the interpretation of purely negative evidence. It is safer to use lipiodol when in doubt.

It should be emphasized that these impressions are formulated when lipiodol has been used for only a short time and when its ultimate results have not yet been demonstrated. Should Sicard's early impressions not be modified, it is quite probable that lipiodol may eventually be used to the exclusion of lumbar punctures and air injections. Our sole objection at the present time is that it requires the unnecessary, even if not obviously harmful, inclusion of a foreign body in the nervous system.

REFERENCES

[1]Froin: Inflammations meningees avec reactions chromatique, fibrineuse et cytologique du liquide cephalo-rachidien. *Gaz. d. hop., Paris, lxxvi*: 1005, 1903.

[2]Marie, P., Foix and Robert: Service que peut rendre la Ponction Rachidienne pratiquee a des etages dierents pour le diagnostic de la hauteur d'une compression medullaire. *Rev. Neurol., xxv*: 712, 1913.

[3]Wegeforth, Ayer and Essick: The Method of Obtaining Cerebrospinal Fluid by Puncture of the Cisterna Magna (Cistern Puncture). *Am. J. Med Sc., clvii*: 789, 1919.

[4]Ayer: Puncture of the Cisterna Magna. Arch. Neur. and Psych., 1920, vol. iv, p. 529. Spinal Subarachnoid Block as Determined by Combined Cistern and Lumbar Puncture with Special Reference to the Early Diagnosis of Cord Tumors. *Arch. Neurol. and Psychiat., vii*: 38, 1922.

[5]Marie, P., Foix and Bouttier: Double punction sus-et-sous-lesionelle dans un cas de Compression Medullaire: Xanthochromie, coagulation massive dans le lequide inferieur seulement. *Rev. Neurol., xxvii*: 315, 1914.

[6]Queckenstedt: Zur diagnose der Ruckenmarkskompression. Deuts. Ztschr. f. Nervenh., 1916, vol. lv, p. 325. Uber Veranderungen der Spinalflussigkeit bei Erkrankungen peripherer Nerven, insbesondere bei Polyneuritis und bei Ischias. *Deuts. Ztschr. f. Nervenh., lvii*: 316, 1917.

[7]Dandy, W. E.: Rontgenography of the Brain after the Injection of Air into the Spinal Canal. *Ann. Surg., lxx*: 397, 1919. Diagnosis and Localization of Spinal Cord Tumors. *Johns Hopkins Hospital Bull., xxxiii*: 188, 1922.

[8]Wideroe, S.: Diagnosis of Spinal Cord Tumors. *Norsk Magazin f. Laegevidenskaben, Christiania, lxxxii*: 491, 1921.

[9]Jacobeus, H. C.: On Insufflation of Air into the Spinal Canal for Diagnostic Purposes in Cases of Tumors in the Spinal Cord. *Acta med. Scand., lv*: p. 555, 1921.

[10]Sicard, J. A., and Forestier: Methode radiographique d'exploration de la cavite epidurale par le lipiodol. *Rev. Neurol.* 28ᵉ annee, 1921 p. 1264. Sicard, J. A., Paraf, J., and Laplane, L.: Radiodiagnostic rachidien Lipiodole. *Presse Med.*, No. 85, p. 885, 1923.

[11]Bloodgood, J. C.: The Pathology of Chronic Cystic Mastitis of the Female Breast. *Arch. Surg., iii*: 445, 1921.

[12]Adson, A. W.: Tumors of the Spinal Cord; Surgical Treatment and results. *Minnesota Med., vii:* 79, 1924.

[13]Dandy, W. E.: The Space-compensating Function of the Cerebrospinal Fluid—its Connection with Cerebral Lesions in Epilepsy. *Johns Hopkins Hospital Bull., xxiv:* 245, 1923.

[14]Adson, A. W.: *Loc. cit.*

[15]Elsberg, C. A., and Stookey, B.: Mechanical effects of Tumors of the Spinal Cord. Their influence on Symptomatology and Diagnosis. *Arch. Neurol. and Psychiat., viii:* 502, 1922.

[16]Dandy, W. E.: Rontgenography of the Brain after the Injection of Air into the Spinal Canal. *A. Surg., lxx:* 397, 1919.

XVIII

STUDIES IN EXPERIMENTAL EPILEPSY *

By Walter E. Dandy and Robert Elman

The ready susceptibility of all animals to convulsions is shown by the fact that they can be produced experimentally in six general ways: (1) by anemia of the brain, (2) by asphyxia (venous engorgement) of the brain, (3) by traumatic stimulation of the central nervous system, (4) by chemical stimulation of the central nervous system, directly or through the vascular system, (5) by electrical stimulation of the central nervous system, directly or indirectly through the skin, (6) by injury to the brain followed by traumatic, chemical, or electrical stimulation, directly or indirectly applied.

ANEMIA AND HYPEREMIA

A splendid bibliography of experimental epilepsy is contained in an exhaustive article by Ito[1]. From this we learn that as early as 1824 Kellie[2], and in 1826 Piorry[3], produced convulsions by bleeding animals; and that in 1824 Ashley Cooper[4] produced convulsions in dogs by depriving the brain of its blood supply through ligation of both internal carotid and both vertebral arteries. Practically the same experiments were repeated by Kussmaul and Tenner[5] (1857) on an extensive scale and with the same results. For reasons which need not now be considered, they concluded that the convulsions originated from stimulation of the medulla, to the exclusion of other parts of the central nervous system. This is probably among the first attempts to establish a "convulsive center"—an ever changing area in the hands of different investigators, who see fit to make overdrawn conclusions from insufficient or uncontrolled experiments. It is clear that from experiments so crude that the entire brain is deprived of its blood supply, conclusions of a specific nature are entirely unwarranted. Victor Horsley[6] long since called attention to the impossibility of placing any great value on these experiments. Leonard Hill[7] with great fortitude compressed one of his own common carotid arteries and a unilateral convulsion followed.

These experiments permit of one conclusion, i.e., that anemia of the brain causes convulsions, and from Hill's experiment on himself, it is safe to conclude that anemia of a cerebral hemisphere may cause convulsions which begin unilaterally. We have no right or reason to infer that cerebral anemia is the source of convulsions which occur in epilepsy. In fact, except in the sudden closure of cerebral vessels from emboli and thrombi, cerebral anemia probably plays no role in the production of convulsions, and subsequent convulsions resulting from these lesions are due to the injured brain tracts rather than to any possible recurring anemia. The oft repeated explanation that local spasm of the cerebral arteries causes convulsions by producing anemia, is purely an assumption, for vasomotor nerves have never been demonstrated in the cerebral vessels. To quote Bayliss and Hill[8]: " . . . . the cerebral vessels are free from any such control (vasomotor); the cerebral circulation passively follows the changes in the general circulation."

*Reprinted from the *Bulletin of the Johns Hopkins Hospital*, XXXVI: 1, January, 1925.

179

Landois [9] (1867) produced convulsions in young dogs by compression of the veins of the neck, the seizures being apparently similar to those brought on by Kussmaul and Tenner by excluding the arterial supply to the brain. Hermann and Escher [10] (1870) repeated Landois' experiments on cats and obtained similar results.

TRAUMATIC STIMULATION

Brown-Sequard [11] traumatized various parts of the nervous system in rabbits and induced convulsions. After section of the spinal cord, partial or complete, or the mere insertion of a needle into it, convulsions developed. Lesions of the medulla, the cerebral peduncles, the corpora quadrigemina, or even injuries of the popliteal or sciatic nerves, were sufficient to cause convulsions. At times convulsions developed spontaneously or from irritation of certain areas of skin which he termed "epileptogenous zones." At this early date, he noted that this epileptogenous zone and the convulsions were on the side contralateral to the lesion when the cerebral injury was in the cerebral peduncles or corpora quadrigemina. Attacks also developed after the cerebrum, cerebellum, and brain-stem had been removed. It was Brown-Sequards view that epilepsy followed from the loss of control of the base of the brain, "principally the medulla," over the excitable reflexes of the cerebrospinal axis. Owing to his prominence, his opinions on epilepsy obtained great weight. Apparently, his views never changed. Many years later, the great Hughlings Jackson [12], whose views were so widely at variance, found Brown-Sequard's opinions on epilepsy still holding sway.

Westphal [13] (1871) showed that convulsions identical with those of Brown-Sequard could be produced in rabbits by lightly striking the head. The convulsions appeared immediately after the trauma, or within a few seconds, and continued over a period of weeks and even months. Rabbits are very susceptible to convulsions, so much so that the most trivial injury to the brain, even to a peripheral nerve, is a sufficient stimulus. This objection makes it difficult to accept any finely drawn conclusions. Nothnagel [14] (1868) produced small focal lesions in the pons. The convulsions which followed were interpreted to be due to stimulation of a convulsive center. He even postulated the seizures to be the result of stimulation of two independent centers situated nearly in apposition— (1) the convulsive center and (2) the vasomotor center, the latter effect causing coma. Binswanger [15] (1886) repeated Nothnagel's experiments and doubted their value as interpreted in human epilepsy. He thought epilepsy to be the result of stimulation of "motor tracts" and not of any center.

CONVULSIONS FROM CHEMICAL STIMULATION

Convulsions due to convulsant drugs are known to all students of pharmacology. Various drugs have been used, among the most effective being absinthe, picrotoxin, cinchonidin, and acid fuchsin. Of these drugs, absinthe has probably been most widely used. There is some question whether it may act only on the brain and not on the spinal cord. First used by Morce [16] (1864), developed into popular use by Magnan [17] (1876), it became the method of choice of inducing convulsions by the great masters, Hughlings Jackson and Victor Horsley. It was their opinion that the convulsions resulting from absinthe more nearly simulated those of epilepsy than those produced in any other way. Although Horsley thought absinthe did not act upon the spinal cord, for after cutting the cord convulsions did not result, Magnan [18] performed the same experiments and convulsions followed. One of the most interesting features of convulsions was disclosed by Horsley (1885) when he showed that the convulsions following absinthe were clonic or tonic, the former depending on the participation of the cerebral cortex and the latter on its absence. Ziehen [19] (1886) also showed that when the cerebral cortex was removed the clonic element of the convulsions disappeared, leaving a tonic spasm. Hill [20] (1900) demonstrated that by shutting off the cerebral circulation after absinthe injection, the convulsions would be transformed at once from clonic to tonic form. From a series of clinical and pathological observations, Hughlings Jackson [21] (1877) had long since made these deductions and the experiments of Horsley were undertaken to test them.

FOCAL CHEMICAL STIMULATION OF THE BRAIN

The use of chemicals as local irritants has been largely confined to the cerebral hemispheres. It probably followed the use of electrical stimulation. Landois [22] (1887) spread kreatin and urinary products over the surface of the brain; Bickel [23] (1898) used bile pigments; Korangi and Tanszk [24] (1890) Liebig's meat extract; and convulsions readily followed all such procedures. Lapynsky [25] (1899) treated the medulla of frogs with urinary products and convulsions followed. The theory that epilepsy was due to auto-intoxication accounted for the stimulants used and acquired considerable support from the results obtained. Pierre Marie [26] (1887) was one of the most ardent exponents of this theory.

By placing on the motor cortex a piece of filter paper saturated with strychnia (a method previously described by Baglioni and Amantea [27] (1914), Amantea [28] (1921) produced focalized convulsions. Following cauterization of the cortex, the same stimulation did not induce convulsions. He found sensitive areas of the skin corresponding to the injured motor area involved, and by light irritation of these skin areas convulsions could be induced at will. These findings correspond closely with those of Brown-Sequard.

ELECTRICAL STIMULATION OF THE BRAIN

The galvanic stimulation experiments of the cerebral cortex of Fritsch and Hitzig [29] (1870) and of Ferrier [30] (1873), which made the greatest contribution of all time to cerebral localization, have also added much to our knowledge of epilepsy. That focal convulsions could be produced in this way was merely a verification of predictions by Hughlings Jackson, who had made such a careful clinical and pathological study of epilepsy. This method was soon to be used as a means of accurate identification of cortical areas in the human brain at operation by Victor Horsley— and with results which were precisely those of animal experimentation.

Munk [31] (1881) showed that convulsions can be produced by stimulation of parts of the cerebral cortex other than the motor area, but that a higher dosage is required.

CONVULSIONS RESULTING AFTER EXPERIMENTAL CEREBRAL DEFECTS ALONE

Luciani [32] (1878) induced spontaneous epilepsy in dogs by excision of the motor cortex. The convulsions, however, did not develop at once, but some time later, the time interval varying between a few days and several months, and began in the side contralateral to the cerebral lesion. In a monkey the seizures developed three days after the motor cortex was excised. The interval between the cortical insult and the onset of convulsions varied from a few days to one and one-half years. The attacks gradually increased in frequency and severity and all but 2 of over 50 dogs and cats so operated upon died in status epilepticus. As the result of his experiments, Luciani thought convulsions were of cortical origin—a view which must always go back to Hughlings Jackson for its origin. Vulpian [33] (1885), conducting similar experiments, obtained the same results.

The well-known extensive cerebral extirpation experiments of Goltz [34] (1892),
also yielded spontaneous convulsions after
the operations, the dogs usually dying in
status epilepticus several months later.
Convulsions were not restricted to those
cases in which the motor cortex was injured, but occurred after artificial defects
of the occipital lobe, the temporal lobe,
in fact, of nearly any part of the cerebral
hemispheres. He looked upon convulsions as a disturbance of a very labile
balance of the nervous system and as induced by an injured brain. It should be
noted in this connection that Ito was unable to observe spontaneous convulsions
in a large series of animals in which he
had introduced foreign bodies extradurally. This was a cause of great concern to
him in view of the results of Luciani and
Goltz. Possibly the extradural situation
of the foreign body may account for the
difference.

Laborde [35] (1891) demonstrated two
frogs before the Biological Society of Paris
in each of which spontaneous convulsions
had followed an injury to the brain; in
one the removal of a large part of the
forebrain, and in the other a mere needle
prick of the corpora restiformia. Convulsions could also be induced at will by
gently rubbing the skin.

Thomas [36] (1921) pricked the brain of
frogs with a needle and convulsions followed injections of sub-normal doses of
acid fuchsin as readily as when extensive
destructions of the brain were made. The
results of these experiments were verified
by Syz [37] (1923).

CONVULSIONS RESULTING FROM CEREBRAL INJURY PLUS STIMULATION

Abel (1910), several hours after a class
demonstration in which a frog's forebrain
had been stabbed, found the animal in
convulsions. This accidental finding impressed Dr. Abel and stimulated one of
the most far-reaching and fundamental
studies on convulsions (Barbour and
Abel [38] (1910). These authors demonstrated that, following injury to the brain
of frogs, convulsions can be readily induced by (a) fatigue, (b) cold, and (c)
much smaller doses of acid fuchsin than
are required to send into convulsions a
frog with an intact brain. Abel [39] (1912)
later observed that the injured central
nervous system stained a deep pink after
acid fuchsin injections, whereas the normal brain remained uncolored in a similar experiment. Syz [37] repeated these
experiments with identical results and
concludes that in some unexplained way
injury to the brain causes an increased
absorption of the dye into the entire central nervous system—a conclusion which,
if substantiated, will be of great significance in the etiology of epilepsy.

Sauerbruch [40] (1913) obtained results
in monkeys and rabbits very similar to
those of Abel, and of Barbour and Abel,
in frogs. Following a puncture of the
motor cortex, or painting the motor cortex with iodine, or the intracerebral implantation of a foreign body, the animals
were studied over periods of two to eight
months, injections of small amounts of
cocaine being used to stimulate convulsions. It required only one-fifth of the
normal convulsive dose to provoke convulsions in these animals.

It should be noted in passing that
Munk [31], working in Horsley's laboratory,
was unable to obtain convulsions after
absinthe injections, if the cortex was
quickly removed. Tsutschaninow's [41]
(1894) results after santonin poisoning,
and Cobb's [42] (1922) after thujone injections, were essentially similar. Cobb
found that decerebrated animals required
two or three times the intravenous dose
of thujone necessary to produce convulsions in an animal with an intact brain,
but that the convulsions are similar.
These latter results—i.e., from the acute
stage of cerebral injury—are hardly applicable to the attacks in epilepsy, for only

the attacks which occur at a later period when the initial defect has healed, are analogous to the convulsions of human epilepsy. They do, however, indicate that the motor tracts of the cerebral hemispheres are more sensitive to systemic toxic stimuli than are the motor tracts in the brain-stem.

The purpose of this communication is to present certain experimental data indicating the importance of defects of the brain in the development of convulsions. It is only fair to state that these experiments were suggested by certain impressions which had been drawn from an analysis of the histories of patients afflicted with epilepsy, from a series of operations on the brains of epileptics, and from a post-mortem study of epileptic brains. Briefly summarized, it appeared from these studies that in most of the cases of epilepsy there were positive evidences of cerebral lesions, which were considered to be the cause of the convulsions. There was nothing specific or uniform about the cerebral lesions; probably the greatest number were congenital maldevelopments or malformations of various kinds; many were acquired defects of vascular, traumatic, or inflammatory origin, and many others were neoplasms and inflammatory new growths [43]. Some lesions were diffuse others were focal. These studies indicated that, although the individual expression of convulsions may vary greatly, they are all fundamentally similar, in that there is an underlying cerebral lesion which in some way lowers the threshold at which convulsions develop.

The accompanying experiments were undertaken to determine if localized traumatic injuries of the brain actually render the animal more susceptible to convulsions, and to learn if, in a general way, the location of the injury is important in their production. These experiments are intended only to determine a principle and they merely scratch the surface of the details of this vast problem.

To bear any trustworthy analogy with human epilepsy, the animals must be tested, not at the time the cerebral defect is produced, but at a later date when healing of the primary lesion has taken place. For epilepsy is a chronic ailment which develops long after the initial injury to the brain.

Nearly all animals are subject to spontaneous convulsions which presumably are analogous to the human convulsions in epilepsy. This is true not only among mammals—dogs, cats, horses, cows, sheep, rabbits, etc.—but also among lower forms —birds, frogs, and others. To interpret experimental convulsions in terms of human epilepsy, it must be possible to produce them at will by artificial stimuli which can be measured. Fortunately, this can be done. Convulsions can be induced at will in any normal animal, just as in a human being, by electrical of chemical stimuli. It then remains to be determined if the measurable amount of these stimuli necessary to induce convulsions—the epileptic reserve—is altered after lesions of the brain have been well healed.

A study of the various experimental methods employed resulted in our adoption of the absinthe method—the old method of Hughlings Jackson and Victor Horsley—as the procedure of choice. These observers considered absinthe to have a fairly specific action on the cerebral cortex. Our experiments add a degree of support to this viewpoint. It is difficult to believe this action is exclusively limited to this part of the brain.

Cats have been used in all of these experiments. A 10 per cent emulsion of wormwood oil in acacia and water was administered through the stomach tube. In order that absorption of the poison might be uniform, the animals were deprived of food for twelve hours. We have chosen an emulsion of wormwood oil (absinthe being the active principle) rather than an alcoholic extract of absinthe in order to avoid any possible mis-inter-

TABLE I

Animal Number	Location of Lesion	Dose per Kilogram of Body Weight																		
		1 cc.	1.5 cc.	2 cc.	2.5 cc.	3 cc.	3.5 cc.	4 cc.	4.5 cc.	5 cc.	5.5 cc.	6 cc.	6.5 cc.	7 cc.	7.5 cc.	8 cc.	8.5 cc.	9 cc.	9.5 cc.
F 2	Motor cortex				+ 12														
F 4	Motor cortex				+ 4														
F 5	Motor cortex				+ 13*					++ 13†									
F 6	Motor cortex		0 8	0 4	+ 16	+ 15	+ 12												
F 7	Motor cortex		0 5		+ 8		0 12												
F 9	Motor cortex		+ 4		+ 3														
K 1	Motor cortex	+ 12	0 6	+ 8	+ 7														
K 3	Motor cortex	+ 8	+ 6	0 5	+ 4														
K 5	Motor cortex			+ 4															
F12	Occipital cortex				0 4	0 5	0 7	0 20	+ 7‡	+ 8									
F13	Occipital cortex				0 4		+ 20	0 12	0 10		+ 16								
F11	Occipital cortex				+ 4§		+ 20	+ 12											
F14	Cerebellar cortex							+ 4											
F15	Cerebellar cortex				0 4														
Normal 1													0	+					
Normal 2														0					
Normal 3																+			
Normal 4																+			
Normal 5																+			
Normal 6																	+		
Normal 7																	+		
Normal 8																		+	
Normal 9																			+ †

Key to table: + = convulsion; 0 = no convulsion; numbers 4, 6, 8, etc. = weeks after operation.
*Death from convulsions. Dose 2.5 cc. per kilogram of body weight.
† Status epilepticus with recovery.
‡ Momentary attack two hours after administration of drug.
§ Animal pregnant.

pretation through the effects of the alcohol. It is quite probable, however, that the intravenous injections of thujone, as used by Cook, may prove superior.

The dose of the drug has been given according to the animal's weight, and the results are so recorded in Table I. The lesions produced in the brain have been simple extirpations of the cortex and sub-cortex over the Rolandic area, the occipital lobe, and the cerebellum. In some experiments a simple incision has been made into the brain and in others a small foreign body has been imbedded below the cortex. The absinthe was given several weeks (four to twenty) after the cerebral injury had been inflicted. The reason for this interval of time was to simulate more nearly the conditions in human epilepsy where the intracerebral lesion is one of months' or years' duration, i.e., where the convulsions develop after the original lesion in the brain has well healed.

SUMMARY AND CONCLUSIONS

The most striking fact contained in these experiments is that one-third to one-seventh of the dose of absinthe required to produce convulsions in normal cats will incite attacks when the motor cortex has been injured several weeks previously. The experiments show conclusively that injury to the cerebellar and occipital lobes is far less effective in making the animal susceptible to convulsions, than is injury to the motor cortex. They also suggest that less absinthe is required to induce convulsions in occipital and cerebellar injuries than in the normal, but since there is some variation of the convulsive dose in normal animals, and from time to time even in the same animal, we are not willing, with the limited evidence at hand, to draw a positive conclusion in these cases.

When the minimal convulsive dose is given to an animal with injured motor cortex, unilateral convulsions will de-velop, and without loss of consciousness. These are comparable to petit mal attacks in human epilepsy. They are not so focal as those seen in human beings; they are evident as a turning of the body in circles, but always in the same direction. If the left motor cortex is removed, the animal will rotate clockwise; if the right motor cortex is affected, the direction of the circles will be counter-clock-wise. Either these unilateral manifestations may terminate without further involvement, or they may pass over into a general convulsion. If the stimulant is of just the right dosage, the seizure remains more or less focal (petit mal), but any increase in the stimulant quickly causes a general convulsion. The inference to be drawn from these observations is that the injured area is the vulnerable point—*locus minoris resistentiae*— which is attacked by the convulsant drug. Another fact which we have observed is the difference in the character of onset of convulsions in cats with motor injury, and those of normal cats. In the normal cats pronounced restlessness and irritability precede a convulsion, as if the whole nervous system were affected by the drug and the convulsions were only a part of this general process. But in cats with healed motor defects, this preliminary irritability does not appear, the convulsions suddenly developing without warning in a placid and normally composed animal. The probable reason for this difference is that the dose of absinthe which causes convulsions in an animal with a motor defect, is far less than the dose necessary to produce general changes in the nervous system. The same difference was observed when the occipital lobe was injured.

REFERENCES

[1]Ito, H.: Experimentelle Beitrage zur Aetiologie und Therapie der Epilepsie. *Deut. u. Ztschr. f. Chir., lii:* 225; 417, 1899.

[2]Kellie, G.: On death from cold, and on congestions of the brain. *Trans. Med.-Chir. Soc. of Edinburgh, i:* 1824.

[3]Piorry, P. A.: Recherches sur l'influence de la pesanteur sur le cours du sang; diagnostic de la syncope et de l'apoplexie, cause et traitement de la syncope. *Arch. gen. de med.,* t. *xii,* annee 4, 1826.

[4]Cooper, Ashley: *Lectures on the Principle and Practice of Surgery.* London, 1824, i.

[5]Kussmaul, Adolf, and Tenner, Adolf: Untersuchungen u. Ursprung und Wesen der fallsuchtartigen Zuckungen bei der Verblutung, sowie der Fallsucht uberhaupt. Moleschott's *Untersuch. zur Naturlehre der Menschen und der Thiere,* Bd. *iii:* 1857.

[6]Horsley, Victor: On the origin and seat of epileptic disturbance. *Brit. M. J.,* i: 693, 1892.

[7]Hill, Leonard: *The Physiology and Pathology of the Cerebral Circulation; an Experimental Research.* London, 1896.

[8]Bayliss, W. M., and Hill, Leonard: On intracranial pressure and the cerebral circulation. Part 1. Physiological, *J. Physiol., xviii:* 1895.

[9]Landois, Leonard: Ueber den Einfluss der venosen Hyperamie des Gehirnes und des verlangerten Markes auf die Herzbewegung, nebst Bemerkungen uber die fallsuchtartigen Anfalle. Vorlaufige Mittheilung. *Centrlbl. med. Wiss.* Nr. 10, 1867.

[10]Hermann, L., and Escher, T.: Ueber die Krampfe bei Circulationsstorungen im Gehirn. *Pfluger's Arch.,* 3, 1870.

[11]Brown-Sequard, Ch. Ed.: D'une affection convulsive qui survient chez les animaux ayant eu une moitie laterale de la moelle epiniere coupee. *Compt. rend. Soc. biol.,* ii: 1851.

[12]Jackson, Hughlings: On the anatomical, physiological and pathological investigation of epilepsy. *The West Riding Lunatic Asylum medical reports. London, iii:* 1873.

[13]Westphal, C.: Ueber kunstliche Erzeugung von Epilepsie bei Meerschweinchen. *Berl. klin. Wchnschr.,* Nr. 38–39, 1871. (Carl Westphal's gesammelte Abhandlungen. Berlin, ii, 1892.

[14]Nothnagel, H.: Die Entstehung allgemeiner Convulsionen vom Pons und von der Medulla oblongata aus. *Virchow's Arch., xliv,* 1868.

[15]Binswanger, Otto: Epilepsie. Eulenburg's *Real Encyclopadie der gesammten Heilkunde.* 2. Aufl., Wien und Leipzig, 1886, vi.

[16]Morce, —: *Compt. rend. Acad. d. sc., lviii:* 628, 1864.

[17]Magnan, V.: *Recherches sur les Centres nerveux.* Manon, Paris, 1876.

[18]Magnan, V.: *Lecons cliniques sur l'epilepsie.* Paris, 1882.

[19]Ziehen, Th.: Ueber die Krampfe infolge elektrischer Reizung der Grosshirnrinde. *Arch Psychol. Nervenh., xvii,* 1886.

[20]Hill, Leonard: *Phil. Tr. Roy. Soc., cxciii:* 106, 1900.

[21]Jackson, Hughlings: *Medical Examiner,* April 5, 1877.

[22]Landois, Leonard: Ueber die Erregung typischer Krampfanfalle nach Behandlung des Centralnervesystems mit chemischen Substanzen unter besonderer Berucksichtigung der Uramie. *Wien. med. Presse,* Nr. 7–9, 1887.

[23]Bickel, A.: Zur vergleichenden Physiologie des Grosshirns. *Pfluger's Arch., lxxii,* 1898.

[24]Korangi, Alex. v., and Tanszk, Fr.: Beitrage zur Physiologie der von der Grosshirnrinde ausgelosten Bewegungen und Krampfe. *Internat. klin Rundschau, 4:* 14, 1890.

[25]Lapynsky, Michael: Ueber Epilepsie beim Frosche *Pfluger's Arch., lxxiv,* 1899.

[26]Marie, Pierre: Note sur l'etiologie de l'epilepsie. *Progres med., 15:* 44, 1887.

[27]Baglioni, S., und Amantea, G.: *Ztschr. biol. Technik Method, iii,* 1914.

[28]Amantea, G.: Uber experimentelle beim Versuchstier infolge afferenter Reize erzeugte Epilepsie. *Arch. ges. Physiol., clxxxviii:* 287, 1921.

[29]Fritsch, G., and Hitzig, E.: Ueber die elektrische Erregbarkeit des Grosshirns. *Reichert-Du Bois' Archiv.,* 1870.

[30]Ferrier, David: Experimental researches in cerebral physiology and pathology. *The West Riding Lunatic Asylum Med. Reports, iii,* 1873.

[31]Munk, Hermann: *Ueber die Funktionen der Grosshirnrinde.* Berlin, 1881.

[32]Luciani, Luigi: Sulla patogenesi dell' epilessia. Studio critico-sperimentale. *Riv. sper. d. frenia., Anno.* 4, 1878.

[33]Vulpian, V.: Recherches experimentales concernant 1° les attaques epileptiformes provoquees par l'electrisation des regions excito-motrices du cerveau proprement dit; 2° la duree de l'excitabilite motrice du cerveau proprement dit apres la mort. *Compt. rend. Acad. sc.,* 17, 1885.

[34]Goltz, F.: Der Hund ohne Grosshirn. 7. Abhandlung uber die Verrichtungen des Grosshirns. *Pfluger's Arch., li,* 1892.

[35]Laborde, J. V.: L'epilepsie experimentale chez la grenouille. *Compt. rend. Soc. biol., iii,* 1891.

[36]Thomas, J. E.: *J. Pharmacol. & Exper. Therap., xvii:* 334, 1921.

[37]Syz, H.: On the entrance of convulsant dyes into the substance of the brain and spinal cord after an injury to these structures. *J. Pharamcol. & Exper. Therap., xxi:* 263, 1923.

[38]Barbour, Henry G., and Abel, John J.: Tetanic convulsions in frogs produced by acid fuchsin, and their relation to the problem of inhibition in the central nervous system. *J. Pharmacol. & Exper. Therap.,* ii: 167, 1910.

[39]Abel, J. J.: On the action of drugs and the function of the anterior lymph hearts in cardiectomized frogs. *J. Pharmacol. & Exper. Therap., iii:* 581, 1912.

[40]Sauerbruch, F.: Experimentelle Studien uber die

Entstehung der Epilepsie. *Verhandl. d deutche Gesellsch chir.*, *xlii*: 144, 1913.

[41]Tsutschaninow, P.: Experimentelle Studien uber den Ursprungsort einiger klinisch wichtiger toxischer Krampfformen. *Arch. exper. Path. Pharmakol.*, *xxxiv*: 208, 1894.

[42]Cobb, Stanley: A case of epilepsy, with a general discussion of the pathology. *Med. Clin. North Am.*, *v*: 1403 1922.

[43]Dandy, W. E.: The space-compensating function of the cerebrospinal fluid—its connection with cerebral lesions in epilepsy. *Bull. Johns Hopkins Hosp.*, *B. xxxiv*: 245, 1923.

XIX

SECTION OF THE SENSORY ROOT OF THE TRIGEMINAL NERVE AT THE PONS *

PRELIMINARY REPORT OF THE OPERATIVE PROCEDURE

In two patients afflicted with tic douloureux the sensory root of the trigeminal nerve was sectioned alongside the pons. The approach to the nerve in this region is through the posterior cranial fossa; in all other operative procedures the sensory root is approached from the middle cranial fossa. Except for the fact that the bony defect is extended laterally and above, a more or less routine unilateral cerebellar exposure is made. The dura is incised almost to the lateral and sigmoid sinuses, both of which are carefully avoided. To facilitate still further a deep exposure in the posterior cranial fossa, much room can be obtained by liberating all the fluid contained in the cisterna magna. This is done by puncturing the membrane. In one case, even more room was obtained by a preliminary intravenous injection of Weed's hypertonic salt solution.

The cerebellar lobe is elevated with a narrow spatula which is gradually pushed mesially under the cerebellum and along the angle formed by the tentorium cerebelli and the posterior surface of the petrous temporal bone, until the brainstem is reached. The acoustic and facial nerves entering the internal auditory meatus are passed *en route* but are not disturbed. The characteristic position of the trigeminal nerve at the apex of the petrous temporal bone, and piercing the tentorium, makes it not difficult of detection. The brain-stem including this part of the trigeminal nerve is surrounded by

the arachnoid membrane and must be opened before the nerve can be divided. In one case the membrane was transparent, the nerve being easily visible through it. In the other, the membrane was so opaque and thick that the nerve could be seen only when the membrane was opened. A fairly large vein lying adjacent to the nerve enters the superior petrosal sinus and must be carefully avoided. In one case another small vein paralleled the sensory root and had to be divided between Cushing "clips" before the nerve could be sectioned. A small hook was passed around the sensory root, which was then gently pulled and divided. In both cases the motor root was uninjured and could be seen intact through the hiatus in the severed sensory root and lying parallel to, behind, and along its superior border.

In presenting this procedure, it is realized that the operations now in use for section of the sensory root through the middle cranial fossa are practically devoid of mortality in the hands of competent surgeons. Although the recovery of these patients was uneventful, the material is too limited to suggest that this operation is either equal or superior to other procedures. Its advantages are: (1) the ease of the approach to the sensory root, due largely to the bloodless intracranial course; after entering the dura a free space without vascular crossings extends directly to the brain-stem; (2) the seemingly easier preservation of the motor root.

Its greatest disadvantage would appear

*Reprinted from the *Bulletin of the Johns Hopkins Hospital*, Vol. XXXVI, No. 2, February, 1925.

to be that the operation is intradural and that for this reason the effects of trauma from any undue retraction of the cerebellum and the difficulties incident to any unexpected bleeding would be serious. Whether those potential dangers prove to be actually greater than in other operations remains to be seen.

XX

STUDIES ON EXPERIMENTAL HYPOPHYSECTOMY *

1. EFFECT ON THE MAINTENANCE OF LIFE

By Walter E. Dandy, M.D., and Frederick Leet Reichert, M.D.

Studies following extirpation of the hypophysis in animals have led to confusion rather than to clearness. One group of investigators arrives at the conclusion that most of the somatic characteristics, normal and abnormal, arise from this structure — even that life depends upon it — whereas another group looks upon it as quite useless or at most unimportant. And strangely enough, these widely divergent results are attained from experiments which, to outward appearances at least, seem very similar. We are, therefore, left with the impression that there must be not only the important element of personal equation in ovedrawing conclusions, but that in the performance of the experiments there must be flaws which have remained hidden.

It is the purpose of this communication to present experimental evidence upon only one phase of alleged pituitary function; namely, Is the pituitary essential to life? We now believe it is easy not only to explain the contradictory results, but also to correlate conclusions which are so far apart.

In view of the fact that the literature on hypophyseal experiments has been so fully and frequently covered, we shall only briefly refer to those reports which bear particularly upon the relationship of the pituitary to the maintenance of life. Victor Horsley, in 1886,[1] published a brief note on the removal of the hypophysis in dogs, using a lateral temporal approach. Two

of the animals lived five and six months and showed nothing that distinguished them from other dogs. Unfortunately, no gross or microscopic necropsy reports were made. For twenty years these results remained unquestioned. In 1908, Gemelli[2] removed the hypophysis of cats, using a buccal route, and obtained results identical with those of Horsley.

Paulesco (1908),[3] slightly altering the operation by opening a vent in the bone and dura of the contralateral side of the skull, arrived at the sensational conclusion that the hypophysis was necessary to life. Out of twenty-two dogs with total extirpations, not one survived longer than forty-eight hours, and all except two died in less than thirty-six hours. From a more extended series there were however, several recoveries which he explained by only "partial" removal of the gland. The object of the second cranial opening was to afford, by dislocation of the brain, a better exposure of the hypophyseal region.

Cushing[4] and his coworkers — Reford, Crowe and Homans — using essentially the same bilateral approach, confirmed Paulesco's findings in every respect. Their experiments have been controlled by gross and microscopic studies of the base of the brain after the death of the animals. The protocols by Crowe, Cushing and Homans[5] have been presented in great detail and with such accuracy that they still offer an unusual opportunity for study and probably different interpretation even at this time.

Stimulated by the above experiments, Handelsmann and Horsley[6] removed the

*Reprinted from *Bulletin of The Johns Hopkins Hospital,* Vol. XXXVII, No. 1, July, 1925.

hypophysis from a larger series of dogs, controlled by extirpations by post-mortem microscopic studies of the base of the brain, and again arrived at precisely the same conclusions which Horsley had originally published, namely, that the hypophysis gave no evidence of any important function.

Since then numerous authors have published results some of which are identical with those of Horsley — Aschner[7] (1912), Sweet and Allen (1913)[8] Benedict and Homans (1912),[9] Camus and Roussy (1913),[10] and Brown (1923).[11] Others, however, have agreed with Paulesco — Reford and Cushing, Crowe, Cushing and Homans, Houssay (1916),[12] Bell (1917),[13] Dott (1923).[14]

That the pituitary is not essential to the life of tadpoles, has been conclusively demonstrated by the extirpation experiments of Smith (1916)[15] and of Allen (1916),[16] and more recently of others. They removed the pharyngeal bud of the hypophysis from very young frog embryos. For the time being we are passing over, as irrelevant to our subject, the profound disturbances of growth and pigmentation which have followed extirpation of this hypophyseal anlage. These results have been consistent in the hands of numerous investigators; they have not been and are not challenged. So far as the alleged relation of the hypophysis to life is concerned, our experiments carry precisely the same conclusion for mammals (dogs) which their experiments have demonstrated for amphibia (frogs) — *i.e.*, that the hypophysis is not concerned with the maintenance of life.

Well secluded at the base of the brain and skull and attached to both almost at the central point, the hypophysis has offered great difficulties of operative approach preparatory to its extirpation. Two methods have been evolved to reach this pea-sized structure: (1) the temporal or intracranial, and (2) the buccal. The former approach used by Horsley (unilateral), Paulesco, Cushing, Sweet and Allen, Bell, Dott, Houssay, Benedict and Homans (bilateral), has the advantage of being an

aseptic route. It is particularly useful in dogs because the sella turcia is shallow and a satisfactory exposure of the hypophysis can be obtained from the side. This method, however, is impracticable in cats, for the sella is deeper and the curved and overhanging posterior clinoid process envelops the posterior half of the hypophysis and hides it from view. The buccal route is also through a septic field, and its use has been attended by a considerable mortality from meningitis and localized infections. It is, however, the only feasible approach for the extirpation of the feline hypophysis. This method was employed in dogs or cats by Gamelli, Aschner, Camus and Roussy, and Brown.

Those who support the view that the hypophysis is essential to life believe that microscopic fragments have been left in the surviving animals and they demand microscopic proof that anterior lobe cells are absent. But Horsley and Handlesmann, Aschner, Gemelli, and Sweet and Allen, have controlled their experiments microscopically to meet this objection.

In attempting an analysis of this maze of contradictory results and interpretations, one lead is striking and probably significant, namely, that of the above mentioned investigators all who have used the buccal route are in agreement that the pituitary body is not essential to life. The only disagreement, therefore, is among those who have employed the temporal (intracranial) route. That the type of operation has much to do with the divergent results, will be shown later.

For several years we have been experimenting with the intracranial approach to the canine hypophysis. At first some of our dogs died just as did those of Paulesco, Cushing, and others, but some lived (adults) and seemed little if any worse for the operation, either immediately or subsequently. Although, to all appearance, precisely the same procedure was used as far as we could judge the extirpation was done with equal care and thoroughness, we were confronted with totally different results. It was at once evident that the life of the animal was not dependent upon "microscopic remnants of the pituitary," for many of our animals were subjected to careful microscopic control. It was also clear that if a few animals survived a total hypophysectomy, there must be an explanation other than loss of "hypophyseal function" for the death of the remainder. The preservation of life in one totally hypophysectomized animal is sufficient denial of the theory that the hypophysis is essential to life.

There seemed but one possible reason for these seemingly paradoxical results, namely, that in some way the operative procedure itself must be held accountable. The fact that death following hypophysectomy usually occurs in less than forty-eight hours (at times after a longer period), is in itself sufficient reason to place the burden of proof on the operator. Moreover, the lassitude, drowsiness, and coma — all not infrequently appearing after a quick recovery from the anaesthetic — the not infrequent convulsions, were precisely like the manifestations (complications) which follow human intracranial operations. They are evidences of pressure (drowsiness and coma) and of local injury (convulsions).

Recently Bailey and Bremer,[17] working in Cushing's laboratory, obtained precisely the same symptoms — lassitude, arched back, coma, convulsions, etc. — described by Cushing as characteristic of the loss of hypophyseal function — by puncture of the tuber cinereum. Though their experiments are mainly concerned with glycosuria and polyuria, the inference is left that the above symptoms are not of hypophyseal origin but are the result of injury to the tuber cinereum — in injury readily associated with hypophysectomy. It is clear that they are also dealing with cerebral trauma and the symptoms are those of intracranial pressure. Proof of this is the entire absence of such symptoms in our experiments in which this entire region was cauterized.

THE OPERATIVE PROCEDURE

Our efforts have been directed toward the development of a method as free from operative complications — trauma and haemorrhage — as possible. We have used only the temporal intracranial route as originally devised by Horsley and, like Horsley, have made only a unilateral bony opening. Almost from the outset it seemed to us that the contralateral subtemporal defect was of doubtful value in providing better exposure, and that the division of both temporal muscles might well be a factor in interfering with the intake of food after operation.

After dividing the temporal muscle parallel to its origin and stripping it from the skull, a large defect is made both of bone and dura. Particularly important is the extension of the opening to the base of the skull. It is also advisable, though not necessary, to remove the zygoma, in order to give the lowest possible entrance to the base of the brain. While the convex inferior surface of the temporal lobe is slightly below a plane between the lower margin of the bony defect and the hypophysis, the spatula can be passed to the region of the sella without undue elevation of the lobe. An exposure of the hypophyseal region sufficient to permit painstaking removal of the pituitary body would, however, demand elevation and retraction of the temporal lobe — a trauma too severe and too prolonged. It is precisely this injury to the brain which has in large measure been responsible for the deaths (usually within forty-eight hours) reported by all investigators who have used this method of approach.

Trauma to the temporal lobe can be avoided or at least greatly reduced in two ways: (1) by inverting the head 100° to 135° so that the brain will fall away from the base of the skull; and (2) by releasing as much cerebrospinal fluid as possible.

After the dural opening has been made, the head is constantly maintained in the dependent position until the hypophysis has been removed. Before attempting an exposure of the hypophyseal region, a small spatula is gently passed to the cisterna interpeduncularis, which is punctured. At once the release of fluid gives much additional room and with the hanging brain but little if any retraction with the spatula is necessary to afford an excellent view of the hypophyseal region and ample room for deliberate and careful removal of the hypophysis. The importance of these details, particularly the hanging brain, can be readily appreciated when it is realized that with the customary position of the head the entire brain must be lifted and held in position during the entire operation — in many of the reported procedures for one and a half to two hours. The effects of this long sustained cerebral trauma are not immediate, but appear some hours later. When sufficient room is obtained by the hanging brain, the spatula seems scarcely necessary except to protect the brain from the wisps of moist cotton which are used to sponge the hypophyseal region. The oculomotor nerve obliquely bisects the view of the hypophysis and, since its function is of no concern, its division at the dural attachment is advisable. An unobstructed view of the hypophysis is then afforded.

The hypophysis is attached at only two points: (1) at the center of the posterior clinoid process where the posterior lobe artery enters, and (2) at the base of the brain by the stalk from which the hypophysis dangles below the cisterna chiasma-

TABLE I
TOTAL HYPOPHYSECTOMY IN ADULT DOGS

Estimated Age	Cauterization of Base	Post-Operative					Duration of Life After Operation	Necropsy Findings
		Glycosuria	Polyuria	Signs of Pressure	Convulsions	Motor Weakness		
1 year	0	0	+	+	++	0	24 days	Distemper. Some cerebral softening
2 years	0	+	+	0	0	0	81 days	Died in country
1 year	0	0	0	0	++	+	16 days	Distemper
1–2 years	+	+	+	+			1 year	Distemper. Emaciated
3 years	+	+	0	++	++	0	19 days	Distemper
1 year	+	0	0	0	0	0	24 days	Died in country
1 year	+	+	0	++	0	0	104 days	Emaciated
2 years	+	0	0	++	++	+	34 days	Died in country
1 year	0	0	0	0	0	0	75 days	Died in country
2 years	0	+	0	0	0	0	8 days	Distemper
1–2 years	0	++	0	0	0	0	144 days	Killed in fight
1–2 years	0	+	0	0	0	0	22 days	Distemper
1 year	+	0	0	0	0	0	69 days	Killed in fight
2 years	++	0	)	0	0	0	237 days	Poisoned in country
7 months	++	0	+	0	+	0	11 days	Cortical injury
8 months	++	+++	0	+	0	0	138 days	Died in country
7 months	+	0	0	0	0	+	27 days	
1 year	+	+	0	+	+	+	1 year	Distemper
2 years	++	+++	+	+		0	32 days	
2 years	+++	+++	+	++	++	0	2 days	Cortical softening; blood clot at base
4 years	0	++	0	0	0	+	138 days	
1 year	0						2 days	Blood clot at base
9 months	0	++	0	++	+	+	5 days	Blood clot at base
3 years	0	+	+	0	0	0	90 days	Poisoned
1 year	0	+++	0	0	0	0	11 days	Pneumonia
2 years	0	0	0	0	0	0	18 days	
2 years	0	0	0	+	++	0	12 days	Distemper
1 year	0	+	0	++	+	0	1 day	Blood clot at base
2 years	0	0	+	0	0	0	10 days	
2 years	0	+	0	0	0	0	2 days	Blood clot at base
1 year	0	+	0	0	0	0	60 days	Poisoned

tis and into the sella turcica. After gently stripping the pituitary body from its stalk with a pair of fine right-angled forceps, a short free zone of the stalk can be clearly distinguished and divided by pinching the accurately approximating blades of the forceps. The attachment to the posterior clinoid process can be separated by the same pinching process with the tweezer blades or by the sweep of an angled hook. A little bleeding which accompanies the liberation of both attachments is easily controlled by two or three gentle applications of moist cotton. The entire intracranial part of the operation can be completed in five to ten minutes and the wound left absolutely dry. It need not be added that bleeding must be absolutely checked, for even the slightest post-operative haemorrhage will compromise the life of the animal. Doubtless haemorrhage has also been an important factor in many of the results of experimental hypophysectomy — as in all human intracranial operations.

Minor differences in the anatomy of the hypophyseal region make the careful extirpation harder or easier, as the case may be. A falciform band of supporting tissue running from the base of the brain to the bridging carotid artery, a shorter hypophyseal stalk, and a posterior lobe attachment more concealed than usual in an anteriorly curving posterior clinoid process, are the variations which have some bearing on the greater difficulties in the

TABLE II
Total Hypophysectomy in Puppies

Estimated Age	Cauterization of Base	Post-Operative					Duration of Life After Operation	Necropsy Findings
		Glycosuria	Polyuria	Signs of Pressure	Convulsions	Motor Weakness		
Without intravenous salt								
3 weeks	0			+			1 day	Slight damage to cortex
3 weeks	0			+			1 day	Slight damage to cortex
3 weeks	0						1 day	Damage to cortex
5 weeks	0			+	++		3 days	Haemorrhage
5 weeks	0			+	+	+	6 days	
5 weeks	0			+	0	0	13 days	
5 weeks	0						1 day	
5 weeks	0			+			1 day	Blood clot
5 weeks	0			+			1 day	Small blood clot
5 weeks	0	+	+				3 days	Killed in fall
5 weeks	0	+	0	++			2 days	Blood clot at base
3 weeks	0						9 months	
With intravenous salt								
5 weeks	0	Trace	0	0	0	0	10 days	Pneumonia. No evidences of damage to cortex or of haemorrhage
5 weeks	0	Trace	0	0	0	0	6 weeks	Died following administration of vermifuge. Marked emaciation. No haemorrhage
7 weeks	0			+	0	0	1 day	Died of haemorrhage following operation
7 weeks	0	++					Still alive	Living and well 3 months after operation
7 weeks	0	Slight					Still alive	Living and well 3 months after operation
8 weeks	0	++	+		++	Walks in circle	8 days	Pneumonia following ether which was given to take x-rays

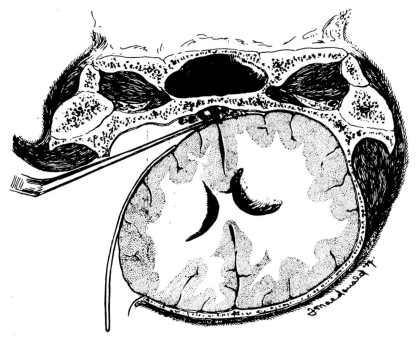

Fig. 1. Diagram to show how the pituitary region is reached. The lateral wall of the skull is removed as far toward the base as possible. The brain volume is reduced by intravenous hypertonic salt solution.

performance of the operation.

OPERATIONS ON YOUNG PUPPIES SHRINKING THE BRAIN BY THE METHOD OF WEED AND McKIBBEN

The operation as outlined above is satisfactory for dogs older than six months, but not for young puppies. In fact it is well nigh impossible to extirpate the hypophysis carefully in puppies from six to ten weeks of age. The cause of death in puppies is precisely that in adults, namely, intracranial pressure resulting from injury to the brain, but there are two outstanding anatomical features of a puppy's brain which render it different from the adult brain and make the operative effects much more rapid and severe. The brain of a puppy is so soft that practically any pressure with instruments will cause destruction, and the amount of fluid which can be withdrawn from the subarachnoid space in an effort to obtain room for the operative exposure is far less, both relatively and absolutely, than in the adult. It is now possible to overcome these handicaps by making use of the brilliant discovery of Weed and McKibben,[18] that intravenous injection of concentrated sodium chloride solution withdraws fluid from the brain and causes it to shrink in an astounding manner and yet without any appreciable injury to the animal (or human being). The dose of hypertonic solution contains 0.33 gm. of sodium chloride per kilo of bodyweight. Half an hour later the volume of brain is so greatly lessened that with the hanging-brain method the hypophyseal exposure is better than that obtainable in the adult animal without the use of concentrated saline (Fig. 1). Since learning the great value of shrinking the brains of puppies, we have also uniformly adopted the method in adults and, needless to say, the approach is immeasurably easier and the results even better.

RESULTS OF TOTAL HYPOPHYSECTOMY

The results of these hypophysectomies are summarized in the accompanying tables. Of thirty-one adult dogs, ranging in estimated age from seven months to three years, five died soon after operation from haemorrhage and cerebral trauma; seven died in the country where they were sent for the summer, and autopsies were not obtainable; distemper caused the largest mortality, ten deaths occurring from eight days to one year after operation. This seemingly excessive toll is, however, essentially similar for unoperated animals which were housed in the laboratory. In seven of the series the base of the brain was sectioned serially and studied for microscopic remnants of the anterior lobe, and in none were any found. In five of the seven so studied, the base had been cauterized at the time of operation. The duration of life in these seven histologically proven total extirpations was thirteen, twenty-two, twenty-seven, sixty-nine, ninety, one hundred and four and one hundred and thirty-eight days. The presence or absence of polyuria, glycosuria, convulsions and evidences of motor weakness immediately after the operation, are included in the tables because they were part of our studies at the time. Some of these results, particularly of polyuria and polydipsia, will have a more direct bearing in a subsequent publication in which the functions of the hypophysis will be considered.

The table of operated young puppies, of three to eight weeks, presents a totally different picture. In the first twelve hypophysectomies in puppies, only one survived longer than two weeks. It lived for nine months. Its post-operative course was difficult and recovery slow. During the operation the temporal lobe was extensively injured and largely sacrificed. Without doubt its stormy convalescence was due to the cerebral injury, but doubtless also its life was preserved by the fact that the deliberate sacrifice of this injured brain prevented an increased intracranial pressure. The table of the post-operative life history of the first eleven puppies might well be that of similar tables in adults by Paulesco and others who claimed the hy-

pophysis to be essential to life. The results are practically indentical. But the series beginning with the use of Weed's hypertonic salt solution is entirely different, because the brain is spared the cerebral trauma incident to the operation. These results are, then, totally at variance with those of the earlier group of puppies and quite like those of the adult dogs — as far as life is concerned. On the day of the operation the animals walk about and on the following day they are almost as playful and lively as the controls.

In order to insure total absence of microscopic remnants of the anterior lobe at the base of the brain, the stump of the infundibulum (to which cells might remain attached) and the region immediately contiguous have been well cauterized with a platinum tip in thirteen adult dogs. The general post-operative course of these animals (possibly excepting polyuria) has not been unlike that of those without cauterization. Microscopic studies (serial sections) of the base of the brain in many of the surviving animals have been made and the sections have been uniformly negative for anterior lobe cells.

With painstaking care and attention to detail there should be a minimal operative mortality in animals over six months, and while our later series of young puppies has been small (six), there seems no reason why the results should be greatly different at this age. All deaths following soon after operation are explainable as the result of trauma, haemorrhage or pneumonia, and deaths appearing later can be readily explained on well-recognized pathological grounds.

SUMMARY

An operative procedure is presented for the safe removal of the canine hypophysis.

We have found no evidence to support, and every evidence to refute, the assumption that the hypophysis is essential to life, or that the group of symptoms which have been described by others as preceding death in hypophysectomized animals are of hypophyseal origin.

REFERENCES

[1]Horsley, Victor: Functional nervous disorders due to loss of thyroid gland and pituitary body. Abstract of third Brown Lecture. *Lancet, i:* 5, 1886.

[2]Gemelli: Sur la fonction de l'hypophyse. *Arch. ital. de biol., L:* 157–174, 1908.

[3]Paulesco, N. C.: *L'Hypophyse du Cerveau*, Paris, Vigot Freres, Eds., 1908.

[4]Reford, L. L., and Cushing, H.: Is the pituitary gland essential to the maintenance of life? *Johns Hopkins Hosp. Bull., xx:* 105, 1909.

[5]Crowe, S. J., Cushing, H., and Homans, J.: Experimental hypophysectomy. *Johns Hopkins Hosp. Bull., xxi:* 127, 1910.

[6]Handelsmann and Horsley, V.: Preliminary note on experimental investigations on the pituitary body. *Brit. Med. J., ii:* 1150, 1911.

[7]Aschner, B.: Ueber die Funktion der Hypophysis. *Arch. f. d. ges. Physiol., cxlvi:* 1, 1912.

[8]Sweet, J. E., and Allen, A. R.: The effect of the removal of the hypophysis in the dog. *Ann. Surg., lvii:* 485, 1913.

[9]Benedict, F. G., and Homans, J.: The metabolism of the hypophysectomized dog. *J. Med. Research, xx:* 409, 1912.

[10]Camus, J. and Roussy, M. G.: Presentation de sept chiens hypophysectomises depius quelques mois. *Soc. de biol., lxxiv:* 1386, 1913.

[11]Brown, C. G.: The effects of complete extirpation of the hyphysis in the dog (preliminary report). *Proc. Soc. Exper. Biol. and Med., xx:* 275, 1922-23.

[12]Houssay, B. A.: Extirpacion de la hypofisis en el perro. First Natl. Cong. Med., Buenos Aires, 1916. Abstr. in *Endocrin, ii:* 497, 1918.

[13]Bell, W. B.: The Pituitary. Bailliere, Tindall & Cox, London, 1919. *Also: Quart. J. Exper. Physiol., xi:* 78, 1917.

[14]Dott, N. M.: An investigation into the function of the pituitary and thyriod glands. Part I. The technique of their experimental surgery and summary of results. *Quart. J. Exper. Physiol., xiii:* 241, 1923.

[15]Smith, P. E.: Experimental abalation of the hypophysis in the frog embryo. *Science, N. S.,* Aug. 25, 1916, p. 280. *Also: Anat. Rec., xi:* 57, 1916.

[16]Allen, B. M.: Extirpation experiments in Rana pipiens larvae. *Science, N. S., xliv:* 1143, 1916.

[17]Bailey, P. and Bremer, F.: Experimental diabetes insipidus. *Arch. Int. Med., xxviii:* 773, 1921.

[18]Weed, L. H. and McKibben: Pressure changes in the cerebrosponal fluid following intravenous injection of solutions of various concentrations. *Am. J. Physiol., xlviii:* 512, 1919; Experimental alteration of brain bulk. *Am. J. Physiol., xlviii:* 531, 1919.

XXI

AN OPERATION FOR THE TOTAL REMOVAL OF CEREBELLOPONTILE (ACOUSTIC) TUMORS *

Potentially benign lesions, usually easy of of recognition, not difficult of operative approach or even of enucleation, nevertheless tumors of the cerebellopontile angle [1] have presented surgical problems which have seemed well-nigh insuperable. Surely few lesions have enticed surgeons with more alluring prospects and have ultimately yielded so little reward for their best efforts for, with few chance exceptions patients have succumbed following total or attempted total extirpation of the tumor. At the beginning of the twentieth century it seems probable that there had been but one tumor of this kind completely and successfully extirpated—one removed by Ballance [2] in 1894 and reported in 1907. Although there is some uncertainty as to the exact nature of this tumor (he terms it a fibrosarcoma), it seems highly probable that it was really one of the true cerebellopontile variety. It was clearly an encapsulated tumor in this region, shelling out readily with the finger, and the patient's survival for many years is alone sufficient evidence to preclude a sarcoma. Moreover, as most of these tumors in earlier years have been recorded as gliosarcomata—a classification well justified by the histological picture—such an entry is evidence in favor of the tumor being of the cerebellopontile variety.

At the beginning of the twentieth century cerebellopontile tumors were recognized by their more or less characteristic signs and symptoms and became a fairly well established clinical entity.

Oppenheim of Berlin, Sternberg of Vienna, v. Monakow of Zurich, Hughlings Jackson and Gowers of London, Babinski of Paris, and Allen Starr of New York, were not only pioneers in the recognition of these tumors but they stimulated a group of surgeons to undertake their removal.

At the International Congress of Medicine in London in 1913, the three great European surgeons—Horsley of London, v. Eiselsberg of Vienna, and Krause of Berlin—who had in such large measure been responsible for the birth and growth of brain surgery, presented their results on the extirpation of cerebellopontile tumors to that date. Horsley had 10 operative deaths in fifteen cases (67 per cent), v. Eiselsberg thirteen deaths in seventeen cases (77 per cent), and Krause twenty-six deaths in thirty-one cases (84 per cent). Krause admitted they yielded the poorest results of all his brain tumors. There seems to have no very great difference in the methods of attacking the tumor. Each used a unilateral cerebellar approach, often little more than an enlarged trephine opening, and the tumor was quickly shelled out with the index finger or spatula. Because of the disastrous results, the operation was often performed in two stages, particularly by v. Eiselsberg and Horsley. Sometimes Krause used suction to draw the tumor from its bed.

The conference ended with no prospect of better operative results in the future. In the hasty and necessarily blind extirpation of these tumors through a totally inadequate exposure, many of these tumors were broken and only partially

---

*Reprinted from Surgery, Gynecology and Obstetrics, August, 1925, pages 129–148.

removed, necropsy revealing more or less tumor undisturbed. Moreover, those few patients who survived were almost without exception badly crippled. So far as I am aware, the ultimate results of the few successes of Horsley, Krause, and v. Eiselsberg were never published, but a fortunately timed publication of Tooth [18] at the same International Congress in London, 1913, presents a comprehensive statistical study of the operative results in all brain tumors from the National Hospital of London to the date of this conference (1913), and appended thereto is a brief summary of each case together with the operator, operation, and, so far as known, the ultimate results. If not including all of Horsley's work, this report at least gives us a fair insight into his results. From this dismal story we learn much concerning the fortitude of these great pioneer brain surgeons who nevertheless persevered to blaze a trail through a forest which must have seemed utterly impenetrable. Looking back, it is clear that they were ill equipped for such a struggle; until the latter part of their work surgery was yet in its infancy. Cranial surgery offered technical problems foreign to those of other tissues; instruments of special character had to be devised; the control of haemorrhage from bone, the brain, and tumors, was unlike that elsewhere. A knowledge of the functions of the various parts of the brain and of the cerebrospinal fluid was only slowly accumulating. The effects on intracranial pressure of the immediate injury to cerebral tissues were at best imperfectly understood; and the avoidance of trauma continued to be almost impossible because technical difficulties prevented sufficient exposure of the desired field. Moreover, sepsis continued to exact a not inconsiderable toll. Though Horsley, v. Eiselsberg, and Krause were all firm adherents of the Listerian principles of combating infection, the avoidance of infection had not been mastered. And, last but not least, neurology was also just developing so that the diagnosis of tumors was usually made when the patient was blind and often *in extremis*. Cerebellopontile tumors, however, had one great advantage over all other brain tumors: not only could fair diagnosis and localization be made with fair accuracy, greater as time passed, but the tumor was known beforehand to be benign and encapsulated. The surgical problem, therefore, was direct.

With a minimum of scientific equipment the struggle for solution of this surgical problem was necessarily in large part through trial and error, but the great Horsley early added to neurological surgery the far reaching and invaluable method of animal experimentation, but shortly before begun by Fritsch and Hitzig in Germany and by Ferrier in England.

One hardly knows whether to admire the indomitable courage of the surgeons or the persisting faith and hope of the neurologist the more. The story contained in these struggles differs only in degree from that of the pioneer efforts in advancing the frontiers of knowledge. It is, therefore, without possible taint of a critical attitude that the statistics of Sir Victor Horsley are studied. Without his contributions, both technical and physiological, to this field of surgery—his bone wax, his method of controlling haemorrhage with pieces of excised muscle, and his introduction of decompressions in order to combat acute post-operative intracranial pressure, etc.— it would not yet be possible to cope with the many problems of intracranial surgery.

Returning to Tooth's analysis of operations for tumor, we find under the heading "Extracerebellar Tumours—Removal of tumour, complete or partial," twelve cases of cerebellopontile tumor operated upon by Horsley. [1] From this group of cases, five (42 per cent) survived the operation for periods of six weeks, two and one-half months, three years, three years+ and eight years+; of these, three died of recurrence at the times stated, one had signs of recurrence at the end of three years (the wound was bulging and tight) and the last case was well and active eight years after the operation. Of the seven deaths (58 per cent), two were from meningitis on the sixth and seventeenth days. It is evident that Horsley has included in his own mortality statistics two deaths which occurred at six and ten weeks, and included in his living cases one which lived eleven months after removal of a tumor on one side and died following extirpation of a second growth in the other angle, a case almost surely of Recklinghausen's disease and not of cerebellopontile tumor. But the most important result in Horsley's series is not his mortality rate but the report of the necropsy findings. Of six necropsies, in only one case had the tumor been totally extirpated, the remaining five showing more or less tumor still undisturbed. In two cases the cerebellar lobe had been very badly damaged.

Tooth's remarks on the results following extirpation of these tumors (including five cases operated upon by other surgeons at the National Hospital without a single recovery), well express the situation and faint degree of hope at that time. "The diagnosis of tumours in this region is so comparatively easy and accurate, and the surgical treatment at first sight so straightforward, that the results in this table are disappointing in the extreme. . . . No doubt the proximity to the vital centres is accountable for great shock, with respiratory and cardiac failure. If the danger of that period can, by any alteration in surgical procedure, be eliminated, there is no reason evident why these cases should not do well."

Nor had this impression of the surgical treatment of cerebellopontile tumors changed in England during the following ten years, if we may judge correctly from the following quotation from Gordon

Holmes [11], when discussing a case presented by Walshe [20] before the Royal Society of Medicine: "It was perhaps presumptuous on his part to refer to the surgical treatment, but so many of his cases had passed through the hands of surgeons that he had had some experience in the matter. He had seen one case recover only after gross removal of the tumour, a man upon whom Sir Victor Horsley operated many years ago, but though he lived for several years he was seriously crippled.[1] The danger seemed to be that total removal necessarily meant a disturbance of the vascular supply on the same side of the pons and medulla; the man to whom he referred had, after the operation, the characteristic symptoms of softening in the lateral side of the pons. He saw a few other cases which had survived operation for a week or so after total removal of the tumour, and all showed evidence of acute bulbar involvement."

The aggregate number of total extirpations of these tumors with recovery to date and freedom from recurrence, is impossible to estimate but with liberal allowance it will probably be less than half a dozen—and we are positive of only two. Foremost of these cases is the one removed by Ballance [2] in 1894. Apparently the only permanent sequelae of the operation many years later were palsies of the fifth and seventh nerves; the former had resulted in corneal ulceration and loss of vision in that eye. The second undoubted cured case is that of Horsley. From Eiselberg's series[9] of four recoveries (including one by his assistant, Clairmont) from the operation, one was able to resume work on the farm but there is no other record noting the ultimate results and freedom from recurrence. Leischner[13] collected from the literature eleven cases which had survived operation. Among these were four from Eiselsberg's Clinic, one of Horsley's (this was before Horsley's report (1913) of five recoveries), Krause[12] one, Poppert[16] one, Baisch[1] one, and Borchardt[3] three. This ensemble, however, is of little significance; they should not be confused with cures, for aside from the cases of Ballance and Horsley, and possibly the one of Eiselsberg's, the subsequent evidence of their cure has not appeared. In the light of the necropsy reports in Horsley's cases, in which but one of six cases was shown to be totally removed, it would appear fair to presume that few if any of these had been totally extirpated and the patients permanently cured. One of the best results reported in this group of tumors was by Willy Meyer of New York (14, 1912). In two stages, four weeks apart, this tumor was removed with a spoon. Three years later he was apparently well, but we have been unable to find subsequent notes on this patient's condition.

The operative method used by all operators was essentially the method of Horsley, v. Eiselsberg and Krause. A two-stage procedure came to be used almost universally and usually the dura was not opened in the first step. It seems probable, however, from Tooth's reports that Horsley always opened the dura and, toward the last at least, his decompression was bilateral. The unilateral exposure of the affected side of the cerebellum was used by Krause and v. Eiselsberg. Krause,[12] it is true, suggested a bilateral cerebellar approach, but it was designed for exploration of the posterior fossa and was not intended to be used when the tumor was known to be in the cerebellopontile angle. It appears that in many instances the opening in the occipital bone was but little larger than necessary to insert the finger or spatula. The tumor was removed by sweeping the finger or spatula around the tumor and making the traction necessary to dislodge it. The finger was preferable for it could better detect the cleavage plane between tumor and brain stem. After such extirpations, furious bleeding must have been inevitable. Always the lobe of the cerebellum was injured, often much of it destroyed, and at times even deliberately removed. Not infrequently the tumor was extirpated through a transcerebellar defect which reached the upper surface of the tumor. Frazier (10, 1905) indeed urged deliberate resection of the outer part of the cerebellar hemisphere and, though a heroic procedure, it probably caused no greater damage to the lobe than that which customarily resulted from these extirpations.

Krause (12, 1903) introduced a very useful procedure to reduce the excessive pressure which was nearly always present with cerebellopontile tumors. A trocar was passed through the tentorium into the lateral ventricle permitting the evacuation of its fluid. This procedure (ventricular puncture), in much more refined form, has come to be a most important item in all operations for tumors below the tentorium.

Perhaps the translabyrinthine approach suggested by the otologist Panse (15, 1904) should be mentioned in passing. At the time this method was proposed, attempts to remove cerebellopontile tumors appeared utterly futile and any suggestion might at least be tolerated. But it was a wholly impractical suggestion. After destroying much of the petrous bone, including the labyrinth and much of the mastoid bone and its contained air cells, and after passing through fields which could not be sterilized and might well harbor dormant infections, the resulting exposure must necessarily have been so meager that it would hardly be possible to do more than nibble at these great tumors. Quix (17,1911) hastily reported the removal of a pea-sized tumor by this method but the patient died a few months later. The usual large recess tumor was present; its surface had only been scratched! The one prerequisite of any operative approach is adequate room to afford thorough inspection of the tumor during its attack in order to permit the deliberate control of haemorrhage. This exposure being lacking in the translabyrinthine approach, other consideration of the procedure is useless.

Inevitably a severe reaction must appear against attempts to remove cerebellopontile tumors, particularly as the gamut of possibilities, both of method and of individual skill, had apparently been run. All of the accumulated technical advances of à quarter of a century had made no improvement in the results. At any rate, the continuance of an operation carrying such an astounding mortality after such an exhaustive trial, was impossible.

The reaction came with the publication, in 1917, of Cushing's[5] important monograph on acoustic tumors, and with it a revolution in treatment. He accepts the only conclusion which the foregoing results and experiences of his own could justify, i.e., "I doubt very much, unless some more perfected method is devised, whether one of these tumors can with safety be totally enucleated." He no longer attempted to enucleate these tumors totally but was content to offer a method by which the tumor could be *partially* removed (intracapsular enucleation).

Cushing's contribution is the only important advance in the treatment of cerebellopontile tumors. For the first time the patient was offered a relatively safe surgical procedure with prospects of temporary relief and prolongation of life, in lieu of a hazardous and desperate effort carrying permanent disability in the wake of the very occasional chance recovery. In the first series of operations his mortality rate was reduced to 35 per cent, and in a subsequent series of about equal number to 11 per cent.

But intracapsular partial extirpation is far from satisfactory, for the growth must always recur. Partial removal of the tumor, even when the growth develops slowly, can never be considered a final operation for a potentially benign tumor.

THE DEVELOPMENT OF AN OPERATIVE PROCEDURE FOR THE TOTAL REMOVAL OF CEREBELLOPONTILE TUMORS

The purpose of this communication is to present an operative procedure by which it has been possible to remove the entire cerebellopontile tumor in a group of cases. Admittedly, it is a procedure of magnitude and carries potentialities of great danger. However, with care and attention to detail the mortality may not be greater, and not improbably even less, than Cushing's partial intracapsular enucleation. The method has been gradually evolved from the failures of other operative procedures. Finally it was forced upon us in an effort to avert an impending death several days following the partial (intracapsular) operation.

Our operations on cerebellopontile tumors cover the past 9 years. At the present writing the series consists of 23 tumors, the results of which are included in Table I under the various methods of operative attack. One case, apparently well on admission, died at stool a few hours before the time scheduled for operation. In a general way the order of the grouping is also chronological, though this is not strictly true. Our operations began at a time (1915) when the results of attempted enucleations were known, but our efforts were necessarily directed along the more or less generally recognized methods of operative attack. The initial attempts at a simple suboccipital decompression met a sharp and entirely unexpected reverse and dispelled at once our pre-existing impressions of the value of this procedure as a palliative measure. Two cases so treated died within twelve hours, postmortem examinations revealing no haemorrhage or other cause in either instance. Although the intracranial pressure was well advanced in both patients, each was conscious and in good physical condition at the time of operation. Disregarding for the moment the explanation of these deaths—now better understood—it is at least evident that this comparatively simple procedure has been accompanied by great danger and has in nowise helped to solve the problem of removing the tumors.

In desperation, our next effort, total extirpation with the finger at one stage, then seemed the only alternative. It was of course, merely a reversion to the well tried and fruitless method of Horsley, Krause, Eiselsberg and others. Nor was there reason to expect better results. After two initial successes, four deaths in succession showed the futility of further attempts. It is of little concern that one case is well five years later, and the fate of the other after leaving the hospital is unknown. The results are of interest and importance only in that their careful analysis did explain the cause of death and therefore suggested methods of avoiding them.

At this time of despair, Cushing's method of intracapsular enucleation was introduced. Its great improvement over other procedures was at once obvious. Despite enthusiastic hopes, however, our first experiences with intracapsular enucleation were unfortunate in being less satisfactory than had been anticipated. Following an uneventful and quick recovery from the effects of the operation, the first patient seven days later became listless and drowsy; vomiting, dysphagia and dysarthria appeared; and during the succeeding three days all symptoms became progressively worse and finally alarming. The late appearance of these symptoms seemed to exclude the postoperative complications which might have been expected, haemorrhage or infection, and suggested that in some way the reaction about the stump of tumor which remained was responsible for the condition. The wound was reopened and the shell of tumor extirpated with the index finger. There was surprisingly little haemorrhage, which was readily controlled. The patient's condition then steadily improved. Diminished drowsiness was at once apparent, the vomiting at once ceased, and five days later she was able to swallow. From the result of this case it seemed logical to infer that if the shell of the tumor could in some way be removed at the first operation, this stormy and dangerous course following subtotal removal might be avoided. In the succeeding cases in which the tumor has been removed at one sitting, the results have amply supported this inference.

THE OPERATION

Needless to say, the success of this procedure is dependant not only upon many technical advances which have been slowly accumulating, but also upon a clearer understanding of intracranial physiology and pathology. Without Horsley's bone wax or Cushing's silver "clips," without Horsley's principle of decompression to take care of post-operative traumatic oedema, without the bilateral cerebellar exposure (probably originated by Cotterill,[4]) which allows more room for exposure and for decompression, and finally without Cushing's intracapsular method of removing the body of the tumor, the removal of the capsule of the tumor could hardly be accomplished.

A bilateral cerebellar approach, which has become more or less a regular practice for all cerebellar lesions, is first made and the bony and dural defect extended laterally and superiorly on the side of the tumor as far as the transverse and lateral venous sinuses will allow. Because of the great depth of the tumor, an ordinary bilateral cerebellar approach alone would not afford the direct inspection and lengthy manipulation which is necessary to dissect the growth from its bed. Indeed, in a survey of Cushing's cases, there are instances in which the tumor was missed at the first operation because of insufficient exposure, and there are other cases in which the tumors were found only by transecting the cerebellar lobe. Attempts to expose the tumor with an insufficient removal of bone causes serious injury to the brain from retraction. Always the mastoid cells are brought into view, but unless the easy exposure of the tumor makes imperative demand, their entrance is avoided. But when opened the cells are at once covered either with a sheet of wet cotton or by reflected dura which is sutured to the galea or trapezius muscle. The history of a mastoid infection would give great concern, and every other possibility of the tumor's exposure would be attempted before yielding to an easier approach which opening hitherto infected cells would provide. The anterior part of the bony extension is carried under the attachment of the trapezius muscle but the continuity of this muscle with the galea is carefully preserved. A good exposure of the entire superior surface of the cerebellum is important in providing a good exposure of one large vein which bridges the space between the superior surface of the cerebellum and the tentorium which it enters en route to the transverse sinus. Unless ligated and divided beforehand, this vessel may easily be stretched and torn in elevating the cerebellar hemisphere and in exposing the tumor. There is less danger of such injury to the contralateral symmetrical vein, and similar precautions against its injury are not necessary. Needless to say, special care is taken to avoid incising either the lateral or sigmoid sinuses, particularly the latter.

Almost without exception, the dura has been so tense that it has been necessary, or at least advisable, to relieve pressure in the dilated ventricles, tapping and withdrawing fluid from the posterior horn of a lateral ventricle. Hydrocephalus invariably results when the tumor has occluded the iter, and few tumors appear for operation before this phase of the tumor's progress is well established. Before removing the ventricular needle, gentle pressure can, if desired, be applied to the intact dura and additional relief of pressure which is exerted upon the posterior fossa will follow the further escape of fluid which is afforded by the upward push of the tentorium. In every case of hydrocephalus from cerebellar lesions, the intracranial pressure above the tentorium can be reduced to that of the atmosphere by this simple expedient and without danger of injury to the brain stem.

After this preliminary measure, gentle elevation of the cerebellar lobe quickly brings the tumor into view, though at a great depth. Another invariable finding in all cases of cerebellopontile tumors is the partial or complete obliteration of the cisterna magna, the cerebellar tonsils projecting through the foramen magnum into the spinal canal. If, however, the cisterna does still contain fluid, its release again contributes that much more room to the all-important exposure of the tumor. An encapsulated bed of fluid (having no communication with the subarachnoid spaces) may or may not crown the outer and superior surfaces of the tumor and, though largely or entirely obscuring the tumor, its presence is almost as characteristic of an underlying cerebellopontile tumor as the direct inspection of the neoplasm itself. Further elevation of the cerebellum brings the unattached outer surface of the tumor into full view and into a position where it can be subjected to an operative attack. Excepting the poles which have passed beyond the confines of the posterior cranial fossa (through the incisura tentorii and the foramen magnum), the entire longitudinal extent of the tumor is brought into full view. The capsule is then incised longitudinally from pole to pole and much of the outer contents removed piecemeal with a curette after the method of Cushing. The capsule is then picked up at the margins of the opening in the tumor, drawn forward with forceps, and the attached surface of the capsule brought into view. The contents of the tumor are then curetted with the brain stem and cerebellum always fully exposed. Continuing this method, the capsule gradually becomes thinner and when drawn forward permits inspection of the cleavage line between the brain stem and capsule of the tumor. When the poles of the tumor have invaded the middle cranial fossa and the spinal canal, removal of their interior allows them to be easily withdrawn into the posterior fossa; such polar extensions of the tumor are least adherent to the brain stem. Gradually in this way the entire capsule is separated from the brain stem. As the capsule is cautiously retracted, several small blood vessels crossing from the brain stem or cerebellum are brought into view and doubly "clipped" and the vessel divided. Practically all bleeding can be forestalled in this way.

Removal of the capsule of the tumor in this way is necessarily very tedious and time consuming. The method employed is but the application of the fundamental surgical teachings of my former chief, the late Professor Halsted. By this great master every operation, whether unusual or commonplace, was performed with the utmost care. All tissues were handled with the greatest gentleness, the field unstained with blood, and a step was never taken blindly. Always his work was painstaking, the field of operation immaculate, and haemorrhage minimal. Time of operation was always subordinate to accurate and thorough performance.

It is clear that as a measure preliminary to removal of the capsule, the intracapsular curettement must be carried out much more thoroughly than when this procedure is the end-result. When the tumor is curetted blindly, i.e., with only the outer aspect of the growth in view, the total amount of tumor removed,

though seemingly great, will be relatively small, for the danger of penetrating the capsule and injuring the brain stem with the curette is always uppermost in the operator's mind, and in avoiding this possibility it is more probable that too little rather than too much will be removed. The more thoroughly the capsule is stripped of its solid contents (up to a certain limit), the easier becomes the final stage of its separation from the brain stem. It should not be inferred that the separation of the capsule is not attended by difficulties. It is always difficult and frequently for some time seems impossible. Only by persistently tugging at the capsule, often gaining but a milli-meter at a step, does its attachment finally yield.

In one of the earlier cases the ultimate release of a fraction of the capsule seemed impossible of accomplishment and was given up. It is quite probable that with increasing experience and confidence this capsule could now be removed. On the other hand, only quite recently the capsule in another case was so delicate that at every attempt at traction it tore and when there seemed no way to overcome this difficulty in desperation the capsule was shelled out with the index finger. There is, however, a marked individual difference in the degree of attachment of the tumor to the brain stem, and there will probably always be instances in which a deliberate and painstaking removal will not be possible.

When the capsule is ultimately delivered, the denuded brain stem should and must be perfectly dry. A fatality will almost surely ensue if even the slightest ooze persists when closure is begun. Drainage has usually been avoided, though in two instances a rubber protective wick was placed in the lateral recess and removed in less than twenty-four hours.

The largest vessels encountered during the operation are the postero-inferior cerebellar and vertebral arteries which wind around the lower pole of the tumor and usually one and at times two branches to the tumor are given off from the former. These arteries are but loosely attached to the tumor and can easily be stripped from it after the branches have been divided. At the other pole of the tumor is a large venous branch of the inferior petrosal sinus. Closely applied to the tentorium and the tumor, from which it emerges, this vein may be very troublesome unless dissected free, ligatured and divided in the operation. Naturally the vessels causing greatest concern are the arteries which cross from the brain stem to the tumor. There are usually three to six of these vessels in addition to two or three from the inferior surface of the cerebellum. Though constituting probably the greatest danger of the operation, there is, however, no great difficulty either in exposing or ligating these vessels.

Removal of the tumor at a single stage is undoubtedly far preferable to two stages. Despite its great length (often three to four hours) the operation is usually well borne, and unless exceptionally difficult can be completed before lowering blood pressure or accelerating pulse gives warning of danger. Only once did the patient's condition necessitate abandoning operation and continuing at a second attempt. In three cases the capsule was intentionally left for a second stage (seven to twelve days later). In the interim the capsule had become so soft, swollen, and friable that the teeth of the forceps were no longer able to retain a grip and the capsule then had to be shelled out with the finger. If the capsule cannot be carefully extirpated at the first stage, its enucleation with the finger can undoubtedly be accomplished with greater safety at a second and not too distant stage, for the oedema of the tumor which remains, doubtless reduces the caliber of the small arteries supplying it and greatly modifies the bleeding.

It is not the purpose of this communi-cation to commend finger enucleation for these tumors. However, in those exceptional cases in which the capsule of the tumor cannot be liberated, I believe the removal of the capsule at a second stage to be superior in the ultimate, and at times in the immediate results, to the subtotal intracapsular enucleation alone. An excellent example of this impression is given in the patient previously mentioned. When, several days after intracapsular enucleation, stupor, vomiting, dysphagia, and dysarthria appeared and progressively increased, not only did she promptly recover and the symptoms quickly disappear after enucleation of the capsule with the finger, but she has since remained as well as any of those patients in whom the operation was completed by careful dissection in one stage.

The bond between the brain stem and tumor may be solely by connective tissue, but in one case at least the tumor has been found at necropsy to be a direct outgrowth of the brain stem. It can hardly be denied that when the tumor is actually continuous with and a direct outgrowth from the brain stem its origin must be from the brain stem and not from the region of the porus acusticus, as has been claimed. But the origin of these tumors is another story which we shall consider at another time. The capsule has always been most adherent at the pons; in the single case in which a line of cleavage could not be followed throughout, the fragment of tumor remained tightly adherent at the pons.

Cerebellopontile tumors are only slightly adherent to the dural covering of the base of the skull, but the separation of the capsule nearly always leaves an oozing, raw surface, and at times an even greater degree of bleeding. At the porus acusticus, however, the attachment is always firm for the auditory nerve is an integral part of the tumor. This attachment has usually been liberated after the tumor has been separated from the brain stem, but in one case the dissection was begun at the meatus and in so doing it was possible to pick up and follow the facial nerve in the capsule, in which it was superficially located, to the brain stem. But in liberating the capsule from the pons, the nerve was accidentally torn. Greatly elongated by its stretch around the tumor, the facial nerve in this case was a very delicate filament scarcely larger than an ordinary cambric sewing needle. In none of the other cases has the facial nerve been seen during dissection of the tumor. Should preservation of the facial nerve with total removal of the growth be ultimately possible, it could doubtless be more easily located at the internal auditory meatus. Its course is probably always, as in this case, on the under surface and toward the lower pole of the tumor.

The trigeminal nerve is always brought clearly in view during the dissection and throughout its intracranial course. Usually it first appears when the upper pole of the tumor is withdrawn from the incisura tentorii or separated from the tentorium. But on one occasion when the dissection from the inferior pole proceeded with unusual ease, the nerve was first exposed at its junction with the pons; its exposure was then continued forward in the direction of the mid-brain. Being tightly squeezed between tumor and brain stem which it parallels the trigeminal nerve has been flattened like a ribbon. Its more distal course is determined by the upper pole of the tumor which pushes the nerve ahead, ofttimes into the middle cranial fossa, causing it to double back upon itself before entering the dural envelope surrounding the gasserian ganglion.

The remaining cranial nerves of the posterior cranial fossa (on the side of the tumor), though pushed aside and even somewhat elongated by the tumor, are much less seriously effected. Before the dissection is started, the spinal accessory nerve, most affected of this group, is often seen bending around the inferior pole of the tumor from behind, but in any case it is quickly brought into view when the inferior pole is drawn forward. The vagus and glossopharyngeal nerves appear in succession when the inferior pole is drawn a little farther forward. Never more than lightly attached to the growth, these nerves are pushed mesially and inferiorly, the distortion of each depending upon the size and configuration of this part of the tumor. In one case a tumor nodule projected between the spinal accessory and vagus nerves. The hypoglossal nerve, having a more mesially placed exit, is less disturbed by the tumor. This entire group of nerves fall away as the capsule of the inferior pole is dislodged. Although the basilar artery has been exposed on two occasions, I have never recognized the abducens nerve.

We have carefully examined every porus acusticus after extirpation of the tumor, but in only two instances was there an appreciable widening of this opening. Not infrequently there was a rather diffuse concavity of the region surrounding the meatus, and in one instance a quite deep pit (about 1 by 1 centimeter and probably 3 millimeters deep) with fairly abrupt walls extended mesially from the porus and included its inner margin, but the outer margin remained unchanged. These findings explain the lack of positive changes in roentgenograms and they also constitute evidence against the theory of origin of the tumor in the internal auditory meatus. When the tumor has extended into the porus, its liberation has not been difficult. Only on one occasion was it necessary to chisel away the outer margin of this opening before this dissection could be completed.

With one exception the operations have been performed under ether anaesthesia. Novocain worked admirably in this exception until the brain stem was reached, when the pain became so severe that ether was given for the capsular dissection. The patients are maintained in the horizontal face-down position. Pulse and blood pressure readings have been the best criteria of the patient's condition and largely determined whether the operation could be concluded in one or two stages.

POSTOPERATIVE COURSE

Few brain tumor extirpations run a more uneventful and satisfactory course than these have done. Without exception, the patients have quickly become conscious, have remained so, and on the following day have appeared free of danger. That two of the series of total enucleations should have survived a super-imposed purulent meningitis (streptococcus viridans and staphylococcus aureus), the symptoms of which appeared forty-eight hours after the operation, indicates the rapidity of recovery from the operation. The postoperative temperature curves of these patients are more or less uniform. The rectal temperature slowly rises to a maximum which is usually reached in ten or twelve hours, and it almost as quickly descends to a level around 101 or lower the next morning. Usually the maximum temperature is about 103.6 to 104.2, though one case reached 104.8. At the end of the operation when the patient is coming out of ether, the quality of the pulse will be at its worst and the rate highest. Despite the gradual post-operative rise of temperature, the patient remains conscious and the pulse slowly falls, usually reaching 100 to 120 on the following morning.

Of the series of five cases in which the capsule was carefully removed (all in one stage), post-operative dysphagia was present in only one patient, and she had been unable to swallow for thirty-six hours before the operation. Five days later nasal feedings were discontinued. In all of the four cases in which the cap-

sule was *enucleated with the finger,* nasal tube feeding was necessary, but in two of these patients inability to swallow had developed 7 and 10 days after a subtotal intracapsular enucleation (first stage) and was therefore not caused by the operation. The one death in this series was from pneumonia (eighth day) and was doubtless induced by aspiration during this period when swallowing was difficult. Surely this death could now be avoided. Fluids are now withheld from patients after operation until they are well able to swallow; in the interim the regular nasal feedings are substituted.

Each of the five cases was able to walk out of the hospital with support, and to some extent alone, the time of departure being sixteen, eighteen, eighteen, twenty-five, and seventy-six days after operation. One patient was unable to walk when she entered the hospital because of a partial hemiplegia (there was also dysphagia) resulting from the tumor's indentation of the brain stem; 22 days after the operation she walked across the room without support. The protracted stay of the patient who remained in the hospital seventy-six days was due to a postoperative streptococcus viridans infection, which was cured by cisternal drainage. Fortunately this patient has retained no ill consequences of the infection.

SUBSEQUENT COURSE OF PATIENTS AFTER REMOVAL OF TUMOR

There has as yet been no recurrence, but the longest time since operation has been only three and one-half years. Every patient is well, free from headache, and has been able to return to work. The one outstanding sacrifice of the operation is the hemifacial paralysis. It has as yet been impossible to preserve the facial nerve, though I am not so sure that this may not eventually be possible. The reason for this hope is that in one case (previously mentioned) the facial nerve was dissected from the porus to the pons but was finally inadvertently torn when the capsular dissection was continued. The patient is informed of the necessary loss of the facial nerve beforehand and is given the choice of an intracapsular curettement of the tumor. With a spinofacial or hypoglossofacial anastomosis, however, the degree of this deformity has been greatly modified. Six of the eight patients have had spinofacial anastomoses and all with returning function. Before attempting an anastomosis, the function of the spinal accessory or hypoglossal nerves must be tested in order to preclude union with a nerve trunk which may have been injured at the time of operation.

The auditory nerve, being incorporated in the tumor and totally paralyzed before the operation, is irretrievably lost. This, of course, holds equally true when intracapsular enucleation is performed. The trigeminal nerve has been injured at operation in each of the 5 cases, but sensation has returned to a more or less degree in every instance. In the three finger enucleations, the trigeminal function has been destroyed in two and only injured in the third. Ulceration of the insensitive cornea is a danger which must be guarded against by shielding the eye. In one of the eight cases enucleation of the eyeball was finally necessary, and in another vision in the affected eye was lost following healing of the ulcer. The danger of this complication is the same as that following resection of the posterior root of this nerve for tic douloureaux. With the improved methods of prevention now in vogue, corneal ulceration should become a less disturbing factor.

In every case there has been dizziness and consequently balance of the body has been disturbed, but always there has been a steady and progressive improvement. It is probable that this disturbance may be the result of retracting the cerebellum—a factor which should be lessened as our skill in removing the capsule improves. A very slight weakness and stiffness of the hand on the homolateral side has persisted in six cases, and in two recent cases (two and six

months) after finger enucleation of the capsule the affection is more pronounced. Soon after the operation there has at times been some slight subjective stiffness of the corresponding leg, but this has soon entirely disappeared except in the above two cases of finger enucleation. Doubtless this slight residual disturbance is the result of injury to the pyramidal tracts in the brain-stem, and for this reason the arm fibers presumably are situated more externally than the fibers for the leg.

Table II indicates in a general way the results obtained in these patients to date. While the time is too short to refer to the absence of recurrence, the encapsulated character of the tumor and its total removal should leave little doubt that they will not recur. It may again be emphasized that the determination of the total removal of the tumor is not by guesswork but by a careful inspection of the site of the growth at the end of the operation. It is at once evident that the results following finger enucleation are incomparable (excepting one case) to those following painstaking removal of the capsule.

EXPLANATIONS OF THE MORTALITY FROM VARIOUS PROCEDURES

At first glance it must been incredible that the total removal of a cerebellopontile tumor can be accomplished with even less mortality than that following the relatively simple currettement of only part of the tumor's interior. It cannot be reasoned that because an operation is simpler, it is better and safer. The simplest operation for these tumors is a cerebellar decompression, but it has been attended by the highest mortality in the hands of nearly every operator. The reason for these seemingly paradoxical results is the simple one of cause and effect. If the patient's condition will justify the additional effort, there is no relief so quick and so complete as that following removal of the cause. There are occasions when the effects of the cause can be relieved by a smaller and less dangerous palliative operation (decompression), but that is only true at times. There are many intracranial tumors which can never be even slightly benefited by any form of palliative procedures, and under such conditions the procedure itself becomes an insult added to an already overstrained intracranial pressure. Cerebellopontile tumors offer seemingly insuperable obstacles to the success of the customary palliative operations in the late stages of the tumor's effects.

The high mortality from the simple enucleation of cerebellopontile tumors with the finger or spatula is now readily understood. Death results from injury to the brain stem when the finger tears the tumor from the brain stem and from packing the denuded brain stem in the frantic efforts to check haemorrhage. An examination of the brain after death in one of our cases showed the lateral margin of the brain stem softened and minute haemorrhages extending almost to the midline in the pons and medulla. This finding is not surprising since immediately after the tumor is shelled out there are always symptoms and signs which serve as telltale indicators that the medulla has been injured. At once respirations cease for many seconds (often a minute or more), after which they reappear irregularly and with serious embarrassment, and after several minutes they usually become more or less normal. However, after a severe injury the respirations may remain irregular, difficult, and ineffective, or apparently they may even fail to reappear, though it has never occurred in our cases. But even when the respirations seem to have become satisfactorily re-established, a secondary phase of embarrassment is almost sure to reappear four to eight hours later. It seems probable that this may be a secondary reaction (oedema) of the tissues to the initial trauma. This phase of secondary reaction is characterized by harsh, slightly irregular, and more rapid respirations; the pulse rate accelerates and diminishes in volume, the temperature rises steadily, the reflexes diminish and the pa-

tient becomes progressively more difficult to arouse. Obviously precisely the same effects are produced when the brain-stem is compressed by haemorrhage.

Why is there such a high mortality following a simple suboccipital decompression in the presence of cerebellopontile tumors? It would often be a great comfort to be able to do a simple bilateral suboccipital decompression and complete the removal of the tumor at a subsequent stage, but for reasons which are only now clear, the mortality is almost as high from this operation alone as from enucleation of the tumor. This danger is shown not only by our own two deaths (100 per cent), but by Tooth's reports which incorporate the results of Horsley's operations. From a series of seven verified extracerebellar tumors, there were four deaths within fifteen hours, a fifth died of respiratory distress on the sixteenth day, and the remaining two of meningitis. It is significant that only one of these tumors was actually disclosed at operation, but all were verified by necropsy. There was, therefore, no trauma to the tumor and the contiguous brain stem to account for the high death rate. More recently Trotter ([19]) has commented upon the dangers as well as the uselessness of suboccipital decompressions for cerebellopontile tumors, a view also voiced by Gordon Holmes. Surely these figures are far too high but the results could never be reduced far enough to make this operation a commendable procedure. In Cushing's series the results following decompression was only one death in ten cases in which a cerebellar decompression was done, but another patient survived only after a desperate struggle in which artificial respiration was maintained for an hour. The reasons for the excessive mortality in decompressing these tumors will be evident if the pathological changes which accompany the tumor's growth are understood, and again those alterations which must suddenly be induced by removal of the occipital bone and dura.

Cerebellopontile tumors not only deeply

indent the brain stem (reducing its bulk as much as one-fourth or even more) but dislocate it to the opposite side causing its normal straight mid-axial line to become a pronounced curve. But this great defect and alteration in the brain stem are tolerated because the changes have been so gradual. It is even remarkable that no appreciable disturbance of function can usually be detected by our clinical tests.

Most cerebellopontile tumors are small in comparison with cerebral tumors or even with other tumors in the posterior cranial fossa. Although the posterior compartment is small, the actual bulk of the tumor is not difficult of compensation by (1) partial obliteration of the cisterna magna, the cisterna pontis, the cisterna beneath the midbrain, and the fourth ventricle; (2) herniation of the tonsils of the cerebellar lobes into the spinal canal (through the foramen magnum); and (3) by pushing the tentorium cerebelli upward. [7] Were it not for a new factor which inevitably supervenes as the tumor grows, life could doubtless be maintained for a much longer time by these adjustments.[1] This new factor is closure of the aqueduct of Sylvius. When this small channel becomes closed by the anterior extension of the tumor, hydrocephalus involving the third and both lateral ventricles inevitably results. It is only with the onset of hydrocephalus that the real intracranial pressure develops. The pressure caused by the hydrocephalus always develops rapidly and soon overcomes the space adaptations which had previously been consummated in the posterior cranial fossa; it also quickly reduces to a minimum nature's remaining reserves of space compensation. Though quite firm, tough, and inelastic, the tentorium cerebelli is gradually pushed backward reducing the space in the posterior cranial fossa.[2] These qualities of the membrane, however, must be of great service in temporarily protecting the contents of the posterior cranial fossa, and to the tentorium is doubtless due the preservation of life pending the advent of surgery. With-

out doubt the danger of cerebellar decompression is proportionate to the degree of hydrocephalus which is present at the time of operation.

What happens when the occipital bone is removed and the dura opened widely — cerebellar decompression? Removal of the occipital bone at once liberates the pressure in the posterior cranial fossa. But this benefit is at once countered, and may be greatly exceeded, by the injurious effects of the backward pressure on the tentorium (hydrocephalus) and its full force is now exerted without opposition upon the delicate brain stem jamming it backward. It would seem that this force must be exerted almost entirely through the incisura tentorii for the tentorium itself would hardly be sufficiently elastic to stretch so quickly as to produce these disastrous results.

It must not be inferred that the results following suboccipital decompression are the same for all tumors in the posterior cranial fossa. Variations result from differences in the character, position, and fixation of the tumor. Almost complete relief of all symptoms will at once follow suboccipital decompression when a cerebellar cyst is evacuated. And ofttimes even when a cyst has not been evacuated or an intra-cerebellar tumor not removed, the same complete but temporary relief will be obtained, for the backward dislocation of the tumor may be great enough to relieve the obstruction at the aqueduct of Sylvius. But cerebellopontile tumors (and some other growths in the posterior fossa) are so firmly fixed to the floor of the skull that dislocation of the tumor cannot occur. Therefore, no relief of the hydrocephalus can be expected from decompression. Moreover, these tumors nearly always extend from one end of the posterior fossa to the other, and are closely attached to the brain stem throughout. Indeed, as noted before, they often extend posteriorly through the foramen magnum into the spinal canal and anteriorly through the incisura tentorii, even at times far enough anteriorly to destroy the posterior clinoid process. Not infrequently, however, a relatively small cerebellopontile tumor produces more severe and fulminating manifestations of intracranial pressure than larger growths because a small projecting nodule of the tumor imbeds itself deeply into the side of the midbrain, causing the aqueduct of Sylvius to be obstructed.

There can be no doubt that many obstructions of the aqueduct and fourth ventricle have a ball-valve action. This can be shown by the fact that at one time the intraventricular pressure will register very high, on a succeeding day it may be normal. In fact, one can easily be misled into assuming the absence of a neoplasm by finding a normal intraventricular pressure; the pressure may be low owing to the particular stage in the cycle of changes resulting from the ball-valve action of the tumor. Such vacillations in pressure are impossible in tumors which have infiltrated the aqueduct; they are most frequent in mobile non-infiltrating tumors; and are of intermediate frequency in fixed non-infiltrating tumors such as the cerebellopontile group. Periodical relief from pressure of this character is doubtless less frequent in occlusions of the aqueduct than of the fourth ventricle because the channel of the iter is so narrow.

It does not seem possible that the hydrocephalus could be relieved by any lateral dislocation of the brain stem away from the tumor in the tentorial opening, for usually the tumor has filled the superfluous space in the incisura tentorii, at least in the lateral aspect; and any anteroposterior dislocation of the brain stem can hardly have any effect other than to make any partial obstruction of the iter complete.

The injury resulting to the brain stem from the supratentorial pressure probably bears a close analogy to that following two other well recognized procedures, often erroneously considered harmless. Severe medullary embarrassment and even death are not rare sequels of a lumbar puncture performed in the presence of high intra-cranial pressure. Death or other injurious effect in these cases is surely due to the injury inflicted upon the brain stem when by the release of the intracranial pressure the cerebellar tonsils are suddenly driven more deeply through the foramen magnum into the spinal canal. One of the patients in our series was in coma from this ill-advised procedure.

The other example of the danger of disturbing established pressure relations is shown when lumbar punctures are performed in the presence of certain spinal cord tumors. In a not inconsiderable percentage of cases, sensory and motor function and sphincter control will be quickly affected, even lost, after lumbar puncture.[8] In nature's effort again to equalize intraspinal pressure after lumbar puncture in the presence of a complete spinal block, the higher pressure above the tumor can only spend its force by jamming the spinal cord against the immobile tumor. Unless the tumor is situated in the high cervical region, these injuries to the spinal cord affect only function, whereas the analogous (though greater) effects of supratentorial pressure on the medulla in the presence of cerebellopontile tumors compromise life as well as function. We believe, therefore, that when the dural and bony support of the occiput is removed (suboccipital decompression), the supratentorial pressure pushes the brain stem backward through the incisura tentorii until its force is spent; also that this injury to the brain stem is probably augmented by the tug on the firmly fixed cerebellopontile tumor. The degree of this damage is probably proportionate to the grade of intracranial pressure and the size of the tentorial opening (the fixation of the tumor is probably fairly constant).

Why should a suboccipital decompression plus intracapsular removal (subtotal) of a cerebellopontile tumor be less dangerous than a suboccipital decompression alone? The fact that the mortality rate in these tumors has been reduced only by the advent of Cushing's intracapsular method of enucleation is ample evidence for the assertion contained in this interrogation. When the interior of the tumor is sufficiently removed, the capsule will be freed of its rigid support, thereby permitting the obstruction of the aqueduct of Sylvius to be released. The supratentorial pressure (of hydrocephalus), which is the real dangerous factor in these operations, will be automatically relieved as effectually for the time being as if the tumor were removed. But one of the greatest defects of subtotal intracapsular enucleation is the difficulty of removing the proper amount of the contents of the tumor to permit this benefit to accrue. Unless the tumor is thoroughly removed so as to leave a fairly empty capsule, the remaining tumor will be essentially as rigid and immobile as the original tumor, and there would then be little if any relief either to the laterally deflected brain stem or to the hydrocephalus. During the removal of the contents of the tumor with a curette, only the outer surface of the growth is brought into view and one has great difficulty in knowing, indeed it is usually impossible to determine, the depth of tumor which still remains imbedded in or projecting beneath the brain stem. The importance of this determination we have learned from completely shelling out the interior of the tumors, as our deliberate total extirpations now necessitate. Curetting the interior of the tumor with the brain stem in the background, necessarily demands caution and, in playing safe, usually more tumor remains than seems possible from the apparent size of the exposed stump. In one of our two-stage extirpations 18 grams of tumor was curetted away and we thought but little was left with the capsule. The remainder of the tumor, when removed at the second stage, weighed 26 grams!

Since hydrocephalus results from occlusion of the iter, and since hydrocephalus is one of the chief factors in the operative mortality, it is safe to infer that the part of the tumor demanding urgent excavation is the upper pole. Otherwise, the hydrocephalus cannot be relieved. One of Cushing's necropsy specimens (Case xix) shows the upper pole of the tumor practically untouched by the intracapsular removal.

The configuration of the tumor also has something to do with the amount of tumor *in situ* after a subtotal removal. Nodules may project into the brain-stem from the inner side of the tumor. It has seemed that these deeply imbedded and invisible localized masses at times cause more symptoms referable to the brain stem and play a greater role in obstructing the aqueduct of Sylvius, than the big bulk of the tumor. The effect of the nodules will not be greatly, if at all, influenced by removal of the outer portion of the tumor with a curette.

Unless one is acquainted with the technical steps in a bilateral cerebellar operation, it would be reasonable to question why the brain stem has not already been injured by the supratentorial pressure during the operation, when the dura is opened widely. This pressure, however, is always under control. Puncture of a posterior horn of a lateral ventricle is always utilized to reduce the supratentorial pressure to that of the atmosphere. The period of great danger to the patient when the hydrocephalus has not been relieved, is in the few hours succeeding the operation — when the intraventricular pressure is again re-established.

Why should there be less mortality after subtotal intracapsular enucleation of the tumor plus removal of the remainder of the tumor, than from the partial removal alone? From this series two deaths were surely impending about two weeks after partial intracapsular enucleation of the tumors and were finally prevented by removal of the remainder of the tumor at that critical period. The defects of the partial operation, therefore, really forced the total removal of the growth. In every case in which a subtotal intracapsular operation has been performed (six in all, if those cases are included in which the intracapsular method was the first stage), the immediate postoperative course has been perfectly satisfactory. It has been several days later when the patient should have been out of danger that the alarming symptoms developed. In some way the stump of tumor caused the important functions located in the brain stem to be seriously compromised. We know from the gross appearance at the second operation that the stump of tumor which remained was swollen and friable — doubtless owing to nature's method of repair — but in all probability these same changes were also present in the contiguous brain tissue and were responsible for the symptoms. Whatever the exact explanation may be, complete subsidence of all symptoms at once followed extirpation of the residual tumor and capsule. No such complication has appeared in any of the cases [5] in which the entire tumor has been removed at one sitting.

A careful survey of the results after various operative attacks, brings us to one general conclusion; with proper care and attention to detail, that operation which at once removes the cause (other things being equal) not only carries the lowest mortality but at the same time offers incomparably the best immediate and permanent results.

OPERATIONS ON PATIENTS IN COMA FROM THE EFFECTS OF CEREBELLOPONTILE TUMORS

There is one exception to the above generalization concerning the removal of the tumor, viz., patients in coma from this type of tumor.

I have excluded from the operative mortality of total extirpations, two patients who entered the hospital when totally unconscious and who were operated upon while in this state. One patient had been unconscious eight hours, the other three, when the operation began, and in each there was Cheyne-Stokes type of breathing. Furthermore, in the first instance the location of the growth was entirely unknown until determined by ventricular estimation. The treatment, if any, for such cases is, I believe, distinctly a different problem from that which obtains when patients are in coma from tumors situated elsewhere in the cranial chamber. When

TABLE I
KIND OF OPERATIONS AND RESULTS

Kind of Operation	Number of Cases	Recovery	Death	Cause of Death
No operation	1	0	1	Died at stool before time set for operation.
Patients in coma at time of operation (intracapsular enucleation and dissection of capsule)	2	0	2	Operation.
Suboccipital decompression. (Tumor not removed)	2	0	2	Operation.
Tumor shelled out with finger (interior not removed)	6	2	4	
Intracapsular enucleation	3	1	2	Both died of meningitis, one on the 46th, the other on the 4th day.
Intracapsular enucleation followed by finger enucleation of the tumor: 3 cases in 2 stages, and the fourth in one stage	4	3	1	Pneumonia, 8th day.
Intracapsular enucleation followed by deliberate painstaking dissection of the capsule (all concluded in one stage)	5	5	0	

patients are comatose from intracranial pressure, it is often possible to restore consciousness by a palliative, properly placed decompression; and at times the tumor may even be safely removed while the patient is still unconscious, all of course depending on the depth and duration of coma and the location and character of the tumor. In many such cases it is incumbent and preferable only to relieve the intracranial pressure immediately and the removal of the tumor can await a second stage, if advisable.

But, as said before, coma from cerebellopontile tumors is not amenable to relief from any form of decompression. Even when the patient is quite conscious and in good condition, a suboccipital decompression is tantamount to a mortality in the advanced stages of intracranial pressure. The realization of the futility of operative palliation in these tumors urged the more radical attempt at removal of the tumor after first curetting the interior. Despite the fact that the extirpation was easy and bloodless in both instances, consciousness was not restored, there was no relief, and death followed within a few hours. In such cases we are dealing with a brain stem already severely injured before the operation began and any operation entailing even the slightest additional injury (such as the removal of the tumor must necessarily exact), could not be tolerated, even with relief of the supratentorial pressure.

Whether the partial intracapsular procedure would ever be successful under such conditions, one can only conjecture. Realizing as we do now the underlying differences between the coma of these and other tumors, it would surely have been wiser to have desisted, though the results would hardly have been different. This particular phase of the problem seems very dismal from our present knowledge and experience. I fear some new and totally different line of attack must be evolved if any results are to be expected in such cases. One great difficulty in these comatose patients is the differentiation beforehand of the kind of tumor, though its location in the posterior fossa may be clear. For tumors other than the cerebellopontile variety (such as intracerebellar tumors), a cerebellar decompression would always be indicated and would frequently prove effective treatment. When the character of the tumor has been determined only by operation, one is faced with the problem of proceeding with operative treatment. And when patients in coma from the effects of cerebellopontile tumors have been subjected to operation, decompression alone will surely be fatal; one can hardly do less than perform the operation devised by Cushing, and surely not more.

SUMMARY

An operative procedure is presented by which cerebellopontile (acoustic) tumors can be completely removed. After a thorough and carefully guarded intracapsular enucleation, the capsule of the tumor is painstakingly dissected from the brain stem.

REFERENCES

[1]Baisch, B.: Ueber Operation in der hinteren Schaedelgrube, *Beitr. z. klin. Chir., lx;* 479, 1908.

[2]Ballance, C. A.: *Some Points in the Surgery of the Brain and Its Membranes.* London, Macmillan Co., 1907.

[3]Borchardt, M.: Zur Operation der Tumoren des Kleinhirnbrueckenwinkels. *Berl. klin. Wchnschr., xlii:* 1033, 1905.

[4]Cottereill: Remarks on the surgical aspects of a case of cerebellopontine tumor by Bruce. *Tr. Med.-Chir. Soc., Edinb., xviii;* 215, 1899.

[5]Cushing, H.: *Tumors of the Nervus Acousticus.* Philadelphia and London, W. B. Saunders Co., 1917.

[6]Dandy, W. E.: An operation for the total extirpation of tumors in the cerebello-pontine angle. A preliminary report. *Johns Hopkins Hosp. Bull., xxxiii:* 344, 1922.

[7]*Idem:* The space compensating function of the cerebrospinal fluid—its connection with cerebral lesions in epilepsy. *Johns Hopkins Hosp. Bull., xxxiv:* 245, 1923.

[8]*Idem:* The diagnosis and localization of spinal cord tumors. *Ann. Surg., lxxxi:* 223, 1925.

[9]Eiselsberg, A. von, and Ranzi, E.: Ueber die chirurgische Behandlung der Hirn- und Rueckenmarkstumoren. *Verhandl. d. deutsch. Gesellsch. f. Chir., xliii:* 514, 1913.

TABLE II

END—RESULTS CASES WITH RECOVERY AFTER CAREFUL REMOVAL OF CAPSULE

	Age	Time Since Operation	Gait	Balance	Arm and Leg on Affected Side	Romberg	Ataxia	VN.	Headaches	Wt.	Remarks
MRW I	49	1 yr.	Walks 1½ miles per day Feels safer with support	Still feels dizzy but is improving	Leg well. Arm and hand stiff	Slight	Neg.	Sensation felt but less acutely	None	+10	Postoperative meningitis (streptococcus virdans) Cisternal drainage.
TH II	56	1 yr.	Walks well	Slightly dizzy	Stiffness hand. Leg normal	Slight	Neg.	Not normal but present	None	-10	
EB III	44	1 yr.	Can walk 4 miles without support. Feels need of assistance only on rough ground and down steep grades	Still slightly affected but gradually disappearing	Hand still slightly affected	Neg.	Neg.	Patch of anaesthesia below eye	None	+8 to +15	Healed corneal ulcer. Little vision remains.
JM IV	29	2½ yrs.	Except narrow plank or down step grade, can walk anywhere without support	Practically normal	Still slight weakness of arm; leg normal	Slight	+	Some loss but sensation present	None	-25	Was unable to walk before operation. Hemiplegia and difficulty swallowing.
IR V	36	1½ yrs.	Can walk a mile without support	Still feels slightly uncertain	Very slightly less than normal	Neg.	Neg.	Not quite normal	None	Same	

CASES WITH RECOVERY AFTER INTRACAPSULAR ENUCLEATION FOLLOWED BY FINGER EXTIRPATION OF CAPSULE

							Neg.		None	+15	Two-stage operation.
EL VI	25	3½ yrs.	Can walk any distance alone	Only occasional loss of balance	None	Very slight swaying		Normal about lower face; diminished above	None	+15	Two-stage operation.
RLB VII	48	6 mos	With support can walk briskly, but requires help except in house	Very marked difficulty in balancing	Good grip but quite shaky	Markedly positive	+	Sensation absent	None	+40	Ulcerated eye removed. Hearing much better. Smallest tumor of series but symptoms of 20 years.
WD VIII	23	2 mos	On discharge from hospital can walk with support. Pt. has been 2 months recuperating from meningitis and a resultant hydrocephalus	Very marked difficulty in balancing	Markedly affected	Markedly positive	+	Sensation absent	None	-10	Postoperative meningitis (staphylococcus aureus); cisternal drainage; resulting hydrocephalus cured spontaneously. Largest tumor of series, wt. 46 gms. Two-stage operation.

NOTE.—As all of the patients live at a distance, this table is compiled from answers to letters of inquiry. Six of the eight cases have had spino-facial anastomoses with returning function in each instance.

[10]Frazier, C. H.: Remarks upon the surgical aspects of tumors of the cerebellum. *New York M. J., lxxxi:* 272 and 332, 1905.

[11]Holmes, Gordon: Acoustic tumours. *Proc. Roy Soc. Med., Sect. Otol., xvi:* pt. iii, p. 40, 1923.

[12]Krause, F.: Zur Freilegung der hinteren Felsenbeinflaeche und des Kleinhirns. *Beitr. z. klin. Chir., xxxvii:* 728, 1903.

[13]Leischner, H.: Zur Chirurgie der Kleinhirnbrueckenyinkeltumoren. *Mitt. a. d. Grenzgeb. d. Med. u. Chir., xxii:* 675, 1911.

[14]Meyer, Willy: Craniectomy for tumor of the acoustic nerve. *Ann. Surg., xlix:* 552, 1909; also 1912, lv, 323.

[15]Panse, R.: Ein Gliom des Akustikus. *Arch. f. Ohrenh. lxi:* 251, 1904.

[16]Poppert: Exstirpation eines Tumors des Kleinhirnbrueckenwinkels. *Deutsche med. Wchnschr., xxxiii:* 613, 1907.

[17]Quix, F.: Ein Acusticustumor. *Arch. f. Ohrenh., lxxxiv:* 252, 1911.

[18]Tooth, H. H.: The treatment of tumours of the brain and the indications for operation. *Tr. XVIIth Internat. Cong. Med., Lond.,* 1913. Sect. vii, Surg. p. 203.

[19]Trotter, W.: Surgical treatment of eighth nerve tumours. *Proc. Roy. Soc. Med., Sect. Otol., xvi:* pt. iii, 37, 1923.

[20]Walshe, F. M. R.: Acusticus tumours *Proc. Roy. Soc. Med., Sect. Otol., xvi:* iii, 32, 1923.

[1]This group of tumors has long been recognized as a distinct clinical and pathological entity. Various other tumors in this region, whether encapsulated or infiltrating, have not been considered. I prefer the designation "tumors of the cerebellopontile angle"—the Kleinhirnbrueckenwinkeltumoren of the Germans—rather than "tumors of the acoustic nerve" for this well known group of encapsulated tumors because it does not include a theory of origin. Both appellations are defective —"cerebellopontile angle" because it merely denotes a location which is the abode of other tumors of varying types; and "acoustic" because the origin of the tumor is still in dispute and also because there are other tumors of the acoustic nerve which, both in structure and position, are entirely unlike those under consideration. Throughout the remainder of the paper the abbreviated term "cerebellopontile tumor" will be used. Though even less accurate, it has attained significance through general usage and has obviated the tendency to use the clumsy and grammatically incorrect expression, cerebellopontile "angle" tumor.

[1]In grouping these cases as cerebellopontile tumors, I have taken the liberty of disregarding Tooth's histological classification of tumors (glioma, fibroglioma and fibroma) and including those tumors which from the history of the patient (early deafness with other symptoms appearing late) and even more the gross appearance of an encapsulated enucleable tumor in the angle, appeared to me probable tumors of this variety. For example, Case 222, entered as a glioma by Tooth, impressed me more as being a cerebellopontile tumor, and two cases of bilateral tumor classified by Tooth as fibroglioma, I have excluded, feeling that they were probably rather examples of Recklinghausen's tumors. I have also included four of Horsley's cases grouped under fibromata. As Horsley refers to fifteen cases at the same meeting, it is fair to assume that he and Tooth (who includes fourteen) refer to the same cases.

[1]Doubtless this reference is to the same patient whom Tooth (1913) mentioned as living and well (with V and VII paralysis) 8 years after operation.

[1]The amazing adaptation of the central nervous system to the steady growth of the tumor is also shown in the trigeminal and facial nerves which become flattened, thinned, and elongated to several times their original intracranial span, and usually without any or at most only an insignificant depreciation of function.

[2]The extent to which the tentorium has been stretched can be roughly estimated by the quantity of fluid which can be recovered from a ventricular needle when pressure is gradually applied to the exposed cerebellar hemispheres.

XXII

INTRACRANIAL TUMORS AND ABSCESSES CAUSING COMMUNICATING HYDROCEPHALUS*

In earlier publications it has been shown that practically all cases of chronic hydrocephalus† are caused by a block at some point in the system of spaces in which cerebrospinal fluid circulates. This block, however, is constant neither in character nor in location. A varied assortment of obstructions includes congenital defects and malformations of or affecting the cerebrospinal spaces, congenital and acquired strictures, inflammatory obliteration of the subarachnoid space, tumors, abscesses, tubercles, etc. But regardless of the intrinsic character of the underlying lesion, and regardless of its location, the effect is always precisely the same — a reduction in the absorption of cerebrospinal fluid. The various clinical and anatomical differences in the expression of hydrocephalus, though interesting, are of no fundamental significance. They are but expressions of an underlying cause.

In every case of hydrocephalus the causative lesion can now be demonstrated not only at necropsy, but during life by clinical tests, and most of them could be found, if need be, at operation. Such being true, there is no longer justification for referring to hydrocephalus as "idiopathic."

*Reprinted from *The Annals of Surgery*, August, 1925.

†The qualification "practically" is used because of a possibility that thrombosis of the vein of Galen, or its closure from other cause, may result in a continuous formation of fluid. We were able to induce a low-grade hydrocephalus in a dog by a ligature so placed on the vein of Galen that an adequate venous collateral circulation failed to develop. If such a venous obstruction occurs without other complications and causes hydrocephalus in human beings, it must be exceedingly rare. In every necropsy we have carefully inspected the vein of Galen and it has always been patent.

It is convenient and useful from the standpoint of therapy to subdivide hydrocephalus into two types: (1) *with* communication and (2) *without* communication, depending upon whether or not the lateral cerebral ventricles are in communication with the spinal subarachnoid space. This differentiation of type is easily made by injecting a cubic centimetre of neutral phenolsulphonephthalein into the spinal canal and testing for the color in the ventricular fluid fifteen to twenty minutes. The presence of the dye in the ventricular fluid at once eliminates the existence of any obstruction within the ventricular system and places it in the subarachnoid space (usually the cisternae) — communicating hydrocephalus. If the dye does not appear in the ventricular fluid the obstruction must be located at some point in the ventricular system (non-communicating hydrocephalus). Fundamentally, of course, these two types are alike; they differ only in the location of the obstruction. It may be noted in passing that occasionally there are two obstructions, both of which may be in the ventricular system, such as at the aqueduct and the basal foramina, or one may be within the ventricular system and the other in the cisterna.

This paper is concerned only with the etiology of the communicating type of hydrocephalus. In previous reports on this subject we have observed only post-inflammatory adhesions and one case of congenital maldevelopment of the subarachnoid space as the cause. In this paper two additional types of lesions are presented — namely tumors and abscesses, or more correctly, the reaction about abscesses. That at least one of the communicating foramina (Magendie and Luschka) at the base of

219

the brain was patent during life, has been shown by the phenolsulphonephthalein test, and at necropsy both by inspection of these foramina and by the passage of ink into the fourth ventricle. In one patient, an infant, an infiltrating glioma (possibly of congenital origin) covered the ventral surface of the pons and medulla; in another, a boy of six, the lesion was also a glioma and quite similarly placed (Figs. 1 & 2); and in a third infant two symmetrically placed abscesses at the tip of each temporal lobe were connected by a dense bridge of inflammatory tissue (Fig. 4). In each instance the location of the obstruction and its impermeability were demonstrated by intraspinous injections of India ink (under pressure) before the necropsy was begun. In no instance did the color pass the block. In cross-section, each lesion involved the entire exposed ventral and lateral surfaces of the brain-stem, thereby obliterating peripheral as well as central portions of the cisternae.

Case I. A baby of five months, referred by Dr. J. G. Lemmon, of Akron, Ohio, exhibited no unusual features of hydrocephalus (Fig. 2). Birth was at term; the delivery was spontaneous and easy. The infant thrived after birth and at three and a half months was able to hold up its head; but at four months it was brought to Doctor Lemmon because "it did not seem so well." The enlargement of the head was first noticed at that time and progressed rapidly, it was no longer able to hold up its head. There had never been a history of an acute illness, of paralyses or convulsions. The anterior fontanelle was large, bulging and tight, all cranial sutures were widely separated. Head measured 46.5 cm., in circumference. No asymmetry or other abnormalities could be seen.

Phenolsulphonephthalein test: one cubic centimetre of phenolsulphonephtalein was injected into the lumbar spinal canal. After twenty minutes fluid was aspirated from a lateral ventricle and showed the dye in concentration which matched a 20 per cent. standard colorimeter solution; two hours later the color had increased so that undiluted it match-

ed an 80 per cent. standard solution. After three hours 8 per cent. of the phthalein was recovered from the urine (spontaneous voiding). A second specimen of urine obtained three hours later contained an equal amount.

It was evident, therefore, that we were dealing with a case of communicating hydrocephalus. There was no reason either from the history, examination, or clinical tests, to suspect a tumor as the obstructing lesion. A few hours following removal of the choroid plexus (through a ventriculoscope) the patient died. When the occipital lobes were exposed no fluid was found in the subarachnoid space of either side.

Necropsy showed a diffuse glioma involving most of the ventral and lateral surfaces of the pons and medulla. Both foramina of Luschka were occluded but the foramen of Magendie was patent. The aqueduct of Sylvia and the third and fourth ventricles were greatly enlarged. The lateral ventricles were greatly enlarged.

India ink injected at the beginning of the necropsy passed freely into the lateral ventricles but stopped sharply at the caudal margin of the tumor underlying the brain-stem.

Case II. A colored boy of six years entered the Johns Hopkins Hospital because of a rapidly developing paraplegia involving only the legs. Prior to his present illness he had apparently been well. He played normally with other children and offered no complaints. His mentality did not appear abnormal. He walked and talked at the usual age. One year previous to our examinations he first complained of a pain in the left leg above the knee and shortly afterward a backache developed in the lumbar region. A scoliosis and kyphosis appeared and increased. Soon a foot-drop developed, then the power of the left leg was affected. Nine months ago he began using crutches. The right leg then became paralyzed and for several weeks he had been bedfast. Control of urine was lost; several times it reappeared only to be lost again. The backache caused him great misery at night.

No complaints had ever been made referable to the head. The objective findings were those of a spinal cord lesion,

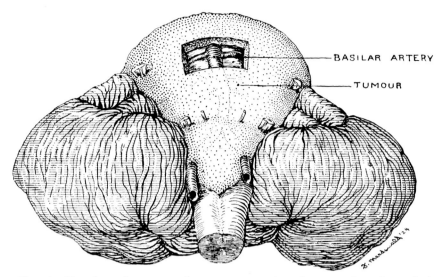

BASILAR ARTERY

TUMOUR

Fig. 1. Drawing of an extensive tumor covering the ventral surface of the brain (Case II). In this case the basilar artery is entirely covered by the tumor and the vertebral arteries are seen entering at its lowermost parts. A window has been made in the tumor by Doctor Macdonald to show the basilar artery beneath.

presumably a tumor because of the gradual progression of signs and symptoms. There was incomplete *flaccid* paralysis of both legs but more marked on the left. However, there was some evidence of spasticity of certain muscle groups of the left leg—notably the hamstrings. A fairly definite bilateral sensory level could be made out at the first lumbar segment. The deep reflexes were normal on the right and absent on the left. A faint ankle clonus could be elicited at times on the left, not on the right. Plantar stimulation produced no response. The first and second lumbar spines were tender to pressure. The above signs and symptoms seemed to clearly indicate that the tumor occupied the lumbar enlargement and roots of the cauda equina.

Another objective but incidental finding in this case caused us much concern in the diagnosis. His head was very large. All the cranial sutures were widely separated (x-ray and Macewen's sign). The x-ray also showed an extraordinary degree of convolutional atrophy of the skull. The sella turcica was three times the normal size, though the posterior clinoid processes were still intact.

The eye-grounds were considered to be negative, though possibly the retinal veins were full but not tortuous. He had not now, nor had he ever complained of headache, dizziness or convulsions. There was no hemianopsia or other disturbance of vision. Our usual neurological examinations failed to find any additional signs by which an intracranial lesion could be located. That he had hydrocephalus could not be doubted, and the deep convolutional markings of the inner table of the skull (rontgenographic findings) indicated that the hydrocephalus was not at a standstill.

Since the paraplegia could only be accounted for by a spinal cord tumor of some kind, it was necessary to assume the existence of a second tumor or other type of lesion to explain the hydrocephalus. Nor did it seem possible that the lesion which had enlarged the sella turcica could account for the hydrocephalus. In the first place, it was too far forward to obstruct the cisternal trunk, and in the second place, the normal vision made it appear that the tumor, if such it were, had broken through the dural envelope of the sella.

A spinal injection of air was made with the hope of obtaining more information concerning the *spinal* lesion. The spinal cord tumor was sharply localized by the level of air in the skiagram, but no air reached the cranial chamber.

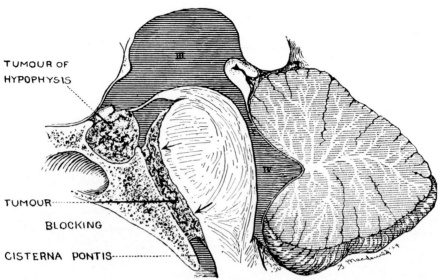

TUMOUR OF
HYPOPHYSIS

TUMOUR

BLOCKING

CISTERNA PONTIS

Fig. 2. A mid-sagittal drawing in semi-diagrammatic form to show the extent and position of the tumor shown in Fig. 1. In both this case and the preceding one a spinal injection of India ink stopped at the lower margin of the tumor, for the cisterna was completely blocked. In this patient the tumor in the region of the hypophysis played no part in the production of the hydrocephalus.

Quite unexpectedly, however, additional proof of the existence of the intracranial lesion and something of its character, was disclosed. Below the level of the tumor the sheath of each spinal nerve was distended into a distinct pouch about one centimetre in length. Such a finding indicated that the intraspinous pressure, which is but a transmitted intracranial pressure, must have been very high prior to the spinal block which had evidently only recently developed.

With proof that a spinal block existed, it was not clear that trepanation for ventricular puncture and phthalein test would throw additional light on the problem. After removal of the spinal cord tumor (a fibromyxoma) cerebrospinal fluid could be withdrawn in very large quantities from the spinal canal, showing that the hydrocephalus was surely of the communicating type. Probably the same occlusion should have been suspected from the dilated nerve sheaths which were demonstrable in the pneumogram. No attempt was made to treat the intracranial condition. The patient later came to necropsy. A diffuse glioma enveloped the entire exposed portion of the brain-stem. Strands of the tumor extended to the sella turcica and possibly joined

by a strand another tumor (the patient's third tumor) in the sella turcica. This sellar tumor seemed an entirely different growth and was attached to the sheath of one optic nerve; the pituitary body was intact and pushed downward and to one side of the sella.

India ink injected into the spinal canal passed through the foramen of Magendie, the fourth ventricle, the iter, third ventricle, and both lateral ventricles, but stopped abruptly at the lower margin of the tumor beneath the brain-stem.

Case III. An infant of six weeks was referred by Dr. J. L. Powe, of Hartsville, S. C., with an obvious diagnosis of hydrocephalus. Labor was difficult, instruments being used. The baby breathed only after heroic efforts had been applied. It was jaundiced during the first week and ran a fever throughout the first two weeks and during this time there was vomiting and great difficulty in feeding. For ten days the mother noticed that the baby's head would frequently jerk and draw far backwards. When three weeks old the head was unusually large. When one month old he had a crying spell in which the head was thrown back. Since then there have been many spells lasting a few minutes in which the body was in strong opisthotonos and he would cry out with pain. It has been impossible to gain weight, the little patient now being greatly emaciated. For a week it had not used either arm or leg normally.

The head was greatly enlarged, measuring 40.5 cm. in circumference. The anterior fontanelle measured 15 x 16 cm. No reflexes were obtainable. Examination of the spinal fluid showed 100 cells per cubic millimetre—all polymorphonuclear cells—and a heavy globulin precipitate.

Phenolsulphonephthalein test (intraspinal injection): Free communication between both lateral ventricles and the spinal subarachnoid in fifteen minutes, the ventricular color (undiluted) corresponding with a standard 40 per cent. tube; 10 per cent. excretion in the urine in two and a third hours.

The diagnosis of an underlying inflammatory lesion seemed certain. Our presumptive diagnosis was hydrocephalus resulting from meningitis.

Necropsy: India ink was injected into the spinal canal. The pathological findings were entirely unexpected (Fig. 3). At the tip of each temporal lobe was a well-encapsulated abscess, which, while attached to the adjacent dura, could be removed, intact, with the brain. The abscesses, each the size of a golf ball, were of almost exactly the same size, 4 x 4 cm., and in precisely the same location. Unfortunately the organism could not be identified as the body had been embalmed with formalin before the brain was removed. Between the two abscesses was a dense broad band of subacute inflammatory tissue, and at the caudal end of this inflammatory band the ink injection had stopped abruptly. The foramen of Magendie and both foramina of Luschka were patent. All of the ventricular channels were unobstructed and greatly dilated. But little brain tissue remained in either hemisphere owing to the great ventricular distention.

From the history of jaundice, fever, and attacks of opisthotonos, all present almost immediately after birth, it seems probable that these abscesses were of intra-uterine origin. The inflammatory band and not the abscesses, *per se,* were responsible for the hydrocephalus.

In each of these three cases the cisterna

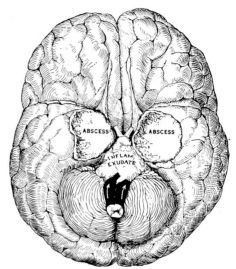

Fig. 3. Sketch of the base of the brain in which an abscess was present at the tip of each temporal lobe. They were adherent to the underlying dura. Between the abscesses is a dense inflammatory mass entirely concealing the underlying vessels, and obliterating the cisternae chiasmatis and interpeduncularis, as well as the cisterna under the pons, and midbrain. The black covering over the medulla has resulted from an injection of ink into the spinal canal at necropsy, the ink stopping at the obstruction in the cisterna caused by the dense, subacute inflammatory mass.

points was completely blocked. In an earlier publication[1] adhesions in this region were found and suspected to be the etiological factor in the production of the hydrocephalus. Later, it was demonstrated by experiments on dogs[2] that when an impermeable band of adhesions was constricted around the pons or mid-brain (occluding the cisterna), hydrocephalus of the communicating type followed. In these experiments and in human cases which have since come to autopsy,[3] the line of obstruction has been graphically outlined by the sharp level at which India ink is arrested when injected intraspinously. To understand why an obstruction in the cisterna pontis should cause hydrocephalus, it is only necessary to know the anatomy of the cerebrospinal spaces, the circulation of the cerebrospinal fluid, the place and manner of formation and absorption of

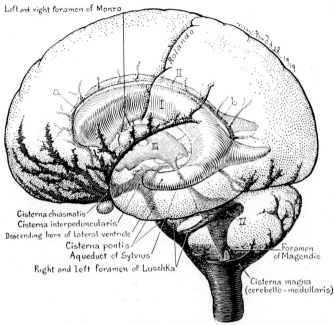

Left and right foramen of Monro

Cisterna chiasmatis
Cisterna interpeduncularis
Descending horn of lateral ventricle
Cisterna pontis
Aqueduct of Sylvius
Right and left foramen of Luschka

Foramen of Magendie

Cisterna magna (cerebello-medullaris)

Fig. 4. Diagram of the circulatory system for cerebrospinal fluid. The obstruction causing the hydrocephalus in each of the three preceding cases was in the subarachnoid space at the cisterna pontis. It is clear that fluid passing out of the ventricle can therefore not pass over the cerebral hemispheres where fluid causes hydrocephalus of the communicating type — that type in which the ventricles communicate with the spinal canal.

cerebrospinal fluid. Briefly summarized, the necessary facts are as follows: Cerebrospinal fluid forms in the ventricular system (from the choroid plexuses) but does not absorb there. Cerebrospinal fluid absorbs in the *subarachnoid* space (directly into the capillaries in every part of the subarachnoid space, and not into the dural sinuses or through special structures such as the Pacchionian granulations). The cisternae beneath the brain-stem together serve as a conduit, which is the only communication between the cistern magna (into which all the ventricular fluid is poured through the foramina of Luschka and Magendie) (Fig. 4). A block in the cisterna pontis or another part of the conduit of cisternae, whether by adhesions, an experimental band, tumors, or an inflammatory band, prevents the passage of fluid to the great absorbing area and causes the fluid to dam back to its source — hydrocephalus.

The long duration of hydrocephalus in Case II without symptoms makes us feel that the hydrocephalus was of slow development — possibly that the obstruction of the cisterna pontis was of gradual formation. When the transverse extent of the cisterna pontis is compared with that of the aqueduct of Sylvius, it is evident that a much longer time may be required for its complete occlusion by a tumor's growth. Under such conditions the manifestations of hydrocephalus would surely be less fulminating. That partial closure of the cisterna pontis may be tolerated without causing hydrocephalus with communication, is demonstrated in cerebellopontile (acoustic) tumors. Often less than half of the transverse extent of the cisterna pontis remains when these tumors are found at operation or necropsy, but hydrocephalus does not result until the tumor has occluded the aqueduct of Sylvius. That the iter is obstructed from these tumors, can easily be demonstrated by injecting indigo-carmin into a lateral ventricle at the beginning of the cerebellar operation; when the cisterna magna is exposed the fluid will be clear. Further proof that the obstruction is at the aqueduct and not in the cisterna pontis lies in the fact that pressure in the posterior cranial fossa can be relieved by tapping the lateral ventricle, whereas if the iter were patent and the cisterna pontis obstructed, all possible relief of pressure in the posterior fossa would be obtained by the release of fluid from the cisterna magna.

SUMMARY

Pathological evidence is offered to show that hydrocephalus of the communicating type may be caused by tumors and abscesses when so situated that they obstruct the cisternal conduit under the brain-stem. Post-mortem injections of India ink proved the cisterna pontis to be completely blocked in each case. The cause of hydrocephalus in these cases is precisely the same as in the more common instances resulting from adhesions after the spontaneous cure of meningitis. All cases of hydrocephalus, whether of the communicating or non-communicating type, have fundamentally the same underlying cause, an obstruction in the system of spaces through which cerebrospinal fluid circulates. The result of any such obstruction is a reduction of the spaces in which cerebrospinal fluid is absorbed.

REFERENCES

[1]Dandy, W. E., and Blackfan, K. D.: Internal Hydrocephalus. An Experimental, Clinical and Pathological Study. Second paper. *Am. J. Dis. Child., xiv:* 424, 1917.

[2]Dandy, W. E.: Experimental Hydrocephalus. *Ann. Surg., lxx:* 129, 1919.

[3]Dandy, W. E.: The Cause of So-called Idiopathic Hydrocephalus. *Johns Hopkins Hosp. Bull., xxxii:* 67, 1921.

XXIII

PNEUMOCEPHALUS (INTRACRANIAL PNEUMATO-CELE OR AEROCELE)*

For at least a century and a half it has been known that under certain pathological conditions — infection and trauma — air can pass through a break in the outer wall of a cranial air sinus into the scalp and, gradually traveling in the loosely attached subaponeurotic layer, form air tumors which at times may be of tremendous size. The two sources of these extracranial aerogenous tumors (recorded as pneumatoceles or aeroceles) have been (1) the mastoid cells and (2) the frontal sinus, the former being much more frequent.[1] It has also long been known that steady pressure on such gaseous tumors caused them to disappear, the air being forced through the eustachian tube or frontal sinus. Swallowing or coughing would again cause the occipital, and coughing the sincipital, variety quickly to reappear. A number of cases of the occipital type have been cured by treating the opening which leads from the sinus into the scalp with iodine or other stimulant, while others have healed spontaneously as granulation tissue gradually choked the fistulous tract.

It is safe to presume that infections and fractures must also have opened the inner wall of the air cells, and at times the dura, and under proper conditions must have passed through these defects not only between the bone and the dura but at times into the cranial chamber. Intracranial air tumors, however, giving no such simple signs of their presence as those of the extracranial variety, have existed without clinical recognition until recent years. The roentgenogram has now made the detection of intracranial air almost as easy and

at least as certain as the direct observation of an extracranial pneumatocele. Apparently only once has the presence of intracranial air that has developed during life been satisfactorily demonstrated without the use of the roentgen ray. This remarkable exception was observed by Chiari[2] in 1884. At necropsy he not only demonstrated that air filled a large cavity in the frontal lobe and the ventricular system as well, but he located a tiny opening leading from an ethmoid cell to the frontal cavity and explained the ingress of air by the explosive force of sneezing. Chiari was confident that no postmortem factors could explain the presence of air and concluded it had surely been present during life. Chiari's brilliant report antedated by many years the advent of roentgenography and by nearly thirty years Luckett's[3] case (1913), this being the first instance in which air was detected by the use of the roentgen ray.

The following year, 1914, Wolff[4] independently discovered air in a German case. Twenty-five cases have been compiled from the literature to date, eleven from the United States, eleven from Germany, two from France and one from Italy. To these we add three more, all of which have been seen in a period of eight months.

The mere annexation of these additional cases is of little concern but the need for better recognition of this condition — symptoms, etiology, pathology and treatment — is best attested by the fact that in only a single instance[5] has intracranial air been suspected before its disclosure at necropsy, operation or by roentgenography. The occurrence of our two cases within a period of six months also indicates that this condition merits consideration in the differ-

*Reprinted from the *Archives of Surgery*, 12: 949–982, May, 1926.

ential diagnosis of cerebral lesions. Treatment moreover is dependent on an early and accurate diagnosis.[6]

There are two sources of intracranial air: (1) a break in the wall of the skull, through which air is forced from the exterior, and (2) the product of gas producing organisms after their entrance into the brain.

After the initial cranial defect, air can be forced into the brain only through an opening in one of the paranasal sinuses or the mastoid cells, for here alone can the air be concentrated by swallowing, coughing or sneezing under a pressure greater than that within the cranial chamber. The bony wall of a sinus can be opened by a fracture, an operation, an infection or by the persistent pressure of a tumor or of the dilated third ventricle of hydrocephalus. In one of the cases here reported, the air entered through a fracture of the frontal bone; in a second, through a fracture through the temporal bone, and in the third, it probably followed an operative defect of the mastoid cells, though the possibility of a bacterial gas product cannot be absolutely eliminated.

REPORT OF CASES

Case 1. A man, aged seventy, referred by Dr. H. I. Thomson of St. Petersburg, Fla., was brought to the Johns Hopkins Hospital, Feb. 20, 1925, in a semi-comatose condition. With strong stimulation by supra-orbital pressure it was possible to get a few disconnected and irrelevant sentences, which indicated complete disorientation as to time, place and persons.

The following story was obtained from relatives: January 6, (forty-five days before admission) he was struck by an automobile and thrown to the pavement, striking his right forehead; he was unconscious for only a few minutes. During a stay of several days in the hospital he was irrational much of the time, but in the second week his condition improved so much that he was discharged from the hospital. Much of the third week was spent at home in bed, but the following week he was up and about most of the time and transacted some business. His

wife, however, noticed that he was careless about financial details, about his clothes and other matters, in all of which he had formerly been particular; but throughout the fourth week there seemed a steady improvement. One afternoon about a month after the accident, the patient was found holding his head in his hands; he said that he would go crazy if he could not get some relief from a terrific headache. During the next few days he was dazed most of the time and again he was taken to the hospital by Dr. Thomson (February 5). He was then in a stupor and, when with difficulty he could be aroused, he was always irrational. Three days later (February 8) he seemed much better, though his condition varied greatly from time to time during the day; on the whole he was much more conscious and often was quite rational. A week before his admission to the hospital (February 11) he had a severe spell of trembling over the whole body which was said to have been more pronounced in the arms and head; a roentgenogram taken February 11 showed a large amount of air in both lateral ventricles (Fig. 4). Again he became irrational and raved on various subjects, jumping from one to another without reason. During much of the time he had to be restrained. His pulse was slow, from 50 to 70; the temperature never rose above 99 F.

He was in this condition on arrival in Baltimore except that restraint was no longer necessary and he was decidedly difficult to arouse, strong supra-orbital pressure being necessary to bring any response. His general physical condition was good; he was stronger and younger than his years would indicate. To the right of the midline the supra-orbital ridge was definitely depressed, though the skin was not broken, nor was this region noticeably tender. There were no extra-ocular palsies nor signs of unilateral motor or sensory disturbance. The eye grounds showed neither engorgement of the veins nor swelling of the optic disks. Examinations of the remaining cranial nerves and regions of the brain were negative. Apparently there had been no disturbance of the gait, and he had not complained of diplopia or cervical rigidity. The reflexes were equal and normally active on the two sides. Plantar stimulation gave plantar flexion. The pulse was 50; temperature, 100 F. The leukocytes totaled 8,000. The systolic blood pressure was 110, diastolic 70.

It was our impression that this lesion was probably a chronic subdural hemorrhage. Doubtless this diagnosis was entertained the more because of another patient who had just been operated on and who had a strikingly similar story. It was quite clear that there was greatly increased intracranial pressure because of his stupor and bradycardia (with normal urinary findings), the negative optic disk notwithstanding. An abscess seemed improbable because fever had been absent throughout his illness; there had never been cervical rigidity and the leukocyte count was now normal. The possibility of a pneumatocele was not considered. In the absence of any localizing signs or symptoms, the depressed fracture was looked on as probably indicating the side of the presumed subdural hemorrhage. Solely on this finding exploration of the right hemisphere was determined.

Being so nearly in coma he was at once prepared for operation. Fortunately, though merely as a matter of routine, stereoscopic roentgenograms were taken en route to the operating room. As nothing significant was expected from the roentgen-ray examination, development of the plates was not awaited. The first intimation of the character of the intracranial lesion was therefore at the operation.

A frontoparietal bone flap of usual size and form was turned down under local anesthesia. The dura was extremely tense and when incised the brain herniated to the maximum degree. There was no subdural hemorrhage but the bulging brain at once indicated a subcortical lesion in the frontal lobe which, being very soft, protruded like a ball from the level of the firmer parietal and occipital lobes. The frontal convolutions were extremely wide and pale. The great pressure from within the brain had squeezed nearly all of the blood supply from the thinned cortex. The sulci were obliterated and entirely free of fluid. Even the larger vessels of the frontal lobe were scarcely visible. We fully expected a big subcortical hemorrhage but when the greatly thinned frontal lobe was incised a strong puff

of air followed. The protruding frontal lobe at once collapsed and instead of the tremendous cerebral hernia which had been present only a moment before, the brain was now sunken far below the dural margins. The frontal lobe was now a great cavity easily as large as a goose egg; the cortex was a mere shell varying from 0.5 to 1 cm. in thickness. Roentgenograms were immediately sent for; these verified the operative findings of intracranial air.

Inspection of the great cavity showed the lining to be everywhere smooth, glistening and avascular. There was no fluid within the cavity. At first nothing unusual was seen, but on the inner (mesial) wall beneath a fold that was readily pushed aside with the spatula, a small oval opening (about 0.5 cm. long) was brought into view. This foramen led directly into the anterior horn of the right lateral ventricle (the upper outer wall) and explained the entrance of air into the ventricles. There was no visible fluid in this part of the ventricle. The foramen of Monro and the choroid plexus were easily seen through the opening. In the anterior tip of the big frontal defect a second opening of smaller size was superimposed on a dural defect. A probe was passed through this opening but it could not find a corresponding defect in the skull, i. e., the probe did not pass into the frontal sinus. Around this dural defect the cortex was rather firmly adherent over an area probably 4 by 4 cm., the adhesions being most dense surrounding the fistula.

The frontal lobe was then dissected free of the adherent dura; the denuded dural opening was again evident but again there was no direct tract into the frontal sinus. There could be no doubt that despite the failure of the probe to enter the frontal sinus, the air must have entered the cerebral defect from that source—an explanation to appear later. Our object in freeing the frontal lobe from the dura was to close the opening from the inside but the great depth of the wound and the close contact between dura and bone made this impractical. The frontal defect was then filled with Ringer's solution, the dura carefully sutured, the bone flap replaced and the wound closed.

A second incision was then made through the shaved eyebrow in order to expose the depressed fracture in the right supra-orbital region. The fragment of bone measuring about 2 by 2 cm. was depressed to a depth varying from scarcely a millimeter on the outer side to probably 5 mm. mesially. The entire fragment was pried from its bed by a periosteal elevator. The line of fracture had passed through the frontal sinus on the mesial side only.

A semilunar tear in the dura (about 3 or 4 mm. in length) was exposed when the bone had been removed. It was situated not directly beneath the line of fracture but at a point corresponding with the center of the depressed piece of bone. As shown in figures 1 and 2, it was necessary for the air from the frontal sinus to be deflected around the posterior surface of the bone before entering the dural defect. This devious passage was in effect a potential valve. The pressure from sneezing or coughing would easily push the dura backward and force the air directly through the dural fistula into the frontal cavity but the increased intracranial pres-

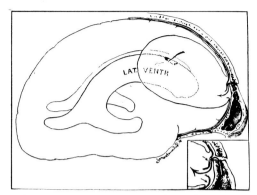

Fig. 2. (Case 1). Lateral view of operative findings.

sure at once sealed the dura against the frontal bone and thus precluded the exit of air.

A small piece of fascia lata was placed over the dural defect and sutured to the dura by a row of silk sutures; the opening was covered with a good margin to spare. This effectually prevented the air from again entering the cranial chamber.

The posterior wall of the frontal sinus was removed in part in order to preclude the accumulation of air extradurally—a seeming possibility—with an inadequate opening for the escape of the air. Healing was by first intention.

The postoperative recovery was rapid and uneventful. When a roentgenogram was taken on the patient's discharge from the hospital, March 3, 1925, thirteen days after the operation, the air had completely disappeared. The frontal defect was filled with Ringer's solution; no other effort was made to replace the air that still remained within the cranial chamber. Experiences with artificial cerebral pneumography[7] have shown that air filling the ventricular system will be completely absorbed in less than twenty-four hours, if the ventricular channels are not blocked. As the air is absorbed the large cerebral defect is automatically filled with cerebrospinal fluid of ventricular origin and at once assumes the aspect of a healed cavity.

In retrospect it is evident that an accurate diagnosis would have made the problem of cure much easier and safer for the patient, i. e., merely closure of the dural opening and possibly enlargement of the

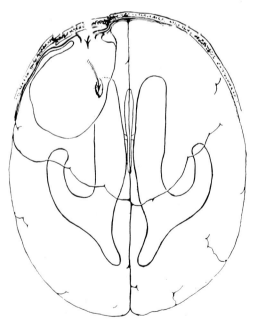

Fig. 1. (Case 1). Findings at operation; the arrows indicate the manner in which air reached the defect in the frontal lobe and by which it passed from this defect into the anterior horn of the lateral ventricle.

posterior wall of the frontal sinus. Had we been even less positive that the lesion was on the side of the fracture — and our reasons were not too free from the possibility of error — a ventricualr estimation test or an air injection would have been in order and the diagnosis might have resulted from the air escaping from the uppermost ventricle, but there is a fair chance that the escape of air might not have been detected. The mistaken diagnosis fortunately permitted an inspection of the anatomic changes of this rare condition and afforded an opportunity to interpret the sequence of events.

Case 2. A man, aged twenty-nine, entered the medical service of the Johns Hopkins Hospital in a state of semicoma, with a temperature of 107.2, pulse 110. One week before admission he came home from work complaining of severe headache and pain in the left ear. A high fever was present on the following day and persisted until his admission to the hospital. Two days previously, however, he felt very much better, took a cold bath, was seemingly refreshed, but toward evening became extremely ill again and for the last eighteen hours had been delirious and unable to eat. Every day since the onset of his illness, except on the day he felt better, he had had a severe chill. His neck had been stiff throughout the week. The left mastoid was definitely tender to firm pressure. Leukocytes totaled 12,000, of which 85 per cent. were of the polymorphonuclear type. The spinal fluid was not under marked pressure (70 mm. of water). Pressure on the left jugular vein caused a rise of spinal fluid to 140 mm. and on the right to 160 mm. The spinal fluid was of ground glass appearance and contained 2,000 cells (96 per cent. polymorphonuclear). No organisms were seen in smears and none grew from cultures.

Examination of the eye grounds showed a slight but definite fulness of the veins; the disk outlines were sharply defined. The paranasal sinuses were not infected. The left ear drum was punctured but pus was not found. Owing to the tenderness over the left mastoid in association with the sharply localized pain in the same region and a history

of otitis media a year before (side not known), it seemed most probable that an old mastoid infection had eroded the bone and produced a subdural abscess, possibly invading the brain. The meningeal changes were interpreted to be "reactive" to a contiguous infection which might be extradural or intracerebral or both.

The mastoid cells were opened by Dr. Chisolm and were not found abnormal until the antrum was reached. Here a collection of pus with extremely foul odor was encountered; it was well walled off from the rest of the mastoid but it had broken through the inner bony wall and communicated with an extradural abscess. From the pus three organisms were grown: (1) a gram-negative rod bacteria, (2) gram-negative cocci and (3) diplocci. They were interpreted by the medical bacteriologic division of the hospital to be (1) *Bacillus coli*, (2) *Staphylococcus albus* and (3) pneumococcus type IV. The sigmoid sinus was inspected and seemed normal and no opening in the dura was detected. The temperature fell to 99 and the pulse to 84 the following morning. However, scarcely any symptomatic improvement was apparent and forty-eight hours after the mastoid operation the temperture had returned to 104 and the pulse to 100. The previous irrational state had not changed.

An intracranial abscess seemed most likely and under local anesthesia a ventricular needle was passed through the dura into the left temporal lobe at a point directly above the mastoid. Probably 2 ounces (59.2 cc.) of a thick, granular, greenish brown pus with a foul fecal odor and mixed with many bubbles of gas slowly escaped under great pressure. The abscess lay immediately beneath the dura. Aside from evacuation of the pus through the needle no other treatment was attempted. Since the infection was presumed to be due to a gas producing organism surgical treatment was considered futile.

When the patient was returned to the ward, a roentgenogram was taken. Unfortunately one had not been taken before. The roentgenogram now showed a small oval patch (2 by 1 cm.) of air in the region of the abscess, another rounded area (7 by 1 cm.) with fringed edges just above and anterior to the first shadow, and finally a third shadow of oval shape, quite sharply outlined as though in a preformed cavity. It was at quite a distance from the other air shadows and suggested, both from its shape and position, the anterior horn of the lateral ventricle.

The puncture of the abscess was followed by no signs of improvement in his condition. On the following day a second series of roentgenograms was taken. The air was still present in the anterior horn of the lateral ventricle and in the temporal lobe, but the size of the air shadows seemed unchanged. There was then reason to doubt the validity of our assumption that the air had been of bacterial origin. It seemed incredible that the volume of air should not have increased if the organisms were responsible.

To meet any question of doubt and leave nothing undone the abscess was drained. The dura was under great pressure. The abscess was entirely within the temporal lobe. From time to time pus could be seen emerging through the dura into the mastoid wound but the fistula could not be seen emerging through the dura into the mastoid wound but the fistula could not be seen owing to its great depth. Again no improvement followed and three days later the patient died. On the day before his death another skiagram showed but little difference in the air shadows—certainly the quantity was not greater. We were therefore confronted with additional evidence which seemed to be against the bacterial origin of the gas. Had bacteria been the source, there should have been an increase in the size of the air shadow. Unfortunately, the possible gas producing property of the organisms was not tested in vitro.

It is my feeling that the air was forced through the mastoid defect produced by the operation into the abscess cavity by swallowing, coughing or sneezing, just as an occipital extracranial pneumatocele has been known to form. Prior to the operation this hardly could have resulted; the abscess was well walled off and there had been no discharge from the ear. Moreover, when the cerebral abscess was drained, a periodic discharge of pus from the abscess into the mastoid defect could be seen, and at that time the dura was

well exposed and there was no extradural abscess.

Necropsy showed a large abscess of the left temporal lobe with a small fistula in the descending horn of the left lateral ventricle; diffuse meningitis; thrombosis of the left lateral sinus (presumably a recent development, since Queckenstedt's test on admission had indicated the sinus to be patent, though the fact that there was 20 mm. less rise of spinal fluid on compression of the left jugular vein may be an indication of a beginning thrombosis of the left lateral sinus).

Case 3. During a consultation with Dr. James K. Corss at Newport News, Va., I was shown a patient whose skull had been fractured a week previously. For two days following the accident, cerebrospinal fluid drained from the right ear. He had since been free of symptoms and was ready to be discharged. Being aware of the possibility of pneumocephalus as a sequel of a cerebrospinal fistula, I at once sought the roentgenograms and found air filling a lateral ventricle, the cisterna chiasmatis and interpeduncularis (in the lateral view), and both lateral ventricles in cross section in the anteroposterior view. The ventricles were small and symmetrical. Dr. Corss kindly obtained another roentgenogram, the air had then disappeared (seven days after the accident).[8]

RESUME OF LITERATURE

In Chiari's case, a chronic infection of the ethmoid cells had weakened the wall, eroded the dura and penetrated the brain. He was able clearly to show at necropsy a tiny fistulous tract leading from an ethmoid cell into a large cavity in the frontal lobe; another opening of larger size led from this frontal defect into a lateral ventricle. Violent sneezing was one of the outstanding symptoms before the onset of severe headaches, which were soon followed by stupor and death. A diagnosis of cerebral abscess had been made. Chiari's case seems to have elicited no comment, and no other cases have been found in a search of the pathologic literature. Even at the present time textbooks either pass over the subject of cranial pneumatocele completely or casually mention only the

ANALYSIS OF CASES OF PNEUMOCEPHALUS REPORTED IN THE LITERATURE

Cases Reported by; Date; Cause	Time Air Was First Detected after Accident or Infection	Cerebro-spinal Fistula	Sneezing	Cranial Air Sinus Involved	Signs and Symptoms	Location of Air In	Operation	Result	Findings	Remarks
1. Chiari 1884 Erosion of sinus wall from chronic infection	Infection of many years' duration	+	+ Severe	Ethmoid	Headache and vomiting	Brain and ventricles	None	Death	Large cavity in frontal lobe; this opens into lateral ventricle, fistula from ethmoid cell	Postmortem examination; excellent drawings of pathologic changes
2. Luckett 1913 Fracture	19 days	+ About a cupful of fluid would immediately follow sneezing	+	Frontal	Headache; periods of confusion; melancholy; choked disks; vomiting; semicoma; Babinski right; white blood cells, 15,600	Brain and ventricles	Decompression needle inserted into ventricle; drainage of cisterna magna for meningitis	Death 4 days later; no organisms seen in ventricular fluid; none from cultures	Diffuse meningitis; at necropsy, air escaped from trocar in ventricle	Earlier roentgenogram of head showed no air; fissure in dura; author thought probably progressive softening took place around the air
3. Wolff 1914 Bullet	7 months	......	..	Frontal	Four months after accident progressive hemiplegia; convulsions 3 months later	Brain (in Rolandic origin) and ventricles	Filled sinus tract with fat	Well	......	Author says there must be communication between the frontal sinus, the cerebral defect and the lateral ventricle
4. Duken 1915 Bullet	5 weeks	......	..	Frontal	Headache and feeling of pressure in left forehead; suggestive unilateral choked disk; skull tympanitic	Brain	Craniotomy; brain under pressure; finger inserted into two cerebral air pockets	Well	Air-fluid level in roentgenogram; yellowish fluid in both cerebral cavities	Author thought of some explosive gas; thought valve action resulted from a flap of bone or periosteum; roentgenray examination showed no air three weeks after operation
5. Duken 1915 Fracture	......	......	..	Mastoid	......	Brain (In temporal lobe beneath mastoid)	None	......	Small bubble of air in roentgenogram	......
6. Gebele 1915 Bullet	6 weeks	......	..	Frontal	Frontal headache; no choked disk; air-fluid noise when head was moved	Brain (two shadows)	Craniotomy; serosanguineous exudate which was sterile; drained; tampon	Death from infection	......	Cultures of fluid at time of operation were negative

7. Kredel . . . . . 1915 Bullet	5 weeks	+	+	Frontal	Headache and pains; no bradycardia; no choked disk	Brain	Frontal sinus opened; hollow sound to tap of knife on dura; air cavity punctured	Well	Cavity size of hen's egg; fluid; serosanguineous; drainage; no tampon; air cavity; back wall of frontal sinus removed	Special mention is made that there was no splashing sound, no changed percussion note, and no valve in fistula
8. Wodarcz . . . . 1915 Shrapnel wound	2 weeks (no roentgen-ray examination)	....	..	Frontal	Rushing noise when head was bent forward first noticed 2 weeks after accident; ceased 1 month later	Brain	Exploration of wound	Well (?)	Splinter of glass in opening; he thought it acted as a valve, as in Duken's case	No roentgen-ray examination; clinical diagnosis from sound of rushing air on change of position
9. Passow . . . . 1916 Bullet	1 month	+ Beginning at 2 months; lasted 7 weeks; reappeared 4 months later	..	Frontal	Headaches; rhinorrhea, 40 to 140 cc. a day; rhinorrhea brought on by bending forward	Brain (egg size)	Enlarged fistula to permit free egress of air; closed opening with fat	Well 5 months after operation; no air in roentgenogram; this was three months after accident	Smooth cavity; small opening into cerebral cavity which was 10 cm. deep	Returned to regiment five months after injury; again headaches and rhinorrhea returned; larger air shadow than on first admission
10. Skinner . . . . 1916, reported by Am. Roentgenol. Soc., 1914 Fracture	4 weeks	....	..	Frontal	Headache and dizziness	Brain	Trephined over air shadow; air pocket punctured	Death from meningitis 20 days after operation	Bulging dura; air and fluid in cavity; collapse of dura after tapping	Air analyzed to eliminate other gas since a gas well was nearby; analysis showed 98.2 nitrogen, 1.8 oxygen
11. Bruning . . . . 1917 Bullet	53 days	....	..	Frontal	Headache and dizziness; no other signs of pressure	Brain (shadow size of a goose egg)	Small bone flap; opening enlarged; tampon and drain; removed bone to fill in defect	Well 18 months later; 1 convulsion since, but back in army	Smooth cavity	Diagnosis of abscess made; bullet entered on left and operation was on right; 14 days after operation there was no more air in the roentgen-ray shadow than before operation
12. Cotte . . . . . 1917 Kicked by horse	10 months	+	..	Frontal	Headache	Subdural space (extracerebral) (probably)	Bone flap; did not open dura; large hernia formed at site of bone defect	Temporarily well; ultimate result not stated	Hollow sound on tapping dura with instrument	Long duration of intracranial air is noteworthy; it would appear to be extracerebral
13. Reisinger . . . 1918 Bullet	5 weeks	+ 18 days	..	Frontal	....	Brain (shadow seems intracerebral but author insists air was extracerebral)	Large bone flap; extradural gauze packs	Well	Dura lying on folds on sunken cavity after puncture; cavity not exposed	Looked on as cyst from the roentgenogram; dura not opened

ANALYSIS OF CASES OF PNEUMOCEPHALUS REPORTED IN THE LITERATURE—(Continued)

Cases Reported by; Date; Cause	Time Air Was First Detected after Accident or Infection	Cerebrospinal Fistula	Sneezing	Cranial Air Sinus Involved	Signs and Symptoms	Location of Air In	Operation	Result	Findings	Remarks
14. Holmes.... 1918 Fracture	At once after accident	....	..	Ethmoid? Frontal?	....	Subarachnoid space (cisterna chiasmatis)	Wall of sinus removed	Death from meningitis one week later		Communication with frontal sinus not disclosed
15. Manasse.... Bullet	5 weeks	....	..	Frontal	....	Brain	Posterior wall of frontal sinus removed	Well	Cavity has smooth wall and contains fine vessels	
16. Glenard and Aimard 1919 Bullet	2 months	+	..	Frontal	Headache on left side, principally noise and bruit in head when moved	Brain	None	Died of pneumonia 6 months later	Necropsy; cavity contained 25cc of yellowish fluid; cavity largely filled by granulation tissue	Air present also at four and a half month, but absent at five months
17. May....... 1919 Fracture	1 day	....	..	Sphenoid	Death in twenty-four hours	Subarachnoid space (cisterna chiasmatis), subdural space (extracerebral)	None	Death from cranial injury	Postmortem roentgenogram	Brief note; air in cerebral suici and anterior to frontal lobe
18. Potter....... 1919 Fracture	1 week	....	..	Frontal	Slight dizziness and slight disturbance with change of position; no more symptoms while air was increasing	Brain (egg size) and ventricles	None	Well (?) spontaneous cure	....	Progressive increase in size of air shadow until fifth week when the lateral ventricle was reached; progressive decrease thereafter
19. Doyle...... (also reported by Spiller) 1921 Fracture	3 weeks	....	..	Ethmoid	Headache; memory defective; convulsions; irrational	Brain	Dura opened	Died next day	Air hissed out when dura was punctured at operation; probe passed through cribriform plate at necropsy	Patient was unconscious three days after accident; for necropsy report comparison should be made with Spiller's article

20. Horrax 1921 Compound fracture	Accidentally discovered 3 months after accident	..	Frontal	No symptoms	Brain	None	Well	....	Lobulated shadow 1 month after accident, but this had disappeared 2 months later when patient sought relief for direct effects of injury, i.e., blindness and deafness on right side of face; loss of smell; strabismus and some mental aberration
21. Teachenor 1923 Fracture	Same day	+	Mastoid	Dizziness; confusion; bilateral Babinski	Subarachnoid space, subdural (extracerebral), ventricle	None	Well	Roentgenograms show both lateral ventricles to be well filled with air	Air disappeared in 18 days; author thought air entered the floor of third ventricle
22. Grant 1923 Compound fracture	2 days	..	Frontal	Confusion; restlessness	Subdural space (extracerebral) (?) (elliptical shadow)	Bone flap nothing seen; pack left to control severe bleedings	Slow recovery	Air escaped after tight dura was tapped	Bone flap was undoubtedly made too high to disclose fistula
23. McCannel 1923 Fracture	4 weeks	:	Frontal	Double vision; congested disks; slight exophthalmos; visual loss though largely the result of the fracture	Brain	None	Well; steady improvement after accident	....	Air was not present eight days after accident (roentgen-ray examination); in less than two more months air gone
24. Imboden Fracture	1 month	:	Frontal	....	....	Air removed			
25. Santoro 1924	Following erosion of floor of skull by a tumor	:	....	....	Ventricle	None	Death from neurositis	....	Original article not obtainable
26. Dandy 1925 Fracture	6 weeks	+	Frontal	Stupor; delirium; bradycardia	Brain and ventricle	Closure of dural opening with a facial transplant	Well	Air cavity filled right frontal lobe and communicated with right lateral ventricle	Potential valve due to dura defect behind depressed fracture; this admitted air and prevented its escape
27. Dandy 1925 Operation on mastoid	1 day	0	Mastoid	Coma; high fever	Brain and ventricle	Puncture of cerebral abscess	Death from cerebral abscess	Abscess contained colon bacilli and micrococci	Air was formed in abscess and ventricle 3 days after mastoid operation; a possibility remains that the air may be of microbic origin
28. Dandy 1925 Fracture	1 day	+ From right ear, lasted 48 hours	Mastoid	Slight headache	Subarachnoid space and ventricle	None	Well	....	Cerebrospinal fistula lasted 2 days

extracranial variety.

Practically all of the cases in the German literature are due to war wounds, the infantry bullet being the usual type of injury. On the other hand, all the American cases followed injuries of civil life. Doubtless cases must have been detected in the American, French and Italian fronts during the war but no reports have been found. And doubtless also many cases have been overlooked in both civil and military life. In only one case (Wodarcz,[3] and this diagnosis was not substantiated by the roentgen ray) has the diagnosis of intracranial air been suspected before its discovery by the roentgen ray, operation or necropsy; usually a brain abscess or meningitis is diagnosed. An analysis of the series shows that air has entered the cranial chamber through all the cranial air spaces, three through the ethmoids (Chiari,[2] Holmes,[9] D o y l e[10] and Spiller[11]), two through the sphenoid (May[12] and Santoro[13]), four through the mastoid (Duken,[14] Teachenor,[15] Dandy,[16] two), and in the remaining cases through the frontal sinus. Mackay[17] (1903) and Hixon[18] (1915) and doubtless others have reported instances of multiple intracranial cavities of air resulting from bacteria (presumably the *Bacillus aerogenes-capsulatus* of Welch), but the findings have been made at postmortem examinations. Since the rapidity of growth of gas from these organisms after death is well recognized, the importance of the findings of gas has been discounted. However, Hixon stresses the fact that in his case necropsy was performed only one hour after death — an interval which should surely warrant the assumption that the air had been present during life. Though gas baccillus infections were rampant during the World War and roentgen rays were employed in detecting the early traces of gas in the soft parts, I have been able to find no record in which air was found or suspected during life; but its disclosure could, of course, have been of only academic interest.

We shall consider only the entrance of intracranial air through clefts in the skull. With the exception of Chiari's case, which was of infectious origin, and Santoro's, which followed erosion of the floor of the sella turcica from local intracranial pressure, (brain tumor), all have followed some form of trauma to the skull. It has been suggested that pneumocephalus is more frequent than the records indicate. Doubtless this is true and more liberal use of the roentgen ray will surely greatly increase the number of cases. But when it is considered that a number of factors must be properly combined before air can enter and remain within the cranial chamber the total number can only be a small fraction of the rapidly mounting number of injuries to the skull.

VARIETIES OF PNEUMOCEPHALUS, THEIR CAUSES AND MODE OF FORMATION

A study of the roentgenograms of the reported cases indicates that air entering the cranial chamber from the cranial air cells may be located in: (1) the subarachnoid space, (2) the subdural space, (3) the brain and (4) the ventricles. Obviously the location of the air is determined by the normal anatomic factors at the site of the fracture, but pathologic and physiologic factors of secondary origin also play a role.

From the published photographs in this series it seems certain that in at least two cases, the air is confined to the subarachnoid space, the cisterna chiasmatis and the cerebral sulci. The anatomy of the cerebrospinal spaces makes it probable that the primary entry of air into the subarachnoid space could be only through the cisterna at the base of the brain and, therefore, only from the posterior ethmoid and sphenoid sinuses. In May's case the sphenoid cells and in Holmes' case probably the ethmoids were opened. Moreover, the close application of the outer layer of the arachnoid membrane to the dura in the region of the cisterna chiasmatis would almost preclude an accumulation of air between the dura and the arachnoid, particularly so when the air can so easily enter the big subarachnoid space. On the other hand a fracture through the frontal sinus would be opposite the cerebral sulci; these are so small and the arachnoid membrane is so tightly clasped to the brain that the entry of air into the subarachnoid space from this source would be almost inconceivable. Here the subdural space, though practically a mere slit under normal conditions, is potentially a space of great size. The fact that compound fractures in the region of the cisterna chiasmatis are less common than elsewhere would seem to explain the relative infrequency of the primary entrance of air into the subarachnoid space. Although cerebrospinal rhinorrhea was not mentioned in either reported instance of this variety of pneumocephalus (May's patient died in twenty-four hours), it would appear to be an almost necessary accompaniment. The danger of meningitis must also be greater in this than in other forms because infection has such easy access to the cerebrospinal spaces. It is noteworthy that the other patient (Holmes' case) who survived the initial trauma died seven days later of meningitis.

The subdural (extracerebral) accumulations of air have exclusively followed compound fractures of the frontal sinus. The roentgenograms of this variety of pneumocephalus appear to be characteristic. An elliptical shadow, conforming in front to the curve of the frontal bone and behind to the curved surface of the frontal lobe which had been pushed backward, defines the shape of the roentgen-ray shadow. It would seem probable that the cases of Cotte,[19] of Grant[20] and of Imboden[21] are of this variety. Reisinger[22] insists on the extracerebral location of air in his case but the round air shadow (characteristic of intracerebral air) makes his claim none too certain, particularly as he did not open the dura at operation.

The intracerebral variety appears to be most common. Usually a shadow of roughly round or oval shape and of varying size projects backward from the frontal bone,

no longer conforming to its contour as does the extracerebral (subdural) form. This defect often fills the entire frontal lobe and extends backward into the parietal lobe. The cavity always communicates with the frontal or ethmoid sinus by a small opening, often so minute as to be easily overlooked. In our case and so far as it is possible to judge in those reported, the dura was tightly adherent to the brain surrounding the fistula. Were it otherwise there would necessarily be a subdural collection of air in the roentgenogram; this has been uniformly absent. An intracerebral enclosure of air must therefore arise relatively late, i. e., after the traumatized brain has become adherent to the dura. It would also seem that a rupture of the cerebral cortex at the time of the accident must be a prerequisite to the formation of an intracerebral pneumatocele. Otherwise adhesions would be unlikely and entrance of the brain tissue would be difficult. The anatomy of this region is favorable to the production of an intracerebral pneumatocele, first, because the dura is so closely applied to the frontal bone that a fracture also readily tears the dura; and second, because the tip of the frontal lobe is in such close apposition to the dura that the cerebral cortex as well as the meninges are easily ruptured. But even so, it is doubtful if an intracerebral pneumatocele or the other forms of pneumocephalus could develop without an added factor, i. e., the increased pressure of the air within the cranial sinuses such as is produced by sneezing, coughing, straining or possibly even of swallowing.

The small size of the sinus tract between the pneumatocele and the sinus has often been commented on; in fact, at operation an opening has not always been found. Moreover, the fact that intracranial pressure has developed is sufficient evidence that a compensatory escape of fluid or air or of both from the cranial chamber is not possible. Because of these facts there has been speculation about a probable valve action in the fistula opening. Wodarcz found a fragment of glass in the communicating tract and considered this to act as a valve. Duken could find no definite valve but thought a piece of granulation tissue or bone must have served this function. Kredel[23] could find no valve and considered a valve unnecessary if the fistula were small. In our case there was a potential valve in that the dural opening was behind the center of the depressed fragment of bone and not, therefore, in a direct line with the fracture. Sneezing would push the dura away from the bone and readily force the air through the relatively large opening of the dura into the cerebral defect; after this the heightened intracranial pressure would seal the dura against the depressed bone and effectively close the opening. But we have every reason to believe that an actual valve is not necessary for the induction of pneumocephalus even when the fistulous tract may be perfectly straight. If the fistula is of just the right size (both length and breadth) and its walls not too rigid it would naturally be widened by the explosive force of sneezing and permit the quick passage of air into the cranial chamber, but the vis a tergo of the lesser and steadier pressure within the cranial chamber, even though above normal, would not be able again to distend the opening and allow the air to escape from the cerebral defect. An opening of an ideal size might also well permit the escape of fluid — cerebrospinal rhinorrhea — and yet prevent the egress of air. The results of three tests may be cited as experiments to prove these statements:

1. An opening may be of such size that fluid can and air cannot pass. Indigocarmin and air were injected into the *right* lateral ventricle of a patient suffering from the effects of a brain tumor that was found to be located in the third ventricle. The dye was at once and freely aspirated through a needle in the *left* lateral ventricle. But the air which had been injected into the right lateral ventricle at the same time failed to reach the left lateral ventricle. The absence of air in the left ventricle was shown not only by the failure of air to be aspirated but also by the absence of an air shadow in the left side of the head, though the right was well filled.

2. Additional evidence that a channel may be patent for fluid and not for air has been included in a recent paper on the diagnosis and localization of spinal cord tumors.[24] It was demonstrated that fluid will often pass freely around a spinal cord tumor (Queckenstedt's test) when air will stop at the lower level of the tumor.

3. Finally, continuing further the test just mentioned, if the intraspinous pressure is increased, the air may be forced beyond the spinal cord tumor which under normal pressure had indicated a complete block under the subarachnoid space. An example of this kind has been reported under the classification of partial obstructions in the same paper on spinal cord tumors. The factors involved in this experiment are precisely the same as those in the development of pneumocephalus.

But the development of an intracerebral pneumatocele is the result of more than the mechanical entrance of air into the brain. Definite pathologic reactions follow the entrance of air into the brain. Definite pathologic reactions follow the entrance of air and these play a big role in the development of the end product as we see it at operation or necropsy. From our experience with cerebral pneumography we know that air is an irritant. After the initial traumatic insult which results to the brain tissue from the explosive entrance of air there is a secondary reaction due to the *irritation* of the air, not unlike, except in degree, the reaction which would follow the introduction of any irritating liquid. One result of the irritation is a serosanguineous fluid which, pouring into the cerebral defect, produces additional local as well as general intracranial pressure. Another result is an edema of the brain tissue contiguous to the defect and resulting both from the traumatic insult and the subsequent irritation of the air. Although life may still be tolerated the loss of much brain tissue must inevitably follow in the wake of these changes. In Luckett's[3] early case it was assumed that a gradual softening of the brain tissue resulted from the effects of the air. We have reasons to believe that the white matter of the brain is much less resistant to trauma than the cortex. The cortex is actually harder to cut; pressure of a spatula quickly produces petechial hemorrhages and edema in the exposed white matter though the same insults will be tolerated by the cortex and its protecting meninges. The white matter, therefore, presumably suffers first and most in the cerebral absorption resulting from pressure and irritation of the air in pneumocephalus.

In many of the recorded cases of intracerebral pneumocephalus a cerebrospinal rhinorrhea has been reported. As long as the cerebral defect is not in continuity with either the ventricles or the subarachnoid space the fluid that escapes must be a serosanguineous reaction product. In some instances (Duken,[14] Gebele[25]) a fluid-air level has been disclosed in the roentgenogram and in one case[26] there is the characteristic story that fluid pours from the nose when the patient bends forward, i. e., when the dependent fluid can pour over the brim of the cerebral cavity as from a cup. A single instance of this kind demonstrates that a valve is neither present nor necessary for the development of pneumocephalus. Duken[14] found a yellow, Kredel,[23] a serosanguineous, and Glenard and Aimard,[27] a lemon yellow fluid. Though there is no evidence contained in this series of cases it seems safe to reason from the known facts that the rhinorrhea of an intracerebral pneumatocele must be less in amount and different in character from that of pneumocephalus of the subarachnoid or intraventricular types in which pure cerebrospinal fluid can escape freely.

Intraventricular pneumocephalus is often but a later stage in the progress of an intracerebral pneumatocele, though the air may enter directly into the ventricles from the subarachnoid space when this variety of pneumocephalus exists. It has been repeatedly shown that air injected into the subarachnoid space through the spinal canal at once passes into the ventricular system. Teachenor's case is an interesting example of the rapidity with which air may reach the lateral ventricles — a few hours. Although Teachenor makes the interesting assumption that the air might have entered the ventricles through a tear in the floor of the third ventricle, I should feel more inclined to believe it entered through the normal channels — the foramina of Luschka and Magendie. This will always be expected when the air is in sufficient quantity in the subarachnoid space. Our case (case 3) is practically a duplicate of Teachenor's.

In the metamorphosis of the intracerebral pneumatocele the frontal defect gradually enlarges and eventually opens into the lateral ventricle of the corresponding size. In our case, and apparently also in Chiari's, the ventricular opening was about as large as the circumference of a slate pencil. Once in the ventricle, the air has free access to every part of the ventricular system and emerges into the subarachnoid space. Precisely as in deliberate cerebral pneumography for diagnostic purposes every part of the ventricular system can then be clearly shown in the roentgenograms.

We also know from experiences with cerebral pneumography that air absorbs almost entirely in the subarachnoid space. It is probable, therefore, that coincident with the rupture of air into the lateral ventricle there may be a transient period of relief from symptoms, i. e., until the cranial chamber is again overwhelmed by a new supply of air from the nasal sinuses. We were interested to pick out if possible any such period in our patient.. Fifteen days before his arrival in Baltimore he rather suddenly and surprisingly came out of a deep stupor. A roentgenogram was not taken, however, until six days later; at that time the ventricles contained air.

SYMPTOMS OF PNEUMOCEPHALUS

Occasionally the symptoms are masked by the greater local disturbances of the fracture as in Horrax's case.[28] Teachenor's patient had surprisingly mild symptoms, doubtless because the fistula through which the air entered was soon closed. On the whole the symptoms of any form of pneumocephalus are severe. With few exceptions they are those of intracranial pressure, headache, vomiting, drowsiness, possibly double vision and dizziness, and finally restlessness, delirium and coma. Papilloedema has been noted in a few cases by Luckett,[3] McCannel,[29] and Duken.[14] It has been noted as absent in other by Gebele,[25] Kredel,[23] Teachenor,[15] and in all of our cases.

It hardly seems possible to make an absolute diagnosis of pneumocephalus from any combination of signs or symptoms except one, sneezing followed by cerebrospinal rhinorrhea. One usually can only suspect this condition and confirm or disprove the suspicion by the pathognomonic roentgen-ray findings. All fractures involving the sinuses should place one on guard for this diagnosis, whether the symptoms of intracranial pressure follow immediately or, as so often happens, at a latter date. A cerebrospinal fistula is probably the sign of greatest significance. Its presence should always make one suspect pneumocephalus. It was solely on the basis of this manifestation that air was suspected and found in our third case. When sneezing follows a frontal fracture with rhinorrhea, the suspicion grows stronger, but when sneezing is followed by a flow of cerebrospinal fluid, as in Luckett's case, one could almost be safe in making a positive diagnosis of pneumocephalus without the roentgen ray. There are practically only four conditions which can appear as late (from several days to weeks after injury) sequelae of a fracture, subdural venous hemorrhage (erroneously called pachymeningitis haemorrhagica), brain abscess meningitis and pneumocephalus. As said before the roentgen ray at once makes or eliminates the

diagnosis of air in the cranial chamber, thus making the differential diagnosis easy.

In Wolff's[4] patient hemiplegia gradually developed and convulsions followed; Doyle's and Spiller's patients also had convulsions; Luckett's patient had a unilateral positive Babinski, Teachenor's bilateral. Other patients have had defects of vision and smell, ptosis, strabismus, etc., all, however, caused by cerebral injury due to the initial trauma and not related to the pneumocephalus. As mentioned before, only one case was suspected from clinical symptoms. In our third case, air was suspected, not from symptoms, but because of the presence of a cerebrospinal fistula. Among the earlier reported cases even the interpretation of the roentgen-ray shadow was most uncertain. Skinner[30] (1916), for instance, thought of the possibility of some gas from nearby gas wells and had it analyzed only to find ordinary air. Duken[14] (1915) thought of some explosive gas, and Bruning[31] looked on the shadow as that of an abscess. Almost without exception headache has been the outstanding complaint and this symptom together with stupor was the combination of symptoms referable to the brain.

In three cases, those of Holmes, May and Teachenor, air was present in the cranial chamber when roentgenograms were taken a few hours after the accident and in Grant's case and in Case 3 of this report it was present in the first roentgenogram, which was taken on the second day. The time at wihch the air was detected in the remaining cases is doubtless always considerably later than the actual appearance time. It is fair to assume that in some instances it must have been present at least soon after the accident and had steadily increased until the cerebral lesion was large enough to cause intracranial pressure. In McCannel's case air was absent eight days after the trauma and present at the next roentgenogram, three weeks later. In my first case air was first detected in the cerebral ventricles five weeks after the accident, and in Potter's[32] case air was in the brain during the first week and in the ventricle when another plate was taken a month later. In eleven cases of the total number the air has been recognized in less than a month after the accident, and in ten instances between the fourth and sixth weeks. In three cases air was recognized only after a longer time, by Wolff in seven months and by Cotte in ten months. Luckett's case (nineteen days) indicates how short a time may be required for air to traverse the frontal lobe and break into a lateral ventricle. On the other hand Passow's case (eight months), Cotte's (ten months) and Bruning's (seventeen months) show how long the air may exist in the frontal lobe and yet not enter a ventricle. It seems probable from Cotte's report that the air in his case was extra-cerebral; if this is true it is an example in which air did not penetrate the brain even after ten months. As cerebral destruction doubtless occurs rapidly both from the irritating effect of air and from the traumatic effects of the explosive force of air, it is difficult to arrive at a conclusion regarding the relative effect of each. The rapidity with which the pneumocephalus develops must also be dependent on such variable factors as the amount of sneezing, the amount of initial cerebral destruction, the size and elasticity of the fistulous tract and also on the presence or absence of a valve. A large opening without a valve is undoubtedly more favorable, other things being equal, because the outflow of fluid and air spontaneously relieves intracranial pressure. Passow's patient was cured by making the sinus larger, thereby preventing retention.

Several cases have been observed over a period of weeks and even months after the air was known to be present in the brain, some with and others without surgical treatment. One of the most interesting of these was Passow's case. One month after a bullet wound in the supra-orbital region, a clear patch was seen in the roentgenogram of the frontal lobe. Although the shadow was absent in the plate taken soon after the accident, the significance of its later appearance was not realized. Five months later the patient was apparently well and returned to his battalion and a pronounced cerebrospinal rhinorrhea, which on the earlier admission had persisted for six weeks, had then been absent two months. However, after a month's activity the same headaches again returned and two weeks later rhinorrhea followed. The air shadow was larger than before. He was then operated on and after another five months, or thirteen months after the accident, the air had disappeared. Potter watched the shadow of air increase in his case over a period of a month; the air finally reached the lateral ventricle after which it soon disappeared.

In Teachenor's case a great quantity of ventricular air disappeared in eighteen days. The importance of a cerebrospinal fistula as a diagnostic sign cannot be over-emphasized. It has been recorded in only nine cases though doubtless it has been overlooked in many, owing to the failure to suspect the diagnostic of pneumocephalus. Overlooked in one of our cases at the time the history was taken, it was later found to be an outstanding and distressing symptom. In Luckett's case about a cupful of clear fluid suddenly *followed sneezing*, the fluid probably being released as the air was driven into the cerebral cavity. Passow's patient drained continuously for two months, at first 140 cc. per day; gradually the flow lessened to 40 cc. per day and ceased, later reappearing after a free interval of four months. Though a history of rhinorrhea could not be elicited in our case, it is difficult to believe it was absent, even with the undoubted valve action in the fistula. Sneezing was recorded and emphasized in the early reports of Chiari and of Luckett, and later of Kredel. It is doubtless the great active factor in the development of this condition.

An instance of rhinorrhea with change of position has been mentioned (Passow's case). This can, of course, appear only in those cases in which the fistula is relatively large and no valve is present. Such an observation, when questioned, should be almost as significant as rhinorrhea following a sneeze. At times the patient heard the gurgling sound in his head on turning, an observation now frequently made in deliberate injection of air into the ventricles. Duken mentions a tympanitic note over the air space, a sign that Kredel was unable to elicit. Wodarcz's patient heard a rushing sound when he moved his head and on this symptom, the diagnosis of pneumatocele was made. This characteristic noise is well known to patients in whom a deliberate injection of air has been made into the ventricles.

THE PROGNOSIS

Excluding May's case, in which death soon followed the accident and was in no way dependent on the pneumocephalus, there are sixteen recoveries and eleven deaths. Of the sixteen recoveries, seven were entirely spontaneous and nine followed operative procedures of various kinds. Undoubtedly several of the postoperative recoveries would have occurred spontaneously for the operation accomplished nothing more than the discovery of the lesion. It is also fair to add that many of the postoperative deaths would have occurred had nothing been done. On the whole the mortality would probably average about 50 per cent if the patients were left untreated. The deaths are due to two factors: (1) intracranial pressure and (2) infection from a compound wound. That air can pass through a paranasal or mastoid air sinus into the brain — even into the cerebrospinal fluid — over a period of weeks and months without infection speaks well for the sterility of the paranasal — principally frontal — sinuses in these cases. But the frequency of meningitis (six cases) and abscess (one case) attests the fact that the sterility of the sinuses is purely a matter of chance. Once an infection develops there is only a bare possibility of spontaneous recovery and a greatly reduced chance from operative treatment.

Nature cures pneumocephalus by closing the fistula with granulation tissue after which the air within the brain absorbs, slowly in the cerebral cavity, much faster from the ventricular system and subarachnoid space. Doubtless some fistulas are prevented from closing by the inclusion of a small foreign body, such as a piece of glass or bone, others because periodic sneezing overcomes the tissue growth, and doubtless others because of infection. It is worthy of note that only in Potter's case[32] has a spontaneous cure resulted after air has reached the ventricle after transit through the frontal lobe. The entrance of air into the ventricle must have been well timed with the closure of the external fistula. When the fistula has finally closed, the cerebral defect remains filled with ventricular fluid if there is a communication with the ventricle; or at first with fluid and ultimately with granulation tissue of the cavity is isolated from the cerebrospinal spaces. The report of Glenard and Aimard shows the result of healing in such a cavity six months after the air shadow has disappeared and the patient was free of symptoms.

OPERATIVE TREATMENT

The attempts to cure this condition have been most varied. In several instances in which a flap has been turned down and the air evacuated after being accidentally found, the communicating fistula has not been treated and the patient has obtained no benefit. Bruning[31] Kredel,[23] Manasse[33] and Passow[26] have removed the posterior wall of the frontal sinus and apparently some of the frontal bone above; they then produced and maintained a large opening between the cerebral cavity and the exterior, the object being to prevent retention of air by providing a large exit. All of these patients recovered. It should be noted, however, that in none was there air in the ventricles. It is hardly possible that any would have recovered with this treatment had the air been in the ventricles at the time of operation for not only would the air become trapped in the ventricles but a cerebrospinal fistula of such size and under these conditions could hardly exist without the development of meningitis. It is of interest that fourteen days after operation Bruning found the air shadow to be larger than before operation. Following a procedure of this kind the cerebral defect must heal from the bottom, filling with granulation tissue. In Passow's case this required five months and in Bruning's case a small shadow still existed fifteen months later. In all of these cases, therefore, the treatment has been directed toward the effect rather than the cause. In addition to producing a large vent for the air cavity, Passow introduced a piece of fat into the fistulous tract hoping to impede the inflow of air from the frontal sinus, but the fate of the fat is not recorded.

It must be remembered that much of the attempted surgical treatment for this condition has been evolved on the spur of the moment and at a time when the underlying pathology was little understood. With an appreciation of the cause there can be little uncertainty in most cases as to the character of the treatment or hesitancy as to its application, namely, in the correction of the cause, i. e., closure of the fistula if it is accessible. This should surely be done as quickly as possible after the character of the lesion has been recognized. The mortality resulting when the fistula is left to the chance of spontaneous cure is too great. The risk of the suggested procedure should be little if anything. Needless to add every effort must be made to learn beforehand the exact location of the fracture, for the dural opening must be directly beneath or at least close by. In depressed fractures of the frontal bone — the most common form — the history, examination and study of the stereoscopic roentgenograms (both lateral and anteroposterior views) should make the site of the opening certain and it should be easy of operative approach.

An operative treatment is here suggested for those cases in which the fistula results from a fracture of the frontal sinus. These are easy of approach and seem to be the most frequent type. The procedure is that which was carried out in our first case. Although this treatment is not proposed for communications into the ethmoid and mastoid sinuses in which the demonstration of the opening by operation will be more difficult, it is not improbable that in some of these, at least, closure of the dural opening in a similar manner may yet be practical.

After the intracranial pressure is relieved by a ventricular puncture (if there is air in the ventricles) or by tapping the pneumatoecle (whether intracerebral or extracerebral), a small incision is made along the line of the shaved eyebrow, the depressed fragment is elevated, and the opening in the dura is located and covered by a transplant of fascia lata which is carefully sutured to the dura. In our case this was particularly easy because of the isolated depressed fracture. Should there be only a crack in the posterior wall or the fragment small and impossible of ready elevation a small bone flap will give ample exposure to permit careful inspection of the dura and suture of the fascial graft. Unless infected, air already in the brain will be taken care of automatically by absorption. This plan of attack should be effective for air accumulations whether extracerebral or within the frontal lobe or, as in our case, within the ventricle. Since the operation is entirely extradural there is no danger of introducing an infection within the cranial chamber. Should a cerebral abscess be present at the time, it should, of course, be handled precisely as an abscess of other origin. If there is meningitis the best chances would appear to follow closure of the fistula, whereby the source of more infection is prevented, and after this, continuous drainage of the cisterna magna through a small catheter.

SUMMARY AND CONCLUSIONS

1. Pneumocephalus may follow in the

wake of any artificial communication between the paranasal or mastoid sinuses and
the cranial chamber. The opening may result from a fracture, from an operative
defect, from the erosion of a chronic infection, from destruction of the floor of
the skull by a tumor or a dilated third
ventricle in hydrocephalus. Pneumocephalus also results directly from infections of
gas producing organisms — *Bacillus aerogenes-capsulatus* (of Welch) and possibly
colon bacillus.

2. Twenty-eight cases of pneumocephalus, including three of our own, have been
compiled from the literature and analyzed.

3. Sneezing, coughing, straining or swallowing is necessary to force the air through
a bony and dural defect into the cranial
chamber.

4. Intracranial air may be subdivided
into four varieties according to location:
(1) subarachnoid, (2) subdural, (3) intracerebral and (4) intraventricular. The
intracerebral variety appears to be the
most frequent.

5. The source of air may be the frontal,
ethmoid, sphenoid and mastoid sinuses.
The variety of pneumocephalus is dependent on the sinus involved, the exact character of the fracture and the duration of
the air in the cranial chamber.

6. The symptoms are mainly those of increased intracranial pressure. Frequently
symptoms follow weeks or even months after a trivial injury of the head. A discharge
of cerebrospinal fluid is usually present;
its presence should always make one suspect
pneumocephalus. Sneezing is a frequent
symptom. Rhinorrhea after sneezing or
after change of position is almost pathogonomonic of this condition.

7. The absolute diagnosis is made by the
roentgen ray.

8. When left to chance the mortality of
pneumocephalus is around 40 per cent.,
infection and pressure being the causes of
death. For fistulas through the frontal
sinuses an operative treatment is proposed.
The dural tear is located and covered by a
transplant of fascia lata, which is carefully

sutured in place.

REFERENCES

[1]Wernher: Pneumatocele Cranii. *Deutsche Ztschr.
f. Chir.,* 3: 381, 1873.

[2]Chiari, H.: Ueber einen Fall von Luftansammlung
in den Ventrikeln des menschlichen Gehirns.
Prag. Vierteljahrsschr. f. Heilk., 5: 383, 1884.

[3]Luckett, W. H.: Air in the Ventricles of the Brain
Following a Fracture of the Skull: Report of a
Case. *Surg., Gynec. & Obst.,* 17: 237, 1913. Stew-
art, W. H.: Fracture of the Skull with Air in the
Ventricles. *Am. J. Roentgenol.,* 2: 83–97, 1913–
1914.

[4]Wolff: Luftansammlung im Rechten Seitenven-
trikel des Gehrins (Pneumocephalus). *Munch-
en. med. Wchnschr.,* 16: 899, 1914.

[5]Wodarcz, A.: Zur Kosnistik der intracranieller
Pneumatozele. *Munchen. med. Wchnschr.,* 62:
968, 1915.

[6]All of the German cases have been reported
under the title intracranial "pneumatocele,"
many of the American and one of the French
as "aerocele." Though equally correct, the
former is to be preferred because it maintains
an association with the long established "extracranial" pneumatocele. However, as the intracranial air is at times not confined to a "tumor"
but may be definitely distributed throughout
the ventricular system or subarachnoid space
or multiple isolated pockets may exist within
the cerebral substance, it seems preferable to
forego both of these appellations and substitute
"pneumocephalus," which connotes only the
presence of intracranial air.

[7]Dandy, W. E.: Ventriculography Following the Injection of Air Into the Cerebral Ventricles. *Ann.
Surg.,* 68: 5 (July) 1918; Roentgenography of
the Brain After the Injection of Air Into the
Spinal Canal. *Ann. Surg.,* 70: 397 (Oct.) 1919.

[8]This case was found as this article was ready to
be sent to press and after the accompanying
figures had been arranged. As the roentgenograms would show nothing additional there
seemed little point in including them.

[9]Holmes, G. W.: Intracranial Aerocele Following
Fracture of the Frontal Bone. *Am. J. Roentgenol.,* 5: 384 (Aug.) 1918.

[10]Doyle, A. S.: Traumatic Pneumocranium. *Am. J.
Roentgenol.,* 8: 73 (Feb.) 1921.

[11]Spiller, W. G.: Aerocele of the Brain. *Med. Clin.
North America,* 5: 651 (Nov.) 1921.

[12]May, R. J.: Report of a Case Showing Air Within
the Cranial Cavity. *Am. J. Roentgenol.,* 6: 190
(April) 1919.

[13]Santoro: Rinorrea cefalo-rachidiana e pneumo-
ventricolo spontanei da tumore della base (ipo-
fisi?), (Spontane Liquorrhinorrhoe und Pneu-
moventrikel bei einer Basis– [Hypophysen–?]

Geschwulst) . *Riv. oto-neuro-oftalmol., 1:* 484, 1924 (original not seen) .

[14]Duken: Ueber zwei Falle von intracranieller Pneumatocele nach Schussverletzung. *Munchen. med. Wchnschr., 62:* 598, 1915.

[15]Teachenor, F. R.: Pneumoventricle of the Cerebrum. *Ann. Surg., 78:* 561 (Nov.) 1923.

[16]Dandy, W. E.: The Treatment of Staphylococcus and Strepococcus Meningitis by Continuous Drainage of the Cisterna Magna. *Surg., Gynec. & Obst., 39:* 760 (Dec.) 1924.

[17]Mackay, M.: A Brain Containing Gas Cyst of Microbic Origin. *Montreal M. J., 32:* 795, 1903.

[18]Hixon: The Gas Bacillus in a Brain Injury. *Brit. M. J., 2:* 905 (Dec. 18) 1915.

[19]Cotte, G.: Hydropneumatocele traumatique du crane. *Bull. et mem. Soc. de chir. de Paris, 43:* 865–867, 1917.

[20]Grant, F. C.: Intracranial Aerocele Following a Fracture of the Skull: Report of a Case with a Review of the Literature. *Surg., Gynec. & Obst., 36:* 251 (Feb.) 1923.

[21]Imboden: American Atlas of Stereoroentgenology *11,* cited by McCannel, A. D.: Aerocele of the Brain with Report of Cases. *Laryngoscope, 33:* 189 (March) 1923.

[22]Reisinger: Ueber intracranielle, aber extracerebrale Pneumatocele nach Schussverletzungen. *Beitr. z. klin. Chir., 109:* 129, 1918.

[23]Kredel, L.: Die Intrazerebrale Pneumatokele nach Schussverletzungen. *Zentralbl. f. Chir., 42:* 649, 1915.

[24]Dandy, W. E.: The Diagnosis and Localization of Spinal Cord Tumors. *Ann. Surg., 81:* 223 (Jan.) 1925.

[25]Gebele: Uber Schussverletzungen Des Gehirns. *Beitr. z. klin. Chir., 97:* 123–145, 1915.

[26]Passow, A.: Ueber Luftansammlungen im Schadelinnern. *Beitr. z. Anat., Physiol., Path. u. Therap. d. Ohres, 8:* 257, 1916.

[27]Glenard and Aimard: Aerocele traumatique du verceau. *Presse med., 27:* 123 (March 10) 1919.

[28]Horrax, G.: Intracranial Aerocele Following Fracture of Skull. *Ann. Surg., 73:* 18 (Jan.) 1921.

[29]McCannel (Footnote 21) .

[30]Skinner, E. H.: Intracranial Aerocele. *J. A. Med. Soc., 66:* 954, 1916.

[31]Bruning, F.: Uebergrosse lufthaltige Gehirncyste nach Schussverletzung. *Beitr z. klin. Chir., 107:* 432, 1917.

[32]Potter, H. E.: A Case of Hydropneumocranium with Air in the Ventricles. *Am. J. Roentgenol., 6:* 12 (Jan.) 1919.

[33]Manasse, cited by Frenzel, K.: Die Pneumatocele des Schadels, Inaugural Dissertation, Breslau, 1919.

XXIV

ABSCESSES AND INFLAMMATORY TUMORS IN THE SPINAL EPIDURAL SPACE (SO-CALLED PACHYMENINGITIS EXTERNA)*

Two recent cases of inflammatory tumors in the spinal epidural space presented a picture then unknown to us from a series of spinal cord tumors. In one of the cases the lesion, a tubercle, developed so rapidly as to suggest an extradural abscess; the other, of several months' duration, was looked on as a tumor, despite the high cell count, until the presumed level of the growth was carefully marked out preparatory to operation. When the predicted level of the tumor was found to be identical with an old scar over the spine of a dorsal vertebra, the diagnosis of some inflammatory lesion affecting the cord, though of ill-defined character, appeared to be a probability. When the history had been taken, the patient expressed the belief that his trouble dated from a severe carbuncle of which this directing scar was the result. About the same time my associate, Dr. Frank Ford, recalled an almost identical case, an inflammatory extradural mass, the symptoms of which followed closely on a carbuncle of the back and continued to increase long after its healing. Curiously, these three inflammatory tumors were situated at almost the same cord level and all were confined to the dorsal side of the spinal canal. These facts seemed to suggest not isolated and bizarre spinal infections but rather examples of a well defined type and doubtless also dependent on an anatomic background.

A search of the literature revealed not only a few additional inflammatory extradural masses but also a greater number of acute purulent infections in the epidural space. Strangely enough most, but not all, of these were confined to the same thoracic level and in each the infection was restricted to the dorsal half of the epidural space. There was, moreover, another fact that defined these primary infections as of a special type; namely, similar extradural infections apparently do not develop in the cranial chamber. These infections, therefore, whether acute or chronic, seemed to occur (1) only in the *spinal* epidural space, (2) only in the dorsal half of the spinal canal, and (3) principally in the thoracic region.

An explanation of these findings was sought in the anatomy of the spinal epidural space. However, the current textbooks of anatomy were of little assistance for in none did the epidural space receive more than brief mention. Dissection of a cadaver shows that the spinal extradural space is present only dorsal to the spinal nerve attachments. Ventral to the nerves the dura is everywhere closely applied to the bones of the vertebrae. Below the second sacral bony segment the epidural space surrounds the dura on all sides. The epidural space is filled with fat and loose areolar tissue containing numerous veins.

Of greatest importance are the variations in the size of the epidural space. In the cervical region the space is only potential, there being only a few strands of fibrous tissue and almost no fat between the laminae and dura. The epidural space really begins to appear at the seventh cervical vertebra and gradually deepens along the thoracic vertebrae, attaining a depth of about 0.5 to 0.75 cm. between the fourth

*Reprinted from the *Archives of Surgery,* 13: 477–494, October, 1926.

and eighth dorsal vertebrae. The space tapers again and becomes shallow between the eleventh thoracic and second lumbar vertebrae. Over the remaining lumbar and the first and second sacral vertebrae the epidural space attains its greatest depth. At the second sacral vertebra the dural envelop ends and a continuation of the epidural tissue fills the caudal end of the sacral canal. Only at the lower terminus of the spinal dura does the extradural space extend ventrally; here for a short distance the dura is encircled by the epidural fat and areolar tissue. The size and shape of the epidural space, therefore, appear to be secondary to the variations in size of the spinal cord. Absent over the cervical enlargement and nearly so over the lumbar swelling the epidural space becomes deepest where the spinal cord or the mass of its roots is smallest, i e., in the upper dorsal and lower lumbar sections. And the space exists only on the dorsal aspect of the dura.

The spinal epidural space is therefore filled with tissues — fat and loose areolar — which offer a foothold for current hematogenous infections, and the intraspinous location of these tissues makes trauma an important inciting agent in the development of hematogenous infections.

Whether the epidural fat performed any normal function other than serving as a padding can hardly be answered unequivocally. It is easy to believe that it acts as a buffer to trauma but such a protective function would appear to be particularly called for in the cervical region, and here the fat is absent. Nevertheless, it would seem to serve some buffer function to direct traumatic insults in the rigid thoracic region. Under certain pathologic conditions the epidural fat is of no little diagnostic and therapeutic value. Practically all spinal cord tumors cause this bed of fat to be absorbed by continuous pressure; in this way the pressure of the tumor on the cord is withheld for a time to a degree commensurate with the volume of the fatty tissue that is destroyed.

During operations for spinal cord tumors the presence or absence of epidural fat, in the thoracic and lumbar but not in the cervical canal, is carefully noted and considered a sign of great value. If fat is present a tumor beneath the dura is unlikely though not impossible, whereas the absence of fat indicates pressure absorption and, therefore, an underlying neoplasm. The recent work of Peters[1] should be mentioned in this connection. He has shown a frequent involvement of the epidural tissues from primary infections of the spinal meninges. We have, however, found no other reports of persisting epidural infections after cures in any form of meningitis.

We are not concerned in this article with the most common extensions of tuberculous infections from the bodies of the vertebrae into the spinal canal. Such infections are easily recognized by the characteristic picture of vertebral destruction in association with the evidences of spinal compression. Moreover, the epidural space is involved in these cases only because it lies in the path of further extension of the tuberculous process and not because of any peculiar characteristic of the space or its contents. Furthermore, in paraplegia associated with Pott's disease surgery is contraindicated; at least up to this time the results obtained by laminectomy have not been helpful and have usually done harm.

Nor shall we consider here those remarkable chronic inflammatory hypertrophies of the cervical region described by Charcot and Joffroy as pachymeningitis cervicalis hypertrophica, nor the more extensive dural hypertrophies, involving the entire length of the spinal dura, described by Mills and Spiller.[2] These proliferations of fibrous tissue, gradually increasing the bulk of the dura on its inner side, grow into and slowly strangle the spinal cord, causing symptoms that are said to resemble syringomyelia. These rare diffuse increments probably arise from the dura; their origin is considered to be syphilitic. Weinberg[3] has only recently described a localized mass of fibrous tissue arising from the inner side of the dura and compressing the cord. Although he makes a probable diagnosis of tuberculosis from the histologic picture of giant cells, the Wassermann reaction in the spinal fluid was positive. It would, therefore, appear justifiable to question whether the lesion might not have been a gumma, the more common primary dural affection.

ACUTE INFECTIONS IN THE EPIDURAL SPACE (I)

Abscesses of the epidural space arise in two ways: (1) by direct extension of a contiguous infection, and (2) by metastasis through the blood stream.

Albers, 1833, from Germany has been credited with first reporting an acute infection of the epidural space. Ducheck, 1853, gave to this condition the name peripachymeningitis, which was later changed to pachymeningitis externa. Cases have been reported under both titles. As will be shown later, both appellations are misnomers for the infections are not of the meninges as was then supposed but of the tissues of the epidural space.

As we have had no patient in whom an abscess of the extradural space has either been suspected during life or found at necropsy we can only assemble and analyze the cases from the literature. Doubtless those which have been compiled are only a small fraction of the actual number of either the acute or chronic infections, for many have received but casual mention or are hidden in obscure or inaccessible publications. Though infections of the epidural space are comparatively rare it is worthy of note that Morowitz[4] had three acute hematogenous abscesses in one year and we had two cases of chronic infection in a somewhat shorter period.

The best bibliography on this subject has been assembled by R. Kaminski (Eine Metastatische Peripachymeningitis und Periostitis spinalis perulenta nach Furunkulose, inaugural dissertation, Griefswald, 1917). Through him we learn that Hasse (three cases) and Ducheck, 1853, have described extradural abscesses secondary to direct extension of an infection from decubitus; Traube, 1863, a case from a psoas abscess and another from an extrapleural abscess. In Mannkopff's case the epidural abscess was an extension of Ludwig's angina. Recently Taylor and Kennedy,[5] 1923, reported an extrathecal lumbar abscess (*Staphylococcus aureus*) which was an extension of an acute pericostal inflammation.

The most interesting extradural infections, and those which present a much more difficult problem in diagnosis, are of hematogenous origin. Quite a series of these has been assembled. In many the infection has been identified as a metastasis from an infection elsewhere in the body, i. e., staphylococcus phlebitis,[6] furunculosis,[7] furunculosis leg[4] (also by Kaminski), furunculosis neck[8] and diplococcus bronchitis.[9]

In three cases, of Lewitzky,[10] Spencer,[11] and Hinz, [12] necropsy revealed no other infection in the body; the abscesses were therefore assumed to be primary in the epidural space. Although Hinz assumed the infection to have probably arisen from a puerperal thrombosis, the extrathecal infection appeared four weeks after a normal pregnancy, the first symptom of the fatal illness being uterine bleeding; no evidence of uterine infection was found at necropsy. Trauma appears to have been an inciting agent in the case of Kaminski and, according to Cassirer, in cases reported by Runge and Pulvirenti.

A study of the accompanying table of acute epidural infections discloses several striking facts. There have been only two recoveries in the entire series of twenty-five cases. (Pulvirenti, Taylor and Kennedy[5]): both of these followed drainage of the infection. Apparently in only the four cases subjected to operation was a diagnosis even suspected before the necropsy findings, and except in Taylor and Kennedy's case there is no evidence to indicate that the nature of the lesion was more than roughly guessed. Without exception the acute infections have been fulminating, death usually resulting in two or three weeks; the minimum duration of life is six days and the maximum thirty days.

How effective operative treatment will be for abscesses of this character can, of course, only be conjectured. Much will necessarily depend on the virulence of the organism, the resistance of the patient and the extent of the infection in the epidural space. Tightly sealed within the vertebral canal, an abscess can hardly rupture into the soft tissues and be spontaneously cured. The only possible avenue of escape would be through an operative defect in the laminae.

At first glance it might appear that the structure of the epidural space would preclude any practical operative drainage. From the high cervical region to the sacral canal the epidural space is continuous, i. e., it is not intercepted by mechanical barriers. But relatively poor as fatty tissue is known to be in combating infections, it is actually able to build a barrier of inflammatory tissue and restrict the acute infection to a small fraction of the epidural space. It is not improbable, in fact it seems more reasonable to believe, that the resistance to infections in the epidural space is largely due to the vascular areolar tissue and not to the fat. In only two (Kaminski, Spencer[11]) of ten cases in which the location of the abscess has been mentioned has the infection spread throughout the length of the epidural space. In such instances operative efforts would necessarily be fruitless. In those cases in which the infection has been walled off, there is every reason to believe drainage would result in a cure.

Doubtless operative results will always be dependent on the stage at which the diagnosis is made. It would appear probable that an abscess though at first walled off must, when increasing rapidly and becoming tense, break its plastic barriers and spread up an down the epidural space. An early diagnosis followed by operation may well prevent diffusion and facilitate restriction of the infection. It is fortunate at least that the epidural space and its infec-

tions are located on the dorsal side of the spinal dura. Were the abscesses situated ventrally drainage would be extremely difficult if not impossible.

There should be little if any difficulty in arriving at a diagnosis of an epidural abscess when the signs of spinal cord compression (accompanied by fever and leukocytosis) develop and the level of the spinal cord injury is contiguous to a preexisting infection. Nor would it appear that the diagnosis of hematogenous abscesses of the epidural space would offer insuperable obstacles. In fact the signs and symptoms of this group (I) seem to be sufficient distinctly to suggest a clinical entity. In practically all of these cases the symptoms of onset is a terrific, almost unbearable and unrelenting pain (1) in the back, or (2) along the course of the spinal nerves (bilateral), or (3) in the legs. In a previous article these types of pain have been attributed, when caused by spinal cord tumors, to involvement of (1) the vertebrae, (2) the spinal nerves, and (3) the sensory paths in the spinal cord. But these pains are much more severe and persistent in inflammations than when due solely to pressure from a tumor. The pain in spinal tumors, or in fact in any other proved lesion, though seemingly of the same kind, cannot approach in severity or persistence the pains of infection of the epidural space.

The next most important impressive evidence of abscesses of the epidural space is the latent period of a few days (from four to nine) between the time of the onset of the excruciating pain and motor, sensory and sphincter loss, has either been sudden or has become complete within forty-eight hours after its onset. In nearly all cases there has been a sharp bilateral sensory level which may or may not have ascended, doubtless depending on whether the epidural abscess has extended upward or has remained localized. In addition to this characteristic story there is always high fever, tachycardia, leukocytosis (18,000 in three cases) and probably always tender-

I. ACUTE INFECTIONS (ABSCESSES)

Reported by	Age and Sex*	Secondary to	Primary Origin	Incited by Trauma	Location of Infection	Symptoms of Onset	Pain; Location	Character of Pain	Paraplegia	Paralysis: Time of Onset; Time Until Complete	Bladder or Rectum
Oppenheim[6] 1910	40 ♀	Phlebitis (staphylococcus)	Metastatic	..	VI dorsal to I lumbar	Sudden pain	+ Lower thoracic vertebrae and legs	Increasing until terrific	+	6th day; rapid increase	......
Hinz[12] 1921	29 ♀	....	Primary ?)	..	IV to VIII dorsal	Backache	+ Back	Backache	+ Flaccid	4th day; sudden	Retention
Morowitz[4] 1919	15 ♂	Healed furunculosis of leg	Metastatic	..	Lower thoracic	Sudden terrific pain	+ Inguinal region bilateral	Spread next day to back and abdomen	+	9th day; 1 day	......
Morowitz[4] 1919	26 ♂	....	Metastatic	..	Lower thoracic	Sudden severe pain	+ Back and legs	Severe, continuous	None	none; none	......
Morowitz[4] 1919	15 ♂	....	Metastatic	..	....	Dizziness and chill	+	Headache	..	....	......
Cassirer[7] 1923	..	Furuncle	Metastatic	..	....	....	....	....	+	....	......
Spencer[11] 1879	..	....	Primary	+	Whole canal	....	....	....	..	....	......
Lewitzky[01] 1877	..	....	....	..	....	....	....	....	..	....	......
Lemoine and Lannois[09] 1882	..	....	....	..	....	....	....	....	..	....	......
Molliere[20] 1897	..	....	....	..	....	....	....	....	..	....	......
Hoestermann[8] 1913	..	Furuncle of neck	Metastatic	..	V to VII dorsal	....	....	....	..	....	......
Kaminiski 1917	15 ♀	Furunculosis of leg	Metastatic	..	Whole length	Sudden pain	+ Knees; then inguinal and finally in back	Terrific	+ Below dorsal II	9th day; sudden	Retention
Schick[9] 1909	40 ♂	Bronchitis (diplococcus)	Metastatic	No	Lower cervical and upper thoracic	Sudden pain in both arms	+ Both arms, shoulder and upper vertebrae	Very severe	+ Weakness of arms later	9th day; sudden	Retention
Traube, 1863, cited by Kaminiski	..	....	Metastatic	..	....	....	....	....	..	....	......
Albers, 1833, cited by Kaminiski	..	....	Metastatic	..	....	....	....	....	..	....	......
Pulvirenti, 1921, cited by Cassirer	..	....	Primary	+	III-IV lumbar	....	....	....	..	....	......
Runge, 1920, cited by Cassirer	..	....	Primary	+	....	....	....	....	..	....	......

I. A. Acute Infections (Abscesses), Resulting fro[m]

Reported by	Age and Sex*	Secondary to	Primary Origin	Incited by Trauma	Location of Infection	Symptoms of Onset	Pain; Location	Character of Pain	Paraplegia	Paralysis: Time of Onset; Time Until Complete	Bladder or Rectum
Taylor and Kennedy[5] 1923	15 ♀	Abscess along ribs	....	..	Lower thoracic and lumbar	Pain and chills	+ Lower ribs	Severe and sharp	Complete	13th day; 2 days	Retention
Mannkopf, 1864, cited by Kaminiski	..	Ludwig's angina	....	..	....	....	....	....	..	....	......
Barth, cited by Kaminiski	..	Puncture wound	....	..	....	....	....	....	..	....	......
Hasse, cited by Kaminiski	..	Decubitis	....	..	....	....	....	....	..	....	......
Hasse	..	Decubitis	....	..	....	....	....	....	..	....	......
Hasse	..	Decubitis	....	..	....	....	....	....	..	....	......
Ducheck, 1853 cited by Kaminiski	..	Decubitis	....	..	....	....	....	....	..	....	......

*In this table ♂ indicates male, ♀ female.

19. Lemoine, G., and Lannois, M.: Perimeningitis Spinale Aigue, Rev. de med. 2: 533, 1882.
20. Moilliere, H.: Note sur un cas de Perimeningite spinale primitive Suppuree, Lyon med., 1887, p. 143.

PRIMARY OR METASTATIC

Sensation	Spine: Rigidity; Tenderness	Kernig Sign	Headache	Leukocytes	Temperature	Reflexes	Spinal Fluid	Duration of Life	Operation	Result	Clinical Diagnosis	Remarks
......	......	..	..	....	Fever	......	....	30 days	None	Death; necropsy	......	Ribs, vertebra; and spinal cord not involved; infection during sixth month of pregnancy
Absent below dorsal VI	+ on 5th day; 5 to 12 dorsal	..	..	....	40 C.	......	Clear no sediment	6 days	None	Dead; necropsy	Thrombosis; embolus puerperal myelitis	Normal pregnancy concluded 1 month before symptoms of onset; uterine bleeding began at time of onset of backache; fever appeared only on third day; organism not determined; cord and vertebrae not involved
Lost	Lower thoracic tender	..	..	18,000	40 C.	......	....	15 days	None	Dead; necropsy	......	Walked home after sudden onset of pain; bedfast next day and thereafter
Hyperesthesia	Lower thoracic and upper lumbar tender	+	..	....	....	......	....	10 days	None	Dead; necropsy	......	Multiple abscesses in lungs and kidneys
Hyperesthesia	Neck rigid	+	+	....	Fever	......	....	19 days	None	Dead; necropsy	......	Many abscesses elsewhere
......	......	..	..	....	....	......	......		+	?	?	Abscess found at operation
......	......	..	..	....	....	......	....	17 days	None	Dead; necropsy	......	Extradural abscess extending from 3 inches (7.6 cm.) below head to sacrum; no mention of dorsal or ventral position
......	......	..	..	....	....	......	....	22 days	......	Dead; necropsy	Meningitis	
......	....	..	..	....		......	......			Dead; necropsy	......	
......	......	..	..	....	....	......	....			Dead; Necropsy	......	
......	......	..	..	....	....	......	....		+	Dead; Necropsy	......	
Diminished	......	..	+ Later	18,000	41 C.	......	Cocci; leukocytes	10 days	None	Dead; Necropsy	......	Gram-positive staphylococcus organism; thick layer of pus in fatty tissue; cord normal; whole length of canal involved
Absent	+ neck and thoracic vertebrae	..	..	....	....	......	Diplococci	28 days	......	Dead; Necropsy	......	Opisthotonus; hiccup continuous for 2 weeks before death
......	......	..	..	....	....	......	....			Dead; Necropsy		
......	......	..	..	....	....	......	....			Dead; Necropsy	......	
......	......	..	..	....	....	......	......	Recovery	+	Recovery	......	Cassirer says healing after operation
......	......	..	..	....	....	......	......			Dead; necropsy	......	

Direct Extension of Contiguous Infections

Sensation	Spine: Rigidity; Tenderness	Kernig Sign	Headache	Leukocytes	Temperature	Reflexes	Spinal Fluid	Duration of Life	Operation	Result	Clinical Diagnosis	Remarks
Absent	......	..	..	18,000	104	......	....	Recovery	+	Recovery	Extradural abscess	Staphylococcus aureus from culture; patient survived and some function returned
......	......	..	..	....	....	......	......	......	......	Dead; Necropsy	......	
......	......	..	..	....	....	......	......	......	......	Dead; Necropsy	......	
......	......	..	..	....	....	......	......	......	......	Dead; Necropsy	......	
......	......	..	..	....	....	......	......	......	......	Dead; Necropsy	......	
......	......	..	..	....	....	......	......	......	......	Dead; Necropsy	......	
......	......	..	..	....	....	......	......	......	......	Dead; Necropsy	......	

II. Inflammatory Tumo[r]

Reported by	Age and Sex*	Secondary to	Primary Origin	Incited by Trauma	Location of Infection	Symptoms of Onset	Pain; Location	Character of Pain	Paraplegia	Paralysis: Time or Onset; Time Until Complete	Bladder or Rectum
Stroubell[13] 1898	86 ♀	....	Syphilis (?)	..	III to VI dorsal	Paraplegia and anesthesia	....	....	Complete	Sudden	......
Schultze[16] 1903	24 ♀	....	Chronic inflammatory tissue	..	V to VII dorsal	Pain	+ Lower ribs and back	Sudden, excruciating	Partial, spastic	3 months; 6 months	Disturb[ed] functio[n] but no [re]tentio[n]
Fischer[21] 1902	44 ♂	....	Syphilis (?)	..	III to VI dorsal	Pain in vertebrae and legs	+	....	+	....	Retenti[on] and inc[on]tinen[ce]
Mendel[17] 1909	..	....	Chronic inflammatory tissue	..	V to IX dorsal	Pain in head, neck and back	+ Head, neck and back	Severe	Partial	2½ years; partial	......
Pelz[22] 1917	67 ♂	....	Tuberculosis	..	Middle and lower thoracic	Pain in back	+ Back and later legs	....	Total	1½ months	Incont[i]nence (2 week[s]
Gampers 1920	..	....	Tuberculosis	..	Lumbar	....	....	....	..	....	......
Lewis and Bassoe 1915	21 ♀	....	....	No	V and VI dorsal	Numbness and pain in legs	Toes	Cramp	Complete	3 weeks	Slight h[esi]tancy i[n] voidi[ng]
Dandy 1926	42 ♂	Direct extension from furuncle on back	Chronic inflammatory tissue	No	V to VIII dorsal	Pain	+ Back and sides	Severe, sharp	Partial	10 months; partial	Incont[i]nenc[e]
Dandy 1926 (Dr. Ford's case)	Middle age ♂	Direct extension from furuncle on back	Chronic inflammatory tissue	No	V to VIII dorsal	Pain	+ Back and waist	Severe, sharp	Partial	3 months; partial	Incont[i]nenc[e]
Dandy 1926	27 ♀ (colored)	....	Tuberculosis	+	III to VI dorsal	Pain	+ Back and sides	Very severe	Complete	8 months; 3 days	Incont[i]nenc[e] then r[e]tentio[n]

*In this table ♂ indicates male, ♀ female.

21. Fischer: Ein Fall von Pacymeningitis chronica externa spinalis, Verhandl. d. Gesellsch. deutsch. *Naturf. u. Karlsbad 2:* 16, 1902.
22. Pelz, A.: Kasuistische Beitrage zur Lehre von den Ruckenmarks Geschwulsten. *Arch. f. Psychiat., 58:* 195, 1917.

No Abscess)—*Continued*

Sensation	Spine: Rigidity; Tenderness	Kenrig Sign	Headache	Leukocytes	Temperature	Reflexes	Spinal Fluid	Duration of Life	Operation	Result	Clinical Diagnosis	Remarks
Absent	......	..	..	......	.....	Absent	....	....	.....	Dead; necropsy	....	Reflexes absent; no clonus; granulation tissue tumor, not like tuberculosis—probably syphilis
sensory el gradally be- he higher	None; V to VI dorsal	..	..	......	.....	Increased ankle clonus	....	10 mos.	+	Dead; necropsy	....	After 5 weeks the pain improved but quickly became worse when numbness of feet ensued; persisted 7 months, then again disappeared but returned for an hour every time he bent over; pain worse on coughing and sneezing; ankle clonus; died of meningitis after operation; tumor dorsal side of dura; grayish red solid mass 12 cm. long, 1 cm. thick; connective tissue strands and cluster of cells
Absent	......	..	..	......	.....	Increased clonus	....	1 yr.	No	Dead; necropsy	....	Mass of fibrinous tissue containing giant cells; thinks it histologically more like syphilis; no evidence of tuberculosis
Partial loss	......	..	..	......	.....	......	....	3 yrs.	+	Dead; necropsy	....	Tumor 9.6 cm. long; granulation tissue without specific character; no necrosis or giant cells
......	......	..	..	......	.....	......	....	16 mos.	No	Dead; necropsy	....	Pain in legs developed only after 4 months; weakness came soon after; tumor 1 cm. long, 1 cm. thick; all on outer side of dura; granulation tissue with many giant cells and tubercles
bsent	......	..	..	......	.....	......	....	....	.....	Dead; necropsy	....	No involvement of vertebrae
bsent	Very little	..	..	......	.....	......	Normal	Well	Spinal decompression	Well	Tuberculous involvement of cord	Patient was in seventh month of pregnancy when symptoms began; was allowed to go to term and labor was successfully completed; 3 weeks later decompressive laminectomy; indurated mass of fat in epidural space (dura not opened); quick return of function; complete restoration of motor power in 3 years.
nsory evel	+; +	+	No	......	No	Greatly increased Babinski reflex +	53 cells; xanthochromia	Well	+	Well	Inflammatory tumor	Pain in back and sides persisted 6 months; since then somewhat diminished; convulsions in legs 1 month; diagnosis of an inflammatory tumor was made before operation; return of function
nsory evel	+; +	..	..	......	No	Greatly increased Babinski reflex +	9 cells; lymphocytes	Well	+	Well	Tumor	This case is presented by permission of Dr. Ford; the operation was performed in Bellevue Hospital, New York; a firm fibrous mass 6 cm. long and 1 cm. thick removed; return of function
al abce be- sen- level	+; +	..	..	......	.....	......	15 cells; lymphocytes	Well	+	Well	Tuberculosis of spine and abscess	Struck back 8 months before; pain had persisted since in that spot; any movement intensified pain; return of function; Wassermann reaction from blood and spinal fluid negative; no tubercles seen

ness and rigidity of the spine. Although there are few records of examinations of the spinal fluid (in two cases organisms were grown in cultures of the cerebrospinal, fluid, possibly because the needle passed through the epidural infection) there must always be an increased cell count (polymorphonuclear cells) as the reaction to an adjacent acute infection. Manometric tests have also not been made in these cases but since the paralyses are evidence of spinal cord compression, a complete block of the spinal canal must surely exist. Such a block was demonstrated in both of our inflammatory tumor cases, in one of which the symptoms of spinal cord involvement developed almost as suddenly as in any of the acute abscesses. Whether an acute epidural abscess may eventually be diagnosed before implication of the spinal cord and before the appearance of a spinal block remains to be seen. At least a pain that appears so distinctive should put us on guard for the earliest sensory or motor changes. Experience has taught us that the more rapidly spinal compression causes paraplegia the more slowly recovery takes place after its relief. Gradual compression of the spinal cord allows a remarkable adjustment to the tumor's bulk; often the spinal cord may be reduced to half its cross sectional volume with little or no loss of function, but after the removal of a slowly growing tumor the recovery of function is very rapid.

The sudden onset of paraplegia in these cases has led to the diagnosis of myelitis or even of thrombosis or embolism. All these conditions should be eliminated by the excruciating pain which for several days precedes paralysis, by the tenderness and rigidity of the spine and by the demonstration of a spinal subarachnoid block. Although meningitis might appear possible because of rigid neck, a positive Kernig's sign, fever and leukocytosis, the sensory and motor level and the cerebrospinal fluid examination, together with the absence of a spinal subarachnoid block, should easily exclude this diagnosis. The possibility of an abscess of the spinal cord might also be considered but the interval of pain that precedes paraplegia in epidural abscesses would doubtless be absent.

INFLAMMATORY EPIDURAL TUMORS (II)

The story in this group of cases is very different. While the pain is of the same general character and extremely severe, it lacks the very sharp onset; it is less fulminating and is prolonged over a period of weeks or months instead of days. The latent period preceding paralysis is far longer and the paralysis is usually slow in developing and usually incomplete. In brief all manifestations are chronic instead of acute. In only two cases (Stroubell,[13] Dandy[14]) did the symptoms of spinal cord compression appear suddenly, and only in these instances and a case of Lewis and Bassoe[15] was the paraplegia complete. In the remaining cases the motor, sensory and sphincter changes developed so slowly (from three months to two and one-half years) as to suggest tumors rather than infections. Four of these tumors have been described as syphilitic or tuberculous because of the histologic demonstration of giant cells and occasional tubercles. Since the histologic differential diagnosis between syphilis and tuberculosis is so often impossible, it is not safe to assume that all of these cases are due either to syphilis or tuberculosis. In our patient syphilis was excluded by the negative Wassermann reaction in both the blood and the spinal fluid. Tuberculosis seemed more probable because of her race (colored), but tubercles could not be definitely demonstrated in sections of the tumor nor was there any other evidence of tuberculosis in the body. She has, moreover, remained well and free of any symptoms or signs of tuberculosis since the operation, over two years ago. In her case trauma seemed to play a definite inciting role; at least she refused to yield from her original story that a pain developed immediately after a blow on the spine and that it persisted in the same spot. And precisely at that spot the tumor was found at operation. A remarkable feature of this case is that an inflammatory tumor probably existed eight months (its gross appearance also supports the slow growth of the tumor) before any symptoms of paralysis and then paraplegia became complete in three days, and without abscess formation.

Four cases of this group would appear to be of staphylococcus origin, those of Schultze,[16] Mendel[17] and Dandy[14] (two). In our two cases the organisms were identified by cultures. In the cases of Schultze and Mendel the infections were probably of metastatic origin. In our two cases the epidural infections were undoubtedly due to the direct extension of the outskirts of deep mid dorsal carbuncles. These two cases strikingly demonstate how differently infections are handled by different tissues. In both of our cases the original carbuncle in the soft tissues of the back had long since healed (five and thirteen months) leaving only a scar, whereas at the end of this time the areolar and fatty tissues of the epidural space were still struggling to wall off the same infections the newly formed inflammatory tissues assumed in the connections of tumors. That living organisms were still present in the connective tissue masses was demonstrated by bacterial stains of the sections, by the presence of minute abscesses in the connective tissue and in one case by the growth of *Staphylococcus aureus* from cultures of the tumor at operation. Moreover, in both these cases the infection was again lighted up by the trauma incident to the operation; the wounds promptly broke down and from one wound *Staphylococcus aureus* was grown in culture.

In all these chronic inflammatory tumors (except in Lewis' case) pain in the back, though far less excruciating than in the epidural abscesses, has been much more severe than from neoplasms whether of intradural or extradural origin. The cell count from the cerebrospinal fluid in our three cases was nine (tubercle), fifteen and fifty-three — all lymphocytes.

The age of the patients afflicted with inflammatory tumors averages higher than of those with abscesses. The series of cases is, however, too limited to warrant conclusions on this point. It is also worthy of note that with one exception[18] these inflammatory tumors have been in the thoracic epidural space and nearly all between the third and ninth vertebrae. Again the series is too small to allow us to consider this too significant. Two facts, however, are suggested as a possible explanation of this greater incidence in the thoracic region: (1) carbuncles and furuncles are more common in the thoracic than the lumbar region; (2) spinous processes are more superficial in the thoracic region and therefore the spine is protected by less soft tissues and is also more susceptible to trauma.

All of the tumors have been well formed and firm. In one of our cases it was of cartilaginous consistency and so tightly bound to the dura that considerable force and sharp dissection with a periosteal elevator was necessary to strip it from the dura. The masses of inflammatory tissue averaged about 1 cm. in depth; the longest was 12 cm. One of ours weighed 15 Gm.

In our three cases the tumor was removed. An equally good result, however, was obtained by Lewis[15] by a simple decompression laminectomy. It is interesting that in his patient operation was delayed over two months to allow the completion of a full term pregnancy. It is also worthy of note that pain was not a conspicuous feature in the case — the sole exception — through the involvement of the fat with inflammatory tissue seemed similar to the other cases in this group.

REPORT OF THREE CASES OF CHRONIC INFLAMMATORY TUMORS OF THE EPIDURAL SPACE

Case 1. A large, well nourished man, aged forty-two, was referred by Dr. L. F. Barker because of gradually progressive paraplegia and anesthesia, suggestive of a spinal cord tumor. The patient persisted in dating his illness from a carbuncle and a series of boils in the back thirteen months before. During this illness he suffered severe pains in the back sides and after healing of the infection of character and the intensity of these pains persisted. For the following six months the pains steadily increased; all efforts to allay them were futile. Since then the pains in the sides has been present only at times but the terrible backache had remained practically unchanged.

Three months previously numbness appeared almost synchronously in both legs. Two weeks later the patient's gait became affected and it was soon necessary to use a cane in walking. Loss of equilibrium and of motor power progressed gradually. One month later both legs became spastic and involuntary jerkings (he aptly termed them "convulsions") appeared. The spastic contractions became so powerful that it was often impossible voluntarily to counteract the muscular pull. At times the legs would be fixed in the extended position and again strongly flexed at the hips and knees. The contractions were very painful. The numbness seemed gradually to extend up the legs and abdomen and finally settled at a level above the umbilicus. Girdle pains and a feeling of constriction developed and persisted in this region. Sneezing produced a queer tingling in his feet.

On admission he was able to walk a few yards with great effort and only when supported, but as attempts at walking brought on the painful clonic contractions he was reluctant to stand. All motor and sensory functions in the upper extremities were normal.

Dr. Barker's examination showed in addition to the motor loss a sharp girdle of hyperesthesia at the eighth thoracic segment with marked loss of sensation to pain, touch and temperature below this level; almost complete loss of muscle sense in both feet; greatly exaggerated knee kicks and Achilles reflexes; a bilateral positive Babinski reflex and ankle clonus. The epigastric reflexes were obtainable but the abdominal and cremasteric reflexes were absent. There had been no incontinence of urine or feces. Examination of the spinal fluid showed xanthochromia, heavy globulin and fifty-three

lymphocytes.

It was Dr. Barker's opinion, in which I concurred, that the patient's condition was due to a spinal cord tumor, the localization of which was quite accurately determined by the sharp girdle of altered sensation. We were disturbed by the high cell count and heavy globulin, neither of which could be satisfactorily explained.

Despite the patient's persistence in associating his symptoms with the series of boils on his back thirteen months before, there seemed to us little possibility of lesion from this source at this late date. However, when according to custom the presumed site of the tumor was scratched by a scalpel for operative localization the marker bisected a round scar over the sixth thoracic spine, obviously the scar of an old carbuncle. The association of the scar and the marker for orientation was too striking to disregard as a coincidence. At once it seemed that there must be some relationship between the old inflammatory process and his tumor. Accordingly I dropped out of the operation to convey this impression to Dr. Barker but both of us felt that the lesion was such as to require exploration.

At operation when the laminae of the sixth and seventh vertebrae were removed a reddish brown mass at once appeared in lieu of the normal extradural fat. The tumor was so fibrous and lacking in cellular elements that an extradural sarcoma, the only likely form of tumor in this location, appeared inconceivable. It was thought to be an inflammatory mass. Frozen sections verified this diagnosis. To get above and below this growth it was necessary to remove extra laminae, the fifth and eighth, i. e., the laminae of four vertebrae in all. Epidural fat was then encountered both above and below the tumor mass and dissection was begun from below upward. The mass was so tightly bound to the dura and it so overhung the lateral margins of the dura that dissection in toto made no progress. The tumor was then bisected longitudinally in the midline, which was the deepest part of the mass; it presented on cross section a semilunar shape. Even then blunt dissection of the tumor was impossible. So tightly was the tumor bound to the dura and so hard was the tumor that

I believe the spinal dura could have been pulled from its attachment before the mass would have separated or the tumor broken. With a sharp periosteal elevator the mass was cut away from the dura, there being scarcely a suggestion of a line of cleavage. The inflammatory mass after removal measured 11 cm. long, 2 cm. deep, and was as wide as the spinal dura which it covered; it weighed 15 Gm. Minute foci of cellular tissue were seen throughout a cut section of the tumor, also little islands of infiltrated fat. There was no evidence of pus. Under the microscope the cellular foci were seen to be miliary subacute abscesses, polymorphonuclear cells predominating. They were surrounded by dense walls of fibrous tissue. Unfortunately cultures of the tissues were not made at operation.

The entire wound quickly broke down from infection. *Staphylococcus aureus* was grown from cultures of the wound, the organisms doubtless liberated from the miliary abscesses of the tumor and stimulated to renewed activity by the operative trauma.

Two months after operation the patient was discharged with the wound healed. Recovery of function, though slow, has been gradual and complete. Two and a half years later he remains perfectly well.

The tumor, therefore, is of inflammatory character. It surely arose from direct extension of the infection of an old carbuncle of the back (thirteen months before operation) into the extradural fat.

Case 2. The second patient was a colored woman, aged twenty-seven. She was admitted to the medical service of the Johns Hopkins Hospital because of a rapidly progressive paraplegia. Eight months before she fell down three or four steps, striking her back in the upper thoracic region. She spent the day in bed because of pain in her back and side. The pain in the back had persisted without remission, but the pain in the side had disappeared at times, though the longest free interval has not been greater than a week. The pain in the back was dull and aching; that in the chest, sharp and cutting. She had not been able to bend forward, even to look down, because any movement of the back intensified the backache. For the last three weeks the pains in the back and chest had been particularly severe; they "cut off her wind" if she bent her body.

Nine days before operation both legs suddenly gave way so that she could scarcely walk. A loss of sensation developed synchronously and rapidly extended upward until a sharp level was reached at the lower costal margin on both sides. She volunteered that she had since been unable to contract her abdominal muscles.

Seven days before admission she developed incontinence and three days later incontinence gave way to retention, catherization being necessary. There had never been spasticity.

Examination showed total flaccid paralysis of both legs; the upper extremities were unimpaired. A sharp sensory level crossed the thorax just below the xiphoid process; below this line there was complete anesthesia to pain, touch and temperature; there was total loss of muscle sense. The epigastric and abdominal reflexes were absent. The left knee kick was feebly present but the right knee kick and both ankle jerks were absent. There was no response to plantar stimulation. Marked tenderness was elicited on deep pressure about the spine of the fourth, fifth and sixth thoracic vertebrae. The spinal fluid examination made on the medical service showed fifteen cells, all leukocytes.

In Queckenstedt's test the cerebrospinal fluid rose 20 mm. from a base level of 115 mm. following compression of both jugular veins; but the level was not restored on release of the jugular pressure. Several times this was repeated with the same results. Roentgen-ray examination of the spine was negative; the Wassermann reaction from the blood and spinal fluid were negative.

Air injection into the spinal canal showed a sharply defined block in the spinal canal at the fourth thoracic vertebra. Immediately on the introduction of the air into the spinal canal her original pain was duplicated and intensified. The injected air did not reach the cranial chamber.

Because of the great rapidity of the paralysis a tuberculous abscess was suspected, probably in relation to a diseased vertebra, though roentgen-ray examination was negative.

At operation a mass of inflammatory tissue was removed from the extradural space between the third and fifth thoracic vertebrae, inclusive. The mass was firm and sharply defined above, below and laterally. It covered only the dorsal aspect of the spinal dura from which it was completely removed. Microscopic sections showed chronic inflammatory tissue containing many giant cells. The pathologic diagnosis was tuberculous granuloma.

Return of motor and sensory functions began two weeks after the operation and progressed slowly. She could walk in three months. It is now two years since the operation and the patient has remained perfectly well. Her gait is absolutely normal.

Case 3. To the foregoing cases I append a third by permission of my associate, Dr. Frank R. Ford. The patient was an Italian laborer who was under Dr. Ford's care at Bellevue Hospital, New York. He had been admitted because of weakness and stiffness of the legs. Five months before his entry into the hospital he was infected with a series of furuncles over the back. These caused severe pain over the back and around the waist. For several weeks after the furuncles had healed, the pain continued severe and the spine was so tender that he could not lie on his back. Three months after the furuncles had healed, the patient noticed weakness and stiffness in his legs. This progressed slowly and a month later he had to give up work.

The patient was a fairly robust man of middle age. Several scars of old boils were seen over the back; one of these was directly over the spinous process of the seventh thoracic vertebra. Though very spastic he could walk without support with difficulty. Cutaneous sensibility was partially lost below a well defined level crossing just above the umbilicus. Sense of position and vibratory sense were greatly diminished. Bladder control was beginning to be affected. All the tendon reflexes were increased in the legs; there was a bilateral positive Babinski reflex; no abdominal reflexes were obtainable. The spinal fluid was clear and colorless, and there were nine cells per cubic millimeter, all lymphocytes.

At operation a firm fibrous mass was removed from the posterior surface of the dura beneath the laminae of the fifth, sixth, seventh and eighth thoracic vertebrae. The mass was about 1 cm. thick and about 6 cm. long. It did not extend under the anterior surface of the dura. The tumor was recognized to be of inflammatory origin. Cultures were taken and *Staphyloccus aureus* grew therefrom. The wound broke down and healed by granulation. A year later the patient walked almost normally. This case is practically a twin to case 1.

SUMMARY AND CONCLUSIONS

1. In three cases of extradural inflammatory tumors, around which a group of acute and chronic cases have been assembled from the literature, the infections arise either from direct extension of contiguous infections of the soft parts or from hematogenous metastasis of an infection in remote parts of the body.

2. We believe the symptoms of these infections to be sufficiently characteristic to represent a clinical syndrome.

3. The spinal epidural space with its content of fat and areolar tissue determines the presence and location of these infections. This space has no prototype in the cranial chamber; it is situated almost entirely on the dorsal half of the spinal dura; its size varies inversely with that of the spinal cord and cauda equina.

4. Although all the acute infections have run a fulminating and fatal course, except two that were drained, it is hoped that with an early and accurate diagnosis, operative treatment (drainage) may be effectual in saving both life and function.

5. The chronic inflammatory tumors of the epidural space are perhaps more difficult of differential diagnosis than ordinary tumors. It should, however, usually be possible. Their treatment is surgical removal as with any other tumor. The dura should not be opened because of the danger of a renewed infection.

REFERENCES

[1]Peters, R.: Ueber die Entzundung der Extradura-

len Gewebes des Ruckenmarks bei der Genickstarre. *Deutsche med. Wchnschr., 32:* 1151, 1906.

[2]Mills, C. K., and Spiller, W. G.: Case of External Pachymeningitis, Implicating the Entire Ventral Surface of the Spinal Dura. *Brain, 25:* 318, 1902.

[3]Weinberg, M. H.: Spinal Cord Tumors; Six Cases Including Tuberculosis of Dura. *J. Nerv. & Ment. Dis., 63:* 23 (Jan.) 1926.

[4]Morowitz, P.: Ueber akute eitrige Perimeningitis (Peripachymeningitis). *Arch. f. klin. Med., 128:* 294, 1919.

[5]Taylor and Kennedy: A case of Extrathecal Abscess of the Spinal Cord. *Arch. Neurol. & Psychiat., 9:* 652 (May) 1923.

[6]Oppenheim, E. S.: Ueber einen Fall von extraduraler spinal Eiterung. *Berl. klin. Wchnschr.,* 1910.

[7]Cassirer: Die Pachymeningitis externa purulenta. *Oppenheim's Lehrbuch der Nervenkrankheiten, Ed.* 7, *1:* 419, 1923.

[8]Hoestermann: Ueber myelitis transversa. *Neurol. Centralbl.,* 1913.

[9]Schick, K.: Pachymeningitis spinalis externa purulenta als Metastase nach Diplokokkenbronchitis. *Wein klin. Wchnschr., 22:* 1185, 1909.

[10]Lewitzky, P.: Ein Fall von Peripachymeningitis spinalis. *Berl. klin. Wchnschr., 14:* 227, 1877.

[11]Spencer, N. H.: Case of Idiopathic Inflammation of the Spinal Dura Mater. *Lancet,* June 14, 1879, p. 836.

[12]Hinz, R.: Ueber einen Fall von Perimeningitis purulenta. *Deutsche med. Wchnschr., 47:* 1229 (Oct. 13) 1921.

[13]Stroubell: Ueber Syphilis der Ruckenmarkshaute. *Neurol. Centralbl.,* 1898, p. 1120.

[14]Dandy, W. E.: The Diagnosis and Localization of Spinal Cord Tumors. *Ann. Surg., 81:* 223 (Jan.) 1925.

[15]Lewis, Dean and Bassoe, P.: Frazier's Surgery of the Spine and Spinal Cord, 1918, p. 922; *Surg. Gynec. & Obst., 20:* 489, 1915.

[16]Schultze, F.: Zur Diagnostik und Operativen Behandlung der Ruckenmarks hautgeschwulste. *Mitt. Grenzgeb. Med. Chir., 12:* 153, 1903.

[17]Mendel, K.: Meningo myelitis unter der Bilde eines Ruckenmarkstumors. *Berl. klin. Wchnschr. 46:* 2239, 1909.

[18]Gamphers, E.: Beitrag zur Pathologie und Therapie der Erkrankungen der Cauda Equina. *Jahrb. Psychiat. Neurol.,* 1920, p. 40.

XXV

A SIGN AND SYMPTOM OF SPINAL CORD TUMORS*

A recent case of spinal cord tumor called to my attention a subjective story and objective findings which would appear to be significant in the differential diagnosis of spinal cord tumors: sudden signs and symptoms of spinal cord compression after straining. These disturbances are emphasized because they are such logical expectations in the light of certain recent observations which have been steadily clearing the mysteries in the diagnosis and localization of spinal cord tumors.

REPORT OF CASE

Clinical History. The patient, a well nourished man, aged twenty-seven, was referred to me by Dr. C. M. Byrnes because of inability to walk, of difficulty in urination and of a heavy dragging sensation in his back. Seven years before when straining at stool he suddenly lost the use of both legs; the arms were unaffected. On awaking the next morning the function had partially returned. At the end of four months his paralysis had improved to such an extent that he could play tennis without handicap. But during the early months of recovery there were several spells—always at stool—in which there was partial loss of function of the limbs, with gradual return to the previous normal during the course of two or three days. The motor weakness was always somewhat greater on the left side. Numbness of the limbs at times accompanied the motor loss, but the patient was never able to recall any occasion when a sensory level existed. At the onset of the paralysis and for several weeks thereafter, he suffered greatly from pain in the lumbar region, but none elsewhere. There was also some difficulty in starting the flow of urine, but no incontinence.

For more than six years after this illness the patient was free of symptoms except at times an urge to urinate and a difficulty in starting the flow. Four months ago, when at stool, partial paralysis of the legs again suddenly appeared and again the weakness of the left leg was a little greater. Numbness and tingling were also present, more on the left. There has since been but little return of function, although many times at stool the paralysis has suddenly increased; however, in twenty-four or forty-eight hours the previous level of function has nearly been restored. Vesical and rectal control has not changed.

Examination.—The neurologic examination by Dr. Byrnes revealed: marked weakness and spasticity of both legs, greater on the left; loss of muscle sense in the toes of the left foot, this was preserved on the right; positive Romberg sign; bilateral ankle clonus and increased patellar reflexes. A vague sensory level was determined about the umbilicus—tenth thoracic segment.

The spinal fluid was clear with four cells, globulin positive and Wassermann test negative.

Quickenstedt's Test: There was no rise of spinal pressure when both jugular veins were compressed.

Spinal Air Test: Thirty cubic centimeters of fluid could be aspirated; no more was obtainable. An equal amount of air was substituted in the spinal canal. Only after several minutes was there a slight headache. But since air could be repeatedly reaspirated from the spinal canal it was evident that it was held below a block in the spinal canal. Roentgenograms of the head disclosed only a small amount of air in the cerebral sulci. We were, therefore, dealing with a spinal block which was nearly but not quite total.

Operation. A simple cyst, measuring about 6 by 2 cm., of oval shape, with a

*Reprinted from the *Archives of Surgery*, 16: 435–441, October, 1926.

rather thick but slightly translucent wall and containing a clear slightly straw colored fluid, was dissected without rupture from the epidural space at the seventh and eighth vertebrae. It was only loosely attached to the dura and could be easily lifted from its bed. It was, however, attached to the sheath of the left seventh thoracic nerve and here alone was sharp dissection necessary for liberation of the tumor. In neither the gross nor the microscopic examinations could any solid element of tumor be found. Microscopic sections of the wall show only a hyaline fibrous tissue, and no nerve elements.

Anatomic Diagnosis. Simple cyst—extradural. It would seem that this tumor was probably of congenital origin.

Result. The patient walked out of the hospital two weeks later and now (after one year) has completely recovered all motor functions and is well in every respect.

COMMENT

The unusual character of this tumor need not detain us, nor shall I dwell either on the unusual history of a series of sudden attacks quickly followed by recovery instead of the characteristic tumor history with signs and symptoms of gradual progression, or on the equally unusual fact that there was a long free interval of seven years between attacks of paraplegia. The character of the tumor — a simple cyst — well explains these seemingly nonharmonizing facts.

We are here concerned solely with the sudden disturbances of spinal cord function associated with straining as a diagnostic sign of spinal cord tumor. In this case the paraplegia occurred so frequently and so consistently when at stool that coincidence cannot be offered as an explanation. The explanation of these changes has been prepared in recent years by the hydrostatic and hydrodynamic studies of Queckenstedt[1] and of Ayer.[2] As a matter of fact precisely the same loss of spinal cord function has quickly followed lumbar punctures in the presence of spinal cord tumors and for precisely similar reasons. This startling and not unusual sequel of a seemingly simple diagnostic procedure has been emphasized elsewhere (Elsberg,[3] Dandy[4]).

From the frequent use of Queckenstedt's test we know that compression of both jugular veins produces: (1) an instant and rapid rise of fluid in the spinal manometer when the spinal subarachnoid space is not blocked; (2) but no change in the column of fluid if the spinal canal is blocked by a tumor or other lesion. Since the jugular veins have no valves, pressure on them causes blood to be held back within the cranial chamber (a closed and inexpansible box), and therefore, the intracranial pressure must at once rise. And because of the normal free communication between the cerebral and spinal subarachnoid space, the intracranial pressure must be transmitted at once to the lumbar spinal canal.

When a spinal puncture is made in the presence of a spinal tumor, the pressure below the tumor is reduced to that of the atmosphere; the pressure above the tumor, always higher, then becomes relatively greater and the full force of this difference is suddenly exerted on the point of obstruction. The result of this pressure is trauma to the spinal cord whose functions are already greatly compromised by the tumor's gradual pressure. This injury is the more readily explainable when one considers the anatomic changes in the spinal cord at the site of the tumor. The spinal cord is always deeply indented by the gradual growth of the tumor to which it must, of course, make an accurate physical adaptation. This involves a marked loss in volume of the spinal cord, though function may still be retained. At the level of the tumor's maximum and the spinal cord's minimum diameter is, of course, the narrowest part of the spinal canal, and through this hour-glass constriction the pressure, now suddenly relatively increased, must try to jam the greater volume of spinal cord as a wedge. The result of this hydrodynamic effort to equalize pressures above and below the tumor is trauma to the delicate spinal cord. The reason an injury of this kind does not always follow is doubtless because the spinal canal may be hermetically closed at the level of the tumor so that the newly established pressure differential can have no effect, or the canal may be still sufficiently patent to permit the ready transfer of fluid, thus equalizing the pressure above and below the tumor.

In our patient a similar pressure differential has been created, but in a different manner. A necessary sequel of straining at stool is increased intracranial pressure from thoracic compression (venous congestion) — the exact equivalent of compressing the jugular veins. Nature has then raised the spinal pressure above the tumor (that below being unaffected). The end-result has, of course, been the same — the spinal cord is driven by the increased pressure into the constriction of the spinal canal at the site of the tumor, and, just as following a lumbar puncture, the spinal cord is traumatized.

In a recent survey of a series of spinal cord tumors no instance of this effect of straining at stool was observed, nor has its mention been noted in a review of the literature on spinal cord tumors.

One of my patients volunteered the statement that frequently when he sneezed or coughed violently, pains and numbness immediately developed in both legs but quickly disappeared. This history was given some time before the other patient's story was known and at the time was passed by as of no significance. The intracranial pressure is, of course, increased by coughing and sneezing in just the same way as by straining at stool and doubtless the pains and numbness of our second patient are explainable in precisely the same way as in our first case. The order in which the signs and symptoms of spinal cord compression develop must, of course, be variable and doubtless dependent on the position of the tumor, i. e., whether dorsal, ventral or lateral. It would, therefore, seem reasonable to expect motor symptoms to be initiated by a ventral tumor, Brown-Se-

quard symptoms by a lateral tumor and possibly sensory symptoms by a dorsal tumor.

At times a localized backache is intensified by coughing, sneezing or straining at stool when the patient is affected with a spinal cord tumor. This was mentioned in the history of our patient. Schultze[5] and Cassirer[6] mention cases in which root pains are intensified by coughing and sneezing. Backache in spinal cord tumors appears to be due to localized intraspinous pressure. An intensification of this pain would, therefore, be expected by the sudden increase of intraspinous pressure above the tumor after sneezing, coughing or straining at stool. Edema of the cord, resulting from the trauma, causes an increased swelling of this local area of the spinal cord and, therefore, a persistence of the backache for sometime thereafter. All forms of pain, which are caused by spinal cord tumors — (1) root pains, (2) tract pains and (3) the pressure pains (backache) — may be intensified by coughing, sneezing and straining at stool. The explanation of the increased pain is precisely that of the sensory, motor and vesical disturbances, i. e., the effect of increased pressure above the tumor.

It is true that the repeated attacks which occurred in our patient will never develop in the usual run of tumors whose growth is progressive, but I am prepared to believe that a history of at least one and possibly even more attacks, of more or less similar character, may at times be elicited if this symptom is suspected by the examiner. And such a story will, I believe, be of great importance in differentiating a spinal cord tumor from other spinal lesions.

As mentioned before, when the spinal canal is tightly closed or when it is yet patent, it is improbable that injury to the spinal cord can result either by lumbar punctures or by straining. In other words the stage, at the tumor's level, must be set to a nicety before the changed intraspinal pressure differential can produce these disturbances of spinal cord functions. The intensified backache, however, should be expected at any time after the original cause of the backache exists; i. e., after the combined volume of tumor and cord is great enough to cause marked intraspinous pressure which can no longer be relieved by nature's method of space compensation.

THE EFFECT OF STRAINING IN THE PRESENCE OF INTRACRANIAL TUMORS

All that has been said concerning the effects of increased intracranial pressure on the spinal cord can be transferred almost verbatim to apply to tumors of the brain, particularly those situated in the posterior cranial fossa. The not infrequent disastrous effects of lumbar punctures on patients with intracranial tumors are too well known to need mention. The deaths and disabilities are likewise explained by trauma to the medulla when the cerebellar tonsils are jammed into the bony ring forming the foramen magnum. The effect is precisely that of injury to the spinal cord following lumbar puncture in the presence of a spinal cord tumor. The result is more serious because the intracranial pressure is much higher, but particularly because injury to the medulla compromises life.

But the increased intracranial pressure caused by straining produces equally disastrous results which have an explanation similar to those following lumbar punctures. During one year, two of our patients suddenly died on the morning of operation when at stool; another passed into coma from which she was rescued by operation. In each of these patients the tumor was of long standing; nor had there been any apparent change in the patient's condition prior to the time of defecation. The sudden, even though transient, increase of pressure was enough to endanger or terminate life — "the straw that breaks the camel's back."

That there may even be a local intracranial pressure effect from straining is shown in a recent patient with a cerebello-pontile tumor. For years she dreaded going to stool because a headache always developed and persisted for several hours in the right suboccipital region (the site of the tumor).

SUMMARY AND CONCLUSIONS

1. In a case of tumor involving the spinal cord, signs and symptoms of spinal cord compression repeatedly and suddenly developed when the patient strained at stool. In another case numbness and pain developed in both legs immediately after sneezing.

2. These signs and symptoms are explained by a sudden increase of the intraspinous pressure above the tumor, and caused by straining at stool, coughing or sneezing.

3. This increased pressure forces the spinal cord downward against the spinal tumor causing trauma of which the disturbed function — motor, sensory and sphincteric — is the result.

4. For similar reasons, root pains, tract pains and backache — the three pains of spinal cord tumors — may follow sneezing, coughing and straining at stool.

5. It seems probable that the sudden onset of any of these disturbances from straining may be a sign of importance in differentiating tumors from other lesions affecting the spinal cord.

REFERENCES

[1]Queckenstedt Zur Diagnose der Ruckenmarkskompression. *Deutsche Ztschr. f. Nervenh.*, 55: 325, 1916 uber Veranderungen der Spinalflussigkeit bei Erkrankungen peripherer Nerven, insbesondere bei Polyneuritis und bei Ischias. *ibid.*, 57: 316, 1917.

[2]Ayer, J. B.: Puncture of the Cisterna Magna, Arch. Neurol. & Psychiat., 4: 529 (Nov.) 1920 Spinal Subarachnoid Block at Determined by Combined Cistern and Lumbar Puncture with Special Reference to the Early Diagnosis of Cord Tumors. *Arch. Neurol. & Psychiat.*, 7: 38 (Jan.) 1922.

[3]Elsberg, C. A., and Stookey, B.: Mechanical Effects of Tumors of the Spinal Cord; Their Influence on Symptomatology and Diagnosis. *Arch. Neurol. & Psychiat.*, 8: 502 (Nov.) 1922.

[4]Dandy, W. E.: The Diagnosis and Localization of Spinal Cord Tumors. *Ann. Surg., 81:* 223 (Jan.) 1925.

[5]Schultze: Zur Diagnostik und operativen Behandlung der Ruckenmarkshautgeschwulste. *Mitt. Grenzgeb. Med. Chir., 12:* 153, 1903.

[6]Cassirer: Die Tumoren des Ruckenmarks. *Oppenheim's Lehrbuch der Nervenkrankheiten, Ed. 7, 1:* 521, 1923.

XXVI

TREATMENT OF CHRONIC ABSCESS OF THE BRAIN BY TAPPING*

PRELIMINARY NOTE

To one who has carefully studied the sequence of events following the customary drainage of chronic brain abscesses, the conclusion is inevitable that many patients so afflicted succumb from the effects of the treatment rather than from the abscess itself. The fact that abscesses in the soft parts are successfully treated by wide drainage, or by drainage and irrigation, is no reason why the same treatment will produce the same results in abscesses of the brain. It is only necessary to compare the structural differences between the brain and the soft parts to understand why drainage affecting the brain is an entirely different problem. The brain being a very delicate and well protected structure and, therefore, unaccustomed to trauma of any kind reacts slowly, weakly and less effectually to the insults of trauma, which drainage must necessarily induce. Proof of this statement is to be found in extirpations of tumors, particularly after the older method of rapid extirpation by the finger. Very quickly after a large tumor has been shelled out in this manner the cavity will be completely filled by the swollen brain — the cerebral edema resulting from injury.

During drainage of a cerebral abscess, the gauze or tubing is constantly injuring the cerebral cortex adjacent to the wall of the abscess. The result of this irritation is precisely the same traumatic cerebral edema, except that it is continuous, which follows a hasty tumor extirpation. Moreover, the surrounding infection quickly invades the injured brain, producing a more or less extensive encephalitis which, in turn, nature must also combat.

In combating brain abscesses, just as brain tumors, nature is constantly hampered by the limited space available. She can indeed take care of a space consuming lesion of surprising size, often as large as a baseball, by eliminating blood, cerebrospinal fluid and the normal watery content of the brain.

Most brain abscesses undoubtedly cause death from increased intracranial pressure. When an abscess is drained, the traumatic edema and inflammatory swelling (resulting in the manner described above) exact an ever increasing additional amount of intracranial room, which soon exceeds the space released by evacuation of pus and which also soon exceeds nature's bounds of compensation.

In still another way the effects of trauma and infection are increased. Through the opening in bone, dura and skin, cerebral cortex must necessarily be extruded by the high intracranial pressure. Subjected to the weight of the head, to the trauma of gauze dressings and to the infections of the skin, this cerebral fungus quickly increases in size, and the infection spreading to the brain still within the cranial chamber causes further intracranial pressure, and then further extrusion of brain — a vicious cycle. There are few lesions offering a less favorable prognosis than such a cerebral fungus.

The dangers of drainage are in direct proportion to the depth of the abscess, the size of the bony and dural defect, and inversely proportional to the size and chro-

*Reprinted from the *Journal of the American Medical Association,* 87: 1477–1478, October 30, 1926.

nicity of the abscess. The cases, therefore, which have the best change of success from continuous drainage are those in which the abscesses are large and are so near the surface that little if any cortex remains. There has recently, I believe, been a tendency to reduce the size of the drainage opening, and in thus avoiding fungus formation there has been an increase in the number of cures.

Several years ago our attention was drawn to the fact that not infrequently brain abscesses were cured spontaneously. We were also impressed by another fact, namely, that quite frequently acute infections had been conquered and a well walled off chronic abscess had resulted. There then followed only a slow increase of intracranial pressure. It seemed to us that in these cases nature really needed but little help to cure the abscess. In other cases it seemed that a little more or rather a little more frequent help would tide the patient along until he could get on with less help and finally with no help at all.

As a result of these observations we ventured to treat chronic abscesses by simply evacuating the pus on one or more occasions. Many times a single release of pus has been necessary on fewer occasions two or more taps have been required. The procedure is as follows: A small perforator opening is made in the bone over the abscess, where it appears to be nearest the dura. A ventricular needle is introduced into the abscess through a tiny nick in the dura. The needle is left in place until pus ceases to drip. The abscess is neither aspirated nor irrigated because of the paramount desire to avoid stirring up the infection by either mechanical or chemical stimuli. The cutaneous wound is tightly closed.

It is, of course, obvious that a chronic abscess cannot collapse; that, if additonal pus is aspirated, either air or fluid must take its place in the rigid cranial chamber. Eventually nature must and will absorb the contents of the abscess and fill the defect gradually either with fluid or with scar tissue, or both. The tiny dural opening precludes both a cerebral fungus and a fistulous tract and thereby prevents the introduction of a secondary infection.

This procedure is of proved value only for chronic abscesses. Acute abscesses present a far less hopeful outlook. While it is possible that a few cases may be helped from the acute to the chronic stage by tapping an acute abscess, many are so virulent and fulminating that a cure is impossible. Certainly the contraindications to continuous drainage — which could only be futile, for there is little to drain — are even greater than for chronic abscesses. If nature cannot wall off an intracranial infection and transform an acute into a chronic abscess, the condition must be hopeless.

In a few cases of epilepsy we had had occasion two and three years later to resect part or the whole of a cerebral lobe containing the scar of the old abscess. Only a cicatrix and single or multiple cysts, surface adhesions and enlarged subarachnoid spaces then remained as gross evidence of the former abscess. By this time the old infection had been so thoroughly eliminated by the cerebral tissue that in no instance was the infection lighted up again by the operative trauma; and in each instance the lateral ventricle was freely opened and resected, giving every opportunity for the rapid development of meningitis if even a trace of the old infection had persisted.

XXVII

GLOSSOPHARYNGEAL NEURALGIA
(TIC DOULOUREUX)*

ITS DIAGNOSIS AND TREATMENT

The pain of trigeminal neuralgia was for many years considered so distinctive in type and severity as to deserve the restrictive designation, "tic douloureaux." Why this particular nerve should alone be subject to this paroxysmal, ticlike type of pain and all the other cranial and spinal sensory nerves be seemingly immune, has never had a rational explanation.

As a matter of fact, pain of the same type does occur in the distribution of the glossopharyngeal nerve, so that the term "tic douloureux" is no longer synonymous with trigeminal neuralgia, but must now include glossopharyngeal neuralgia. Whether similar pains of the facial, vagus and possibly of other sensory nerves will eventually be found to be of similar kind, remains to be seen.

Weisenburg[1] was apparently the first to direct attention to the resemblance of an unusual pain of the ninth nerve to the so-called idiopathic pain of tic douloureux of the trigeminal nerve. In his patient, however, the paroxysms of pain were caused by a tumor in the cerebellopontile angle, but in many ways the pain was analogous to that of tic douloureux of the trigeminal nerve. In fact, it was first mistaken for trigeminal neuralgia, but the pain was not influenced by a partial removal of the gasserian ganglion. The pain was always at the "root" of the tongue, and extended down the throat and to the ear. There was a burning feeling and dryness in the throat, and frequently the sensation of flies and roaches crawling. At times the paroxysms

were excruciating, and usually were brought on by eating. During the last year of the patient's life, contact of food with a sharply defined trigger zone at the base of the tongue caused terrific paroxysms of pain. Actual chewing movements did not induce this pain.

Ten years after Weisenburg's report, three cases of "algie velopharyngee essentielle" were described by Sicard and Robineau.[2] In each case the pain was paroxysmal, was induced by swallowing, chewing, speaking and often spontaneously, and was referred to one side of the pharynx, soft palate and tonsil. Doubtless because the pain was of long duration and not accompanied by other manifestations of tumor, the condition was considered to be "essential" or idiopathic. It is hardly probable that they recognized the pain as an involvement solely of the glossopharyngeal domain, for their treatment, as practiced and recommended, consisted in sectioning in the neck and branches of the glossopharyngeal nerve, the pharyngeal branches of the vagus and the superior cervical ganglion. Since the appearance of these publications, a number of cases have accumulated rapidly.

Doyle[3] reported four and Adson[4] three other cases from the Mayo Clinic. Harris,[5] in his splendid book, "Neuritis and Neuralgia," adds six cases from his own service in London. As this paper was written another case was appended by Goodyear.[6]

Although all of these have been reported as cases of glossopharyngeal neuralgia, the doubt lurks that the pain is confined exclusively to the distribution of the glossopharyngeal nerve. For this reason, the

---

*Reprinted from the *Archives of Surgery, 15:* 198–214, August, 1927.

suggested treatment of Sicard and Robineau was followed in the cases of Doyle and Adson, i. e., the branches of both the vagus and glossopharyngeal nerves were divided. They seem to have been misled by an uncertainty of the sensory nerve supply to the pharynx, believing branches of the sphenopalatine ganglion and vagus nerve to be the source of its supply. Harris is "uncertain whether the vagus has any share in the production of this (glossopharyngeal) neuralgia, and whether section of the pharyngeal branch of the vagus is also necessary." It appears probable that the unorthodox and faulty conclusions by Vernet[7] (referred to by Sicard and Robineau and by Doyle) on the nerve supply to the pharynx by the glossopharyngeal and vagus nerves is largely responsible for this confusion. The sensory distribution of the ninth nerve will be considered later.

In addition to the foregoing series of cases assembled from the literature, two more are reported. Curiously, these cases appeared six weeks apart. Both were recognized as glossopharyngeal neuralgia by the characteristic history of the attacks before the patients were actually seen. These cases are presented not only to emphasize the clinical picture of this remarkable and not uncommon condition, but also to present a simple form of treatment, practically devoid of danger, and productive of permanent cure without disability.

Case 1. *History.*—A strong, healthy man, aged 45, but looking much older, was first seen in the neurologic dispensary by Dr. Frank Ford, who at once recognized the pain to be that of glossopharyngeal neuralgia. Seldom have we seen a man in greater agony, even in the most severe cases of trigeminal neuralgia. He was then having paroxysms of terrific pain in rapid succession, some induced by swallowing or talking and some even occurring spontaneously. Afraid to swallow or to talk, he sat in terror, with his head hanging forward and directed toward the right in order to allow the saliva to drool from his mouth and away from the affected side. He dared to eat only after his tongue had been cocainized over

its base, and particularly, as he so strongly emphasized, over one spot about the size of a dime, near the junction of the tongue with the left tonsil. This 'trigger zone," so real to him, did not show anything on examination. For three and one half years he had endured this pain at varying intervals. It had begun in September, 1923, with a severe knifelike thrust at the base of the tongue immediately after taking a drink of cold water; it lasted a few seconds, but for three weeks it occurred several times a day and ended as abruptly as it began. During the attacks, the left ear drum felt as though it were being pushed out and "were ready to burst." In one severe attack just before his operation, the patient felt as if all the teeth in the lower jaw on the affected side were "jumping out of their sockets." For more than two years he was free from pain when asleep; but during the six months before admission to the hospital, he had been frequently wakened from a sound sleep by the knifelike pains, particularly when lying on the left side. The attacks were due, he thought, to the accumulation of saliva on the trigger zone. His tonsils had been removed in September, 1926, and again in November, 1926, in the vain hope of effecting a cure. During the latter operation, the throat was extensively burned with a cautery. The pain was decidedly worse afterward, and from then until his admission to the Johns Hopkins Hospital in April, 1927, the pains became more and more frequent and severe. He said it seemed to him that a red hot poker was being jabbed through the tongue. At first the attacks were of only two or three seconds' duration, but during the past six months each had lasted about ten seconds. He had the impression that the attacks were more frequent when he talked a great deal, but in his occupation as a missionary there was little opportunity to get complete rest for any length of time. He had obtained relief for a few days by local application of cocaine.

Results of all examinations, including tests for taste and sensation in the domain of the ninth nerve, were entirely negative. The Wassermann reaction was negative.

Operation.—On April 6. 1927, I performed an intracranial section of the ninth nerve, in the posterior cranial fossa.

The patient made an uneventful recovery, with immediate and subsequent complete relief from pain of any kind. There was no disturbance of swallowing afterward. He was unable to detect any symptoms due to the loss of function of the ninth nerve. Objectively, however, there was total loss of sensation and of taste over the back of the tongue and pharynx. No motor impairment of any kind could be detected by examination.

Case 2. A man, aged fifty-six, well developed and strong, but pale and sallow from lack of nourishment, was referred by my associate, Dr. S. J. Crowe, on May 10, 1927. Fifteen years before, while talking with a friend, the patient had been suddenly seized with an excruciating pain in a spot at the back of the tongue and near the right tonsil. It lasted only a few seconds, but during the following years similar pains in the same location struck him suddenly without warning; after they had disappeared, he was entirely free of pain. It seemed as though a red hot iron were being thrust through the tongue at this spot. At first he was unable to discover any inciting cause for the attacks. The free intervals were as long as a year and a half, but the pain always recurred in the same spot. Since November, 1926, the attacks had become more frequent and severe and of longer duration, often lasting several seconds. During this time, the attacks have been induced consistently by drinking, eating and talking. For two weeks before I saw the patient, he had been almost without food or drink and had scarcely dared to speak. Sneezing and coughing also brought on the paroxysms. For the two days before he consulted me, one attack had followed almost immediately on the other, giving the patient almost no interval of relief longer than a few minutes, despite hypodermic injections of morphine. During my brief examination the patient had three paroxysms, each lasting about five seconds. Immediately after each attack, he could swallow with impunity for a few seconds, but this period of immunity was soon over. He could direct the examiner to the spot on the base of the tongue which seemed to him so well defined, but nothing was objectively evident. Results of all examinations, including tests for taste and sensation, in the distribution of the ninth nerve were negative.

Operation.—On May 11, 1927, under local procaine hydrochloride anesthesia, the glossopharyngeal nerve was divided intracranially in the lateral cistern. Postoperative convalescence was uneventful. All pain immediately disappeared and had remained absent up to June 1, 1927. The patient was unable to detect any abnormal sensations incident to the loss of sensation. There were no signs or symptoms of injury to the vagus nerve. Motor loss could not be observed. The patient was a public speaker, and, despite his terrible pain, was most reluctant to have anything done unless assured that his voice would be unimpaired; there was no change.

THE OPERATION

The glossopharyngeal nerve is divided intracranially, a unilateral cerebellar approach being used. It is the same exposure that I have used for the past three years as the method of choice in dividing the sensory root of the trigeminal nerve. The glossopharyngeal nerve is, however, much easier of access. It is one of the simplest of intracranial operations, and can readily be performed with either local or general anesthesia. An incision is made which begins at a point about 2 centimeters below the inion, gently curves upward, reaching slightly above the line of attachment of the trapezius muscle to the occipital bone, and then turns more abruptly downward along the mastoid bone until within from 1.5 to 2 centimeters of its tip. The trapezius muscle is divided just below its attachment and retracted downward and outward. The bone is removed over much of the corresponding side, at least far enough to the midline to afford access to the cisterna magna, which is punctured to release fluid and to provide additional room. The bone is rongeured laterally to the mastoid, but not far enough to enter the mastoid cells. The dura is opened in stellate fashion. Gentle elevation of the cerebellar lobe then allows ample exposure of the cerebellopontile angle. The cisterna lateralis is quickly brought into view, and, when pricked, the lining arachnoid membrane collapses. The fifth, eighth, ninth, tenth and eleventh cranial nerves then appear. The auditory nerve is probably the best landmark. The glossopharyngeal nerve is, of course, next in succession in a caudal direction and is probably from 0.75 to 1 centimeter caudal to the auditory nerve. A relatively tiny nerve, about the size of the lead in a pencil, always single and free from contact with the vagus, which lies immediately caudal—the glossopharyngeal nerve—can be readily lifted with a blunt hook without touching the vagus or any other nerve. A knife or a pair of scissors cuts the suspended nerve in an instant. The patient whose nerve was sectioned under procaine hydrochloride anesthesia (applied only extracranially) did not experience any sensation when the glossopharyngeal nerve was divided. The operation should be devoid of danger. There is no reason for even touching the vagus, auditory or facial nerves. There can, of course, be no question about the permanency of a cure, for precisely the same problem has long since been solved in trigeminal neuralgia. After section of the sensory root of any nerve central to its ganglion, regeneration is impossible.

The operations heretofore employed in glossopharyngeal neuralgia have been of the peripheral type, either section or avulsion of the nerve. Besides the local difficulties of isolating and dividing the ninth nerve high up in the neck without injuring the sympathetic trunk and particularly the vagus (a difficult task), the objection remains that regeneration of the nerve is likely to follow its division peripherally. As noted before, Sicard and Robineau introduced this manner of division of the nerve for glossopharyngeal neuralgia, and in all cases the sympathetic and pharyngeal fibers of the vagus were intentionally included. Adson avulsed the glossopharyngeal nerve in the hope that at least the petrous ganglion would be included, but the vagus, being closely associated, was injured. He regretted that he had not tried intracranial section of the nerve and hoped to do so in his next case. In a patient afflicted with an extensive carcinoma of the tongue and pharynx, Fay,[8] in 1926, sectioned the ninth nerve, together with three upper cervical nerves, in an extensive occipital and cervical exposure. The vagus nerve was injured, and, doubtless because

of inadequate exposure, the pulse rate immediately dropped from 125 to 80. He also planned a unilateral cerebellar approach if a patient with glossopharyngeal tic douloureux should come for operation. Harris, in 1926, attempted to inject the glassopharyngeal nerve (in the neck) with alcohol, but failed to reach the nerve. Injections of alcohol could hardly be successful. Injury to the contiguous jugular vein, the internal carotid artery, the sympathetic, spinal accessory and vagus nerves would seem more probable than a successful injection into the glassopharyngeal nerve.

In passing, it is well to note the importance of section of the glossopharyngeal nerve in inoperable carcinomas of the tonsil and nasopharynx. Should the domain of the fifth nerve also be invaded by the growth, the sensory root of the trigeminal nerve can easily be divided at the same time and with little added time. As mentioned before, this approach has been my method of choice for section of the sensory root in tic douloureux for the past few years.

CLINICAL FEATURES

The close similarity between glossopharyngeal neuralgia and tic douloureux of trigeminal origin has been commented on by Sicard and Robineau, Doyle, Adson and Harris. Surely both varieties of this fearful pain equally deserve the appellation, tic douloureux. The characteristic sudden, ticlike paroxysms of excruciating pain and the induction of pain by external stimuli are common to each.

In the twenty cases of glossopharyngeal neuralgia assembled from the literature and epitomized in the accompanying table, the clinical picture is strikingly uniform. The paroxysms of pain always strike some part of the glossopharyngeal sensory area — the tonsil, back of the tongue or the pharynx; the pain is always unilateral and induced by liquids or solids passing over the sensory endings of the ninth nerve in the mouth or pharynx. The pain is always excruciating; it is variously described as lancinating, knifelike or like stabs of a red-hot iron. Each individual pain usually lasts only a few seconds, rarely over a minute; the duration of the paroxysm, is, therefore, usually less than that of trigeminal neuralgia, but it would seem more severe, if possible. There is a strong tendency for the paroxysms to occur in a series over a period of time varying from a few days to a few weeks; in nearly every case intermissions of several months have occurred. The longest period of relief was three and three-fourths years in one of Adson's cases. But the identical pain always returns in precisely the same location. In a few cases there has been some tendency for the pain to shift from an initial point more remote and eventually to reach the central area of the glossopharyngeal sensory domain; for example, in two of Doyle's cases the original pain was in the ear, and in one of Adson's cases it was in the lobule of the ear and the angle of the mandible, but the pains were brought on by swallowing or other stimuli of the tongue and pharynx. In early all cases pain radiates to the ear, i. e., the meatus, the concha, the lobule or in front of or behind the ear, and not infrequently it begins there either before the more central pain or almost simultaneously with it. Rarely does the pain radiate elsewhere than to the ear or its environs and to the affected side of the throat. It seems probable that Jacobson's nerve is responsible for this aspect of the pain, but as there is no external sensory supply by the glossopharyngeal nerve, pain to the mandible and outer ear must be looked on as referred. At times, as in two of Doyle's cases, in one of Adson's and in one of Harris', the ear was actually tender to touch. In the latter two instances, touching or washing the ear would precipitate the characteristic attacks. Although the method par excellence of starting attacks of glossopharyngeal neuralgia is to drink hot or cold liquids — cold is more effective than hot — the attacks are also induced in many other ways. Other recognized causes are: swallowing (solid foods seem to be less effective than liquids), talking yawning, coughing, shouting, sneezing, touching the ear, suddenly turning the head, and in one instance touching the angle of the mandible; often the attacks seem to occur spontaneously. A trigger zone was present in both of the cases reported (the base of the tongue, near the tonsil), in one of Adson's cases (pharyngeal wall) and in Goodyear's case (tonsillar pillar). Harris remarked on the absence of a "trigger zone" in cases of glossopharyngeal neuralgia, and considered its absence to be almost the only essential difference between glossopharyngeal neuralgia and trigeminal neuralgia; the four cases in which there were trigger zones have appeared since the publication of his book.

Like trigeminal neuralgia, glossopharyngeal neuralgia usually appears in the later half of life, and usually after the age of 50. Whether significant or not, one observation stands out strikingly in this early series; there are only three cases (10 per cent) in women.

I have placed in the same group the cases in which the glossopharyngeal neuralgia was caused by a tumor and those in which it has been considered essential or idiopathic. As a matter of fact, the only reason for having assumed that the condition is idiopathic was the analogy of the features of the pain with those in trigeminal neuralgia. Necropsy was performed only in Weisenburg's case; and an intracranial exposure of the ninth nerve has been made only in my two cases. From the latter cases alone, positive objective proof is furnished of the essential nature of glossopharyngeal neuralgia. As a matter of fact, the proportion of tumors that have been demonstrated is high, compared with their incidence in trigeminal neuralgia. Three of the series of patients are known to have had tumors: Weisenburg's patient with cerebellopontile tumor and two of Harris' patients who had carcinoma of the tonsil. It seems probable that tumors were present in two more instances. One of Harris' patients lost twenty-two pounds (10 Kg.) in weight in two months, indicating a serious wasting underlying cause.

Another victim had convulsions induced by the pain, in fact, a cerebral exploration had been made for a tumor of the brain, though with negative results. This patient died a year later, presumably from the intracranial lesion (tumor?). There is, therefore, a known incidence of 15 per cent of tumors in this group and a probable incidence of at least 25 per cent. Weisenburg's case, taken in conjunction with the well known slow, insidious growth of tumors in the cerebellopontile angle, as well as the frequently obscure malignant lesions of the tonsil and nasopharynx, should make one always alert to the possibility that an underlying tumor may be the cause instead of an idiopathic neuralgia. Moreover, a careful survey of the histories in the cases here assembled seems to indicate no discernible difference in the character or location of the pain or its provoking influences, whether there is an underlying tumor or not. One additional great advantage of the intracranial operation for glossopharyngeal neuralgia is that automatically any intracranial lesion is discovered and may be eliminated. If a tumor is causing the condition, no treatment is, of course, rational which does not deal with the removal of the tumor if that is possible.

The diagnosis of essential glossopharyngeal neuralgia is made solely from the history and from observation of the attacks. In many of the cases from the literature a diagnosis of trigeminal neuralgia was made, but this was before the glossopharyngeal neuralgia was recognized. The pain of glossopharyngeal neuralgia was so characteristically located in the region of the ninth nerve that in none of the cases collected here should there be any doubt of the diagnosis. One might possibly think of trigeminal neuralgia when the ear is tender and when touching the ear incites attacks, but even then the pain is mainly induced by stimuli in the back of the mouth, and the pain is always in this region.

Neuralgia of the seventh nerve (geniculate ganglion) has been described by Hunt as accompanied by pains largely localized in the ear.

Geniculate herpes is a well recognized condition but geniculate neuralgia is none too securely established; at least it remains to be proved that a ticlike neuralgia of the seventh nerve occurs without more spasms. A tic of the facial nerve, described by Cushing as "tic conouloif," is characterized by spasms of the facial muscles, and cannot be confused with glossopharyngeal neuralgia.

GLOSSOPHARYNGEAL NERVE SUPPLY

Isolated loss of function of the glossopharyngeal nerve apparently has not been known. Pope,[9] in describing a case of thrombosis of the vertebral artery pressing on the glossopharyngeal nerve, quotes Gowers as saying: "There is no recorded case in which the roots of the glossopharyngeal nerve alone have been diseased." Cassirer,[10] writing in Oppenheim's Lehrbuch makes a similar statement. Cases of tumor on traumatic injuries to the nerves at the base of the skull have paralyzed the glossopharyngeal nerve, but this paralysis has never been purely and solely of the glossopharyngeal nerve. Indeed, Pope's case seems more probably an aneurysm and not a thrombosis, for there was a fusiform mass. In addition to the incomplete injury to the glossopharyngeal nerve, there was partial facial paralysis and some disturbance of the trigeminus, both subjective and objective; moreover, it is difficult to understand how the vagus, which is in such close proximity, could have been spared. It is almost inconceivable that any neoplasm could be so small and so isolated as to cause a pure glossopharyngeal paralysis, and it is equally incredible that any effect of trauma could induce an isolated paralysis of this nerve. Vernet's conclusions on glossopharyngeal function, as noted, which have received much more consideration than they deserve, have been derived from observations of tumors, inflammations and fractures affecting all of these structures in the jugular foramen. From such a source it is impossible to separate disturbances of the ninth and tenth nerves, which are so intimately related over such a long distance. The only possible way to cause pure glossopharyngeal destruction and, therefore, to test the function of this nerve is by intracranial section at operation. Section of the nerve in the neck has always been accompanied by injuries of the vagus and usually of the sympathetic nerve. The entire nerve can never be sectioned or avulsed in the neck, for branches — notably Jacobson's nerve — cannot be reached. The two cases here reported are presented as pure isolated lesions of the glossopharyngeal nerve; there were no other involvements of the cranial nerves. The after-effects of division of the glossopharyngeal nerve intracranially were almost the same in both cases.

Motor Changes. Symptomatically, there was absolutely no subjective or objective motor disturbance in either instance. Swallowing was unaffected. The constrictors of the pharynx were unimpaired. The soft palate moved normally and equally on the two sides. Most textbooks of anatomy agree that the stylopharyngeus muscle is the only muscle supplied by the glossopharyngeal nerve. I do not know of any test that will demonstrate its loss of function; apparently its absence (if the nerve is affected) is not noticeable to the patient. These cases, I believe, effectually contradict the claims of Vernet that the important middle constrictor of the pharynx is supplied by this nerve; its nerve supply is from the vagus.

Alterations of Taste. The nerve supply of taste will shortly be the subject of a more detailed study in conjunction with Dr. Dean Lewis. For this reason, only cursory mention will be made here of the part played by the ninth nerve in the supply of taste to the tongue as a whole.

In both of the cases reported there was complete loss of taste in the posterior third of the tongue. This confirms the usual conception of the nerve supply of taste for this part of the tongue. It opposes the rather unusual view long taught by Gowers and others that the trigeminal nerve supplies taste to the whole tongue. In one of the cases reported here, no change occurred in the perception of taste in the anterior two thirds of the tongue. In the other case there was a slight, but definite, alteration to the degree that on the normal side, sweet, sour, bitter and acid were all recognized more quickly (a few seconds) and registered with greater intensity than on the side with the cut glossopharyngeal nerve; but all tests for taste were accurately registered on the affected side (anterior two-thirds). The interpretation of these minor alterations of taste in one case and none in the other will be discussed in the forthcoming paper. At least, it is evident that the ninth nerve supplies taste for the posterior third of the tongue, but does not supply taste to the whole tongue, a view long held by Luciani and by his followers even at present.

Sensory Changes. The results in both cases are best shown in the accompanying sketches. For the examinations of the sensory loss in the pharynx and nasopharynx and the base of the tongue I am indebted to Dr. S. J. Crowe. The only differences noted in the two cases were that in one patient sensation was perceived in the eustachian tube for a few millimeters below the pharyngeal orifice; in the other, there was no sensation for a distance of about 2.5 cm. In one patient the sensory deadline exactly bisected the uvula; in the other, almost the entire uvula was anesthetic. In both patients, a cap of sensation remained at the vault of the nasopharynx, doubtless being supplied by the trigeminal nerve. The remainder of the pharynx, anterior, posterior and lateral, down to the epiglottis (including the posterior aspect), the vellecula and the pyriform sinus, was anesthetic. Anteriorly and posteriorly, the line of anesthesia ended sharply at the midline. The soft palate is supplied by the glossopharyngeal nerve

TABLE OF CASES OF GLOSSOPHARYNGEAL NEURALGIA ASSEMBLED FROM THE LITERATURE

Author and Year	Age and Sex	Duration of Pain	Nature of Pain	Location of Pain	Radiation of Pain	What Induces Pain	Duration of Paroxysm	Pain in Ear	Tenderness of Ear	Trigger Zone	Pain Unilateral	Pain Has Intermission	Cause of Pain	Treatment
Weisenburg 1910	35 ♂	......	Sharp shooting; dry burning feeling in throat	Root of tongue	Throat and ear	Eating, drinking	....	+	....	+	+	..	Tumor of cerebello-pontile angle	Gasserian ganglion
Sicard and Robineau 1920	Young soldier ♂	Several years	Severe paroxysm	Pharyngeal wall	....	Swallowing, talking, chewing	....	..	....	..	+	+	None	Peripheral section of ninth, pharyngeal branches of tenth, and sympathetic nerves
Sicard and Robineau 1920	Young soldier ♂	Several years	Severe paroxysm	Pharyngeal wall	....	Swallowing, talking, chewing	....	..	....	..	+	+	None	Peripheral section of ninth, pharyngeal branches of tenth, and sympathetic nerves
Sicard and Robineau 1920	51 ♀	......	Severe paroxysm	Pharyngeal wall	....	Swallowing, talking, chewing	....	..	....	..	+	+	None	Peripheral section of ninth, pharyngeal branches of tenth, and sympathetic nerves
Doyle 1923	63 ♂	5 yr.	Severe paroxysm	First in ear, later in tonsillar region	Ear	Eating, drinking, talking, yawning	....	+	+ of auricle	..	+	+	None	First gasserian, later peripheral section of ninth and tenth nerves
Doyle 1923	52 ♂	3 wk.	Severe paroxysm	First in ear, later in throat	Ear	Talking, swallowing, spontaneous	20 to 40 seconds	+	+ over tragus after paroxysms	..	+	..	None	Injection in third branch of fifth and auricular temporal nerves
Doyle 1923	57 ♂	1 yr.	Paroxysms; feeling of choking	Side of pharynx	Angle of mandible	Drinking	1 to 2 seconds	..	....	..	+	+	None	None
Doyle 1923	61 ♂	9 yr.	Excruciating paroxysms	Side of pharynx	External auditory meatus	Movements of head, talking, drinking, swallowing, fright	2 to 50 seconds	+	....	None	+	+ pains in series	None	None
Adson 1924	61 ♂	9 yr.	Severe paroxysm	Lobule ear and pharynx	Ear and angle of mandible	Movements of head, swallowing, talking, spontaneous	....	+ lobule	+ Excessive, auricle	None	+	+ longest 3¾ years	None	Attempted peripheral avulsion of ninth nerve, but nerve later found intact; vagus injured
Adson 1924	52 ♂	4 yr.	Severe stabbing pains	Tonsil and ear	Ear	Drinking, washing ear	....	+	+	+ on pharyngeal wall	+	+	None	Avulsion of ninth nerve; vagus injured

Author / Year	Age / Sex	Duration	Character of pain	Location	Radiation	Exciting causes	Duration of attack		Trigger (ear/touch)	Trigger point			Associated conditions	Treatment
Adson 1924	38 ♂	17 yr.	Knifelike spasms	Pharyngeal muscles	Ear	Drinking, eating, talking, pressure on maxilla	Few seconds to few minutes	+	··	None	+	+ longest 6 mos.	None	Avulsion of ninth and part of tenth nerves
Harris 1926	87 ♀	12 yr.	Severe paroxysms	Left side of throat	Ear	Swallowing	....	+	Concha intensely tender to touch	None	+	+	None	Injection in mandibular branch of trigeminal nerve
Harris 1926	53 ♂	6 mo.	Severe paroxysms	Root of tongue	Ear and back of jaw	Swallowing, eating, yawning	....	+	··	None	+	+	None	Attempted injection in ninth nerve not successful
Harris 1926	50 ♂	5 yr.	Excruciating paroxysms	Throat	Ear, back of jaw and neck	Swallowing and touching ear	....	+	Touching ear started attacks	None	+	+ longest 1 year	None; but had convulsions and died 2 years later (brain tumor?)	Injection in mandibular nerve
Harris 1926	65 ♂	6 yr.	Severe paroxysms	Tonsil	Ear	Yawning but not swallowing	20 seconds	+	··	None	+	+ longest 1 year	Carcinoma of tonsil	Local removal of carcinoma
Harris 1926	59 ♂	.....	Pain on swallowing	Tonsillar region	......	Eating, swallowing, hot drinks especially	....	··	None	None	+	··	Carcinoma of tonsil	Local removal of carcinoma
Harris 1926	54 ♂	.....	....	Side of throat	......	Excitement, muscular exertion; not swallowing	....	0	None		+	+	Possibly carcinoma; great loss of weight	None
Goodyear 1927	74 ♂	.....	Excruciating spasms	Throat and tonsil	Anterior to ear	Talking, swallowing, not chewing	+	··	··	+ tonsillar pillar	+	+	None	None
Dandy 1927	45 ♂	3½ yr.	Excruciating paroxysms	Back of tongue and tonsil	Ear drum feels as if pushed out	Swallowing, talking, spontaneous	Few seconds	+	None	+ base of tongue near tonsil (very striking)	+	+ longest 2 years	None	Intracranial section of ninth nerve
Dandy 1927	56 ♂	15 yr.	Excruciating spasms like thrust of hot iron	Base of tongue and tonsil	......	Swallowing, talking, sneezing, coughing, spontaneous	2 to 5 seconds	··	None	+ base of tongue near tonsil (very striking)	+	+ longest 1½ years	None	Intracranial section of ninth nerve

only in a narrow rim on its oral surface and over a greater extent on its nasal surface. The tonsil and eustachian orifice were insensitive in both cases. The epiglottis was anesthetic on its posterior aspect; the line of demarcation of the area with the normal sensation of the anterior surface from that supplied by the vagus is a sharp line along the rim of the epiglottis. The precise line of demarcation between the area of normal and of lost sensation was difficult to determine in two places — above at the vault of the nasopharynx and below at the beginning of the esophagus. These two narrow zones are therefore shown in dots in contrast to the cross-hatch which denotes the absolute loss of sensation. The anterior wall of the sphenoid and the posterior end of both the middle and interior turbinates were sensitive. There was no area of anesthesia in the nasal cavity. It could not be determined whether there was any loss of sensation along the posterior border of the vomer.

Secretory and Sympathetic Nerves. No disturbance of salivary secretion could be detected after the glossopharyngeal nerves had been sectioned.

I am aware that the small superficial petrosal nerve is a continuation of Jacobson's nerve through the tympanic plexus. It has received much attention as an important link in the chain of certain theories of taste; it has been supposed also to carry sensation to the nasal cavity. even to the pharynx. I have not been able to adduce evidence of either function.

SUMMARY AND CONCLUSIONS

1. Glossopharyngeal neuralgia is a type of tic douloureux exactly like trigeminal neuralgia. Its clinical picture is so characteristic and the history of the attacks so vivid that the diagnosis is easy and unmistakable.

2. Two cases are reported and appended to eighteen others which have been assembled from the literature. The clinical features of this condition are analyzed and tabulated.

3. The treatment of glossopharyngeal neuralgia is purely surgical. An operation by which the ninth nerve is sectioned intracranially was carried out in both cases. The superiority of this operation over section of the glossopharyngeal nerve in the neck is due to the fact that other nerves are not injured and the nerve is cut above the ganglion, thereby precluding return of the malady. The operation is practically without danger to life and leaves no subjective or objective disturbance in its wake.

4. These isolated glossopharyngeal lesions afford an excellent opportunity to study the function — —sensory, motor and gustatory — of this nerve. It is probable that these cases are the only instances of pure, unmixed and total loss of function of the ninth cranial nerve.

REFERENCES

[1]Weisenburg, T. H.: Cerebello-Pontile Tumor Diagnosed for Six Years as Tic Douloureux: The Symptoms of Irritation of the Ninth and Twelfth Cranial Nerves. *J. A. M. A., 54:* 1600 (May 14) 1910.

[2]Sicard, R., and Robineau: Communications et presentations: I. Algie velopharyngee essentielle. Traitement chirurgical. *Rev. neurol., 36:* 256, 1920.

[3]Doyle, J. B.: A Study of Four Cases of Glossopharyngeal Neuralgia. *Arch. Neurol. & Psychiat., 9:* 34 (Jan.) 1923.

[4]Adson, A. W.: The Surgical Treatment of Glossopharyngeal Neuralgia. *Arch. Neurol. & Psychiat., 12:* 487 (Nov.) 1924.

[5]Harris, W.: *Neuritis and Neuralgia.* New York, Oxford University Press, 1926.

[6]Goodyear, H. M.: Tic Douloureux of the Glossopharyngeal Nerve. *Arch Otolaryng., 5:* 341 (April) 1927.

[7]Vernet, M.: Syndrome du trou dechire posterieur (Paralysie des nerfs glossopharyngien, pneumogastrique spinal). *Rev. Neurol., 34:* 117, 1918.

[8]Fay, T.: Intracranial Division of Glossopharyngeal Nerve Combined with Cervical Rhizotomy for Pain in Inoperable Carcinoma of the Throat. *Ann. Surg., 84:* 456, 1926.

[9]Pope, F. M.: Thrombosis of Vertebral Artery Pressing on Glossopharyngeal Nerve Unilateral Loss of Taste at Back of Tongue. *Brit. M. J., 2:* 1148, 1889.

[10]Cassirer: Die Lahmung des N. Glossopharyngeus, in Oppenheim. *Lehrbuch der Nervenkrankheiten, 1:* 775, 1923.

XXVIII

REMOVAL OF RIGHT CEREBRAL HEMISPHERE FOR CERTAIN TUMORS WITH HEMIPLEGIA*

PRELIMINARY REPORT

In the gradual evolution of resections of frontal, temporal and occipital lobes for the cure or attempted cure of invasive and otherwise incurable cerebral tumors, it has been found that the right temporal lobe, either frontal lobe or either occipital lobe (the left posterior to the supramarginal gyrus) could be completely removed without apparent mental impairment. It therefore seemed a logical expectation that the right cerebral hemisphere might be removed with little, if any, change in the mentality of a right handed person. At times patients already paralyzed on the left side from the inroads of cerebral neoplasms and without any prospect of its correction are eager to live, even at the price of permanent loss of function on that side of the body, if only the mind remains undisturbed. Five times during the past five years patients in this condition have urged every effort to save their lives, regardless of the physical disability. In four of these patients the tumors (gliomas) had been found at operation but their removal could not be accomplished without inducing a hemiplegia. The pressure symptoms had been relieved at the time of the first operation by a large decompression (removal of the bone flap). In each case the paralysis of the right side subsequently became complete.

The first of these patients was seen five years ago when in coma. The tumor was located by ventricular estimation and found at operation to be a glioma occupying much of both the right frontal and right temporal lobes. It seemed probable that the middle cerebral artery was incorporated in the tumor, and the ligation of this vessel would have caused a left hemiplegia. Several weeks later, when the left side was paralyzed, the right hemisphere was removed, but in the region of the carotid artery the tumor had invaded the dura and this small portion could not be excised. The patient died three and one-half years later from recurrence of the tumor. He was repeatedly examined before leaving the hospital and there did not seem to be any obvious mental impairment. He was always happy and grateful for his extension of life.

In a second patient, also in coma, a solid glioma was found to occupy the right parietal, temporal and frontal lobes. The bone flap was removed, and relief from pressure was afforded. At the insistence of his family, the right hemisphere was removed; but since the tumor had deeply invaded the corpus striatum, its complete removal was impossible. He died three months later of recurrence. An extensive infection had followed the operation, precluding any accurate estimate of his mental capacity.

A third patient died from hemorrhage forty-eight hours after the hemisphere had been extirpated for a recurrent glioma of the temporal, frontal and parietal lobes. A silver clip had slipped from the middle cerebral artery. Since consciousness was never regained, mental examinations were not possible.

A fourth patient died of pneumonia two weeks after excision of the right hemisphere. During all of the first week after the operation he was perfectly conscious

*Reprinted from the *Journal of the American Medical Association*, 90: 823–825, March 17, 1928.

and answered every question promptly and accurately. He was always perfectly oriented as to time, place and person. We could not detect any mental impairment from these cursory tests.

The fifth patient, a woman, aged thirty-five, is still under observation. Her case was different from any of the preceding in that she had never had a headache; her only symptoms were gradual but rapid loss of sensation and motor power in the left side. These changes could hardly be due to any lesion other than a tumor in the internal capsule. An air injection showed obliteration of the right ventricle and slight obliquity of the third ventricle to the left. Slight movement of the left leg was still possible but she could not stand. Her brother, a physician, had anticipated the diagnosis and the eventual outlook if operation was performed. Both he and the patient were eager for a cure by immediate excision of the hemisphere rather than to have her submit to any partial effort, which would surely be followed by a recurrence of the tumor and doubtless prevent a subsequent cure. Any attempt to resect the tumor at such great depth could be done only by sacrificing the middle cerebral artery, and the results of this vascualr loss, except for the absence of a homonymous hemianopia, would be essentially the same as those following removal of a hemisphere. The right cerebral hemisphere was extirpated in a single mass. The tumor, a glioma measuring about 3 by 3 cm., was so well surrounded by normal brain tissue that it was not seen until the specimen was cut later. Unfortunately, this patient, too, has been the victim of an infection, but she has now (two months after the operation) apparently recovered from its effects. During the high fever she was delirious off and on for several weeks. Gradually the periods of delirium have lessened, and she is now rational at all times. She is always well oriented as to time, place and person, has a good sense of humor and seems normal mentally.

The hemiplegia in these cases is always complete in the arm and leg but only partial in the face. In one patient, the facial movements seemed almost unchanged after the removal of the hemisphere. The other patients showed varying degrees of asymmetry much like the variations that follow involvement of the motor cortex by the tumor's growth. In the patient who lived three and one-half years after the hemisphere was removed, slight flexion and extension of the knee and thigh subsequently developed, but there was never enough function to be of any service. His days were spent in a wheel chair. No movements were ever observed in the arm.

The degree of rigidity in the extremities has also been variable. It has always developed more slowly and less intensely than we had anticipated. A complete flaccidity supervenes for at least several hours after the operation, and at the same time a suggestive positive Babinski reflex first makes its appearance. In none of the patients was there more than a mild rigidity during the postoperative stay in the hospital. The patient, now in the hospital, two months after the operation, only at times shows any resistance whatever on passive movements of the leg. One could scarcely say that there is any degree of rigidity of the leg. The arm shows slightly more resistance, enough to be definite, but as yet there are no signs of contracture. Both the arm and the leg lie in any position in which they have been placed. The patient, who lived three and one-half years, had a markedly contracted arm but no contracture of the leg.

Epicritic and protopathic sensation are completely lost over the arm, trunk and leg. Deep sensation is well preserved. Movement of the joints in painful, and squeezing the muscles causes pain. The patient can tell when the thigh, knee or foot is flexed or extended, or even which toe is manipulated, but is unable to tell whether the toes are flexed or extended. Painful stimuli induced by squeezing the muscles of the thigh or calf cause the leg to draw up in a rather vigorous reflex movement.

Another feature of interest is the preservation of sensation in the face. Epicritic sensation, such as very light touch and differentiation of degrees of temperature, is lost, but a heavier touch and stronger differences of temperature, the proper localization of stimuli and their doubleness are recognized accurately. The corneal reflex is diminished somewhat but preserved. The motor function of the fifth nerve is intact. The tongue protrudes with slight, if any, deviation. Taste over the anterior two thirds of the tongue is apparently preserved but lessened. Hearing is normal in both ears. This we have noted by gross test in all of the cases reported, and in the last patient audiometer readings are normal in both ears. This disposes of the assumption that there is cortical representation for hearing in the right temporal lobe. A complete left homonymous hemianopia has, of course, followed the removal of a hemisphere.

The success of the operation is dependent on painstaking care in hemostasis. The middle and anterior cerebral arteries are ligated just above their origin from the carotid either with silk ligatures or with silver clips, and the vessels are divided between the ligatures. The elimination of the arterial supply of blood at once causes a considerable lessening of the cerebral bulk and makes the next step — ligature of the many cerebral veins that enter the longitudinal and transverse sinuses — much easier. Every vein that enters these sinuses must be carefully ligated before the hemisphere is removed. In the earlier cases the veins were "clipped" at the point of entrance to the sinuses, but in the last case they were carefully tied in the cortex with transfixion sutures of silk and a small triangular wedge of cortex containing the venous stubs was left attached to the longitudinal sinus. This method of handling the venous trunks is, I think, superior to that of clipping the unprotected veins; but much depends on the confidence which can be reposed in the clips. The recent use of "flat clips" makes for a feeling of greater security.

After all the arterial and venous channels have been isolated, ligated and divided, the hemisphere is gently liberated from its attachment to the falx, to the opposite hemisphere in the frontal region below the falx, and to the base of the skull. We have found it better when the whole hemisphere is thus liberated from all peripheral attachments first to section the frontal lobe, which requires only a sweep of the scalpel, and then, entering the anterior horn of the lateral ventricle with the index finger, to use this as a lever. The corpus callosum is then divided at a distance from the falx (in order to avoid possible injury to the left anterior cerebral artery, which is closely adjacent). With scissors or the edge of a spatula, the internal capsule is divided flush with the ventricle. The cerebral incision is then carried through the depth of the temporal lobe to a line just external to the inner dural margin in the middle fossa. The only bleeding encountered in the removal of the entire hemisphere is through very small vessels in the cut surface of the internal capsule (requiring only a moist tampon) and several small vessels which emerge from the under surface of the temporal and occipital lobes, doubtless from the posterior communicating and the posterior cerebral arteries.

In one patient, the tumor had grown so deeply that the cleavage line through the internal capsule passed through the lower fringes of the tumor. A second excavation was then made into the corpus striatum. It was this patient who subsequently died of hemorrhage due to a faulty clip. Obviously, one cannot tell from the surface inspection of the tumor whether the entire tumor can be included in the mass extirpation. In one case the tumor was not seen until the hemisphere was subsequently sectioned. This patient should be cured. In three instances the tumor had invaded the dura. In two of these the tumor subsequently recurred. In the third, a section of dura was excised with the adherent nodule of tumor; but the patient later died of pneumonia.

This is an operation of magnitude, but it should carry a relatively low immediate mortality owing to the relatively small amount of bleeding on which shock is so largely dependent. Except for the accidental slipping of a silver clip in one case there would not have been any immediate operative mortality in the series. Although this is scarcely an operation to be advised, it nevertheless offers to those desirous of living under adverse conditions a much longer extension of life than is possible in any other form of treatment, when the tumor cannot be completely removed; and in certain tumors situated within the confines of the hemisphere, it offers a cure otherwise not obtainable.

XXIX

MENIERE'S DISEASE*

ITS DIAGNOSIS AND A METHOD OF TREATMENT

The purpose of this communication is to present the results of an operation which I believe will permanently cure the symptoms of Meniere's disease. Briefly stated, the treatment is section of the auditory nerve intracranially. It is attended with almost no risk of life, and since there is always subtotal deafness on the affected side before the operation, section of the nerve adds little of practical importance to the deafness. Other symptoms do not result when the auditory nerve is severed.

In its usual form, Meniere's disease has a well defined and well recognized symptom complex. The patient is suddenly seized with a violent attack of dizziness, at once associated with nausea, vomiting and unilateral tinnitus referred to an ear which is progressively growing deafer. These attacks are repeated from time to time, usually with increasing frequency. The patients are well between the attacks, though eventually they may recur so frequently as to be almost continuous. At such times, as for example in case 1, the patient for weeks may not be able to take food or to retain it when it is taken. The attacks are of such violence and come on with such suddenness that the patient lives in terror of their reappearance. They last from a few hours to several weeks. The symptoms have been known and described for more than a century, but it was Meniere who first suspected their aural origin. Whether or not his impression proves to be correct, he at least rescued a clinical entity from a hopeless confusion of symptoms which had not implied any pathologic significance. At the time of Meniere's pub-

lication, the symptoms of this condition, and of epilepsy, also, were considered evidence of cerebral congestion or apoplexy. Indeed, the sudden nature of the attacks of Meniere's disease might well appear at first glance to be apoplectiform.

It is necessary to understand the beliefs current at that time in order not to be misled by the title of Meniere's paper, "Maladies de l'oreille interne offrant les symptomes de la congestion cerebrale apoplectiforme." There is even yet the erroneous impression (perhaps atrributable to the title) that Meniere thought this condition was due to cerebral hemorrhage or to hemorrhage into the semicircular canals. He made it clear that the symptoms are considered by all authorities to be due to cerebral congestion, but he repeatedly emphasized his belief that they are surely due to a disease of the internal ear. Elsewhere he said "The signs of cerebral congestion, so called, are not too well established; and — the signs of cerebral congestion and apoplexy will have to be revised." Meniere referred to the work of Itard (published in 1825) in his paper. At times, Itard is unjustly given credit for the discovery of Meniere's syndrome, but, according to Meniere he assembled cases of epilepsy, hysteria and other conditions with those of aural vertigo and classified all of them as "cerebral apoplexy." It is interesting that at the meeting of the Academy of Medicine of Paris when Claude Bernard was almost unanimously elected to be a member, the subject of cerebral congestion was discussed at length, and Meniere's work was cited as argument in opposition. It was the sense of the meeting that since "there was so much contradiction, confusion and exag-

*Reprinted from the *Archives of Surgery, 16:* 1127–1152, June, 1928.

281

geration on this subject it was better to separate epilepsy and confine the attention to true cerebral congestion." Meniere maintained that there could not be any possible relationship between epilepsy and aural vertigo, because epileptic persons do not have unilateral deafness, and patients with aural vertigo do not lose consciousness nor have the mental stigmas so common to persons with epilepsy.

Meniere's belief in the site of the lesion in the disease which has since borne his name was largely due to the well known experiments on extirpation of the semicircular canals by Flourens (1842). Meniere also reported gross observations made at necropsy in one case with acute symptoms, which persisted until death occurred five weeks later. The semicircular canals were found to contain "serosanguineous lymph." The brain did not show any abnormality. The observations made at necropsy by Meniere are obviously those of some acute aural condition and are not those of Meniere's disease which is now known as a chronic disease. The necropsy report of Meniere cannot be used to support his clinical syndrome, unless it be to show that such symptoms may be present in an acute form and may be referable to a lesion of the inner ear and not to the brain.

There is, in fact, no available material to indicate the character of the underlying lesion of Meniere's disease. A few cases have been reported, but all are complicated by other lesions. Politzer's patient had a tumor of the brain, Voltolini's had meningitis; Gruber's patient died of typhus and had blood tinged lymph in the semicircular canals.

Evidence that Meniere's disease is due to a lesion of the inner ear is based almost entirely on the presence of deafness. In the absence of proof, it is permissible to doubt that the pathologic process is actually in the semicircular canals. In fact, by analogy with other conditions, it is easier to believe that the nerve itself and not the end-organ may be primarily involved. It is evident from histories of Meniere's disease that infections of the middle ear have no etiologic relationship. Meniere early called attention to the absence of otitis media and of hereditary factors in the explanation of an underlying case.

TREATMENT IN MENIERE'S DISEASE

Charcot (1874), who frequently demonstrated cases of Meniere's disease at his clinics, admitted the utter hopelessness of all forms of treatment then in vogue. He noted that when deafness became complete the disease stopped spontaneously. This observation prompted him to wonder if surgical intervention might not at some future time offer the solution by dividing the auditory nerve. But this suggestion was made when antiseptic surgery was just beginning and several years before the dawn of brain surgery. With one exception the attempts at surgical treatment have been directed toward the semicircular canals.

Frazier (1912), following a suggestion by Mills (1908), divided the auditory nerve intracranially in a single patient and precisely as in the operation here described, but the dizziness was not relieved. A study of Frazier's case leads one to doubt that the diagnosis of Meniere's disease was correct; the characteristic "attacks" of dizziness, nausea and vomiting were not present. Rather there was a chronic state in which dizziness could be induced by postural change. The patient also was unable to lie in comfort on the contralateral side. These symptoms would seem to indicate involvement of the cerebello — brain stem — vestibular paths by a neoplasm or inflammatory process. Furthermore, there was a history of influenza quickly followed by deafness — an etiologic relationship not recognized in Meniere's disease.

Section of the eighth nerve for persistent tinnitus was then tried by Frazier (1913), but the ultimate success is not known. He stated that "the intense roaring sound" had disappeared at the time of the patient's discharge from the hospital. The results in the cases reported in this paper make one wonder how far section of the eighth nerve can control noises referred to the ear.

Other surgical attempts at treatment in cases of Meniere's disease have been directed toward direct attacks on the inner ear after chiseling through the mastoid. Houtant trephines the labyrinth; Portmann incises the saccus endolymphaticus. Aboulker exposes the dura behind the mastoid and expects to "decompress" the auditory nerve "either with or without opening the dura." The assumption of Aboulker that an increase of pressure of the cerebrospinal fluid in the posterior cranial fossa was responsible for Meniere's disease was due to Babinski's claim that lumbar punctures relieved the symptoms. At a meeting of the International Congress of Otology in 1922, this theory was supported by Nylen (Stockholm) and Quix (Utrecht). In refutation of this assumption it is only necessary to say that Meniere's disease is never seen when the intracranial pressure is really increased as in tumors of the posterior cranial fossa. An increase of pressure around one auditory nerve, aside from being pure conjecture, is impossible because the cisterna lateralis which surrounds the auditory nerve is freely open in three directions. In none of my operative series was there the slightest evidence of increased intracranial pressure, either local or general.

REPORT OF CASES

Case 1. *History.* A well nourished man, aged fiifty-three, was referred by Dr. G. H. Barksdale, of Charleston, W. Va., in September, 1924, because of vertigo, nausea, vomiting and buzzing in the left ear. The symptom of the onset was a unilateral buzzing in the ear which began two and one-half years previously. Impairment in hearing was noticed at the same time and had progressed gradually. Two months before examination a, headache began in the morning; later in the day, the patient became very dizzy. He went to bed, but the vertigo continued throughout the day. There were severe nausea and persistent vomiting. Everything seemed to move to the left. He said that he believed he would have fallen to the left if he had not gone to bed. Other attacks occurred but they did not last longer than a day. Three days before admission he had the most severe attack which wakened him out of a sound sleep. He saw objects moving to the left, and was greatly nauseated for five hours. Numerous attempts to vomit were ineffectual. A friend who saw him in this attack said that the temperature was 97 F. and the pulse rate, 60. For the past few months he had had a little headache over the occiput. The headaches were never severe, but were much worse during the attacks. Ringing in the left ear had been present since the onset of the condition. It was more intense during an attack. There had never been infection of the middle ear or mastoid.

Neurologic and Physical Examination.— With the exception of a questionable positive Romberg test (with tendency to fall to the left) and the disturbance referable to the eighth nerve, the results of the neurologic examination were negative. The patient had a bradycardia (60) during the attack. The Wassermann reaction of blood was negative. According to the tests the hearing in the left ear was moderately impaired; a watch tick was not audible. C 64 was not heard in the left ear; C 128 was heard only one fourth of normal time. C 1024 and C 2048 were not greatly changed. Bone conduction was greater than air conduction.

Vestibular tests showed that spontaneous nystagmus was not present. There was a normal response to caloric stimulation of both ears, but the left ear (affected side) was more quickly induced than the right.

Operation.— The left eighth nerve was divided intracranially under local anesthesia. The patient did not experience any sensation when the auditory nerve was dissected and divided. The postoperative course was uneventful.

Three and a half years after the operation, the patient was in perfect health and has been actively at work for the past three years. He has never had the slightest suggestion of an attack since the operation.

Case 2. *History.* A well nourished woman, aged fifty-four, was referred to me by Dr. Julian Chisolm, on Nov. 10, 1924. For three or four years the patient had had occasional attacks of dizziness and vomiting. At first they were not severe. One year before admission, she had a severe attack associated with ringing in the left ear and some impairment of hearing in the left ear. She was confined to bed for four days and found that she was much more comfortable when lying on the left side. Two months later, an even more severe attack prostrated her. It was like the preceding one, except that there was pain in the left occipital region and occasional tingling and numbness of both hands. There were also zig-zag flashes of light. For the past three months before consulting me there had been a constant tinnitus in the left ear, some unsteadiness of gait and a constant dull ache in the region of the left mastoid. There was no history of otitis media.

Examination.— The results of the physical examination and the Wassermann reaction of blood were negative. The results of the neurologic examination were negative, except for changes referable to the auditory nerve.

The hearing test revealed total deafness in the left ear; the right ear was normal.

The colonic test did not show any response to irrigations of the left ear; the right was normal.

Operation.—The left auditory nerve was sectioned intracranially on Nov. 12, 1924, under ether anesthesia. The patient was discharged from the hospital ten days later.

She has not had any attacks since operation. She complains of a drawing, tight feeling in the occipital region at the operative field, and zigzag flashes in the eyes; this sensation has been present for more than twenty-five years. Sometimes there is a little dizziness with the flashes of light (migraine?).

Case 3. *History.* An undernourished woman, aged fifty-five, was referred by Dr. Barker on Jan. 11, 1927, because of Meniere's disease. She was exhausted from prolonged vomiting. Her skin was sallow and pale. Eighteen months before, she was suddenly seized with dizziness, nausea and vomiting. The attack lasted all night. The vomiting was described as projectile. She did not have any fever, chills or pain. She had never been well since the onset of the condition. Six weeks later, she had another attack precisely like the first.

The interval between attacks gradually lessened, until the patient was admitted to the hospital. Each attack lasted one or two days. Only hypodermic injections of morphine gave any relief. Six months before coming to the hospital, she had a prolonged attack during which she did not take food for five weeks. A diagnosis of gallstones had been made in her home town, and the gallbladder had been drained. Gallstones had not been present. The appendix had also been removed at the operation. Her attacks of dizziness, nausea and vomiting persisted as before, though possibly with some moderation. Five weeks before admission her most severe attack began and still persisted. Since the attack began, she had had scarcely any food. She said she felt as if she were going round, first one way, then another. The attacks were not brought on by change of position, but during an attack she could not lie on either side. Sudden movements of the head then intensified the attack. There had been a gradually progressive loss of hearing in the right ear since the onset of the present illness. At the time of consultation, she could hear but little on the right side. There was also a continual ringing in this ear which became much worse during attacks. Recently, there had been some ringing in the left ear. An occasional slight pain was experienced in the right ear. There had never been an infection of either ear or mastoid. Nothing in her past history appeared to have any bearing on her condition. An attack of rheumatism, localized to the right hip, was noted thirty-five years before. During the menopause, two or three years previously, cyanosis of the fingers had been noted. She had always been nervous. Since her trouble began (eighteen months before), she lost twenty-six pounds (11.8 Kg.).

Examination.— The patient was in Dr. Barker's medical service for one month. There were few days during this time when the dizziness, nausea and vomiting were not present. The vomiting was often projectile. During most of this time she could retain nothing by mouth and was given fluids by rectal, subcutaneous and intravenous methods.

Except for the disturbed functions of the eighth nerve, the results of the neurologic examinations were entirely negative.

Examinations of auditory and vestibular functions were made by Dr. Baylor. All tuning forks were heard on the left side within normal limits. On the right, there was marked shortening with all forks. Vibrations of tuning fork C 128 were barely heard to C 2048.

Irrigation of the right ear produced a rotary nystagmus to the left, but no subjective dizziness. Irrigation of the left ear caused a rotary nystagmus to the right, but no subjective vertigo.

The audiometer test showed loss of hearing in the right ear and of some of the high tones in the left ear. The vestibular function was not abnormal.

The Wassermann reaction of the blood was negative. The blood pressure was 110 systolic and 70 diastolic.

Operation.—On Jan. 11, 1927, intracranial division of the right auditory nerve was performed under local anesthesia. The patient was not conscious of any sensation either when the auditory nerve was being liberated or when it was being divided. The postoperative course was uneventful.

Fourteen months after the operation, there had not been the slightest evidence of an attack. She had regained her original weight and more and was well.

Case 4. *History.* A large robust man, aged forty-seven, was referred in April, 1927, by Dr. F. C. Schreiber of Washington. One year before, the patient had felt dizzy when he awoke and raised his head. He vomited, but was not nauseat-ed. He was bedfast for three days. He felt dizzy every time he moved his head and vomited nearly as often. It was three weeks before the dizziness entirely disappeared. Four months later, he had another attack exactly like the first but this lasted only a week. Seven months before, tinnitus and deafness developed in the left ear; both appeared suddenly during an attack of dizziness and vomiting. The attacks of dizziness were not associated with moving objects. Headaches were not present. The patient reeled and staggered when walking during an attack. During the past month, there had been no additional attacks, but the patient was always dizzy, he complained of poor memory during the recent attacks.

Physical and Neurologic Examinations.— A positive Babinski sign and ankle clonus were present on the left side. The only other positive symptoms were the disturbed function of the eighth nerve. Unfortunately, the audiometer and caloric records of the functions of the vestibular and auditory divisions of this nerve were lost. It was recorded, however, that air conduction was less than bone conduction in the left ear, and that hearing was lost for the high tones and diminished for the low tones.

The blood pressure was 125 systolic and 85 diastolic. The Wassermann reaction of blood was negative.

The unilateral Babinski sign and ankle clonus made the diagnosis of Meniere's disease rather uncertain.

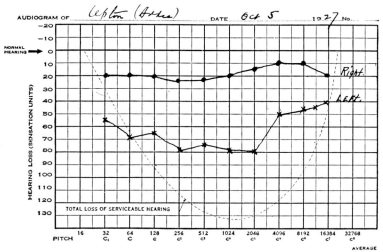

Fig. 1. Audiometer chart showing the loss of hearing in a typical case of Meniere's disease.

Operation.—In March, 1927, the left acoustic nerve was divided intracranially under local anesthesia. Thorough exploration of the cerebellopontile angle did not disclose a tumor. The entire intracranial course of the eighth nerve was in full view. Later, the symptoms did not clear up, and it was found by caloric tests that vestibular function was still present, though there was total deafness. Apparently, in an effort to avoid the facial nerve, the vestibular division of the nerve had not been divided. Two weeks later, the wound was reopened and this branch sectioned. The facial nerve was also injured despite caution. This was the only injury to the facial nerve in the series. It was later corrected by a spinofacial anastomosis.

The patient had not had attacks of dizziness and vomiting one year after the operation, but it is only fair to recall that for seven months prior to the operation he had had no attacks. After the operation he still complained of the constant dizziness which he described as lightheadedness and which was also present before operation. This steadily diminished after operation, until it was barely noticeable. The patient insisted that this dizziness was always worse in damp weather. It did not seem probable that it was caused by the disturbance of the eighth nerve, for it was unaffected by its section and seemed entirely independent of the attacks.

Case 5. History. A well nourished man, aged thirty-three, was referred to the hospital in June, 1927, because of dizziness. Two years before, he had suddenly become dizzy while at work. He continued at work but after an hour it was necessary to stop. A month later, a similar attack of dizziness had occurred while he was at work, and it had lasted all day. Nausea or vomiting were not associated with the attack. Objects always rotated from right left, i. e., toward the deaf ear. During an attack he could not lie on the affected side; the dizziness was less when he was lying on the opposite side. At first the attacks recurred about every month, but there had been one free interval of seven months. During the past year there had rarely been an interval of longer than a week between attacks. In an effort to obtain relief, the nasal sinuses had been operated on, and the gallbladder had been

drained. There were some left-sided headaches from the beginning, but they were always more intense just before an attack. A year and a half before admission, loss of hearing was noticed in the left ear; it had steadily progressed. Buzzing and ringing in the left ear had been present constantly for about the same length of time.

Examination.—The results of the physical and neurologic examinations were negative, except for tests of hearing and vestibular function. The audiometer test showed a 58 per cent loss of hearing in the affected (left) ear and 27 per cent in the right ear. In the vestibular tests, caloric irrigations to the left ear did not give any response; they were normal to the right ear.

Operation.—On June, 1927, under ether anesthesia, the left auditory nerve was sectioned at the internal auditory meatus. The patient had an uneventful recovery.

Ten months after the operation, there were no signs of recurrence of the attacks. There was occasional tinnitus.

Case 6. *History.* A highly nervous, well nourished woman, aged fifty-four, was referred by Dr. P. S. Sisco of Baltimore. For six years she was subject to violent dizzy spells which came on without warning and were accompanied by nausea and vomiting. The duration of the attacks varied from a few miutes to eight hours. During the attack she was afraid to move, for any change of position exaggerated her symptoms. Her first attack had occurred when she awoke from a sound sleep. Objects moved from left to right, i. e., away from the lesion. The attacks averaged two or three a month. Vomiting was persistent and exhausting. There was also a distressing desire to micturate and defecate and, since she lay motionless to reduce the dizziness as much as possible, she had to remain on the bedpan throughout the attack. After a seizure she fell asleep, and on awakening felt well again. The attacks had greatly increased in frequency, until she had several each day. A gradual loss of hearing in the left ear had occurred until she thought she was totally deaf on that side. The other ear had not been affected.

She said that for about a year she staggered like a drunken person, but without a definite tendency to fall to either side. During the past month, she had felt dizzy almost constantly. Recently any sudden motion of the head precipitated an attack. For years she had been unable to lie on the affected (left) side. Tinnitus—a ringing noise—had been present in the left ear since the onset of the condition six years before. She thought her memory was affected. Occasionally before an attack, she noticed that everything seemed bright, but she did not have a definite visual aura. She also had a vague impression of "smelling something" before an attack, but she could not give any better description of the sensation. There was no history of otitis media.

Examination.—The results of the physical examination were negative. The Wassermann reaction of the blood was negative.

The results of the neurologic examination were negative, with the exception of the changes referable to the eighth nerve.

The hearing test showed a 70 per cent loss of hearing in the left ear and 30 per cent in the right.

The left ear did not show any response to the caloric test; the right ear was normal.

Operation.—On Aug. 16, 1927, the left eighth nerve was divided under ether anesthesia.

The patient left the hospital ten days later. Eight months after the operation, she was well and had had no sign of her old attacks. Only an occasional trace of tinnitus remained.

Case 7. History. A woman, aged thirty-five, was referred by Dr. T. P. Sprunt of Baltimore in April, 1927, because of attacks of dizziness. Ten years before a thyroidectomy had been performed by Professor Halsted because of marked symptoms of exophthalmic goiter. She had never been in robust health since the operation, but she had continued to work steadily and had not had any serious illness.

She dated the onset of her condition to a sudden attack of dizziness fifteen months before when she was about to leave home. She had a violent sensation of turning to the right. Shortly afterward she was nauseated and vomited. The attack wore off during the day. Since then, similar attacks had occurred rather frequently, until she had them about every two or three weeks. The dizziness never caused her to reel or fall, but there was the sensation that she was rotating to the right, i. e., away from the lesion. The symptoms were accentuated when she lay on the left side. As long as she kept still and kept her eyes closed, she was better. Between the attacks she was free from any disturbance. Since the beginning of her dizziness, the hearing in the left ear had been impaired. This had been progressive. Tinnitus was present almost constantly throughout her illness, but was worse, perhaps, at the time of the attacks. Her past history did not shed any light on the cause of her illness. She had never had otitis media or mastoiditis. The blood pressure was 128 systolic and 82 diastolic. The Wassermann reaction of the blood was negative.

Examination.—The results of the physical and neurologic examinations were negative, with the exception of the local alteration in the function of the acoustic nerve.

The audiometer test showed a 56 per cent loss of hearing in the left ear; the right was normal. The caloric tests showed a normal response in both ears.

Operation.—The left auditory nerve was divided intracranially under local anesthesia. When the acoustic nerve was being manipulated and divided, the patient complained of the same sensation of rotation and of nausea as during an attack. It promptly dissappeared when the nerve was severed. The postoperative recovery was uneventful.

One year after the operation, the patient had not had any sign of her former attacks. For several months, she had had a feeling of dizziness and uncertainty when walking and was hesitant about crossing the street. This has now disappeared almost entirely. The noises in the ear persist as before. They have become less noticeable as she pays less attention to them. It is my impression that the tinnitus is neurogenic.

Case 8. *History.* A well nourished woman, aged thirty-two, was referred from the medical dispensary. Five years before she was suddenly seized with a severe attack of dizziness accompanied by severe nausea and vomiting. She felt as though she were "falling forward or backward," and it was necessary for her to hold on to something to keep from falling. The next attack occurred three weeks later. Since then, the attacks had recurred with increasing severity and greater frequency, until they averaged about two or three a week. The attacks occurred without apparent cause and were not induced by movements of the head or body; they often occurred when the patient was sitting or recumbent. Objects moved before her but with indefinite direction; they seemed to whirl in a general confusion. Three years later, she first noticed that the hearing in the left ear was impaired; this progressed until she was practically deaf in that ear. There was no tinnitus. Recently, there were some dull frontal headaches, but they were not important. She said that occasionally, during the most severe attacks, she thought that she lost consciousness, momentarily, and that she had a tendency to stagger to the right during the dizzy attacks; during the free intervals, the gait was normal. Later a new feature was added to the attacks, in that there was a "queer feeling" in the head just before the attack began. She took this as a warning signal to lie down promptly. There was no history of otitis media or mastoiditis and no known cause for her distress.

Examination.— The results of the physical and neurologic examination were negative except for the local condition.

The hearing tests showed a marked reduction of hearing for all tones in the left ear. Air conduction was greater than bone conduction. Hearing on the right side was essentially normal; there was about 65 per cent loss of hearing on the left by the audiometer test and 18 per cent on the right.

In the caloric tests, irrigation of the left (affected) ear with ice water caused rotary nystagmus. The response of the right ear was more active.

Dr. Crowe had observed this patient for more than a year, and had made several audiometer examinations. The tests showed a steady increase in deafness.

*Operation.—*The left auditory nerve was divided intracranially under ether anesthesia. The postoperative course was uneventful. Four months after the operation, there had been no suggestion of an attack. It is worthy of note that one year before the operation, the eighth nerve was explored and an anomalous artery lying on the nerve was "clipped." A unilateral decompression resulted. No improvement followed.

Case 9. *History.* A greatly undernourished woman, aged forty-seven, was referred by Dr. J. Heyward Gibbes of Columbia, S. C., on Jan. 2, 1928. Five years before, she was suddenly seized with an attack of dizziness while walking. She did not fall, but probably would have done so if she had not sat down. She was nauseated and vomited. Since then, similar attacks, lasting from three to five hours, had occurred every few weeks, but not infrequently they had occurred every two or three days. After many spells, she remained very weak for several days; at times it would require two weeks to recuperate. During the attacks, everything seemed to be turning around from right to left, i. e., toward the affected side. She could lie comfortably only on the back of her head. There was one free interval of six months, and for the past nine months nausea and vomiting had been absent during the attacks. She fell during three seizures. She said that the attacks occurred so suddenly that she fell before she realized she was dizzy. The seizures varied considerably in severity. Diminution of hearing was first noticed in the left ear at the time of the first attack. The hearing steadily diminished, until she was practically deaf in that ear, but the hearing was unchanged on the other side. Tinnitus had been present almost continuously in the left ear since the first attack of dizziness but was never present in the right ear. She described the sensation as a buzzing sound; at other times it was like a whistle. It was always after a dizzy attack. She did not think that the hearing was worse after the spells. Headaches did not occur. She had not had otitis media.

*Examination.—*The results of the physical examination were negative. The Wassermann reaction of the blood was negative.

The neurologic examination showed the following positive symptoms: The left corneal reflex was greatly diminished; the Romberg sign was positive, the patient falling to the left. Left facial weakness (but doubtful) was suggested by the fact that blinking seemed a little tardy. There was no ataxia or adiadokokinesis. The eyegrounds were normal.

The audiometer test showed 90 per cent deafness in the left ear. Bone conduction was absent for tuning forks 128 to 512. Hearing in the right ear was normal. Weber's test referred to the right ear.

The caloric test did not show any subjective or objective response whatever on the left; the right ear was normal.

The absence of response to caloric stimulation, the positive Romberg sign and the diminished corneal reflex made me entertain the diagnosis of a cerebellopontile tumor, though the character of the attacks seemed more like Meniere's disease.

Operation.— Cerebellar exploration was performed on Jan. 4, 1928. There was no tumor in the cerebellopontile angle. The auditory nerve was clearly visible from the pons to the internal auditory meatus. There was no sign of pressure in the posterior cranial fossa. The auditory nerve was divided.

The patient made an uneventful recovery and was discharged two weeks after the operation. There have been no attacks to date (three months after operation). The patient wrote that she was in better health than for many years. Occasional tinnitus occurred.

SYMPTOMS AND DIAGNOSIS OF MENIERE'S DISEASE

There has not been the semblance of an attack since operation in any of the nine cases. There was reason to question the cure by the operation in only one case (2). This patient is the only one of the nine who had total loss of both vestibular and auditory function (at least to our tests) at the time of the operation. It is, therefore, open to question why she had attacks if the nerve was totally out of commission. We are thrown on two possible explanations: (1) that some slight nerve function might still have been present and have evaded the tests, or (2) that since the last attack before operation the deafness had become complete, and if this were true, the cure should and might well have been spontaneous and not dependent on surgical division of the nerve.

It may be asked how it can be certain the nine cases are Meniere's disease. The diagnosis was made on the objective symptoms of unilateral subtotal deafness, and in each instance, inspection of the entire intracranial course of the auditory nerve excluded a tumor or other localized space-occupying lesion. Perhaps the most important single diagnostic feature of Meniere's disease is the sudden, fulminating onset of "attacks" without warning and without recognizable inciting cause; and after the attack has subsided, the patient is again in perfect health with only a residual unilateral loss of hearing and persisting tinnitus. It will be seen from Table I that while there are differences in detail, the general character of the attacks is much the same. Dizziness and unilateral tinnitus are the only two absolutely constant symptoms in the cases of this small series. In one patient nausea and vomiting were absent in all attacks, and in another, the nausea and vomiting, though present in early attacks, later disappeared. The character of the dizziness varies. Usually but not invariably objects rotate or whirl. Objects may seem to turn in one direction as in case 1, to the left; they may turn first one way then another (case 3), or in no definite direction (cases 7 and 9). In one case (7), the patient seemed to be turning to the right, and in another case (3), she seemed to revolve first one way then another. It is interesting to note that in three cases objects seemed to rotate toward the affected side and in two toward the opposite side.

During an attack, movements of the head intensified the dizziness in all cases. In one case, increase of symptoms resulted from the movement of the eyes so that the patient had to keep her eyes shut during the seizure. Nearly all patients are at once forced to seek the recumbent position. One patient dared not move from the flat of her back or turn her head until the attack wore off. Two other patients could not lie on either side and obtained relative freedom only when lying on the back of the head. One patient was not conscious of any difference in symptoms owing to position. Without exception, movements

TABLE I

DATA SHOWING GENERAL

Case	Sex*	Age	Side Involved	Duration of Symptoms	Duration of Hearing Loss	Dizziness	Tinnitus	Nausea	Vomiting	Self or Objects Turning	During Attacks Dizziness Made Worse by Lying on	
											Affected Side	On Opposite Side
1	♂	53	Left	2½ yr.	2½ yr.	+	+ Buzzing and ringing	+	+	Objects turn to left	....	....
2	♀	54	Left	3 yr.	1 yr.	+	+ Ringing; constant 3 months	+	+	......	More comfortable on affected side	+
3	♀	55	Right	1½ yr.	1½ yr.	+	+ Continual ringing, worse just before each attack	+	+++	+ Objects turn first one way then another; also feels as if she is turning	Comfortable only when lying on back of head	Cannot lie on either side
4	♂	47	Left	6 mo.	1 yr.	+	+ Tinnitus began six months after first attack	+	+	No	No	No
5	♂	32	Left	1½ yr.	2 yr.	+	+ buzzing and ringing	No	No	Objects right to left	Made dizziness worse	More comfortable on opposite side
6	♀	35	Left	6 yr.	6 yr.	+	+	+	+++	+ Objects turn without consistent direction though often left to right	For years had been unable to lie on affected side (left)	....
7	♀	54	Left	15 mo.	15 mo.	+	+ Worse in attacks	+	+		Changes make dizziness worse	No difference
8	♀	33	Left	5 yr.	2 yr.	+	+ But only in later months; never a conspicuous symptom	+	+	Sensation that she was rocking back and forth; objects also whirl but without definite direction	Position makes no difference, all comfortable	No difference
9	♀	47	Left	5 yr.	5 yr.	+	+ Almost continuous	+ But recently absent	..	Objects turn from right to left	Can lie only on back of head	Can lie only on back of head; between attacks can lie with comfort only on opposite side

*In this column, ♂ indicates male; ♀, female

CHARACTERISTICS OF MENIERE'S DISEASE

Do Symptoms Increase by Movement of Head	On Affected Side		Other Signs and Symptoms	History of Otitis Media	Wassermann	Remarks	Time Since Cutting Eighth Nerve	Result
	Caloric Test	Hearing Test						
....	Normal	Marked impairment	Headache during attacks	No	Negative	Tinnitus increased in attacks; bradycardia (60) in attacks	3½ yr.	Well; no attacks
....	Total absence of response	Total deafness	Zigzag flashes of light, migraine? pain in left occipital region; tingling and numbness of hand; unsteady gait	No	Negative	....	3½ yr.	No attacks; well, except for attacks of migraine which have been present for 25 years
+	Normal	Marked impairment	....	No	Negative	Some ringing and slight loss of hearing in opposite ear	14 mo.	No attacks; well; ringing in ear when she gets tired
++	Normal	Diminution of hearing	Left Babinski sign; left ankle clonus	No	Negative	Patient has constant dizzy sensation between attacks	1 yr.	Well; no attacks; constant tinnitus persists
+	No response	58% loss (also 27% loss in good ear)	Some left sided headaches in attacks	No	Negative	....	10 mo.	Well; no attacks; occasional tinnitus
++ Must lie on back and perfectly still	Total absence of response	75% loss (also 30% in good ear)	Distressing desire to urinate and defecate during attacks; tendency to stagger; sees lights before attacks	No	Negative	....	10 mo.	Well; no attacks; no tendency to stagger now; tinnitus at times
Symptoms improved by keeping eyes closed	Normal response	50% loss	Patient had some residual symptoms of exophthalmic goiter	No	Negative	Sensation of whirling and nausea when acoustic nerve was divided (under procaine hydrochloride)	1 yr.	Well; no attacks; tinnitus persists
+	Response is less acute than in other ear	Loss 65% (18% loss in good ear)	Patient though there was momentary loss of consciousness in attacks; "queer" feeling in hand became premonitory symptom	No	Negative	....	4 mo.	Well; no attacks; no tinnitus
+	No response	90% loss	Left corneal reflex diminished; Romberg sign, falls to left	No	Negative	Tinnitus was always worse after dizzy spell; attacks come so suddenly does not realize she is dizzy until after she has been thrown to the ground; exhausted for a week or more after attacks	2½ mo.	Well; no attacks; tinnitus persists, but is not so annoying as before operation

of the head or body failed to induce dizziness after the attack had passed, though one patient always slept on the opposite side because she feared an oncoming attack.

Tinnitus was uniformly present and always in the affected ear. In one case (8), however, it did not appear until five years after the onset of the attacks and even then was a minor symptom. Usually it persists in the free interval between the attacks. At times intensification of the tinnitus seems to usher in an attack and is worse during and for sometime after the seizure has passed. Tinnitus is described as a ringing or buzzing sensation. In one case, tinnitus did not develop until six months after the first attack and was synchronous with deafness.

Hearing was diminished in one ear in every case, usually to the point of rendering the ear almost useless for practical purposes. In recent cases in which audiometer tests were made, the loss of hearing was 75,65 and 90 per cent. It is noteworthy that although the loss of hearing was noticed synchronously with the first attack, this is not necessarily true. In case 2 deafness was not noticed until two years after the first attack; in case 4, five months, and in case 8, three years after the first initial seizure. It is, of course, possible that the early stages of deafness were not observed by the patients. It has been noted already that total deafness was present in only one patient from this series. In the other cases, the losses of hearing were 56, 58, 65, 75 and 90 per cent. In three cases there were losses of 18, 27 and 30 per cent in the good ears. These losses may or may not have any relationship to the other ear, which is the participant in Meniere's syndrome.

One of the most surprising observations is the great variability in the results of tests of vestibular function. If Meniere's disease is really a primary lesion of the semicircular canals, it is fair to expect the vestibular function to be profoundly and uniformly disturbed; at least, it should be more disturbed than the auditory function. On the contrary, the acuity of response from caloric stimuli is found undiminished in three cases, and only slightly diminished in another.

Three of the patients in the foregoing case reports had headache during the attacks. In two cases, the headache was on the side of the lesion and more in the occipital region than elsewhere. In another instance, the headache was general. One patient had a "queer" feeling in the head just before an attack. She looked on this as an infallible warning sign.

One patient thought there might have been on one occasion momentary loss of consciousness. In none of the remaining cases was there a suggestion of loss of consciousness. The preservation of conciousness is indeed one of the striking characteristics of Meniere's disease. A distressing desire to urinate and defecate during an attack made it necessary for one patient to lie on the bedpan until the attack was over. Two patients complained of some general dizziness or "light headedness" between the seizures. In both of these cases the dizziness persisted for several months after the eighth nerve was divided; it gradually abated and in less than a year it had almost completely disappeared. Nystagmus, which is occasionally reported in cases of Meniere's disease, was not observed in any of the cases from this series.

PSEUDO-MENIERE'S ATTACKS

The question has often been asked whether unilateral deafness is a necessary sign of Meniere's disease. Frankl-Hochwart suggested the term "pseudo-Meniere's" to apply to cases which seem similar but lack the unilateral deafness. The following history is presented as an instance of so-called pseudo-Meniere's disease because the attacks seem similar, yet without any subjective or objective evidence of impaired hearing, and no unilateral signs.

A man, aged fifty-nine, referred by Dr. S. J. Crowe, for the past eight or nine years had been having recurring dizzy spells associated with nausea and vomiting. During the attack everything whirled about him. He could not lie on the left side or on the back of the head. The attacks averaged about two a year. There was some tinnitus in both ears. At the onset of his trouble, attacks appeared almost daily for over a month, gradually disappearing. Other spells lasted only a few days, but they were fearful, and he lived in terror of their reappearance. The whirling objects continued with his eyes shut, but not so severely. Between attacks he was well in every way. Hearing was not impaired and there were no headaches. The results of the physical and neurologic examinations were negative in every respect. Hearing tests were normal in both ears. Caloric tests gave normal response in both ears.

Although pseudo-Meniere's attacks are usually considered to be of hyterical origin, Politzer suggested that in some cases the organic evidence of disturbed hearing may be late in appearing. The analysis of my cases might seem to give support to this view for in three cases the loss of hearing (subjective) was not observed until long after the onset of the dizzy attacks. In the foregoing case, however, the attacks have been present for eight or nine years — far longer than the hearing-free interval in any of my cases. The patient did not have any unilateral manifestations during the attack except that he could not lie on the left side or back of the head. Such a history would seem to preclude a hysterical attack. It is hardly possible that dizziness of this type could be simulated. Moreover, the patient is a practical, placid and unemotional person.

The following report is from the most severe case of dizziness in my experience and differed from all others.

Edema (Encephalitis [?]) of Cerebellum Producing Extreme and Unremitting Dizziness, Also Severe Nausea and Vomiting. History.—A well nourished woman, aged forty-three, was referred by Dr. Harry Slack of Baltimore. For three weeks, she had been bedfast with dizziness which was almost constantly present. It was least when she was on her back; became greatly intensified with every movement of the head to either side. Any attempt to raise the head off the pillow instantly brought on such intense dizziness that the patient feared she would pass into coma. She was almost always nauseated and vomited many times. This illness came on suddenly, and without any antecedent illness or infection. She complained of a feeling of pressure in the suboccipital region.

Examination. The results of the physical and neurologic examinations were normal. There was no ataxia or nystagmus. There was no disturbance of hearing in either ear. Caloric tests gave a normal response on both sides. Cervical rigidity was not noted. The temperature was never elevated. The leukocyte count was 13,400 and 15,800. Lumbar puncture was performed hesitatingly. The pressure was subnormal, the fluid dripping only slowly; the rate of flow was not increased by jugular compression. Examination of the spinal fluid was negative; there were 3 cells and no globulin. The Wassermann reaction of the blood and spinal fluid was negative. The eyegrounds had been closely watched. but always seemed normal until the last four days, when the veins became definitely fuller; the disk margins were unchanged.

Course. All forms of medical therapy proved unavailing. The patient's condition was rapidly growing worse, presumably because of the ability to take food.

Operation. On March 17, 1927, a bilateral cerebellar exploration was finally performed because the subjective localized pressure sensation and the type and severity of dizziness made this localization seem most probable. The dura was exceedingly tight. The cisterna magna—a good index of pressure in the posterior cranial fossa—was obliterated. The tonsils of the cerebellum had herniated into the spinal canal completely filling the foramen magnum. To liberate them, the dura was split in the midline to the atlas. The lateral ventricle was tapped in an effort to decrease the pressure, but there was no hydrocephalus. The cerebellar lobes were equal in size and looked alike; both appeared much smaller than normal. There was no apparent cause of the great pressure. There was no surface appearance of a tumor, and the short duration of such fulminating symptoms seemed to make the presence of a tumor unlikely. An extended search was not made for a tumor. There was no evidence of an inflammatory process. It was difficult to close the muscles owing to the pressure. A bilateral cerebellar decompression remained and constituted the only therapy resulting from the operation. The dizziness at once disappeared and had not returned one year after operation. It is also noteworthy that after the operation the patient could lie in any position without inducing dizziness.

Comment. The swelling of the cerebellum was undoubtedly due to edema, but the cause of the edema remains obscure. A few months after the operation the decompression was soft and did not protrude. The swelling of the brain, therefore, must have subsided. If a tumor had been present, the decompression would have become progressively tighter. Perhaps in the absence of any recognizable cause the lesion may be considered a form of encephalitis. The cerebellar edema does not suggest in any way angioneurotic edema described by Oppenheim as a not uncommon cause of Meniere's disease. The absence of increased pressure by spinal puncture was due to the fact that the cerebellar tonsils had filled the foramen magnum and prevented the transmission of cranial pressure. The symptoms in this case differ from Meniere's disease in the constancy of the symptoms and the absence of attacks with associated deafness. They differ from pseudo-Meniere's also in the absence of attacks. The symptoms are associated with organic cerebellar lesions, which will be considered shortly.

MENIERE'S ATTACKS DUE TO A LOCALIZED LESION ON THE AUDITORY NERVE

That attacks with the characteristic symptoms and signs of Meniere's disease may be due to a localized lesion involving the auditory nerve is shown by the following case report:

History. A rather feeble woman, aged sixty-six, was seen in consultation with Dr. Leslie Gay of Baltimore. Her first symptoms were gradually progressive deafness and tinnitus of the left ear (the right ear was almost deaf from an old infection during childhood). One year later she was suddenly and without warning seized with a terrific attack of dizziness during which there was nausea and repeated vomiting. The room seemed to jump around, the bed to tilt up and the walls to move in every direction. There was no definite revolving sensation. The attack lasted about thirty minutes. Brief spells of much the same character have since occurred almost daily. Any quick movement will induce dizziness. The deafness varied greatly from time to time. Tinnitus was constant in the left ear. Her eyesight became so poor that she could not read. She never had headache. Her systolic blood pressure varied greatly during Dr. Gray's observations over a period of several months. Usually it ran from 160 to 190, but has been as low as 110. Her hands and feet were swollen at times, even when in bed; at other times, the swelling was absent.

One month before operation her symptoms became much more severe. Roaring was nearly always present throughout the head, and was often referred to both ears. The hearing became much worse. Her gait was unsteady and uncertain. The left corneal reflex was diminished.

Caloric response on affected side was normal. Irrigations started mild attacks of dizziness and nausea.

The audiometer test showed 63.5 per cent loss of hearing in the right ear (old deafness), and 65 per cent loss in the left (affected side).

Operation. On Nov. 22, 1927, a section of the left auditory nerve was performed. An aneurysm was found under the eighth nerve. It was traced downward and was continuous with the vertebral artery. Two days after operation, the old noises returned. One week later, it was noted that she could not lie on the left side (nerve cut on this side) for any length of time because nausea and vomiting would start, but dizziness had not been present since operation. The patient's condition became slowly worse and the noises became unbearable. She was unable to stand. Three weeks later, the left vertebral artery was tied in the neck. At the same operation, the right vertebral artery was exposed and pinched between the blades of the forceps; death resulted apparently simultaneously and instantly.

Immediate release of the forceps was unavailing.

This case is presented as an illustration of a tumor (aneurysm) pressing on the eighth nerve and giving symptoms which, until later neurologic symptoms appeared, did not seem different from those of true Meniere's disease. It will be noted also that the basilar aneurysm was so situated that the vestibular function was not affected, at least as indicated by caloric tests. The case also illustrates the fact that a primary lesion of the semicircular canals or of the cochlea is not necessary for the induction of attacks of the Meniere's type; and that a lesion of the nerve itself and more specifically of the cochlear branch alone can cause them. I am reminded of the analogy with trigeminal or glossopharyngeal neuralgia, in either of which, in their usual form, a satisfying cause is not demonstrable; but occasionally a cerebellopontile tumor causes identically the same paroxysmal ticlike pains.

In this case, moreover, the dizzy spells which were present daily before the operation appeared to stop just as abruptly and as completely after section of the eighth nerve as in the cases of Meniere's disease. It is also worthy of note that noises referred to the ear did not cease. In fact they became distressing and almost unbearable. Noises, therefore, must at times at least, have an explanation other than by the nerve transmission.

Another point is brought out in the analysis of the symptoms of this case i.e., that while at first the onset of the attacks was abrupt without warning and not due to postural change, at a later date attacks of dizziness, nausea and vomiting were brought on by quick movements of the head. In other words, the real difference, if any, between the dizziness in the attacks of Meniere's and that of tumors in the cerebellum and brain stem, need not be great, for one type of dizziness can seemingly merge into the other and either may be induced by the same lesion.

OTHER TYPES OF DIZZINESS FROM KNOWN LESIONS

In order to compare the dizziness during an attack of Meniere's disease with that associated with other known lesions of the brain, and to determine if possible the significance of differing kinds of dizziness, the analysis in Table II has been made.

It will be seen that seven of these lesions are located in the posterior cranial fossa; only one was found in the right temporal and occipital lobes. It was formerly my impression that if severe dizziness, nausea and vomiting are induced or greatly accentuated when the position of the head is changed, or if the patient is practically unable to lie with the head in certain positions, the lesion, whatever its character, is probably located in the posterior cranial fossa. The fact that this is not absolutely true is shown by case 8 in which the lesion is exclusively cerebral, but there is no doubt that tumors and other lesions in this general region produce dizziness as a symptom much more profoundly and in much more distressing form than tumors located in the cerebral hemisphere.

I had hoped that such a startling symptom as the inability to lie on one side without starting dizziness or without making it worse and the relative or complete immunity from dizziness by lying on the other side might prove to be a valuable localizing sign, or at least indicate the side of the lesion. But this does not appear to be true. From the patients in whom this character of the dizziness has been analyzed and checked with the strictly unilateral lesions, it will be seen that three could lie with comfort on the side of the lesion but could not lie on the contralateral side; and five (one cerebral) could lie in comfort on the contralateral but not on the ipsolateral side. One must, therefore, conclude that this symptom has no importance in deciding the side of the lesion. I believe, however, that this type of dizziness is a most important indication that an organic lesion — a tumor or inflammatory process — does exist in or on the cerebel-

TABLE II

ANALYSIS SHOWING DIFFERENT KINDS OF DIAGNOSIS IN MENIERE'S DISEASE

Patient	Location of Tumor	Kind of Tumor	Patient Can Lie in Comfort on		Dizziness Made Worse by Lying on the			Does Movement of Head Precipitate Dizziness	Do Objects Turn	Does Patient Seem to Turn	Is Onset of Dizziness Sudden or Gradual	Are Attacks Accompanied by			Caloric Test	Hearing	Remarks
			Opposite Side	Side of Lesion	Side of Lesion	Opposite Side	Back					Tinnitus	Nausea	Vomiting			
1	Aneurysm of basilar artery	Aneurysm	+	No	+	Improved	No	Yes	...	...	Sudden	+ Later became roaring and on other side (to lesser extent)	+	+	Normal	65% loss, but varies from day to day	Cutting auditory nerve stopped dizzy spells, but did not stop tinnitus and old noises in ear; diminution of left corneal reflex; blood pressure varies from 110 to 190; gait finally became unsteady, though unaffected at first
2	Left lobe of cerebellum to the left of the center	Sarcoma	+	No	+	Improved	No	Yes	...	...	...	...	0	0	Normal	Normal	Tended to fall to right in attacks (i.e., to opposite side)
3	Right lobe and vermis	Glioma	+	No	+	Improved	...	Yes	...	...	...	...	...	...	Normal	Loss equal on both sides	Tended to fall and stagger to the right
4	Right cerebellopontine angle and lobe	Glioma	No	+	Improved	+	+	Yes	No	No	Sudden	No	...	...	...	Total deafness in right ear	Dizziness was described as a swimming sensation, objects did not move; raising head off pillow brought on dizziness; total deafness of right ear
5	Right extra-cerebellar	Sarcoma	No	+	Improved	+	...	Yes	...	...	...	No	No	No	Normal	Normal	Tended to fall to the right
6	Left cerebellar lobe	Small tubercle 1.5 by 1.5 cm.	No	+	Improved	+	+	Yes	...	...	...	No	+	+	...	Normal	Unable to turn off left side for five weeks; staggered toward the right; necropsy showed no other tubercles in brain
7	Right cerebellopontine angle	Gumma	No	+	+	Improved	+	Yes	+	0	Sudden	+ Right ear, never left	+	+	Normal	Both ears affected equally	
8	Right temporal and occipital lobes	Cyst with intracystic angioma	No	+	No	No	No	Yes	+	...	Sudden	No	No	No	Normal	Normal	

lum or brain stem and possibly certain parts of the cerebral hemispheres. Dizziness does not seem to be different whether tumors are within or without the brain stem and cerebellum. When dizziness is present, there does not appear to be any special feature to differentiate that in Meniere's disease from the dizziness associated with tumors of the cerebellum and brain stem, or perhaps of the cerebral hemisphere. In any of these conditions objects or even the person may move; and in either case change in position of the head may increase the dizziness. On the whole, the dizziness, nausea and vomiting are much more fulminating and profound in Meniere's disease. Moreover, Meinere's is characterized by "attacks" and in the free interval the patient is almost symptom free; whereas from tumors a more or less chronic state of dizziness exists, or at least the patient remains in a potential dizzy state. In true Meniere's disease there is an associated loss of function of the auditory nerve, and this does not obtain in tumors unless this nerve is directly compressed as was true in two of the foregoing cases or in occasional cases of cerebellopontile tumors.

It is in the cases of direct involvement of the auditory nerve by tumors that the differential diagnosis from Meniere's disease becomes more difficult. In the later stages of a tumor's growth there are other signs of pressure and of contiguous nerve ininvolvement making the diagnosis easy, but in the earlier stages these manifestations are absent. In neither of the two cases just mentioned were there signs of pressure or of implication of other cranial nerves. On the other hand, in one of the reported cases of Meniere's there was a positive Romberg sign and a diminished corneal reflex, both presumptive signs of a tumor, but a tumor was not present. In another case there was a positive Babinski sign and ankle clonus on the side of the deafness, but seemingly neither was significant. One of the important features of the operation here described is that a tu-

mor if present will be disclosed and if not present the only alternate diagnosis would seem to be Meniere's disease; and for this section of the eighth nerve is the rational treatment.

At times one is confronted by Meniere's disease affecting the only good ear. A case in point was seen by me several months ago and was recently explored. There was some variation from the usual story of Meniere's disease in that the hearing varied greatly from time to time, often suddenly and without apparent explanation. On the chance that a gross lesion might account for this phase of the symptoms — the basilar aneurysm heretofore referred to gave a similar story and was in fact the only case of either series with such variation in hearing — the nerve was explored but there was no tumor. Since it did not seem justifiable to sacrifice his hearing, the auditory nerve was not divided.

In one of the patients from this series, the vestibular and cochlear branches of the auditory nerve were separate and distinct; such an anatomic variation would lend itself to division of the vestibular nerve without injuring the cochlear nerve and the hearing. Even when the two branches are inseparable, an artificial though necessarily inaccurate division should easily be possible with preservation of at least the major part of the cochlear branch. Such a procedure was contemplated but was not carried out in the patient who was deaf in the other ear. Perhaps it may yet be advisable though there is no precedent on which a cure could be assured. Other experiences have shown how sensitive the auditory nerve is to trauma and even though the injury seems slight, the hearing never returns. An artificial cleavage between the two branches of the nerve, if attempted, must, therefore, be made with the least possible trauma.

IS MENIERE'S DISEASE "AURAL" VERTIGO?

Grouping of symptoms into a syndrome without an underlying pathologic basis always carries much uncertainty and a burden of proof. On the one hand, it is possible that the same symptoms may be attributed to different causes and on the other hand, different symptoms may have the same underlying cause. It is difficult to know on the basis of what particular symptoms cases may be included or excluded from Meniere's disease.

Apparently no case of Meniere's disease in its chronic form has been subjected to careful pathologic studies after death. This being true it is permissible to doubt that Meniere's disease is really "aural vertigo." There are certain data which at least make it probable that a lesion of the semicircular canals is not the cause. It cannot be reasoned that the lesion is primary in the semicircular canals because movements of the head stimulate dizziness. The examples, par excellence, that dizziness need not be from this source are given in the cases of dizziness due to verified tumors of the brain and allied lesions in the cases already reported. In these cases changes in posture induce dizziness and here the semicircular canals are known not to be involved. Probably stimulation of the semicircular canals induces the dizziness, but the source of the stimulus is elsewhere. It is known to be at a distance and in the nervous pathways, i. e., the cerebellum, brain stem and auditory nerves. These pathways together with the internal ear form a system which when working properly controls equilibrium, and when disturbed induces dizziness. That the semicircular canals do not harbor the primary lesion of Meniere's disease is also strongly indicated by the fact that in one third of the cases reported in my series there was no appreciable alteration of vestibular function as tested by the caloric reaction. I have not felt justified in using other tests of presumed vestibular function, such as the rotation experiments, because of the patient's great dread of inducing attacks.

On the other hand, it may be reasoned that the cases of so-called pseudo-Meniere's disease are precisely like those of true Meniere's except that unilateral deafness is absent, and that in these cases the primary lesion is probably in the semicircular canals and not in the cochlea. Against this argument is the absence of any change in the caloric reactions in the foregoing case. Cases in which there is loss of vestibular function with cochlear function unimpaired have not yet been demonstrated. However, in the absence of positive objective evidence, the location of the offending lesion cannot be assumed.

On the other hand, since in six of nine cases of true Meniere's disease there is loss of both vestibular and cochlear functions, it seems more reasonable to expect the lesion — in these cases at least — to be primary in the nerve itself rather than in the peripheral end-organs. Given the objective evidence of unilateral deafness without vestibular alteration, there are only two possible sources of the offending lesion, namely, the cochlear nerve of the cochlear end-organ. For practical purposes, the exact location does not matter. Section of the acoustic nerve should produce the same result in either point of origin. It is not improbable that the character and location of the cause may not always be the same.

COMPARISON OF MENIERE'S DISEASE WITH TIC DOULOUREUX AND EPILEPSY

In the symptomatic expression of Meniere's disease one is strongly reminded of other human ills, such as trigeminal neuralgia, glossopharyngeal neuralgia, and possibly of epilepsy. In all there is the same periodicity of attacks, coming on without warning and without apparent cause — all suggesting lesions of nerves or of nerve tracts or systems. In cases of neuralgia, the symptoms remain confined to the domain of the affected nerve, but in epilepsy whole systems, i.e., those controlling consciousness, motor and sensory function, speech, taste and others, may be and usually are involved by the spread of the stimuls. It has been learned from experiments on animals that any cerebral defect is a potential source of epilepsy; that although the cells of the motor cortex are responsible for the remarkable phenomenon of clonic convulsions, lesions of the connecting fibers even far removed from the motor cortex, may induce attacks of precisely the same general character as when the motor cortex is involved directly. Are not Meniere's attacks in reality like seizures of epilepsy (or of trigeminal or glossopharyngeal neuralgia) differing only in that a different part of the nervous system is affected? In either case any defect in the nerve circuit is always a locus minoris resistentiae removing the inhibition which holds functions under control and permitting their explosion as it were. It may be asked whether such a comparison of Meniere's disease with epilepsy is justified because in the former there is always a progressive objective loss of function (hearing). In cases of epilepsy there may or may not be progressing loss of function; the actual result depending on the character of the underlying cause; but regardless of the kind of lesion the expression of the convulsion is just the same. The same is true of trigeminal or glossopharyngeal neuralgia. The characteristic ticlike pain is precisely the same whether a tumor is the offending cause or whether the cause escapes the present inadequate tests.

It is useless to speculate further concerning the character of the leison causing Meniere's disease, or its precise location within the limits just defined. Frankl-Hochwart mentioned leukemia, syphilis, rheumatism and trauma as predisposing causes and reported cases to support this statement. Recently I saw a patient (not included in this report) afflicted with Meniere's disease and with proved syphilis of the nervous system. In none of the nine cases in this report has there been any of the predisposing causes mentioned by Frankl-Hochwart. The uniform absence of a history of otitis media or of mastoid infection or of a positive Wassermann reaction from the blood is worthy of note.

It would seem that the treatment in cases of true Meniere's disease by section of the eighth nerve has precisely the same rationale as section of the sensory root of the trigeminal or glossopharyngeal nerves in tic douloureux. If the attacks begin either in the eighth nerve or in the cochlea — and they begin in one or the other — and if the lesion is strictly unilateral, impulses can no longer be transmitted after section of the nerve. It is then hardly conceivable that future attacks are possible after section of the eighth nerve. Moreover, since section of the nerve is central to the ganglionic cells in the semicircular canals and cochlea, regrowth of the nerve and recurrence of the attacks should be precluded. If these impressions and deductions are correct, section of the eighth nerve should serve as a therapeutic test of Meniere's disease just as section of the trigeminal sensory root or of the glossopharyngeal nerve are tests for tic douloureux of these nerves.

SUMMARY AND CONCLUSIONS

1. Intracranial section of the affected eighth nerve is suggested as a cure for Meniere's disease. This operation has been performed on nine patients, none of whom has had a subsequent attack. The elapsed time since operation varies from three months to three and one-half years.

2. The operation should be attended by no mortality and with no after-effects, since the patients are practically deaf in the affected ear before operation.

3. Although the series of cases is small, the results suggest that section of the acoustic nerve should stop Meniere's attacks just as absolutely as intracranial section of the glossopharyngeal nerve or of the sensory root of the trigeminus stops the attacks of tic douloureux in these two nerves.

4. The symptoms and signs of Meniere's disease are analyzed. The dizziness of Meniere's and pseudo-Meniere's diseases are compared with that of other known lesions — tumors, inflammations and aneurysms — in the cerebellum and brain stem.

5. There appear to be reasons to doubt that the cause of Meniere's disease is primary in the semicircular canals. A primary lesion of the acoustic nerve seems a more primary source of the attacks.

REFERENCES

[1]Aboulker, H.: Pathogenesis and Surgical Treatment of Meniere's Disease. *Presse med., 35:* 1412, 1927.

[2]Barany, in Lewandowsky: *Handbuch der Neurologie.* Berlin, Julius Springer, 1912, vol. 3, p. 817.

[3]Cassirer, in Lewandowsky: *Handbuch der Neurologie,* 1914, vol. 5, p. 265.

[4]Charcot: *Progres med.,* Jan. 1874, nos. 4 and 5 Dec., 1875, no. 50.

[5]Dandy, W. E.: Section of the Sensory Root of the Trigeminal Nerve at the Pons. Preliminary Report of the Operative Procedure. *Bull. Johns Hopkins Hosp., 36:* 2, 1925.

[6]Dandy, W. E.: Glossopharyngeal Neuralgia (Tic Douloureux); Its Diagnosis and Treatment. *Arch. Surg., 15:* 198 (Aug.) 1927.

[7]Frankl-Hochwart: Der menieresche Symptomenkomplex, in Nothnagel: *Specialle, Pathologie und Therapie,* 1897, vol. 2, p. 11.

[8]Frazier, C. H.: Intracranial Division of the Auditory Nerve for Persistent Tinnitus. *J. A. M. A., 61:* 5, 327 (Aug. 2) 1913.

[9]Frazier, C. H.: Intracranial Division of the Auditory Nerve for Persistent Aural Vertigo. *Surg. Gynec. & Obst., 15:* 524 (Nov.) 1912.

[10]Gruber: *Lehrbuch der Ohrenheilkunde,* Vienna, 1870, p. 617.

[11]Hautant: *Arch. internat. d'laryngol. otol. rhinol., 28:* 781, 1922.

[12]Leo, H.: *Contribution a l'histoire de la maladie de Meniere.* These, Paris, 1876.

[13]Meniere, M.: Sur une forme particuliere de surdite grave dependant d'une lesion de l'oreille interne. *Gazz. med. de Paris, 16:* 29, 1861.

[14]Meniere, M.: Nouveaux documents relatifs aux lesions de l'oreille interne characterisees par des symptoms de congestion cerebral apoplectiforme. *Gazz. med. de Paris, 16:* 239, 379 and 597, 1861.

[25]Meniere, M.: Maladies de l'oreille interne offrant les symptoms de la congestion cerebral apoplectiforme. *Gazz. med. de Paris, 16:* 29, 55 and 68,

[16]Meniere, M.: *Bull. Acad. de med.,* Paris, 26: 241, 1861.

[17]Nave, F.: *Die Meiniere'sche Krankeit.* Inaug. Diss., Braslau, 1877.

[18]Oppenheim, cited by Cassirer in Lewandowski: *Handbuch der Neurologie,* vol. 5.

[19]Politzer: *Arch. f. Ohrenh.,* 1865, p. 88.

[20]Portmann, G.: Le traitment chirurgical des vertiges par l'ouverture du sac endolymphatique. *Presse med., 34:* 1635, 1926.

[21]Voltolini: *Monatschr. f. Ohrenh.,* 1869, p. 109.

XXX

ARTERIOVENOUS ANEURYSM OF THE BRAIN*

The intracranial arteriovenous aneurysms here described are not peculiar to the brain. With the exception of differences of detail due to environment, they are essentially the same as arteriovenous aneurysms situated elsewhere in the vascular system.

The discovery of an arteriovenous aneurysm is always credited to William Hunter.[1] Enthusiastic phlebotomists of that period prepared two perfect examples of arteriovenous aneurysm for Hunter, which he was quick to recognize. His description of the signs and symptoms left little to be added, even at the present time. At the point of the communication between the artery and the vein, he recognized a loud hissing murmur and a strong tremulous thrill; large tortuous venous sacs were seen to pulsate; the brachial artery was greatly enlarged and serpentine cephalad to the arteriovenous fistula, but distal to it, the artery became smaller than on the other side. He was able to reduce the size of the veins, stop their pulsation and eliminate both the murmur and the thrill by pressing on a localized spot, which he recognized to be the opening between the artery and the vein. It was Hunter who first suggested the term "anastomosis" to denote the union of the two vessels.

To arteriovenous aneurysms of traumatic origin have since been added a great group with precisely the same clinical features, but in which the characteristic vascular changes have been present since birth. Virchow[2] referred to cases of Krause (Wm.) and Breschet as demonstrating beyond doubt the congenital origin of such cases. He also mentioned a case which Langier watched during the patient's life and in which he performed dissection after the patient's death; a free communication was found between the posterior auricular artery and a nearby vein. There are now many cases in which dissections of these aneurysms at operation or necropsy have demonstrated communication between a large artery and a contiguous vein by one or more aberrant vessels which could have arisen only as errors of vascular development in the embryo. In recent years, remarkable examples of these anomalous congenital communications in the neck and extremities, as disclosed at operation, have been reported by Halsted,[3] Rienhoff[4] and Reid.[5]

Finally, there is a third group of cases in which an arteriovenous communication is established through the medium of a mass of abnormal vessels which take the place of the usual capillary bed, erroneously known as angiomas because of the impression that they are new growths; the true character of these lesions has long been obscured. The component vessels may be atypically arterial or venous, or both may be combined. Virchow discussed these tumors at length, and with some hesitation classified them under the heading "angioma racemosum arteriale." The following excerpt from his "Krankhaften Geshwulste" shows his grasp of the real underlying pathologic process:

Finally there remains that form of angioma, in which the vascular enlargement is outspoken and in which the character of the tumor is more in the background. Many of these forms are not to be understood in the light of oncology. They are often classified with angiomata and one cannot make a true line of demarcation between them and angiomata. Their difference lies principally in the fact that the process is diffuse, and that dilatation of both arteries and veins is present. These tumors have recently been called by

*Reprinted from the *Archives of Surgery, 17:* 190-243, August, 1928.

301

John Bell aneurysma per anastomosin, and by Walker perhaps better, aneurysma anastomoseon.

Another group of vascular tumors so well known, even at the present time, as angioma cavernosum, were included by Bell under his aneurysms per anastomosin. Virchow referred to Dupuytren's experiments to prove that in these tumors injections of colored substance passed freely from the artery into the veins through the intermediary tumor. Virchow, though not conceding the arteriovenous communication, noted the fact that in some cases of cavernous angiomas (venous tumors) the artery is dilated and tortuous just as in true arteriovenous aneurysms.

It was Virchow's view that these arteriovenous aneurysms (or angiomas) were not new growths in the usual sense, but were of congenital derivation. Subsequent embryologic and pathologic researches demonstrated that no other explanation is tenable.

Professor Halsted,[3] whose interest in this subject extended over a period of several years, and who stimulated the splendid researches and publications of Callender,[6] Reid,[5] Holman[7] and Reinhoff,[4] approached the origin of arteriovenous aneurysms from the vascular anlage in the early embryo. It is known that the adult system of arteries and veins is derived from a general capillary network; that both arteries and veins form from this capillary network; that the final arterial and venous systems are derived by extensive evolution of a vastly different primitive system. This metamorphosis is accomplished by shifting, consolidating and eliminating not only capillaries but even the great venous and arterial trunks of the early embryo. It is evident that the retention of the original vascular connections between arteries and veins will readily explain the origin of the adult arteriovenous aneurysms. Dr. Halsted had in mind the arteriovenous aneurysm with aberrant congenital connecting channels. But it would seem that the maldevelopment of the original vascular bed would similarly explain the nests of abnormal vessels which are interposed between the arteries and veins and which replace the normal capillary bed.

Arteriovenous fistulas of traumatic origin are practically impossible in the brain, because the principal arteries and veins are not in juxtaposition as are the vessels of the head, neck and extremities. Arteriovenous aneurysms between the internal carotid artery and the cavernous sinus are exceedingly common, but as they are really outside the cranial chambers, and as they are in point of origin rather laws unto themselves, they need not be considered here. They are dependent on an anatomic arrangement which is not duplicated anywhere in the body. As the internal carotid arteries traverse the cavernous sinus in their passage through the base of the skull, a traumatic rupture of one of the arteries by a fracture of the base of the skull must inevitably result in an arteriovenous fistula, unless or until the arterial opening is repaired. The nomenclature of lesions which should really be included under arteriovenous aneurysms is most confusing. Being so dependent on the personal equation for the interpretation, they are reported under many titles, i.e., angioma cavernosum, varix aneurysmaticus, angioma arteriale racemosum, angioma plexiforme, aneurysma cirsoidea, aneurysma serpentina, aneurysma anastomotica, arteriovenous aneurysm, tumor cirsoidius, and particularly by the Germans as Rankenangiom — a term first applied by Virchow. Reinhoff[4] suggested a simple and sensible revision of the nomenclature of all vascular dilatation and communications into (1) venous, (2) arterial and (3) arteriovenous aneurysms, thereby discarding the term hemangioma as least for major lesions. This classification meets my full approval. In the group of arteriovenous aneurysms, the various terms "cavernous," "racemose," "cirsoid" and "serpentine," whether applied to arteries or veins, are merely descriptive of a superficial expression of a lesion and not of the fundamental pathologic process. A long as the term hemanigioma is employed when an arteriovenous connection exists, there must always be uncertainty as to whether the tumor is arterial or venous. As a matter of fact, they may be either or both, but regardless of these superficial differences there is a direct communication through the vascular abnormality which has replaced the normal capillary bed. Moreover, the outward expression of an arteriovenous aneurysm, i.e., the arterial tortuosity and dilatation and the engorgement of the veins leaving the tumor, are doubtless identical whether the communicating channels are exclusively arterial or venous or predominantly one or the other.

In attempting to gather the cases of arteriovenous aneurysms of the brain, the records of venous aneurysms and the various subdivisions of angiomas have been reviewed, and most of them have been collected from these groups. For example, there is no more perfect example of an arteriovenous aneurysm than the one pictured in Krause's colored plate,[8] but which he calls a venous angioma. On the other hand, cases reported as Rankenangioma and cirsoid aneurysma, and therefore presumably arteriovenous aneurysms, have been excluded from this group because the absence of changes in the arteries and veins leading to and from the tumor has suggested a pure venous lesion. Other cases reported as venous, which undoubtedly seem to be arteriovenous, are those of Astwazaturoff,[9] Steinheil,[10] Durck, Kalischer,[11] Muhsam,[12] Eiselberg,[13] Campbell and Ballance[14] and others. Doubtless the teaching of Oppenheim and Krause was in large part responsible for the interpretation of these vascular lesions as venous.

FREQUENCY OF ARTERIOVENOUS ANEURYSMS OF THE BRAIN

The first arteriovenous aneurysm of the brain was reported by Steinheil[10] in 1895, or 138 years after William Hunter's[1] first reported arteriovenous aneurysms in the arm.

A total of twenty-two cases which seemed to represent this type of intracranial aneurysm have been collected from the available records. Two additional cases of Struppler[15] and Simmonds[16] (second case) have been included, though the status of both is doubtful because the description of the venous outlets is inadequate. Several cases heretofore classified as cases of angioma, and usually assumed to be similar to those collected here, have been excluded. Among them are the cases of Oppenheim,[17] Sweasey-Powers,[18] Lewandowsky and Selberg,[19] Cassirer and Muhsam,[20] Uyematsu,[21] Creite, Abrikosoff,[22] Lechner,[23] Verse,[24] Rossolimo[25] and Bruns. It has also not been possible to include the cases of Isenschmid,[26] because neither observations made at operation nor those made at autopsy establish the clinical diagnosis. In one of his cases at least, the diagnosis is almost surely correct for, in addition to a well defined extracranial arteriovenous aneurysm, Jacksonian epileptic attacks were of long standing. The symptoms that I have considered essential for the diagnosis of an arteriovenous aneurysm have been, first and foremost, marked fulness and enlargement of the veins of exit; second, an increased size and tortuosity of the artery entering the snarled mass of vessels. Without the enlarged veins on the cortex or elsewhere one cannot assume the existence of an arteriovenous fistula.

The seeming infrequency of this lesion cannot be judged by the small number of cases assembled from the literature. Were this true, the lesion would be rare indeed. The eight cases which occurred at the Johns Hopkins Hospital among about 600 cases of verified tumors of the brain during a period of five years, are perhaps a better index of its relative frequency. In clinics on which neurologic material is concentrated, arteriovenous aneurysms apparently occur in from about 0.5 to 1 per cent of the cases. It is clear that more cases will be disclosed at operation than at necropsy, because the symptoms (usually epilepsy) are not such as to require prolonged hospitalization. Most of the necropsies were obtained on patients who were brought to the hospital in coma resulting from cerebral hemorrhage. This number obviously represents but a small proportion of the afflicted persons.

CASES OF INTRACRANIAL ARTERIOVENOUS ANEURYSM

Case 1. *History.*—A well nourished, well built, muscular man, aged fifty-two, an army officer, was suddenly and without warning seized with a severe clonic convulsion lasting about fifteen minutes. This attack occurred six years prior to examination, just after his return from France, where he actively participated in the World War. He had never had any kind of an attack before. For the next three years similar attacks occurred about once every two months; then for two years there was no attack, but for the past year they have appeared about every month. Recently, there have been petit mal attacks with loss of consciousness for from forty to sixty seconds, but no muscular contractions. One week ago he had a violent generalized headache; following this, a pain persisted in the right frontal region. His head turned to the left during the convulsions, but there was no other focal sign. At times he had had a dull aching pain in the fingers of the left hand and had complained of some stiffness in this arm. The attacks usually occurred in the early morning. He has had some trouble with his memory; he said that he often forgot most important things.

Examination.—A tenderness to deep pressure was revealed over the right parietal region. The patient said that there was a localized sore spot in this region (not over the tumor as later discovered). The neurologic examination did not reveal anything. The eyegrounds were normal. The roentgenogram of the head was negative. The Wassermann reaction of the blood was negative.

While he was in the hospital, an attack was observed by the nurse, but focal signs other than by turning the head to the left were not seen. Urine was lost. Motor weakness did not follow the attack.

The injection of air into the cerebral ventricles showed dislocation of the ventricular system to the left side. The third ventricle was also bent obliquely to the left. The anterior horn of the right ventricle was smaller than the left. A diagnosis of right frontal tumor was made.

Operation.—Right craniotomy was performed. A group of tremendous engorged and tortuous veins covered the anterior half of the right temporal lobe, and to a much lesser extent the frontal lobe. They emptied into a huge sylvian vein, joined at right angles a large anomalous vein which crossed the frontal lobe in a vertical direction and continued downward across the temporal lobe. There was no well defined rolandic vein. The network of veins dipped over the anterior margin of the temporal lobe, entirely obscuring the anterior pole. The largest venous trunk was over 1 cm. in diameter. The veins were a definite pink and were in striking contrast to the black veins elsewhere in the brain. One could easily see the blood rhythmically (with each heart beat) passing through the dilated thin walls of the veins. On palpation, a distinct thrill could be detected in the veins. Since any attempt to treat the aneurysm surgically appeared to involve a risk greater than my co-workers and I were justified in assuming, the dura was closed and the bone flap was replaced.

Second Operation.—Two weeks later the wound was reopened, the frontal lobe retracted and the inferior surface of the frontal lobe and the anterior pole of the temporal lobe well explored. Search was at once made for an arterial communication. A large anomalous branch passed from the middle cerebral artery (immediately distal to its origin) directly into the mass of engorged serpentine vessels. It was thick-walled and definitely arterial at its origin, but less than 0.5 cm. distally there was an abrupt transition to a thin-walled vein. This vessel was almost as large as the middle cerebral artery at this point. The arterial portion of the vessel was well isolated, surrounded by two silk sutures and ligated. The venous tumor immediately collapsed. We did not see any suggestion of a central tumor mass such as was present in other cases of the series from which the veins emerged. It was our impression that the condition was a pure arteriovenous fistula, produced by an anomalous vessel passing directly from the middle cerebral artery into a large venous trunk, which ultimately reached the sylvian vein. The great veins could be seen to connect with the sylvian vein.

Postoperative Course.—When the patient was coming out from under the effects of the ether, he complained of severe headache and weakness of the contralateral part of the arm and the leg. During the ensuing twenty-four hours, this side slowly became completely paralyzed, and his pulse rate steadily dropped to 60. Since the patient was somewhat drowsy, we suspected an extradural hemorrhage, but elevation of the bone flap did not show any collection of blood. The paralysis puzzled us, for our manipulations were entirely under the frontal lobe, too far afield from the motor tract to cause weakness, and seemingly remote from the middle cerebral artery. If the middle cerebral artery had by some chance been injured, why did the paralysis develop so gradually? We have also wondered whether the drop in the pulse rate might not be similar to the bradycardia noted by Holman as a constant sequel to the closure of arteriovenous fistulas in his series of dogs. Five days after the operation, recovery of function began in the left side and steadily progressed. Still unable to explain the cause of the hemiplegia, it is equally difficult to explain the recovery. Aside from a slight residual weakness of the left arm and hand and a slight limp, the patient was well three and a half years after the operation. Two and a half years after the operation, he had one convulsion; since then there have been no other seizures, either petit or grand mal, nor have there been any headaches or soreness corresponding to the old "localized tender spot." The spells of forgetfulness have disappeared.

Case 2. *History.*—A well nourished, normal looking boy, aged nineteen, sought relief from convulsions (1922). At the age of 15, he was seized with numbness in the left corner of his mouth. A "pricking sensation as of pins and needles" quickly followed and spread over the left side of the face. The tongue was pulled to the left, and it also had a similar "sensation as of pins and needles." The left side of the face twitched. The sensation spread to the left arm, but the arm did not twitch. The attack lasted only about one minute. The hand was weak for several minutes after the attack; consciousness was lost. Five months later,

he was attacked by a convulsion while asleep. He foamed at the mouth, and urine was passed. During the following two months there were four more such attacks, all occurring during sleep, then a free interval of several months.

One year ago, a unilateral (left side) convulsion was not accompanied by loss of consciousness, and similar attacks have since occurred about once a month, always with the warning aura of numbness at the corner of the mouth. There has been only one unconscious spell during the past year; the hand and arm are always weak after such a spell.

Examination.—The results of the examination were negative. There was no objective evidence of motor weakness on the left side. The reflexes were normal and equal on the two sides. The roentgenogram was negative. The Wassermann reaction of the blood was negative. The preoperative diagnosis was probable cerebral tumor causing jacksonian epilepsy. A tumor was suspected because motor weakness followed in the wake of the convulsion.

Operation.—Feb. 11, 1922: Right craniotomy was performed. On the dural side of the bone flap, the inner table of the skull was eroded in a circular area about 1 by 1 cm. The roentgenogram, however, was negative. There was a corresponding localized bulge of the dura. Both abnormalities corresponded with, and were produced by, the underlying bulge in a hugh vein. A remarkable cluster of serpentine veins was concentrated on the surface of the parietal lobe just below the arm area and extending alongside the rolandic vein and the sylvian vein. Both the rolandic and the sylvian vein were tremendously dilated; each was as large as a little finger. The central dilatation in the vein was doubtless close to the maximum point of entry of the arterial circulation. It was about 2.5 by 2.5 cm. in diameter. A cluster of smaller veins of varying size resembled a mass of angle worms. The superficial area of the group of veins was roughly circular (measuring 4.5 by 4.5 cm.) and completely obscured the underlying brain. Running anteriorly from the vascular plexus and then coursing mesially over the frontal lobe into the superior longitudinal sinus was another abnormally large vein, though smaller than the rolandic. The main trunk of the sylvian vein which skirts the upper margin of the temporal lobe and empties into the tranverse sinus was also greatly enlarged.

All of these veins pulsated like arteries. Through the thin walls of the rolandic vein the pulsing, swirling red arterial blood could be seen. The palpating finger could readily detect a thrill, not only in the large veins, but in the serpentine cluster composing the tumor. Everything indicated that the lesion was an arteriovenous aneurysm.

After consultation with the patient's brother, who realized the great danger involved, an attempt was made to extirpate the mass. It was hoped that the surface vessels might be ligated and the tumor undermined and included in a mass dissection of brain tissue, without actually coming in contact with the vessels of the tumor. As this was our first experience with this type of lesion, we little realized its extreme difficulties and dangers. The sylvian vein was tied with two silk ligatures and the vessel divided. We hoped to work through the cortex from this point mesially, but as there was not sufficient room, the line of attack was shifted to the mesial aspect of the tumor. The rolandic vein was doubly tied and divided. A remarkable resistance was encountered in ligating the vein. Usually a vein offers almost no resistance to the sliding knot, but in this instance the knot could be slipped down only step by step because of the pressure within the vein. Ligation and division of the rolandic vein were accomplished without incident. A few minutes later, however, while a subcortical dissection was being performed and preparation was being made to ligate additional vessels, a sudden burst of blood flooded the operative field. The rolandic vein had burst, not at the points of ligature but in the bulge of the vein about midway between the ligatures on its now isolated segment. The closure of the venous outlets had taken away too many of the channels of exit for blood from the tumor and the thin-walled rolandic vein, no longer able to withstand the added extra strain of increasing arterial pressure, burst at its weakest point. The bleeding became profuse. Pressure with cotton and gauze accomplished little more than to check the bleeding temporarily. A rapid extirpation of the mass was at-

tempted, but the bleeding vessels multiplied. There was no cerebral tissue, only a skein of wormlike vessels which bled furiously. The carotid vein was tied in the neck, and while this reduced the bleeding so that tampons of cotton controlled it, shortly afterward the renewed pressure established by collateral again lifted the cotton pack, and the bleeding began anew. When it was again stopped, the patient's condition was so seriously affected that he died a few hours later.

Case 3. *History.*—A healthy looking man, aged thirty-five, was referred by Dr. Ralph Greene, of Jacksonville, Fla., on Jan. 25, 1925, because of a general mental and physical breakdown, headache, double vision, periods of somnolence, slurring speech and staggering gait.

The patient's condition was said to have begun two years before examination with a staggering gait and a tendency to swerve to the left. He said that he would fall to the left any time when his eyes were shut. Diplopia had been present more or less continually for the past two years. Dizziness was frequent and disturbing. A thick slurring speech had been noticed for a month. Headaches had occurred irregularly, but were noticeable when the patient was constipated. There was also pronounced mental impairment with paranoid trend. He was irritable and suspicious and adopted a superior attitude. His insight and judgment were poor. His speech was slurring and he quickly rambled over a number of subjects without cohesion and without meaning. He had formerly studied medicine and apparently did well until he stopped because of a dislike for the subject. His memory was uncertain. Convulsions, loss of consciousness, motor or sensory disturbances or difficulty in swallowing were not noted.

Examination.—The neurologic examination showed bilateral choked disk of 3 diopters in each eye. There were no obvious extra-ocular palsies to explain diplopia; coarse nystagmoid jerks of the eyeballs occurred when the patient looked far to the right or left. There was dysarthria; greatly diminished hearing in the left ear; slight ataxia in the heel to knee test, but not in the finger to nose test; staggering gait; positive Romberg sign, the patient falling constantly to the left and no adiadokokinesis. He walked with a broad base.

There were bilateral positive Babinski and Oppenheim signs; otherwise the reflexes were normal. There were no motor or sensory changes. The Wassermann test of the blood was negative. A roentgenogram of the head was negative.

A tentative diagnosis of cerebellar tumor was made, but the pronounced mental changes were unexplainable.

Ventricular estimation showed both ventricles to be large and in free communication with each other (indigocarmine test). The fluid was under greatly increased pressure.

Operation.—A cerebellar exploratory operation was performed. When the cerebellum was exposed, six large tortuous veins stood out in strong relief about equally on both cerebellar lobes. They converged to two large trunks at the border of the superior surface and dipped

out of sight onto the tentorial surface of the cerebellum. The danger of injury to the unusual veins made it seem inadvisable to attempt to follow the veins on the tentorial surface. Neither a thrill nor arterial pulsation was detected. Exploration of the under surface of the left cerebellar lobe brought into view two remarkable conditions: 1. The whole inferior surface of the cerebellum was covered with a venous sinus completely hiding this part of the cerebellum. 2. The vertebral artery, which usually is small and seen only after a search was much enlarged and displaced outward. It lay alongside as well as under the brain stem. Further inspection could not be made because it was fraught with too much danger. The usual bilateral cerebellar decompression was left to relieve pressure.

After the operation, the occipital region

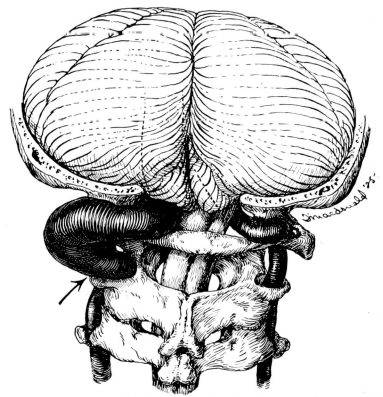

Fig. 1. (case 3). Sketch of aneurysm showing the tremendous vertebral artery on this side. This diagrammatic sketch is intended to show the difference between the vertebral arteries on the two sides. The sketch is not accurate in that the bulge of the artery was between the atlas and the axis, but from the artist's view at the operation it might well have looked as it does. The artery was doubtless also enlarged below this point, though it could not be inspected at the operation.

was examined with a stethoscope. A loud to and fro murmur was heard in front of and back of the ear and over the cerebellar decompression, but it appeared to be just as audible over the right as over the left side.

The impression gained from the operation was that undoubtedly a congenital arteriovenous aneurysm existed between the left vertebral artery and unknown veins.

Second Operation.—Two weeks after the first operation, the left vertebral artery was ligated between the atlas and occiput. The artery was perhaps three times its normal size. It was with great difficulty that it could be surrounded by a ligature and tied. Before the vertebral artery was ligated, the cerebellar wound was bulging and tight; immediately afterward it became soft and somewhat sunken, and remained so during the remainder of the patient's stay of a month in the hospital. A discharge note by Dr. Deryl Hart states that the bruit, formerly heard so strongly over both temples, could be heard only over the right (contralateral) temple. The gait was much improved; the Romberg, Babinski and Oppenheim signs were negative. Subjective diplopia still persisted.

Two and a half years later, the patient wrote that he had remained well and free from headaches, but judging by his letter, there had not been any mental improvement.

Case 4. *History.*—A sparely nourished man, aged forty-seven, was referred by Dr. L. S. Stubbs and Dr. H. W. Curtis, of Newport News, Va., on Oct. 1, 1925, because of frequent jacksonian convulsions and some motor weakness. Six years before this, he was suddenly seized with a cramp in the left hand; this was immediately followed by weakness of the legs, loss of consciousness and a convulsion. He regained consciousness an hour and ten minutes later, but was so weak that he could not leave the bed for three days. A month later, he was seized with an attack similar in origin but less severe; consciousness was lost for only a few minutes. During the next three years, such attacks occurred with fair regularity about every two months. Three years before coming to Dr. Stubbs and Dr. Curtis, he had the first attack in which he was conscious throughout. A cramp

attacked the left hand, causing his hand to close into a fist; the arm quickly became rigid and drew up above the head. He had a sensation of being unable to catch his breath; he thought it grew dark about him, and it seemed as if his heart had stopped beating; profuse perspiration broke out. He thought he was going to die. He thought his left leg was paralyzed, for he could not move it; the muscles of his trunk did not seem to be affected. This attack lasted half an hour, gradually passing away. For the next two years, there were no more attacks (he was taking phenobarbital); then followed an attack like the last one. Since then similar attacks, without loss of consciousness, had occurred at intervals of about two months. After one attack the left arm and leg were paralyzed for half an hour, the function gradually returning. In addition, the left arm steadily became weaker, until it was considerably disabled. There had been only one attack at night, and no petit mal attacks. Severe headaches occurred after the attacks; with these exceptions, he did not have headaches. The attacks appeared to be induced by constipation, but not by exercise or excitement. Phenobarbital was definitely helpful; he ascribed the two years' free interval from attacks to this drug. There was no history of trauma.

Examination.—The neurologic examination showed that there was some motor weakness of the left side of the face and of the left arm, but not of the leg. Sensation was not changed. Biceps and triceps reflexes were markedly increased on the left side. The knee jerks were slightly greater on the left; the Babinski sign was negative. The Wassermann reaction of the blood was negative.

A roentgenogram of the head showed a group of calcified areas in the right frontoparietal region. In the anteroposterior view, these extended almost from the surface to the midline. The shadows were linear and circular, and in one place there was a definite whorl. The shape of these shadows suggested a vascular pattern, and from the roentgen-ray observations alone, a vascular tumor was suspected.

Operation.— On Oct. 3, 1925, a left craniotomy was performed over the region so clearly defined in the roentgenograms. The inner table of the bone was much thinner. These changes of pressure were due to a localized dilatation along the course of a large tortuous cerebral vein in front of and below the face portion of the rolandic area. From this venous center four large tortuous veins radiated as from the hub of a wheel. This venous dilatation was also situated almost in the center of an indurated subcortical mass, sharply defined by palpation and measuring about 5 by 5 cm. The large venous dilatation could be seen to pulsate, and when partially obliterated a thrill was imparted to the palpating finger. At each heart beat, the swirling red (arterial) blood could be seen through the walls of the vein. There seemed no hope of a successful surgical intervention for such a vicious arteriovenous lesion. A subtemporal decompression was made; it remained fairly full and tight after the operation.

Second Operation.—Three weeks later, it was decided to ligate the right common carotid artery. Because of the danger of this procedure at the patient's age, a partial occlusion was first made with a rubber band. Twelve days later, the wound was reopened, the artery was ligated above and below the band, and the intervening tissue (including the band) was excised. There was a rather extensive reaction of all the tissues contiguous to the rubber foreign body. The carotid artery was already completely occluded with firm fibrous tissue within its lumen. It was our impression at the time that this was a satisfactory method of inducing a gradual occlusion of the carotid. It would however, be dangerous if eventual total occlusion of the internal carotid artery could not be tolerated. No untoward symptoms were noted at the time of partial ligation or subsequently when it became total.

When the carotid artery was exposed for ligation, a lumbar puncture was performed, and the height of spinal fluid was measured. On each temporary closure of the carotid artery (to test for possible symptoms of cerebral anemia), the spinal pressure became reduced from 280 to 225 mm. and returned to the previous normal level when the lumen of the carotid artery was again restored. The blood pressure rose from 168 to 175 each time the carotid artery was closed.

For five days after the operation, the decompression was markedly sunken, then becoming flush with the skin.

The convulsions disappeared for more than a year. They then returned in mild form, but after eighteen months had again become like the former attacks.

Case 5. *History.*—A well nourished man, aged forty-eight, was first seen in coma in the medical service of the Johns Hopkins Hospital, on Jan. 21, 1925. During the past ten years, he had had four convulsive seizures with loss of consciousness and with involvement of the left arm and leg. He did not rouse from the attack he had just before his admission to the hospital. He had incontinence of urine and feces, a pulse rate of 44 and rapid, stertorous breathing. Gradually, the coma disappeared. A residual partial hemianesthesia, hemiplegia and homonymous hemianopsia were present on the left side when consciousness was restored. Eventually, all of these signs disappeared almost entirely. Bloody fluid was obtained from several lumbar punctures. He convalesced slowly, and when discharged from the hospital six weeks after the onset of coma, he was mentally confused and forgetful. There was no history of trauma.

Six months later (July, 1925), he had another attack, with unconsciousness, but it lasted only three or four minutes. Shortly afterward, he returned to the hospital for treatment. During the time since his comatose spell he had done some work, but had been morose and gloomy. After dinner he sat alone or went to bed, always shunning company. He was forgetful and at times confused.

Examination.—A slight homonymous defect was found in the left visual field; the left knee jerk was obtained only on reinforcement; the right, not at all. No motor or sensory disturbance remained on the left side. The blood pressure was 125 systolic and 85 diastolic. The Wassermann reaction of the blood was negative.

It was evident that the patient had had a cerebral hemorrhage in the parieto-occipital region. At his age, and with negative vascular signs, it was safe to assume the existence of an underlying tumor or aneurysm from which the hemorrhage had arisen.

A ventriculography showed that in the right postrolandic region there was a great defect which was in free communication with the body of the lateral ventricle. The loss of cerebral tissue was interpreted to be the sequal of the hemorrhage which had occurred seven months before. The actual tumor or aneurysm did not show, but was assumed to be alongside the cerebral defect.

Operation.—On July 21, 1925, a right craniotomy was performed. A plexus of large, tortuous veins obscured the brain just above the sylvian vein and below and posterior to the motor face area. The rolandic vein, which skirted the mass of superficial veins, was two or three times its normal size; the sylvian vein was also much enlarged. This circumscribed mass of veins dipped into the cerebral cortex. Red arterial blood could be seen swirling in the rolandic vein with each heart beat. A thrill could not be felt.

About 1 cm. behind the venous plexus the meninges were transparent in an oval area about 1 by 1.5 cm. A cystlike dome was bulging upward from below. When this was opened, it proved to be the big ventricular dilatation (cerebral defect) indicated by the ventriculograms. The cerebral defect became larger below the surface and was nearly as large as a hen's

egg. Its size was little reduced where it opened into the lateral ventricle.

In the anterior wall of the defect, several small, hard, dark gray nodules, from about 1 to 2 mm. in diameter, protruded into the cavity. Poorly covered by the white matter of the brain, they were recognized as vascular buds and as the outposts of a vascular tumor. Extirpation of the mass seemed possible and was attempted after ligation of the vessels on the surface of the brain. We were not unmindful of our earlier tragic experience in ligating the superficial veins, but this tumor looked far less vicious from the surface. After the tumor was circumvented by ligatures, extirpation was begun from the cyst forward. The cortex was first incised below the tumor in order to get the entering arterial trunks. A dense mass of intertwined serpentine red vessels of more uniform size was encountered.

A detour of the incision was made downward, and in this way the vascular mass was divided. Three fair-sized arteries were isolated near their entrance into the cluster of vessels. After ligation of the arterial supply, the vascular tumor was

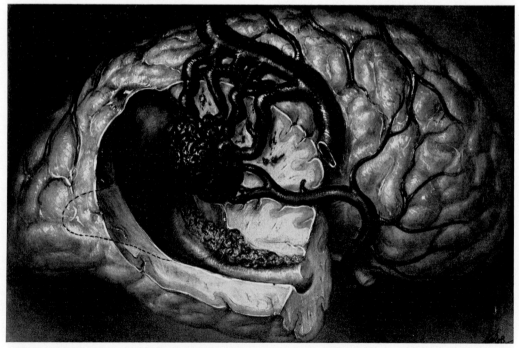

Fig. 2 (case 5).—Reconstruction of arteriovenous aneurysm from the necropsy specimen. The large middle cerebral artery terminates in the mass of vessels—the so-called angioma—whereas on the opposite side the middle meningeal artery continues on posteriorly. The vascular bed protrudes into the defect which has resulted from the cerebral hemorrhage and which communicates freely with the lateral ventricle.

removed without difficulty. Bleeding was entirely stopped when closure was begun. However, despite a prompt recovery from the anesthetic, the patient died six days after the operation from a slowly developing intraventricular hemorrhage. During the operation the opening into the lateral ventricle had been carefully packed to preclude bleeding into it.

Necropsy showed three branches of the left middle cerebral artery clipped at the margin from which the tumor had been excised. Had it not been for the open ventricular system, this patient would surely have survived, for the hemorrhage would have been far less significant and easily handled. Our reasons for excising this tumor were: 1. The tumor was back of the rolandic area, and a hemiparesis could probably be avoided. 2. Owing to the protrusion of the arterial units into the cerebral defect, a cerebral hemorrhage would probably occur again and by flooding the ventricular system cause death.

The middle cerebral arteries of both sides were dissected after death. The right was from one-third to one-half larger, even to its origin at the carotid artery. The affected middle cerebral artery turned upward and terminated in the branches which entered the nest of vessels. The left artery, however, took an entirely different course in this region and for some distance continued backward toward the occipital lobe.

Case 6. *History.*—A well nourished young man, aged thirty-one, complained of loss of vision, progressive weakness of the left arm and leg, headache and convulsions.

The first symptoms of onset, dating back fifteen years, were intermittent spells of blurred vision and headache across the forehead on the right side. These spells occurred once or twice a week. Limitation of vision to either side was not noticed at that time. In 1916, a decompression and puncture of the corpus callosum were performed at the Mayo

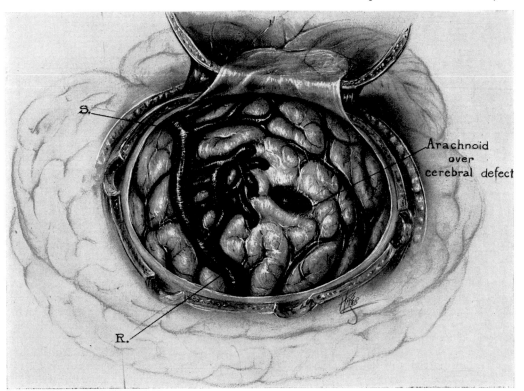

Fig. 3. (case 5). The cluster of veins overlying and draining the mass of vessels below the surface of the vein. These veins abnormal in position empty into the tremendous rolandic vein which is continous with an equally large sylvian vein. Arterial blood could clearly be seen in the veins. The cyst just posterior to the cluster of veins is the outer part of the defect which resulted from the cerebral hemorrhage which occured several months previously.

Clinic. The patient was benefited for a short time, but the symptoms gradually returned.

In 1918, while on duty in France, he fell from a horse; a severe headache developed, but lasted only for several days. Craniotomy was performed at the Mayo Clinic in 1920. At that time, a choked disk was reported, and at the operation, usually large cortical vessels were noted. For the past six years, he has steadily become worse. His vision has steadily diminished; since 1920, he has been unable to see to the left side (left homonymous hemianopsia). The sense of pressure in the head, and particularly in the right temple, has become more and more intense. Numbness and weakness in the left hand, arm and leg began about 1921, and have gradually increased.

Epileptic attacks appeared soon after the sensory and motor symptoms. They were initiated with numbness in the left arm and leg and a drawing sensation in the left side of the face, but consciousness was not lost. The attacks usually came while he was asleep and awakened him. A painful headache always followed. In some of the attacks, only part of the left side was involved. The epileptic attacks steadily increased from two or three a month in 1920 to fifteen a month. The later attacks began with numbness and stiffness of the fingers of the left hand and the toes of the left foot. The right side was never involved. Diplopia appeared recently. During the past three years the vessels over his face and head, particularly on the right side, have become much larger and more conspicuous.

Examination.—Over the occipital region of the right side was a diffuse bulging mass about 5 by 5 cm. but without sharply defined boundaries; it pulsated strongly with each heart beat. The superficial temporal, posterior auricular and occipital arteries were tortuous much enlarged and easily visible. When all three of the arteries were compressed, the swelling in the scalp subsided and ceased to pulsate. A bony opening could be palpated just mesial to the right mastoid process and in the normal position of the mastoid vein. This opening, which also showed clearly in the roentgenogram, was about 1 by 1 cm. in diameter. Another small opening in the right frontal region was all that remained of a gradually clos-

ing decompression (performed ten years before). When the patient stooped, the veins of the head and face became enormous. A loud systolic murmur was heard over the entire head, but much more over the right parietal and occipital regions.

The positive neurologic observations were: high grade papilledema (6 doipters) in both fundi; hypesthesia for pain, touch and temperature over the left side of the face and of the left arm and leg; slight weakness of the left facial muscles. The patient walked with a decidedly spastic hemiplegia gait; the left hand and arm were weaker than the right; sharply defined and complete left homonymous hemianopsia was present.

The corneal reflex was less active on the left; the knee jerks, biceps, triceps and achilles reflexes were exaggerated on the left; there was ankle clonus on the left; the Babinski sign was negative.

A roentgenogram showed a circular opening (1 by 1 cm.) in the occipital bone just mesial to the right mastoid process.

Operation.—June 20, 1926: Since the extensive pulsating mass in the left occiput seemed to be dependent on the patency of the superficial temporal, the posterior auricular and the vertebral arteries, these were first ligated, although it was evident that the intracranial lesion (presumably also an arteriovenous aneurysm) was much more extensive, since there was hemianopsia, partial hemianesthesia and hemiplegia. The mass of vessels in the scalp was carefully dissected, and at the time the branches of the external carotid artery were exposed for ligation. All three of the vessels entered the extracranial vascular mass, and through the large, bony opening which corresponded in position to the mastoid vein, a vein of corresponding size entered, filling the opening, and carried the blood from the vascular tumor. The angioma was dissected from the scalp and its entering arteries carefully marked for later study. The huge vein was carefully ligated at the bony opening with a transfixion suture of silk. Immediately after the operation, each vessel was carefully traced. The occipital artery passed directly into the big mastoid vein. This continuity was demonstrable by a probe which passed without interruption from the artery into the vein. Likewise a probe in the posterior auricular artery passed directly into the occipital artery just before it entered the big mastoid vein. A third small artery, presumably a branch of the superficial temporal, could not be traced accurately. There was, therefore, an arteriovenous fistula between the occipital artery and the mastoid vein and another interarterial fistula between the posterior auricular and the occipital arteries. The position of the great mastoid vein suggested that it entered the lateral venous sinus; it, therefore, seemed probable that the external arteriovenous fistula was separate and distinct from the arteriovenous aneurysm within the cranial chamber. Whether they were in communication through the lateral sinus could not be determined.

Second Operation.—July 20, 1926: The patient's signs and symptoms had been unchanged after the external operation. Feeling that an attack on the intracranial aneurysm would be too hazardous, a large right subtemporal decompression was performed in order to relieve the intracranial pressure. It was hoped that the patient might be relieved, at least to the extent of stopping the headaches and preserving the vision which was being menaced by a high papilledema.

When the dura, which was excessively bloody, was cautiously opened, several tortuous vessels lying in the subdural space were found attached to the inner side of the dura. Most of these vessels could be stripped away from the dura, but others entered it and had to be ligated. These extremely tortuous vessels were red and pulsated strongly. All that were visible were clearly arterial channels.

These arteries, which formed free loops in the subdural space, could be compared only to a tangled mass of angle worms; they were also about that size and fairly uniform. This vascular tumor was situated along the posterior part of the temporal lobe. Everywhere this part of the brain was completely hidden from view. Three tremendous veins emerged from this cluster of vessels. A fourth vein of about the same size paralleled the anterior part of the decompression and could not be seen to enter the angioma. Pulsation could be seen and a thrill palpated in these veins.

When the vessels were freed from the dura, furious bleeding resulted. It was possible to control the hemorrhage only by a cotton pack. The next day, careful removal of the pack was again followed by arterial bleeding, through somewhat less severe. A piece of muscle then controlled it.

The headaches were entirely relieved by the operation, but the symptoms and signs have remained as before. The decompression has since bulged at times, but at other times has been sunken.

Case 7. *History.*—A normal looking boy aged fourteen, was referred to by Dr. Ralph Greene, of Jacksonville, Fla., because of jacksonian epilepsy (Oct. 27, 1926). His trouble dated back to the age of seven years, when his mother handed him a glass of water; he dropped it and said his hand was weak and that he could not hold it. He was conscious throughout the attack. A few weeks later when cutting paper, he complained that he could not use his right hand. Three months later, when at school, he had the first convulsion. After the attack, he recalled that his tongue felt queer and that he could not swallow. It was observed that his right hand was drawn in the convulsion. A second convulsion occurred a year later; it resembled the first. A month later, the right side suddenly became completely paralyzed. Though he was unable to talk, he understood everything. There was some fever for three or four days and severe headache. A week later, the function began to return in the leg and arm, and in three weeks speech began to return. In three or four months, his speech was again normal, but there has since remained a slight residual weakness of the arm and leg. Further symptoms did not appear until two weeks before he came to the Johns Hopkins Hospital (October, 1926), when another attack began in the right hand. He had headaches only after attacks. There was no history of trauma.

Examination.—The neurologic examination showed the following positive symptoms: definite weakness of the facial muscles, the right hand, arm and leg; some atrophy of the right side; increased deep reflexes on the right; no ankle clonus, and a positive Babinski sign on the right.

The roentgenogram was negative. The Wassermann reaction of the blood was negative.

A diagnosis of tumor or aneurysm was made, more probably the latter because of the old history of a cerebral hemorrhage and with so little progression of signs or symptoms over a period of seven years.

A filling defect nearly obliterated the anterior part of the body of the left lateral ventricle. In the background of air, a linear calcified shadow was clearly visible, whereas in the roentgenogram without air, this shadow could not be seen.

Operation.—On Oct. 29, 1926, left craniotomy was performed. When the dura was exposed, a localized bluish swelling was evident toward the mesial part of the bony defect. The dura over this region had been unusually bloody; it was also thinner than elsewhere. The localized bulge was due to an underlying venous diltation which appeared to come out of the brain tissue and which passed into a large vein that coursed mesially to the superior longitudinal sinus. It

corresponded in position with the rolandic vein, which it undoubtedly represented. A second smaller vein passed downward from the mass to the sylvian vein. The large rolandic vein was distinctly red, and through its thin walls the pulsing red blood could be seen rhythmically mixing with the darker venous blood. No other enlarged veins were present on the surface of the brain. Palpation of the brain revealed an indurated area beneath the face area, but no attempt was made to expose the underlying tumor or to treat the lesion in any way. Its position in the important part of the leading cerebral hemisphere precluded any further effort.

A year later, his condition was practically unchanged.

Case 8. *History.*—A well nourished man, aged thirty-five, in good general health, complained of generalized convulsions (May 5, 1925). His first attack had occurred fourteen months earlier. It was described as a generalized convulsion which came without warning and lasted

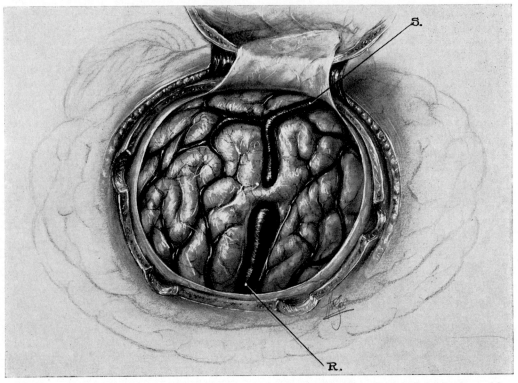

Fig. 4. (case 7). The large rolandic vein can be seen coming directly out of the brain and has arisen from the vascular mass situated beneath. Arterial blood could be seen pumping into it. It will be noted that it has no connection with the group of veins below and which also comes out of the depth of the brain. The convolutions separate these two ends of the vein. The lower branch is continuous with the sylvian vein which is also large.

about half an hour. He frothed at the mouth, bit his tongue but did not have incontinence of urine. The attack came on during sleep. A few hours later, he had another attack which seemed to be similar to the first, and two hours later another. Three months later, he had another attack at dinner, and was told that his left side had been rigid (probably incorrect). This attack lasted from twenty to thirty minutes. Additional attacks occurred six, ten and fifteen months later. Unilateral features were not noted in any of them except the one just quoted, but he has been told that his head usually turned to the right. There was no history of trauma.

Neurologic and Physical Examinations.— The results of the neurologic and physical examinations were negative. The Wassermann reaction of the blood was negative.

The ventricular system was dislocated to the right side, indicating a cerebral tumor on the left. The ventricular fluid was normal.

Operation.—On July 21, 1925, left craniotomy was performed. Five greatly dilated and somewhat tortuous veins stood out in strong relief on the surface of the brain. The rolandic and sylvian veins formed a relatively enormous continuous channel from the sylvian fossa to the superior longitudinal sinus. An almost equally large offshoot of the sylvian vein paralleled the rolandic vein and entered the longitudinal sinus, and two other branches of similar size passed downward from the sylvian vein to enter the transverse sinus. The latter veins, running closely together, formed en route a plexus over the temporal lobe. The red blood could be seen swirling in these veins with each pulse beat and mixing with the darker venous blood. The arteriovenous connection was deeper in the brain and could not be seen or palpated. The wound was closed without any attempt to treat the aneurysm.

Second Operation.—Two weeks later, the left common carotid artery was exposed under local anesthesia. After several transient compressions of the carotid without subjective of objective noticeable change, the artery was ligated just below the junction of the internal and external carotid arteries. Manometeric readings of the spinal fluid were made at the time of compressions of the internal carotid artery (lumbar puncture was performed at this time). With each temporary closure of the common carotid artery, the pressure of the spinal fluid fell from 240 to 215 mm. The pressure returned to its former level when the arterial compression was released. The blood pressure rose from 104 to 110 immediately after the ligation.

It should be noted that for several days before the ligation, the carotid artery was compressed on many occasions by pressure on the neck and without symptoms; the results indicated that the operative ligation would probably be safe.

The patient has remained free from both petit and grand mal attacks to date (two and a half years). There have been no untoward symptoms as a result of the closing of common carotid artery.

Extracranial Arteriovenous Aneurysm— the Portotype of the Intracranial Lesion.— A well nourished, healthy woman, aged twenty-nine, was referred by Dr. A. E. Pagan, of Washington, D. C., because of deforming veins of the scalp. Since early childhood (at least since she was two years of age), a lump had been present in the midline of the scalp and between the parietal eminences. It had always pulsated, but had been soft and painless. It had not given her any trouble, and had not grown in later years. Nine years before, when her first child was born, a lump thought to be a big vein, appeared in the middle of the forehead. This swelling grew forward and became larger spasmodically; during each of seven pregnancies, it increased in size until it overhung the bridge of the nose and extended over to the inner canthus of each eye. Many other large tortuous veins filled the scalp and became steadily larger until they began to encroach on the outer canthus of both eyes. The patient again became pregnant and was anxious about the vein increasing in size at the time of delivery. There had been no signs of intracranial pressure, though intermittent general headaches had been present for four or five years. On one occasion she had had an attack of numbness involving the right hand and lasting two weeks, but consciousness was not lost. There was no motor weakness during the attack, or at any other time. Noises in both ears had appeared recently and were

TABLE I.—ANALYSIS OF AUTHOR'S EIGHT

Case, Age, Sex*	Location of Vascular Tumor	Duration of Symptoms	First Symptom	Principal Symptoms	General Pressure Signs and Symptoms	Focal Symptoms	Roentgen-Ray Observations	Eyegrounds
I 52 ♂	Right temporal lobe	6 yr.	Convulsion (general)	Convulsions (grand and petit mal); headache (1 week); soreness right temple (1 week)	Headache (1 week)	Head turns to left in convulvulsion; some subjective numbness in fingers of left hand	Negative	Normal
II 19 ♂	Right parietal lobe	4 yr.	Convulsion	Jacksonian convulsions often followed by weakness of left hand	None	Jacksonian convulsions beginning in left side of face	Negative	Normal
III 35 ♂	Cerebellar left vertebral artery	2 yr.	Staggering gait	Staggering gait, diplopia, headache, dizziness, dysarthria; mental impairment	Headache; choked disk; hydrocephalus	Staggering gait, Romberg, deafness	Negative	Choked disk
IV 47 ♂	Fronto-parietal right	6 yr.	Focal convulsions	Convulsions; motor loss on left side	None	Left hand, arm and leg involved in convulsion; motor weakness left arm	Extensive shadows in right fronto-parietal region	Normal
V 48 ♂	Parieto-occipital right	10 yr.	Convulsion	Convulsions; cerebral hemorrhage, moody and forgetful	None, except during cerebral hemorrhage from which he recovered	Left side involved in attacks; left paresis, anesthesia, and hemianopsia after cerebral hemorrhage, later disappeared	Negative	Normal
VI 31 ♂	Temporo-occipital	15 yr.	Transient visual disturbances	Headaches, convulsions, hemiplegia, hemianesthesia, hemianopsia, diplopia	Choked disk; headache	Hemiplegia, hemianesthesia, hemianopsia, focal convulsions (left side)	Large circular hole in right occiput	Choked disk
VII 14 ♂	Parietal	7 yr	Attack of weakness in right hand	Convulsions (jacksonian); weakness right side of body; symptoms for cerebral hemorrhage on one occasion	None	Weakness right side of face, right arm and leg; attacks beginning in right arm; motor aphasia and hemiplegia after cerebral hemorrhage	Linear calcified shadow	Normal
VIII 35 ♂	Left parietal	14 mo.	Convulsion	Convulsions	None	Head turns to right	Negative	Normal

*In this table and the following tables, ♂ indicates male; ♀ female.

CASES OF ARTERIOVENOUS ANEURYSMS

Head-ache	General Epilepsy	Focal Epilepsy	How Diagnosed	Diagnosis before Operation or Autopsy	Operations and Observations	Conditions at Necropsy	Remarks
1 week only	+	Head turns to left	Ventriculography and craniotomy	Tumor of the brain	Anomalous branch of right middle cerebral artery supplied vascular mass; after its ligation, mass of venous vessels collapsed	Living	Patient has had but one attack since operation (3½ years); never had headache; general health excellent
None	..	+ begins in left face and arm	craniotomy	Tumor of the brain	Mass of serpentine vessels with large emerging veins; attempted extirpation; vessel burst between the ligatures	.....	Patient died of hemorrhage
+	None	None	Neurologic signs of localization; cerebellar exploration	Tumor of the brain	(1) Cerebellar exploration; (2) ligation left vertebral artery	Living	Patient's general pressure and neurologic signs and symptoms largely dissappeared, but mental changes persisted
None	..	+ left arm	Roentgenogram	Aneurysm of the brain	(1) Exploration of aneurysm; (2) internal carotid later ligated	Living	Attacks returned after a year's absence following operation; the shadow in the roentgenogram was the important diagnostic sign in this case
None	+	+	Ventriculography	Tumor or aneurysm (because of cerebral hemorrhage)	Excision of vascular tumor	Shows arterial trunk from middle cerebral supplied tumor	Cerebral hemorrhage from the vascular mass
Severe	..	+	By external arteriovenous vascular bed	Arterio-venous aneurysm	(1) Extracranial arteriovenous aneurysm (dissected out); (2) mass of angle worms in temporo-occipital region; big veins (in cortex) with arterial propulsion	Living	Two separate arteriovenous aneurysms present, one in the scalp, the other in the brain
None	..	+	Ventriculography, history and exploration	Tumor or aneurysm	Big venous dilation in which arterial blood could be seen	Living	Patient gave history of a cerebral hemorrhage, one year after first symptoms
None	+	Head turns to right	Ventriculography	Tumor of the brain	(1) Large distended rolandic and sylvian veins; arterial blood seen (through wall of vein) to be pumping into venous blood; venous plexus over temporal lobe; (2) internal carotid artery ligated	Living	Has had no attacks to date (2½ years)

Examination.—A pulsating tumor about as large as a lemon was palpable in the midline of the head between the parietal eminences. When the whole head was shaved, this mass was easily visible. From this tumor, as from the hub of a wheel, a number of enormous, tortuous veins coursed posteriorly, laterally and anteriorly. Pressure on the jugular veins promptly caused them to become tight and much fuller. Pressure on certain veins caused the distal portion to collapse, but the collapsed portion nearly always filled up slowly from collateral channels; when the collateral channels also were compressed, the distal part of the veins remained collapsed and did not fill. Particular reference is made to this point because of the large midline vein which extended to the nasion. When the collapsed venous space was palpated, it felt rough and one received the impression that there was a groove in the bone; until this test was made we wondered whether there might not be communication with the superior longitudinal sinus situated immediately beneath. The possibility of this communication was, therefore, eliminated by the test. Palpation of the veins failed to disclose an arterial pulsation. A slight murmur could be heard over the veins when examination was made with a stethoscope. A thrill could be definitely made out over the large median vein and in other veins near the tumor. The greater the distance from the tumor, the less distinct the thrill became. The degree of pressure must be just right to elicit the thrill. All of the veins were easily compressed. The tumor mass itself gave a strong expansible pulsation. The tumor was fairly soft and partly compressible, giving the impression of a mass of angle worms. When the mass was compressed firmly, it became painful and induced headaches. Compression could not be tolerated for more than a few minutes, nor could a number of veins be compressed at one time without causing pain and headache—doubtless for the same reason. Temporary occlusion of the veins caused the central tumor to become full and tight.

The roentgenogram showed large grooves of the middle meningeal artery on both sides; both grooves extended to the midline and appeared to end directly beneath the tumor of the scalp, otherwise the roentgenogram was negative.

The results of the neurologic examination were negative. The Wassermann reaction of the blood was negative.

A diagnosis of arteriovenous aneurysm of the scalp was made. The large channels of both middle meningeal arteries and the focal numbness of the hand made it seem probable that there was an intracranial extension of the aneurysm.

Operation.—The tumor itself was not removed, for intracranial extension was feared, because of the numbness of the hand which had been present for two weeks. The superficial temporal, internal maxillary and occipital arteries were ligated on both sides of the neck. On the left side, the external carotid artery was also ligated at its origin. After ligation of the arteries, the veins responsible for the tumor on the forehead were ligated. The veins responsible for this part of the swelling had previously been determined by compression with the fingers. The disfiguring part of the venous bed at once disappeared and has not returned. The redundant part of the skin disappeared and no sign of the old deformity remained. A few days after the operation, all of the veins in the scalp became hard and tender and were no longer compressible. Apparently they had thrombosed, and when the patient was seen six months later, all trace of them had disappeared. The central tumor mass had greatly diminished in size and no pulsation could be detected. The tinnitus had ceased. The patient had been well in every respect.

In retrospect, there is reason to believe that removal of the mass might have been safely performed without ligation of the branches of the external carotid. The result, however, would not have been different.

SEX AND AGE AND TIME OF APPEARANCE AND DURATION OF SYMPTOMS IN CASES OF ARTERIOVENOUS ANEURYSM OF THE BRAIN

In the literature, twelve of the cases of arteriovenous aneurysms of the brain reported occurred in men and eight in women. Curiously, the eight patients in the cases reported in this paper were men, but there seems to be no reason to lay emphasis on this point or to expect any differences due to sex.

The time of appearance of convulsions or the other more occasional symptoms is one of the most surprising features of this lesion. Being surely of congenital origin, it would be logical to expect symptoms soon after birth. Data on this point are available for eighteen of the thirty cases as follows: The first symptoms appeared in seven patients between the ages of one and ten; in three patients between eleven and twenty; in three patients between thirty-one and forty; in five patients between forty-one and fifty; there was no record of first symptoms for patients between twenty-one and thirty years of age.

In 44 per cent of the patients, therefore, the first symptoms did not appear until after the age of thirty and in 30 per cent, symptoms began after the fortieth year. The latest time of appearance was at the age of forty-eight.

The duration of symptoms ranged from a few hours to fifty years. In four of eighteen cases, symptoms had been present for more than twenty years.

LOCATION OF INTRACRANIAL ARTERIOVENOUS ANEURYSMS

The aneurysms are located in almost every part of the brain. Three are in the cerebellar region (Leunenschloss,[27] Znojemsky,[28] Dandy). In one case (Znojemsky) there were two separate and distinct aneurysms: one in the right cerebellar lobe, the other in the cerebral hemisphere. In two instances, there were arteriovenous aneurysms in the scalp, apparently independent of the intracranial lesion (Muhsam, pulsating exophthalmos; Dandy, occipital artery and mastoid vein).

An overwhelming proportion of the aneurysms are located in the paracentral region and have arterial connection with a branch of the middle cerebral artery. In two cases, the corpus callosal artery supplied the arterial connection (Deetz,[29] Steinheil[10]).

THE GROSS APPEARANCE OF ARTERIOVENOUS ANEURYSMS

The venous trunks draining the aneurysms (when located in the cerebral hemisphere) nearly always connect with the external venous circulation through the rolandic and sylvian veins, and when these form a continuous channel, as they usually but not always do, both show the maximum effect of the arteriovenous connection. This is evidenced by their dilatation throughout their course. The degree of involvement of the contiguous veins varies in individual cases; at times other nearby veins may be almost unaffected. In a single case, the venous outlet was through the internal venous system (Steinheil); one small vein of Galen and the great vein of Galen were dilated and tortuous throughout their course to the sinus rectus. In addition, a sacculated aneurysm with a long pedicle was present on the vein of Galen.

Because the external venous system carries the outflow of blood from most of the arteriovenous connections, the characteristic venous changes are on the surface of the brain. This makes it possible to detect these cases so easily at operation. And since the veins are free from all accessory coverings, it is also possible to see through their walls and detect the pulsing red, arterial blood against a background of black venous blood. This opportunity does not exist elsewhere in the body. So far as I am aware, attention has not been directed to this point — so essential to the diagnosis — heretofore.

In many of the cases of arteriovenous aneurysms located in the cerebral hemispheres, there are congenital abnormalities of the venous system on the exterior part of the hemisphere. In one case the rolandic vein arose directly out of the brain substance, having its origin in the aneurysm. In two other cases, the rolandic vein did not exist as a well defined venous channel.

The degree of venous engorgement is dependent on the size of the arterial supply and on the size of the mass of vessels, or rather on the size of their lumina, forming the arteriovenous communication. A large angioma with many vessels takes some of the brunt of the arterial force off the venous channels of exit. A small angioma or a short connecting link throws all the arterial force directly into the veins. The smaller the artery and the smaller the lumen of the arteriovenous communication (i.e., the larger the number of vessels intervening between the artery and veins), the smaller will be the venous channels which drain the aneurysm. And conversely, the larger the artery and the larger the lumen of the arteriovenous connection (i.e., the smaller the mass of vessels between the artery and vein), the greater will be the effect on the veins emerging from the aneurysm. Many large veins, therefore, indicate a small angioma or a free end to end communication between an artery and vein. Smaller veins indicate a larger angioma and an arteriovenous communication which is relatively well compensated, i. e., nearer the function of the capillary system. Doubtless there are many smaller arteriovenous aneurysms with a small arterial inlet and relatively small veins of exit which could not be established as abnormal. A thrill could not be felt in them, nor could arterial blood be seen pumping into them. There have been several cases at the Johns Hopkins Hospital which showed definite vascular abnormalities and which were thought to be arteriovenous aneurysms, but these have been excluded from all consideration because the absolute evidence was lacking.

Kaiserling's[30] case and case 1 in my series are excellent examples of excessively large and tortuous veins which result when no barrier is interposed between an artery and a vein. In Kaiserling's case, a tortuous elongated artery could be seen emptying directly into a huge venous chamber. In case 1, a short anomalous branch of the middle cerebral artery, and with normally thick arterial coats, abruptly passed into a vein. The transition between the thick arterial and the thin venous coats was clearly seen during the inspection of the vessel. Reid's case[31] of an arteriovenous aneurysm between the subclavian artery and veins in the neck seems in every way an exact duplicate of this case in the brain.

A mass of vessels forming the connection between the artery and veins, i. e., the so-called angioma, when such is present, is usually in the depths of the brain, but this is not necessarily true. In case 6, the mass was external, at least in large part. The gross character of the mass of entwined vessels is also variable; some look exactly like arteries, some like veins, and some like a combination of arteries and veins.

The arteries supplying the mass of vessels have always been larger than normal; some have been very tortuous (Deetz,[29] Simmonds,[16] Kaiserling[30]). In the only case of my series in which the artery was observed, the middle cerebral artery was enlarged all the way to the internal carotid artery. It was not tortuous, nor was its enlargement excessive — perhaps from one-third to one-half larger than the corresponding vessel of the opposite side. The arterial change, while always definite, is never comparable to that of the veins, which is really the characteristic part of the picture of arteriovenous aneurysms.

HISTOLOGIC APPEARANCE OF THE VESSELS IN SO-CALLED ANGIOMA

The histologic appearance of the vessels comprising the vascular skein is varied. The vessels show extreme differences in size, even in the same section. The walls are at times thin, suggesting veins, and others alongside are thicker, suggesting arteries. The intima may be narrow, but frequently it is greatly thickened and at times irregularly so. Many vessels are entirely occluded by thrombus formation. The elastic fibers are shown in special stains to be present in the intima of many vessels but not in others. Rarely is the elastic tissue a well defined layer; usually a strand is present here and there. The media is usually poorly developed, with much hyaline degeneration or calcification. These changes, while doubtless varying considerably in detail, are essentially similar in all microscopic reports in the literature. They indicate abnormal, poorly developed vessels with debilitated walls, which render the person the victim of vascular rupture long before the allotted time for normal vessels. The extensive thrombosis has been commented on by several authors (Emmanuel,[32] Therman,[33] Leunenschloss,[27] Astwazturoff,[9] Kaiserling[30]). It is doubtless one of the important reasons for the progression of the lesion in the later years of life. Each thrombosed vessel throws an additional strain on the venous system and on the angiomatous mass. Doubtless it is this added strain which is also responsible for many of the hemorrhages. The intercommunication of the vessels within the vascular nest has been described. I have been unable to learn whether or not this was true in case 2 which came to necropsy, for the mass was mutilated during its removal. Simmonds[16] reported evidence of canalization of thrombi.

SIGNS AND SYMPTOMS OF ARTERIOVENOUS ANEURYSM OF THE BRAIN

(*a*) *Convulsions.* With four exceptions, the first symptom in this group of cases was a convulsion, and most of these (all but two) were of the jacksonian type. The starting point of the seizures, i.e., the aura, when present, varied with the exact point at which the motor or sensory tracts were involved. It is, of course, not necessary that the attacks show the jacksonian march; at times even the focal or unilateral character of the attacks may be none too clear, though probably in all cases there will at least be turning of the head to the opposite side. Jacksonian attacks are present only when there is a direct infringement on the motor tracts. Those aneurysms at a distance from the motor tracts will give

less conspicuous unilateral signs in the attack, and usually no aura. In two of the cases reported here, there were no warning signs (aura). In both of the cases without jacksonian convulsions the head turned away from the side of the aneurysm and eventually in each other unilateral features presented.

In a number of instances, consciousness was not lost in the attacks even when the seizure involved an entire side of the body. (Deist,[34] Laves,[35] Steinheil,[10] Dandy). Later, as the attacks became more severe, the other side of the body also became involved and consciousness was lost.

Indeed convulsions need not occur even though the motor or sensory areas are involved. Only two cases in which the cerebral hemispheres were involved failed to cause epilepsy (Simmonds,[16] Struppler[15]). Two cases of cerebellar arteriovenous aneurysms involving the cerebellum failed to produce convulsions (Leunenschloss,[27] Dandy), but tumors in the cerebellum or the posterior cranial fossa rarely cause epilepsy,

(*b*) *Motor and Sensory Disturbances.* Another important and frequent sequel of the convulsions is a transient sensory or motor paralysis. This occurred in nearly all of the cases which have been reported. Sensory or motor weakness following a convulsion is strong evidence in favor of a tumor of some kind. When the same motor involvement occurs repeatedly with such precision of attack and over a period of so many months or years and with little or no permanent progression, an arteriovenous aneurysm would appear to be the most probable lesion. The paralysis often does increase slowly in these cases, for the volume of the vascular network must slowly increase, especially in later life. It will be remembered that the degenerative and proliferative changes (calcification and thrombosis) which occur prematurely in the angiomatous mass must from time to time demand readjustments and always the volume of the network of vessels must expand in this process, thereby causing increased paralysis.

Sudden hemiplegia or hemianesthesia are the results of hemorrhage, which is so prone to occur at any age, but particularly during advancing years. Usually the paralysis disappears, in part or whole, the amount of recovery depending on the proximity of the aneurysm to the motor or sensory tracts.

(c) *Other Focal Signs and Symptoms.* Other focal manifestations are at times present. Transient attacks of aphasia occurred in the cases of Ranzel[36] and Sterzing.[37] Homonymous hemianopsia was noted by Steinheil[10] and was present in two of the cases in my series, one permanently, the other only transiently after a cerebral hemorrhage. Simmonds[16] reported blindness in one eye and loss of smell and taste. The reflexes on the contralateral side of the body are, of course, always increased when a motor weakness exists; often ankle clonus and usually a positive Babinski sign, even though motor weakness was not apparent.

Mental changes have been uncommon. Steinheil's patient became demented. One of the patients in my series became moody and was forgetful after recovery from a cerebral hemorrhage.

(d) *Cardiac Changes.* Hypertrophy of the heart has been shown to occur in dogs after the production of arteriovenous fistulas (Reid,[5] Holman[7]). Some of the cases reported by Reid and Holman also showed cardiac hypertrophy and even decompensation, for which they assumed the arteriovenous fistula to be responsible. Since enlargement and tortuosity of the arteries always follow a fistula, it is easy to believe that the heart too must suffer. Holman produced measurements to indicate that the size of the heart was actually reduced after the cure of an arteriovenous fistula. Emanuel,[32] Isenschmid[26] and Laves[35] found cardiac enlargement in their cases and attributed it to the effects of the aneurysm. The heart was not found to be enlarged, or its function disturbed in any of the cases reported here.

(e) *Signs and Symptoms of General Pressure.* In only seven of the thirty cases was there a history of headaches (Muhsam,[12] Simmonds,[16] Eiselsberg,[13] Emanuel,[32] Dandy, [three]). This is noteworthy when the great size of the lesion is considered. The space adjustment, however, has occurred in early life and only gradual changes usually occur thereafter, excluding, of course, the always overhanging possibility of a sudden hemorrhage. In one of my patients, a man of 52, a headache had been present for only a week prior to the patient's admission to the hospital; his headache was sharply localized to the right frontal region owing to the fact that the vascular bed was in contact with the meninges. The headaches in other cases have been generalized. The patient of Campbell and Ballance and three of the patients in my series had severe headaches after each attack. Emanuel's patient was excused from military duty because of severe headaches which persisted throughout youth and finally disappeared; his head was also large.

Few examinations of the eyegrounds are reported in the assembled cases. A papilledema is reported only by Muhsam. The eyegrounds were carefully examined in all of our cases. In six, there was no change; in two, a well advanced choked disk. The pressure in one of these was due to an obstructive hydrocephalus; the cerebellar lesion had blocked the aqueduct of Sylvius. In the other case, a choked disk had been present for more than ten years. After a subtemporal decompression, the decompression was at times full and tight, again soft and even sunken. The great variations in pressure may account for the preservation of vision even with such a long-standing swelling of the eyegrounds.

Diplopia as a sign of pressure was reported only twice (Muhsam, Dandy).

(f) *Cerebral Hemorrhage.* The premature degenerative vascular changes which have been commented on explain the frequency of cerebral hemorrhage in this group of cases. It is a fairly safe, but not absolute, rule that when a cerebral hemorrhage occurs during youth or middle age, i.e., before the time when vascular accidents are to be expected, there must be an underlying tumor or aneurysm, either of which will contribute defective vessels. In the twenty-two cases collected from the literature, nine patients, or 41 per cent, died of cerebral hemorrhage (Drysdale,[38] Kaiserling,[30] Borchardt,[39] Ranzel,[36] Simmonds,[16] Sternberg,[40] Sterzing,[37] Wichern[41] and Leunenschloss[27]). Only two of the eight patients whose cases are reported herewith had a cerebral hemorrhage, one known and the other presumed from the history, but both patients recovered. The probability of death from cerebral hemorrhage from these lesions is also increased because in many instances the nest of vessels frequently projects into the lateral ventricle. A hemorrhage of smaller size may develop in the tumor or the contiguous brain tissue and may not induce coma, as in one of the eight cases; the hemorrhage seemed certain because of the sudden complete hemiplegia with slow recovery. Sterzing's case is a remarkable example of the capricious character of the defective vessels in the vascular network. His patient, who died of cerebral hemorrhage at the age of thirty-two, had suddenly developed hemiplegia with disturbance of speech (presumably due to a cerebral hemorrhage) twenty-two years earlier when ten years old. After a slow return of function, there had been no motor change until a year and a half before death, when the same side again became paralyzed; curiously, jacksonian convulsions did not develop until after this late attack of paralysis. Childbirth was an inciting cause of the cerebral hemorrhage in Borchardt's case.

Roentgenologic Evidence. The results of the roentgen-ray examination were of great importance in two cases. In one case, a probable diagnosis of an intracranial aneurysm was made principally on the basis of the roentgen-ray examination. A series of calcified shadows covered an area roughly circular and about 5 cm. in diameter;

all were beneath the surface of the brain. While most of the shadows had no unusual shape, circular or spiral, the shape of three of this group suggested calcium deposition in the walls of the blood vessels. In fact, such shadows could hardly be produced in any other lesion (excepting of course calcified blood vessels in tumors).

In a second case, a linear shadow, 1.5 cm. long, could be seen along the anterior horn of the lateral ventricle. This shadow, however, was visible only after the ventricle had been filled with air, which afforded an excellent contrast medium for the background. In a third case, a circular hole about 1 cm. in diameter, located alongside the mastoid, was clearly shown in the roentgen ray. The importance of this roentgenographic evidence, however, was minimized because it was readily palpable, being large enough to admit the tip of the index finger.

The large middle meningeal grooves (bilateral) commented on in the history of the extracranial arteriovenous aneurysm cannot be used as positive evidence because a cranial exploration was not made. As almost all of the intracranial aneurysms are located within the brain, there is little possibility of any vascular burden being referred to the middle meningeal arteries, and therefore the arterial vascular changes which are usually sought from this source in roentgenograms of the skull will be lacking. The positive roentgen-ray observations in cases of arteriovenous aneurysms of the brain will be largely confined to the calcified deposits in the abnormal vessels of the brain, or perhaps to localized areas of erosion. It is noteworthy that in two of the cases reported here, there was a localized erosion of the inner table of the skull, but the roentgenograms failed to disclose it.

VENTRICULOGRAPHY

The use of the air contrast medium in the cerebral ventricles is always important when the existence or even the character of an intracranial lesion is in doubt. Even though arteriovenous aneurysms only occasionally produce signs and symptoms of intracranial pressure, the lesion is one which occupies intracranial space, and therefore will usually give the positive evidence of a deformed ventricular system. Mention need not again be made of the calcified deposit which could be observed only with an air background, but such a condition is of less importance than the deformation of the ventricular system.

In two of the cases in my series in which the unilateral character of the attack was rather uncertain, the ventriculogram showed the entire ventricular system to be dislocated to the opposite side. The roentgenographic changes do not, of course, make the diagnosis of an arteriovenous aneurysm; they only denote a space occupying lesion. In another case, the ventriculogram indicated a large defect communicating with a lateral ventricle. Since the patient had previously had a history of cerebral hemorrhage, the ventricular hernia was assumed to be due to the localized hemorrhage which occurred on that occasion. But this cranial defect did not indicate the location of the aneurysm or tumor which had caused the hemorrhage.

Ventriculography yields much invaluable information in cases of epilepsy. It at once separates those lesions which are space-occupying. It will also demonstrate those lesions which are due to loss of brain tissue; also many of the congenital cerebral deformations. Even in cases of well defined focal or jacksonian epilepsy, ventriculography often yields most important information prior to a cranial exploration, for many lesions are below the cortex and would escape detection by inspection or palpation of the brain were the ventriculographic evidence not known at the time.

THE DIAGNOSIS OF ARTERIOVENOUS ANEURYSM OF THE BRAIN

The signs and symptoms of arteriovenous aneurysms show striking uniformity when taken as a whole. The outstanding complaints are: (1) jacksonian convulsions usually followed by (2) a transient motor or sensory disturbance, and (3) a gradually progressive and permanent motor or sensory paralysis coming on over a period of years and not directly depending on convulsions. When to these are added the long time element, the data are sufficiently characteristic at least to suggest the diagnosis of an arteriovenous aneurysm above other lesions affecting the brain. The transient paralysis following a convulsion and particularly the gradual permanent paralysis (not related to convulsions) makes a tumor formation of some kind an almost certain diagnosis. The accurately repeated jacksonian convulsions, involving such a sharply restricted part of the rolandic area and particularly when covering a period of so many years, should make a true neoplasm very unlikely. When the convulsions begin in early life and extend into the adult life, a neoplasm can almost be excluded. But when the epilepsy begins in later life and the time interval is still short, slowly growing tumors such as the meningiomas are important lesions to be differentiated; likewise they may show pressure symptoms late. Venous angiomas must always enter into consideration. They too will cause transient motor and sensory losses after the jacksonian seizures, but the permanent motor and sensory changes are far less possible, and when they do occur they are less progressive than in the arteriovenous variety. With symptoms, such as those described in the typical cases, the diagnosis of arteriovenous aneurysm should at least always be strongly suspected.

Moreover, given sharply defined jacksonian convulsions, appearing in youth and continuing into adult life, with a gradually progressive paralysis and then a superimposed cerebral hemorrhage such as afflicted so many of these patients, one could almost venture an absolute diagnosis of an arteriovenous aneurysm.

In those cases with the less well defined jacksonian convulsions developing in adult life and without a slow paralysis, one would have little reason to suspect an arteriovenous aneurysm; rather the diagnosis of a cerebral tumor would be considered most probable.

The roentgen-ray evidence, as in one of the cases which I have reported, may, unaided be sufficient for diagnosis. The presence of calcified shadows in circles or whorls, is, I believe, almost pathognomonic of vascular degeneration. When taken in conjunction with the clinical data, the diagnosis should be unequivocal.

Not infrequently a well defined extra-cranial arteriovenous aneurysm is demonstrable in patients who also have the intracranial signs and symptoms described for cerebral arteriovenous aneurysms. With such symptoms, an intracranial lesion of the same type is to be expected. An intracranial arteriovenous aneurysm was diagnosed in one of the cases reported here by this method of reasoning (case 6).

THE TREATMENT FOR ARTERIOVENOUS ANEURYSMS OF THE BRAIN

Occasionally spontaneous recovery in cases of arteriovenous aneurysm has been reported, but there is little real hope for such a successful outcome either in the brain or elsewhere in the body. The only way to cure an arteriovenous aneurysm is to ligate the entering artery or to excise the vascular tumor. But the radical attempt at cure is attended by such supreme difficulties and is so exceedingly dangerous as to be contraindicated except in certain selected cases. It has never seemed fair to make this attempt except on the insistent demand of the patient who fully understood all phases of the situation. Moreover, there are ways of helping the condition with little if any risk, and this in many cases at least seemed more to be recommended than the attempted extirpation of the vascular mass.

As in most cerebral lesions, however, each case should be considered a law unto itself. There are large aneurysms and small ones; those which are mostly arterial, others mainly venous; some are superficial, others deep; some are in highly important areas of the brain, others in portions largely silent. All of these factors, and finally the patient's wishes in the matter, must be weighed. An aneurysm in the left cerebral hemisphere in a right-handed person is surely noli me tangere under all conditions. Any attempted cure, even if successful, would almost surely result in disturbances of speech or motor power, or of both. Aneurysms of the corpus callosal arteries do not offer any greater surgical possibilities.

There is more reason to attempt to cure a patient who has arteriovenous aneurysms in the right cerebral hemisphere. In most of these cases, the arterial connections with the lesions are provided by branches of the middle cerebral artery. Should the aneurysm be postrolandic, the arterial connection can be ligated without injury to the motor function. In one case, we were able to do this without great difficulty. After ligating the arteries supplying the angioma, excision of the vascular bed was easy and relatively bloodless. In another case, in which the anterior pole of the right temporal lobe was covered with great tortuous and distended veins, the anomalous vessel was located and ligated with a silk ligature. It arose from the middle meningeal artery just beyond its origin from the internal carotid; following this the mass of distended venous trunks collapsed. This patient has remained well for three and one-half years; he has had only one convulsion (a year ago), whereas before the fistula was closed, convulsions occurred every month. There is no assurance of a permanent cure of epilepsy even after the cure of an aneurysm. The cerebral defect will always remain at the site of the old lesion and any lesion of the cerebral hemisphere will always remain a potential source of convulsions. However, the convulsions will be far less and more easily controlled with an inactive lesion than with one which is active.

TABLE II—ANALYSIS OF THE CASES OF ARTERIOVENOUS

Author	Date, Sex, Age	Location	Duration Symptoms	First Symptom	Principal Symptoms	Sign or Symptom of General Pressure	Focal Symptoms	Eye-grounds
Bergmann[42]...	....	Fossa of Sylvius and paracentral fossa	..	....	....	....	....	.....
Borchardt[39]...	1925 ♀ 27	Paracentral	..	....	Convulsions; paralysis	....	....	.....
Campbell and Ballance[14]	1922	Paracentral	..	Weakness of arm and leg; and fits	Mild degree hemiplegia and anesthesia; convulsions	None	Hemiplegia and hemianesthesia; increased reflexes; ankle clonus	.....
Deetz[29]	1902 ♀ 56	Right side of corpus callosum	..	Convulsion	convulsions; paritial hemiplegia	None	Left hemiplegia; jacksonian convulsions	.....
Deist[34]	1922 ♂ 56	Paracentral (left)	12 yr.	Convulsion	Convulsions;	None	Jacksonian convulsions; Babinski+	Negative
Drysdale[38]	1904 ♀ 26	Prerolandic (right)	11 yr.	Convulsion	Convulsions; weakness	....	....	.....
Eiselsberg[13] ...	1913 ♂ 39	Paracentral	..	Convulsion	Convulsions; headaches	Headaches	Jacksonian convulsions	.....
Emanuel[32]....	1898 ♂ 36	Paracentral	30 yr.	Headaches when a boy	Convulsions	Headache; large head	Jacksonian convulsions	.....
Kaiserling[30]...	1913 ♂ 26	Most of hemisphere	..	....	....	....	....	.....
Kalischer[11]....	1897 ♂ 7	Sylvian fossa and frontal lobe	1 yr.	Convulsion	Convulsions; hemiplegia gradually became complete	None	Convulsions and hemiplegia	Negative
Krause[8]	1908 ♂ 46	Paracentral	..	....	....	....	....	.....
Laves[35].......	1925 ♀ 53	Paracentral and post-rolandic	12 yr.	....	....	....	....	.....
Muhsam[12]	1924 ♀ 25	Occipital region	..	....	Diplopia; headache	Diplopia; headache	....	Large tortuous vessels; slight choking
Ranzel[36]......	1909 ♂ 36	Left occipital lobe	2 yr.	Convulsion	Convulsions; some motor and speech disturbance	None	Jacksonian convulsions, hemiplegia, aphasia	.....

ANEURYSM COLLECTED FROM THE LITERATURE

Head-ache	General Epilepsy	Focal Epilepsy	How Diagnosed	Diagnosis Before Operation or Autopsy	Operation and Observations	Conditions at Necropsy	Remarks
..	..	..	Operation and necropsy	Brain tumor	Large veins on surface of brain	Walnut sized knot of vessels beneath surface of brain, very tortuous	Puncture of dura blindly; terrific hemorrhage, uncontrollable, death; diagnosed cavernous angioma
..	+ right	..	....	......	....	Section shows aneurysm	Old specimen from Virchow Krankenhaus; patient died in childbirth of cerebral hemorrhage
After attacks	..	+ left toes	Operation	Tumor	Large veins on surface	Living	Hemiplegia and hemianesthesia were gradually progressive
..	..	+ left-sided	Necropsy	......	....	Right corpus callosal artery large and tortuous; mass of vessels plunged into frontal lobe	Very extensive tumor covers mesial surface of hemisphere, fills frontal lobe and reaches anterior horn of ventricle and corpus striatum
None	.	+ right leg	Necropsy	......	....	Large veins on surface	
..	..	+ arm and leg	Necropsy	......	....	Anterior cerebral artery very large; hemorrhage	Large veins on surface obscured brain; patient gradually become more and more deeply comatose following fit 10 days previously
+	..	+ right side	Operation	......	Large veins on surface	....	Very large veins on surface of brain; ligated; condition of patient unchanged
In youth only	..	+ arm	Necropsy	......	....	Large surface veins; mass of vessels in brain grown into ventricle and choroid plexus, also extended to pulvinar	Patient died in coma following attack; was excused from military duty because of headache; vessels are thrombosed and calcified; no mention of cerebral hemorrhage
..	..	+	Necropsy	......	....	Large surface veins	No history, except that patient died in comma following attack; this is a remarkable specimen, the veins and arteries being sharply defined; the communication is shown in the photograph; the venous channels are larger than in any other case; there is no network of vessels
None	..	+ right corner of mouth	Necropsy	......	....	Large veins on surface and mass of vessels in frontal lobe	No change in big arteries at base of brain; Virchow said it was an unusual case
..	..	+	Operation	......	Ligated some veins, says they then distended like sausages	Large surface veins; smaller vessels of the tumor just reach the surface	Typical surface appearance of lesion shown in painting
..	..	+ left hand	Operation and autopsy	......	Large veins on surface; no thrill or pulsation	Cluster of entwined vessels below surface	No loss of consciousness in earlier attacks; at operation brain was punctured, severe bleeding which was uncontrollable; branch of middle cerebral artery (containing small sacculated aneurysm) enters vascular tumor which protrudes into ventricle; hypertrophy of heart
+	..	..	Necropsy	......	....	....	A pulsating tumor near inion connects with veins of brain and longitudinal sinus; also pulsating exophthalmos; very large veins in dura and in the brain and on its surface
..	..	+ right arm	Necropsy	......	....	Small knot of vessels in left occipital lobe	Patient died of hemorrhage in an attack

TABLE II—ANALYSIS OF THE CASES OF ARTERIOVENOUS

Author	Date, Sex, Age	Location	Duration Symptoms	First Symptom	Principal Symptoms	Sign or Symptom of General Pressure	Focal Symptoms	Eye-grounds
Simmonds[16]	1905 ♀ 13	Right occipital lobe	6 yr.	Headaches	Headaches, hemiplegia, loss of touch and smell; blindness right eye	Headache	Hemiplegia	. . . .
Astwazaturoff[9] . .	1911 ♀ 35	Right fronto-parietal	. .	Convulsion	Convulsions; headache	Headache	Jacksonian convulsions	. . . .
Simmonds[9]	1905 ♂ 55	Right parietal	Since childhood	Convulsion	Convulsions	. . . .	. . . .	. . . .
Steinheil[10]	1895 ♂ 49	Right frontal	Since childhood	Convulsion	Convulsions; progressive paralysis and hemianopsia (left homonymous)	. . . .	Hemiplegia hemianopsia (left homonymous); jacksonian convulsions	Normal
Sternberg[40]	1905 ♀ 25	Temporal lobe	. .	. . . .	. . . .	. . . .	. . . .	. . . .
Sterzing[37]	1908 ♂ 32	Corpus striatum	22 yr.	Weakness right leg	Hemiplegia; convulsions; some motor aphasia	No	Hemiplegia; jacksonian convulsions	. . . .
Struppler[15]	1900 ♀ 48	Paracentral	Few hours	Coma	None until coma	No	None	. . . .
Wichern[41]	1912 ♂ 32	. . . .	. .	Hemiplegia	. . . .	No	Hemiplegia; jacksonian convulsions	. . . .
Leunenschloss[27] .	1914 ♀ 24	Right cerebellar lobe	15 yr.	Headache	Headache; hemiplegia; deafness; dizziness	Headache	Deafness	. . . .
Therman[33]	1910	Parietal lobe	. .	. . . .	. . . .	. . . .	. . . .	. . . .
Znojemsky[28]	1910	Parietal lobe also cerebellum	. .	. . . .	. . . .	. . . .	. . . .	. . . .

ANEURYSMS COLLECTED FROM THE LITERATURE—*Continued*

Head-ache	General Epilepsy	Focal Epilepsy	How Diagnosed	Diagnosis Before Operation or Autopsy	Operation and Observations	Conditions at Necropsy	Remarks
+	None	None	Necropsy	......	......	Enormous dilated veins on surface; tumor of entwined blood channels	There was much thrombosis with some evidence of canalization; patient died of cerebral hemorrhage from attack
+	..	+ left side	Necropsy	......	......	Mass of vessels size of dove's egg below cortex right fronto-parietal region; enlarged veins on surface of brain	Patient died of meningitis; calcareous deposits in vessels of vascular mass
..	..	..	Necropsy	......	......	Specimen shows a large coiled vessel with many pouching dilations; no note about veins	It is open to question whether this case is an arteriovenous aneurysm; patient died of cerebral hemorrhage (into ventricle)
..	..			Epilepsy; later, aneurysm	......	Left corpus callosol artery large and tortuous; right vena galeni magna large; tumor consists of mass of entwined vessels	Patient finally became demented; vessels of tumor did not seem either like normal veins or arteries; they were large cavernous spaces
..	..	..	Necropsy	......	......	Mass of blood vessels in brain	Drawing of vessels suggests arteriovenous aneurysm
..	..	+ right	Necropsy	......	......	Mass of vessels deep in corpus striatum; extends into ventricle at caudate nucleus; connection with choroid plexus vessels	When 10 years old patient suddenly developed weakness of right arm and leg; then improved and became stationary for 20 years when paralyzed anew; 1½ years later coma and death from cerebral hemorrhage
None	None	None	Necropsy	......	......	Mass of small vessels in rolandic area	Patient died of cerebral hemorrhage; this lesion may or many not be an arteriovenous aneurysm; it has been described as a cavernous angioma
..	..	+ right side	......	......	......	Hemorrhage into ventricle and subarachnoid space; tumor of vessels 6 by 3 cm. in frontal region	When 10 years old hemiplegia suddenly developed on the right side with speech disturbance; gradual return of function and stationary condition for 21 years when paralysis and later convulsions developed
+ localized in back	No	No	Necropsy	......	......	Vascular bed of vessels in right cerebellar lobe, anterior and posterior inferior cerebellar arteries run into angioma	Death from hemorrhage; much calcification and thrombosis in vessels
..	..	..	Necropsy	......	......	Large surface veins; collection of vessels in parietal lobe projects into ventricle	Accidental finding at necropsy following operation for sarcoma of jaw; extensive thrombosis of cortical veins even of longitudinal sinuses; dilated venous trunks are localized to region draining angioma
..	..	......	Necropsy	......	......	....	This article is written in the Russian language but apparently there are two independent intracranial arteriovenous aneurysms; photogrhaphs appear to establish the lesions as arteriovenous

A third and only other attempt at radical cure by extirpation of the angioma was our first experience with a lesion of this type. Thinking at the time that it was a venous angioma, its extirpation after careful ligature of all the superficial veins seemed possible. The huge rolandic vein was doubly ligated and divided both above and below the great mass of cortical vessels and another vein was being sutured when suddenly the rolandic vein burst, not at the site of the sutures, but midway between them. It was then evident that the bleeding was arterial, and that with the venous outlets closed, the arterial pressure within the veins was greater than the wall of the vein would stand. The vein ruptured at the localized swelling shown in the drawing, i. e., at the weakest point and probably where the main force of the artery is projected. This accident demonstrated the danger of closing the veins while the arteries supplying the aneurysm are intact. When the second ligature was being placed on the big rolandic vein it was observed that considerable force was necessary to tighten the knot and occlude the vessel, and it could be done only step by step; the arterial pressure was responsible for this difficulty. Krause's case is interesting in this connection. He, too, ligated some veins on the surface, thinking the angioma to be venous and hopnig to benefit the patient by reducing the number of veins. Fortunately nothing happened. He commented on the fact that the ligated veins "ballooned out like sausages." Bergman's[42] patient died from uncontrollable bleeding; assuming a localized bulge in the dura to be a cyst, a blind puncture into it was followed by terrific bleeding. Laves' patient also was lost on account of hemorrhage following an exploratory puncture of the brain. Once there is a tear in such a nest of vessels, their defective walls almost preclude all chance of controlling the bleeding. Each attempt at hemostasis is promptly followed by more bleeding.

In two of my cases in which the aneurysm was located in the rolandic and prerolandic areas, palliative treatment was tried, the internal carotid artery being ligated in the neck. In one case there have been no attacks, either petit or grand mal, since the operation (two and one-half years). The other patient, roentgenograms of whom showed the extensive calcification, was free from attacks for a year, after which they gradually recurred with practically the same intensity and frequency as before operation. The latter patient being 47 years old, the carotid was at first only partially ligated with a band of rubber tissue. Three weeks later, it was found to be totally occluded by a thrombus.

A subtemporal decompression and excision of the extracranial aneurysm (of the scalp) were performed in another patient who was losing vision because of a longstanding papilledema. His headache was relieved, but his condition otherwise was unchanged.

The cerebellar arteriovenous aneurysm had caused hydrocephalus. This was relieved by the bilateral cerebellar decompression which, as a routine, remains after a cerebellar exploration. The decompression remained full and tight until it was later relieved by ligation of the left vertebral artery in the neck. At operation, the intracranial portion of this artery was found to be several times its natural size, and this led to the belief that it supplied the arterial connection to the aneurysm. When exposed between the atlas and occipital bone, this great tortuous artery was just as large as the intracranial portion. Following its ligation, the bulging decompression subsided and has remained in this condition. Although his neurologic symptoms have greatly improved or disappeared, the mental disturbance still persists.

Ligation of the vessels, whether internal carotid or vertebral, can hardly result in a cure. Only an amelioration of the signs and symptoms can be expected, and doubtless even this cannot be permanent. The precedent for such ligations is the treatment of arteriovenous aneurysms between the carotid artery and the cavernous sinus. Following ligation of the internal carotid for these traumatic aneurysms, there is much improvement but usually not a cure. The collateral supply through the circle of Willis militates against a cure; it is fair to presume the same free collateral circulation will preclude the cure of the intracranial aneurysms.

SUMMARY AND CONCLUSIONS

1. Eight arteriovenous aneurysms of the brain are presented from a series of tumors of the brain. Twenty-two additional cases have been assembled from the literature.

2. Arteriovenous aneurysms of the brain are similar to those of the vascular system elsewhere in the body, except that traumatic arteriovenous aneurysms probably do not occur in the brain, because large arterial and venous trunks are not in apposition.

3. There are two other types of arteriovenous aneurysms, one in which an anomalous vessel of congenital origin establishes a direct end to end communication between an artery and vein; the other in which a network of vessels — a so-called angioma — is interposed between an artery and one or several veins. A capillary bed between the artery and vein is lacking in both types; the arterial blood, therefore, passes directly into the veins.

4. Both types are evident by the large, full and tortuous veins on the surface of the brain. A thrill can usually be felt, and red arterial blood can be seen pumping into the dark venous blood. The observations make the diagnosis absolute. There are usually congenital abnormalities of the surface veins of the brain.

5. Arteriovenous aneurysms of the brain are not uncommon, occurring in about 1 per cent of a series of tumors of the brain. They are located in almost every part of the brain.

6. The symptoms are fairly uniform and characteristic. Jacksonian convulsions, followed by transient loss of sensation or motor power in the part affected by the convulsion, and a gradually progressive sensory or motor hemiplegia on the affected side, are the symptoms common to most of the aneurysms affecting the cerebral hemispheres. The symptoms are usually of many years' duration, often beginning in childhood and continuing into adult life; again, they frequently do not begin until after the thirtieth or fortieth year.

7. General pressure symptoms, like those of a tumor of the brain, do occur, but in a minority of cases.

8. Cerebral hemorrhages occurred in about 40 per cent of the cases. It is the principal cause of death.

9. Changes shown by the roentgen ray are at times helpful in making a diagnosis and occasionally are pathognomic. Ventriculography helps to determine the existence of a space-occupying lesion.

10. The treatment is of two types: (1) ligation of the entering arteries, with or without extirpation of the mass of vessels — so-called angioma; (2) ligation of the internal carotid artery (for cerebral aneurysm) or of the vertebral artery (for cerebellar aneurysm). Occasionally, a subtemporal or cerebellar decompression (depending on the location of the aneurysm) may be indicated.

Radical ligations or extirpations alone are curative, but are exceedingly dangerous to life and function and indicated in the minority of cases, when the aneurysm is posterior to the motor tracts.

REFERENCES

[1]Hunter, W., cited by Callender: *Bull. Johns Hopkins Rep., 19:* 260, 1920.

[2]Virchow: *Die Krankhaften Geschwulste,* Berlin, 1863, vol. 3.

[3]Halsted, W. S.: Congenital Arteriovenous and Lymphaticovenous Fistulae. *Tr. Am. S. A.,* 1919.

[4]Rienhoff, Jr., W. F.: Congenital Arteriovenous Fistula. *Bull. Johns Hopkins Hosp., 35:* 271, 1924.

[5]Reid, M. R.: The Effect of Arteriovenous Fistula upon the Heart and Bloodvessels *Bull. Johns Hopkins Hosp., 31:* 43, 1920.

[6]Callender, C. L.: Study of Arteriovenous Fistula with an Analysis of Four Hundred and Forty-Seven Cases. *Johns Hopkins Hosp. Rep., 19:* 260, 1920.

[7]Holman, E. F.: Physiology of an Arteriovenous Fistula. *Arch. Surg., 7:* 64 (July) 1923.

[8]Krause, F.: *Chirurgie des Gehirns und Ruckenmarks,* vol. 1, p. 88, 1908, English trans., New York, Rebman Company.

[9]Astwazaturoff, M.: Ueber die kavernose Blutgeschwulst des Gehirns (zur Kasuistik der Pseudomeningitis). *Frankfurt. Ztschr. f. Path.,* 1911, vol. 4.

[10]Steinheil, S. O.: *Ueber einen Fall von Varix aneurysmaticus im Bereit der Gehringefoesse.* Inaug. Diss., Wurzburg, 1895.

[11]Kalischer, S.: Demonstration des Gehrins eines Kindes mit Teleangiektasien der linksseitigen Gesichtskopfhaut und Hirnoberflache. *Berl. klin. Wchnschr., 34:* 1059, 1897.

[12]Muhsam, R.: Ueber Varicen und Angiome des Zentralnervensystems. *Arch. f. klin. Chir., 130:* 522, 1924.

[13]v. Eiselsberg, A. F., and Ranzi, E.: Ueber die chirurgische Behandlung der Hirn– und Ruckenmarkstumoren. Ligatur von Angiomen. *Arch. f. Klin. Chir., 102:* 341, 1913.

[14]Campbell, H., and Ballance, C.: Case of Venous Angioma of Cerebral Cortex. *Lancet, 1:* 10, 1922.

[15]Struppler: Ueber das Cavernose Angioma des Grosshirns. *Munchen. med. Wchnschr., 37.* 1269, 1900.

[16]Simmonds, M.: Ueber das Angioma racemosum serpentinum des Gehirns. *Virchows. Arch. f path. Anat., 180:* 280, 1905.

[17]Oppenheim, H.: Die Geschwulste und die syphilitischen Erkrankungen des Gehirns, in Nothnagel's *Practice,* vol. 9, p. 20.

[18]Sweasey-Powers, W. J.: Ein Fall von Angioma cavernosum des Gehirns. *Ztschr. ges. Neurol. & Psychiat., 16:* 487, 1913.

[19]Lewandowsky, M., and Selberg, F.: Ueber Jacksonsche Krampfe mit tonischem Beginn und uber ein kleines Angiocavernom des Gehirns. *Ztschr. ges. Neurol. & Psychiat., 19:* 336, 1913.

[20]Cassirer and Muhsam: *Berl. klin. Wchnschr., 17:* 755, 1911.

[21]Uyematsu, S.: A Case of Haemangioma Cavernosum of the Cerebrum. *J. Nerv. & Ment. Dis., 52:* 388, 1920.

[22]Abrikosoff, A. S.: Ein Fall von Angiona arteriale racemosune der Arterial basilons und der beiden arterial communicans posterior. *Zentralbl. f. allg. Pathol., 22:* 210, 1911.

[23]Lechner, Ellen: Ein Beitrag zur Kasuistik der Hirnangiome. *Beitr. z. klin. Chir., 125:* 174 1922.

[24]Verse: Demonstration eines in die Substanz des Kleinhirns eingebetteten Aneurysma serpentinum et sacciforme der Arteriae Cerebri posterior Sinistra. *Munchen. med. Wchnschr., 58:* 544, 1911.

[25]Rossolimo, G. S.: Zum Ausgang von Gehirnoperationen. *Deutsche Ztschr. f. Nervenh.,* vol. 6; *Neurol. Zentralbl., 15:* 714, 1896.

[26]Isenschmid, R.: Die klinische Symptome des cerebralen Rankenangioms. *Munchen. med. Wchnschr., 59:* 243, 1912.

[27]Leunenschloss, O.: Ueber das Angioma arteriale racemosum des Gehirns. *Studien zur Pathologie der Entwicklung, 2:* 21, 1914.

[28]Znojemsky, J.: Angioma arteriale racemosum arteriae cerebelli inferior, anterior, sinistrae et Angioma racemosum arteriae cerebri mediae sinistrae. *Rev. v neulorl. psychiat., fig. a diaetet. therap., v Praze, 7:* 207, 1910.

[29]Deetz, E.: Ueber ein Angioma arteriale racemosum in Bereich der Arteriae corpus callosi. *Virchows Arch. path. Anat., 168:* 341, 1902.

[30]Kaiserling: Ueber ein ungewohnliches Aneurysma kortikaler Hirnarterien. *Verhandl. d. Patholog. Ges., 16:* 220, 1913.

[31]Reid, M. R.: Studies on Abnormal Arteriovenous Communications, Acquired and Congenital. *Arch. Surg., 10:* 601 (March) 1925, fig. 12; *10:* 996 (May) 1925 *11:* 25 (July) 1925; *11:* 237 (Aug.) 1925.

[32]Emanuel, C.: Ein Fall von Angioma arteriale racemosum des Gehirns. *Deutsche Ztschr. f. Nervenh., 14:* 288, 1898.

[33]Therman, E.: Ein Fall von Angioma racemosum cerebri. *Arch. path. Inst. d. Univ. Helsingfors, 3:* 67, 1910.

[34]Deist, H.: Ein Fall von Angioma racemosum der linken Lobus paracentralis in seiner klinischen und versicherungsrechtlichen Bedeutung. *Ztschr. f. d. ges. Neurol. u. Psychiat., 79:* 412, 1922.

[35]Laves, W.: Ein Fall von Angioma arteriale racemosum des Gehirns. *Jahrb. f. Psychiat. u. Neurol., 44:* 55, 1925.

[36]Ranzel, F.: Zu rKasuistik kombinierter Hirnaffektionen ein Fall von Rankenangiom des Gehirns mit tuberculous Meningitis. *Wein. klin. Wchnschr., 22:* 1214, 1909.

[37]Sterzing, P.: Ein Fall von Angioma arterial racemosum im Gehirn. *Zentralbl. allg. Path.., 19:* 278, 1908.

[38]Drysdale, J. H.: Report of Case, Pathological Society of London. *Lancet,* 1904, p. 96.

[39]Borchardt, M.: Die chirurgische Bedeutung der Gehirnaneurysmen. *Beitr. klin. Chir., 133:* 429, 1925.

[40]Sternberg, C.: Demonstration eines Falles von Angioma arteriale racemosum des Gihirns. *Verhandl. deutsch. path. Gesellsch., 7–9:* 308, 1905.

[41]Wichern, H.: Klinische Beitrage zur Kenntnis der Hirnaneurysmen. *Deutsche. Ztschr. f. Nervenh., 44:* 220, 1912.

[42]Bergmann: Zur Kasuistik operativer Hirntumoren. *Arch. klin. Chir., 65:* 935.

XXXI

VENOUS ABNORMALITIES AND ANGIOMAS OF THE BRAIN*

Essentially all lesions common to the blood vascular system are found in the brain. In an article in a recent number of this journal,[1] the arteriovenous aneurysms or fistulas in the brain were analyzed. In this communication, the venous and capillary tumors, aneurysms and abnormalities will be considered. Although the relative frequency of vascular tumors and aneurysms of the brain is difficult to estimate, the actual number is rapidly increasing, owing to the more intensive development of neurosurgery and of the means by which the accurate diagnosis and localization of intracranial lesions can be made. In a series of about 600 verified tumors of the brain, the vascular tumors and aneurysms of the brain (excluding vascular anomalies) were 5 per cent. Eight of these tumors were arteriovenous; fifteen were referable to the venous and capillary system, and seven were arterial.

The vascular lesions most favorable for treatment are those arising from the veins and capillaries. Taken as a whole, they perhaps offer less danger and better results from complete extirpation than tumors of any other type in the brain.

VENOUS ABNORMALITIES IN THE BRAIN

Among a series of cerebral explorations for jacksonian epilepsy, the accompanying seven examples of abnormalities of the venous system were encountered and drawn at the time of operation. In one case, the observations were amplified by necropsy. In every instance, the marked venous irregularities were associated with malformations of the brain, some of which were primary, others secondary.

The venous irregularities were of varied form. In five instances, the sylvian vein was the site of the abnormality. In most of the cases, a number of anomalous veins were spread over the frontal, temporal and parietal lobes and were tributaries to the sylvian vein. It is not an infrequent condition in presumably normal brains for the rolandic vein to be either absent or relatively insignificant, instead of being the outstanding vein of the hemisphere. Such conditions merely indicate the great normal variations of the venous system that occur in the brain and that still appear to be of no significance.

In case 3, one sees a relatively enormous vein over the frontal lobe. This vein is continuous with the sylvian vein as the rolandic vein should be, but it is 4 or 5 cm. anterior to a small rolandic vein which emerges from the brain tissue just below the facial center. In case 5, the rolandic vein passes from the sylvian as it normally should, but sweeps backward in a crescent, and finally, when approaching the falx, bends sharply forward at a right angle and then again mesially at another right angle. Both of these rolandic variations, however, are only a small part of the composite venous and cerebral abnormalities.

In none of the venous deformities is the size of the vessel abnormal (possibly excepting case 3); rather, it is the number, shape and distribution of the vessels that are abnormal. In this respect the venous changes differ from those of the arteriovenous aneurysms in which the size of the vessels is so striking. In addition to the great size, the venous component of arterio-

*Reprinted from the *Archives of Surgery, 17:* 715–793, November, 1928.

venous aneurysms also show great abnormalities in shape, number and distribution. One can always be sure that the lesion cannot be arteriovenous if the veins are of normal size. Moreover, in venous anomlaies, aneurysms or tumors, one never sees in the veins exposed at operation pulsating red blood, which is characteristic of arteriovenous aneurysms.

In some instances, the deformation of the cerebral convolutions is even more striking than that of the veins. Many of the convolutions are of relatively enormous size and lack the characteristic shape. They appear like masses of brain tissue, improperly formed. In such cases, doubtless both the veins and the brain tissue are wrapped up in the same fundamental maldevelopment. Case 4 is another example of a vascular abnormality being dependent on the primary embryonic cerebral defect; the sylvian vein received a branch from each side of the cyst and passed along the sylvian fissure as a bifid trunk. In this case the temporal lobe did not have any attachment to the parietal lobe, except in the depth of the brain.

In case 7 (Fig. 1) there was a venous plexus in the sylvian fissure of each side and eight or ten additional small plexuses in the piaarachnoid over both cerebral hemispheres. In this patient there were two other associated cerebral deformations: (1) absence of the corpus callosum, (2) stricture of the aqueduct of Sylvius with resulting hydrocephalus. The child was an imbecile.

Cerebral and vascular deformations are, therefore, commonly associated. The one may cause the other, or, as in case 5, they may be entirely independent and referable to a faulty general development in the embryo. In cases 2, 5, and 6, tremendous vascular deformations were present, in that many vessels of fairly uniform size radiated from the sylvian vein. In such cases the vascular bed becomes a space occupying lesion of considerable size and doubtless acts as a tumor, for in each instance the epileptic seizures were focal and

began in the face, i. e., the part of the motor area nearest the tumor. Surrounding this vascular bed, there is always a pool of fluid in the subarachnoid space, and usually the leptomeninges over the affected areas are thickened and often opaque. The brain tissue beneath is also softened and the convolutions atrophied as compared with the surrounding unaffected brain tissue. In case 6 ventriculograms demonstrated that the vascular bed had indented the body of the lateral ventricle. As seen at operation, the network of vessels was so dense that the underlying brain was entirely obscured.

Another abnormality not infrequently seen is the tortuosity of veins. This is shown in a series of anomalous veins in case 1. Not infrequently one sees many of the smaller terminal veins tortuous when the larger trunks are not affected. In a recent case of congenitally deformed brain, a series of eight or ten such venules diverged from the center of the frontal lobe, some going to trunks entering the sylvian, rolandic veins, and others to frontal veins passing to the longitudinal sinus. This tortuosity of some of the smaller veins was also present in case 5. In this case there was also a diverticulum (venous aneurysm of the superior longitudinal sinus).

CLINICAL FEATURES OF VENOUS ABNORMALITIES

With two exceptions (cases 1 and 7) these patients were operated on to find the cause of jacksonian epilepsy. The patient in case 7 was operated on for hydrocephalus; the vascular tumors therefore were incidental. Operation was performed in case 1 because of blindness, and the vascular changes were also incidental. Three of the patients (cases 2, 4 and 7) had varying grades of mental retardation. Another was too young to judge the mental status (case 6).

Two patients (cases 2 and 3) had some slight evidence of motor weakness of the opposite side of the body. In both of these patients the motor weakness was increased for a short time after the epileptic seizures. In one patient (case 5), the epileptic seizures did not begin until he was twenty-eight years old, and in another patient (case 3) the attacks began when he was thirteen years of age. The other patients developed convulsions at five months, eight months and two and one-half years of age. The time at which convulsions develop from a cerebral lesion is most variable, as these results indicate. The remarkable fact is that a lesion can exist for twenty-eight years without causing trouble and then without apparent reason convulsions will suddenly appear. In arteriovenous aneurysms, the time of onset of attacks may be delayed until much later in life. Perhaps there is more reason for a later origin in arteriovenous lesions, for they have a definite tendency to increase in size. One can conclude only that any cerebral lesion is always a potential source of epilepsy, and that the time element is uncertain for reasons that are not known.

REPORT OF CASES OF VENOUS ABNORMALITIES OF THE BRAIN

Case 1. *Venous Anomaly of the Brain.*

A boy, aged three and one-half years, was referred by Dr. Rosenberger of Milwaukee because of blindness. Two weeks before admission to the Johns Hopkins Hospital, the patient had begun to stumble over objects, apparently because he did not see well. He was unable to recognize pictures which he had known perfectly before this time. Since then he had been unable to see at all. There had never been convulsions or any other symptoms. The results of the neurologic examination were entirely negative with the possible exception of the eyegrounds. There seemed to be pallor of the optic disks, though perhaps this was questionable. The x-ray examination of the head was normal.

A suprapituitary tumor was suspected because of the blindness and questionable optic atrophy as suggested by the ophthalmoscopic examination.

The right ventricle was uniformly smaller than the left.

Operation.—Right craniotomy was performed to expose the optic chiasm. A

series of four tortuous and somewhat enlarged veins converged from the frontal and parietal lobes of the sylvian vein. Except that the sylvian vein was larger than usual and bifid for some distance, it was not abnormal. The cisterna chiasmatis was so large that there was a question at the time as to whether this could have caused the blindness. During his stay in the hospital the blindness persisted, but a report two years later stated that his vision was normal again.

Viewed in retrospect, the operative observations did not explain the blindness, nor had the vascular conditions which are here reported caused trouble. They were merely evidences of a congenital maldevelopment in the brain.

Case 2. *Venous Anomaly of the Brain.*

A girl, aged three and one-half years, was referred by Dr. Walter Cox of Winchester, Va., because of focal epilepsy. Birth had been normal and easy, and had occurred at full term. When the infant was five months of age, it had first been noticed that the normal mental response, evidenced by smiling and holding up the head, had not appeared. When she was eight months old, definite signs of retardation had been noted. When one year of age, the right arm and leg had attempts to hold up the head had been been less developed than the left, and unsuccessful. When eighteen months old, she had seemed to see things, but did not fix her attention on objects or persons for any length of time. She has never learned to walk or talk. When two and one-half years of age, she had had the first convulsion, which had lasted about a minute. The eyes rolled up at the onset of the attack, the right hand drew up, then the leg and soon the entire body was involved in a clonic convulsion. She was unconscious about an hour. Numerous convulsions of similar type had since recurred. On one occasion, six or seven attacks had followed in quick succession. Incontinence of urine and even of feces had been noted. There had been many attacks of petit mal type, evidenced by a momentary staring expression.

Examination.—The child could not stand or talk. She responded with a silly grin when questions were asked. The right side of the body was relatively underdeveloped, though the arm and leg moved freely. There was also slight facial asymmetry. The deep reflexes were increased on the right side.

A probable diagnosis of a congenital lesion of the left cerebral hemisphere was made.

Operation.—Left craniotomy was performed. A large collection of fluid (subarachnoid) covered the anterior half of the exposed area of brain. Over the frontal region, the fluid was at least 1 cm. deep. Through this fluid, and better after its evacuation, five separate interlacing veins (a venous plexus) were seen which filled the sylvian fissure. From this series of veins, twelve or thirteen parallel branches passed across the frontal and parietal lobes to the superior longitudinal sinus. The convolutions of the frontal and parietal lobes were pale, soft, depressed and irregular. The convolutional markings of the temporal lobe were much less affected, but strikingly abnormal also. The subsequent course of the patient was unimproved.

Anatomic Diagnosis.—There was an extensive congenital maldevelopment of the brain. In this, the vascular system shared extensively forming a bed of vessels which almost obscured the frontal lobe.

Case 3. *Venous Anomaly of the Brain.*

A boy, aged fourteen, entered the Johns Hopkins Hospital because of convulsions. Since birth the left side of the body had been smaller and weaker than the right. Mentally, he had been somewhat precocious. One year before admission to the hospital, he had had the first convulsion, which had begun in the left side and which had quickly become generalized. For two years previously, he had had spells of tickling sensation in the left side of the face. No attention had been given to these attacks, but later they had been an aura of a convulsion. The seizures came on about every two weeks. After a convulsion, the left side was partially paralyzed for several minutes.

Operation.—A right craniotomy was performed on Feb. 19, 1927. The striking observation was the large vein which came out of the posterior part of the frontal lobe about midway between the falx and the sylvian vein. It passed downward into the sylvian vein. A small inconspicuous rolandic vein was about 4 cm. posterior to this anomalous vessel and it had no visible connection with the sylvian vein. The size of the big frontal vein raised the question as to whether an arteriovenous aneurysm might not be beneath, but the blood in the vein was not definitely redder than normal; pulsation could not be seen in the blood stream; nor could a thrill be felt. Even more striking than the venous abnormality was the great deformation of the convolutions in the frontoparietal region. Several were of enormous size and markedly irregular. Nothing could be done to help the patient. The presence of the old hemiplegia still leads one to wonder if a deep vascular lesion may not be present.

Case 4. *Venous Anomaly of the Brain.*

A physician's child, aged three years, was mentally backward, unable to raise the head and had frequent convulsions. When eight months old, he had had convulsive twitchings in the left side of the mouth and face. A month later, there had been a series of generalized convulsions lasting several hours. For the next two years he had had two or three convulsions daily, but for six months before operation they were absent. There has been practically no mental development. For several months he had been getting weaker and had taken food poorly.

When three months of age, the patient had had a high fever and a rigid and retracted neck; examination of the spinal fluid revealed seventy-six cells. Shortly after this attack, his right eye had become crossed, and he had lost the use of his left arm and leg. He had become emaciated and had been unable to move the head for some time. Gradual improvement had followed during the next few months, and the function of the left leg had returned entirely, but the arm had remained spastic and was not used much. It was five months after this illness when the first convulsion developed, beginning in the left side of the face (the affected side).

Physical and neurologic examinations revealed only the slightly spastic left arm which the patient used much less than the right.

The history suggested an old inflammatory lesion, perhaps an old healed abscess.

Ventriculography showed a large cavity in the region of the right temporal lobe, filled with air and communicating with the lateral ventricle.

Operation.—The right cerebral hemisphere was explored. A large cyst was found between the temporal and parietal lobes, and opened into the body of the lateral ventricle. A branch of the sylvian vein passed on each side of the cyst. The whole temporal lobe as far back as the occipital lobe did not have any superficial attachment to the rest of the branch. The bifurcated sylvian vein surely represented a congenital malformation. The separation of the temporal lobe from the rest of the brain was surely due to a congenital defect and doubtless the big cyst with its communication with the lateral ventricle was another malformation. There were no signs of an old inflammatory process on the surface of the brain (adhesions and meningeal thickening). Moreover, if an acute abcess had broken into the ventricle, death undoubtedly would have been the outcome. The failure of the child to develop mentally doubtless denoted other congenital cerebral malformations in the left hemisphere. The child survived the operation, though benefit did not result.

Case 5. *Venous Anomaly of the Brain; Also Venous Aneurysm of the Longitudinal Sinus.*

A large, strong miner, aged twenty-nine years, was referred because of jacksonian convulsions. Eight months before admission to the hospital, when picking berries, he had had a severe headache in the left temple. This had lasted a few days, when he had had the first generalized convulsion. There was an aura of pain in the teeth on the right side. He had had nine other major attacks since then, in all of which his right hand and face first began to contract. Mental change, dizziness or vomiting was not noted.

The results of the physical and neurologic examinations were entirely negative. The Wassermann reaction of blood was negative.

Operation.—A left craniotomy was performed on March 14, 1928. Aside from two little arachnoid villi which had perforated the dura and formed small knoblike papillomas between the dura and bone (the cause of their formation and their significance, if any, is not clear), nothing abnormal was encountered until the brain was exposed. A striking, congenitally malformed brain was disclosed.

The arachnoid was thickened and the subarachnoid fluid formed a large pool over much of the exposed brain. This bed of fluid was particularly deep over a greatly widened sylvian fissure into which nineteen veins of varying size converged from the frontotemporal and parietal lobes. They passed into the sylvian and rolandic veins. The rolandic vein was very large and abnormally placed. It made a big bend posteriorly after leaving the sylvian vein and when about 3 cm. from the longitudinal sinus suddenly turned forward at right angles, and after a course of 4 or 5 cm. again turned abruptly at right angles to enter the longitudinal sinus. No thrill could be felt in the enlarged rolandic vein, nor was there evidence of red arterial blood in the vessel. Over the frontal lobe another series of veins (about eight in all) converged to three larger trunks which entered the longitudinal sinus anterior to the point of entry of the rolandic vein.

After the subarachnoid fluid had been evacuated, the convolutions were seen to be badly misshapen and malformed. Many were large and pointed instead of having the normal well rounded surface. In addition to these abnormalities, a venous diverticulum from the longitudinal sinus was found with the characteristic anatomic conditions described under the cases of this type. This was removed and a fascial transplant sutured in the dural defect. It was not thought that this aneurysm was causing the attacks because they began in the face, but rather that they were caused by the congenital vascular and convolutional ensemble contiguous to the facial center. Nothing could be done to help this.

The postoperative course was uneventful.

Case 6. *Venous Anomaly of the Brain.*

An infant, aged five months, was referred by Dr. J. W. Amesse, of Denver, because of jacksonian convulsions beginning in the right side of the face but quickly becoming general. The first attacks had begun a month before admission to the hospital. They had steadily increased in number and severity, and many attacks occurred daily.

The results of the physical and neurologic examinations were negative; also the Wassermann reaction of blood. The family history was negative.

Operation.—A small left-sided cranio-tomy was performed. The sylvian fissure was wide and a roughly circular area extended mesially from it. This area was covered with fluid, beneath which a mass of veins could be seen. After the fluid was evacuated, this cluster of vessels, not unlike a pampiniform plexus of tortuous entwined veins, was more distinct. The vessels completely obscured the underlying brain. They covered Broca's convolution. A second smaller plexus was situated on the temporal lobe about 2 cm. from the large plexus. Several veins bridged the intervening gap and connected the two vascular beds. The vessels were all veins. Palpation did not reveal a thrill nor was pulsation visible. The shape and size of the convolutions were irregular and markedly abnormal.

The operative observations indicated a congenitally malformed brain with venous anomalies.

Case 7.—*Venous Anomalies of the Brain: Venous Plexuses.*

An infant, aged two and one-half years, was referred by Dr. J. B. Sidbury of Wilmington, N. C., with the diagnosis of hydrocephalus. The head was large at birth; ptosis of left upper lid also dated from birth. At the age of three months, the head had grown rapidly, then measuring 18½ inches (47 cm.). Jerky movements of the extremities had been frequent during the first three months, but there had not been any convulsions. The child had held up her head when she was six months of age, and had laughed

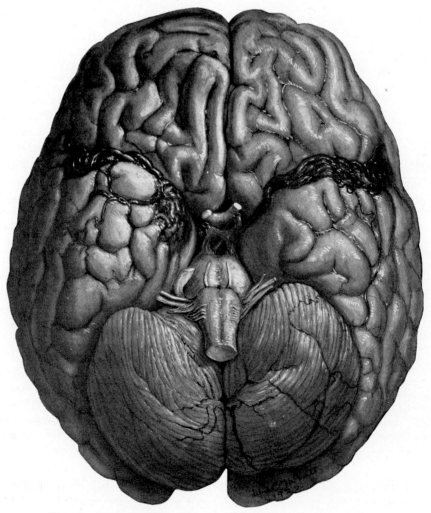

Fig. 1. Congenital plexiform agioma in each sylvian fissure.

a month later. She could not sit up alone, though she used her hands and legs in playing. The head did not grow so rapidly after the first six months. At one year of age, it measured 21½ inches (54.6 cm.); at present (2½ years of age) it is only 22½ inches (56.8 cm.). When the child was 5½ months of age, the first tooth had appeared; at 1 year there had been twelve teeth. Her condition had remained more or less stationary for the past eighteen months. She could not sit or stand alone, could not feed herself, and could not talk. She gritted her teeth a great deal, particularly when she lost her temper. The fontanels were entirely closed. An obstruction in the ventricular system was shown by the fact that phenolsulphonphthalein injected into the spinal canal did not appear in the ventricular fluid.

Operation.—The floor of the third ventricle was removed for hydrocephalus. The fissure of Sylvius contained a venous plexus (angioma). The angioma was made up of cerebral tortuous veins which were entwined. Tributaries converged to the venous plexus from the frontal and parietal lobes.

The child died forty-eight hours after operation. Autopsy showed another venous plexus on the other side of the brain and in precisely the same position, which was almost an exact duplicate of the one found at operation. In addition, there were eight or ten little venous collections of much the same character in the pia-arachnoid membranes over both hemispheres. Each little vascular mass of veins measured from 1 to 2 cm. in diameter, and was flattened on the brain and not elongated like those in the sylvian fissure. They were free in the meninges and could be dissected from the brain. In addition to these vascular abnormalities, the corpus callosum was absent and the aqueduct of sylvius obliterated (Fig. 1).

VENOUS ABNORMALITIES IN THE DURA: VENOUS ANEURYSMS?

In a group of four venous aneurysms with focal epilepsy in which the attacks began in the leg or arm, and anatomic observation was so uniform and so striking that I venture to suggest an etiologic relationship. The lesion is a diverticulum of

the superior longitudinal sinus — a venous aneurysm. My attention was first drawn to this condition in a patient who had bilateral symmetrical elevation of the skull, to either side of the longitudinal sinus and slightly anterior to the rolandic area. Although superficially the bony prominence suggested an osteoma, the x-ray examination showed this diagnosis to be incorrect, for the bone was greatly thinned in addition to being pushed definitely outward. On exploration of this part of the skull, the sudden thinning of the bone was found to be striking and the dura immediately beneath to be exceedingly bloody, owing to the presence of a well localized dural vascular bed. On turning back the dura, this same localized area was found to be densely attached to the brain tissue by pacchionian granulations which were absent both in front of and behind the affected area. Moreover, after the fibrous attachments had been separated the underlying brain tissue was distinctly soft. The palpating finger sank into this part of the brain to a greater depth than elsewhere. There was, therefore, a localized softening of the brain immediately beneath a localized vascular bed in the dura, and a localized erosion of the inner table and bulging of the outer table of the skull directly over the same lesion. It was not difficult to believe that any lesion which could produce such striking changes in the bone could also damage the brain and thereby cause epilepsy. Moreover, its location directly in the prerolandic leg and arm centers suggests the correlation of the pathologic and clinical data.

In excising this vascular dural mass, which bled freely because the dura was thinned and attached to the bone, it could be seen that it was fed by several channels from the longitudinal sinus, and that it did not have a single wide communication with the sinus. There was no arterial communication with the middle meningeal artery, although the bleeding was so severe as to make one wonder if it might not be an arteriovenous aneurysm. It is also worthy of note that the rolandic vein does not enter into this vascular bed in the dura; it passes into the longitudinal sinus, immediately posterior to it.

This patient had only two attacks during the year following the operation and none in the next six years. The capricious results following any form of treatment in cases of epilepsy make any claims hazardous. Moreover, even though the venous aneurysm is removed, the cerebral defect remains and is in itself always a potential source of convulsions. It is, of course, always advisable to remove the primary cause even if the secondary cerebral defect cannot be altered. The attacks will improve even if the patient cannot be cured.

In the two other cases (9 and 10) which I have classified under this group, the clinical and pathologic observations were such exact duplicates of those in the case just described that additional comment is not necessary. Since the operation in these cases has been performed only during the three months prior to the time this paper was written, too little time has elapsed to consider the results. All patients have made uneventful recoveries after removal of the lesion.

There is perhaps reason to deny the existence of this lesion. X-ray examinations of the skull frequently show in this location a degree of rarefaction which must be looked on as a normal observation — usually it is called a venous lake. But in the cases here described, the normal x-ray changes are exaggerated. Where the normal changes end and the pathologic begin must vary in different persons. In fact, in the case just described (case 8), a seemingly identical lesion, and of the same size, remains on the opposite side and has not caused any symptoms. If the x-ray change is in association with focal convulsions that begin in the leg or arm, and if another lesion in the prerolandic cortex is absent, the existence of the lesion and its casual relationship would seem to be definite.

Brief mention is made of a case in which there was an enormous occipital sinus (case 11). Whether it has any clinical significance is doubtful, but it is an example of a venous anomaly, which may offer great surgical difficulties and dangers if not recognized before it is opened. This sinus, while normally present, may be and not infrequently is entirely absent, and when present its size is most variable, though rarely over 1 cm. wide. In one patient, a hydrocephalic infant, the occipital sinus was proportionately larger than in this patient; it was not the cause of the hydrocephalus but was merely another manifestation of a congenital anomaly. In both of these cases, the occipital sinus bifurcated near the foramen magnum and each branch passed laterally in the dura to enter the internal jugular vein at the jugular foramen.

REPORT OF CASES OF VENOUS ABNORMALITIES IN THE DURA

Case 8. *Venous Aneurysm from a Longitudinal Sinus.*

A large, strong man, aged 24, was referred by Dr. W. L. Brown, of El Paso, Texas, in May, 1921, because of recurring jacksonian convulsions. The family and past histories were negative, except for one incident which will be included in the story of his present illness.

The first attack had occurred suddenly six years before admission to the hospital, when the patient was eighteen years old. Since that time, they had averaged about two a month, with a tendency gradually to become more severe and more frequent. Every attack came at night just as he was dozing off to sleep. A queer feeling "like a chill" awoke him. In a few seconds the right arm and face began to jerk and then became numb. He then lost the power of speech but was still conscious. He passed into coma as the convulsions became clonic and bilateral. Following the convulsion, he had a queer sulphur taste in his mouth (uncinate attack?). An interesting fact in his history was that when 11 years of age he complained of attacks of numbness of the right arm over a period of nearly a year. This disappeared until the advent of convulsions seven years later.

The results of the physical and neurologic examinations were negative, except for a bony prominence situated in the midsaggital line and extending on each side of the midline; the left side was distinctly a little larger. In the midsaggital plane it was a trifle less than midway between the nasion and the inion. The bony prominence measured about 7 cm. from side to side (bilateral) and 3½ cm. anteroposteriorly. The roentgenograms showed a marked localized bulge of the skull in this region with great thinning of the bone from within.

Operation.—On May 28, 1921, left craniotomy was performed, approaching the midline. The brain appeared normal except for the region of the arm and leg centers where the brain was firmly attached to the dura by a mass of pacchionian granulations. In front of this restricted area which corresponded exactly with the eroded bone in the roentgenogram, the pacchionian granulations and attachments to the dura were absent. The lesion was strikingly localized. The bone was then rongeured away over the affected area. The skull became progressively thinner as the longitudinal sinus was approached, where it was about 3 mm. thick. The denuded dura bled furiously from several perforations of the dura which was closely attached to the area of eroded bone. These venous channels were not continuous with the veins which cross from the cerebral hemisphere and are en route to the longitudinal sinus. Rather they were off-shoots from the longitudinal sinus, and seemed to communicate with a common vascular bed, for it was necessary to ligate all the channels as they entered the longitudinal sinus before the bleeding in the dural vascular bed could be controlled. The rolandic vein passed just posterior to the venous aneurysm to enter the longitudinal sinus. It was not injured. The other interesting feature of the lesion was the firm and dense attachment of the aneurysm to the brain by pacchionian granulations. These had to be severed with a knife or scissors. Contiguous to this local area both anteriorly and posteriorly, these attachments were entirely absent. The leptomeninges were greatly thickened and opaque for some distance beyond the aneurysm and the brain was distinctly softer than the surrounding normal brain. Such observations make it difficult to believe that pacchionian granulations are other than

protective formations against the pressure of large venous channels. In the later years of life, the pacchionian granulations develop normally along the rim of brain which lies along the wall of the longitudinal sinus. Doubtless the explanation of these granulations is similarly a reaction to the trauma incident to the flow of blood through the longitudinal sinus.

The entire area of dura containing the venous diverticulum was removed and replaced by a transplant of fascia lata. The dura was divided close to the longitudinal sinus by placing a series of clamps at the base and closing the dural margin with a series of transfixion sutures of silk.

As the convulsions had never primarily attacked the left side of the body, no attempt was made to remove the right-sided lesion, which was a duplicate of that removed from the left.

The immediate postoperative recovery was uneventful. During the first year following operation, the patient had two attacks and has had none in the following six years.

Case 9. *Venous Aneurysm from Longitudinal Sinus.*

A highly nervous woman, aged 27, was referred because of frequent jacksonian convulsions. The family and past histories were entirely negative. One year before admission to the hospital, she had suddenly felt dazed for a few seconds (petit mal). Several days later, she had experienced the same sensation. Two or three weeks later, numbness and stiffness had appeared in her right arm and leg in association with the dazed spells. For several seconds after an attack she could not speak or write, and there would be a transient weakness and numbness of the hand and leg. She had not lost consciousness in attacks at this time. In some attacks, the right side of the face twitched. The numb feeling was associated with the sensation of an electric shock passing through the right side of the body. There had not been generalized convulsions. On one day, a few weeks prior to operation, the attacks had come every ten or fifteen minutes. A day seldom passed without the occurrence of severe attacks. Headaches were never present.

The results of the physical and neurologic examinations were entirely negative.

X-ray examination showed an area of erosion in exactly the same position as in the preceding cases.

A probable diagnosis of venous aneurysms from the longitudinal sinus was made.

Operation.—On Jan. 24, 1928, a left craniotomy was performed as in the preceding case. The bone was very thin over a restricted area about as large as a half dollar. The same venous lakes bled freely and had to be controlled by pressure of the finger. The dura was pulled mesially. The same dense area of pacchionian granulations was separated from dense opaque leptomeninges. The same softened zone of brain was immediately beneath. Elsewhere pacchionian granulations could not be seen. A fascial transplant was used to replace the dura which was excised and carefully sutured close to the longitudinal sinus.

The postoperative course was uneventful.

Case 10. *Venous Aneurysm from the Longitudinal Sinus.*

A well nourished boy, apparently normal mentally and physically, except for convulsions which began in the right leg, gave a past history which was negative except that glands of the neck had been removed eight years before the present examination. There was no history of epilepsy on either side of the family.

The convulsions began three years before admission to the hospital, when he was 11 years of age. There was no antecedent history of trauma or illness which seemed to have any bearing on the onset of the attacks. From the beginning the seizures were of jacksonian character always beginning in the right leg, and almost simultaneously, but a trifle later, in the right arm. Frequently, a numbness of the right leg and at times of the right arm was an aura. A residual weakness of the right leg and less of the arm followed the attack and persisted for several minutes. The convulsions lasted from one to two minutes, were clonic and became general as consciousness was lost. He had never bitten the tongue or lost sphincter control. There was usually sufficient warning to allow him to sit down before the attack came on. The attacks became more frequent, averaging about two a month. Most of the convulsions occurred just after wakening in the morning.

The results of the physical and neurologic examinations were entirely negative. There was no objective weakness of the right arm and leg. The roentgenogram showed a marked thinning of the inner table of the skull along the midsaggittal line and about midway between the nasion and inion. The area of erosion was about 3 cm. long. There was a slight bulging of the outer table over this region.

The combination of this erosion of the skull and the focal attacks beginning in the leg suggested that the probable lesion was a venous aneurysm—diverticulum of the longitudinal sinus.

Operation.—Precisely the same operation was performed and the same observations were disclosed as in the first case of this group.

The immediate postoperative recovery was uneventful. The operation was performed only a month before this paper was written.

Case 11. *Abnormality of Occipital Sinus.*

A well nourished man, aged 34, was referred by Dr. W. S. Thayer because of headaches in the occipital region. Throughout boyhood, the patient had had periodical headaches, always localized to the back of the head, at times radiating to the eyes. The headaches had increased with age. They were always intensified by work or exercise, and improved when the patient was in a recumbent position or by the application of cold to the head. During the past year, the patient had several attacks of weakness and numbness of the left arm and leg, but the motor power was never entirely lost.

The patient's head has been abnormally large since childhood, but has not grown in the past fifteen years. The large head suggested a spontaneously healed hydrocephalus.

The results of the physical, serologic, roentgenologic and neurologic examinations were negative. Two diagnoses were suggested: (1) a cerebellar lesion which might have been responsible for the old hydrocephalus and was now causing attacks affecting the left side of the body; (2) a neurosis. The patient was very introspective, and had always feared paralysis.

Operation.— A cerebellar exploration was made after ventricular estimation had shown large ventricles. An enormous occipital dural sinus 2.5 cm. in width was found and ligated. The cerebellar region was normal. The foramen of Magendie was as large as the circumference of a lead pencil. The patient's headaches persist unchanged five years after the operation. The occipital sinus therefore had no bearing on the causation of the headache.

ANGIOMAS

Luschka (1854), who described the first angioma of the brain, divided angiomas into two types: (1) those arising by sequestration of a small portion of the embryonic capillary vascular system; (2) "true tumor" formation from vascular tissue. His case was of the latter type — a true tumor. The first type corresponds to the vascular nevi or telangiectases of the skin. Before Luschka's report, tumors of both types were well known elsewhere in the body, and because of their cavernous structure Rokitansky referred to them as "cavernous angiomas," a name by which they have since been known. It is questionable whether this classification is pertinent at the present time. There is, it is true, the type in which there is little connective tissue between the vascular spaces, and another type in which the connective tissue predominates and the vascular spaces are of microscopic size; but there seems little, if any, fundamental difference between the two types. Certainly both types grow like tumors. Whether one arises de novo and the other is always of congenital origin has not been proved. At the present time it seems preferable to avoid classification based on conceptions of origin and to group them all as cavernous angiomas. When the stroma is in abundance and the vascular spaces microscopic, this type of angioma is frequently known as hemangiomendothelioma or perithelioma. In addition to cavernous angiomas, there is another type which should be added — venous plexus or angioma plexiforme.

ANGIOMA PLEXIFORME

A lesion of this character has been described among tumors of the spinal cord, where they are not uncommon. In a series of seventy-five tumors of the spinal cord, I had four angiomas of this character. In a review of the literature on angiomas of the brain, I did not see any reference to similar observations, unless the case of D'Arcy Power is of this type. From the brief note and the accompanying sketch, this appears unlikely; more probably the tumor in Power's case was an arteriovenous aneurysm.

There seems to be no reason why a venous plexus should occur in the spinal cord and not in the brain. In the present series of angiomas of the brain, there are four examples of this lesion. A remarkable example of bilaterally symmetrical venous plexuses in the sylvian fossae is shown in case 7 (Fig. 1), reported under venous anomalies. In addition, there are several smaller circumscribed plexuses over both cerebral hemispheres. This patient was only two and one-half years old, and since the vascular lesions were accompanied by other congenital cerebral defects, it is fair to conclude that the angiomas were of congenital origin also. Cases 2 and 6 of the venous anomalies are also examples of this lesion, although in case 2 the form was perhaps less pure, since numerous large veins ran into the plexus, making it less sharply defined. These three cases show how insensibly venous anomalies and venous angiomas of this type blend into each other. In a final analysis they are probably identical.

A fourth example (case 12) of this lesion is presented with reservations, since the entire extent of the lesion was not seen. Although the tumor displayed the exact gross appearance of an angioma of the venous plexus type, it is not impossible that an underlying solid tumor may have been beyond operative exposure. Although solid tumors may cause a plexiform assembly of veins, it seems incredible that one so extensive could arise from this source. At the time of the operation, an extensive exposure was made in search of a solid growth. This patient was the only one of the series who was an adult. His symptoms were those of a slowly growing tumor in the hypophyseal region. The sella turcica was destroyed; there was a first bitemporal hemianopsia and later primary atrophy of one optic nerve with retention of vision only in the nasal half of the other eye. There was also in addition, pain in the trigeminal domain on both sides, probably explainable by the overflow of the angioma laterally. In retrospect, it is difficult to see how the character of the lesion could have been determined from signs and symptoms. One should still have had to be content with the preoperative diagnosis of a hypophyseal tumor.

There has not been any occasion to remove a venous plexus of the brain. In one patient (case 7), it appeared to have no bearing on the hydrocephalus, for which relief was sought. Should one be more favorably situated over the cerebral cortex and at the same time be more circumscribed, it should not be difficult to remove. I have removed completely four of these from the dorsal side of the spinal cord, with only one death, which occurred several days later from meningitis. Although the hemorrhage might at first appear to be a formidable danger, there is actually little to be feared. The loops of veins are bound loosely with arachnoid connective tissue, and when carefully separated, the whole network of venous loops becomes disengaged, much like a skein of yarn, and becomes resolved into two or three long veins which communicate with each other and with other veins on the surface of the cord. In the case which came to necropsy, the venous channels had entered into the spinal cord. The venous spaces within the spinal cord occupied a considerable volume of the cord and probably accounted for the symptoms more than did the great plexus of vessels on the surface.

REPORT OF CASES OF ANGIOMA PLEXIFORME

Case 12. *Angioma Plexiforme.*

A physician, aged forty-four, was referred by Dr. Carl Henning of Washington with the diagnosis of a hypophyseal tumor. His chief complaints were continuous ocular neuralgia and bitemporal hemianopsia. He had always had headaches. Due to severe paroxysms of pain in the eyes, he had became a morphine addict, finally taking from 10 to 12 grains (0.65 to 0.78 Gm.) a day. The addiction to morphine dated back six years, when the pains had become unbearable. Only through the use of this drug was he able to keep at his work. The pain first began in the right eye and often radiated to the cheek and teeth on the right side. Two years before admission to the hospital, diplopia had appeared and had been present at varying intervals until this report was written. At that time, an x-ray examination showed erosion of the posterior clinoid processes. Two years before, pains of the same character had extended to the left eye, face and teeth. A bilateral temporal hemianopsia had then been found by Dr. Henning. Teeth on both sides had been extracted, at patient's insistence, in an effort to get relief from the pain. Eighteen months before, a subtemporal decompression had been performed elsewhere, but without appreciable benefit.

Neurologic examination revealed the following: 1. A bitemporal hemianopsia was noted which was not sharply demarcated, there being some slight vision in the temporal fields near the center. The visual acuity was greatly reduced, more in the right eye, with which fingers could not be counted at a distance of 20 cm. 2. There was the characteristic pallor of primary atrophy in the temporal side of both disks. The nasal margin of each disk was hazy. The retinal veins were moderately engorged and tortuous. 3. There was complete destruction of the posterior clinoid processes (x-ray examination); the sella turcica was deep. Otherwise, the results of the examination were negative. There was no objective, sensory or motor disturbance referable to either trigeminal nerve. The Wassermann reaction of the blood was negative.

Operation.—In March, 1922, an anterior right craniotomy was performed for exploration of the hypophyseal region. A bluish tumor protruded anteriorly between the optic nerves (Fig. 2). When the arachnoid membrane was opened

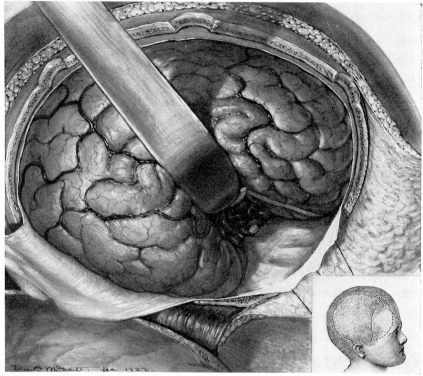

Fig. 2. (case 12). Plexiform agioma in the region of the hypophysis. It caused all the symptoms of a hypophyseal tumor.

and the cerebrospinal fluid allowed to escape, the tumor was seen to be a mass of entwined veins, each about as large as a slate pencil. Pulsation could not be observed. There was no evidence of arterial blood such as one sees through the wall of distended veins in an arteriovenous aneurysm. Treatment of the lesion being hopeless, the wound was closed. The patient died thirty-six hours after operation, presumably from restriction of morphine, though possibly from an extradural hemorrhage. He was conscious until shortly before death. Necropsy was not permitted, so that further observations on the origin and distribution of the angioma cannot be added to the operative notes.

CYST WITH ANGIOMA IN THE WALL

Of all the tumors of the vascular system of the brain, angiomatous cysts offer the best prognosis. It may almost be said that as a type and eliminating individual exceptions, they offer more than any other

tumor of the brain. Usually the cyst is large and the tumor small. The tumor is embedded in and projects from some point in the wall of the cyst. Always relatively small, compared to other tumors, it may actually be so small as to escape casual observation. There can be no doubt that in many of the so-called simple cysts a tiny angioma will be found on more careful inspection. The solid tumor is flat or rounded; it varies in size from a few millimeters to 2 or 3 cm. in diameter. Its surface is smooth and appears to be covered by the smooth lining of the cyst, but the cyst is not lined with epithelium. On sectioning the wall, a minute, insignificant looking, reddish brown lesion will frequently be found to cause the relatively enormous cyst. In the gross appearance, the intracystic angiomas are usually mistaken for gliomas. A careful gross inspection will usually make the differential diagnosis. An angioma is fibrous and acellular and the larger tumors are usually compressible and spongelike. In the fixed specimen, the tumor has changed from reddish brown to black, because of the old fixed blood in the tumor. A glioma is softer, more cellular and consequently more friable. Cells of the latter easily scrape off on the edge of a scalpel. It is noncompressible and its color a more uniform brown in the fresh specimen and a less intense brown or black when fixed. The content of cysts, whether of angiomatous or of gliomatous origin, is apparently the same. In either type, the fluid is clear lemon or orange yellow and a white coagulum is present at the bottom of the cyst. The reason for the cyst formation in these tumors it not known.

In an intensive study of cysts of the cerebellum, Lindau assembled fifteen cases, including a case reported previously by Schloffer, and another by Friedrich and Stiehler. This number is many more than the combined total number of all the cases, both cerebral and cerebellar, in the literature.

Other cases of angiomatous cysts were reported by Luzzatto, Bielschowsky, Baum, Bruns, Koch, Newmark and Schweyer. Four of these (Bielschowsky, Baum, Bruns and Schweyer) were in the cerebral hemispheres; two in the cerebellum and one (Luzzatto) in the brain stem. Koch's patient had bilateral angiomas. In Newmark's case, the tumor was in the meninges and the cyst was extracerebellar. Including my seven cases, there have now been reported twenty-nine cases of angiomatous cysts, twenty-four cerebellar, four cerebral, and one in the brain stem.

It is of interest to note that Lindau found angiomatous cysts to be almost twice as frequent as those of gliomatous origin. He doubtless refers to the large cysts with small single intracystic papilloma. Lindau's statements are supported by careful histologic studies with differential stains to detect glia fibers. From operative experience, the histologic evidence indicates the angiomatous and gliomatous cysts to be about equally divided. However, there are

three cases diagnosed gliomatous cysts which I feel confident, because of the gross description in the operative notes, are angiomatous cysts; the sections have been lost. If these are really angiomatous cysts, the results would be similar to those of Lindau. On a restudy of the histologic material, it is surprising to find how many tumors have previously been diagnosed gliomas when they are sharply defined angiomas. There are many exceedingly vascular gliomas which in the gross or microscopic examinations might be mistaken for angiomas, but a careful study of the vascular spaces of a glioma show well defined vascular coats which are absent in the angioma. Moreover, even with a hematoxylin eosin stain, the reticulated stroma of a glioma has little resemblance to that of an angioma.

Lindau's intensive study demonstrates anew the fact that when supposedly rare lesions are better known they are frequently found to be common. All seven of my cases of intracystic angiomas were in the cerebellum. As indicated in the accompanying sketches, the solid tumors were located at divergent parts of the wall of the cyst. All have reached the surface of the cerebellum and have been in contact with the pial vessels, but whether this is significant in their origin, I am not prepared to suggest.

Clinical Features. — There is nothing characteristic about the signs and symptoms produced by angiomatous cysts. Other types of cysts in the same position and of the same size give identically the same disturbances. All produce intracranial pressure, usually but not invariably evidenced by headache, nausea, vomiting and papilledema; they therefore compromise life. In most instances they also induce symptoms of localization, but this is not always true. If the cyst occupies a silent area of the cerebral hemisphere, localizing symptoms will be absent until it has grown alongside cerebral tracts with function — speech, motor, sensory, visual, uncinate, etc. All of the cases of cerebellar cysts collected from the literature showed outspoken so-called cerebellar disturbances — staggering gait, often with the tendency to swerve to one side, positive Romberg sign, and often nystagmus, ataxia, adiodokokinesis, stiffness of the neck and dizziness. One of my patients did not have any symptoms or signs of localizing import. Another had symptoms which were suggestive, but not positive. In these cases, ventriculography and ventricular estimation made the location absolute.

Clonic convulsions probably never occur with cerebellar cysts, but frequently with cerebral cysts. Convulsions resulting from cerebral cysts are often of local character and may have the jacksonian characteristics. In the cerebral cases reported, in those of Schweyer, Bruns and Baum the patients had jacksonian seizures; Bielschowsky's patient alone did not have convulsions. None of the twenty-four cerebellar cysts produced clonic convulsions. On the other hand, tonic spasms may occur in the late stages of cerebellar cysts. Such attacks are, in fact, characteristic of a tumor in the posterior cranial fossa; they result from compression of the motor tracts in the brain stem. This phenomenon was seen in cases 14 and 15. Newmark's patient had momentary losses of consciousness without convulsions.

Although a genuine hemiplegia or hemianesthesia is usually referable to lesions of the cerebral hemisphere, a few of the cerebellar angiomatous cysts induced paralyses, though usually in transient attacks. One of Lindau's patients had attacks in which both legs were paralyzed; another lost the use of the left arm and leg at times. Two of my patients had attacks of pain and numbness in one side of the body (cases 13 and 18). One of Lindau's patients and one of mine had trigeminal pain; in both instances the cerebellar cysts were unilateral. Luzzatto's case of a cyst in the medulla gave symptoms suggesting syringomyelia, and in its gross appearance the cystic cavity was like that found in syringomyelia. Recently several cases of

syringomyelia with cysts of the spinal cord have been reported in which tiny angiomas have been secreted in the walls of the cysts.

The reflexes are altered according to the relationship of the tumor to and the degree of injury of the motor tracts. Among the cerebellar cysts, reflex changes are usually not great, though not infrequently ankle clonus, a positive Babinski reflex and increased deep reflexes are present on one or both sides — constantly or transiently. The corneal reflex is frequently diminished and at times absent on the side of the unilateral tumor and on both sides from a midline tumor of the cerebellum.

The age at which symptoms first appear is essentially the age of greatest frequency of tumors of the brain in general, i. e., between the ages of 25 and 50.

The time of the initial symptoms in eighteen cases of cerebellar angiomatous cysts is as follows: between the ages of 20 and 30, three cases; between 30 and 40, nine cases; between 40 and 50, four cases; between 50 and 60, two cases.

In half of all the cases, symptoms first appeared in the third decade. The youngest patient was 21, the oldest, 52 years.

The duration of symptoms before death or operation is surprisingly short in most cases of cerebellar cysts. In six, the symptoms had been present less than six months; in four, less than one year or more than six months; in four, two years or less; and in one each, three, four, five and eight years. In approximately half of the cases, therefore, the symptoms began less than one year before death or operation. Only two cerebral angiomatous cysts have data concerning the duration of symptoms; Bielschowsky's patient had symptoms for fourteen months and Schweyer's for twelve years. It is obvious that the rapid onset of symptoms is due, not to the size of the comparatively insignificant tumor, but to the growth of the cyst which forms with relatively great rapidity.

Four of my patients were males and three were females. From the cases in the literature there are more males, fifteen to eleven. The frequency is probably not influenced by sex.

By using this analysis of signs and symptoms, it appears possible to make at least a tentative diagnosis of an angiomatous cyst — an absolute diagnosis seems impossible. Given a cerebellar tumor appearing in a patient between the ages of 25 and 40, symptoms rapidly progressive (less than one year) with variations in them from time to time and the absence of profound disturbances of a primary lesion of the brain stem a cyst, angiomatous or gliomatous, should be suspected.

Treatment of Patients with Angiomatous Cysts. — Angiomatous cysts are usually among the easiest and safest intracranial lesions to extirpate. Extirpation of the little tumor embedded in the wall of the cyst is sufficient. The extirpation must be done painstakingly, and a good margin of tissue must be included with the angioma. The danger is minimal when the tumor is small and situated near the surface. It increases somewhat when the tumor is larger and is located far forward over the midbrain. The larger tumors are usually vascular and for this reason offer difficulties in removal. A most important factor in the safety of the operation lies in the early diagnosis. In the late stages, the subtentorial pressure is so high that the dura cannot be safely opened because the cerebellum will herniate through the dural defect and rupture. Puncture of a lateral ventricle will relieve the supratentorial pressure, but not enough to prevent injury to the cerebellum. Puncture of a cerebellar lobe with a hollow, blunt needle will eliminate this hazard when a cyst is reached.

It is hardly necessary to add that as methods of treatment in an effort to cure tapping or completely evacuating a cyst by a transcortical incision, or treatment of the tumor by Zenker's solution or some other fixative are perfectly futile. They are inexcusable, for they have left uncured a lesion which can be so easily removed and permanently cured.

The operative efforts reported in the cases compiled from the literature have not been numerous. The first extirpation of a tumor of this type was performed by Bruns in 1897, but his patient died of meningitis. Baum's (1911) patient was in coma at the time of the operation, recovered, and died a year later of pneumonia. Schloffer's (1926) patient recovered after an extensive resection of a cerebellar hemisphere. One of my patients died nearly ten years ago, without exposure of the tumor. At that time there was no means of locating the tumor (she was in deep coma at the time) and the then routine subtemporal decompression was performed, of course, without relief. From careful inspection of the autopsy specimen, it is doubtful whether at that time the cyst could have been found for there was no surface evidence of its presence when the brain was removed. The tumor was 4 cm. beneath the surface of the cerebellum. I have also wondered whether the solid part of the tumor would have been detected had it been possible to locate and open the cyst. At the present time, however, the methods of accurate localization of tumors would make the disclosure of the cyst possible regardless of its depth. The five patients on whom the extirpation of the tumor in the wall of the cyst has been performed have made uneventful and complete recoveries and are now living and well. They are without any signs of recurrence of the tumor. One patient is well seven years after operation (April 13, 1921). At the time of the operation, he was in deep coma. The operation was performed only after the tumor was localized by ventriculography. Another patient is well after five years. Her vision, which was lost due to retinal hemorrhages caused by the intracranial pressure, has returned to normal. Another patient who was nearly comatose quickly became conscious after operation (sixteen months ago).

The seventh patient died en route to the hospital, though in good condition when he left home. The sudden development of coma, and the comparatively short duration of the intracranial signs and symptoms, make an early diagnosis of paramount importance, if cures are to be obtained. Often warning is not given that death impends.

The only safe way to relieve intracranial pressure due to a cerebellar cyst is to evacuate the cyst. The relief is then prompt and complete for the time being; it becomes permanent when the tumor — the cause of the cyst — is removed. The evacuation of the cyst relieves not only the direct pressure on the brain stem, but also the hydrocephalus. Relief of the latter is almost as important as the former, for the hydrocephalic ventricles gradually push the tentorium backward and exert great pressure on the structures — including the medulla — in the posterior cranial fossa. A subtemporal decompression may or may not effect temporary relief depending on whether the tumor can be lifted from the foramina of Luschka. The only safe and certain attack therefore is to open the cyst and extirpate the tumor. This same principal of relief by the direct operative attack on tumors holds true for all intracranial neoplasms. There could not be better proof of this statement than the prompt recovery from coma after removal of the cause of the intracranial pressure in the foregoing cases.

REPORT OF CASES OF CYST WITH ANGIOMA IN THE WALL

Case 13. *Angiomatous Cyst.*

A well nourished woman, aged thirty-two, blind and unable to stand, was referred by Dr. George Price of Spokane, Wash. Her symptoms dated back only seven months, when she had noticed stablike pains in both eyes which had lasted only a few seconds and had disappeared when she lay down. There was also some headache in the frontal region and sides of the head. They had become more severe and more persistent; for the two months prior to operation they were

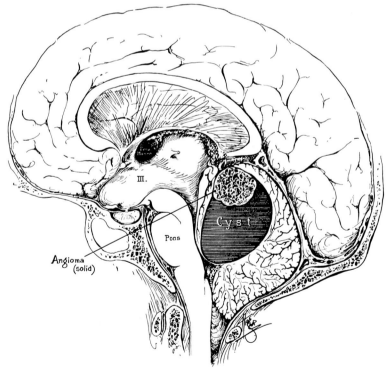

Fig. 3. (case 13). The operative observations in an angiomatous cyst. The solid tumor was situated directly over the midbrain.

constant.

Sudden fainting spells, lasting from ten to fifteen minutes, and without loss of consciousness, had occurred nearly once a week for the past five months before operation. She felt dizzy during these spells; her "thoughts were paralyzed" and "everything seemed to rush to the head" and she would fall to the floor. Staggering gait had been present two months; she swayed from side to side and had a tendency to bear to the right. She had had occasional attacks of numbness of the right arm and leg, and the neck had been rigid.

One month before admission to the hospital, her vision suddenly had become blurred and since that time she had been blind. Attacks of nausea and vomiting had been present for the past three months. It is of interest that two years ago an ovarian tumor, said to be a carcinoma, had been removed by Dr. Terry in San Francisco.

Neurologic examination elicited the following positive observations: 1. There were tremendous bilateral choked disk (6 diopters); each nerve head was covered with dozens of hemorrhages. Much of the contiguous retina was also obscured by the hemorrhages. 2. The patient could not see fingers with either eye. 3. She showed a positive Romberg sign and fell to the right. 4. Staggering gait and 5. Hyperactive but symmetrical reflexes were present. The Wassermann reaction of the blood was negative. X-ray examination of the head was negative. A metastatic tumor was suspected.

Ventricular estimation (at time of operation) showed that the lateral ventricles were large and communicated freely with each other (indigo carmine test). The pressure of the ventricular fluid was very high.

Operation.—On Jan. 6, 1923, cerebellar exploration was performed. A large cyst was struck with a hallow needle 3 cm. below the surface of the vermis (Fig. 3). A transverse transcortical incision was then carried into the cyst, which was larger than a walnut. Straw colored fluid escaped, and a gelatinous coagulum was removed. A small, rounded, firm papilloma about the size of a hazelnut projected from the wall of the cyst at its anteriormost part and lay just under the great vein of Galen. Its removal was attended by such profuse bleeding that its angiomatous character was at once apparent. Though its base was only about 0.75 by 0.75 cm., every attempt to dissect it free was followed by a brisk hemorrhage. After it was removed the bleeding surface was temporarily packed with moist cotton under pressure, and later the use of silver clips completely stopped the bleeding. The unopened fourth ventricle bulged into the floor of the cyst.

Microscopic examination showed that the tumor was made up of endothelial lined, blood-containing spaces of varying size. Abundant connective tissue interposed between the vascular sinuses was the only other feature of the tumor.

The patient made an uneventful recovery. Five years later, she was well; her vision had returned; her gait was unaffected, and she was able to do her own housework.

Case 14. *Angiomatous Cyst.*

A poorly nourished woman, aged thirty-six, was referred by Dr. F. H. Kliefoth, of Schertz, Tex., on Feb. 20, 1928. Six months before, suboccipital headaches had first appeared with nausea and vomiting. Dizziness and staggering gait, dimness of vision and diplopia had soon developed and had increased. Later, the patient had been subject to "nervous spells" in which numbness extended upward from the fingers and toes of both sides. During these spells, which lasted from twenty to thirty minutes, the arms were flexed, the legs extended and she was unable to move. Until the attack passed, she was unable to speak, although she was conscious.

Examination showed an extremely ill woman. She was drowsy in spite of the severe headaches to which she had been subject. It was evident that she was bordering on coma.

The Romberg sign was positive; she promptly fell to the left; ataxia and adiadokokinesia were positive on the left; there was lateral nystagmus. High grade papilledema of both eyegrounds was observed.

Operation.—The diagnosis of a cerebellar tumor was confirmed by ventricular estimation, and a bilateral cerebellar exploration made. A cyst of the left cerebellar lobe was found and evacuated. The cyst was about as large as a walnut, and contained clear orange-yellow fluid. The fourth ventricle bulged into the mesial side of the cyst. A small smooth reddish-brown tumor, about as large as a split pea, could be seen in the wall of the cyst; it was located in the left cerebellar tonsil which had herniated into the foramen magnum. It was necessary to liberate the tonsil in order to reach the tumor and permit its extirpation. The tumor was excised with a zone of normal cerebellar tissue on all sides. Histologically, the tumor was a typical cavernous angioma.

The patient made a complete recovery and is now well. There are no residual cerebellar symptoms.

Case 15. *Angiomatous Cyst.*

A well nourished woman, aged forty-four, entered the hospital in coma, in October, 1918. For two months she had complained of dizziness after exertion, and some suboccipital headaches associated with vomiting nearly every day. At first, when perfectly quiet she had been comparatively free from both headache and dizziness, but gradually the headaches had become much more intense and were not affected by resting. She staggered like a drunken person and had shaking of both hands (but more the right), so that at times she was scarcely able to lift the cup to her mouth. She had several attacks in which her whole body became rigid like a board, but consciousness was not lost nor were there any clonic convulsive movements. A month prior to operation, she had had periods of mental cloudiness, some hallucinations and had been disoriented. Later she had alternately laughed and cried and had ceased to take interest in her surroundings.

The physical and neurologic examination showed the following:

A coarse tremor of the right hand and arm was frequently observed. The veins of the forehead and eyelids were very full. The eyegrounds showed fulness of the veins and a beginning bilateral papilledema. The Babinski reflex was positive on both sides; the corneal reflex and knee jerks were normal, and ankle clonus was not noted.

At the time this patient was seen, the stereotyped treatment for such patients was a subtemporal decompression—now known to be useless. Through the operative defect a large lateral ventricle was tapped, reducing the supratentorial pressure to normal. She died twenty-four hours after the operation.

When the brain was examined at necropsy, evidence of the tumor was not found on the surface of the brain. Section of the cerebellum, at a later date, showed a cyst about 3 by 3 cm. in diameter. At first evidence of a solid tumor was not present, but later a small circular thickened area about 3 mm. in diameter was detected. Microscopic examination of this area showed a typical angioma.

Case 16. *Angiomatous Cyst.*

A young engineer, aged twenty-eight, was seen, in consultation with Drs. Julius and Harry Friedenwald of Baltimore, at another hospital on April 13, 1921. He was then comatose despite a subtemporal decompression which had been performed two weeks before.

The following history was obtained from Dr. Friedenwald: The symptom of onset was an attack of headache, lasting three or four hours, and beginning six months before admission to the hospital. At first, the attack recurred about every ten days, but for the three months before admission they had been continuous and frequently associated with nausea and vomiting. For three months he had been troubled with dizziness and staggering gait. The dizziness was always worse when he was lying on the right side. Diplopia had been present at times for three or four months.

The results of the neurologic examination were negative, except for a bilateral papilledema of high grade. The decompression in the right subtemporal region was full and tight.

Operation.—On April 13, 1921, an injection of air was made; the tumor was localized to the posterior cranial fossa, and a cerebellar operation was performed. A large cyst of the left lobe was first tapped, then evacuated through a transcortical incision. Clear, yellowish fluid escaped from the cyst. On the posterior lateral wall of the cyst was a smooth, reddish-brown solid tumor about as large as a pea. It reached the surface of the cerebellum. The solid tumor was removed with a zone of normal cerebellar tissue.

Recovery was prompt and complete. The patient has since carried on his occupation and has remained entirely well.

Case 17. *Angiomatous Cyst.*

A poorly nourished man, aged thirty-five, was referred with the diagnosis of a tumor of the brain on June 3, 1924. His symptoms dated back only three months, when he had suddenly been seized with a severe occipital headache, dizziness and vomiting. The attack had lasted two days. Similar attacks had recurred in increasing frequency. Three weeks after the onset of his illness, staggering gait had developed. Vomiting had become so intense that he lost thirty pounds (13.6 Kg.) in weight. Occasionally, there had been roaring in the right ear. From time to time, dark spots had appeared before the eyes, and for six weeks before operation his vision had been blurred. He had been bedfast for four weeks fearful of turning his head because of the certainty of precipitating dizziness. Diplopia had not been present.

Neurologic Examination.— The patient could only see enough to count fingers. There was a marked papilledema of both optic nerves. Many hemorrhages obscured the region of the disks. There was a positive Romberg sign, with tendency to fall to the left and backward; retropulsion, unsteady gait, cervical rigidity and ataxia were present. The reflexes were normal. A Babinski reflex or ankle clonus was not noted.

*Operation.—*On June 4, 1924, ventricular estimation showed marked hydrocephalus, with free communication between the lateral ventricles—indigo carmine passed quickly from one ventricle to the other.

Because of the patient's poor physical condition, the operation was performed under local anesthesia. A large cerebellar cyst was tapped in the left lobe; clear lemon-yellow fluid escaped. A smooth, reddish tumor, as large as a cherry, protruded slightly into the cavity of the cyst at the outer aspect near the midline. It also penetrated through the remaining cerebellar tissue to reach the surface. The tumor was easily excised with contiguous cerebellar tissue. The patient made an uneventful recovery, and has since been well (nearly four years).

Case 18. *Angiomatous Cyst.*

A large, strong man, aged thirty-four, was referred by Dr. Malcolm Campbell, of Malvern, Ia., on Oct. 20, 1927, with the diagnosis of a tumor of the brain. His symptoms had begun two years before, when he had first noticed pain in and behind both eyes and radiating to the occipital region. Eighteen months later, severe occipital headaches had begun, and had persisted up to the time of operation. During the month before operation, he had had spells of numbness and tingling in the right arm and leg. Dizziness, vomiting or unsteadiness of gait were not noted.

The neurologic examination showed a bilateral papilledema measuring 5 diopters in each eye. There were no other positive neurologic observations. The Romberg sign was negative; ataxia, or nystagmus was not noted. There were no signs by which the localization of the tumor could be made.

Ventriculography showed that the lateral ventricles were much enlarged; they communicated freely; the third ventricle was enlarged and mesially placed; the aqueduct of Sylvius was patent throughout and also the fourth ventricle until an abrupt vertical line was reached 2 cm. back of the aqueduct. This line marked the anteriormost part of the tumor.

*Operation.—*On Nov. 2, 1927, a bilateral cerebellar exposure was made. The bone was exceedingly bloody, despite the release of pressure by a ventricular puncture. The dura was still so tight that it seemed unsafe to expose the cerebellum. Puncture of the left and right cerebellar lobes yielded nothing; on puncturing the vermis, a yellow fluid spurted. With the dural tension relieved, the dura was evacuated. A colorless, gelatinous clot was pulled out of the bottom of the cyst. The outer surface of the cyst contained only meninges, the cortex having been entirely atrophied. The cerebellar tonsils were herniated far into the spinal canal. After the cyst was evacuated, the tonsils could readily be withdrawn from their incarcerated position; as they were withdrawn, one could see a cluster of little yellowish cystic nodules much like a bunch of grapes. They occurred as much in one tonsil as in the other. They were attached to the meninges. The fourth ventricle bulged into the cyst. The anterior part of the solid tumor was attached to the wall of the cyst, where it was inseparable from the fourth ventricle. The entire solid tumor was removed with a good margin of cerebellar tissue. This procedure necessitated the removal of both tonsils and part of the roof of the fourth ventricle. The tumor and brain tissue weighed 9 Gm.

The postoperative course was uneventful. The patient is now well (six months after the operation).

Case 19. A man of about forty years of age was referred by Dr. R. R. Snowden, of Pittsburgh, with the diagnosis of an unlocalized tumor of the brain. For about a year he had been having head-

aches, which had gradually increased in intensity. For a few months prior to death they had been almost continuous. He had loss of vision, hiccups, projectile vomiting and inability to maintain his balance. With the exception of a double papilledema, Dr. Snowden did not make any positive observations on examination.

The patient died en route from the station to the hospital.

Necropsy showed a large cyst of the left cerebellar lobe with a small flat circumscribed tumor embedded in the cerebellum and wall of the cyst.

Microscopically, the tumor was a typical cavernous angioma.

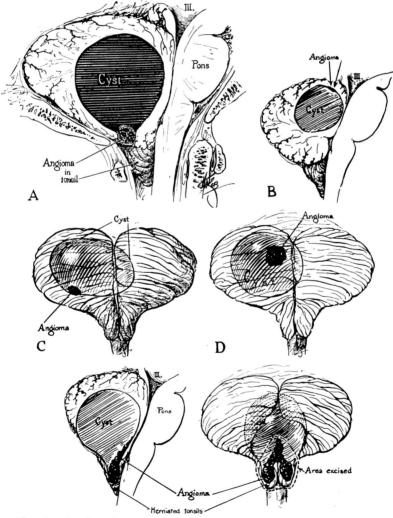

Fig. 4. Sketches showing the location of the small solid tumors in a series of cysts: (*a*) case 14; (*b*) case 15; (*c*) case 16; (*d*) case 17, and (*e*) case 18.

CAVERNOUS ANGIOMA

Cavernous angiomas differ from the foregoing group of tumors principally in the absence of a cyst and in the larger size of the vascular spaces which are usually on the range of unaided vision. The five cases here reported differ greatly from each other in the gross appearance of the tumors. On one extreme, they seem to fuse insensibly with the angiomas associated with cysts, and on the other with the plexiform angiomas. In general, it may be added that they lack the hyperplastic character of the former and the gross venous make-up of the latter. The tumor in case 20 showed a gross cavernous character, and in case 23, hyperplastic stroma. It has already been noted that the angioma plexiforme fused insensibly with the venous anomalies. It would seem therefore, that other types of lesions of the venous and capillary systems blend with each other. Perhaps it may be preferable to subdivide the cavernous angiomas into two types according to the early proposal of Luschka, but for the present I am inclined to disregard the differences and group them all together. Although many of the lesions of both the embryonal vascular type and of the angioplastic type (that so-called "true tumor" of Luschka) are small and apparently dormant, others with seemingly the same histologic and gross appearance and undoubtedly growing. Either, therefore, may or may not act as a neoplasm. Probably the most rapidly growing and much the largest tumor of my series was one of the primitive vascular — presumably the least active — type.

Until Lindau's publication, the overwhelming percentage of angiomas was cavernous. With the addition of his great number of angiomatous cysts, the latter have come to assume a less subordinate position. The cavernous angiomas are far less concentrated to one locality in the brain, in contrast to the favored cerebellar habitat of the angiomatous cysts.

Forty-four cases of cavernous angioma have been found in the literature. The number reaches forty-nine, with addition of the five cases included in this report. In nine of these cases (18 per cent), multiple tumors of the same character were scattered throughout the brain. In most of them, there were two or three angiomas (Finkelnburg, Jakob, Malamud, Muller and Ohlmacher), but in Creite's case there were eight, in Kuf's twelve, and in Huebschman's thirty; in Kalischer's case, the brain was studded with angiomas.

The distribution of these tumors is as follows: frontoparietal lobes, thirty-two; brain stem and fourth ventricle, fourteen; cerebellum, eight; in depth of cerebral hemisphere and third ventricle, nine; occipital lobe two.[2]

The gross appearance of a typical cavernous angioma is characteristic. It is spongelike and compressible because of the large spaces which one can usually see with the naked eye. It is always well circumscribed, but never encapsulated; its color is reddish brown because of the contained blood. Some of the tumors are soft, others firm, depending on the size of the blood spaces and the amount of connective tissue. Although they have a good venous and arterial blood supply, neither is excessive, and neither is disproportionate to the other. When opened at operation, they bleed freely and in proportion to the size of the cavernous spaces and the entering arterial supply. The bleeding is principally venous, though on the confines of the tumor the arterial bleeding may give some trouble. The tumors do not pulsate. The size of these tumors varies from minute areas to a mass larger than one's fist. The largest tumor in my series occurred in a baby, 1 month old. It was both intracranial and extracranial. Both portions were directly continuous through numerous small defects in the bone and dura.

Microscopically, these tumors show endothelial blood spaces with scant or not supporting coats, with a minimal amount of connective tissue between the blood spaces.

Thrombosis and calcification, principally the former, frequently occur, but apparently to a far less extent than in an arteriovenous aneurysm. Lindau has stained the tumors with glial stains to exclude the diagnosis of a glioma. Microscopic studies have been made exclusively with hematoxylin and eosin stains, from which the diagnosis is easily made on the grosser aspects of the histologic picture.

Signs and Symptoms of Cavernous Angioma. There is a striking uniformity in the symptoms when viewed as a whole. Occasionally, as in Kuf's patient who died at the age of eighty-one, symptoms were not present. Other patients did not show symptoms until one of the vascular spaces suddenly ruptured and the patient died of a cerebral hemorrhage. Three patients from the group died in this way. This is a far smaller proportion of deaths from hemorrhage than in the group of arteriovenous aneurysms, probably owing to the arterial pressure in the defective walls of the latter.

A spontaneous cerebral hemorrhage occurring during the period of youth and middle age in a person without hypertension must nearly always indicate an underlying tumor or aneurysm. Most instances of so-called spontaneous "subarachnoid hemorrhage" arise in this way. At times the lesion is so small that it may be overlooked, or in the vascular break may be a tumor of the spinal cord as in Lorenz's case. It is not fair to make a final anatomic diagnosis of primary "arachnoid hemorrhage" unless the spinal cord has been searched for angiomas, for these tumors are common throughout the central nervous system. Cases of angiomas of the spinal cord have been reported by Gaupp, Hadlick, Barenbruch, Lorenz, Roman, Pinner, Tannenberg, Lindau and Ritter. For the literature on this subject, the reader is referred to the publication of Tannenberg and Ritter.

The accompanying tables show at least three striking differences between cavernous angiomas and angiomatous cysts. 1. Most of the symptoms of cavernous an-

giomas are focal, and few are of general intracranial pressure. 2. The duration of symptoms is much longer. 3. The symptoms begin at an earlier age. Assuredly, these generalizations have their exceptions.

The clinical disturbances obviously depend on the location of the tumor as well as on its character. Tumors in the brain stem cause the most profound loss of function and affect life long before tumors in the silent lobes of the cerebral hemispheres. The symptoms in some of the cases of cavernous angioma occurring in early life are of short duration because the children so affected soon die.

In one of my patients, a tremendous cavernous angioma was present at birth. An external portion resembled an occipital meningocele; an internal portion pushed the cerebellum far forward and caused hydrocephalus. This tumor developed early in embryonic life, for at birth it was larger than one's fist. It doubtless developed early also because both the dura and occipital bone were honeycombed with parts of the tumor which connected the nerves within and without the skull. Kalischer's patient had convulsions soon after birth and died when he was $1\frac{1}{2}$ years old. In thirty patients, the age of onset of the symptoms could be computed. In eleven or about one-third, symptoms began before the tenth year; in eighteen, or 60 per cent, before the twentieth year, and in twenty-five, or 83 per cent, before the age of 30. (Only 16 per cent of the angiomatous cysts showed symptoms before the thirtieth year.)

The duration of the symptoms shows a contrast almost as striking. Six patients had symptoms for less than one year (three of these died of cerebral hemorrhage and one of operation); four had symptoms for two years; five for three years; and five, for from five to ten years; seven, for from ten to twenty years, and four, for from twenty to thirty years. In the group of patients with angiomatous cysts, 50 per cent had symptoms less than one year, whereas 80 per cent of those with cavernous angiomas had symptoms longer than one year, and

50 per cent had symptoms longer than five years.

By far the most common symptom of cavernous angioma is epilepsy, and usually the attacks are jacksonian. This is largely due to the fact that most of the tumors are in the cerebral hemispheres and near the rolandic area. It is highly improbable that a cavernous angioma located solely in the cerebellum will cause epilepsy. Many of the patients have had motor or sensory weakness, some slight, some transiently after an attack and others of severe grade.

Headache, vomiting and choked disk are infrequent in cerebral cavernous angiomas because the tumor rarely attains sufficient size to cause intracranial pressure. Rupture of a vessel in the tumor may at once induce intracranial pressure. One of my patients (case 24), with an angioma of the occipital lobe and a big cerebral hemorrhage, had a bilateral papilledema of high grade. Lewandowsky and Stadelmann reported a case presumably of angioma, in which a big cerebral hemorrhage was encountered by a puncture. The patient recovered.

Cavernous angiomas in the cerebellum and brain stem may cause hydrocephalus by closing the aqueduct of Sylvius or fourth ventricle, intracranial pressure then following. A high grade of hydrocephalus was present in all four of my cases of cerebellar cavernous angiomas. In one of these cases, the angioma was small and caused intermittent or recurring hydrocephalus, the tumor acting in ball-valve fashion. It is interesting that over a period of ten years the patient's attacks were intensified in three successive pregnancies. Finally, as the tumor grew, the ball-valve action was largely overcome, for her symptoms rarely abated. In another patient (case 20), slight trauma — presumably causing hemorrhage in the tumor, on several occasions, precipitated paralyses and general intracranial pressure. The first instance of this relationship occurred when the patient was 14 months old. The early age also indicates the probably congenital origin of the tumor. The relationship of trauma and cerebral hemorrhage from vascular tumors was considered in the paper on arteriovenous aneurysms.

Two of my four cerebellar cavernous angiomas would easily have been tolerated in the cerebral hemispheres without symptoms of pressure. The other two were large. One had grown tightly into the brain stem. The changes in the reflexes in this group of tumors are usually of little help in making a diagnosis; the deep reflexes

TABLE I—ANALYSIS OF SYMPTOMS

Author	Date of Publication	Age	Sex	Type of Angioma			Tumor		Location of Tumor	Duration of Symptoms	Age at First Symptom	First Symptom	Signs and Symptoms of Intracranial Pressure	Focal Signs and Symptoms
				Cavernous	Small Solid Tumor with Cyst	Single	Multiple							
Dandy........	1928	44	M	Plexus	.....	+	..	Hypophyseal region	6 years	38 years	Pains in eyes	Erosion of posterior cilnoid process	Bitempora hemianops and destru tion of sella
Dandy........	1928	2½	F	Plexus	.....	..	+	Sylvian fossa of each side	Since birth	Since birth	Large head	Yes, but not from angioma	....
Dandy........	1928	5 mo.	M	Plexus	.....	..	+	Sylvian fossa	1 mo.	4 mo.	Convulsions	None	Convulsions begi in face

are increased along with motor disturbance; an ankle clonus and Babinski reflex are at times present, at other times absent. In midcerebellar tumors, bilateral reflex changes may be found.

X-ray examinations have not been helpful in my cases, for calcified lesions were not present in any of them; nor has any case from the literature been diagnosed from the roentgenograms. In one case, the convolutional atrophy of hydrocephalus was excellently demonstrated, but the large head and Macewen's sign (of separated sutures) had made the evidence given by the roentgenograms unnecessary.

Ventriculography was indispensable in making a diagnosis in two of my cerebellar cases, and ventricular estimation was useful in clinching the localization in another. These methods should always be used when the slightest doubt is entertained either of the existence of a tumor or of the location of a tumor that is known to exist.

Treatment of Cavernous Angioma.—Just as is true of angiomatous cysts, or for that matter any kind of tumor, the only satisfactory treatment is extirpation, when this is possible. Some tumors lend themselves readily to removal; others present difficulties which are insuperable. One of my pa-

tients, a baby 1 month of age (case 21), died of shock when a bloody suboccipital angioma (the continuation of an intracranial tumor) was removed. Bleeding had to be controlled by plugging the big venous spaces in the bone with wax. A second patient, a boy, aged sixteen (case 20), died one month after removal of a large cerebellar angioma which had grown into the brain stem. Death was not due to the tumor's removal which he survived, but to closure of the fourth ventricle caused by the formation of a cicatrix between the raw surfaces of the cerebellar lobes and pons from which the tumor had been removed. In this case, the foramina of Luschka had long been sealed by the tumor.

A third patient died before operation. This should have been much the easiest tumor of the group to have extirpated, had it been found at operation. There was a huge blood-filled cavity in the parieto-occipital lobes. The walls of the cavity were rough, having been carved out of the white matter of the brain which hung in shreds in the cavity; in this respect, it was entirely unlike the smooth cyst associated with an intracystic angioma.

Two of the cavernous angiomas were entirely removed, and the patients are apparently well. In one patient (case 22),

ASES OF PLEXIFORME ANGIOMA OF THE BRAIN

Epilepsy			Motor or Sensory Symptoms	Other Symptoms	Mentality	Operation	Cause of Death	Necropsy	Remarks	Studied Microscopically
Focal	Petit Mal	Grand Mal								
0	0	0	Pain in cheek and teeth	Diplopia	Normal	Tumor exposed, but inoperable	Operation	0	Patient was morphine addict; tumor was made up of coils of veins and resembled the well known venous plexus angiomas of the dorsal surface of the cord; the entire tumor could not be seen, nor could necropsy be obtained	0
0	+	0	Cannot sit up but uses both arms and legs	Failure to develop mentally and to coordinate muscular movements	Imbecile	+ Third ventriculostomy for hydrocephalus; angioma disclosed in sylvian fissure	Operation	+	Bilateral plexus of veins (angioma) in each sylvian fissure; several other small plexuses over both hemispheres; absence of corpus callosum; the angiomas did not cause the mental or physical disturbances, they were merely incidental conditions; stricture at iter caused hydrocephalus	0
+	+	+	None	None	Infant	Exploration	Operation	+	Two typical venous plexuses about 2 cm. apart; they were connected by communicating branches and emptied into the sylvian vein	+

TABLE II—ANALYSIS OF SYMPTOMS IN CASE

| Author | Date of Publication | Age | Sex | Type of Angioma | | Tumor | | Location of Tumor | Duration of Symptoms | Age at First Symptom | First Symptom | Signs and Symptoms of Intracranial Pressure | Focal Signs and Symptoms |
				Cavernous	Small Solid Tumor with Cyst	Single	Multiple						
Baum	1911	21	M	..	+ cyst contained yellow fluid	..	..	Left parietal	.....	.....	Convulsions and coma	Coma	Jacksonian attacks
Bielschowsky	1902	24	F	..	+ small solid tumor in large cyst	+	..	Right frontal lobe	14 mo.	23 yr.	Headache and dizziness	Choked disk, vomiting, headache	Facial weakness, positive Romberg, increased reflexes
Bruns	1897	24	M	..	+	..	..	Left parietal	.....	.....	Convulsions	No	Jacksonian attacks
Friedrich and Stiehler	1922	41	M	..	+	..	+	Cerebellum	2 yr.	39 yr.	Pain in neck	Headache, vomiting, loss of vision	....
Koch	1913	47	M	one side	other side	..	+	Each cerebellar lobe	3 yr.	44 yr.	Glycosuria	+	....
Lindau	1926	26	F	..	+	+	..	Cerebellum	5 yr.	21 yr.	Headache	Headache; vomiting, choked disk	Staggering, ataxia, nystagmus, loss of corneal reflex
Lindau	1926	50	M	..	+	+	..	Cerebellum	6 mo.	49 yr.	Headache	Headache, vomiting; choked disk	Staggering gait and Romberg, nystagmus
Lindau	1926	42	F	..	+	+	..	Cerebellum	4 yr.	38 yr.	Headache	....	....
Lindau	1926	37	M	..	+	..	..	Cerebellum	8 yr.	29 yr.	Headache	Headache, vomiting, choked disk	Staggering to right, nystagmus
Lindau	1926	28	F	..	+	+	..	Cerebellum	1 yr.	27 yr.	Headache and stiff neck	Headache, vomiting	None
Lindau	1926	46	M	..	+	+	..	Cerebellum	6 mo.	45 yr.	Headache	Headache, choked disk	Romberg, falls to right
Lindau	1926	40	F	..	+	+	..	Cerebellum	1 yr.	39 yr.	Dizziness and staggering	Headache, lumbar puncture	Romberg and staggering
Lindau	1926	33	F	..	+	+	..	Cerebellum	2 yr.	31 yr.	Weakness	Headache, vomiting, choked disk	....
Lindau	1926	..	..	..	+	+	..	Cerebellum	.....	.....	....	....	....
Lindau	1926	52	M	..	+	+	..	Cerebellum	.....	.....	....	....	Loss of left facial and trigeminal functions
Lindau	1926	33	M	..	+	+	..	Cerebellum	.....	.....	....	Choked disk	....
Lindau	1926	32	M	..	+	+	+	Cerebellum and medulla	.....	.....	....	....	....
Lindau	1926	38	F	..	+	+	..	Cerebellum	.....	.....	Headache	Choked disk	....
Luzzato	1925	..	..	..	+	+	..	Medulla		.....	....	....	Paresis left face, disturbance of speech and gait

—CYST WITH ANGIOMA IN THE WALL

Epilepsy			Motor or Sensory Symptoms	Other Symptoms	Mentality	Operation	Cause of Death	Necropsy	Remarks	Studied Microscopically
Focal	Petit Mal	Grand Mal								
+	..	+	....	No	Good	+ with finger extirpation	....	+	Patient in coma when operated on; no previous symptoms; solid tumor size of walnut; died one year later of pneumonia	+
0	..	0	Dizziness; diplopia	....	......	0	Intracranial pressure	+	Large cyst with hazelnut sized solid tumor; cerebellar tumor suspected	+
+	..	+	Weakness in right leg also paresthesia	....	......	+	Meningitis, postoperative	+	....	+
..	..		....	....	......	0	Intracranial pressure	+	Small angioma in cerebellum, another in pons and one in medulla	+
..	..	..	....	Diabetes	Normal	0	....	+	Patient had von Hippel's disease; cysts of pancreas (with diabetes); cysts and angiomas of liver	+
0	..	0	Left facial paralysis	....	Normal	0	Intracranial pressure	..	Cyst with angioma—hydrocephalus; cysts of pancreas, cysts of kidneys; hypernephroma	+
0	..	0	Weakness left arm and leg; trigeminal pain	Babinski + loss of corneal reflex	Normal	Decompression	Intracranial pressure	+	Cyst 3 by 2 by 1.5 cm.; tumor 1 by 2 by cm. in upper part of cysts; hydrocephalus	+
0	..	0	....	......	......	0	Intracranial pressure	+	Cyst 5 by 6 by 2 cm.; smooth wall; tumor 1 by 1 cm.	+
0	..	0	....	Loss of corneal reflex	......	0	Died 24 hours after spinal injection of air	+	Cyst 6 by 4 by 2 cm.; tumor 1.5 by 1.5 by 0.7 cm.; adenoma of both suprarenal glands; hydrocephalus	+
0	..	0	....	Both corneal reflexes diminished	......	0	Intracranial pressure	+	Cyst 3 by 2 by 2 cm.; tumor 1 by 1 cm.	+
+	+	+	....	Rigid neck	......	0	Intracranial pressure	+	Cyst 4 by 5 by 2 cm.; tumor 1 by 0.5 cm.; hydrocephalus	+
..	..		....	Adiadokokinesia	......	0	Intracranial pressure	+	Cyst with angioma; hydrocephalus	+
..	..		Weakness both legs	Blindness	......	0	Tonic convulsions	+	Small angioma in cyst.........	+
..	..		....	....	......	....	....	+	Museum preparation.........	+
..	..		....	Nystagmus blindness	......	Trephine	Intracranial pressure	+	Cyst 4 by 4 by 1.5 cm.; tumor 1 by 0.5 cm.	+
..	..		....	....	......		Intracranial pressure	+	Cyst with angioma in the wall	+
..	..		....	....	......		Intracranial pressure	+	Large cyst with angioma; also several small angiomas in cerebellar lobes (largest size of pea) one in medulla	+
..	..		....	Tremor of fingers of both hands	......	....	Intracranial pressure	+	....	+
0	..	0	Weakness of left face	....	Suggestive of a neurosis	0	....	+	Patient had a cavernoma of medulla with cyst formation like a syringomyelia	+

the tumor was excised from the left lobe of the cerebellum with a margin of cerebellar tissue. It is now over two years since the operation. She is entirely well and without residual cerebellar symptoms.

The other successful extirpation was a tumor laying on the pons and medulla (case 23). During the dissection, the tumor was thought to be a "venous aneurysm," because there seemed to be a single sac with several large venous outlets and because it was so compressible. After removal and section of the tumor, it was seen to be a typical solid cavernous angioma. The mass was dissected with great care after ligating the large venous outlets

as shown in the accompanying drawings (Fig. 6). No artery of size was seen to enter the tumor. There was no injury to the brain stem or cerebellum during the dissection. The patient also is well, one year after operation.

REPORT OF CASES OF CAVERNOUS ANGIOMA

Case 20. *Cavernous Angioma of the Cerebellum and Brain Stem.*

The patient was a very well nourished boy, aged sixteen, with a large head. He had been bedfast for sometime and sought relief for headache, disturbance of vision, disturbance of gait and projectile vomiting. His symptoms dated

TABLE II—ANALYSIS OF SYMPTOMS IN CASES—

Author	Date of Publication	Age	Sex	Type of Angioma		Tumor		Location of Tumor	Duration of Symptoms	Age at First Symptom	First Symptom	Signs and Symptoms of Intracranial Pressure	Focal Signs and Symptoms
				Cavernous	Small Solid Tumor with Cyst	Single	Multiple						
Newmark.....	....	32	F	..	+	+	..	Cerebellum	1½ yr.	30 yr.	Pain in back of head	Headache, vomiting, diplopia, choked disk	Occipital pain, buzzing left ear
Schlaffer......	1926	40	M	..	+	+	..	Cerebellum	9 mo.	39 yr.	Headache	Headache, choked disk	Staggering gait, falls backward to left
Schweyer	1914	23	M	+	+	+	..	Frontoparietal lobe	13 yr.	12 yr.	Convulsions	No	Jacksonian attacks
Dandy........	1928	32	F	..	+	+	..	Vermis of cerebellum	7 mo.	31 yr.	Headache	Headache vomiting, choked disk with tremendous retinal hemorrhages	Staggering gait and positive Romberg,
Dandy........	1928	36	F	..	+	+	..	Cerebellum	6 mo.	35 yr.	Headache	Headache, vomiting, choked disk	Staggering gait, Romberg, ataxia, nystagmus, adiadokokinesia
Dandy........	1928	44	F	..	+	+	..	Cerebellum vermis	2 mo.	44 yr.	Dizziness and headache	Headache, vomiting, choked disk	Staggering gait, ataxia
Dandy........	1928	28	M	..	+	+	..	Cerebellum, left lobe	6 mo.	27 yr.	Headache (in attacks)	Coma, choked disk	Staggering gait
Dandy........	1928	35	M	..	+	+	..	Cerebellum, left lobe	3 mo.	35 yr.	Occipital headache	Headache, vomiting, choked disk	Staggering gait, Romberg, ataxia
Dandy.......	1928	34	M	..	+	+	..	Vermis of cerebellum	2 yr.	32 yr.	Pain in eyes and occiput	Headache, vomiting, choked disk	None
Dandy........	1928	40	M	..	+		..	Left cerebellar lobe	1 yr.	39 yr.	....	Headache, vomiting, choked disk	Staggering gait

back to the age of fourteen months, when he had fallen a distance of four feet, striking the back of the head on a brick. He had been unconscious for only a few minutes, but immediately afterward had become paralyzed on both sides. The father, who is a physician, insisted that both sides were paralyzed at that time. After three weeks, the paralysis had gradually cleared up; both sides had improved about the same time. The father said further that the child had been talking for about three months prior to the injury, and that after the blow on the head speech had been lost but had returned with the motor function. His head had always been large, but the father explained that this was

a family characteristic; all of the father's brothers had large heads. The boy, however, wore a 7¾ hat, while the size of his father's hat was 7½; his grandfather wore a No. 8. During the convalescence from the injury to the head, the patient had vomited a great deal and had cried much after the initial drowsy period wore off. Even after six weeks, the vomiting and crying had persisted. The patient had continued to have headaches and spells of vomiting up to the age of 6 years; at this time he had been thrown from a horse and had been unconscious for about an hour. During the next two days, he had been unable to stand. He had always been more clumsy than the other children, and his movements were

‌YST WITH ANGIOMA IN THE WALL—*Continued*

Epilepsy			Motor or Sensory Symptoms	Other Symptoms	Mentality	Operation	Cause of Death	Necropsy	Remarks	Studied Microscopically
Focal	Petit Mal	Grand Mal								
0	+	0	....	Attacks of moment's loss of consciousness	Normal	0	Intracranial pressure	+	Pea sized tumor in extracerebellar; collection of yellow fluid (left cerebellar lobe)	+
..	..	..	Bilateral Babinski	Dizziness	....	Extirpation with lobe of cerebellum	Living	..	Large part of cerebellum removed with tumor	+
+	..	+	None	None	Normal	0	Status epilepticus	+	Cyst size of cherry, filled with blood; tumor size of small walnut alongside; some calcification	+
0	0	0	Occasional attacks of numbness of right arm and leg	Stiff neck dizzy attacks	Normal	Removal	Living and well, 5 years	..	In a large cyst filling the vermis was a small papilloma (angioma); it lay over the midbrain; totally removed; vision has returned to normal	+
‌onic spasms of ‌hole body; no loss ‌ consciousness			Transient ankle clonus on right	Dizziness; stiffness of neck; diplopia	Normal	Removal of angioma in the wall	Living, 2 mo.	..	A half pea-sized angioma was located in the tonsil of cerebellum	+
‌onic spasms but ‌ loss of con‌iousness			Positive Babinski	Dizziness	Mental cloudiness	....	Intracranial pressure	+	Cyst in vermis of cerebellum tiny plaque of angioma over region of the midbrain	+
0	0	0	Reflexes normal	Dizziness diplopia	Normal	Removal of angioma	Living; 7 years since operation	..	Localization of tumor by ventriculography	+
0	0	0	Reflexes normal	Blind; dizziness; stiff neck	Normal	Removal of angioma	Living; 4 years	..	Ventricular estimation test substantiated cerebellar localization	+
0	0	0	Numbness and tingling in right arm and leg	....	Normal	Removal of angioma	Living; 6 months	..	Localization of tumor made solely by ventriculography	+
		..		....	Normal	....	Intracranial pressure	+	Patient died before reaching hospital	+

TABLE III—Cases of Multiple Cavernous

Author	Date of Publication	Age	Sex	Type of Angioma		Tumor		Location of Tumor	Duration of Symptoms	Age at First Symptom	First Symptom	Signs and Symptoms of Intracranial Pressure	Focal Signs and Symptoms
				Cavernous	Small Solid Tumor with Cyst	Single	Multiple						
Creite........	1903	21	F	+	..	..	+	See under remarks	19 yr.	2 yr.	Convulsions	No	No
Finkelnburg ..	1905	14	M	+	..	..	+ two	See under remarks	2½ yr.	11 yr.	......	Choked disk	Staggering gait, left abducens palsy
Huebschamann	1921	39	M	+	..	..	+ about 30 in all	Scattered	......	.....	Convulsions		....
Jakob	1924	34	F	+	..	..	+	See under remarks	20 yr.	10 yr.	Convulsions	Pains in head	Weakness left side; jacksonian attacks
Kalischer	1897	1½	..	+	..	..	+	See under remarks	1 yr.	6 mo.	Convulsions	No	Jacksonian attacks and later paralysis
Kufs	1928	81	M	+	..	..	+	Both hemispheres pons	No symptoms	.....	None	None	None
Malamud.....	1925	51	F	+	..	..	+	See remarks	22 yr.	39 yr.	Headache	Diplopia, headache, dizziness	Symptoms like paralysis agitans 3 years before death
Muller	1923	17	M	+	..	..	+	Caudate nuclei (both sides)	5 days	17 yr.	Headache	Pain in head, coma, bradycardia	....
Ohlmacher ...	1899	..	..	..	..	..	+	See under remarks	......	.....	......	....	....
												Cases of Cavernous Angioma in	
Astwazaturow .	1911	35	F	+	..	+	..	Right frontoparietal	2 yr.	33 yr.	Headache	+	Attacks in face, arm and legs
Astwazaturow .	1911	23	F	+	..	+	..	Right temporal lobe	13 yr.	10 yr.	Convulsions	No	Jacksonian epilepsy
Bail..........	....	10	M	+	..	+	..	Left rolandic area	2 yr.	8 yr.	Convulsions	+ choked disk	Jacksonian epilepsy
Bremer, d'Antona	Ref. Lechner	20	M	+	..	+	..	Parietal	......	.....	Convulsions	....	Jacksonian attacks beginning in thumb
Bremer and Carson	Ref. Lechner	23	..	..	..	..	..	Subcortical	......	.....	Convulsions	....	....
Cassirer and Muhsam	1911	22	M	+	..	+	..	Right parietal postcentral	5 yr.	17 yr.		Headaches since youth	Jacksonian attacks sensory type, beginning in left hand

ANGIOMA OF THE BRAIN FROM THE LITERATURE

Epilepsy			Motor or Sensory Symptoms	Other Symptoms	Mentality	Operation	Cause of Death	Necropsy	Remarks	Studied Microscopically
Focal	Petit Mal	Grand Mal								
0	..	+	No	....	....	0	Convulsions	+	Eight isolated tumors—all of same small structure; six are scattered through both cerebral hemispheres, another is in the cerebellum and one in the pons; vessels greatly calcified	+
0	..	0	....	Diplopia, difficulty in urination, pains in back and limbs	....	0	Pressure	+	Small tumor in corpora quadrigemina; larger one in fourth ventricle and extends into spinal cord; tumor causes hydrocephalus	+
..	..	+	....	....	....	0	Convulsions	+	About thirty tiny angiomas were scattered throughout brain	+
+	..	+	Weakness left side	Intention tremor, ataxia, dysarthria	....	0	Convulsions	+	Three tumors were present—all small: (1) in fundibulum, (2) in pons, (3) in fourth ventricle	+
+	..	+	Weakness right side	....	....	0	Convulsions	+	Left hemisphere studded with small tumors on all surfaces; hemiplegia gradually developed	+
0	..	0	None	....	Senile dementia	0	Senility	+	Nevi in skin presumably related; daughter had apoplexy (recovery) at age of 17; dozen small tumors scattered throughout white matter of brain, one in posterior horn, another in pons; multiple cavernomas in liver	+
										+
0	..	0	....	Extra ocular palsides, queer feeling in both hands	Attacks of euphoria, depression and apathy	0	....	+	Tumors (1) in region of infundibulum and third ventricle (1.5 by 2.75 cm.); (2) in right pallidum (3 by 5 mm.); (3) in pons, and medulla (4) several others scattered in left hemisphere	
..	..	..	....	Extra-ocular palsies, cervical rigidity	....	....	Hemorrhage	+	Small tumor in caudate nucleus of each side; patient died five days after first symptoms of hemorrhage	+
..	..	..	....	....	....	0	....	+	Three angiomas were present—all small; (1) collosal gyrus; (2) optic thalamus; (3) spinal cord; an osteoma and a fibroendothelioma were also present	+

Fronto-Parietal Region of the Brain

Epilepsy			Motor or Sensory Symptoms	Other Symptoms	Mentality	Operation	Cause of Death	Necropsy	Remarks	Studied Microscopically
Focal	Petit Mal	Grand Mal								
+	..	+	....	Loss of memory	Retrograde amnesia	0	Meningitis	+	Tumor size of "mark"; vessels thrombosed and calcified	+
+	..	+	....	Loss of memory	Loss of memory	0	Convulsions	+	Tumor extends deeply into hippocampus	+
										+
+	..	+	....	....	....	0	Convulsions	Large tortuous mass of veins or surface	Attacks followed two weeks after slight head injury; possibly an arteriovenous aneurysm	
+	..	+	....	....	....	+	....	..	....	+
..	..	+	....	....	....	+	....	..	Tumor size of a nut.........	+
+	+	+	Loss of touch eventually	Weakness of hand after attacks	Slow at school	+ removed	Living	..	Patient complained of headache after exertion; no difficulty with hemorrhage when tumor excised	+

TABLE III—Cases of Multiple Cavernous Angioma

Author	Date of Publication	Age	Sex	Type of Angioma		Tumor		Location of Tumor	Duration of Symptoms	Age at First Symptom	First Symptom	Signs and Symptoms of Intracranial Pressure	Focal Signs and Symptoms
				Cavernous	Small Solid Tumor with Cyst	Single	Multiple						
Worster-Drought and Dickson	1928	31	M	+	..	+	..	Fronto-parietal	3 yr.	27 yr.	Convulsions	Severe head pains	Jacksonian attacks in left side of face
Engelhardt....	1904	26	M	+	..	+	..	Right parietal 4x3x3 cm.	23 yr.	3 yr.	Convulsions	No	Jacksonian attacks
Krause	1911	18	M	+	..	+	..	Left parietal	17 yr.	1 yr.	Convulsions	No	Paralysis of right arm after attacks when 1 year old +
Krause	1911	10	M	+	..	+	..	Left parietal	1 yr.	9 yr.	Convulsions	Choked disk	
Leischner.....	1909	39	M	..	..	+	..	Left parietal	10 yr.	29 yr.	Convulsions	Headaches	Attacks begin in right side of face
Lewandowsky and Selberg	1913	45	F	+	..	+	..	Right frontal	.....	.....	Convulsions	No	Jacksonian attacks
Luschka......	1854	40	M	+	..	+	..	Left frontal	.....	....	....	....	
Pean.........	....	15	M	+	..	+	..	Parietal lobe	.....	.....	Convulsions	....	Jacksonian attacks
Poirer........	....	34	M	+	..	+	..	Right parietal lobe	3 yr.	.....	Headaches	Headaches	Jacksonian attacks
Powers	1913	45	F	+	..	+	..	Right frontal	6 mo.	44 yr.	Convulsions	None	Head to left in convulsions
Starr and McCosh	1894	21	M	+	..	+	..	Left frontal	16 yr.	5 yr.	Pain in head	Pain and headache	Pain left side of head
Strominger ...	1903	Infant	..	Mass of vessels in meninges	..	+	..	Meninges left side	Infancy	.....	....	....	....
Struypler	1904	48	F	+	..	+	..	Left rolandic area	Few weeks	48 yr.	Convulsions	None	Attacks in right foot
Volland	1913	..	..	+	..	+	..	Falx surface of right hemisphere	.....	.....	....	....	....

Cases of Cavernous Angioma in

Author	Date of Publication	Age	Sex	Cavernous	Small Solid Tumor with Cyst	Single	Multiple	Location of Tumor	Duration of Symptoms	Age at First Symptom	First Symptom	Signs and Symptoms of Intracranial Pressure	Focal Signs and Symptoms
Herman	1928	40	F	+	..	+	..	Right occipital lobe	10 yr.	30 yr.	Coma	None	Jacksonian attacks
Dandy........	1923	34	M	+	..	+	..	Right occipital lobe	2 yr.	31 yr.	Pain in leg, and vertigo	Headache, choked disk	None

Cases of Cavernous Angioma Situated Deeply in

Author	Date of Publication	Age	Sex	Cavernous	Small Solid Tumor with Cyst	Single	Multiple	Location of Tumor	Duration of Symptoms	Age at First Symptom	First Symptom	Signs and Symptoms of Intracranial Pressure	Focal Signs and Symptoms
Stief	1924	22	M	+	..	+	..	Third ventricle	.....	.....	....	....	Disturbance of gait and speech
Uyematsu.....	1920	..	..	+	..	+	..	Corpus callosum	.....	.....	....	....	....

OF THE BRAIN FROM THE LITERATURE—*Continued*

Epilepsy			Motor or Sensory Symptoms	Other Symptoms	Mentality	Operation	Cause of Death	Necropsy	Remarks	Studied Microscopically
Focal	Petit Mal	Grand Mal								
+	..	+	Hemiplegia	Sudden hemiplegia	....	0	Intracranial pressure	+	Coma followed ten days after hemiplegia	+
+	..	+	....	....	....	0	Convulsions	..	First convulsions at age of three years; then no more until sixteen years old; steadily increasing; tumor largely calcified	+
+	..	+	Weakness right side	....	....	Removal +	....	No	....	+
+	..	+	Weakness right side after attacks	....	....	Removal +	....	No	....	+
+	..	+	Right side weak after attacks	Dizziness aphasia	....	Removal +	....	No	Paralysis after early attack; function largely returned but weakness increased after attacks	+
+	..	+	....	Suggestive left Babinski	....	Removal +	....	No	....	+
..	..	..	....	....	....	0	....	+	....	+
+	..	+	....	....	....	+	....	..	....	+
+	..	+	Weakness of left side	....	....	0	....	..	....	+
0	0	+	None	None	....	+	Convulsions	+	Angioma is sharply outlined in brain; walls of blood spaces are made up of connective tissue and not neuralgia	+
0	..	0		....	Excitable; often violent; not balanced	Removal +	....	No	Patient unconscious twelve hours after a blow at age of 5; pain in left side of head since; another period of unconsciousness after blow at age of 16; eager to study but excitable; gives way easily to emotions; fairly bright	+
..	..	..	Hemiplegia	....	....	0	....	+	Angioma of meninges—pushed brain away; patient had nevus on face	+
+	..	+	....	....	....	0	Convulsions	+	Tumor size of hazelnut; no convulsions until age of 48; then seventy-five in twelve hours	+
..	..	..	....	....	....	0	....	+	Tumor size of hickory nut....	+

Occipital Region of the Brain

Epilepsy			Motor or Sensory Symptoms	Other Symptoms	Mentality	Operation	Cause of Death	Necropsy	Remarks	Studied Microscopically
+	..	+	....	....	....	0	Convulsions	+	At age of 30 patient had first convulsion; no more until ten years later when she had three more; died in status epilepticus	+
0	0	0	Pain in arms and legs	Stiff Neck vertigo, diplopia	Normal	0	Hemorrhage from tumor	+	Patient died the day before the time set for operation; a large hemorrhaege had resulted from a small cavernous angioma in the occipital lobe	+

the Brain and in the Region of the Third Ventricle

Epilepsy			Motor or Sensory Symptoms	Other Symptoms	Mentality	Operation	Cause of Death	Necropsy	Remarks	Studied Microscopically
0		0	....	....	Normal	0	....	+	Tumor size of walnut grew upward from region of infundibulum into both hemispheres to corpus callosum and projected into both lateral ventricles	+
..	..	..	....	....	....	0	....	+	....	

TABLE III—CASES OF MULTIPLE CAVERNOUS ANGIOMA
CASES OF CAVERNOUS

Author	Date of Publication	Age	Sex	Type of Angioma		Tumor		Location of Tumor	Duration of Symptoms	Age at First Symptom	First Symptom	Signs and Symptoms of Intracranial Pressure	Focal Signs and Symptoms
				Cavernous	Small Solid Tumor with Cyst	Single	Multiple						
Levick ...	1914	9	F	+	..	+	..	Cerebelum	Rapid progression	.....	Paralysis	Headache	Cerebellar symptoms
Lindau...	1926	48	M	+	..	+	..	Cerebellum	6 yr.	42 yr.	Headache	Vomiting, headache, choked disk	....
Lindau...	1926	..	..	+	..	..	+	Cerebellum and pons	......	.....	....	....	....
Dandy ...	1928	16	M	+	..	+	..	Vermis of cerebellum	15 yr.	1 yr.	Paralysis bilateral after slight trauma	Large head, choked disk, convolutional atrophy of skull, headache, vomiting	Hydrocephalus; staggering gait; Romberg
Dandy ...	1928	1 mo.	M	+	..	+	..	Suboccipital intra and extracranial	Before birth	Tumor was present at birth	Tumor	Hydrocephalus with large head	Tumor resembles meningocele
Dandy ...	1928	35	F	+	..	+	..	Left cerebellar lobe	10 yr.	25 yr.	Headache	Headache, choked disk	Partial deafness on left

Cases of Cavernous Angioma in

Author	Date of Publication	Age	Sex	Cavernous	Small Solid Tumor with Cyst	Single	Multiple	Location of Tumor	Duration of Symptoms	Age at First Symptom	First Symptom	Signs and Symptoms of Intracranial Pressure	Focal Signs and Symptoms
Berblinger	1922	27	M	+	..	+	..	Medulla	13 yr.	14 yr.	Paralysis	+	Paralysis first one arm, then other
Enders ...	1908	60	M	+	..	+	..	Left side of pons	......	.....	Convulsions	No	Attacks begin in right side of body
Leyser....	1922	20	F	+	..	+	..	Pons 1 by 3 mm.	20 days	20 yr.	Coma	Coma	....
Nalin	1928	11	M	+	..	+	..	Fourth ventricle	9 mo.	10 yr.	Headache	Coma (no choked disk)	Staggering gait, nystagmus, ataxia, adiadokokinesis
Nambu...	1907	63	..	+	..	+	..	Pons			....	....	....
Schuback .	1927	28	F	+	..	..	+	Fourth ventricle	5 yr.	23 yr.	Headaches	Headache, loss of vision	Staggering gait, nystagmus, ankle clonus and Babinski
Tophoff ..	1925	28	F	+	..	+	..	Pons		.....	....	....	....
Wohlwill .	1927	28	F	+ with von Hippel's	..	..	+	Fourth ventricle spinal cord	5 yr.	23 yr.	+	+	Weakness left leg
Dandy....	1928	31	M	+	..	+	..	On pons and medulla	2½ yr.	29 yr.	Stiffness of right leg in spells	Headache, choked disk, dimness of vision	None, diagnosis by ventriculography

OF THE BRAIN FROM THE LITERATURE—*Continued*
ANGIOMA IN CEREBELLUM

Epilepsy			Motor or Sensory Symptoms	Other Symptoms	Mentality	Operation	Cause of Death	Necropsy	Remarks	Studied Microscopically
Focal	Petit Mal	Grand Mal								
0	..	0	Weakness of left leg and face	Occipital pain, reflexes increased on left	....	Removal +	....	No	....	+
..	..	..	....	....	....	....	Intracranial pressure	+	Large solid angioma in cerebellar lobe, mostly capillary spaces, others larger	+
..	..	..	....	....	....	....	....	+	Three angiomas, one in pons and two in cerebellum; all very small—museum specimen	+
0	0	0	Bilateral at times	Strabismus	Normal	+ Removal of tumor	Hydrocephalus	+	This angioma had grown into the medulla and pons; on several occasions slight trauma induced signs and symptoms suggestive of hemorrhage into the tumor	+
0	0	0	None	None	Baby	Removal of extracranial tumor	Shock	+	Very large tumor outside the skull and another even larger inside and directly beneath; both were continuous by extension of tumor directly through occipital bone	+
0	0	0	Numbness of left side after spell of headache	Anosmia	Normal	Removal	Living and well	..	Tumor was removed with zone of normal cerebellar tissue; complete recovery; localization made by ventriculogrophy	+

Brain Stem and Fourth Ventricle

Epilepsy			Motor or Sensory Symptoms	Other Symptoms	Mentality	Operation	Cause of Death	Necropsy	Remarks	Studied Microscopically
Focal	Petit Mal	Grand Mal								
0	..	0	Paralysis	Urinary incontinence	Normal	0	....	..	Associated with von Hippel's disease	+
+	..	+	No	....	....	0	Convulsions	+	Tiny tumor in pons, more to left side	+
0	..	0	Paralysis	....	....	0	Hemorrhage (?)	+	....	+
0	..	0	....	....	....	0	Intracranial pressure	+	Tumor filled fourth ventricle, pushed into pons; hydrocephalus	+
..	..	..	....	....	....	....		+	Small tumor	+
0	..	0	Left-sided paralysis	Difficulty in urination	....	0	Intracranial pressure	+	(1) tumor size of walnut in fourth ventricle; (2) another in dorsal spinal cord; (3) retinal angioma (von Hippel's disease); (4) cysts of pancreas and kidney	+
..	..	..	....	....	....	0	Apoplexy	+	Patient died of apoplexy	+
0	..	+	Weakness left side of body	....	....	0	Intracranial pressure	+	Tumor size of hazelnut in roof of fourth ventricle; another tumor (2 cm.) in dorsal cord; von Hippel's tumor of retina; cysts of pancreas and kidney	+
	0	0	Numbness and weakness of left side, increased at times	Loss of vision, uncertain gait, but not staggering	Normal	Removal	Living and well	..	Tumor completely removed (by dissection) from floor of fourth ventricle	+

slower and less sure. After the age of six, the clumsiness had increased. When he was two and one-half years old, it had been noticed that a crossed eye had developed without warning; the right eye drew in toward the nose. For some-time after the injury to the head (at the age of six,) the eyeball had not moved; this condition had improved gradually during the next six months, some weakness of the external rectus muscle persisting. Until the age of twelve, there had been little change in his condi-tion. He could not read well because of the extra-ocular palsies; his clumsiness seemed to increase, and he became weaker and had a tendency to deviate to the right side while walking.

At the age of twelve, he had tripped and fallen on the right side of the head while running at school. He had been unconscious for twenty minutes and drowsy for several days; during this time he had had a fever and his tempera-ture had been as high as 103 F.; he had complained of a severe headache. Again he had been unable to walk for a period of sixty-one days, and during all of this time he had complained of severe head-aches. After two months he had begun to walk, but only with support. Two weeks later, he had been able to stand alone. For the following two years, nothing unusual had happened, and then without warning the headaches had re-appeared and had occurred more or less constantly; they were always severe and occurred every two or three weeks.

A year before operation, the boy's father had noticed that his disturbance of gait, awkwardness and clumsiness were still persisting. At this time, it had been noticed that he staggered definitely toward the right. Two months before operation, the patient had become pro-gressively worse, and during all of this time he had been confined to bed.

Examination showed a rather sallow, fat boy with a large bony frame and poor musculature. He complained of severe headache. His large head was dis-proportionate to the development of his body, and showed a marked cracked pot sound on tapping along the fronto-parietal sutures. The veins of the eye-lids and scalp were prominent and full. The eyegrounds showed a slight chok-ing of both disks, perhaps a little more

marked on the right; the temporal margins, however, were still visible. Weakness of both external rectus muscles produced an evident strabismus. There was slight but definite weakness of the right facial muscles. His hearing was impaired on both sides, but air conduc-tion was better than bone conduction. The entire right side of the body was definitely weaker than the left. There was a marked positive Romberg sign, and he always fell to the right. Ataxia was present in both hands, but more on the right. There was adiodokokinesis on both sides, more on the right, and nystagmus in both directions. Reflexes were equal and active. The Babinski sign was absent. X-ray examination show-ed separation of the suture.

It was evident that the patient had a cerebellar lesion and presumably a tu-mor. It was also evident that this lesion had been present since the age of four-teen months, so that it must have been congenital. As the symptoms of localiz-ation and those of general pressure in-creased after slight trauma, it seemed probable that the lesion must have been a tumor which was readily susceptible to hemorrhage. The diagnosis of a cere-bellar tumor was made.

Operation.—On June 19, 1925, a bilat-eral cerebellar exposure was made. The lesion was at once evident in the vermis and the mesial side of both cerebellar lobes; it presented a brownish discolor-ation and was extremely hard and in-elastic. Although sharply circumscribed, it was not encapsulated. In order to gain a better impression of the lesion, the foramen of Magendie and the fourth ventricle were exposed. The cerebellar lobes were separated in order to reach the tumor in the fourth ventricle. After proceeding about 2 cm. along the floor of the fourth ventricle, several large veins were encountered running directly out of the brain stem into the hard in-durated mass of tumor, which was con-tinuous with the mass described on the surface. The entire fourth ventricle was obliterated at its level by the tumor, which did not give any outward evidence of being more than dense fibrous tissue. As large veins were present everywhere and were coming directly out of the medulla, extirpation seemed hopeless. The wound was closed.

The patient's condition remained practically unchanged for the next ten days. After further thought and in view of the hopeless nature of the lesion, I was persuaded to make an attempt to remove the tumor, though it was clear that it would be necessary to carve the tumor from the brain stem, into which it had grown.

Second Operation.—On June 30, 1925, the cerebellar wound was reopened. The entire vermis and the inner margin of each cerebellar lobe was then prepared for resection with the tumor. Preparatory to this section, the veins on the surface were ligated, and the large veins which ran from the surface of the cerebellum to the tentorium were doubly ligated and divided. The incision was then carried through the cerebellar cortex beyond the confines of the tumor. Much to my surprise, no vessels of moment were encountered during this part of the dissection. The hemispheres were retracted to either side. The tumor then remained attached only to the floor of the fourth ventricle, i. e., the pons and medulla.

The anterior surface of the mass was found to be well defined and ended just posterior to the aqueduct of Sylvius. The portion of the fourth ventricle between the aqueduct and the obstruction was greatly dilated, and the aqueduct was as large as one's little finger. The release of this fluid greatly facilitated the operation. The dissection was then begun along the floor of the fourth ventricle. There was no line of cleavage; the mass of fibrous tissue was densely adherent to the brain stem, and from this source the large veins were seen to enter, as at the previous operation. There seemed to be no alternative than to deliberately cut through the mass just above the floor of the ventricle, and to control the bleeding with silver clips and with packs. It now seemed fairly certain that the lesion was not an arteriovenous aneurysm and that the struggle with hemorrhages would be mainly with veins. Much to my surprise, however, these enormous veins bled relatively little, and many of them were thrombosed; it was possible to cut through the entire scar with little bleeding, and this was readily controlled. The mass of tumor was then lifted out of its bed. The wound was closed without drainage.

Recovery from the immediate effects of the operation was uneventful. The patient did not have any immediate effects from the removal of the tumor mass. He lived one month after the operation. About ten days after the operation, it was evident that the hydrocephalus still persisted, for there was steadily increasing pressure on the cerebellar wound.

Necropsy showed that the three sides of the raw surface produced by the extirpation of the tumor had closed together and had again completely closed the fourth ventricle. All of the vascular fibrous mass had been removed, except the portion which was deliberately left on the floor of the ventricle.

The microscopic diagnosis was cavernous angioma. It doubtless was of congenital origin.

Case 21. Cavernous Angioma in Posterior Cranial Fossa and Extracranial Suboccipital Region.

An infant, aged one month, was referred by Dr. W. P. McDowell, of Norfolk, Va., because of a lump in the back of the head, presumably an occipital meningocele (Fig. 5). The tumor had been present since birth and was then about double the size at birth. The whole head had also been rapidly increasing in size during the three weeks before operation. Before this time, the head had not seemed unusually large. Convulsions had not occurred, neither had there been nausea or vomiting. The swelling was exactly in the midline in the suboccipital region; it was of oval-shape and measured about 5 by 5 by 7 cm. It was everywhere covered by normal skin, and did not show any evidence of nervous tissue. It was compressible and seemed to pulsate. At the time of operation, the diagnosis of meningocele was made, though doubtless had the light transmission test been made it would have changed this diagnosis. X-ray examination would also have excluded a meningocele, for there was no opening in the center of the occipital bone. Advanced obstructive hydrocephalus was diagnosed by ventricular estimation.

Operation.— At operation, the lesion was quickly recognized as a tumor. It was intimately attached to the skull and was so bloody that at every attempt to separate it from the skull applications

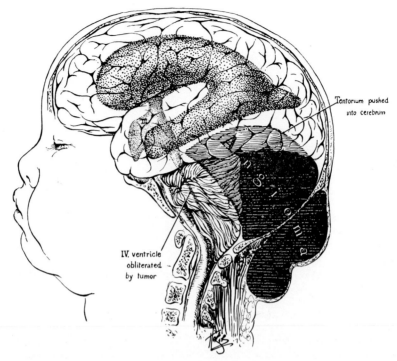

Fig. 5. (case 21). The position and relative size of the tremendous anigioma. The tumor pushed the cerebellum far forward thereby causing the tentorium to bulge. It has completely occluded the fourth ventricle causing a hydrocephalus of high grade.

of wax were necessary to stop bleeding. The periostium was everywhere absent, the bone rough and irregular from the extensive adherence of the tumor and the many vascular channels which penetrated it. Nowhere was an opening seen to penetrate the bone. For this reason, it was evident that the tumor was not causing the hydrocephalus. It was equally evident that another tumor, presumably of the same angiomatous type, must be present in the posterior cranial fossa, and causing the hydrocephalus. Necropsy proved this assumption to be correct. An equally large tumor was present in the posterior cranial fossa. It was attached to the inner surface of the occipital bone, and lay immediately beneath the external tumor. The internal and external tumors were directly continuous through the bone by angiomatous extensions of microscopic size.

Both intracranial and extracranial tumors were alike; they were soft, sponge-like and compressible. Blood could be expressed from the spaces which were of

varying size up to nearly 1 cm. in diameter.

The microscopic appearance showed the tumor to be a cavernous hemangioma.

Case 22. *Cavernous Angioma of Left Cerebellar Lobe.*

A well nourished woman, aged thirty-five, was referred by Dr. Walter B. Martin, of Norfolk, Va., with the diagnosis of an unlocalized tumor of the brain. Her symptoms had begun ten years before when during a pregnancy she had had severe headaches in the frontal and temporal regions of both sides. The headache had shifted slowly to the back of the head. Since this time, she had had headaches of the same character about every six months; each attack lasted about from six to eight weeks. The headaches began gradually, increased steadily, reaching a maximum usually in about six weeks. She was then forced to stay in bed. They then disappeared gradually. The disappearance of the headaches could not be accounted for any more than their beginning. Nausea and vomiting accompanied the headaches. During one of these attacks of headache, she had partially lost the hearing in the left ear. Eight months before operation, in one of these spells, she had lost the sense of smell and taste, and since then had constantly smelled a nauseating odor of "burnt celluloid." Her last attack of headache had begun about twelve weeks before operation and persisted until that time. In this attack she felt some numbness in the left arm and leg and stiffness in the neck. There was no diplopia.

Neurologic examination showed the following positive conditions: (1) double choked disk, about equal on the two sides; (2) complete loss of smell; (3) 50 per cent loss of hearing—bone and air conduction in left ear.

It is noteworthy that except for a subjective cervical rigidity and the possible disturbance of hearing, there were no indications of a cerebellar lesion. The loss of smell and the possible uncinate attacks suggested a lesion in the uncinate gyrus (temporal lobe).

Ventriculography showed a bilateral hydrocephalus with a large third ventricle.

Operation.—On Dec. 29, 1925, cerebellar exploration was performed. A tumor appeared in the left cerebellar lobe. It reached the surface beneath the lateral sinus, to which it was attached by filmy adhesions. Two tortuous veins passed over the cerebellum and entered the tumor. A large artery also passed into the tumor from below. A third vein skirted the tumor. After the vessels on the surface of the cerebellar lobe had been tied, the tumor was removed by resecting a good margin of cerebellar tissue around it. The subcortical part of the tumor was not seen at any time until the resected mass was sectioned for study. The tumor was then seen to be composed entirely of a meshwork of blood-containing spaces with some interposed connective tissue. A diagnosis of cavernous angioma was made.

The postoperative course was uneventful. The patient did not suffer any noticeable ill effects of the loss of the cerebellar tissue. She has remained well to date, over two years after operation.

Case 23. *Cavernous Angioma of the Fourth Ventricle.*

A healthy looking man, aged thirty-one, was referred by Dr. Samuel Key of Austin, Tex. Two years before admission to the hospital, his right leg had occasionally dragged and become stiff. For seven or eight months, there had been some weakness in the fingers of

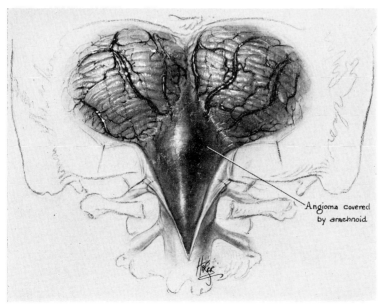

Angioma covered by arachnoid

Fig. 6. (case 23). Bulging tumor between the cerebellar lobes over the medulla. It is covered with arachnoid which must be split before the tumor can be exposed.

the left hand. The fingers on the right hand had also become numb and stiff, but less than those on the left hand.

Six months before operation he had begun to have attacks of blurred vision; since this time, he had had several such attacks daily. Dimness of vision would last half an hour or more after each seizure. Later his vision had been greatly limited "on both sides." He had never had headache, but in the morning when getting up there had frequently been pain back of the right ear. When he held his neck stiff, this pain seemed to dissappear.

About four months before operation, he had suddenly fallen to the floor unconscious. When he awakened, he was in bed but felt well. He did not bite his tongue and was not incontinent. Three weeks before operation, he had had a similar attack. He did not know whether he had had a convulsion.

The positive neurologic observations were: (1) bilateral choked disk (4 diopters in each eye); (2) visual fields greatly reduced; visual acuity 20/100 in each eye; (3) definite motor loss in left arm and leg; (4) definite hypo-esthesia in left arm and leg; (5) uncertain gait, but not staggering (Romberg sign negative); (6) slight nystagmus in right lateral fixation. It is noteworthy that all of the reflexes were normal. The x-ray picture showed destruction of the posterior clinoid processes.

Ventriculography showed high grade bilateral hydrocephalus with large third ventricle.

Operation.— On July 28, 1927, bilateral cerebellar operation was performed. A strictly midline tumor was found between the cerebellar lobes and resting directly on the medulla and pons (Fig. 6). When first seen, it was covered with arachnoid and was thought to be a glioma, but after the membranes had been split, it was seen to be a well encapsulated tumor. There was an oval, smooth, bluish, fluctuant central mass closely attached to the brain stem. From this tumor, which had every appearance of a venous aneurysm (it did not pulsate and imparted no thrill), three large veins, larger than slate pencils, emerged. One vein came from the vault of the tumor and passed over the right side of the pons and was lost to view; the second emerged

from the vault of the tumor and passed over to the left side of the medulla, and the third passed from the lower pole of the tumor, down the center of the spinal cord and at the level of the axis (the atlas had been removed posteriorly), two branches passed over the right side of the spinal cord and one over the left. All of these veins were carefully ligated, after which the central tumor mass was carefully elevated from its bed in the brain stem. One other vein, slightly smaller than the one already mentioned, emerged from the exact center of the under surface of the tumor and passed directly into the medulla near its junction with the pons.

The patient promptly recovered from the operation which was without incident, except that there was some increase in the incoordination in the left hand. This disturbance soon improved, and when seen seven months later he was perfectly well except for a very slight weakness—far less than in the left hand on admission.

Case 24. *Cavernous Angioma of Occipital Lobe with Hemorrhages.*

A normal looking man, aged thirty-two, was referred by Dr. T. P. Sprunt, of Baltimore, in October, 1926. In February, 1926, the patient had had a spell of severe pain in the legs and arms, more on the left side. The pain had not been constant, but had occurred in waves. He had continued at work for ten days, when persistent nausea and vomiting had developed. He could not retain food. After two weeks in bed, he had felt well enough to be up and about, but for five months he had felt groggy and tired. He had then returned to work. A month later, when arriving at the office, he had suddenly had an attack of severe vertigo, and two hours later had experienced violent nausea and vomiting, all of which had lasted for twelve hours; objects had seemed to whirl about him. Diplopia had also appeared at that time. There had been a queer feeling in the eyes, and his neck had been stiff. He said that he thought he had staggered at times, but that the dizziness may have accounted for this. He had improved gradually, and eight days later had again left the bed. For the next year and a half, he had done little work and had rested a great deal.

He had again been referred by Dr.

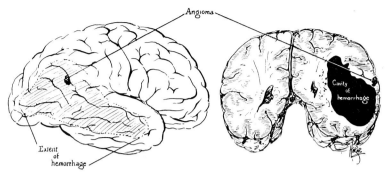

Fig. 7. (case 24). Sketch of the brain (at necropsy) showing the position and extent of a large hemorrhage and small angioma. The patient died before operation.

Sprunt, in March, 1928, because bilateral choked disks had been discovered. He did not complain of headaches and felt that his recovery, though not complete, had been steadily progressive. He said that the dizzy feeling was still present when his head was suddenly turned to the right.

Except for a bilateral papilledema of four diopters in each eye, the results of the physical and neurological examination were negative. It was my impression that the patient had a tumor of the brain, probably a cyst with an intracystic papilloma. The long duration of the symptoms with periods of marked improvement would seem to indicate a cyst. The sudden symptoms on several occasions suggested hemorrhages from the tumor. Because of the rigidity of the neck and the outspoken dizziness,[3] particularly on turning the head to the right, a presumptive localization of the tumor was made in the cerebellum.

An injection of air into the cerebral ventricles was advised for the accurate localization of the tumor, to be followed by the exploration of the tumor in anticipation of its removal if possible.

The patient was scheduled to enter the hospital a week later, on March 17, 1928. Suddenly, on March 16, 1928, he complained of violent dizziness and headache. A few minutes later, he was deeply comatose and had Cheyne-Stokes respirations. He was rushed to the hospital, but became cyanotic and died as he entered the operating room. In an attempt to resuscitate him, a ventricular puncture was performed quickly in first aid fashion. A spurt of dark blood (hemorrhage) followed the right occipital puncture, but his pulse did not beat again and respiration did not commence. It was then clear that he had had a cerebral hemorrhage in the right occipital lobe.

Necropsy showed a large, oval cavity (as large as one's fist) in the right occipital lobe and extending into the temporal lobe (Fig. 7). The cyst was about from 1 to 2 cm. below the surface of the brain. At first a tumor could not be seen, but on more careful inspection, a small, smooth swelling was noted in the region of the angular gyrus. At first it was thought to be merely the indentation of a convolution, but cross-section demonstrated a small mass of loose, spongy tissue measuring about 1 by 1 cm.; it replaced the cortex and connected with the pia-arachnoid. It was clearly an angioma.

The microscopic diagnosis was cavernous angioma.

Relationship of Angiomas of the Brain to Angiomas and Other Congenital Lesions Elsewhere in the Body.—The frequency of multiple angiomas in the brain must prepare one to believe that the same lesions must occur concomitantly elsewhere in the body, especially when it is recognized that these lesions are peculiar to the vascular system and not to the brain. Strominger (1903) demonstrated one of the early cases of cavernous angioma of the brain and called attention to an associated extensive nevus of the face which he considered highly significant. Finkelnburg's (1905) patient had a cyst of the cord in addition to angiomas of the corpora quadrigemina and fourth ventricle. Koch's (1913) patient had diabetes mellitus, and at necropsy, cysts of the pancreas, cavernous angiomas of the liver, an angiomatous cyst of one cerebellar lobe and a cavernous angioma of the other lobe were found. In addition, his patient had von Hippel's disease, i.e., so-called angiomatosis retinae. This was the first instance of the association of the vascular lesion in the retina (assumed to be an angioma) and an angioma of the brain. In 1913, Oppenheim presented to the medical society four patients, in each of whom he suspected an angioma of the brain because congenital nevi of the face and body existed in association with longstanding symptoms of cerebral origin, mainly paralyses and convulsions. Although none of his diagnoses were checked by necropsy or operation, Oppenheim said, "An angioma of the brain must always be considered when vascular naeve of the face are present." Berblinger (1922) reported another case of von Hippel's disease in a patient who had a cavernous angioma of the body.

The association of angiomatosis of the central nervous system with angiomatosis retinae (von Hippel's disease) and cysts of the pancreas, liver and spine attained new importance with Lindau's splendid publication. He thinks that cysts or cavernous angiomas in the cerebellum occur in 20 per cent of all cases of angiomatosis retinae. In half of his cases of angiomatous cysts of the cerebellum, there were cysts of the pancreas; and in two-thirds, cysts of the kidneys. Lindau considered these disturbances of the brain, retina, pancreas and kidneys a congenital maldevelopment complex. Since Lindau's publication, Schuback (1927) and Wohlwill (1927) have published reports of cases of angiomas of the brain in which cysts of the spinal cord, pancreas and kidneys and angiomatosis retinae existed. Kufs (1928) reported a remarkable case of the angioma of the brain with nevi of the body and many cavernomas of the liver. This patient's daughter had had a cerebral hemorrhage

(from which she had recovered) at the age of 17. Kufs looked on this hemorrhage as a rupture of an angioma, and thought that the family indicated a hereditary basis for the angioma.

In none of my cases has von Hippel's disease been observed, although the eyegrounds have always been carefully examined. The retinal picture is so striking and characteristic that, once seen, it could not be missed. As most of the pathologic material was obtained at operation, nothing can be contributed toward a better knowledge of the relationship between angiomas of the brain and cysts of the abdominal organs.

SUMMARY AND CONCLUSIONS

1. A series of cases of venous anomalies, plexiform angiomas, angiomatous cysts and cavernous angiomas of the brain are reported. The additional cases of similar types are collected from the literature, and their clinical features are analyzed.

2. The venous anomalies are of congenital origin. Their clinical symptoms are usually epilepsy and disturbances of mentality. They are frequently associated with other deformations of the brain.

3. Three cases of angioma plexiforme are reported. They resemble a similar lesion well known in the spinal cord.

4. A network of venous spaces in the dura and communicating freely with the longitudinal sinus is offered as a cause of focal epilepsy beginning in the leg or arm. Its constant location suggests that it is probably the congenital remains of an embryonic dural circulation.

5. Angiomatous cysts exist throughout the brain, but with greatest frequency in the cerebellum. The size of the tumor embedded in the wall of the cyst is relatively insignificant. Intracranial pressure develops rapidly because of the cyst formation and the resultant hydrocephalus. Localizing symptoms are usually, but not always, present. These tumors cannot be differentiated clinically from other types of cysts of the brain.

6. Cavernous angiomas assume many gross appearances. They are scattered throughout the brain, but appear to occur with greatest frequency in the frontoparietal region. The predominating symptom of this type of tumor is jacksonian epilepsy with or without transient or permanent motor weakness. Pressure symptoms will develop if the tumor is situated near the ventricular channels or outlets. The typical tumors begin early in life; they grow slowly, and the symptoms endure for many years. A clinical diagnosis can be made at times.

7. Hemorrhage from the tumor is always a potential danger in all types of angiomas, though to a less degree than in arteriovenous aneurysms of the brain.

8. Both the cavernous angiomas and the angiomatous cysts should be treated surgically by complete removal of the solid tumor together with a margin of contiguous brain tissue. Both of these types of tumor offer good prospects of complete cure and with relatively little risk. The tumors in the cysts are among the easiest tumors of the brain to extirpate.

REFERENCES

[1]Dandy: Arteriovenous Aneurysms of the Brain. *Arch. Surg., 17:* 190 (Aug.) 1928. Since the article on arteriovenous aneurysms of the brain was sent for publication, nine additional probable cases have been found (Blank, Durck, Federoff and Bagorad, Heitmuller, Herzog, Klimesch, D'Arcy, Power, Shoyer, Wichnewski).

[2]Where multiple tumors were present they have been entered in each location.

[1]Astwazaturow, M.: Beitrag zur Kasuistik der Kavernose Blutgeschwuelste des Gehirns. *Neurol. Zentralbl., 30:* 363, 1911; Frankfurt, *Ztschr. f. Path., 4:* 3, 1911.

[2]Bail: Ein Fall von seltener Hirngeschwulst; Angiom der Piavenen. *Zentralbl. f. Chir., 31:* 768, 1904.

[3]Baum: Kavernoses Angiom des Gehirns mit Erfolg Operiert. *Munchen. med. Wchnschr., 58:* 411, 1911.

[4]Berblinger, W.: Zur Auffassung von der Sogenannten von Hippelschen Krankheit der Netzhaut. *Arch. ophth., 110:* 395, 1922.

[5]Von Bergmann: Zur Kasuistik operativer Hirntumoren. *Arch. f. klin. Chir., 65:* 936, 1902.

[6]Bielschowsky, M.: Zur Histologie und Pathologie

der Gehirngeschwulste Angioma Cavernosum im Stirnpol. *Arch. Ztschr. f. Nervenh., 22:* 54, 1902.

[7]Brandt, R.: Zur Frage der Angiomatosis retinae. *Arch. f. ophth., 106:* 127, 1921.

[8]Bremer, D'Antona: Quoted by Lechner from Bergmann.

[9]Bremer and Carson: Quoted by Lechner; Chipault: *Chirurgie operatoire du system nerveux.*

[10]Bruns: *Die Geschuwulste des Nervensystems.* Berlin, S. Karger, 1897.

[11]Bruns: L.: Demonstration eines durch Operation gewonnent cystischen Tumoren (angioma cavernosum) des Grosshirn. *Neurol. Centralbl.,* 1895, p. 125.

[12]Cassirer and Muhsam: Ueber die Exstirpation eines grossen Angioms des Gehirns. *Berl. klin. Wchnschr., 48:* 755, 1911.

[13]Creite: Zur Pathogenese der Epilepsie (Multiple Angiome des Gehirns mit Ossifikation). *Munchen. med. Wchnschr., 50:* 1767, 1903.

[14]Worster-Drought, C., and Dickson, W. E.: Venous Angioma of the Cerebrum. *Zentralbl. Neurol. u. Psych., 48:* 562, 1928 Orig. *J. Neurol. & Psychopathol., 8:* 19, 1927.

[15]Enders: Ein Angiom in der Bruckengegend. *Munchen. med. Wchnschr., 2:* 1648, 1908.

[16]Engelhardt: Zur Frage der Dauerheilung nach operativer Behandlung der traumatischen Jackson' schen Epilepsie. *Deutsche med. Wchnschr., 1:* 98, 1904.

[17]Fabritius: Ein Fall von cystic Kleinhirntumor. *Beitr. path. Anat. u. allg. Path., 51:* 311, 1911.

[18]Finkelnburg: Zur Differentialdiagnose zwischen Kleinhirntumoren und chronischen Hydrocephalus (Zugleich ein Beitrag zur Kenntnis der Angiome des Zentralnervensystems). *Deutsche Ztschr. f. Nervenh., 29:* 135, 1905.

[19]Friedrich and Stiehler: Ein Hamangioendotheliom der Medulla Oblongata. *Deutsche Ztschr. f. Nervenh.,* 1922, vol. 73.

[20]Fuchs, A.: Zur Pathogenese und Anatomie de Netzhautcysten. *Arch. f. Ophth., 105:* 333, 1921.

[21]Gaupp, J.: Zwei Neurofibrome und ein Angiom der Cauda equina. *Beitr. path. Anat. u. allg. Path., 2:* 510, 1888.

[22]Heine: Ueber Angiogliosis retinae mit Hirntumor (Capillares Hamangiom), *Ztschr. f. Augenh., 51:* 1, 1923.

[23]Herman, E.: Cavernoma Cerebri Haemorrhagica Spinalis meningealis epi, intra et subdural. *Deutsche Ztschr. f. Nervenh., 79:* 34, 1923.

[24]Huebschmann: Ueber einige seltene Hirntumoren *Deutsche Ztschr. f. Nervenh., 72:* 205, 1921.

[25]Jakob, A.: Ueber einen seltenen Fall von multiplen Hamangiom des Centralnervensystem. *Zentralbl. ges. Neurol. u. Psychiat., 40:* 118, 1925.

[26]Kalischer: Demonstration des Gehirns eines Kindes mit Teleangiektasien der linksseitigen Gesichtskopfhaut under Hirnoberflache. *Berl. klin.*

Wchnschr., 1897, p. 1059.

27Koch, K.: Beitrage zur Pathologie der Bauchspeicheldruse. *Virchows Arch. path. Anat., 214:* 180, 1913.

28Krause, F.: *Chirurgie des Gehirns und Ruckenmarks,* Berlin, 1911, p. 361.

29Kufs, H.: Ueber Heredo familiare Angiomatose des Gehirns und der Retina, ihre Beziehungen zu einander und zur Angiomatose der Haut. *Ztschr. ges. Neurol. u. Psychiat., 113:* 651, 1928.

30Lannois and Bernoud, quoted by Kalischer, 1898.

31Lechner, Ellen: Ein Beitrage zur Kasuistik der Hirnangiome. *Beitr. z. klin. Chir., 125:* 174, 1922.

32Lehocsky: Zwei Falle von Angioma racemosum im-Kleinhirn, Hirnpathologie: Beitrage aus dem Hirnhistologischen Institute der Universitat Budapest, 1924.

33Leischner, H.: Zur chirurgie Behandlung von Hirntumoren. *Arch. klin. Chir., 89:* 542, 1909.

34Levich, I. U.: Diagnosis of Brain Tumors in Children. Pediatra, *10:* 317–447, 1914; abstr., *J. A. M. A., 62:* 1517 (May 9) 1914.

35Lewandowsky, M., and Stadelmann, E.: Ueber einen bemerkswerten Fall von Hirnblutung. *J. Psychiat. u. Neurol., 11:* 249, 1908.

36Lewandowsky, M., and Selberg, F.: Ueber Jaksonsche Krampfe mit tonischem Beginn und uber ein Kleines Angiocavernom des Gehirns. *Ztschr. ges. Neurol. u. Psychiat., 19:* 336, 1913.

37Leyser, E.: Ein Angiom der Brucke. *Monatschr. f. Psychiat. u. Neurol., 51:* 83, 1922.

38Lindau, A.: Studien uber Kleinhirncysten. *Acta path. et microbiol. scandinav.,* 1926, supp. 1.

39Lorenz: *Kavernoses Angioma des Ruckenmarkes mit todlicher Blutung.* Inaug.-Diss., Jena, 1901–1902.

40Luschka, H.: Kavernose Blutgeschwulste des Gehirns. *Virchows Arch. path. Anat., 6:* 449, 1854.

41Luzzatto, A. M.: Cavernoma des Bulbus verbunden mit Syringobulbie. *Zentralbl. ges. Neurol. u. Psychiat., 39:* 243, 1925.

42Malamud, W.: Ueber einen Fall von Multiplem Hamangiom des Zentralnervensystems mit bemarkenswerten Klinischen Verlauf. *Ztschr. ges. Neurol. u. Psychiat., 97:* 651, 1925.

43Muller, H. H.: Ueber einen Fall von Multiplem Hirnangioma. *Monatsschr. Psychiat. u. Neurol., 53:* 243, 1923.

44Nalin, E.: Ueber einen Fall von Angioma cavernosum am Boden des IV Ventrikels. *Zentralbl. ges. Neurol. u. Psychiat., 48:* 563, 1928.

45Nambu, T.: Hamangiom im Pons Varoli. *Neurol. Zentralbl., 26:* 1162, 1907.

46Newmark, L.: An Angioma of the Cerebellum. *J. Nerv. & Ment. Dis., 42:* 286, 1915.

47Ohlmacher: Multiple Cavernous Angioma, etc., in a Case of Secondary Epilepsy. *J. Nerv. & Ment. Dis., 26:* 395, 1899.

48Oliver, T., and Williamson, G. E.: Cerebral Tumors Successfully Removed by Operation. *Brit. M. J., 2:* 1607 (Nov. 26) 1898.

49Oppenheim: *Lehrbuch der Nervenkrankheiten.* Berlin, *2:* 1384–1449, 1913.

50Oppenheim, H.: Geschwulste des Gehirns. *Spec. Path. u. Therap.,* 1897, vol. 9

51Pean, quoted by Bergmann: also Lechner.

52Poirer, quoted by Bergmann; also Lechner.

53Powers, W. J.: Ein Fall von Angioma cavernosum des Gehirns. *Zentralbl. ges. Neurol. u. Psychiat., 16:* 487, 1913.

54Ritter, O.: Spinal Cord Compression from Vascular Changes in Meninges. *Beitr. z. klin. Chir., 138:* 339, 1926.

55Roman, B.: Hamangiom des Ruckenmarks. *Centralbl. f. Path., 24:* 993, 1913.

56Scarlett, Hunter W.: Angiomatosis of the Retina *Arch. Ophthal., 54:* 183, 1925.

57Schloffer, H.: Ausgedehute Abtragrung einer Kleinhirnhemisphare. *Med. Klin., 41:* 1521, 1925.

58Schuback, A.: Ueber die Angiomatosis des Zentralnervensystems (Lindausche Krankheit). *Ztschr. ges. Neurol. u. Psychiat., 110:* 359, 1927.

59Schweyer, H.: Zur Kasuistik seltenen Gehirntumoren. *Arb. a. d. Geb. d. path. Anat. und Bakteriol., 8:* 145, 1914.

60Starr, A., and McCosh, A. J.: A Contribution to the Localization of the Muscular Sense. *Am. J. M. Sc., 108:* 517, 1894.

61Stief, A.: Zur Kasuistik der Kavernome des Gehirns. *Ztschr. ges. Neurol. u. Psychiat., 93:* 181, 1924.

62Strominger, L.: Ausgebreitetes Angiom der linken Hirnhalfte. *Zentralbl. f. Chir., 30:* 755, 1903.

63Struppler, T.: Ueber des Cavernose Angioma des Grosshirns. *Munchen. med. Wchnschr., 47:* 1267, 1900.

64Tannenberg, J.: Ueber die Pathogenese der Syringomyelie, zugleich in Beitrag zum Vorkommen von Kapillarhamangiomen in Ruckenmark. *Ztschr. ges. Neurol. u. Psychiat., 92:* 119, 1924.

65Tophoff: Ein Fall von Cavernoma Cerebri. *Deutsche Ztschr. Nervenh., 86:* 285, 1925.

66Turner, F. C.: A Case of Cystic Growth in the Cerebellum and Right Adrenal. *Tr. Path. Soc. London, 39:* 9, 1888.

67Uyematsu, S.: A Case of Haemangioma Cavernosum of Cerebrum. *J. Nerv. & Ment. Dis., 52:* 388, 1920.

68Virchow, R.: Ueber Naevi vasculosi des Gehirns. *Virchows Arch. path. Anat., 30:* 272, 1864.

69Volland: Ueber Zwei Falle von Cerebralem Angioma nebst Bemerkungen uber Hirnangioma. *Zitschr. Erforsch. u. Bhandl. d. jugendl. Schwachsinns., 6:* 130, 1913.

70Wohlwill: Ein Fall von Angiomatosis des Zentralnervensystems (Lindausche Krankheit), *Zentralbl. ges. Neurol. u. Psychiat., 46:* 456, 1927.

[71]Zajaczkowski, A.: Ein Fall von Angioma cavernosum des Stirnbeines. *Zentralbl. Chir., 28:* 507, 1901; Original, Przeglad hirurgiezny, vol. 4, no. 3.

The following are references to additional cases of probable arteriovenous aneurysms of the brain not included in the article.

[72]Bland: Ueber ein Rankenangioma des Gchirns. *Munchen med. Wchnschr., 57:* 465, 1910.

[73]Durck: Ueber ein grosses plexiformes venoses angiom der weicher Hirnhaute. *Munchen. med. Wchnschr., 54:* 1154, 1907.

[74]Federoff and Bagorad: Zur Klinik der Angiome des Grosshirns. *Ztschr. ges. Neurol. u. Psychiat., 94:* 497, 1925.

[75]Heitmueller: Hildebrand, Jahresherichte, 1905, p. 168; Jahreshericht uber die Fortschrilte auf dem Gebiete der Chirurgie, Wiesb.

[76]Herzog, E.: Angioma racemosum venosum des Schadels und Gehirns. *Zentralbl. ges. Neurol. u. Psychiat., 48:* 419, 1928.

[77]Klimesch, E.: Ueber einen Fall von Angioma arteriale racemosum in der Balkengegend. *Wein. klin. Wchnschr., 39:* 358, 1926.

[78]Power-D'Arcy: Angioma of the Cerebral Membranes. *Tr. Path. Soc. London, 39:* 5, 1888.

[79]Shoyer, A. F.: An Angioma of Broca's Convolution. *J. Ment. Sc., 46:* 775, 1900.

[80]Wichnewski: *Zentralbl. f. Chir.,* 1913, p. 694.

XXXII

AN OPERATION FOR THE CURE OF
TIC DOULOUREUX

PARTIAL SECTION OF THE SENSORY ROOT AT THE PONS*

Steadily improved by many technical advances, the original intracranial attack on the branches of the trigeminal nerve, independently and almost simultaneously suggested by Hartley[1] of America and Krause[2] of Germany, has gradually evolved from a procedure of questionable merit and great danger into one of the safest and most successful of major surgical procedures. There are, indeed, few greater triumphs in the history of surgery, for the obstacles at that early period of cranial surgery must have seemed insuperable. But the operation in its most approved form is still far from perfect, largely because of certain disturbances which follow in its wake. With the belief that these defects are now, in a large part, avoidable and with no greater risk to life, another operation for the permanent cure of tic douloureux is proposed.

Although tic douloureux has been recognized as a clinical entity for centuries, its relationship to the trigeminal nerve was long unsuspected because the course and function of the cranial nerves were unknown. In his book, "Die Neuralgie der Trigeminus," Krause[3] said that Avicenna (A.D. 1000) gave an accurate description of this disease; that Schlichtung (1748) first cut the infra-orbital nerve for the pain that was called "face neuralgia," and that Nicolous Andre (1756) first introduced the appellation, tic douloureux. Fothergill (1773) described "a painful affection of the face" with great accuracy, but the disease was then too well known to justify

the designation "Fothergill's neuralgia."

Through Galen's period until Meckel's careful dissections of the fifth nerve (1748), the facial nerve was believed to supply not only motor but also sensory function to the face. The fifth nerve was thought to be the nerve of taste (Eckhard). Experimental proof of the sensory function of the fifth nerve and the motor function of the seventh nerve was produced almost simultaneously by Magendie[4] and Sir Charles Bell,[5] about 1821. Despite his accurate anatomic studies and his knowledge that tic douloureux was referable to the domain of the fifth nerve, Sir Charles Bell thought that the origin of tic douloureux was in the sympathetic nervous system: "The painful affection of the face called tic douloureux is seated in the fifth pair and for the most part in the second division of the trigeminal nerve; and so convinced am I that it is the more direct connection established betwixt the sympathetic nerve and the fifth that produces the pain that I would wish to divide the sympathetic in the neck, if I thought it could be done with safety, which it cannot." Though on one occasion he divided the supra-orbital nerve, his great efforts were directed toward the medical treatment of this condition. He frequently referred to successful results with croton oil and colocynth — an accidental discovery — though he later admitted that the results "were not always so happy as in the cases mentioned."

It was the experimental contributions to nerve function which permitted the first rational therapy for tic douloureux. Prior to the experiments of Bell and Magendie,

*Reprinted from the *Archives of Surgery, 18:* 687–734, 1929.

division of a nerve was performed from time to time, but usually the facial nerve was divided. Krause said that in 1778, Langier cut the facial nerve at the stylomastoid foramen, of course without material benefit to the patient, and that Lizars (1821) first cut the inferior dental nerve. It is not impossible that section of the facial nerve might at times have been followed by an appreciable reduction of the pain owing to the absolute rest induced by paralysis of the facial muscles. Neurectomy of the peripheral branches of the trigeminus quickly became the recognized treatment even though the pain always recurred. The general acceptance of this operation is shown by the fact that Wagner, in 1869, had done 135 peripheral neurectomies.

Further progress awaited the advent of anesthesia and aseptic surgery. Perhaps the first suggestion of a more radical treatment was made by Mears[6] in 1884, who stated:

If in any case I believed.... that the morbid condition had invaded the Gasserian ganglion I would not hesitate to enlarge anteriorly the oval foramen by the application of a burr to the surgical engine and by traction draw down the ganglion from its position in the fossa upon the anterior surface of the apex of the petrous bone and proceed in a cautious manner to break it up or remove it by sections with the small blunt scissors.

Mears was thinking along the line of attack soon to be proposed and carried out by Rose[7] (1892), who was in consultation with Ferrier.[8] Bland Sutton[9] (1886) had previously resected the ramus of the mandible and divided the inferior maxillary nerve at the base of the skull but had not made an effort to enter the cranial chamber. Rose's mutilating operation, in which the ramus of the mandible was removed and the floor of the skull trephined at the foramen ovale, was employed in five cases and the pain relieved. Pieces of the gasserian ganglion were curretted away rather blindly. The amount of ganglion actually removed or destroyed must have been small, for he made the following comment:

It is interesting both from clinical and physiological aspects to observe the rapid diminution of the anaesthetic area, and it would appear that the distribution of sensation is taken up by neighboring branches much in the same way as arterial anastomosis takes place in the vascular system.

It is now clear that the ganglion was not removed but the initial loss of function was due to its injury by trauma. Andrews[10] of Chicago was also working independently on a precisely similar attack about this time. He had published his studies on the cadaver (1891) a year before the appearance of Rose's paper, but he had not performed any operation on the living. Rose's operation received little recognition. It yielded at once to the superior method which appeared the same year.

Reports of the new intracranial operations of Hartley and Krause were published only a month apart. They were practically identical in conception and execution. Each of these men performed a craniotomy and stripped the dura from the middle fossa of the skull until the second or third branches of the trigeminus appeared. But the efforts of each were then directed toward intracranial section of the peripheral branches of the gasserian ganglion and not to the ganglion itself. As such the procedure was really little superior to the more superficial operations then in vogue. The priority[11] of the approach undoubtedly belongs to Hartley, whose publication appeared in March, 1892 (the operation was performed on Aug. 15, 1891), more than a month before the appearance of Krause's paper. The real contribution to the treatment of this condition, however, was the removal of the gasserian ganglion, and the credit for this belongs to Krause[12] (1893). True, it was only a step from intracranial section of the branches of the ganglion to the removal of the ganglion itself, but it was the one big factor in the treatment for tic douloureux. The importance of this step is further emphasized by the prevailing belief (shared by Victor Horsley) that removal of the ganglion was impossible because of its close attachment to the wall of the cavernous sinus.

Antedating the publications of both Krause and Hartley was Victor Horsley's[13] description (1891) of an unsuccessful operative attack on the sensory root of the trigeminus. The operation was performed four years earlier. Horsley also stated that Macewen independently tried a similar attack on the ganglion, but that as it was unsuccessful a report of it was not published. Horsley's conception of treatment in trigeminal neuralgia by section of the sensory root of the trigeminal nerve with complete disregard of the gasserian ganglion was many years ahead of his time. It was Horsley's belief not only that division of the sensory root would stop the pain just as effectively as removal of the ganglion but that the root would not regenerate; moreover, as already mentioned, as a result of dissections on the cadaver, Horsley thought that the gasserian ganglion was too tightly adherent to the cavernous sinus to permit its separation. Ferrier[8] shared his views, but there was no evidence at that time to support the assumption. For many years after operations on the gasserian ganglion had been successful, the possibility of merely dividing the sensory root was considered but not carried out because of the absence of proof of its nonregeneration. In a paper with W. W. Keen, who was one of the great pioneers in this field of neurological surgery, Spiller[14] (1898) wrote:

> If it could be shown that the sensory root of the Gasserian ganglion does not unite after its fibers are divided, we should have a fact of great importance. Division of this root would probably be a less serious operation than the removal of the entire ganglion and might have the same effect in the relief of pain, but the surgical difficulties might be insurmountable.

Three years later Spiller and Frazier[15] reported the first successful case of intracranial division of the sensory root of the trigeminus, a procedure which has since become more or less a routine. At that time Spiller[16] brought forward, in support of this operation, the literature on nonregeneration of the pathways in the spinal cord after division and thought that after section of the sensory root of the trigeminus the results would be the same.

Horsley[17] reached the sensory root by an intradural approach, retracting the temporal bone. Although the root was easily found and avulsed, the patient died seven hours later without regaining consciousness. At autopsy neither hemorrhage nor any other cause of death was found. Despite the fact that his patient was emaciated and in poor condition when the operation was attempted, Horsley was quick to see the superiority of Krause's operation. Frazier later succeeded where Horsley failed because he approached the sensory root extradurally and doubtless also because the surgical advances of a decade made the task much easier. It must be remembered that cerebral surgery was just beginning when Horsley attempted to divide the sensory root.

A number of improvements have been added to the original operation on the gasserian ganglion and its posterior root. These have not only made the operation almost devoid of mortality, but have greatly minimized the postoperative sequelae. Horsley (1900) created a small permanent bony defect instead of turning down a bone flap as originally done by Hartley and Krause. This makes the operation shorter and less formidable; it reduces the frequency of extradural hemorrhage, and it allows a more inferior and therefore more direct and easier approach to the ganglion. Tiffany[18] (1896) recommended an intentional incision of the dura in order to evacuate cerebrospinal fluid. This seemingly minor point of technic adds greatly to the ease and safety of the operation. The additional room obtained not only facilitates manipulation in a restricted operative field, but it also reduces the trauma to the temporal lobe (from traction). Moreover, it at once reduces the venous oozing which often impedes the operator's progress.

In his pioneer publication, Rose (1891)

suggested preservation of the ophthalmic division of the ganglion as a possible means of preventing postoperative keratitis. Tiffany [19] (1896), too, expressed a hope that deliberate partial section of the gasserian ganglion (the lower two thirds) might be available. Tiffany also suggested the possibility of saving the motor root of the trigeminus and emphasized its importance in the rare cases of bilateral tic douloureux.

A great improvement in the operative treatment of tic douloureux was made by Spiller and Frazier [15] (1901) when they disregarded the gasserian ganglion and exposed and divided the sensory root behind it. Also, for the first time, they were able to preserve the motor root which lay alongside and mesial to the sensory root. Frazier [20] (1925) added still another improvement—perhaps the most important of all—namely, subtotal resection of the posterior root. From morphologic studies, he [21] concluded that the peripheral branches of the gasserian ganglion were represented in a well defined order in the posterior root. His procedure of choice has since been to segregate and preserve those fibers of the posterior root which correspond to the ophthalmic branch. I shall later comment on this point in considering the function of the trigeminal nerve.

During the past twenty-five years, the operative mortality for all types of operative treatment has been reduced to a low point, i.e., from 0.5 to 1 per cent in the hands of experienced operators who specialize in cranial operations. For reasons which are not clear, the mortality in Germany is still reported around 10 to 12 per cent (Gutnikoff, [22] Hartel [23]), with operators of the greatest experience. With such a prohibitive operative mortality, it is not surprising that alcoholic injections are in great favor abroad.

It is worthy of note that at the present time all methods of attack on the gasserian ganglion or the sensory root are extradural. Except for Horsley's unsuccessful experience, an intradural attack has not been proposed. The safety of an extradural operation is at once apparent. Not only is the danger of hemorrhage during the operation minimal when the attack is outside the dura but when prolonged retraction is necessary the dura and not the brain receives the brunt of the trauma. It seems probable that the death in Horsley's case was due to traumatic edema.

But with all the technical improvements which have been added, the operation is not without its liabilities. To quote from Frazier [20] who, by testing Spiller's beliefs, has introduced nearly all the important additions to Krause's original operation:

But chiefly because of the possibility of corneal complications following the radical operation, the frequency of which has been under-rather than over-estimated, we must admit of the treatment of trigeminal neuralgia, that the last word has not been said.

First and most important of the postoperative liabilities are the disturbances in the eyes; second, the muscles of mastication are commonly lost on the affected side, which interferes with opening the mouth and with mastication; third, the side of the face becomes sunken due to atrophy of the masseter and temporal muscles; fourth, not infrequently, varying degrees of facial paralysis result, and fifth, epilepsy occasionally follows in the wake of an extradural hemorrhage.

These complications are indeed gradually becoming less frequent owing to the improvements in the operative procedure and to the skill of the experienced surgeons, but they continue to appear even with the best operators. Patients so affected are greatly handicapped, at times even to the point of invalidism. If by other methods it is possible to eliminate these disturbances in part or in whole, the factor of operative safety being equal, the improvement would be most acceptable.

In 1925, I [24] presented in a preliminary note an operation by which the sensory root of the trigeminus was divided at the pons, a unilateral cerebellar approach being used. At the time, I entertained little enthusiasm for the procedure as a routine measure in treating persons with tic douloureux because the method then in use was so safe. Moreover, at that time the advantages of the operation, aside from the greater ease of performance, were not appreciated. In certain conditions as, for example, when pain was induced by the invasion of the gasserian ganglion by a malignant tumor, it was indispensable. But at that time there appeared to be no reason to expect any material advantages in the treatment for tic douloureux. However, as the number of cases increased it was observed that the complications of the old method did not appear; there were no corneal disturbances and the motor root was never injured. Moreover, for reasons which will be considered later, after section of the posterior root, sensation of varying amount was usually but not always retained in the face, and without return of the pain. Although there did not seem to be the same need of perserving the fibers of the first branch of the trigeminus since the cornea was not affected after complete section, it was usually just as easy to make a subtotal section of the root as its complete division.

Owing to the great advantages of the subcerebellar route, all patients (88) have been treated by this method during the past two years.

THE OPERATION

A somewhat crescent shaped incision is made in the occipital region on the affected side (Fig. 1). The incision begins near the midline and extends in transverse direction just below the origin of the trapezius muscle. Laterally the incision turns sharply downward in a straight line to the tip of the mastoid. The trapezius muscle is divided transversely, stripped from the occiput, and retracted downward and somewhat mesially. An area of bone, perhaps 4 by 4 cm., is removed and two extensions of this central defect are made—one toward the cisterna magna, the other toward the mastoid. The latter extension must be carefully made so that the utmost room can be obtained. Cautiously, the bone is

nibbled away toward the mastoid cells and the transverse and sigmoid venous sinuses. The mastoid cells are, of course, carefully avoided because of the danger of infection. Occasionally they have been opened accidentally, but with no untoward effect. The opening, however, is always covered with a flap of dura which is sutured to the periosteum. In the region of the transverse sinus and its junction with the sigmoid sinus, the lateral bony extension can be made larger because the mastoid cells usually stop at a lower level. This extension is really the most important part of the bony defect, for it is from here that the subcerebellar approach is made. The dura is then incised in stellate fashion, and at once the cisterna magna is sought and opened. The release of this fluid provides ample room for exploration.

The cerebellar hemisphere is then elevated with a narrow spatula directed upward and inward (Fig. 1 B). The thin membranous covering of the cisterna lateralis, which extends the entire length of the posterior fossa and lines the brain stem, is opened between the auditory nerve and the tentorium (Fig. 1 A). After the collapse of the cisterna lateralis and removal of the loose arachnoid membrane between the auditory nerve and the tentorium, the sensory root of the trigeminus stands out sharply in the depth (Fig. 1 B). At the incisura tentorii, the petrosal vein crosses from the inferior surface of the cerebellum to the petrosal sinus (Fig. 1 B and C). It lies in and is attached to the outer lining of the cisterna lateralis. The arachnoid membrane must therefore be cautiously removed from the vein to avoid tearing it.

The petrosal vein and the auditory nerve are the two most important landmarks, and between them—they are about 1 to 1.5 cm. apart—the spatula is introduced. The sensory root of the trigeminus is then in full view throughout its course from the tentorium to the pons, a span of from 1 to 1.5 cm. The sensory root lies probably 1 cm. deeper than the petrosal vein. A small blunt dissector at an angle with its long shank is passed between the sensory root and the pons in order to free the nerve. A small angled knife also on a long flexible shank then follows up the free space between the

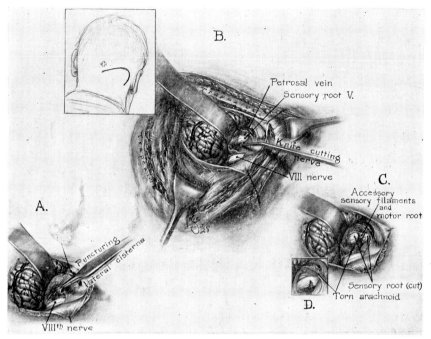

Fig. 1. A, the cisterna lateralis, which is being opened to obtain additional room and to expose the sensory root of the trigeminus; B, exposure of the fifth nerve with the blade of the knife inserted beneath the sensory root. Anterior to the sensory root is the petrosal vein, and posterior to it is the eighth nerve; C, fifth nerve totally divided with the intact accessory branches anteriorly and beneath; D, subtotal section of the sensory root.

nerve and the pons and by gentle traction on the blade of the knife, the nerve is severed either in part or whole as desired (Fig. 3 B). Section of the nerve is usually bloodless; occasionally a tiny bleeding is suppressed by the application of a moist cotton pledget.

The operation is much easier and quicker to perform than the temporal method, for the route is bloodless. Only a few minutes are usually required to elevate the cerebellum, open the cisterna lateralis and aspirate the cerebrospinal fluid and complete the section of the nerve. There are times when the petrosal vein causes trouble because of its inconstant position and size. Occasionally it may obscure the nerve in part or even almost entirely. It is then necessary to retract the vein with the spatula. On two occasions the vein was torn by retraction, but the bleeding was controlled by packing gently with the moist cotton or by application of a silver clip. Recently when the vein has obscured

the sensory root or rendered its exposure difficult, it has been doubly clipped and divided at once. This is made much easier and safer by using flat clips in a long clip holder specially made with the handle bent at right angles to the shaft. The petrosal vein has, in addition, other abnormalities; at times it bifurcates, again it may be double throughout this part of its course, and on two occasions it was absent. In two of the earlier cases the auditory nerve was traumatized by the spatula in trying to avoid or retract the petrosal vein. In neither of these cases did the hearing return, although the nerve was intact. In one of these cases the facial nerve also was paralyzed, but the function returned three months later. Only once has the facial nerve actually been seen at the operation. It is usually so well covered by the auditory nerve that it is entirely out of sight. Injury to the auditory nerve must be considered a potential danger of the operation. It should hardly occur again when one can, if necessary, so easily dispose of the petrosal vein. In a recent case, I felt sufficiently secure in this regard to perform the operation despite the fact that the patient was totally deaf in the other ear.

On two occasions, the posterior surface of the cerebellum has been injured but without any subsequent appreciable disturbance of gait or equilibrium. In one of these cases, a vein running between the tentorium and the cerebellum was torn when the cerebellum was being cautiously elevated. By quickly enlarging the bony defect it was possible to locate and close the bleeding point, evacuate the hematoma and proceed with section of the nerve. In the other case the cerebellum bulged so tightly, despite the release of fluid, that the operation could not proceed until a subsequent stage when the bony opening was enlarged to give more room. Swelling of the brain is a not uncommon sequel of ether anesthesia, but only in this instance has the swelling of the cere-

bellum been a serious handicap. However, in the last thirty operations, rectal ether has been used, with great benefit. The greater available space in the posterior fossa is most striking in all cases and makes the operative procedure easier. There has not been the slightest postoperative disturbance in this series.

Except in the case just mentioned evacuation of the cisterna magna has provided ample room in which to work. Elevation of the cerebellum does not require any force except that necessary to overcome the weight. In fact, care must be taken to obtain room by retraction. It must be obtained by removing bone and fluid. If the bony exposure is not ample, efforts to retract the brain to obtain more room will be injurious to the cerebellum and may cause a crossing vein to tear along the tentorial surface.

In only one instance has a slight extraocular palsy been present, and this—a weakness of the sixth nerve—steadily lessened during the following two weeks. Another patient complained of seeing double,

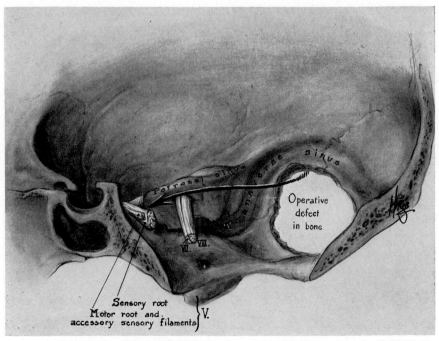

Fig. 2. Interior of skull, showing route by which the fifth nerve is divided, the cerebellar approach being used.

but as the ocular movements were not limited, it was difficult to tell what muscle was involved. Before the patient left the hospital, the vision was greatly improved.

There has been but one death due to the operation; this was due to hemorrhage from a vein along the sensory root. Three patients died of intercurrent diseases before being discharged from the hospital. One patient died of meningitis a week following the operation from a source now known and now preventable. A second patient died of intestinal obstruction which developed ten days after the operation. He had been sitting up and had recovered from the effects of the operation. A third patient died of cerebral thrombosis two weeks after the operation. She was a questionable operative risk because of hypertension (240). Albumin was found in the urine. Total occlusion of one radial artery indicated the presence of an obliterative process within the arteries. She had twice been refused operative relief at another clinic because of her general condition. Beginning a week after the operation, when she, too, was sitting up, weakness of he left side appeared and gradually increased. Two days before death, signs of intracranial pressure developed, causing the cerebellar wound to bulge. Necropsy showed a diffuse thrombosis involving practically the entire right cerebral hemisphere. The cerebral cortex was swollen and hemorrhagic throughout the entire right hemisphere. The right lateral ventricle was collapsed; the third and left lateral ventricles were dislocated to the left. Since the entire hemisphere was involved, there seems no possible relationship between this process and the remotely removed field of operation.

In the entire series of eighty-eight cases, not a trace of redness of the conjunctiva was found during the first week after the operation. In one case the conjunctiva became reddened ten days after operation, doubtless due to trauma of some form. Subsequently there is, of course, no great-

er protection of an insensitive cornea following these operations than by the temporal route. Never has the cornea looked dry and lusterless, changes indicative of impending corneal ulceration. Tears have been observed to flow just as freely from the affected as from the other side. Since this method has been adopted, only once has it been necessary to employ the temporal route. In this case a low, congenitally misplaced, transverse venous sinus prevented access to the region of the trigeminal nerve.

A second outstanding result of the series has been that in not a single instance has there been even a transient weakness of the muscles of mastication. The explanation of this fact is that the motor root of the trigeminus is so far removed from the sensory root that there is little occasion to damage it. Usually, the motor root is not seen. The motor root is always mesial and anterior to the sensory division. Obviously, therefore, there has been no instance in which the suprazygomatic and infrazygomatic regions have become atrophied and sunken.

The danger of postoperative hemorrhage is always far greater in the temporal region because the branches of the middle meningeal artery and the other arteries supplying the dura are stripped from the bone. Postoperative hemorrhages in that location are indeed not uncommon even after the middle meningeal artery has been ligated, for there is an extensive arterial supply derived from the sphenoidal fissure. The only source of late bleeding in the subcerebellar approach would be from the exposed trapezius muscle, and this should not cause concern if closure is carefully made.

Jacksonian epilepsy occasionally follows in the wake of an extradural hemorrhage owing to the injury to the brain by the clot. This most dreaded of all complications cannot occur if the posterior approach is used, because this approach is far removed from the motor cortex.

Finally, from the standpoint of the surgeon, the operation is much easier. After the bone is removed there is no hemorrhage to combat, and only a few moments are required to expose and divide the nerve. By the temporal route the struggle with bleeding may be long, difficult and exhausting to the operator.

In a short paragraph in a long article on the treatment for tic douloureux by the injection of alcohol, Von Dollinger [25] (1912) mentioned the fact that on three occasions he had divided the sensory root beneath the cerebellum. Although this was easier than by the lateral route because of the absence of the tedious bleeding from the cavernous sinus and the middle meningeal artery, he advised giving up all operative treatment in favor of Schloesser's injection of alcohol. A year after my report, Clairmont [26] (1926) reported a case in which the operation was by this approach but in which death occurred two days later. He encountered severe bleeding which was eventually controlled, but the patient doubtless died from the effects of trauma.

For the success of the operation one must have a narrow spoon spatula, a tiny knife at right angles to a long flexible shaft, long, thin, angled forceps, perfect electrical illumination, a dry field and at the moment of division of the nerve absolutely smooth, even and unobstructed respiration under anesthesia. Trauma to the cerebellum must be avoided. Unless one has the utmost extension of the lateral bony defect and unless the cisterna magna is opened before the cerebellum is elevated, the exposure will be inadequate and any attempt to retract the cerebellum to overcome a defective approach will surely be followed by injury and hemorrhage, which will be not only destruction of function but highly dangerous to life. With an adequate exposure, the operator does not place any pressure on the cerebellum other than the force necessary to counteract its weight. The operation is certainly dangerous unless the operator is perfectly equipped and unless he is well

acquainted with the anatomy of this region.

In those patients who were operated on earlier in this series, the sensory root was totally severed. Later, when it became evident how much sensory function was carried by a small accessory filament, a small fragment of the sensory root itself was deliberately left, thereby making it unnecessary to depend on chance accessory fibers. Later, a larger portion (from one-third to one-fourth) of the sensory root was left intact after partial radiculotomy. Partial section of the sensory root was found to be just as easy of performance and much more consistent in superior results. By this method, almost normal sensation is permanently retained over the whole side of the face, even though the pain for which the patient was operated on has been abolished. In effect, the operation appeared to do little more than cut pain fibers and to produce essentially the same result in the domain of the trigeminal nerve as chordotomy for pain in the extremities. In the last twenty cases, partial division of the sensory root has been used exclusively. However, as the original procedure of total division of the sensory root throws much light on the structure and function of the trigeminal nerve, these results have been recorded first and the results of the operation in its present form—partial section—appear later in the paper.

PRESERVATION OF SENSATION IN THE FACE AFTER PRESUMABLY TOTAL DIVISION OF THE SENSORY ROOT BY THE CEREBELLAR ROUTE

Since the frequent preservation of sensation in the face and cornea is one of the important features of the cerebellar route, the following sensory examinations following division of the sensory root are presented in some detail.

I. *Cases Showing Total Anesthesia*

Case 1. In a woman, aged fifty-nine, examination on discharge showed complete loss of sensation for touch, pain and temperature over all three branches of the nerve. The corneal reflex was abolished.

Case 2. In a woman, aged sixty-three, examined six months after operation, there was total loss of perception of touch, pain and temperature over the entire domain of the fifth nerve. Deep sensation was lost. The corneal reflex was absent.

Case 3. In a woman, aged seventy, tests made ten days after operation showed complete loss of all forms of sensation. The corneal reflex was absent.

Case 4. In a woman, aged fifty-one, examination on discharge ten days after operation showed absolute loss of all forms of sensation over the domain of the severed trigeminal nerve. There was no recognition of deep pressure sensation until tests were made near the periphery of the affected zone. Movement of the skin having normal sensation then made tests for deep sensation impossible. The corneal reflex was absent. Muscles supplied by the motor branch of the trigeminus functioned normally. Vasomotor response was apparently normal. When ice was placed on both lips simultaneously, blanching occurred at the same time on each side, and when the ice was removed the color returned synchronously. When a pin was scratched across both sides of the forehead, upper lip or chin, dermatographia or wheal formation did not develop on either side.

II. *Preservation of Touch Only (the Entire Domain of the Fifth Nerve Apparently Being Similarly Affected).*

Case 5. In a woman, aged seventy, sensory examination on discharge, fifteen days after operation, showed complete loss of perception of sharp and dull stimuli and of heat and cold. Perception of light touch was present everywhere, though it was less acute than on the normal side. All branches were equally affected. Doubleness of objects was recognized accurately.

Case 6. Sensory tests, after section of the sensory root of the trigeminus at the pons, showed that the patient could detect and localize light touch (with cotton) at all points over the trigeminal area. She was unable to differentiate between sharp and dull stimuli at any point, nor could she differentiate between heat and cold. There was an active corneal reflex.

III. *Preservation of Touch Only and Over the Second and Third Branches Only (Total Anesthesia of First Branch).*

Case 7. In a man, aged fifty-six, examined at the time of discharge, eleven days after operation, all forms of sensation were abolished over the area of the first branch; touch was preserved over the second and third branches. Heat and cold and sharp and dull stimuli were not perceived. The corneal reflex was absent.

IV. *Preservation of Touch and Temperature Only (Anesthesia for Sharp and Dull Stimuli). All Three Branches Were About Equally Affected.*

Case 8. In a woman, aged fifty-four, in whom sensory tests were made ten days after operation, there was marked hypoesthesia for all forms of sensation over the affected side. Perception of light touch was everywhere present; heat and cold were detected after delay; sharp and dull stimuli were differentiated though with some uncertainty. A diminished corneal reflex was present.

Case 9. In a woman, aged forty-two, examined one week after operation, all three branches were equally affected. Perception of light touch was everywhere present. Heat and cold were recognized everywhere. Sharp and dull stimuli could not be differentiated. Sharp stimuli registered only as touch. The corneal reflex was abolished.

Case 10. In a woman, aged forty-eight, examined on discharge, perception of light touch was everywhere preserved. Heat and cold were accurately recognized, though the acuity was greatly diminished. Sharp and dull stimuli were not recognized except when the stimulus was extreme. The corneal reflex was present but diminished. Doubleness of objects was registered correctly.

V. *Preservation of All Forms of Sensation Over the Second and Third Branches Only (the First Branch Was Anesthetic).*

Case 11. A man, aged forty-six, had multiple sclerosis. Sensory examination at the time of discharge from the hospital, nine days after operation, showed anesthesia for all forms of sensation over the first branch and part of the second. Some sensation was present over the remainder of the second branch, touch, pain and temperature all being recognized. Over the third branch, all forms of sensation were practically normal. The corneal reflex was absent.

VI. *Preservation of Touch Over all*

Three Branches but of Heat and Cold and of Sharp and Dull Stimuli Over the First Branch Only. (Anesthesia for All Sensations, Except Touch, Over the Second and Third Branches).

Case 12. Sensory examination showed slightly subnormal sensation for all types over the distribution of the first branch. Over the second and third branches touch was distinguished, but the perception of heat and cold and of sharp and dull stimuli was absent.

VII. *Preservation of All Forms of Sensation in All Three Branches, But With Greatest Acuity Over the First Branch and Less Over the Second and Third Branches. Usually the Sensation Over the Third Branch was Still Less Than the Second. In Many Instances the Sensation Over the Forehead Was Only Slightly If At All Subnormal.*

Case 13. In a man, aged sixty-nine, examined at the time of discharge, sensation over the first branch was practically normal. Light touch, pain and temperature were registered accurately everywhere, but with less acuity over the second and third branches. The corneal reflex was normal.

Case 14. A man, aged thirty-eight, examined on discharge, seven days after operation, did not notice the sensory loss. Light touch with a wisp of cotton was perceived promptly over the entire domain of the fifth nerve; it felt a little keener over the forehead. Heat and cold and sharp and dull stimuli were correctly and promptly recognized everywhere but with greater acuity over the forehead. Sensation over the forehead was little less than on the normal side. The corneal reflex is no less active than that of the normal side.

Case 15. Touch was accurately perceived over the entire affected trigeminal domain, though it was less acute than on the other side. Heat and cold were accurately differentiated over all three branches but better over the first branch. Sharp and dull stimuli were also perceived, though with more difficulty than heat and cold. For all forms of sensation the acuity was less than on the normal side. In the supra-orbital region of the side operated on, the acuity was somewhat greater than over the two lower branches. The corneal reflex was present and quite active. Doubleness of objects was accur-

ately recognized.

Case 16. Lightest touch was recognized over all three branches. Perception of heat and cold seemed normal over the first branch and was present but greatly diminished over the second and third branches. When two objects were touching the face at any point, their number was correctly noted. Perception of sharp and dull stimuli was normal over the first branch but was poorly differentiated over the second and third branches. There seemed to be patches where sharp stimuli could not be detected. The corneal reflex was as acute as on the normal side.

Case 17. In a man, aged fifty-five, examined at the time of discharge, eight days after operation, light touch with cotton, sharp and dull stimuli, deep pressure, heat and cold were appreciated over the entire distribution of the affected trigeminal area, but the acuity of recognition progressively diminished from the forehead to the chin. The left corneal reflex was present but slightly less active than on the other side.

Case 18. A man, aged fifty-five, examined one week, and again five months, after operation, had some sensation over the entire affected side. Sensation was greatest over the forehead, less over the cheek and still less over the chin. Light touch was promptly recognized over all three branches, though less than on the normal side. Sharp and dull stimuli were correctly differentiated over all three branches, though with diminishing acuity from above downward. Cold was accurately registered over the entire side of the face. Heat was promptly noticed when applied over the forehead, but not over the cheek and chin. The corneal reflex was nearly as active as on the normal side.

Case 19. In a man, aged sixty, examined on the eighth day after operation and again ten months later, the results of the tests remained the same on both examinations. Light touch was everywhere recognized, though a little less sharply than on the normal side. Heat and cold and sharp and dull stimuli were recognized over the entire side but somewhat less acutely than the other side. There was slightly greater sensory acuity over the first branch than over the cheek, and still a little more than over the chin. The corneal reflex was active, but slightly less than on the other side.

Case 20. In a woman, aged forty-nine, examined on discharge, the ninth day after operation, there was no complete sensory loss. Sensation over the forehead was little if any less than over the side not operated on. Hypo-esthesia for all forms of sensation was present over the second and third branches. The corneal reflex was normal.

VIII. *Preservation of All Forms of Sensation and of About Equal Degree Over All Three Branches. Although There Was Always Some Hypo-esthesia, It Might be so Slight as to be Detected Only With Delicate Tests.*

Case 21. Examination two and one-half months after operation showed the sensation to be but little affected. Light touch, sharp and dull stimuli and slight differences of heat and cold were promptly perceived. The acuity of sensation was definitely a little less than on the normal side. There was no apparent difference in sensation in the three branches. The corneal reflex was practically as active as on the normal side.

Case 22. In a man, aged forty-four, examined on discharge, eight days after operation, all forms of sensation were impaired but present over all three branches. Except for the distribution of the second branch (which had previously been injected with alcohol) the sensory loss was about the same over all branches. The corneal reflex was present but less active than on the normal side.

Case 23. In a woman, aged fifty-five, bilateral section of the sensory root was performed at a single operation. She said that feeling on both sides of the face was "natural". Perception of light touch with cotton was intensified everywhere. Heat and cold and sharp and dull stimuli were accurately recognized on both sides. The domain of the fifth nerve could not be mapped out, for the patient said that the sensation was the same as over the area of the cervical nerves. Examination was made at the time of discharge, ten days after operation. The corneal reflex was present on both sides.

The foregoing sensory examinations [27] show such greatly variable differences in both the quantity and the quality of the retained sensation that one's credulity might well be tested. At times all forms

of sensation are totally abolished. Again all forms of sensation, i. e., light touch, corneal reflex, heat and cold, sharp and dull, may be retained and approximate though never quite equal to those on the normal side. The difference may indeed be so slight as not to be noticeable to the patient. But regardless of the degree or kind of preserved sensation never has there been a single instance in which a suggestion of the old pain reappeared.

From the cases in which sensation is preserved the only uniform result is the retention of touch, though even this is of varying acuity. At times, touch alone is preserved; at other times touch and temperature only, and in one instance at least cold was accurately recognized when heat was not appreciated (case 18). That heat and cold require separate conduction paths would appear to be indicated by this observation. But it is not fair to place great emphasis on an unsupported single test.

The sensation which remains may be uniformly acute over the whole domain of the fifth nerve; or, again, in other instances it may be more intense in one part than in another. The most frequent observation is greater sensation over the forehead, less over the cheek and still less over the chin. But the variation may obtain in the reverse direction. There appears to be no general plan.

In the foregoing case reports, reference has been made to sensation corresponding with the first, second and third branches. This has been done for convenience only. Such designations, when one is speaking of fractions of the sensory root, may indeed be misleading for it is doubtful if the retained sensation is referable except in a general way to the three peripheral divisions of the nerve. The transition between the shading zones of retained sensation is usually too insensible to make out a sharp line of demarcation. The gradations of sensations conform only in a general way to the three branches of the nerve.

In explanation of these bizarre and seemingly paradoxic sensory sequelae, one might naturally infer that the sensory root had not been completely divided. But the nerve is easy to inspect after its division, and the stumps can be seen. Analysis of the sensation which remains would seem to preclude such an explanation, for why should all branches of the nerve retain sensation if the nerve should have been only partially divided? One would at least expect some part of the face to be rendered totally anesthetic to all forms of sensation. If, on the other hand, the claim is conceded that the sensory root is totally severed, how could the results be explained? And why should division of the sensory root at the pons yield results different from those obtained when it is divided in the dural envelop near the gasserian ganglion? Also why, in so many instances, is the retained sensation greater over the general domain of the first branch than of the other branches of the trigeminus? And why is one form of sensation retained and another lost, and perhaps another only diminished?

In a publication with May (1910), Victor Horsley [28] expressed the belief that the motor root carried sensory fibers and adduced both clinical observations and histologic studies to prove his point. In support of their claim, these authors quote Bregmann's [29] studies of wallerian degeneration and the discovery of sensory ganglionic cells near the motor nucleus. Van Loudon [30] (1907) brought similar evidence to prove that the motor root contained sensory fibers. Van Gehuchten [31] thought all sensory fibers were in the mesencephalic root.

Sensory fibers in the motor root could not explain the results, for the motor root runs behind the gasserian ganglion and usually blends with the third branch at some distance distal to the ganglion. Therefore, it could not send fibers to the first branch and often not to the second branch. If sensory fibers were carried in the motor root, the third branch would

surely contain the most, if not all, sensation, whereas the reverse is usually true, i. e., the ophthalmic branch usually contains most of the sensation which is preserved.

It has been suggested that the gasserian ganglion might function without a central sensory connection, or possibly through the central connection established by the superficial petrosal nerves. Spiller mentioned this possibility when he first suggested division of the posterior root instead of removal of the ganglion. It will be remembered that during the approach to the sensory root by the temporal route, the petrosal nerves are often injured, whereas in the cerebellor approach they are not encountered. It might be assumed that the preservation of this connection might be of value in retaining some function for the ganglion. However, the total anesthesia which results in some cases from section of the posterior root by the cerebellar route must eliminate this theory of independent sensory function of the gasserian ganglion. And because of the total anesthesia, one can also say that the motor root, at times, at least, does not carry sensory fibers. The evidence, however, is not sufficient to disprove, but it does place a burden of proof on, the theory that sensory fibers are contained within the motor root.

If the sensory observations are correct, as I believe they are, there can be but one explanation, namely, that there must be some anatomic feature of the sensory root which has not been recognized. And if this is true, that feature must be subject to considerable variation.

Examination of the sensory root of the trigeminal nerve reveals a number of accessory branches on which I believe the preservation of sensation depends. Either before or after the dura is reached, they join the main sensory trunk. When the sensory root is divided at the pons, these fibers remain intact and, as is true of the motor root, they may or may not be seen during the operation, being frequently hidden by the tentorium. It is therefore probable that this variable and intact sensory supply explains the differing results which obtain after the operation. The remarkable fact remains that these fibers apparently never carry pain fibers, if this may be assumed from the fact that the old pain of tic douloureux has instantly ceased and has not reappeared. Moreover, since there is evidence of dissociation of sensation, there must be specificity of the nerves as carriers. In support of this is the absence of perception of heat and cold with preservation of touch; the retention of temperature sense with the absence of perception of sharp and dull objects; and again the ability to perceive sharp and dull stimuli and at the same time the elimination of the pain of tic douloureux.

On the other hand, it is difficult to understand how the small accessory fibers can often assume so much sensory control and over all three branches of the face. From their anterior position one would be prepared to believe that if they should carry sensation it would be only to the domain of the first branch of the nerve. It would seem to explain the greater preservation of sensation in the first branch than in the others, but the fact remains that the other branches retain sensation. One other anatomic observation is noteworthy, i. e., that the accessory branches join each other and also send branches to the fibers of the posterior root before losing their identity.

It is, of course, important to trace the microscopic course of the accessory fibers within the brain stem. Although their position would appear to indicate their destination in the mesencephalic root of the trigeminus rather than in the spinal root, this can as yet only be an inference. The seeming absence of pain fibers in the accessory roots would also appear to be evidence against their participation in the spinal root which is usually presumed to carry the pain fibers.

It is interesting that in two of the four cases of total anesthesia, deep pressure sensation was totally abolished: in the other two cases, deep sensation was not tested. The pathways of deep sensation have been claimed for both the trigeminal (Davis [32]) and the facial (Maloney and Kennedy [33]) nerves. These results indicate that deep sensation goes along with other sensations through the trigeminal nerve.

Vasomotor response was tested in two patients in whom all forms of sensation were abolished. It was found to be unchanged. When ice was firmly placed over both sides of the lip simultaneously, the degree of blanching of the mucous membrane was identical on both sides and the red color returned in percisely the same time. A scratch across the forehead or on both cheeks did not cause dermatographia or formation of wheals on either side.

ANATOMIC VARIATIONS OF THE SENSORY ROOT AND THE ACCESSORY BRANCHES AND OF THE ADJACENT BLOOD VESSELS

In an occasional case, the motor root is isolated and leaves the pons unaccompanied. But in most specimens there are additional branches of approximately the same size as the motor root and lying alongside. It is, in fact, impossible to tell by gross inspection of the nerve roots which is the motor root and which are sensory branches. That they are sensory is shown by following them in the dural envelop extending toward the gasserian ganglion; the nerves join freely with the sensory root and eventually the motor root runs alone behind the gasserian ganglion to enter the inferior maxillary nerve. The number of these little accessory sensory branches varies up to ten or twelve. The branches on the two sides may or may not be symmetrical. They send filaments to, and receive other filaments from, the main sensory root, forming at times a network of interchanging fibers. The accessory sensory fibers are grouped together at the pons at the point of emergence of the motor root, and an appreciable interval of space—usually 2 or 3 mm.—separates them from the point of entry of the main sensory root. There are, however, variations in this respect, too. In some instances the accessory fibers enter the pons in a continuous line between the motor and sensory root, making all fibers practically continuous. In one instance the line of accessory fibers ran ventral to the sensory root. The accessory branches are never consolidated into a compact root but run individually, having, however, loose, delicate, fibrous attachments to each other.

The main sensory root of the trigeminus also has variations. The size of the root varies greatly; a large root may be three times as large as the smallest. The shape of the root at the pons also varies. Usually it is oval or flat from its close relation to the pons; toward the gasserian ganglion it becomes more rounded. The long diameter of the nerve root is usually parallel to the pons, but it may be rotated up to 45 degrees. Its directional plane is important in facilitating the fractional division of the root. When it is lying flattened against the pons, as it usually does, partial section of the nerve is relatively easy, but when it is lying at an angle, the anteriormost part of the root is not visible from the operator's point of view. I have seen this rotation only twice, and in each instance it was the posterior border of the root which was rotated outward. In both instances, section of the entire nerve was necessary.

Variations in the gross structure of the sensory root alongside the pons are also important from an operative standpoint. Usually the nerve is compact and closely bound together by a semblance of a sheath. At times, however, the fibers are quite loosely bound and easily separated, or at least permit the nerve to be split into several parts. This is of importance in permitting partial section of the nerve. Since the blunt instrument which is used to liberate the nerve from the pons may find such an easy line of separation in the nerve, a partial division of the nerve not

infrequently results after which the extra fasiculus of the nerve must be separately isolated and divided if total section is desired. In one necropsy specimen the main sensory root was divided into two nearly equal parts by a longitudinal cleft; the one half (posterior) was covered by a sheath; in the other half, the individual roots were loosely held together. Usually evidences of a nerve sheath are absent in the passage through the dural canal.

Vascular variations in this region are important in facilitating or rendering more difficult the operative procedure. Only occasionally does an artery concern the operator, but in two or three instances an arterial loop projects freely in the subarachnoid space and encircles the sensory root. At these times the free loop must be carefully avoided, and the part of the artery between the pons and the sensory root is cautiously isolated from the nerve by blunt dissection before its division with the knife. In one instance it was necessary to depress the free arterial loop, and a small wet cotton pack was used to cover and keep it out of reach during the manipulation of the nerve. This vessel is a branch of the basilar artery.

It is, however, the variation of the neighboring veins which is of chief concern at operation. The petrosal vein offers the only real problem in the operation. If it is normally placed, there is ample room and it can be disregarded. But there are frequent variations in this vessel. In two operations, the vein was absent. In others, the vein is situated more posteriorly than usual and so partially obscures the nerve. It is then necessary either gradually to elongate and dislocate the vein or to ligate it with silver clips. At times the vein is formed by the junction of two smaller veins midway between the cerebellum and the petrosal sinus, and the vein may occasionally be double. At times the nerve is sectioned when the surgeon is working anterior to the petrosal vein and occasionally between its branches. In a recent case one half of a bifid petrosal vein ran external to the auditory nerve, which it entirely concealed, and then coursed over the petrous temporal bone from the internal auditory meatus to the petrosal sinus. It was therefore necessary to work in a small opening entirely surrounded by large veins.

Division of the sensory root is usually not attended by bleeding, but on one occasion a vein of some size was divided when the nerve was sectioned and bled quite freely until controlled by a small cotton pack. Examination of several specimens obtained at necropsy revealed in one instance a small branch of the petrosal vein running in the sheath of the nerve. In other cases the nerve seemed free of any vessels of appreciable size. To insure the brain stem against the effects of gentle packing for hemorrhage, which might occur, a small wet cotton pack may be inserted between the pons and sensory root before it is divided.

PARTIAL SECTION OF THE SENSORY ROOT

From embryologic and anatomic studies, Frazier and Whitehead concluded that each branch of the trigeminal nerve was represented by a well defined subdivision of the sensory root, and on that basis Frazier introduced subtotal section of the sensory root in the dural envelop just posterior to the gasserian ganglion, still using the lateral approach. His main object was to spare the nerve supply to the cornea and avoid corneal ulceration. However, the immediate postoperative corneal ulceration is probably not so much dependent on the loss of corneal sensation as on other factors which will be considered later under keratitis. Although there is seemingly less need than formerly to preserve sensation to the eye, it is much better to retain it, other things being equal.

For a technical standpoint, the sensory root can be partially divided at the pons (the cerebellar approach being used) with just as much ease and safety as a total resection of the nerve. Moreover,

structural features (the flat oval shape and relative immobility) of the sensory root at the pons make partial section of the sensory root much easier and more expeditious than in the dural envelop where Frazier divides it.

The sensory root is almost round when leaving the gasserian ganglion and in its transit through the dural conduit, but it becomes flattened alongside the pons with the flat surface usually in full view. Fortunately, the sensory root is firmly welded to the pons by a ring of fibrous tissue derived from the inner layer of the pia arachnoid membrane. This layer forms the inner wall of the subarachnoid space. The outer layer is occasionally attached to the fifth nerve at a point near the dura, but usually continues alongside the dura to the gasserian ganglion, which it partially surrounds, thus permitting much of the ganglion to be covered with cerebrospinal fluid. Division of the sensory root alongside the pons is, therefore, always within the subarachnoid space. It is the fibrous attachment at the pons which permits avulsion of the sensory root (the temporal route being used) with no greater danger of injury to the pons than did its simple division with a knife. Likewise, it is this strong fibrous fixation (together with the paucity of fibrous tissue in the nerve root) which makes it possible partially or totally to divide the sensory root at the pons (by the cerebellar route) without producing injury of the pons.

In fifteen instances the sensory root has been subtotally sectioned, only the anteriormost fibers being left intact (Fig. 1 D). The sensory results in the first five cases of partial resection are typical of the others.

Case 24. In a man, aged fifty-five, subtotal section of the sensory root was made for pain in the third branch of the nerve. The anteriormost fibers were preserved. A fair estimate of the fibers in the trunk remaining would probably be about one tenth of the whole. Five days later, the sensory examination showed the following: All forms of sensation were perceived almost as sharply as on the sound side. Sensation seemed equally acute over all three branches. The corneal reflex was no less active than on the other side.

Case 25. In a woman, aged sixty-two, the posterior fourteen-fifteenths or more of the sensory root was divided for pain in the third branch of the nerve, only a fine strand remaining. At the time of discharge from the hospital, the only sensory change that was subnormal was a small area in the lower lip and chin, and here the lessened sensation was for sharp and dull objects only; perception of heat and cold and light touch was just as normal as elsewhere. Aside from this hypo-esthesia, there was no greater acuity of sensation of any form over the first division than elsewhere. The acuity of all forms of sensation was the same on both sides of the face. The corneal reflex was present and undiminished. Tears flowed from the affected eye.

Case 26. In a woman, aged thirty-two, the posterior four fifths of the sensory root was sectioned at the pons for pain in the second and third branches of the nerve. When leaving the hospital one week later, the patient had almost normal sensation over the entire domain of the trigeminus. Subjectively, the patient was unaware of any change in sensation. Objectively, the lightest touch was promptly detected everywhere; there was no appreciable difference in intensity of the sensation according to branches, nor was there any difference between the affected and the normal sides. Sharp and dull were instantly and accurately registered. The slightest difference was not observed according to branches of the trigeminus, nor was the acuity of sensation less than on the normal side. Slight differences of heat and cold were promptly recognized over all three divisions of the nerve, without any appreciable difference over any branch and with no less acuity than on the normal side. When more intense heat was used a slight difference was noted—the only subnormal sensory change—over part of the domain of the second and third branches but not over the first branch. The difference was slight but definite. An attempt was made to map out with some degree of accuracy the exact limits of this lessened sensation, but the transition was not great enough to permit its demarcation. Greater degrees of cold did not produce a different sensory response in the two sides. Sensation of touch, temperature and sharp and dull objects was just as normal over the affected side of the tongue and the mucus membrane of the mouth as on the other side. The corneal reflex was undiminished.

During the patient's stay in the hospital, it was noticed that on three occasions tears flowed only from the eye on the normal side. When this was disclosed to the patient, who was a nurse, she stated that this condition obtained before the operation and followed two unsuccessful attempts to inject the third branch of the nerve one month earlier. After neither injection did the slightest alteration of sensation follow in any of the face. That this loss of tears was present before operation is shown by the fact that she told her family physician of the absence of tears after the injections of alcohol. Until this disclosure, it was difficult to believe that partial section of the sensory root could have been the cause, though there seemed no other explanation. It is, in fact, none too clear how the injections of alcohol could have caused this loss of tears. However, there can be no doubt of the unilateral flow and scarcely a doubt of the time of occurrence.

Case 27. In a woman, aged forty-eight, subtotal section of the right sensory root was performed for pain in the third branch. About one tenth of the root along the anterior border was left intact. Sensory examination the next morning showed that, subjectively, the patient could detect a slight difference in the two sides, the right being slightly numb over the second and third branches externally, but not in the mouth or on the tongue.

The lightest touch with a wisp of cotton was everywhere promptly perceived. Sharp and dull objects were immediately and accurately differentiated. Heat and cold were at once recognized. The patient detected a slight but definite difference in the intensity of a sharp object and of heat and cold—sensation on the affected (right) side being less acute. There was, however, no appreciable difference over any part of the right trigeminal area; i. e., the same slight hypo-esthesia was present to the same degree over all three branches and within the mouth and over the right side of the tongue. The corneal reflex was present but somewhat diminished.

Case 28. In a man, aged sixty-two, with pain in the supra-orbital branch of the trigeminus, the posterior three fourths of the sensory nerve was divided.

After operation, sensation for heat and cold was slightly diminished over all three branches. Light touch everywhere was as acute as on the normal side. The corneal reflex was preserved. Operation was performed one month before this paper was sent for publication.

This is the only instance of the series of partial radiculotomies in which the pain was in the first branch of the nerve. A case of this type puts to the most severe test the claim that there is a separate bundle of pain fibers. If pain fibers to the branch of the trigeminus were carried in the anterior border of the nerve, as formerly supposed, the operative procedure in this case would have had no effect on the pain.

The sensory examinations after thirty instances of partial division of the nerve show surprisingly little difference from the normal. But the same almost perfect results have also been occasionally obtained when, as I have believed, the entire main sensory root has been divided. If the latter results had not been known the former would surely have been considered impossible, but with the background of the persistent sensory function after presumably total section of the sensory root, the results after partial section do not appear so disturbing and inconsistent. One naturally wonders how it is possible to correlate these results with Frazier's claim that certain parts of the sensory root accurately represent the three peripheral division of the trigeminal nerve. But again the same doubt appeared after total division of the nerve, for the small accessory roots supplied all three branches of the nerve, though often with inequality of sensation in the various branches. It is doubtful whether, because of the network of fibers and accessory branches near the pons, subtotal division of the sensory root at the pons may or may not produce sensory results

differing either in quantity or in quality from those following fractional division immediately back of the gasserian ganglion. It is to be regretted that sensory examinations after Frazier's method cannot be offered in comparison. As far as I know, Frazier has not presented postoperative sensory examinations to uphold his views.

If the sensory examinations after either partial or total section of the sensory root are as represented, the conclusions seem inescapable; (1) that after partial division of the sensory root there is no sharp and absolute differentiation of the sensory root into three divisions representing the three peripheral branches, and (2) that a small fraction of the sensory root or even the small accessory sensory branches alone are able to dominate the entire sensory domain of the trigeminal nerve with varying degrees of perfection. It would seem that most, at least, of the peripheral representation of sensation for the trigeminal nerve must lie in the gasserian ganglion.

The results of this study lead to the belief that pain fibers do not leave the main sensory root by any of the branches anastomosing with the accessory fibers. If it were permissible to use logic instead of experiment, it would be reasoned as follows: If Frazier does not find any recurrence of pain after subtotal retrogasserian division of the sensory root, using his anatomic divisions as a guide, the same results should be obtainable by dividing the root at the pons. There is, however, no proof that the position and distribution of the pain fibers may not have shifted in the distance intervening between the point of retrogasserian section and that near the pons. The determination of this point will be possible only by carefully observing a long series of cases of subtotal section.

Since in the cases reported, subtotal section has only been performed recently, the evidence of permanent relief of pain cannot be established. However, the immediate cessation of pain has been just as absolute as after total section of the sensory root. It is necessary to leave such a tiny filament of the nerve to insure sensation approximating the normal that I feel justified in recommending its preservation. However in the more recent operations I have felt safe in leaving from one-quarter to one-third of the sensory root. There has been no return of pain in any case. It should be emphasized that in all of the cases of subtotal section of the sensory root the anteriormost fibers have been retained. Gradually the results have seemed to indicate that the fibers for pain were located in the posterior part of the root.

In estimating the sensation which remains after subtotal division of the sensory root, it must be remembered that the results include the variable accessory fibers in addition to the persisting fraction of the sensory root. The sensation which remains may therefore not always be exactly the same, although apparently it always approaches the normal.

In all but one of the patients in whom subtotal section of the sensory root has been performed, the pain has been located in the third or second and third branches. If one works on the original hypothesis that the anterior fibers of the sensory root supplied all forms of sensation to the first peripheral branch of the nerve, this procedure does not appear unorthodox for pain in the second and third branches. But the postoperative sensory results not only seemed to preclude this hypothesis but suggested that the pain fibers for all three divisions of the trigeminal nerve were in the posterior border of the sensory root (in cross-section). In case 28, therefore, the same subtotal section (of the posterior three fourths of the cross-section of the sensory root) was performed, although the pain was in the supra-orbital branch. This patient's pain stopped immediately (it is now one month since the operation) just as it did in those whose pain was in the second or third branches.

If it is true that pain fibers occupy a separate bundle in the posterior border of the sensory root, the operative treatment has been wholly empiric and successful only by a fortunate chance in the location of these fibers. Had the position of the pain fibers been located along the anterior border of the nerve, all partial sections would have been uniformly unsuccessful.

WHY DOES KERATITIS (CORNEAL ULCERATION) DEVELOP AFTER SECTION OF THE TRIGEMINAL NERVE?

That corneal ulceration (keratitis) promptly followed section of the sensory root of the trigeminus was shown by Magendie over a century ago, when for the first time he divided this root in rabbits and dogs. When the first operations on the human gasserian ganglion were performed by Rose (1892) precisely the same distressing corneal ulcerations resulted.

At first at a loss to explain the changes, Magendie finally concluded that they must be of trophic origin. He also believed that his experiments justified the claim that the corneal changes developed more rapidly and more intensely when the section was made through the ganglion or in front of it than when the posterior root was divided.

Magendie's illustrious pupil Claude Bernard was also greatly interested in this experiment and accepted Magendie's trophic explanation. To show that contact with the air and the resulting dryness was not responsible for the ulceration, Bernard[34] (1858) cut the facial nerve in rabbits and obtained entirely negative results.

Numerous experiments have since brought forth greatly differing conclusions concerning the etiology of this condition. In support of the trophic theory of Magendie were the experiments of von Graefe[35] (1854), who excised the lids and lacrimal glands without inducing keratitis. Von Graefe, however, was still cautious in explaining the experiments on a neuropathic basis for which there were so few known facts. Virchow[36] (1855), too, though impressed with von Graefe's experiments, still retained an open mind concerning the cause of the corneal disturbance.

Schiff[37] (1855) looked on the vascular dilatation of the conjunctiva and sclera as vasomotor changes and thought the keratitis to be of similar origin. Snellen[38] (1857) sutured the eyelids together before dividing the trigeminus and prevented keratitis; when the lids were opened ten days later ulceration followed. He naturally concluded that keratitis is of purely traumatic origin. After incomplete section of the trigeminal root, Samuel[39] (1860), Buttner (1862) and Meissner[40] (1867) did not find ulceration of the cornea, even when it was insensitive, and at times ulceration developed when the cornea remained sensitive. From these discordant results, the observers independently concluded that intact fibers were "trophic" and maintained the nutrition of the eye. They even tried to define the exact part of the sensory root carrying trophic fibers. Samuel (1860) was able to produce keratitis in dogs merely by stimulating the gasserian ganglion with an electric current. He considered this evidence entirely opposed to any mechanical theory.

From microscopic studies, Senftleben[41] (1875) concluded that the changes in the cornea were "necrotic" and of traumatic origin. Von Hippel[42] (1889) and Hanau[43] (1896) concluded from experiments on closure of the lids that the keratitis is due to drying. Gaule[44] (1892) found "trophic" pitting of the cornea within a few hours after section of the gasserian ganglion, and in spite of closure of the lids. Hanau kept a dog's eyelids closed for a year after section of the trigeminus. During this time the condition of the eye was perfect, but on the day after the lids were opened ulceration appeared. He said that Gaule's corneal pits could be seen after the cornea was dried from local applications of cocaine. Turner[45] (1895) found keratitis in only two of eighteen canine experiments in which the sensory root was cut. He did not find evidence to support trophic changes.

Facing nearly every theory are facts which are seemingly but not actually contradictory. It has been noted by several writers that nearly all ulcerations appear within a few days after the operation. If the cornea is clear on discharge from the hospital ten days or two weeks after the operation, the great danger is past. This does not mean that later ulcerations do not develop. Any insensitive cornea, not having a warning sign, is always susceptible to injury from a foreign body, but there is no evidence that an equal stimulus over an equal time would not produce the same degree of ulceration in the normal eye. It is to prevent the later ulcerations from trauma that the retention of corneal sensation by a partial radiculotomy is important. For the prevention of the immediate postoperative ulcerations with which surgeons have been principally concerned, there is probably little, if any, advantage.

The first successful operations on the gasserian ganglion by Rose[7] (1892) were followed by ulcerations in three of his five cases. In one case the eye was lost and in two others the eyes "were very, very bad for a time." . . . "The effect upon the nutrition of the eye is decidedly serious." And in his cases sensation in the ophthalmic branch remained intact. Horsley[13] thought that corneal ulceration was due to irritation by chloroform and as a preventive closed the lids by suture before the operation. That his reasoning was incorrect is shown by two experimental facts: (1) earlier experiments on animals were conducted without anesthesia, and (2) the normal eye was never affected.

Horsley found four cases of keratitis (one eye was lost) in his first twenty-five cases. Cushing[46] reported three corneal ulcerations in his first twenty-one cases, and in one case the eye was lost even though sensation of the ophthalmic branch was retained.

One gains the impression that keratitis is becoming less frequent and less severe since the sensory root is divided than when the ganglion was removed. Frazier, Beule,[47] Bagozzi[48] and Bastianelli[49] have reported improved results with this method. However, despite the improvements in subtotal resections of the root, Frazier reported two cases of keratitis in his first twenty-five operations of this type. With Frazier's subtotal radiculotomy, Grant [50] (1920) gave the percentage of cases of keratitis as about 10.

That corneal ulcerations can be prevented by closure of the lids is indubitable. Moreover, severe ulcerations will heal when the lids are closed. This method, learned from experiments on animals, was early adopted by Krause, Horsley, Keen and others. The fact that keratitis will not develop when the eyelids are closed has been one of the strongest arguments in favor of a pure mechanical theory. Proponents of this theory argue that there must be traumatic insults to the unprotected eye even though they cannot be observed. Opponents of the mechanical theory ask why the onset of keratitis is unusual except immediately after the operation—a fact early demonstrated by Rose and Krause, [51] Keen, [52] Cushing [53] and others hoped to obtain the same protection by using Buller's shield, sealed to the face and nose by adhesive tape. They also looked on the retention of moisture as an important feature of the glass shield.

Krause and others had found loss of lacrimation after section of the ophthalmic branch of the eye; Cushing verified his observation. Corneal dryness has since been considered one of the important factors in the causation of keratitis. There is no doubt that the cornea has a telltale, dull, dry and lusterless appearance just before keratitis develops; but, although the eye may be kept moist by the closed chamber with the Buller shield, this has little, if any, value in preventing the onset of keratitis, and there is reason to question whether under its protection ulcers once formed do not develop with greater rapidity owing to the formation of more ideal conditions for bacterial growth. The nerve supply to the lacrimal glands has long been studied without as yet conclusive results.

The lacrimal branch of the ophthalmic division of the trigeminus undoubtedly supplies the lacrimal gland, and Krause, Cushing and others have commented on the absence of lacrimal secretion after gasserian operations. The lacrimal gland is also believed to be supplied by the great superficial petrosal branch of the facial nerve. But repeated extirpations of the lacrimal glands have failed to induce corneal ulceration. Even extirpation of the lacrimal glands plus the removal of the eyelids (von Graefe) have failed to produce it.

If the gasserian ganglion or the sensory root is attacked along the temporal fossa, both the great and the small superficial petrosal nerves are almost necessarily sacrificed when the dura is stripped from the base of the skull. Dixon [54] (1897) early called attention to this fact. It would therefore appear probable that the entire supply of these two nerves would be lost to the lacrimal gland by this operation. By the cerebellar approach the petrosal nerves are not disturbed, and it has been frequently observed that lacrimation is unaffected after this operation in contrast to the observations of Krause and Cushing after the temporal approach. It is not improbable that the loss of the petrosal nerves instead of the division of the fifth nerve explains the difference in the diametrically opposite results. On the other hand, I recently saw a patient from whom a cerebellopontile tumor had been removed one year before. The facial nerve was sacrificed, as is always necessary when the tumor is completely removed. There is no disturbance of function of the fifth nerve, but she has never had tears from this eye since the operation. This observation needs checking with more cases before the conculsion is drawn that the seventh nerve (through the petrosal branch) alone is responsible for lacrimation; but at least the importance of the nerve is indicated. The more anterior temporal approach of Cushing [55] and Lexer [56] may at times spare the petrosal nerves, but this is doubtful for this part of the temporal fossa is difficult to avoid when the ganglion is exposed.

That the absence of lacrimation alone should be responsible for the keratitis does not appear probable: first, because the incidence of keratitis should be much higher, perhaps nearly constant, if the petrosal nerves are always sacrificed, as seems probable, and second, because removal of the lacrimal gland alone does not produce keratitis. It will be recalled that in the experiments of Magendie and Claude Bernard, in which keratitis almost always followed section of the fifth nerve (in rabbits), the approach to the nerve was intradural; injury to the petrosal nerves was therefore precluded.

That keratitis does not develop when the eyelids are sutured together does not mean that extraneous or nonphysiologic trauma to the eye is responsible for the keratitis. It doubtless does mean that the trauma of the movements of the lids causes the ulceration, but this is equivalent to a confession that there is an underlying pathologic condition in the cornea rendering it liable to injury by stimuli which are physiologic and are acceptable to the normal eye.

After every operation on the gasserian ganglion or the sensory root, the eye is carefully protected so that all external trauma can be absolutely excluded. But with this protection, the cases of keratitis continue. It may be argued that this protection reduces the number, but even this is highly questionable. There must, therefore, be some other reason why the cornea is frequently affected in the anesthetic eye and never in the normal eye.

The question of trophic function to any nerve is still being debated without an acceptable conclusion. To anyone who has sectioned the gasserian ganglion or the sensory root, the frequent herpes located in the mucous membrane of the upper and lower lips on the side operated on and always developing from twenty-four to seventy-two hours after operation, must in-

dicate an etiologic relationship to the simple traumatic division of the nerve. Similarly, in herpes zoster the cutaneous changes conforming to the peripheral distribution of the nerve, although the primary lesion is in the ganglion or sensory root of the nerve, must be evidence of a function of the nerve other than that of simply transmitting sensory or motor stimuli. At a recent meeting of the Missouri-Kansas Neuropsychiatric Society, Dr. A. L. Skoog [57] demonstrated a remarkable case of lancinating pains associated with cerebrospinal syphilis. Following every attack of pain there appeared, two or three days later, an extensive herpetic eruption in the peripheral distribution of the nerves which were causing the pain.

The end product (herpes) of these inflammatory attacks both in its character and in its distribution seems precisely similar to the post-operative herpes following central operations on the trigeminal nerve. Is not, therefore, the herpes of traumatic origin and an indication or a traumatically disturbed trophic function? During the period when the gasserian ganglion was being removed or the sensory root divided by the temporal route, the occurrence of keratitis seemed to defy all explorations until the conclusion was forced on me that the cases in which the ganglionic dissection was most difficult and prolonged (usually due to hemorrhage) seemed more susceptible to keratitis. This empiric conclusion appeared not to offer any explanation unless trauma to nerves could affect the tissues in the eye in some manner possibly analogous to the production of herpes in the lip, i.e., a traumatic herpes. More and more the conviction has developed that the disturbances of the eyes after trigeminal operations are due to trauma to the ganglion or the sensory root.

WHY SHOULD NOT KERATITIS DEVELOP AFTER SECTION OF THE SENSORY ROOT AT THE PONS (CEREBELLAR APPROACH)?

That postoperative keratitis can be almost, if not entirely, eliminated by the cerebellar approach here reported is, I think, assured. In explanation, the only important difference (other than the preservation of the petrosal nerve already referred to) appears to be the avoidance of trauma to the ganglion or sensory root. When the temporal approach is used, the ganglion is traumatized before and after the dura is opened; by the cerebellar route, it is only necessary to encircle and divide the nerve. Certain clinical evidence seems to support this explanation. Perhaps the most severe and relatively the greatest number of corneal changes followed the first operations on the gasserian ganglion by Rose. Through an inadequate opening in the floor of the skull, he attempted with only partial success to gouge and scrape away the ganglion. The disastrous corneal changes also occurred despite the fact that sensation of the cornea was always retained. Trauma and not loss of sensation was seemingly responsible for the keratitis.

That keratitis may now be less severe and occur less frequently than formerly would appear to be explained by the technical improvements in operations and the greater skill of the surgeons.

CAN KERATITIS FOLLOW INJURY TO THE SENSORY ROOT?

Whether keratitis can follow injury to the sensory root has been answered in the affirmative in animals, at least, by Magendie's original experiments, but, as already mentioned, he thought that keratitis more readily followed section of the ganglion than of the sensory root. Bernard's experiments also confirmed Magendie's results.

From another line of the operative material, it is possible to transport results which offer an answer for man. When cerebellopontile tumors are completely extirpated—including the capsule—there was such a high percentage of corneal disturbances that now as a routine the eyelids are closed at the end of the operation. In this operation the facial nerve is always destroyed, but the trigeminal nerve is always preserved, though frequently there is an appreciable diminution of sensation. Again it is thought that the trauma to the sensory root instead of the gasserian ganglion. The facial paralysis undoubtedly predisposes to the development of the corneal change, but as experiments on animals and ample clinical material have shown, facial paralysis alone will not cause keratitis.

It should be noted that herpes of the lips follows the procedure perhaps just as frequently as when the temporal approach is used. Owing to the great frequency of keratitis following the trauma incident to removel of cerebellopontile tumors and to the frequency of herpes after section of the nerve at the pons, it is safe to say that injury to the sensory root produces keratitis just as readily. But in this operation of sectioning the sensory root, far less trauma is inflicted than by the temporal route. If it were necessary to use the same amount of trauma, the results would probably not be any better.

In application of this hypothesis is a recent case in which a cerebellopontile tumor was removed. Dissection of the trigeminal nerve from its attachment to the tumor would have necessitated more than the usual amount of trauma. To avoid this, the nerve was promptly sectioned below the tumor. Despite the coexisting facial paralysis, not the slightest redness of the cornea appeared after the operation.

WHY DOES FACIAL PARALYSIS FOLLOW THE TEMPORAL APPROACH?

Since a temporary facial paralysis resulted in one of the early cases in which the cerebellar route was employed, a complete immunity to this complication cannot be claimed by the new operation. When the temporal approach is used, the frequency of facial paralysis has been reported by Adson [58] to be about 7 per cent. It is always a discouraging sequel because its avoidance has seemed purely a matter of chance. Three explanations have been offered: (1) the nerve is injured by traction at a point in the face; (2) the nerve is injured at the brain stem when the sensory nerve is avulsed, and (3) the geniculate ganglion is injured by traction on the superficial petrosal nerves when the dura is stripped from the base of the skull. That the facial nerve could be injured in the face is incredible because of the high position of the operative incision. That it is not injured there is easily shown by the test for taste proposed by Dean Lewis in one of my cases. If the injury is peripheral, taste will be unaffected; if it is central, taste will be lost. In one of my patients (operated on by the temporal route), the taste was entirely lost. That the facial nerve cannot be injured at the pons by avulsion of the sensory root is evident when the distance between these nerves is appreciated.

Dixon [54] first called attention to the possibility of injuring the facial nerve at the geniculate ganglion by traction on the petrosal nerve. In opposing the conclusions of Krause [51] that taste was carried from the anterior two thirds of the tongue by the fifth nerve, Dixon reasoned that the facial nerve had probably been traumatized in this way and that the facial injury accounted for the loss of taste. More recently, Alfred S. Taylor [59] of New York and later Kanaval and Davis [60] have expressed views similar to those of Dixon. Taylor advised division of the petrosal nerves to prevent traction on the geniculate ganglion.

In one of my patients operated on by the temporal route, a relatively large anomalous, obstructing band was cut with a scalpel when the progress of stripping the dura from the roof of the petrous temporal bone had been temporarily halted. The nervous character of the structure was recognized as soon as it was cut. In this unusual position the nerve could not be other than the geniculate ganglion, and the prediction was made that the patient would wake up with a facial paralysis. The paralysis was complete at first; a year later, perhaps 75 per cent of the motor function had returned but there remained a tic-like facial movement in addition. During this operation it was also found that the roof of the petrous temporal bone was defective at the point where the geniculate ganglion was cut. Later, a number of skulls were examined, and in two a similar defect was present in the same spot in the root of the petrous temporal bone; in both cases the defect was bilateral. Undoubtedly, therefore, the geniculate ganglion projects through this occasional hiatus in the bone and attaches itself to the overlying dura, from which it can be separated only with varying degrees of injury. Spee [61] (1896) mentioned the fact that such defects occasionally are present in adult skulls and always in children. This he called the "hiatus spurius canalis facialis."

In most instances, the facial paralysis resulting from these injuries is of a mild grade. It is probable that in these cases the geniculate ganglion is injured when the petrosal nerves are torn out of the ganglion during the dissection of the dura. The weakness may indeed not be apparent until twenty-four hours or more after the operation, doubtless owing to the slow onset of the effects of edema. Doubtless if the dura in this region were separated from the bone by sharp dissection and the petrosal nerves cut (Taylor's suggestion) instead of torn, the facial nerve would escape injury, unless the ganglion itself actually protruded.

OPERATION FOR BILATERAL TRIGEMINAL NEURALGIA

Fortunately, bilateral tic douloureux is rare. Krause early called attention to it. Because of a possible later development

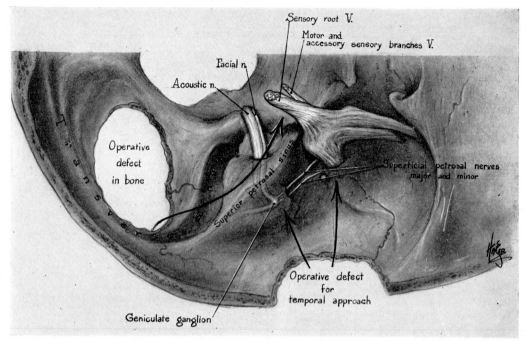

Fig. 3. When the temporal route is used, facial weakness and paralysis not infrequently follow. Injury to the facial nerve results from trauma to the geniculate ganglion. When the dura, to which the superficial petrosal nerves are frequently attached, is elevated to expose the gasserian ganglion, the petrosal nerves are torn. At times they are pulled out of the geniculate ganglion. Occasionally, the geniculate ganglion protrudes through a congenital defect in the roof of the petrous temporal bone and is attached to the dura. Direct injury to the geniculate ganglion then causes a more profound facial paralysis.

of tic on the opposite side, Tiffany [19] first suggested that an effort be made to spare the motor branch at the operation. He thought it possible to do so. I have seen but three cases of bilateral tic douloureux. One case came under observation a number of years ago when it was not thought justifiable to suggest any operative relief because the motor branch of the trigeminus had been lost in an earlier ganglionectomy when the pain had been unilateral. The other two patients came for treatment with both sides affected. On each side the characteristic agonizing ticlike paroxysms were being discharged independently, but with greater frequency on the one side than the other. At times there would be a short free interval on one side or the other and occasionally on both, but usually both sides were in pain. Both had been badly mutilated by peripheral operations, but the masseter and temporal muscles still retained function.

Since the motor branch of the trigeminus can be preserved with certainty by the cerebellar approach, it was possible to suggest section of both sensory roots at the same operation. The patients were prepared as for a routine bilateral cerebellar approach. The bony defects toward the mastoid were made on both sides and after the fluid in the cisterna magna was evacuated, each cerebellar hemisphere was lifted in turn and each sensory root divided. The postoperative course of both patients was uneventful. Anesthesia was total over the domain of both trigeminal areas in one case and partially preserved on both sides in the other. In one case taste was impaired at first but returned to normal during the ten days the patient was in the hospital. In the other case, taste was unaffected. The muscles of mastication were not disturbed; there was no difficulty in swallowing.

Frazier[62] recently reported a case of bilateral trigeminal neuralgia in which operation was successful, first on one side and several years later on the other. But the patient had a close call from difficulty in swallowing after the operation. The motor branch of one nerve had been sacrificed at the earlier operation, thus placing a heavy burden of responsibility on the preservation of the remaining motor branch. Fortunately the dysphagia was only transient, the motor branch doubtless being merely traumatized.

In a consideration of the treatment for bilateral tic douloureux, the results of Harris[63] following injections of the gasserian ganglion with alcohol should be mentioned. He reported two cases of bilateral tic douloureux in which an apparent cure was effected by injections. He found it possible to inject the ganglion with alcohol and still avoid injury to the motor root which lies in apposition. His results appear to have justified his confidence.

NEED OF THIS APPROACH TO RELIEVE PAIN WHEN THE GASSERIAN GANGLION IS INVADED BY CARCINOMA

In one of the cases reported, the gasserian ganglion was invaded by carcinoma which had entered from the nasopharynx. This patient was suffering from the characteristic paroxysmal pain superimposed on a steady burning pain in the two lower branches of the trigeminus. The presence of a tumor seemed probable because of a partial loss of sensation over the domain of the second and third branches. This patient came for treatment when only two or three operations had been done by the cerebellar route and at a time when the favorable points of the operation were not yet in evidence. Exposure of the branches of the gasserian ganglion, the ganglion itself, or the sensory root, though attempted by the temporal route, was impossible because of the extensive growth of the tumor

between the dura and the floor of the middle fossa. Since the patient was unable to take morphine, the new cerebellar approach seemed the only solution. As the tumor had not invaded the posterior cranial fossa, division of the posterior root by the cerebellar route did not offer any difficulties.

TRIGEMINAL NEURALGIA CAUSED BY CEREBELLOPONTILE TUMORS

Another important reason for using the cerebellar approach for tic douloureux or trigeminal neuralgia is that occasionally a cerebellopontile tumor may be the underlying cause of the pain. By this approach the tumor can then be discovered and removed. In one patient in the series reported, a typical cerebellopontile (acoustic) tumor was accidentally disclosed in this way.

A man, aged sixty-five, complained of and was observed in typical severe paroxysms of pain along the second and third branches of the fifth nerve. He was totally deaf in the corresponding ear, but the deafness was not considered significant for it had been present for several years and other symptoms had not been present. There was no sensory change, subjective or objective, in the distribution of the trigeminus; the corneal reflex was unchanged. The masseter, temporal and pterygoid muscles functioned equally on the two sides. Other cranial nerves were unaffected. The usual unilateral approach was made. There had been no evidence of pressure; the cisterna magna was large and when evacuated there was ample room to explore the cerebellopontile angle. A typical cerebellopontile tumor—about as large as a pigeon's egg—filled the angle normally occupied by the cistern lateralis. The tumor was much the smallest (6 Gm.) of a large series of cerebellopontile tumors. It shelled out with ease and without the need of a bilateral bony defect which is usually so urgently needed. The sensory root of the fifth nerve curved around the anterior pole of the tumor. As it was feared that the tic might not cease, the sensory root was then divided. The patient made an uneventful recovery.

While it is uncommon to find tumors of

this kind causing trigeminal neuralgia, they do occur occasionally and will be missed by the lateral approach. Tumors of this type are among the most favorable tumors of the brain, and when so discovered by accident at an early stage of their growth their removal becomes easier and the subsequent results should be better.

In addition to this tumor, two aneurysms of the basilar artery were unexpectedly disclosed. There is no evidence that the aneurysms had any etiologic bearing on the neuralgia. The fifth nerve was slightly higher than the aneurysm in each instance.

Weisenburg [64] (1910) reported a case which in a negative way emphasizes the advantage of the cerebellar route. Unimproved by section of the sensory root by the Hartley-Krause lateral approach, his patient came to necropsy six years later. A cerebellopontile tumor was found. It was the condition post mortem in this case which led Weisenburg to the discovery of the closely allied tic douloureux of glossopharyngeal neuraliga.

OPERATIVE TREATMENT VERSUS INJECTIONS OF ALCOHOL FOR TIC DOULOUREUX

Patients affected with the trigeminal tic douloureux are not infrequently advised to accept injections of alcohol either into the peripheral branches or into the gasserian ganglion as superior treatment instead of operative section of the sensory root. One's view on this subject must be guided by the relative merits and liabilities of each procedure. When operations carry an appreciable mortality, injections of alcohol have every right to paramount consideration. When the operative mortality reaches 12 or 15 per cent, as reported in some clinics, operative treatment should not be considered. But when the mortality is reduced to a fraction of 1 per cent, which obtains with many operators at the present time, any method of surgical treatment demands consideration because it offers a permanent cure. Injections of alcohol never cure. They relieve pain over a

period varying from two or three months to two years, the latter period of relief being exceptional. Patients, therefore, must look forward to injections during the remainder of life. As these injections are always painful, by no means uniformly successful and not infrequently unsuccessful, patients often endure the return of pain for weeks or months before being willing to undergo again the next extremely painful and dreaded ordeal. Succeeding injections tend to become less effective and more difficult, and usually in the late years of life patients finally seek permanent relief by operation.

But much has been said in favor of injections of alcohol, and surgeons have indeed been the first to weigh the liabilities of operative treatment and to suggest injections of alcohol in their stead. Even Frazier, who has reduced the operative liabilities to a minimum, frequently advises insection of the sensory root. It is the dangers of corneal ulcertion and occasional facial paralysis which still confront even subtotal section of the sensory root. I feel strongly that with these difficulties eliminated and with the preservation of sensation to the face—not infrequently almost normal— that operative permanent relief of pain by the cerebellar route is always indicated, provided, of course, the patient's general condition is satisfactory and if the expectation of life may be several years.

I have not given any consideration to injections of alcohol into the gasserian ganglion because I consider it an indefensible procedure. Easy to perform and theoretically superior in that it offers destruction of the ganglion cells and permanence of relief, it nevertheless leaves a most terrible train of signs and symptoms in its wake. A few years ago the arguments in its favor sounded so plausible that it seemed an easy solution of this dreadful malady. But in two of four injections the patients went through a terrible ordeal—paralysis of all the homolateral cranial nerves in the posterior cranial fossa and, in addition, dizziness, nystagmus, ataxia, vomiting and staggering gait. Others have had exactly similar experiences. In fact it seems impossible that anyone who uses this method can escape these sequelae. The explanation can be readily understood by injecting 1 cc. of colored solution into the gasserian ganglion of a cadaver. Quickly the color passes around the brain stem and cerebellum. The inner two thirds of the gasserian ganglion is surrounded by cerebrospinal fluid. An extension of the subarachnoid space usually reaches the outer third of the ganglion, and within the subarachnoid space the ganglion is without a sheath. An injection of alcohol into the ganglion therefore readily passes through the nerve into the cerebrospinal fluid, or it may be injected directly into the cerebrospinal fluid. The alcohol then almost instantly attacks the brain stem and the attached cranial nerves.

Many who speak freely of injection of the gasserian ganglion are really performing only a peripheral injection. It is not unusual for alcohol so injected gradually to spread up the third branch and deaden sensation (though to a lesser degree) in the second branch and even at times in the first branch. In introducing this criticism of injections of the ganglion, I am not unmindful of the superior reports of Harris by this method. His caution in using only a few drops of alcohol seems to indicate his fear of these dreadful experiences.

SUMMARY AND CONCLUSIONS

1. A new operative attack on the sensory root of the trigeminus is presented for the cure of trigeminal tic douloureux. The sensory root is reached at the pons through a bloodless path beneath the cerebellum.

2. The sensory root can be divided either partially or totally. At first, total division of the sensory root was performed. Gradually it was found that by partial section of the root the pain is cured and, at

the same time, the sensation to the entire domain of the fifth nerve is little disturbed.

3. Partial section of the sensory root at the pons is now advocated exclusively.

4. The advantages of partial section of the sensory root by the route here proposed are:

(a) Immediate postoperative corneal disturbances are uniformly absent.

(b) The motor root is always preserved.

(c) Sensation, approaching the normal, is retained over the entire domain of the trigeminus, irrespective of the branch involved in the pain.

(d) The corneal reflex is usually preserved.

(e) The approach is bloodless after the dura has been exposed.

(f) The operation is much easier and quicker to perform.

5. The operation is, in effect, essentially that of a cordotomy, in that only pain fibers are sacrificed and all forms of sensation are retained.

6. Observations herein described deny the hypothesis that the periperal branches of the trigeminus are accurately represented by subdivisions of the sensory root.

7. Some postoperative sensory observations suggest that there are separate nerve fibers for various types of sensation.

8. Pain fibers appear to travel separately and to be located exclusively in the posterior part of the sensory root (in cross-section).

9. Even when the sensory root is totally divided, varying degrees of sensation are retained in the face. At times, this sensation approaches the normal. This is due to the fact that accessory sensory branches usually accompany the motor root and later join the sensory root. When the accessory branches are absent, anesthesia of the face is complete.

10. The accessory branches of the sensory root apparently never contain pain fibers, nor are pain fibers brought to them by anastamoses with the fibers of the sensory root.

11. The motor root is always preserved because it is at a safe distance from the sensory root.

12. Bilateral tic douloureux can be cured at a single operation by this method because the motor roots are not injured. Two patients have been cured by the bilateral operation.

13. Certain facts seem to indicate that postoperative keratitis is due to trauma of the gasserian ganglion or of the sensory root—traumatic neuritis.

14. Deep sensation to the face is carried through the trigeminal nerve and not the facial.

15. Vasomotor changes do not develop when the fifth nerve is divided.

16. Lacrimation continues after division of the fifth nerve.

17. Facial paralysis results in the temporal approach because the geniculate ganglion is injured, either directly or by tearing the superficial petrosal nerves. These nerves are not injured by the cerebellar approach.

18. Occasionally, tumors in the cerebellopontile angle cause tic douloureux. By this approach, they will be disclosed. The chances of a successful removal are enhanced because the tumor is found earlier. By the temporal route, these tumors would be missed. In the series described, one (unsuspected) tumor was found and successfully removed. Two aneurysms of the basilar artery—presumably not having any bearing on the neuralgia—were found at operation.

19. When malignant tumors invade the gasserian ganglion, relief cannot be obtained by dividing the sensory root by the temporal route. The cerebellar route is indispensable in such cases.

REFERENCES

[1]Hartley, F.: Intracranial Neurectomy of the Second and Third Divisions of the Fifth Nerve. *New York M. J., 55:* 317, 1892.

[2]Krause, F.: Resection des Trigeminus innerhalf der Schadelhohle. *Arch. klin. Chir., 44:* 821, 1892.

[3]Krause, F.: *Neuralgie des Trigeminus.* Leipzig, F. C. W. Vogel, 1896, p. 103.

[4]Magendie, F.: *Textbook of Physiologie.* 1822, English trans. by Revere.

[5]Bell, Sir Charles: *The Nervous System,* Ed. 3. London, 1844.

[6]Mears, J. E.: Study of the Pathological Changes Occurring in Trifacial Neuralgia. *Am. Surg. A., 2:* 469, 1884.

[7]Rose, W.: Surgical Treatment of Trigeminal Neuralgia. *Lancet, 1:* 295, 1892.

[8]Ferrier, D.: On Paralysis of the Fifth Cranial Nerve. *Lancet, 1:* 1, 1888.

[9]Sutton, J. B.: *Neurotomy of the Third Division of the Fifth Nerve.* M. Chir. Tr., 71: 107, 1888.

[10]Andrews: Paper read before the Section of Surgery and Anatomy, at the American Surgical Association, 1891, p. 153.

[11]Because of this almost simultaneous appearance of the papers of Hartley and Krause, Victor Horsley suggested that both be given equal credit. Though the procedure was frequently known as the Hartley-Krause operation, the divided honor was quite naturally not acceptable to either. (Krause: A Question of Priority in Devising a Method for the Performance of Intracranial Neurectomy in the Fifth Nerve. *Ann. Surg., 18:* 363, 1893. Hartley: Intracranial Neurectomy of the Fifth Nerve, *Ann. Surg., 17:* 571, 1893).

[12]Krause, F.: Entfernung des ganglion gasseri und des Central davon gelegenen Trigeminusstammes. *Deutsche med. Wchnschr., 19:* 341, 1893.

[13]Horsley, Victor: Remarks on the Various Surgical Procedures Devised for the Relief or Cure of Trigeminal Neuralgia. *Brit. M. J., 2:* 1139, 1191 and 1249 (Nov. 28, Dec. 5 and Dec. 12) 1891.

[14]Keen, W. W., and Spiller, W. G.: Remarks on Resection of the Gasserian Ganglion. *Am. J. M. Sc., 116:* 503, 1898.

[15]Spiller, W. G., and Frazier, C. H.: The Division of the Sensory Root of the Trigeminus for the Relief of Tic Douloureux. *Univ. Pennsylvania M. Bull., 14:* 341, 1901.

[16]Spiller, W. G., and Frazier, C. H.: An Experimental Study of the Regeneration of Posterior Spinal Root: Contributions from the William Pepper Laboratory of Clinical Medicine. *Univ. Pennsylvania M. Bull.,* 1903, p. 4.

[17]Horsley, V.: An Address on the Surgical Treatment of Trigeminal Neuralgia. *Practitioner, 65:* 251, 1900.

[18]Tiffany: Intracranial Neurectomy and Removal of the Gasserian Ganglion. *Ann. Surg., 19:* 47 (Feb.) 1894.

[19]Tiffany: Intracranial Operations for the Cure of Facial Neuralgia. *Ann. Surg., 24:* 575, 1896.

[20]Frazier, C. H.: Subtotal Resection of Sensory Root for Relief of Major Trigeminal Neuralgia. *Arch. Neurol. & Psychiat., 13:* 378 (March) 1925.

[21]Frazier, C. H., and Whitehead, E.: The Morphology of the Gasserian Ganglion. *Brain, 48:* 458,

1925.

²²Gutnikoff, B.: Treatment of Trigeminal Neuralgia. *Arch. f. klin. Chir., 135:* 79 (April) 1925.

²³Hartel, F.: Surgery of Trifacial Neuralgia. *Munchen. med. Wchnschr., 71:* 1089, 1924.

²⁴Dandy, W. E.: Section of the Sensory Root of the Trigeminal Nerve at the Pons: Preliminary Report of the Operative Procedure. *Bull. Johns Hopkins Hosp., 36:* 105 (Feb.) 1925.

²⁵Von Dollinger, Julius: Die Behandlung der Trigeminusneuralgien mit den Schloesserschen Alkoholeinspritzungen. *Deutsche med. Wchnschr., 38:* 297 (Feb. 15) 1912.

²⁶Clairmont, P.: Zur Behandlung der Gesichtsneuralgia; die Durchtrennung des Nervus trigeminus in der hinteren Schadelgrube. *Deutsche med. Wchnschr., 15:* 609, 1926.

²⁷Taste in the anterior two thirds of the tongue has also been carefully tested in a number of these cases. The results have been included in a paper with Dr. Dean Lewis, and will shortly appear in the *Archives of Surgery.* Taste is not carried by the sensory root or peripheral branches of the tigeminus. It is carried by the facial nerve.

²⁸May, O., and Horsley, V.: The Mesencephalic Root of the Fifth Nerve. *Brain, 33:* 175, 1910.

²⁹Bregmann in Obersteiner's *Arbeiter, 1:* 82, 1892.

³⁰VanLoudon: Untersuchungen betreffend den zentralen Verlauf des Nervus trigeminus nach intracranialer Durchschneidung seines Stammes, Petrus Camper. *Nederl. bijdr. t. anat., 4:* 285, 1907.

³¹Van Gehuchten: De l'origine du pathetique et de la racine superieure du trijumeau. *Bull. Acad. roy. Belgique, 29:* 417, 1895.

³²Davis, I. E.: The Deep Sensibility of the Face. *Arch. Neurol. & Psychiat., 9:* 283 (March) 1923.

³³Maloney, W. J., and Kennedy, F.: The Sense of Pressure in the Face, Eye, Tongue. *Brain, 34:* 1, 1911.

³⁴Bernard, C.: *Lecons due systeme nerveux.* Paris, 1858, vol. 1, p. 192.

³⁵Von Graefe, H.: Neuroparalytische Hornhautaffection. *Arch. f. Ophth., 1:* 306, 1854.

³⁶Virchow, R.: *Virchows Arch. path. Anat., 8:* 33, 1855.

³⁷Schiff, M.: Untersuchungen zur Physiologie des Nervensystem. 1855, vol. 1, p. 91.

³⁸Snellen, in von Hippel: *Arch. Ophth., 35:* 217, 1889.

³⁹Samuel, S., in von Hippel: *Arch. Ophth., 35:* 217, 1889.

⁴⁰Meissner, G.: Ueber die nach der Durchschneidung des Trigeminus am Auge des Kaninchens eintretende Ernahsungsstorung. *Ztschr. f. rationelle Med., 29:* 96, 1867.

⁴¹Senftleben: Ueber die Ursachen und das Wesen der nach Durchschneidung des Trigeminus auftretenden Hirnhautaffection. *Virchows Arch. path. Anat., 65:* 69, 1875.

⁴²Von Hippel, E.: Zur Aetiologie der Keratitis neuroparalytica. *Arch. Ophth., 35:* 217, 1889; Diss. Gottingen, 1889.

⁴³Hanau, H.: Experimentalkritische Untersuchungen uber die Ursache der nach Trigeminusdurchschneidung entstehenden Horn hautveranderungen. *Ztschr. Biol., 16:* 146, 1896.

⁴⁴Gaule, J.: Die Veranderungen der Hornhaut nach Durchschneidung des Nervus trigeminus. *Cor.-Bl. f. schweiz. Aerzte, 22:* 350, 1892.

⁴⁵Turner, W. A.: The Results of Section of the Trigeminal Nerve with Reference to the So-Called "Trophic" Influence of the Nerve on the Cornea. *Brit. M. J., 2:* 1279, 1895.

⁴⁶Cushing, H.: The Surgical Aspects of Major Neuralgia of the Trigeminal Nerve. *J.A.M.A., 44:* 773 (March 11) 1905 cont., 860 (March 18) and 1002 (April 1) 1905.

⁴⁷Beule: Resection of the Gasserian Ganglion, Foreign Letter (Belgium). *J.A.M.A., 82:* 721 (March 1) 1924.

⁴⁸Bagozzi: Un caso di neurotomia retro-gasserina (Ein Fall von Wurzeldurchsechneidung des Gasserchen Ganglions). *Thirty-first congr. di chir., Milano 26:* 29, 1924; *Riforma med., 40:* 1111, 1924.

⁴⁹Bastianelli: *Thirty-first congr. di. chir., Milano,* 1924, p. 26; *Riforma med. 40:* 1111, 1924.

⁵⁰Grant, F. C.: Trigeminal Neuralgia, *M. J. & Rec., 121:* 206, 1925.

⁵¹Krause, F.: Die Physiologie des Trigeminus nach Untersuchungen an Menschen bei denen das ganglion gasseri entfernt worde ist. *Munchen. med. Wchnschr., 42:* 577, 1895.

⁵²Keen, W. W., and Mitchell, J. K.: Removal of the Gassarian Ganglion as the Last of Fourteen Operations in Thirteen Years for Tic Douloureux. *Proc. Philadelphia County M. Soc.,* 1894.

⁵³Cushing, H.: The Major Trigeminal Neuralgias and Their Surgical Treatment Based on Experiences with 332 Gasserian Operations. *Am. J. M. Sc., 160:* 157, 1920.

⁵⁴Dixon, S. F.: On the Course of the Taste Fibers. *Edinburgh M. J., 1:* 395, 1897.

⁵⁵Cushing, H.: A Method of Total Extirpation of the Gasserian Ganglion for Trigeminal Neuralgia *J.A.M.A., 34:* 1035 (April 28) 1900.

⁵⁶Lexer, E.: Zur Operation des Ganglion gasseri nach Erfahrungen an 15 Fallen. *Arch. f. klin. Chir., 65:* 843, 1902.

⁵⁷Skoog, A. L.: Case Presented at Missouri-Kansas Neuropsychiatric Society, Kansas City, Oct. 19, 1927. *J. Nerv. & Ment. Dis., 67:* 275, 1928.

⁵⁸Adson, A. W.: Preservation of the Motor Root of the Gasserian Ganglion During the Division of the Sensory Root for Trifacial Neuralgia. *Surg., Gynec. & Obst., 35:* 352, 1922.

[59]Taylor, Alfred S.: Personal communication to the author, 1926.

[60]Kanaval, A. B., and Davis, L. E.: Surgical Anatomy of the Trigeminal Nerve. *Surg., Gynec. & Obst., 34:* 357 (March) 1922.

[61]Spee: Skeletlehre; in Kopf: *Handbuch der Anatomie des Menschen* 1896, vol. 1, p. 215.

[62]Frazier, C. H.: Division of Sensory Root on Both Sides. First Experience in a Series of 432 Radi-

cal Operations for Major Trigeminal Neuralgia. *J.A.M.A., 87:* 1730 (Nov. 20) 1926.

[63]Harris, W.: *Neuritis and Neuralgia*. New York, Oxford University Press, 1926, p. 418.

[64]Weisenburg, T. H.: Cerebello-Pontine Tumor Diagnosed for Six Years as Tic Douloureux: The Symptoms of Irritation of the Ninth and Twelfth Cranial Nerves. *J.A.M.A., 54:* 1600 (May 14) 1910.

XXXIII

WHERE IS CEREBROSPINAL FLUID ABSORBED? *

In most textbooks of physiology and many of anatomy it is stated as an accepted fact that cerebrospinal fluid passes from the subarachnoid space into the great venous sinuses through the pacchionian granulations. This statement was based on the results of injections of prussian blue suspensions into the spinal canal of cadavers by Key and Retzius. The color was found in the superior longitudinal sinuses and could be seen to pass through the pacchionian granules. But the observations were valueless in physiologic interpretations because cadavers instead of living animals were used and because the pressures used in the injections were far beyond any possible normal figures. It has since been repeatedly demonstrated that under normal conditions granules of prussian blue never pass through the pacchionian bodies.

Moreover, the hypothesis that cerebrospinal fluid is absorbed by the pacchionian granulations is instantly shattered by the fact that these structures are acquisitions only of age. They do not exist in infants and young children, nor do they exist in many animals.

Recently Weed [1] has somewhat modified the details of this hypothesis, though accepting it fundamentally. He recognized the absence of true pacchionian granulations, as has been noted here, and in their stead proposed so-called subarachnoid villi, which are of microscopic size and the forerunners of the pacchionian granulations of later life.

Weed [1] has brought forward a type of experimental evidence which he thinks is proof that fluids—not granules—pass directly through microscopic villi into the longitudinal sinus. His experiment was to introduce solutions of potassium ferrocyanide and iron ammonium citrate into the subarachnoid space and subsequently fix the central nervous system in an acid medium; salts of prussian blue resulted as a precipitate and he assumed that the pathways of absorption were directly laid down by the precipitated granules and extended directly through from the subarachnoid space to the longitudinal sinus.

That the exit for cerebrospinal fluid is not through the pacchionian granulations (or through Weed's arachnoidal villi) can be conclusively demonstrated by the simple experiment of separating both cerebral hemispheres of dogs from all attachments to the longitudinal, transverse and circular sinuses (Figs. 1 and 2). It then becomes impossible for any arachnoid diverticula of either gross or microscopic size to maintain direct connection between the subarachnoid space and the great venous sinuses. As a matter of fact, in young dogs in which the operation is performed there is usually — aside from venous connections—only one small area on each side suggesting a pacchionian granulation and forming an attachment between the extensive subarachnoid space and the longitudinal and transverse sinuses of each side. This small attachment is fairly constant in position and lies in the anterior fourth of the longitudinal sinus. The experiment is not difficult to perform, and when the four animals in which it was undertaken were killed four, five and six months later, in not one was there the slightest increase in the size of the cerebral ventricles or in the size of the extracerebral subarachnoid space. These results prove that it is impossible for cerebrospinal fluid to pass directly into the

*Reprinted from *The Journal of the American Medical Association*, 92: 2012–2014, June 15, 1929.

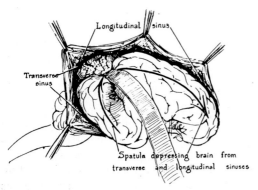

Fig. 1 Method of separating the cerebral hemisphere of a dog from the longitudinal and transverse sinuses. By this method all possibility of communication between the subarachnoid space and the venous sinuses by way of pacchionian granulations or other openings is eliminated.

large venous spaces through a medium of any type.

An average sized dog, about 6 to 8 months old, was anesthetized with ether. One-half hour before the operation, concentrated sodium chloride solution (25 per cent) was injected intravenously to reduce the cerebral volume and facilitate the operative manipulations. A large bony defect was created by ronguering away the vault of the skull. The longitudinal sinus was bared over nearly its entire extent and the defect carried laterally and posteriorly on both sides. After the dura had been incised on each side, it was retracted to the superior longitudinal sinus and the transverse sinus. The spatula was then inserted between the anterior part of the longitudinal sinus and the cerebral hemisphere, and the latter was depressed about 1 to 1.5 cm. This separation was continued backward to the torcular herophili and continued laterally along the lateral sinus to the sigmoid sinus. The cerebral hemisphere was then elevated by the spatula and the ventral surface of the brain separated from the circular sinus for an equal distance. In identically the same way the other cerebral hemisphere was separated from the same venous sinuses of the opposite side. The muscle, galea and skin were then closed (the dura remaining open).

The dog did not experience any immediate or subsequent distress. The wound never bulged. Had there been pressure from accumulated fluid, whether within the ventricles, the brain or the subarachnoid space, the decompression would have protruded. Six

months later the animal, which had every appearance of being perfectly normal, was killed. There was no accumulation of cerebrospinal fluid on the surface of the brain. The brain was hardened in situ and sectioned three weeks later. There was not the slightest enlargement of the lateral ventricles.

Three other dogs were operated on in precisely the same manner. The survival periods were four, five and six months. Exactly the same negative results were present in each instance. As a matter of fact, the separation of the hemispheres from the venous sinuses was, practically speaking, little more than a gesture because, except for a large anterior cerebral vein and a single fibrous attachment just anterior to it, the cerebral hemispheres were nowhere attached to any of the three large sinuses. The brain fell away on the slightest pressure of the spatula. However, disregarding the fact that normal pacchionian granulations or arachnoid villous attachments do not exist, the separation of both cerebral hemispheres from all the great venous sinuses renders any such communications impossible. With he entirely negative effects on the cerebrospinal fluid and its spaces, the claim that such structures are absorbing agents for cerebrospinal fluid becomes untenable.

As a matter of fact, it would seem not

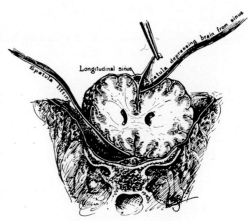

Fig. 2. Cross-section of the separation of the hemisphere from the longitudinal sinus and the elevation of the hemisphere from the circular sinuses. This procedure is carried out on both sides of the brain.

to require an experiment of such extended -character to arrive at this conclusion. That pacchionian granulations do not absorb cerebrospinal fluid has been shown by the absorption of various dyes in solution — indigo carmine. Methylene blue (methylthionine chloride-U. S. P.) and phenolsulphonphthalein. When these dyes are injected into the spinal canal they can be detected in the blood stream in less than two minutes. On the other hand, it takes practically an hour for the dyes to reach that part of the subarachnoid space where the pacchionian granulations are presumed to exist. In that time, i. e., before the pacchionian granulations have been reached, from 20 to 25 per cent of the dye has been both absorbed and excreted in the urine. Moreover, if the spinal canal is closed by a ligature in the lower cervical region, the same dyes, when injected into the closed spinal canal (below the ligature), pass into the blood and are excreted by the urine just as promptly. There are no pacchionian granulations in the spinal canal. [2]

How? then, and where does cerebrospinal fluid absorb? That it passes directly into the blood is shown by the prompt detection of the dye in the blood (two minutes). That the lymphatics do not play a part is shown by the absence of dyes in a fistula that collects all the lymph from the thoracic duct. A trace of color appears in approximately an hour, but by this time the body is well saturated with the dye. In addition to this physiologic evidence is the fact that the lymphatics have never been demonstrated in the brain.

There has not appeared any reason to change the view which I expressed in an article written in collaboration with Blackfan; namely, that the fluid passes into the subarachnoid space. The cerebrospinal fluid is in contact with the capillaries of the pia-arachnoid. As a matter of fact there are few places in the body where fluids will not rapidly absorb into the blood. The curve of subarachnoid absorption is not greatly dissimilar from that of the peritoneal, pleural cavities, the muscle or the subcutaneous tissue, and in none of these cavities is it necessary to call on specialized structures to explain the absorption of fluid.

REFERENCES

[1]Weed, L. H.: The Cerebrospinal Fluid. *Physiol. Rev., 2:* 171 (April) 1922.

[2]Dandy, W. E., and Blackfan, K. D.: Internal Hydrocephalus: An Experimental, Clinical and Pathological study. *J. A. M. A., 61:* 2216 (Dec. 20) 1913 Internal Hydrocephalus. *Am. J. Dis. Child., 8:* 406 (Dec.) 1914. Dandy, W. E.: Experimental Hydrocephalus, *Ann. Surg.,* 70: 129 (Aug.) 1919

XXXIV

OPERATIVE RELIEF FROM PAIN IN LESIONS OF THE MOUTH, TONGUE AND THROAT*

The recent development of an operative attack on the trigeminal and glossopharyngeal nerves at the brain stem for the cure of trigeminal and glossopharyngeal tic douloureux[1] at once suggested the permanent relief from pain in which the peripheral distribution of both of these nerves are responsible, namely, in chronic ulcers, burns from radium or malignant lesions of the tongue and throat.

The exact form of treatment by which relief from pain is to be sought will necessarily depend on the character, location and rate of growth of the lesion and the general state of the patient's health. At times morphine or other strong sedatives may be the treatment of choice. For the relief from pain confined to the inferior or superior maxillary nerves an injection of alcohol into the peripheral branch may be indicated. Obviously, the operative relief from pain is intended only for a selected group of patients whose general condition and expectancy of life is such as to make it seem advisable.

Since the tongue and pharynx are supplied by two sensory nerves, the glossopharyngeal and the trigeminus, chronic lesions frequently overlap from the domain of one nerve into the other. Under such conditions, the exclusion of only one nerve will have little effect on the intensity of the pain. Both nerves must be divided to give relief.

The trigeminal nerve supplies all of the inner side of the mouth, most of the roof and the floor of the mouth, the anterior two thirds of the tongue and the nasal sinuses. The glossopharyngeal nerve supplies sensation to the posterior third of the tongue, the uvula and the posterior part of the soft palate, the posterior wall of the pharynx and the posterior surface of the epiglottis. Pain is always greatly intensified in ulcerations of the mouth and pharynx because of the passage of liquids and food over the exposed nerve endings. The pain may also be much increased by applications of radium.

The proposal, therefore, for the relief from pain (in selected cases) when the sensory fibers of both nerves are involved or will later probably be involved is the intracranial division of both the fifth and the ninth nerves. Since the intracranial positions of the trigeminal and glossopharyngeal nerves are in such close proximity, precisely the same approach (subcerebellar) has been used in each procedure. It is possible to divide both nerves at the brain stem almost as easily as either. The sensory root of the trigeminal nerve can be severed with much greater ease and with far less time by this new procedure, which has been used exclusively for the past two years at the Johns Hopkins Hospital and University, than by the older approach along the floor of the temporal fossa (Hartley-Krause). After a small unilateral bony defect has been made, only a few minutes are required to divide the sensory root of the fifth nerve either entirely or in part, and only a few additional seconds are needed to resect the glossopharyngeal trunk. Other great advantages of this route for section of the trigeminus are (1) the constant absence of injury of the motor branch of this nerve and (2) the

*Reprinted from the *Archives of Surgery, 19:* 143–148, July, 1929.

almost complete absence of corneal redness and ulceration—the two principal
deterrent features of the Hartley-Krause
method. (3) For reasons not yet definitely
ascertained, some sensation to the face is
usually but not always retained.

REPORT OF A CASE

A sallow, undernourished man, aged
forty, was suffering terrific pain in the
region of an old ulcer on the right side
of the tongue; the pain radiated to the
back of the throat, the right ear, the lips
and teeth on the right side, the inside of
the cheek and the right half of the hard
palate. The pain was present almost
constantly, and though always severe, the
intensity varied from time to time. Exacerbations of the pains always resulted
from rubbing the mustache and shaving
or lightly rubbing the lower part of the
face on the right side. The inside of
his mouth burned like fire on the right
side. Chewing and swallowing so greatly
increased the pain in the mouth and ear
that he was afraid to eat or drink. The
pain was not relieved by any sedative.
It was finally necessary to resort to morphine, and many strong doses were required to bring relief. During the three
weeks before operative relief was obtained,
it had been necessary to give 130 doses
of morphine. The patient became desperate and belligerent until the large
amounts of morphine reduced the pain
to a point of toleration. Most of the
right half of the tongue had been removed several months previously for a chronic
ulcer, presumably carcinomatous. A few
weeks later, the glands of the neck were
removed on the right side. Microscopic
sections, however, failed to show carcinoma, either in the ulcer of the tongue
or in the glands of the neck. Since the
ulcer followed in the wake of a healing
Vincent's angina, it is more probable
that the original ulcer was benign. Six
weeks after the operation on the tongue,
radium needles were implanted, and
thereafter the pain became violent and
unrelenting. On the lateral border of
the tongue was a contracture due to the
healed lesion. It was covered with epithelium and was not indurated. Actual
ulceration was not now visible.

Operation.—Sept. 18, 1927: A unilateral cerebellar exposure was made on the
right side. The bony defect extended to
the mastoid cells, which, however, were
carefully avoided. The cisterna magna
was punctured, releasing a large amount
of fluid and thereby affording ample
room for a subcerebellar exposure. The
cerebellum was lifted with a spatula until the cisterna lateralis was brought into
view. After evacuation of the fluid of
the lateral cistern, one could at once
see the series of cranial nerves on this
side. The ninth and the fifth nerves were
easily isolated and divided, the former
with scissors, and latter with a tiny knife
at right angles to a long flexible shaft.
The division of both nerves after their
exposure probably did not consume more
than five minutes, the entire operation
taking about forty minutes.

The postoperative course was uneventful. The patient was immediately relieved from all pain, and despite the large
doses of morphine which had been given
before operation, there has been no further
need or desire for the drug. His color,
general appearance, weight and behavior
rapidly improved. At the time this report
was written (Feb. 1, 1928) the patient
was back at work and in perfect health.
He has gained 30 pounds (30.6 Kg.) in
weight, and has been entirely free from
all pain since the operation.

AFTER-EFFECTS OF OPERATION

The after-effects of the operation are
confined to the loss of sensation incident
to the loss of the two sensory nerves.
However, in not one of three patients in
whom the glossopharyngeal nerve alone
was divided has there been any appreciation of this sensory loss, nor has the
loss of taste over the posterior third of
the tongue been noticed, although the
objective sensory loss was absolute. Loss
of sensation over the trigeminal area is
only partial as obtained in seven of ten
cases after division of the sensory root at
the pons. The sensation over the forehead is only a little impaired; that over
the second branch is somewhat more affected, and over the third branch, the
loss is a little more. Touch is preserved
over all branches, but most acutely over
the first branch. Heat and cold can be

differentiated over all branches, but most keenly over the first branch. The corneal reflex is retained. This seeming paradox, i. e., preservation of sensation, is the usual story and greatly reduces the subjective feeling of great numbness which obtained after the old operation. It is not due to partial severance of the nerve as might be suspected. Perhaps there are sensory fibers accompanying the motor branch of the nerve which is always preserved intact.

INDICATIONS FOR AND ADVANTAGES OF THE OPERATION

When the sensory domain of the glossopharyngeal nerve is invaded by carcinoma or a chronic or incurable lesion, relief can be obtained only through section of the ninth nerve.[2] Alcoholic injections of the nerve are practically precluded because of the intimate relations between the peripheral fibers of the vagus, and also because of the fact that the glossopharyngeal nerve lies in the sheath of the jugular vein and close to the internal carotid artery. Peripheral section of the glossopharyngeal nerve in the neck is much more dangerous than intracranial section of the nerve because of the intimate association with the vagus nerve, injury to which induces profound disturbance of deglutition. The vagus has always been injured when section or avulsion of the glossopharyngeal nerve has been attempted in the neck. Moreover, intracranial section of the central fibers of the ninth nerve makes their regrowth impossible, whereas after peripheral division, the pain would doubtless return. Intracranial section is easier and almost devoid of danger.

Should the domain of the trigeminal nerve alone be involved, and the involvement be only on one side, the relief from pain offers the choice of two methods, (1) injection of alcohol and (2) intracranial section (either partial or total) of the sensory root of the trigeminus. If the lesion is a carcinoma and so rapid in its growth that the duration of life is probably a matter of few months, the injection of alcohol into the inferior or superior maxillary branches of the trigeminus would be preferable.

However, should the probable duration of life be many months or years, or should the lesion be such that the duration of life is not directly affected, division of the trigeminal nerve intracranially by the cerebellar route is far superior to the repeated and painful injections with the added loss of the muscles of mastication.

But when with the same expectancy of life the lesion is such that the sensory domains of both the ninth and the fifth nerves are involved, injections of alcohol will be futile. Intracranial section of the ninth nerve alone will give relief in its distribution; and, as previously noted, when this is done the sensory branch of the fifth nerve is already in view and can be easily divided. It need not be emphasized that when the sensory root of the fifth nerve is divided through the temporal route (Hartley-Krause operation) it is not possible to section the glossopharyngeal nerve at the same time, for it is far afield of this exposure. Moreover, there is far less hesitancy in advising division of the sensory branch of the trigeminal nerve by the cerebellar route than by the temporal approach since trophic disturbances of the eye are eliminated and injury to the motor branch of the trigeminal nerve (muscles of mastication) never occurs; finally, the operation has not been attended with mortality.

There remain the possibilities of relieving pain when the lesion is in the midline of the tongue, mouth or pharynx, and involves the sensory fibers of both trigeminal, or of both ninth, or even perhaps of all four nerves. The cerebellar approach to the intracranial part of these nerves is easily extended to a bilateral exposure by enlarging the unilateral into the bilateral approach which is more or less routine in operations for cerebellar tumors. Whether both glossopharyngeal and both trigeminal nerves could be sacrificed, one can only infer. In a case of bilateral trigeminal neuralgia, the sensory roots of both trigeminal nerves have been divided by this approach at one sitting and with no added operative difficulties other than the greater time consumed in making a bilateral instead of a unilateral cerebellar exposure. The additional division of both ninth nerves, while not difficult technically, might well be inpracticable because of the loss of the gag reflex.

Whether chronic lesions of the tongue or nasopharynx would ever present the need of such operative relief, I am not prepared to say. In such cases, bilateral alcoholic injections of the inferior maxillary nerve would be precluded because both motor branches of the trigeminus would be paralyzed and swallowing made impossible. Relief from such pain could hardly be obtained safely except by section of the sensory roots at the pons where the motor roots are safely removed.

Whether both glossopharyngeal nerves could be divided for the relief from pain cannot be answered by precedent. Though technically easy and safe, the absence of the gag reflex on both sides would probably make it impractical. Division of either the ninth or the fifth nerve, or of both on one side, may also be of advantage in permitting the application of radium to a malignant lesion without pain, immediately or subsequently.

SUMMARY AND CONCLUSIONS

An operation is presented for the complete and permanent relief from pain associated with chronic, benign and malignant lesions of the mouth, nose, tongue and throat. When the pain is referable to the sensory domain of both the glossopharyngeal and trigeminal nerves on one side, there is no other way of permanent relief. Under such conditions the glossopharyngeal nerve and the sensory root of the trigeminus can be divided at the brain stem (subcerebellar approach), both nerves being exposed simultaneously in the same operative field. Both nerves can be divided easily, quickly and with little danger to life or function.

NOTE: Since this article was sent for publication, three additional cases of combined fifth and ninth nerve divisions have been performed. In two of the patients the upper three cervical sensory roots have also been divided intradurally because the malignant lesions had extended into the domain of the cervical nerves.

REFERENCES

[1]Dandy, W. E.: Section of the Sensory Root of the Trigeminal Nerve at the Pons.—Preliminary Report of the Operative Procedure. *Bull. Johns Hopkins Hosp.*, *36:* 2, 1925; Glossopharyngeal Neuralgia (Tic Douloureux). *Arch. Surg.*, *15:* 198 (Aug.) 1927.

[2]T. Fay recently divided the ninth nerve intracranially and the upper three spinal sensory roots by a combined laminectomy and cerebellar exposure. He thought it necessary to divide this group of nerves because the more distant skin areas of the neck had been invaded by an ulcerating carcinoma which was primary in the neck. (Intracranial Division of the Glossopharyngeal Nerve Combined with Cervical Rhizotomy for Pain in Inoperable Carcinoma of the Throat. *Ann. Surg.*, *84:* 456, 1926.)

XXXV

AN OPERATIVE TREATMENT FOR CERTAIN CASES OF MENINGOCELE (OR ENCEPHALOCELE) INTO THE ORBIT *

Pulsating exophthalmos may arise from: (1) arteriovenous aneurysms of the brain, orbit or cavernous sinus; (2) arterial and arteriovenous aneurysms of the orbit and (3) defective roof of the orbit. The treatment for pulsating exophthalmos, therefore, is dependent on and directed to the underlying cause. In the case here reported, the pulsating exophthalmos was due to an orbital meningocele of congenital origin. It would perhaps be more correct to speak of congenital absence of the roof of the orbit, for doubtless this defect was primary, the cerebral meningocele following in its wake as a necessary mechanical sequel. The differential diagnosis of the cause of the pulsating exophthalmos was based on the positive roentgenologic evidence that the roof of the orbit was in large part missing on the affected side. The explanation of the exophthalmos was that the unopposed pressure of the brain or the meningeal contents was gradually forcing the orbital contents outward. The pulsation was due to the direct transmission of the pulsation of the brain to the eyeball.

For such a cause the obvious treatment is reconstruction of the orbital roof, preferably by an autotransplant of bone. In this patient, a measured graft was taken from the outer table of the skull, giving much the same slight curvature that obtains in this portion of the normal orbital roof.

The approach for this exposure was through a small anteriorly placed bone flap, extending from the orbital ridge to the anterior hair line or slightly beyond. This approach is used as a routine for the operative attack on hypophyseal tumors and is suitable for all explorations of the roof of the orbit A few years ago a much more extensive cranioplasty[1] was advocated as an approach to prechiasmal tumors involving the optic nerves and extending into the orbit, or for tumors arising in the orbit and extending into the cranial chamber. Experience, however, has shown that in most instances the restricted exposure serves equally well and has the other advantages of being a less formidable procedure and of reducing the incidence of postoperative extradural hemorrhage. Had an encephalocele been encountered instead of a meningocele, its removal should not have been difficult owing to the ample room provided by the operative approach.

The bone transplant was obtained along the posterior line of incision and back of the hair line. The entire thickness of bone was removed, then split by chiseling through the diploe. The outer table was used for the graft.

A search of the literature on meningocele, encephalocele and congenital malformations of the orbit indicates that the lesion is rare. No record was found of an operative procedure directed toward a cure.

REPORT OF A CASE

History.— A bright girl, aged sixteen, was referred by Dr. Alan C. Woods because of a unilateral pulsating exophthalmos due to a defect in the roof of the orbit. She had previously been seen by Dr. Arnold Knapp of New York. From a series of x-ray pictures, Dr. Knapp had

*Reprinted from the *Archives of Ophthalmology,* 2: 123–132 August, 1929.

first made the diagnosis of congenital absence of the left roof of the orbit.

Soon after the birth of the child the mother noticed that the left eye protruded slightly and was a little lower than the right. Slowly the eye became more prominent, and a definite internal strabismus developed. One year before examination the exophthalmos seemed to increase rather abruptly and at the same time the vision was affected. There had been no headaches or other symptoms.

Examination.—Aside from the local condition and related functions, a minor congenital deformation of the ear and marked thinning of the skull in the frontal region (lateral view), the physical and neurologic examinations revealed nothing. Her general condition was excellent.

The report of Dr. Woods' examination was as follows: "Exophthalmometer readings: Right 19 mm., left 24 mm. The best vision on the right is 20/30+; on the left 20/100. There is a slight concentric contraction of the left visual fields though the change is not great (Fig. 1). In addition to the exophthalmos, the left eye deviates downward and inward. A fine vertical nystagmus is present. The optic disc is normal in outline; the physiological cup is a little blurred; the disc is flat with slight overfilling and rather marked tortuosity of the veins. The pupils are equal and react normally to light and accommodation."

On looking at the eye from a lateral position, a pulsation, synchronous with the pulse, was easily seen. It was also palpable, but there was no thrill. No murmur was audible. X-ray pictures of the skull taken laterally and anteroposteriorly (both stereoscopic) showed that the posterior half of the roof of the orbit was missing. There was a small shelf internally and externally. All of these observations had previously been made by Dr. Knapp.

Operation.— On July 15, 1927, a transplant of bone from the outer table of the skull was bridged across the roof of the orbit. The curvature of this bone was essentially the same as the arch of the orbital roof. Moreover, the external and internal margins of the orbit were adequate to give a base on which the graft could rest and to which it should ultimately unite. A bed was chiseled from the external rim of the orbital roof where it joins the side of the skull, and into this notch the outer margin of the transplant fitted accurately and firmly. The graft was passed through a tunnel between the dura and the orbital contents. The inner margin of the transplant rested on the inner rim of the orbital plate. from which the dura and periosteum had been scraped to permit the transplant to lie in apposition with bare bone. The ends of the graft fitted so accurately that it was not necessary to wire the graft in place. The new superior orbital fissure was probably a little wider than normal but the difference was not great.

Other Details of the Operation and Abnormal Observations.— The outer surface of the brain was covered with large pools of fluid in the subarachnoid space; the leptomeninges were opaque and great-

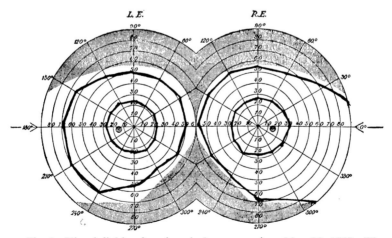

Fig. 1. Visual fields of patient before operation, May 28, 1927. The best vision on the right was 20/30, that on the left, 20/100.

ly thickened. The release of this fluid yielded adequate room to permit elevation of the brain without producing trauma. It was not necessary to puncture the lateral ventricle or to withdraw spinal fluid by lumbar puncture, as is the custom when intracranial room is at a premium. On retraction of the frontal lobe the defect in the posterior two thirds of the orbital roof showed precisely as in the x-ray picture. The bony defect was everywhere covered by dura which was firmly attached to the eyeball. The dura extended backward with a gradual decline to and across the floor of the middle fossa. An isolated small fragment of bone lay between the dura and the eyeball.

The tip of the temporal lobe was covered by tremendously dilated subarachnoid spaces, with opaque membranes—changes not unlike those on the surface of the brain, except in degree. Superficial examination might well give the impression that the tip of the temporal lobe, which was entirely hidden from view, was covered by an actual cyst. These large subarachnoid spaces were continuous through the sylvian fossa with similar spaces over the frontal and parietal lobes. The maximum depth of fluid was about 2.5 cm. The intact temporal lobe lay beneath the bed of fluid.

Three small veins crossed from the external surface of the temporal lobe to the orbital tissue piercing the dura enroute. They were doubly ligated with silver clips and divided. With these veins out of the way and the bed of fluid evacuated, the view of the entire anterior and middle fossa was unobstructed. A tremendous anomalous vein lay along the inner side of the middle fossa and outside the dura. It was formed by the confluence of two large veins—doubtless the superior and the inferior orbital veins—which also pierced the dura covering the orbital contents. It doubtless represented an extradural cavernous sinus. Posteriorly, the ultimate destination of the vein could not be traced.

The left optic nerve was bent to the right, due to the pressure of the large cup of fluid on the tip of the temporal lobe. Search was made for the carotid artery which always stands out conspicuously alongside the optic nerve, but it could not be found. It is interesting that both the internal carotid artery and the cavernous sinus were absent. Knowing that the carotid artery in its transit through the skull passes through the cavernous sinus, I was led to wonder if the absence of the cavernous sinus might not lead to the loss of the internal carotid artery. No attempt was made to disclose the other nerves (III, IV and VI) entering the orbit. The anterior clinoid process on the left side was absent.

Postoperative Course.— Immediately after the operation there was perhaps a tiny exophthalmos of the affected eye, though the difference between the position of the two eyes was slight. During the succeeding two or three weeks there was some protrusion, doubtless from edema of the orbital tissues. This gradually subsided, and the eye has since been in almost normal position in the anteroposterior direction.

The following observations on the eye were recorded by Dr. Woods, subsequent to the cranial operation:

Sept. 27, 1927 (Ten Weeks After the Orbital Transplant) : A marked edema of the orbit and further protrusion of the eye which occurred after the operation had disappeared. To protect the eye, a median tarsorrhaphy was done (by Dr. Woods). The dergee of exophthalmos was 19 mm. right and 21 mm. left. The eye still showed 10 per cent of internal strabismus with 5 per cent of deviation downward. The media and fundus were unchanged. Slight nystagmus still persisted.

Nov. 27, 1927 (Nineteen Weeks After the Orbital Transplant) : There was no relative exophthalmos. Exophthalmometer readings were 19 mm. for both eyes. The internal strabismus of the left eye measured 25 degrees; the downward deviation was 5 per cent. Corrected vision remained 20/30+ right, and 20/100 left.

Operation on the External Rectus Muscle by Dr. Woods.—The extra-ocular palsy was, of course, not changed by the orbital operation. Seventeen months later (Dec. 6, 1928), Dr. Woods operated to correct the internal strabismus and vertical deviation. His note on the operation was as follows:

Resection and advancement of the external rectus muscle on the left side was performed. The upper fibers of the tendon were advanced slightly more than the lower fibers in order to get some correction of the vertical deviation. The eye healed without complications, and the deep sutures were removed a month later. The eyes were entirely straight so far as lateral deviation was concerned, and there was no vertical deviation downward. The left eye, however, appeared to be on a lower level than the right, being about 2 mm. lower in the orbit. For this condition I do not think anything could possibly be done, nor do I think anything should be attempted.

Final Results.—A slight downward displacement of the eyeball still remained. There was no exophthalmos or pulsation of the eyeball. The eyes focused well. The extra-ocular movements were nearly perfect five months later. There was no diplopia.

SUMMARY

1. A case of pulsating exophthalmos, due to congenital absence of the orbital roof, is reported.

2. The pulsating exophthalmos was cured by covering the orbital defect with a transplant of bone taken from the outer table of the skull.

3. Other associated congenital deformations were encountered at operation: (1) a meningocele, (2) a large extradural vein which apparently replaced the cavernous sinus and (3) an absence of the internal carotid artery on the affected side.

REFERENCE

[1]Dandy, W. E.: Prechiasmal Intracranial Tumors of the Optic Nerves. *Am. J. Ophth.*, 5: 169 (March) 1922.

XXXVI

LOOSE CARTILAGE FROM INTERVERTEBRAL DISK SIMULATING TUMOR OF THE SPINAL CORD *

The two loose cartilages here reported were disclosed at operation for persumed tumors of the cauda equina. In each instance the spinal canal was completely blocked as shown by the shadows of iodized oil 40 per cent. The signs and symptoms were so rapidly progressive and the pain in the spinal column so severe that presumptive diagnoses of carcinoma of the vertebra were made. The fact that the two cases appeared only a few months apart leads me to believe that the lesion may not be so infrequent, although a review of the literature has failed to disclose other cases of their kind. The lesion is a completely detached fragment of cartilage from an intervertebral (lumbar) disk and is surrounded by serum. It bulges dorsally into the spinal canal as a tumor, and by compressing the roots of the cauda equina causes motor and sensory paralysis, loss of reflexes and of rectal and vesical control. The lesion is undoubtedly of traumatic origin.

REPORT OF CASES

CASE 1. A sparsely nourished man, aged forty-seven, was referred by Dr. Lewellys F. Barker. Whether or not the past history was relevant to the present illness was not clear at the time. Three years earlier a tumor had been removed from the hand; a microscopic diagnosis of a sarcoma was made. The scar on the hand, the regions of the epitrochlear and axillary glands, had since been treated intensively with radium. Subsequently an axillary gland was removed, but no sign of malignancy was discovered. Two years later, he consulted Dr. Barker because of convulsions which dated back two years.

*Reprinted from the *Archives of Surgery, 19:* 660–672, October, 1929.

The patient was readmitted to Dr. Barker's service on May 15, 1928, with an entirely different complaint. Ten weeks before admission he had a severe attack of pain in the lumbar region and both hips; there was more pain in the right hip. The pain radiated down the back of both legs, with more pain in the right leg. After two months of excruciating pain, it was necessary to resort to morphine for relief. Six weeks before admission to the hospital, a "dead feeling" developed in both legs and gradually increased. Two weeks before, he was barely able to stand alone. Assistance was necessary to walk a short distance. One week before, retention of urine and feces developed; after that time he was catheterized twice daily. He lost forty-two pounds (19.1 Kg.) in weight, fifteen pounds (6.8 Kg.) of which were lost in the last two months before admission. Pain in the lumbar region, hips and legs steadily became more severe.

On admission to the Johns Hopkins Hospital, the patient was found to have a total flaccid paralysis below the knees. Except for feeble flexion and extension of both legs at the hips, the legs were useless. Sensation was impaired though not entirely lost; sharp and dull stimulation were not differentiated. Vibratory sense was lost. Flexion and extension of the toes could not be differentiated, though the patient could tell which toe was touched. There was loss of sphincter control of feces and urine. (retention of urine was complete). Marked tenderness, even to light pressure, was noted over the spine of the third and fourth lumbar vertebrae. The lumbar muscles were in continuous strong spasm. Movements of the spine were painful, and even coughing intensified the pain. The patient was averse to any movement, and flexion of the knee was painful.

The abdominal reflexes were normal; the cremasteric reflexes were not obtained, and the knee jerks were subnormal.

420

The Achilles jerks were not obtained, and there was no ankle clonus. The Babinski, Gordon and Oppenheim tests were negative. The Wassermann reaction of the blood was negative. Roentgenograms of the lumbar spine were negative.

Through a cisternal puncture, 0.5 cc. of iodized oil was injected. It stopped abruptly at the level of the third lumbar vertebra.

*Preoperative Impression.—*The rapidly progressive paralysis, sensory, motor and sphincter, the severe pain and tenderness in the back, the great loss of weight and finally the history of a malignant lesion of the hand (doubtless incorrect) led me to suspect a metastic lesion of the third lumbar vertebra, despite the absence of signs of destruction in the roentgenogram.

*Operation.—*It was decided to explore the lesion to be sure of its character, and if it was malignant to perform a chordotomy. The laminae of the third and fourth lumbar vertebrae were removed. No change in the amount of extradural fat was observed. When the dura was opened, the roots of the cauda equina herniated markedly. The nerves were greatly injected, and because of this increased vascularity, oozing followed when they were touched. It was seen that there was a sharp knuckle of the roots protruding backward. Above and below this knuckle, there was a sharp drop. Palpation revealed a hard tumor lying beneath the roots and pushing them through the dural opening. The roots were then retracted to the left, and a bulging tumor mass was seen. It was round, about as large as a big hazelnut (about 1.5 by 1.5 cm.) and entirely covered by dura. It seemed semifluctuant when touched with the point of the forceps. The lesion was still thought to be malignant, even though the ventral dura was intact. After some hesitation I thought it advisable to incise the dura, and much to my surprise a border of loose cartilage protruded through the opening. With forceps, the cartilage was picked up and delivered without resistance. It was roughly oval, but crumpled. When straightened, it measured 2 by 0.8 by 0.3 cm. Its edges were very irregular, almost serrated. It had no attachments to the vertebral cartilage. Exploration of the cavity with a small curet revealed no additional sequestrums either of cartilage or of bone. A few drops of fluid escaped with the "floating cartilage." On gross inspection, there was no evidence of bone.

*Microscopic Report.—*A few scattered cartilage cells in varying states of degeneration were scattered through a pink-staining hyaline mass which was not entirely homogeneous, but in places was broken up by scattered fibrils longitudinally arranged. There were no inflammatory changes. No round or polymorphonuclear cells appeared in the sections, and there were no bone cells or deposits of calcium.

*Postoperative Course.—*Recovery from the operation was uneventful. The pain, though immediately relieved, was not at once abolished. Gradually it became less and less, and in a few weeks ceased. Vesical control was regained in two weeks and rectal control four weeks after operation. Return of motor power began seven weeks after the operation (three weeks after leaving the hospital). In a letter written six months after the operation, the patient stated that he could walk long distances without support, and every week improvement continued.

Subsequent History.— After the nature of the lesion was known, the recent history was again reviewed for trauma. The patient then recalled a severe, sharp lumbar pain which came with a sudden jolt when he was riding horseback three months before, or about two or three weeks before the onset of his present illness. He had forgotten the pain, since it disappeared after a few hours and had not returned during the succeeding days.

CASE 2. A large man, aged sixty-one, was referred by Dr. Eugene V. Parsonnet of Newark, N. J., because of paralysis of the lower limbs. He had been in perfect health until twelve weeks before, when he pushed his automobile out of the driveway. Immediately afterward, a dull, heavy pain developed in the small of the back. He went about his duties, and in a few days the pain abated. A week later, without appreciable cause, a sudden excruciating pain struck the lumbar region and radiated down the posterior aspect of both thighs. The pain was so severe that he had to remain in bed for two or three days. Movement of the spine caused severe pains. A few days later, he was again relieved, and returned to work. Ten days after the second attack, he was siezed with a third and even more severe pain at the same site and with the same referred distribution.

At this time (about a month after the first pain), he was seen by Dr. Parsonnet, who noted the following: 1. The normal anterior lumbar curve was missing. 2. There were definite scoliosis of the lumbar spine to the right. 3. Marked spasm of the erector spinae muscles. 4. Moderate tenderness at the third and fourth lumbar spinous processes. 5. The right knee jerk was diminished and the right ankle jerk absent. The patient was able to stand, but any movement elicited great pain.

An orthopedic consultant was called who advised stretching the sciatic nerves. This was done under deep anesthesia with ether. A plaster jacket was applied with the back in hyperextension. The spica extended to the toes of the right foot; the left leg was left free. On recovery from the anesthesia the patient was unable to void, but this was considered a sequel of the anesthesia. Three days after application of the cast, loss of power developed in both feet; he was unable to flex the toes. A slight edema of the left ankle (not included in the cast) developed. Two days later (five days after the cast had been applied), he could not move his left leg (the right was in the cast) and there was incontinence of feces. On the following day, the cast was removed.

A neurologist who was called in consultation noted the following: 1. There was loss of deep and superficial sensation from the toes to the hips and loss of sensation around the anus. 2. The patient was unable to make any movements of either foot or leg below the knee. He could flex and extend the leg at the hip. This was some improvement, for two days earlier he was reported to be unable to make any movement of the leg. Paralysis was of the flaccid type. 3. Examination of the reflexes showed the ankle and right knee reflexes absent, the left knee reflex was diminished, and the abdominal and cremasteric reflexes were normal. 4. There was loss of vesical and rectal control. 5. Tenderness persisted over the third and fourth lumbar vertebrae. A lumbar puncture was done; the fluid was clear and colorless and registered 10 mm. of pressure with the mercurial manometer; jugular compression (Queckenstedt test) caused the pressure to rise instantly to 30 mm., and on release of jugular pressure, the fluid promptly fell to the former level. The cell count was normal and there was no increase of globulin.

The patient was referred to me twelve weeks after the strain in the back and three weeks after the sciatic nerves had been stretched and the cast applied. The physical and neurologic observations were essentially the same as those just reported: 1. Sensation of every form was absent below the third lumbar segment but it was normal above this segmental level. 2. Flexion, adduction and extension of the leg at the hips were possible but decidedly weak while abduction was absent; there was no movement at the knee, ankle and toes. 3. All reflexes were abolished at and below the knee. 4. There was complete loss of vesical and rectal control. Lumbar puncture showed definite xanthochromia, the fluid having a greenish-yellow tint. The cell count was 10. The Queckenstedt test was negative, the column of fluid rising and falling with application and release of jugular compression. Iodized oil was injected; it descended only the distance of half a vertebra, lodging at the level of the fourth lumbar vertebra.

The only abnormality that could be detected in the roentgenograms (anteroposterior view only) was a supernumerary lumbar vertebra. The intervertebral disks appeared normal in size and shape.

Preoperative Impression.—That a tumor completely blocking the spinal canal was present at the level of the third lumbar vertebra seemed certain. That there was a definite relationship to the "stretching" of the sciatic nerves because of the sensory, motor and sphincter loss that occurred promptly thereafter could hardly be questioned. But it was necessary to admit that there was a preexisting lesion which had caused the severe pain in the back and down the legs. Though a metastatic lesion of the vertebra was suspected, no destruction of bone could be seen in the roentgenogram and no primary carcinoma could be found, though carefully sought. The true nature of the lesion was not suspected.

Operation.—Laminae of the fourth and fifth lumbar vertebrae (corresponding to the normal third and fourth) were removed under rectal ether anesthesia. Before the dura was opened, one could feel a hard mass about 1.5 cm. long, but when it was opened no tumor was visible. The roots of the cauda equina covered the exposed field. However, a sharply defined hillock of the cauda equina pushed backward, and under it one could still feel tumor of bony hardness. The roots of the cauda equina were definitely reddened and swollen. The cauda equina was retracted from the right side with a blunt dissector and a well circumscribed bulging extradural mass was at once visible; it crossed the midline posteriorly but was more on the right than the left. The mass was white, being covered with intact dura. When pressed firmly with the end of the forceps it seemed to fluctuate; at least it was soft in the center where it gave evidence of pointing. At once the picture of case 1 was recalled to mind for the gross appearance of the swelling was the same in both cases. The dura was slit longitudinally for a distance of about 1 cm. It was entirely avascular. A piece of loose cartilage projecting into the dural opening was picked up with the forceps and easily delivered. It was entirely unattached and no force was required to withdraw it. A few drops of fluid escaped with the floating cartilage. Further exploration of the cavity was not attempted. The borders of the cartilage were irregular; there was no sign of infection, no redness of the cartilage and no redness of the dura which covered the tumor. No fragments of bone were found attached to the cartilage. The cut edges of the dura sank back into the cavity from which the cartilage was removed. The knoll of the cauda equina entirely disappeared. The alinement of the vertebrae was normal.

Microscopic Report.—Exactly the same microscopic picture presented as in the preceding case. A few scattered cuts of cartilage were present, though in varying degrees of preservation. There was no cellular reaction indicative of an inflammation.

Subsequent Note.—The patient's recovery from the operation was uneventful. Urinary control returned ten days, and rectal control one month, after operation. Some sensation had returned within a month. He was beginning to walk four months after operation. Doubt of eventual complete recovery of motor function as in case 1 can scarcely be entertained, for the nerves are intact and apparently uninjured.

ANALYSIS OF CASES

In each case a large fragment of the intervertebral cartilage had become detached and was acting as a sequestrum. The reaction to the "foreign body" caused a swelling which bulged dorsally into the spinal canal. Pressure on the roots of the cauda equina then produced paralysis of all function below the nerve level of the tumor and through edema some function was lost for distance above the tumor.

The detached cartilage is almost certainly the result of trauma, but a relatively trivial trauma. In the first case no history of trauma was given voluntarily; it was elicited only after trauma was suspected. The trauma in the second case was almost surely the slight wrench caused by pushing an automobile. Several attacks of pain identical in both character and location were again induced by slight trauma before the advent of paralysis, and the location of the pain remained the same after the paralysis developed. The severe trauma incident to "stretching the sciatic nerves" and to placing the body in the cast with the lumbar region flexed undoubtedly caused the lesion to fulminate and promptly to reach the stage of tumor formation some time in advance of the normal course of events.

The preoperative diagnosis of a lesion in the vertebra could hardly be questioned in either case, because the slightest movement of the lower part of the spine always brought on or intensified the pain. Moreover, the tense spasm of the erector spinae muscles and the sharply localized severe tenderness of the spinous process offered supporting evidence of the strongest kind. In these respects the lesion is hardly different from carcinoma of the vertebra. In either condition, only the recumbent posture could long be tolerated.

In both patients, the pain radiated down

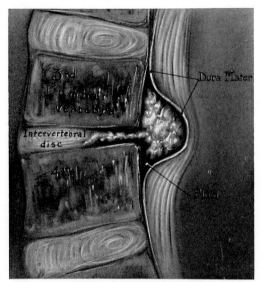

Fig. 1. Sketch to show conception of position and manner of formation of loose cartilage projecting into the spinal canal and compressing the cauda equina.

the back of both legs but usually down one more than the other. The side most involved proved to be the side of the greater bulge of the tumor. These facts lead one to wonder whether bilateral sciatic pains do not in most instances indicate a lesion affecting the spinal cord or cauda equina, more frequently the latter. These cases at least offer pathologic evidence of a definite lesion inducing symptoms of so-called sciatica with its all too meager pathology.

That the floating cartilage in each of these cases was in the lumbar region is doubtless significant. The maximum effects of shocks and of torsion of the body are transferred to the lumbar spine. As protection against shocks, the intervertebral disks attain their greatest size in the lumbar region. That the lesion occurs about the middle of the lumbar spine is probably also because of an additional point of least resistance, for here the maximum part of the anterior lumbar curve is attained. Certainly moveable vertebrae on a curve offer the maximum opportunity for localized effects of trauma.

That the lesion occurs on the posterior instead of on the anterior aspect of the lum-

bar vertebra is probably also significant. The normal anterior curvature of the lumbar spine would be expected to throw greater localized effects of trauma on the posterior side of the disk. In other words, the cartilage should be more readily pinched posteriorly than anteriorly. Then, too, the relatively thin and incomplete posterior ligaments of the lumbar spine should more readily permit protrusion of a tumor in the intervertebral disk than the stronger and complete anterior ligament. Whether a loose cartilage could push through the strong and firmly attached anterior ligament can only be conjectured. There is as yet no evidence that a loose cartilage forms only in the posterior part of the disk though it may well be possible. From the size of the extended cartilage as seen at operation, it is hardly possible that more than a third or at most a half of the anteroposterior diameter of the disk can be involved.

Finally, in both instances the tumor presented not in the midline but to one side. Doubtless the explanation for this fact is that the posterior common ligament is defective laterally along the lumbar spine. Since the lesion is of traumatic origin it is probably not without significance that both of these patients are men. It is also not improbable that the additional lumbar vertebra in one patient may have had some part in making the lumbar spine susceptible to injury.

Emphasis has been placed on the seemingly trivial injuries that cause the cartilaginous sequestrum formation. It is not improbable that the repetition of minor traumas may, at times, at least, be an important factor. The history of the repeated attacks in case 2 suggests this possibility. There must be many instances in which the intervertebral cartilage sustains the degree and character of injury experienced in these two cases, and yet subsequently heals instead of going on to sequestration. It is difficult to believe that the complete detachment of the cartilaginous fragment does not require considerable time, and that with proper rest and fixation of the spine this outcome may be avoided. A remarkable contrast in the disposition of fragments of intervertebral cartilage is presented by severe fracture dislocations of the spine. There the cartilage is badly torn and frequently fragmented, but in the process of healing it is organized with bone and fibrous tissue into a solid mass.

The x-ray has disclosed nothing in either of these cases. After the character of the lesion was known, the roentgenograms were again inspected, with negative results. However, only anteroposterior views were taken before operation, and positive signs would hardly be expected from this view. However, shortly after operation on the second patient, lateral stereoscopic views of the affected part of the spine were taken, and not the slightest defect could be seen. The absence of bone in the sequestrum might well preclude the delineation of the tumor.

DIAGNOSIS

It is not difficult to arrive at the diagnosis of a tumor of the cauda equina because of the progressive paralysis—sensory, motor and sphincter—and loss of reflexes. The rapid progression of these signs and the severe pain in the back, the rigid lumbar spine due to spasm of the erector spinae muscles and the marked tenderness over the spinus processes and laminae of the lumbar vertebrae are such as to make metastatic carcinoma of the body of the vertebra the most likely diagnosis. The absence of roentgenologic changes in the body of of the vertebra would appear to carry much importance in the differential diagnosis between this lesion and metastatic carcinoma or sarcoma of the body of the vertebra. The malignant lesions are almost the only ones that offer difficulties in differential diagnosis.

Aside from the negative roentgen changes in the body of a vertebra, there seems to be no absolute differential objective evidence.

Even the clinical and microscopic examinations of the cerebrospinal fluid may show no differences, for both lesions are extradural. Each may give a mild degree of xanthochromia and globulin increase. Both give a negative reaction to the Queckenstedt test if the block is caudal to the point of entry of the needle, and both show a complete block at the upper level of the tumor when iodized oil is injected.

In the differential diagnosis two considerations are all-important: (1) to make the clinical diagnosis of carcinoma only on absolute evidence, i. e., microscopic or roentgenologic, and (2) to accept the operative diagnosis of a malignant condition only on positive evidence. My willingness to accept suggestive evidence of malignancy nearly deprived the first patient of the opportunity of having the lesion explored. In fact, had he not been eager to grasp the faint hope which an operation offered, the lesion would not have been disclosed. Even at operation the bulging mass from the body of the vertebra was at first considered so surely malignant that there seemed little reason to open the tumor.

The order of return of the various functions is most interesting. In both cases the vesical control returned completely in about ten days. Rectal control returned in about one month in each instance. Sensation gradually returned in about a month, but motor power made no improvement whatever until from seven to eight weeks after the operation in the first case, and at the end of the second month the motor power had not yet returned in the second patient. In the first case the motor improvement came slowly and continued for several months.

RESEMBLANCE OF THIS LESION TO OSTEOCHONDRITIS DISSECANS OR TRAUMATIC JOINT-MICE

Superficially at least, the loose vertebral cartilage appears to resemble the loose cartilage of the knee, elbow and ankle joint following osteochondritis dissecans described by Konig in 1888. They differ in that fragments of bone were not attached to the cartilage in either of my cases. The environment too is greatly different in that there is no cavity—even potential—as in the knee and elbow joints. More common in the knee joint than elsewhere, this condition has come to be recognized as a clinical entity, but the dividing line between osteochondritis dissecans and other joint-mice appears to be none too sharp. The distinction is usually made that in osteochondritis dissecans the loose bodies occur singly or at most in pairs, and that there is no evidence of inflammatory joint involvement elsewhere. Konig[1] could find no evidence of traumatic or constitutional origin and for that reason considered them to represent a distinct pathologic process. Barth[2] thought they were purely of traumatic origin. Ludloff, who first diagnosed them by roentgenograms and treated them surgically, thought that they were due to occlusions of end-arteries. Other authors (Freiberg and Wooley,[3] Ridlon,[4] Codman,[5] Weil,[6] Anglin [7] and Troell [8]) have come to no more definite conclusion. Budinger [9] (1907), Axhausen [10] (1914), Kappis [11] (1920) and Brackett and Hall [12] (1917) were more positive of their purely traumatic origin. They also called attention to the fact that the injury may be slight and repeated. The present trend of opinion seems to be that the term osteochondritis dissecans is a misnomer (for there is no evidence of inflammatory character), and that it is better to classify these loose bodies under traumatic joint-mice.

SUMMARY

1. Following slight (or repeated) trauma a fragment of an intervertebral disk may become detached, and eventually bulge into the spinal canal as a tumor. The "tumor" is composed of the cartilage and fluid formed by reaction to the foreign body.

2. Two instances of this lesion are reported, both being disclosed at operation. Both are in the midlumbar region, and both occurred in men during the latter half of life.

3. The trauma at onset is relatively trivial and perhaps repeated. The lesion is probably similar to osteochondritis dissecans or traumatic joint-mice of the elbow and knee joint.

4. The early symptoms are those of localized vertebral pain plus bilateral sciatica—one side being affected more than the other. Later, the symptoms are rapidly increasing paralysis, sensory and motor paralysis and loss of urinary and vesical control and of reflexes—all due to compression of the cauda equina.

5. The signs and symptoms suggest carcinoma of the vertebra. This preoperative diagnosis was made in both cases.

6. This lesion offers a pathologic basis for cases of "so-called sciatica," especially bilateral sciatica.

7. The lesion is cured by operative removal of the cartilage.

REFERENCES

[1]Konig: Ueber freie Korper in den Gelenken. *Deutsche Ztschr. Chir., 27:* 90, 1888.

[2]Barth: Die Entstehung und das Wachstum der freien Gelenk–Korper. *Arch. klin. Chir., 56:* 507, 1898.

[3]Freiberg and Wooley: Osteochondritis. *Am. J. Orthop. Surg., 8:* 477, 1910.

[4]Ridlon: Osteochondritis Dissecans. *J.A.M.A., 61:* 1777 (Nov. 15) 1913.

[5]Codman, E. A.: Formation of Loose Cartilages in the Knee Joint. *Boston M. & S. J., 149:* 427, 1903.

[6]Weil, S.: Ueber doppelseitige symmetrische osteochondritis dissecans. *Beitr. klin. Chir., 78:* 403, 1912; *Ztschr. Chir. Mech. Orth.,* July, 1912.

[7]Anglin, R. H.: Loose Bodies in the Knee, with Special Reference to Their Etiology and Growth. *Brit. J. Surg., 1:* 650 (April) 1914.

[8]Troell, A.: The Origin of Free Bodies in the Knee with Special Reference to Osteochondritis Dissecans. *Arch. klin. Chir., 105:* 399, 1914.

[9]Budinger: Ueber tranmatische Knorpelrisse im Kniegelenk. *Deutsche Ztschr. Chir., 92:* 510, 1907.

[10]Axhausen: Die Entstehung der freien Gelenk–Korper und ihre Beziehungen zur Arthritis deformans. *Arch. f. klin. Chir., 104:* 581, 1914.

[10]Kappis: Osteochondritis dissecans und traumatische Gelenkmause. *Deutsche Ztschr. Chir.,* *157:* 187, 1920.

[12]Brackett, E. G., and Hall, C. L.: Osteochondritis Dissecans. *Am. J. Orthop. Surg., 15:* 79, 1917.

XXXVII

AN OPERATION FOR THE TREATMENT OF SPAS-MODIC TORTICOLLIS *

It would seem that spasmodic torticollis had run the gauntlet of therapeutic efforts, surgical, medical and psychic. With one exception, the surgical methods have appeared after one or two trials and after an all too brief test of time. And, with this exception, the lack of later reports by the authors is in itself almost adequate evidence that the procedures have ended in failure, as indeed they must. Again, with this one exception, the surgical procedures have been unilateral. Regardless of one's interpretation of the underlying spasmodic contractures, one fact is incontrovertible, i. e., the disease is never restricted to an isolated muscle or to a single group and never to the muscles of one side.

To one not acquainted with the subsequent history of cases of this type, it is indeed difficult to understand why the simple excision of a preponderant, rigid, sternomastoid muscle, which dominates the clinical picture, or better still, the division of the spinal accessory nerve supplying it and the trapezius muscle, will not correct the condition. But these efforts have long since been found to do little more than to afford at best a brief respite. Soon the muscles on the contralateral side pulled the head just as strongly, and when a similar procedure was carried out there, other muscles quickly produced spasmodic contractures just as severe and unrelenting as the original. Attempts of this character were more or less in vogue, though unsuccessful, when Keen,[1] America's pioneer neurologic surgeon, realizing the more widespread involvement of the cervical muscles of rotation, first (18-91) divided on one side the posterior divisions of the first, second and third cervical nerves at their points of emergence from the vertebrae. It is interesting that Keen's surgical effort was advised by Wier Mitchell, from whom a functional basis for spasmodic torticollis would not have been unexpected. Taylor[2] (1915) reported unilateral division of the upper four sensory cervical nerves by the first intraspinal attack for this condition. His procedure was proposed on the basis of Foerster's treatment in Little's disease by reduction of the incoming sensory stimuli. McKenzie[3] (1924) carried the intraspinal divisions of the nerves a step farther, sectioning the upper three motor and sensory nerves and the spinal accessory nerve—all on one side only.

In the following year (1925), Finney and Hughson[4] reported the first bilateral operation. It had been used in thirty-one cases over a period of twenty years; twelve patients were cured, sixteen were improved and three were unimproved. Both spinal accessory nerves and the posterior divisions of the upper three cervical nerves on both sides were divided. The former were sectioned alongside the sternomastoid muscles, the latter at the points of emergence from the spinal vertebrae. The operation was, in effect, a bilateral Keen's operation plus division of both spinal accessory nerves. These were the first cases of torticollis in which cure was reported, the reason doubtless being that for the first time a number of nerves had been sectioned bilaterally. Moreover, they were the first cases in which the operative results were adequately tested by time. That cure was not obtained in all cases was due to a number of factors, principally, no doubt, to the individual vari-

*Reprinted from the *Archives of Surgery, 20:* 1021–1032, June, 1930.

*From the Johns Hopkins University and Hospital.

ations in the extent of involvement of the cervical muscles.

The etiology and pathology of spasmodic torticollis are not known. The explanation of the disease is beset with many theories which it is needless to repeat. None is satisfying. I have nothing to contribute to this phase of torticollis; my only strong conviction is that spasmodic torticollis is undoubtedly of organic and not of functional origin. Certainly in the group which I have observed there has been no greater evidence of a psychogenic background than in any other group of lesions subjected to surgical treatment. This, I am sure, is also Finney's strong impression in his larger series of cases. Even could a functional basis be entertained, certainly no treatment along these lines has offered results at all comparable with those obtained by the operation of Finney and Hughson.

AUTHOR'S OPERATION

Greatly impressed by the ultimate results of Finney's long struggle with torticollis, it occurred to me that much the same results could perhaps be obtained more simply and easily by attacking the same nerves centrally, i. e., alongside the spinal cord rather than at the periphery. Seven patients have been operated on by this method. Through a high cervical laminectomy in which the laminae of the upper three vertebrae are removed, the sensory and motor roots of the first, second and third cervical nerves are resected (Fig. 1). Until recently, both spinal accessory nerves were divided alongside the medulla, and the higher medullary branches were also divided independently with a tiny knife. But recently, this part of the operation has been discarded because it is not always possible to get the anteriormost filaments. It has, therefore, seemed better to divide the spinal accessory nerve intraspinally at the level of the foramen magnum only in order to expose better the first cervical motor branch. When the operation is concluded, the patient is turned on the back, and

through two small incisions in the neck the spinal accessory nerves are exposed and divided, and the central ends are reversed and sutured in this position to avoid regeneration. Separate section of the spinal accessory nerves requires only a few moments and is, I think, much better than intracranial division of these nerves at the jugular foramen as carried out by McKenzie in his unilateral procedure. To divide this nerve at the jugular foramen, an extra bony defect of considerable magnitude must be made in the occipital bone.

In earlier cases, the outcome of function of the sternomastoid and trapezius muscles was awaited, and at a later date the spinal accessory nerves were divided, when necessary, under local anesthesia. Although the upper three cervical sensory roots had been sacrificed and the cutaneous sensation abolished, there is usually some pain in exposing the spinal accessory nerves. Doubtless this pain is of sympathetic origin. It is quite variable, however, in one case there was no sensation throughout the dissection of both nerves; in another there was some but not much pain, and in a third the pain was quite severe throughout. In the latter case and two others, the postoperative function of the sternomastoid muscle had persisted on one side only.

Intradural division of the sensory and motor nerves is easy to perform and is practically devoid of danger to life or function. Loss of function in the affected muscles and in sensation of the skin are absolutely total and permanent, because neither the motor nor the sensory nerves can possibly regenerate.

I am not convinced that cutaneous anesthesia is of any value in determining the course of toricollis. In one of the earlier cases, the fourth, fifth and sixth sensory roots were also sectioned in a longer laminectomy. It has appeared necessary to divide the upper three sensory roots in order to have access to the motor roots. However, it is quite possible that sufficient retraction of the sensory roots may be obtain-

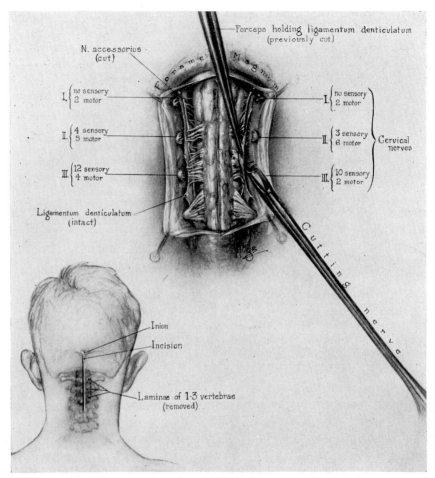

Fig. 1. Operative procedure by which the upper three cervical sensory and motor nerves are divided on both sides intraspinally. The instrument shown cutting the nerve was devised by Dr. Trimble. It is a combination nerve hook and scissors.

ed to permit sacrifice of the motor roots only. An effort will be made to determine the practicability of subsequent cases attaining this end. It will doubtless be difficult, because the sensory roots are short, run transversely and are directly over by the motor roots. The first cervical sensory root is variable and probably of little concern. In three of our cases it was absent on both sides, and in one case it was present on one side only.

Although the perverted function of chief concern in spasmodic torticollis is rotation of the head and neck, there may be associated strong flexion, extension or lateral traction. Practically all of the muscles per-

forming rotation when acting singly also produce flexion or extension when acting together. There are, in fact, few muscles attached to the head and neck which do not in some degree perform either flexion or extension in addition to rotation, or inversely they perform some degree of rotation in addition to the predominant function of flexion or extension. The exact amount of rotation at any time depends on the leverage obtainable by the attachment of the muscle to the head or neck. Muscles such as the longus colli, and the scalenus medius are too strictly median to permit of more than a minimal degree of rotation when acting singly. The larger semispinalis capitis (complexus) muscle, though mesially placed, has such a wide attachment to the skull that when acting singly a fair degree of rotation must result in addition to its predominant function of extension. Even the group of small suprahyoid muscles must play a minor role in rotation, flexion and extension of the head and neck.

In looking at the problem of torticollis from an anatomic standpoint, it is, therefore, evident that practically all the muscles of the head and neck must be taken into consideration. It is, of course, entirely unpractical to put them all out of commission in order to obtain a cure. Fortunately, this is unnecessary. Finney's proposal, which has proved so successful, has demonstrated that if the functions of the major rotators are eliminated, in whole or in part, the remaining muscles are for all practical purposes adequate to take care of the required movements of the head and neck, and by their training subsequent to the operation, the torticollis can be overcome entirely or nearly so. Fortunately, also, the empiric results of Finney and Hughson have shown that it is only necessary to divide the spinal accessory nerves and the upper three cervical motor roots to attain this.

In most cases, at first, the head seems a little insecure and lacking in support, but this deficit is gradually overcome when the intact or partially preserved muscles are

MUSCLES INVOLVED IN TORTICOLLIS

Group I:	Muscles	Nerve Supply	Function After Operation
Small muscles between the atlas, axis and the occiput	Rectus capitis anterior		
	Rectus capitis lateralis		
	Rectus capitis posterior major	First and second cervicals	Abolished
	Rectus capitis posterior minor		
	Obliquus capitis inferior		
	Obliquus capitis superior		
Group II:			
Larger muscles of neck (arranged in order of importance	Sternomastoid	Spinal accessory, second and third cervicals	Abolished
	Trapezius		Abolished
	Splenius capitis	Second and third cervicals	Abolished
	Splenius cervicis	Fourth to eighth cervicals	Unaffected
	Levator anguli scapulae	Third and fourth cervicals	Only partially lost
	Longissimus capitis	Second to fifth cervicals	Partially lost
	Longissimus cervicis	Fifth to eighth cervicals	Unaffected
	Semispinalis capitis (Complexus)	Second to eighth cervicals	Partially lost
	Longus capitis	First, second and third cervicals	Abolished
	Scalenus anterior	Second to seventh cervicals	Slightly affected
	Scalenus medius		
	Scalenus posterior		
Group III:			
	Digastric	Fifth and seventh cranials	Unaffected
Muscles of deglutition, many of which play a minor role in rotation of the head and some are affected by section of the cervical nerves	Stylohyoid	Seventh cranial	Unaffected
	Mylohyoid	Fifth cranial	Unaffected
	Geniohyoid	Twelfth cranial	Unaffected
	Geniohyoglossus	Twelfth cranial	Unaffected
	Hyoglossus	Twelfth cranial	Unaffected
	Thyrohyoid	Twelfth cranial	Unaffected
	Sternohyoid	First, second and third cervicals and twelfth cranial	Affected
	Omohyoid	First, second and third cervicals and twelfth cranial	Affected
	Sternothyroid	First, second and third cervicals and cranial	Affected

used as a result of training. After a few months scarcely any residual musclar loss can be detected, subjectively or objectively. A glance at the accompanying table will show exactly how far the removal of this nerve supply affects these muscles. The function of the entire group of small muscles between the occiput, atlas and axis is entirely abolished. The remaining muscles are entered in their probable importance as rotators of the head and neck. It will be seen that some of the larger muscles retain part—even a large part—of their nerve supply after the operation and therefore function in restricted degree. Of the more important muscles of rotation, only the functions of the sternomastoid and trapezius and splenius cervicis, the longissimus capitis and cervicis, the semispinalis capitis and the levator angulae scapulae and the group of scaleni muscles are affected only in part.

The retention of muscular function obviously explains the failure to obtain complete cure in all cases of torticollis; in some cases the result has fallen just short of complete cure and in practically all tremendous improvement has been secured. This statement is based on the results in the cases of Finney and Hughson and my own.

The limits of intraspinal section of the cervical nerves are reached by the operation here reported. Since the fourth cervical nerves give rise to the phrenic nerves and the remaining cervical nerves to the branchial plexus, they must be left intact. In those more refractory cases which retain some degree of imperfection after operation, it is possible to pick out more readily a single or small group of offending muscles and remove their nerve supply by a minor peripheral operation. In one of my cases the head is entirely quieted, but the levator angulae scapulae muscle continues to act. As this muscle receives its nerve supply from the third and fourth cervical nerves, its function is partly retained after the intraspinal operation. Improvement should be anticipated by peripheral division of the branch of the dorsalis scapulae

nerve.

REPORT OF CASES

Group 1: Cases in Which Cure is Reported.

CASE 1. A physician, aged forty, four years before being operated on for spasmodic torticollis, experienced a slight aching pain in the lower cervical vertebrae, which tended to be transmitted around both sides of the neck. At that time, she paid little attention to it. During this attack, the head began to draw to the right and backward, both steadily and spasmodically. Relief was obtained by allowing the head to hang over the edge of the bed. Over a period of two years, the symptoms gradually disappeared—the shaking first, the pain later. For a year and a half, she was quite well. Four months before operation, the head again began to draw to the left instead of to the right, as in the first attack. This state of powerful contraction of the rotator muscles persisted without signs of relenting. If the head was forcibly drawn to the other side, it returned in a few seconds. At times, there was numbness in both arms. Until two months before, there was a sore spot at the base of the neck on the left side.

Examination.—Aside from the local condition, there were no objective signs. The head was strongly drawn to the left and slightly backward. The sternomastoid muscles seemed to preponderate.

Operation.—April 11, 1928: The spinal accessory, the first, second and third motor roots and the upper five sensory roots (the first sensory root was absent on both sides) were sectioned intraspinally.

Subsequent division of the left spinal accessory nerve in the neck was necessary in this case.

Result.—After operation, there were minor jerkings of the head. These were gradually overcome during the next few months. Since then, the patient has been free from symptoms.

CASE 2. An army officer, aged forty, had torticollis, with turning of the head to the left, for the past two years. Previous to the onset of this trouble, he had had two or three attacks of "crick in the neck" each year. Sixteen years before, one of these attacks kept him bedfast for several days; four years before another equally severe attack was followed three days later by an excruciating "neuritis" in the left arm, lasting for a month. Throughout the duration of the torticollis, the head had drawn steadily to the left. He could counteract it only by holding the hand on the head. There were no spasms. The examination revealed nothing except the local condition. The head was drawn strongly to the left; efforts to correct this position caused the head to jerk. The left sternomastoid muscle was drawn like a tight cord across the neck.

Operation.—Nov. 26, 1928: Laminectomy of the upper three cervical vertebrae was performed. The spinal accessory nerves and the upper three cervical motor and sensory nerves on both sides were sectioned intradurally. Subsequent division of the spinal accessory nerves in the neck was unnecessary.

Result.—Immediately after the operation, the same tendency to draw the head to the left was evident at times; there was also some unsteadiness of the head. The patient spent several months abroad and returned free from all symptoms and has so remained to date. He has resumed his occupation.

CASE 3. An accountant, aged forty-seven, had been troubled with a stiff neck for eight years. One year earlier (nine years before operation), a dull pain persisted along the right side of the neck for several months, finally disappearing. One year before, his head began to draw to the right. Six months before, the head began to draw to the left and the left shoulder began to elevate.

The results of the examination were negative, except for the outspoken torticollis with rotation to the left.

Operation.—March 20, 1929: Cervical laminectomy was performed. The spinal accessory and the first, second and third sensory and motor roots on both sides were sectioned intradurally. Before the patient left the hospital, the left spinal accessory nerve was divided in the neck.

Results.—Unsteadiness of the head persisted in slight degree for two or three months, gradually abating. Immediately after operation, the patient complained of some subjective difficulty in swallowing, but aside from some tardiness there was no objective evidence of dysphagia. There has since been improvement but not entire correction.

CASE 4. A sparely nourished woman, aged sixty-one, presented a most remarkable picture of torticollis. When lying in bed, her head was quiet and could be maintained in any position, but immediately on assuming a sitting posture her head would snap with great violence. Although the most common direction of the sudden thrust of the head was to the right, it was frequently to the left; at other times, backward and forward. She was never able to swallow when sitting or standing unless the head was strongly supported. With the head at rest in the recumbent position, there was no dysphagia. She dated her trouble to a so-called nervous breakdown five years before. She had been weak and nervous and unable to carry on any longer. Two months later, pain and jerking appeared in the neck. It was intermittent at first, but recently had become incessant when she was not in a recumbent position.

Operation.—Oct. 31, 1929: Tribromethyl-alcohol anesthesia was administered by rectum. Both spinal accessory nerves and the first, second and third sensory and motor nerves on both sides were sectioned intraspinally. Two weeks later, both spinal accessory nerves were divided without any anesthesia and absolutely without pain, except when the spinal accessory nerves were handled. This pain was referred to the ear and angle of the jaw.

Result.—The patient remained in the hospital one month. She was practically devoid of involuntary movements of the head or neck at all times after the operation.

CASE 5. A fairly well nourished man, aged fifty-nine, referred the onset of his trouble to a spell of constant pressure and stiffness in the back of the neck. This occurred four years before operation for torticollis, lasted six months and disappeared completely. Soon thereafter, sudden attacks of intermittent spasms of the muscles of the neck caused rotation of the head to the right every two or three minutes. Gradually, the attacks fused and strong rotation of the head persisted to the right. Shortly after the onset of his trouble, he had difficulty in swallowing. This became so severe that he could scarcely take any nourishment, and in two weeks he lost twenty pounds (9 Kg.). Without apparent reason, swallowing gradually improved and finally became normal. It was, however, always necessary to steady the head with his hand in order to permit swallowing. The contractions were said to cease during sleep, but the rotation of the head to the right persisted. The platysma contracted during the attacks, and athetoid-like movements of the hands and arms participated.

Operation.—April 20, 1925: The spinal accessory, first, second and third cervical and sensory nerves on both sides were sectioned intradurally.

This was one of the most severe cases of the series. Three months before this operation, the patient had been operated on by Dr. Finney. He seemed so little improved that at Dr. Finney's suggestion I cut the nerves intradurally for the first time. On discharge from the hospital three weeks later, the patient was considerably improved though far from well. I have not seen him since then and was fully prepared to be told, in response to an inquiry, that he was still affected. The following excerpts from his letter (Dec. 1, 1929), however, lead me to include him with the patients cured: "I have been doing very well. My neck does not pull or jerk any more. . . . I weigh 143 lbs.; the best I ever weighed was 153."

This case well emphasizes the importance of time and practice in overcoming the traces of the malady which still linger after the operation. I am, therefore, not at all sure that the same results might not well have followed Dr. Finney's operation had he been given the advantage of the same period of time for recovery.

Group 2: Cases in Which Great Improvement but Not Cure Is Reported

CASE 6. A school teacher, aged forty-one, had severe tension of the head to the left and downward. Although the head was always strongly rotated, there were frequent superimposed spasms. Voluntary efforts increased the unsteadiness of the head. She dated her trouble to a "nervous strain" a year before. Soon thereafter, the head began pulling to the left. Recently, the character of the attacks changed. The head drew to the right and backward. A rest cure of eight weeks seemed to bring some improvement, but it was slight and very transient. A brace between the head and shoulders was worn for two weeks without appreciable benefit. Contractions were worse when she was lying down. Her voice was greatly affected for some time, and she was able to talk only in a whisper for several weeks.

Operation.—Nov. 14, 1928: Both spinal accessory, the first, second and third cervical sensory and the motor roots on both sides were sectioned intradurally. Three months later, with the patient under local anesthesia, the right spinal accessory nerve was divided in the neck. Although the skin was anesthetic from the loss of sensory nerves, it was necessary to use procaine hydrochloride freely in the deeper approach to the spinal accessory nerve. Section of this nerve produced a sharp deep pain in the ear and at the angle of the lower jaw.

Result.—The head is perfectly still, but the neck continues to draw to the left and to rotate slightly. The muscle involved is undoubtedly the levator anguli scapulae; perhaps the scaleni are also involved. The end-result of this strong muscular pull is a curvature of the neck. The patient has subconsciously overcome the curvature by a counter pull and holds the head erect without conscious effort. She feels so well that she is unwilling, for the present at least, to have the nerve to the levator anguli scapulae muscle divided in the neck. She is again teaching school. Her voice, though still not normal, is greatly improved and carries without apparent effort.

CASE 7. A sparely nourished man, aged fifty-four, a bookkeeper and accountant, first noticed jerking of the right shoulder upward and forward when writing two years before operation. Sixteen months before, his head drew downward and to the right, remaining there all day. A few days later this contraction was repeated, and since that time the head had remained almost constantly down in that position when the patient sat or stood. Partial relaxation occurred when he was in a recumbent position. Jerking developed only when he attempted to correct the position of the head. Relief was obtained when his mind was diverted; it was intensified by nervous strain.

Operation.—Oct. 9, 1928: The spinal accessory, first, second and third cervical sensory and motor roots on both sides were sectioned intradurally. Ten days later, with the patient under local anesthesia, the right spinal accessory nerve was divided in the neck.

Result.—This is the only case in the series in which unsatisfactory results were obtained. Objectively, the patient is tremendously improved, certainly more than the patient in the preceding case. Indeed, with very little effort on his part, the slight rotation which exists could easily be overcome by voluntary effort. He is the only psychoneurotic patient of the series. His chief complaints now are sensory rather than motor, the most serious trouble being a sensation of a steel bar that is constantly separating his shoulders and holding them apart. Pains were constantly present in the neck and head. Being most introspective, he is continually striving to find an underlying cause for his symptoms, experimenting with medicines and seeking the advice of numerous physicians. A background of serious family and financial troubles has added greatly to the somatic psychosis. He cannot be induced to make any effort to readjust himself to his family or to renew his work.

RESULTS OF THE OPERATION

Of the eight patients included in this effort, five appear to be practically cured; two fall short of a complete cure but are greatly improved; the remaining one is not living. In four of the cases in which cure has been recorded, the patients have been personally examined from time to time since the operation. The lapse of time since the operation is twenty, fourteen, nine and two months. These patients have consistently improved since the operation, and without exception have had no recessions. All patients, with the exception of the one operated on recently, have returned to work. Perhaps it is not justifiable to include the last case in which only two months have elapsed since operation. My reasons for doing so are that this case was the most severe in the group, and the patient was more perfectly relieved immediately after the operation than any of the others. The fifth patient considered as cured has not been seen since the operation. The inclusion of this case in the group in which cure was obtained is based on the patient's letter in which he stated that his head no longer jerks and draws. He was the first patient operated on by this method.

The two patients who were not completely cured are greatly improved. Perhaps a conservative estimate of the improvement in these patients, whom I have observed from time to time, would be about 85 per cent. The degree of objective improvement is about the same in each instance, and in each the levator anguli scapulae muscles (possibly the scaleni are partly at fault) seem to be the cause of failure to obtain complete cure.

There has been no operative mortality in the series. The single death occurred three weeks after operation, and was due to pneumonia contracted ten days after the operation. During the first ten days the patient was entirely free from fever, a fact which eliminates the anesthetic as the cause. He was a very bad surgical risk, having auricular fibrillation and advanced myocarditis, but he was so miserable that we were prevailed on to accede to his urgent wish for the operation.

In only one instance has there been entire freedom from minor jerking or drawing of the head immediately after the operation. The movements, however, lack the tremendous force of the preoperative state. Nevertheless, the mere existence of the same muscular effects after the operation will have a severe psychologic effect on patient and surgeon alike if its existence and import are not realized. The patient should be prepared in advance to know that the resultant cure will not be instantaneous. After convalescence from the operation, the patient should be induced, if possible, to spend from three to six months in rest and in graduated exercises which will strengthen the muscles of the neck. Finney and Hughson emphasized the importance of the postoperative period of training in eliminating the last traces of muscular incoordination.

Mention should be made of a minor degree of dysphagia which was noticed in two of my patients. It is noticed principally in swallowing solids. The act of deglutition is always possible, but more effort is required. Since dysphagia was not present before operation, it must be due to loss of the nerve supply to some muscle of deglutition. But since this disturbance was absent in five cases, one is led to wonder whether the muscles involved may not have a variable nerve supply. The table (group III) showing the muscles involved in deglutition and their nerve supply indicates that three of the infrahyoid muscles—sternohyoid, sternothyroid and omohyoid—partially lose their nerve supply by the operation. Each of these muscles also receives a partial nerve supply from the hypoglossal nerve, i. e., through the ansa hypoglossi, and this remains intact. The remaining infrahyoid muscle—the thyrohoid—is supplied exclusively by the hypoglossal nerve. The partial loss of the infrahyoid muscles leaves the many suprahyoid muscles, to a degree, unopposed. The varying degree of nerve supply to the infrahyoid muscle, i. e., whether from the cervical or the hypoglossal nerves, probably explains the difference in results with respect to deglutition.

DIFFERENCE BETWEEN THE AUTHOR'S OPERATION AND THAT OF FINNEY AND HUGHSON

In the operation of Finney and Hughson, only the posterior divisions of the first three cervical nerves are divided, the anterior divisions being inaccessible. By their operation, therefore, the following muscles of rotation remain intact or in part as indicated: (1) rectus capitis lateralis; (2) rectus capitis anterior; (3) longus capitis; (4) sternomastoid (branches from the second and third cervicals) ; (5) trapezius (branch from the third cervical) ; (6) levator anguli scapulae (branch from the third cervical) .

I am not sure that the muscles retained by their operation and sacrificed by mine will eventually make any difference in the ultimate result. It is my impression that the principal difference, if any, would lie in the partial preservation of function in the more powerful muscles, i. e., the sternomastoid, trapezius and levator anguli scapulae muscles.

SUMMARY AND CONCLUSIONS

1. An operative procedure is presented for treatment in spasmodic torticollis. The first, second and third sensory and motor roots on both sides are sectioned intradurally, and the spinal accessory nerves are divided peripherally, small incisions in the neck being used.

2. Eight patients have been operated on by this method with the following results: (*a*) five appear to be cured; (*b*) two are greatly improved but not cured; (*c*) one died of pneumonia (not contracted at the time of operation) three weeks after operation.

3. Torticollis is cured by removing the nerve supply from the major muscles of rotation. The remaining muscles will overcome in time and by training the lost motor function and in most instances any remaining traces of the condition.

NOTE.—Since this article was submitted for publication I have sectioned the upper three motor cervical nerves on both sides without sacrificing any sensory fibers. There was no difficulty in avoiding the sensory roots, and the preservation of sensation should make a worth while improvement in the procedure.

REFERENCES

[1]Keen, W. W.: A New Operation for Spasmodic Wry Neck–Namely Division or Exsection of the Nerves Supplying the Posterior Rotator Muscles of the Head. *Ann. Surg.,* 13:44, 1891.

[2]Taylor, A. S., in Johnson: *Surgical Therapeutics.* 1915, vol. 1, p. 525.

[3]McKenzie, Kenneth G.: Intrameningeal Division of the Spinal Accessory and Roots of the Upper Cervical Nerves for the Treatment of Spasmodic Torticollis. *Surg., Gynec. & Obst.,* 39: 5, 1924.

[4]Finney and Hughson: Spasmodic Torticollis. *Ann. . .Surg., 81:* 255, 1925.

XXXVIII

CHANGES IN OUR CONCEPTIONS OF LOCALIZATION OF CERTAIN FUNCTIONS IN THE BRAIN *

From a series of cerebral operations of varying character several conclusions have been reached:

1. It is possible to remove all of the right cerebral hemisphere above the basal ganglia with no appreciable disturbance of mentality; this procedure has been carried out on several occasions for the removal of extensive tumors in the right hemisphere.

2. On one occasion both frontal lobes have been completely extirpated for the treatment of a bilateral frontal brain tumor, and following this there has been no appreciable disturbance of mentality. The patient is perfectly oriented as to time, place and person; the memory is unimpaired; he reads, writes and conducts mathematical tests accurately; his conversation is seemingly perfectly normal.

Furthermore, by the excision in other cases of the left occipital lobe and of the lower third of the left temporal lobe, we can be sure that none of these regions are responsible for intelligence. The intellect, therefore, is concerned with the remaining portion of the left cerebral hemisphere and is doubtless closely related to the speech mechanism.

3. It has been found after ligation of the anterior cerebral artery on the left side that consciousness is completely and forever lost. This does not result when the same vessel is ligated on the right side. There is, therefore, within the limits of the distribution of this vessel an area specifically concerned with consciousness. The same result follows when this vessel is occluded at the middle of the corpus callosum, indicating that the seat of consciousness is posterior to this point in the vessel.

4. The entire body of the corpus callosum may be split in the midline without any appreciable disturbance of function. This structure is, therefore, eliminated from participation in the important functions which hitherto have been ascribed to it.

*Reprinted from *The American Journal of Physiology, 93:* 2, June, 1930.

XXXIX

THE COURSE OF THE NERVE FIBERS TRANSMITTING
SENSATION OF TASTE *

Dean Lewis, M.D. and Walter E. Dandy, M.D.

In 1822, Francois Magendie after dividing the trigeminal nerve within the skull in dogs made the following statement: "The question of taste, formerly so obscure, no longer presents any difficulty. Physiological experiments and pathological observations have solved it. If the trunk of the fifth nerve is divided in the skull, taste is completely lost, even for sour and bitter substances. This total loss of taste has been noticed in persons in whom the fifth nerve has been compressed or altered." The problem of taste was not, however, to be settled so simply and unequivocally.

As it has been impossible to expose the nerves concerned in the mediation of taste sensations throughout their courses, indirect methods of study, such as the following, have been employed: (1) clinical studies checked by pathologic observations, (2) experiments on animals and (3) postoperative observations on human beings. From the evidence which has accumulated, one theory remains constant: the role of the chorda tympani in the transmission of sensations of taste. All observers admit that it does transmit these sensations, but there is no agreement as to the route of the taste fibers in this nerve from the terminal sense organs to the central nucleus.

At the time Magendie performed his experiments, little was known concerning the function of the chorda tympani. A few years before, Bellingeri (1818) described it as the sensory part of the facial nerve and assumed that it transmitted sensations

of taste to the brain. The significance of this assumption seemed, however, to have been little appreciated until Claude Bernard, Magendie's successor, made his contributions to the studies of taste. Montault, a pupil of Romberg, and Bernard presented a thesis (1831), in which three cases of facial paralysis accompanied by loss of taste over the anterior two thirds of the tongue were reported. In 1843, Bernard reported four more cases, in which the facial palsy was caused by acute infections and fractures. He noted that the general sensitivity of the side involved was not affected and that taste lost during the paralysis returned with recovery. Section of the nerve, earlier performed by Magendie, was repeated by Bernard with a knife especially designed for this purpose by Magendie. After division of both facial nerves intracranially he noted loss of taste similar to that which followed section of the chorda tympani in animals. He believed, however, that the loss was not complete, but that the acuity of taste sensation was markedly lessened.

Bernard must have tested for loss of taste after section of the trigeminal nerves in dogs—an experiment frequently made by him—but there is no mention of any such tests in his protocols. He was particularly interested in the trophic changes that followed section of the fifth nerves and these are frequently mentioned, but curiously enough no mention is made concerning the effect of such division on taste. He accepted the views of Magendie, his preceptor, that the fifth nerve transmitted sensations of taste, and sought to explain

*Reprinted from the *Archives of Surgery, 12:* 249–288, August, 1930.

alterations in taste following division of the facial nerve as due to lack of "motor control" over the taste buds. He stated, "The chorda tympani should be considered a motor nerve, which by its action upon the papillary lingual tissue regulates and renders instantaneous the transference of a rapid stimulus to the sensory nerve which conducts it to its center." When paralyzed, it affects taste, "not as a nerve of sensation, but by a special inertia of the gustatory organs."

It was not then generally conceded that the chorda tympani played an important role in the conduction of sensations of taste. Tests which confirmed this view were shortly to be made. Duchenne (1850) and Blau (1879) took advantage of fistulas of the middle ear to make observations on the function of the chorda tympani. They found that by stimulating the internal wall of the tympanum by irrigations, cautery and faradic current, they could produce sensations of taste in the anterior two thirds of the tongue, but not in the posterior one third. At times the sensation so produced was sweet, at other times sour, while at still other times a prickly sensation was produced. Blau stated that Troltsch had previously produced much the same sensations by pinching granulations over the chorda tympani on the internal wall of a chronically inflamed middle ear. Since these experiments were made, ample opportunity has been afforded to study the effect on taste of division of the chorda tympani nerve during operations on the mastoid and middle ear.

Guzot and Cazalis (1839) were credited by Luciani, and Biffi and Morganti (1846) by Lussana with discovering that the chorda tympani carries taste sensations from the anterior two thirds of the tongue only and that the glossopharyngeal nerve serves the same function for the posterior one third. As previously stated, however, Montault appears to have called attention to this dual supply several years before (1831).

It is now generally accepted that the chorda tympani conducts all taste fibers from the anterior two thirds of the tongue, but there is no unanimity of opinion as to the path that these fibers pursue from the geniculate ganglion in the facial to their central nucleus. The attempts to determine the course of these fibers may be assigned to three periods which, in a general way, confirm to three types of investigation. The first period, one in which animal experimentation predominates, covers the first two thirds of the nineteenth century. This period was dominated by Magendie, Bernard and Schiff. The second period, largely one of clinical and pathologic studies, supplemented now and again by animal experimentation, covers the remaining one third of the nineteenth century. The third period, beginning a few years before the close of the nineteenth century and extending to and including the present time, is concerned with tests on patients in whom the cranial nerves have been divided intentionally for the relief of painful tic or some definite lesion.

Several different pathways of the fibers of the chorda tympani from the geniculate ganglion of the facial nerve to the central nucleus have been proposed. These proposals have been based on experimental, clinical and operative observations.

PATHWAY PROPOSED BY SCHIFF

Schiff (1867) made a radical departure from the teachings of Magendie and Bernard. We have already noted that it had been conceded by most observers that the chorda tympani contained all the fibers of taste from the anterior two thirds of the tongue. Schiff made the following experiments:

1. He cut the fifth nerve in animals between the brain stem and the gasserian ganglion and found that the sense of taste was lost. He found that if he cut the facial nerve at the pons, taste was not affected, and therefore concluded that the sensations of taste must pass to the brain

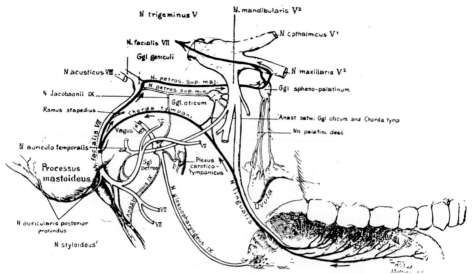

Fig. 1 Pathway for taste fibers suggested by Schiff.

through the sensory part of the fifth nerve.

2. He found that when he cut the facial nerve at the geniculate ganglion or distal to it the sense of taste was destroyed, and concluded that these fibers must be deflected to the fifth nerve at the geniculate ganglion.

3. He then cut the third branch of the fifth nerve at the foramen ovale without influencing taste, but found that taste was lost when the second branch of the fifth nerve was divided at the foramen rotundum.

He concluded, therefore, that the fibers of the chorda tympani which carried sensations of taste passed by way of the great superficial petrosal nerve from the geniculate ganglion to the sphenopalatine ganglion, by way of the second division of the fifth nerve to the gasserian ganglion and then through the sensory root to its central nucleus.

The validity of Schiff's experiments and the entire conception of the course of the taste fibers suggested by him were quickly questioned. His results also differed markedly from those of Claude Bernard, who found that taste was profoundly changed after intracranial division of the facial nerve.

However, some early clinical reports appeared to support Schiff's views. Erb reported a case in which the second branch of the fifth nerve was destroyed by a "mass of inflammatory" tissue; Senator (1882) and Salomonsohn (1886), cases in which the nerve was involved in a "chronic inflammatory mass in the middle fossa," and Heusner (1886), another case of the tuberculous caries of the bone (but there was no autopsy). In these cases taste was lost over the anterior two thirds of the tongue. These lesions were too diffuse to warrant the conclusions that were made concerning the course of the nerves involved in taste.

For a long time, Schiff had considered it probable that not all the taste fibers passed through the chorda tympani, but that part of the fibers at least passed through the lingual. He thought, however, that these fibers did not pass directly to the gasserian ganglion, but that they were deflected to the tic ganglion, then to the geniculate by the lesser superficial petrosal nerve and back again to Meckel's ganglion by way of the great superficial petrosal nerve, and by branches from Meckel's ganglion to the second branch of the trigeminus.

LUSSANA'S OBSERVATIONS AND PATHWAY PROPOSED BY HIM

Two years after Schiff suggested the route just described, Lussana (1869) made an impressive contribution to the study of the course of the fibers of taste. He assembled a well selected group of clinical cases, and from a study of these arrived at a new conception of the course of taste fibers. He concluded that the nervus intermedius (Wrisberg) was the only nerve which transmitted sensations of taste from the anterior two thirds of the tongue.

Lussana's first case was seen with his associate Renzi. The patient had complete loss of sensation over half of the face and tongue (fifth nerve), with no impairment of taste. At autopsy the seventh and eighth nerves were found intact, the fifth destroyed.

His second patient had facial neuralgia. The lingual nerve, including the chorda tympani, had been divided by an operation—"the first time such a procedure had been done in the history of science." Taste was completely lost over the anterior two thirds of the tongue, but pain sense was not affected. This experiment was used by him to eliminate the glossopharyn-geal nerve as the nerve of taste for the anterior two thirds of the tongue.

His last and crucial case was again "the only case of its kind in science." In this patient the chorda tympani had been divided, and there had been no injury to the fifth nerve. The patient, a man aged 48, had gradually become deaf in one ear, and in seeking relief had fallen into the hands of a charlatan who, in the presence of many onlookers, attempted to demonstrate his skill. Three times a long, narrow lance was thrust deeply into the ear. The patient fell to the floor in great agony, a convulsion followed and hemiplegia developed. The charlatan fled in haste from the angry mob. Lussana found this patient two years later. The paralysis had cleared, sensation in the face was normal, but taste for the anterior two thirds of the tongue was still lost. The chorda tympani had been divided.

Lussana supported his unique clinical observations by experiments on animals. After cutting the inferior maxillary nerve above the entrance of the chorda tympani into the lingual or intracranially, he found no alteration in taste. When the chorda tympani was divided in the tympanum,

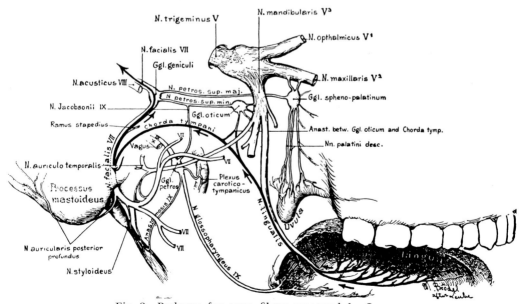

Fig. 2 Pathway for taste fibers suggested by Lussana.

taste was permanently lost. Three years later he published additional data supporting his original contention and referred to the "remarkable" earlier work of Stich (1851), who had collected from the literature many cases of facial paralysis accompanied by loss of taste. Lussana's earlier paper provoked much adverse criticism on the part of Schiff, Vulpian and Vizioli.

PATHWAY SUGGESTED BY ZIEHL

Ziehl (1889) proposed still another pathway, thus adding to the confusion which already existed. He too believed that the taste fibers entered the brain by way of the fifth nerve, but thought that they passed by way of the third branch into the gasserian ganglion instead of by the second as Schiff had suggested. This course was based on the observations of Romberg, confirmed by autopsy which was "performed by Henle in the presence of Johannes Muller." In this case taste was lost over the anterior two thirds of the tongue on one side, and at autopsy a mass of granulation tissue was found which compressed the third division of the fifth nerve at the foramen ovale. Ziehl believed that the observations in this case indicated that sensations of taste were carried to the brain

by the third branch of the fifth rather than by the second as thought by Schiff and Erb. Accepting the view that all taste fibers pass up the chorda tympani to the geniculate ganglion, he assumed that they then passed by way of the small superficial petrosal nerve directly or by detour through the tympanic plexus, probably in both ways, to the otic ganglion and then by its communicating branches to the third division of the fifth through the gasserian ganglion to the brain.

Many of Ziehl's views were based on the none too definite results of animal experiments made by Vulpian, who claimed that taste was lost after the fifth nerve was divided intracranially, but was unaffected when the seventh and ninth were divided within the skull.

Ziehl's theory was the one that later become most generally accepted. It received support from a new line of evidence: the effects on taste of operations on the gasserian ganglion performed by Krause. Ziehl's theory also seemed to be supported by a case reported by Ferguson, who found at autopsy in a patient in whom taste to the anterior two thirds of the tongue had been lost, an exostosis which compressed the vidian nerve.

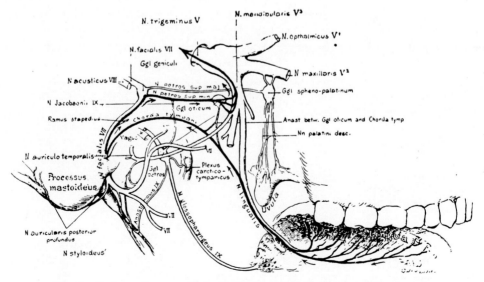

Fig. 3 Pathway for taste fibers by Ziehl, and later supported by the operative results of Krause on human subjects.

Gowers (1885 and 1897) ardently championed the theory that the fifth nerve was the pathway, without indicating preference for either the second or third branch. He not only accepted the circuitous pathway proposed by Schiff, but, as the result of the examination of three patients in each of whom taste was lost over the entire half of the tongue, was convinced that "taste impressions reach the brain solely by the roots of the fifth nerve and that the doctrine that the roots of the glossopharyngeal nerve had anything to do with taste is a curious myth, due to too wide an induction from certain anatomic facts and from dubious experiments on animals." And again, "It is possible that nerve fibers for taste on the back of the tongue may be distributed with the ninth nerve, reaching there from the otic ganglion of the trigeminus by the small petrosal nerve and the tympanic plexus. This course, I confess, seems strangely circuitous, but it is scarcely more circuitous than that which is certainly taken by taste fibers of the front of the tongue." Although Gowers' publications were twelve years apart, his views on taste remained unchanged. However, despite Gowers' standing in the medical world, his claim that the fifth nerve conducted taste fibers from the posterior one third of the tongue gained few supporters. Too many cases were observed which proved that his conclusions were incorrect.

Dixon strongly opposed the views of Gowers and became the outstanding champion of the route through the facial nerve. Dixon's impressions are summed up in the following quotation: "We must remember that we are not forced to accept these complicated courses (for taste innervation) for the geniculate ganglion is the homologue of the spinal ganglia just as is the gasserian of the fifth nerve. The nervus intermedius is considered to be continuous with the chorda tympani and so would represent a continuation of these fibers to the ganglion cells of the brain." He also emphasized the fact that in the human embryo, the chorda tympani is a direct branch of the facial nerve and in the early stages of development is not connected with the lingual nerve.

PATHWAY FOR TASTE THROUGH THE GLOSSOPHARYNGEAL NERVE

At least as early as 1834, the glossopharyngeal nerve was considered the nerve of taste for the entire tongue (Lussana). Biffi and Morganti (1846) determined the lingual supply to the anterior two thirds of the tongue and the glossopharyngeal supply to the posterior third. As previously indicated, Montault had already anticipated these observations. Despite the support favoring the fifth or seventh nerve supply for taste, there are those who believe that other evidence indicates that the ninth nerve supplies taste fibers to the entire tongue.

Eulenburg (1871), after obtaining negative results following section of the fifth and seventh nerve in animals, suggested that there must be a communication between the geniculate ganglion and the ninth nerve through the small superficial petrosal nerve, the tympanic plexus and Jacobson's nerve. Landois (1880) also taught that taste was carried by the ninth nerve, possibly by the route suggested by Eulenburg or by a branch passing directly from the facial nerve in the fallopian canal to the ganglion petrosum of the glossopharyngeal nerve.

Lehmann (1884) reported a cerebral injury with paralysis of the ninth nerve and none of the fifth; taste was reported lost over the entire one half of the tongue. Luciani (1915) in his textbook of physiology supported the glossopharyngeal theory. Recently Doyle (1923) cited a case in which taste was lost over one half of the tongue after peripheral avulsion of the ninth nerve, but the sensory root of the fifth had previously been avulsed. Although this case is cited to support the glossopharyngeal theory of taste, taste was not

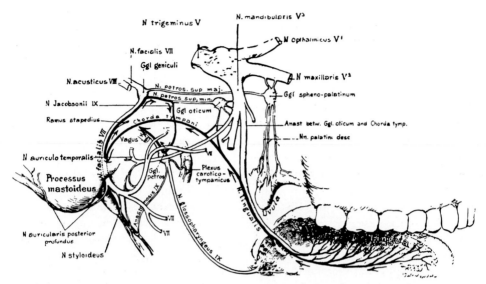

Fig. 4   Pathway for taste fibers suggested by Eulenburg and Landois.

tested either before or after division of the trigeminus or before avulsion of the glossopharyngeal nerve. This evidence is therefore inconclusive as far as the anterior two thirds of the tongue is concerned.

It can readily be understood from the foregoing comment that tumors, inflammatory lesions, and cranial injuries have almost always affected more than one nerve and have therefore rendered any conclusions untrustworthy. The results of animal experimentation are so variable that no conclusions can be drawn.

OPERATIONS ON PATIENTS

With the development of cranial surgery, a better opportunity was afforded to determine the effects on taste of section of the different cranial nerves. Krause (1895) divided intracranially the second division of the fifth nerve. Taste was not affected. Krause's observations did not support the views of Schiff and Erb, for taste was not affected when the great superficial petrosal and vidian nerves and the branches of the sphenopalatine ganglion were divided. Later the ganglion was removed from the same patient, and taste was lost. It seems natural, therefore, that Krause should have concluded that the third branch of the fifth

conducted the fibers of taste.

Krause's work was quickly criticised by Dixon, who believed that the results were due to injury of the geniculate ganglion when the dura was stripped from the floor of the middle fossa. Dixon believed that both petrosal nerves might be stripped from their bed during exposure of the ganglion and that this ganglion might be pulled on or injured. Weakness of the facial muscles, even paralysis of these muscles in Krause's cases, seemed to support this contention.

Other surgeons began to report cases but with varying conclusions. Tiffany (1894) reported loss of taste after division of the second and third branches of the fifth nerve. Finney and Thomas reported loss of taste after extirpation of the ganglion in one case; in another, taste was preserved. Gowers cited the observations made on five patients operated on by Sir Victor Horsley and Ballance. Taste was lost in four and preserved in one. Horsley's results and views much like those of Krause. Cushing in 1903 reported twenty cases of operation on the gasserian ganglion. In four, taste was impaired. Davies (1907) added twenty cases, the results almost duplicating those of Cushing. Taste was lost in one case, impaired in three and unchanged in sixteen. Krause later reported six cases, taste being lost in two, impaired in three and unchanged in one. Krause finally came to the conclusion, because of the variable observations, that taste fibers must pursue different courses in different individuals, and Oppenheim, Germany's leading neurologist at that time, concurred in this view. Harris (1926) published a series of eighty-six cases of tic douloureux in which alcohol had been injected into the third division of the fifth nerve or the gasserian ganglion. Taste was lost in eighty of these. Such an injection probably produces a more localized lesion than operations on the gasserian ganglion when approached in the usual way through the middle fossa. He was surprised to find, as were others before him, that although in a few cases taste was totally lost at first, it sometimes returned later, even when the tongue remained anesthetic. The objection can no longer be raised in these cases that the geniculate ganglion was injured in stripping the dura from the middle fossa. Harris, like Krause, expressed the belief that taste fibers have different courses in different persons, but that the fifth nerve is the principal nerve of taste. In explanation of these differences, he cited the work of Nageotte, in which it was shown that the fifth and sensory parts of the seventh and ninth nerves have a common nucleus which is continuous caudalward.

MATERIAL OF PRESENT STUDY

We have presumed to add to the lengthy literature on the course of taste fibers because we have material which has hitherto been unavailable. Pure isolated divisions of the fifth, seventh and ninth nerves have been performed subtentorially for the relief of surgical conditions. Combined division of the fifth and seventh has also been performed. The fifth nerve has been divided intracranially at the pons for trigeminal neuralgia. The subtentorial operation has the advantage of not disturbing the petrosal nerves or geniculate ganglion or any other cranial nerve. Division of the seventh nerve alone has occurred during the removal of tumors of the cerebellopontine angle in a method recently described. As yet it has been impossible to extirpate these tumors without dividing the seventh nerve. As the fifth and ninth nerves are usually pushed aside by these tumors, they may not be injured when the tumor is removed. There is also an instance of a pure lesion of the seventh nerve which was accidentally injured when the auditory nerve was divided for relief from Meniere's disease. There was no disturbance of the fifth or ninth nerve in this case.

NECESSITY OF CONTROL OBSERVATIONS

Before presenting our evidence concerning the course of taste fibers derived from cases in which pure isolated lesions have been produced, it may be well to state something concerning (1) the methods of testing taste and (2) the necessity of making control tests. An appreciation of these two things may explain to some extent the divergent views held by different observers.

For a long time we were unable to understand why members of our own staff obtained different results. Three examiners would obtain results as variable as those reported in the literature. Even in a patient whose taste was found to be lost by one examiner, normal or subnormal taste would be found by another. Different results may be obtained for the following reasons: 1. Patients confuse touch and taste. 2. When patients are allowed to withdraw the tongue, taste will quickly be perceived by oral and posterior glossal taste buds. 3. At times, saliva coming in contact with the solution would carry the substance to be tested to the back of the mouth. 4. Patients are prone to guess, particularly when sensation is present. 5. By the sense of smell, patients may tell before tasting whether the solutions offered them are acid or bitter; solutions should therefore be used which do not stimulate smell.

In testing taste, the tip of the tongue should be covered with gauze and held by the examiner until the taste has been accurately identified in one of two ways: (1) The patient points to one of four tastes printed on a card, or (2) he nods when the examiner mentions the taste. The tongue is not to be drawn into the mouth until the taste has been definitely determined. If this method of examination is employed, the results will be accurate and uniform. Preoperative observations should be made as control experiments. Deviations from the normal occur frequently and either unilaterally or bilaterally. Therefore unless taste is carefully tested before the operation, erroneous conclusions may be drawn. The acuity of taste varies considerably in different patients, as is indicated by the following observations.

CASES 1 AND 2. Two patients, both men, suffered with tic douloureux. Examination showed that neither had taste perception over the anterior two thirds of the tongue on either side when tested before operation.

CASE 3. A man, aged forty, had a painful malignant ulcer of the tongue. He had no taste perception over the anterior two thirds of the tongue (either side) when tested before the operation.

CASE 4. A man, aged fifty-six, had had the gasserian ganglion removed seven years by the temporal route before the test was made. This patient had no sensation of taste on the anterior two thirds of the tongue on either side.

CASE 5. A man, aged sixty-five, entered the hospital for treatment for tic douloureux. When tested for taste perception before operation, it was found to be absent on the side of the neuralgia, but normal on the other side (anterior two-thirds). No cause for loss of taste on the affected side could be determined.

CASES 6 AND 7. A man, aged forty-nine, and a woman, aged sixty-two, were afflicted with tic douloureux. Before operation neither sugar nor salt could be detected on either side of the tongue (anterior two-thirds). Acid and bitter substances could be tasted, but perception was delayed.

CASE 8. A woman, aged forty-five, was afflicted with tic douloureux. She could not taste sweet or bitter substances. She could taste sour substances after thirteen seconds and salt after twenty-three seconds. The observations on both sides were identical.

CASE 9. A man, aged sixty, with tic douloureux could not taste sugar, salt or bitter substances on either side of the tongue (anterior two-thirds). Sour substances could be tasted after eight seconds.

CASE 10. A man, aged sixty-three, afflicted with tic douloureux could not taste sugar or bitter substances. Perception of salt and sour were present but were delayed eight seconds.

It will be seen from the observations given that it cannot be assumed that taste is normal in any person. Each one should be tested before operation, for the incidence of defective taste is high and the character of the change is variable. Although loss or diminution in acuity of taste is usually symmetrical, this is not necessarily so, as is indicated by the hemigeusia in case 5. Had not taste been tested before operation in this case, section of the sensory root of the fifth nerve would have been regarded as the cause of the loss of taste.

There is still another possible cause of error. If alcoholic solutions of bitter substances are used diffusion occurs, and after a minute or more, taste may be perceived on the other side. The patient may or may not know on which side the taste perception occurs.

In all of our observations one minute has been the upper limit for taste determinations. Substances not detected within this time will not be appreciated at all.

PURE EXPERIMENTAL NERVE LESIONS

The material has been grouped under the following headings: (1) pure fifth nerve lesions, (2) pure ninth nerve lesions, (3) combined pure fifth and ninth nerve lesions, (4) pure seventh nerve lesions (intracranial) and (5) pure seventh nerve lesions (peripheral).

Group 1: Pure Fifth Nerve Lesions

CASE 1. A sparely nourished woman, aged sixty-three, sought relief from trigeminal neuralgia. Pain like a pin prick began eleven years before examination, in the right side of the face below the eye. At first the attacks were not severe, but gradually they became more so and occurred more frequently; six years before, they became excruciating. They were induced by eating drinking or touching the lip. Four injections of alcohol afforded relief over varying periods of time. The neurologic examination gave entirely negative results. Gustatory tests were not made before operation.

On Sept. 17, 1927, the right sensory root was divided by the subcerebellar route. Total anesthesia resulted for all forms of sensation in the domain of the trigeminal nerve.

Five months after operation, the results obtained by one of us (W. E. D.) in tests for taste were:

	Right (Affected Side), Seconds	Left Side
Salt	0	40 seconds
Acid	15	Instantly
Bitter	10	5 seconds
Sugar	0	0 seconds

CASE 2. A rather obese woman, aged seventy, sought relief for tic douloureux on the right side. Two years before consulting us she experienced sudden attacks of sharp pain, like needle pricks, in the right molar region. The pains became progressively more severe and more frequent. Gradually also the involved area of the face spread to the eye and the forehead. Eating, drinking, cold and touching the face precipitated the pain. The physical and neurologic examinations gave entirely negative results. Gustatory tests were not made before operation.

On March 30, 1927, the sensory root of the right trigeminal nerve was divided at the pons, by the subcerebellar route. Complete anesthesia for all forms of sensation followed in the domain of the trigeminal nerve.

Eight days after operation, the following results were obtained by one of us (W. E. D.) in a test for taste:

	Right (Affected Side), Seconds	Left
Sugar	15	Instantly
Salt	50	Instantly
Acid	20	Instantly
Bitter	60	Instantly

Eleven days after operation, the following results were obtained by another examiner:

	Right (Affected Side), Seconds	Left
Sugar	0	Instantly
Salt	0	Instantly
Acid	20	Instantly
Bitter	3	Instantly

Nine months after operation, the following results were obtained:

	Right (Affected Side), Seconds	Left, Seconds
Sugar	0	0
Salt	0	0
Acid	2	2
Bitter	2	2

The results of a recent test, two and one-half years after operation were:

	Right (Affected Side), Seconds	Left, Seconds
Sugar	0	30
Salt	2	2
Acid	2	1
Bitter	2	2

CASE 3. A slender, emaciated woman, aged fifty-one, was referred by Dr. John Gilmore, of Wheeling, W. Va., for relief from tic douloureux. Ten years ago a slight pain began in the lower teeth and the lower lip on the left side, without known cause. Gradually the pain became more severe and spread to the upper two branches of the nerve, thus involving the entire area of the right trigeminal nerve. The pain was paroxysmal and of terrific intensity. A draught of cold air, eating and drinking induced the attacks. All of the teeth on the left side had been extracted in a futile effort to abolish the pain. She had lost a great deal of weight because eating was painful. Physical and neurologic examinations yielded negative results. Section of the left sensory root of the trigeminal nerve at the pons (subcerebellar route) was performed on Feb. 7, 1928. Total anesthesia for all forms of sensation resulted in the domain of the affected nerve.

Before operation the following results were obtained by an associate in a test for taste on the affected side only:

	Left (Affected Side)
Sugar	7 seconds
Salt	15 seconds
Acid	8 seconds

Bitter .... Not identified;
called "sweetish"

Three days after operation, the following results were obtained by one of us (W. E. D.):

	Left (Affected Side), Seconds	Right, Seconds
Sugar	10	10
Salt	0	2
Acid	10	2
Bitter	10	2

Ten days after operation, the following results were obtained by an associate:

	Left (Affected Side), Seconds	Right, Seconds
Sugar	5	5
Salt	20	10
Acid	18	10
Bitter	15	12

CASE 4. A large robust man, aged forty-two, was referred by Dr. John Gilmore, of Wheeling, W. Va., for treatment for tic douloureux. Six years before, tenderness was first noticed along the lower branch of the trigeminal nerve. Paroxysms of pain soon developed at the site of tenderness. The pain gradually increased in severity, and finally it involved all three branches of the nerve, though the starting point was in the mandibular branch. Never a day passed without several attacks of terrific pain. Eating, drinking and touching the face induced the pain. Physical and neurologic examinations gave entirely negative results.

On Feb. 7, 1928, the sensory root of the left trigeminal nerve was sectioned totally at the pons. Complete anesthesia over the domain of this nerve resulted.

Before operation the results of a gustatory examination on the affected side only, made by an associate, were as follows:

	Left (Affected Side)
Sugar	10 seconds
Salt	12 seconds
Acid	20 seconds
Bitter	15 seconds

Seven days after operation, the following results were obtained by one of us (W. E. D.):

	Left (Affected Side), Seconds	Right, Seconds
Sugar	30	20
Salt	Not recognized	5
Acid	2	2
Bitter	2	2

Ten days after operation, the following results were obtained by an associate:

	Left (Affected Side), Seconds	Right, Seconds
Sugar	25	15
Salt	12	5
Acid	5	7
Bitter	20	10

CASE 5. A well nourished woman, aged fifty-nine, was referred by Dr. H. Klinzing, of Pittsburgh, for treatment for pain in the right side of the face. Fifteen years before she was seen by us the type of pain of which she complained began in the right temple, soon passed to the eye, where it became more intense, and persisted for about twelve hours. There was some radiation of the pain to the upper and lower teeth on the same side, also to the back of the head and ear on the right side. The pain never spread to the left side, not did it ever arise there. It was present almost every day and generally lasted about twelve hours. It usually began about four o'clock in the afternoon. Acetylsalicylic acid and a brand of amidopyrine relieved the patient only partially and for about two hours. Eating, drinking and rubbing the face did not induce the pain nor did anything else of which she knew. Physical and neurologic examinations yielded entirely negative results.

Because of the radiation of the pain to the teeth, a diagnosis of an unusual form of trigeminal neuralgia was made.

Complete section of the right sensory root at the pons was performed on July 28, 1927. Total anesthesia resulted for all forms of sensation in the affected nerve. Complete section of the sensory root was made because of the unusual type. There has not been a suggestion of the former pain to the time of this writing, two years later.

Before operation, the following results were obtained by an associate in examinations for taste:

	Right (Affected Side)	Left
Sugar	Instantly	Instantly
Salt	Instantly	Instantly
Acid	Instantly	Instantly
Bitter	Instantly	Instantly

Seven days after operation the following results were obtained by the same associate:

	Right (Affected Side), Seconds	Left
Sugar	2	2
Salt	2	Instantly
Acid	2	Instantly
Bitter	Instantly	Instantly

CASE 6. A well nourished woman, aged forty-eight, was referred by Dr. Louis Hamman. Her complaint was attacks of pain in the right eye. Since the age of 15, the patient had had occipital headaches extending to the vertex. About nine years before she consulted us this headache seemed to change to a single pain localized in the right eyeball. At first the pain occurred about every six weeks. Gradually it increased to once a week and became more intense. It began gradually, at first being scarcely perceptible; it continued steadily to become more severe, reaching its maximum intensity in about twelve hours, and then gradually subsided. Each attack lasted about forty-eight hours. Codeine deadened the pain slightly. There was no pain in the face. Nothing induced the pain or modified the attack. At times there was a sensation of cold in the eyeball. The pain did not radiate to any part of the sensory domain of the trigeminal nerve. There was no known history of similar pain in any member of her family. The results of physical and neurologic examinations were normal.

The pain was suggestive of migraine. Relief from pain of seemingly similar character had been given by section of the sensory root in three other cases; this operation was performed on the right side on July 9, 1929. Total anestheia resulted for all forms of sensation in the right terminal area.

Before operation, taste was found by an associate to be normal on both sides.

After operation (eight days), the following results were obtained by an associate:

	Right (Affected Side), Seconds	Left, Seconds
Sugar	3	2
Salt	4	2
Acid	2	2
Bitter	2	2

CASE 7. A sparely nourished man, aged fifty-eight, was referred by Dr. Le Grand Guerry, of Columbia, S. C., because of bilateral tic douloureux. For twenty-one years he had suffered with trigeminal neuralgia of the right side; apparently all three branches were involved at the onset. The left side became involved six years before we saw him, but only the second and third branches were painful. The pains on both sides had all the characteristics of tic douloureaux. They were paroxysmal, and were brought on by eating, drinking, cold air or touching the face. He had had numerous peripheral operations and injections of alcohol, with short periods of temporary relief. Usually when the pain began on one side (either side) it spread to the other side, though there were periods when the attacks affected one side only.

The diagnosis was bilateral trigeminal neuralgia.

On April 30, 1926, both the right and left sensory roots of the trigeminal nerves were sectioned at the pons (subcerebellar route) at the same operation.

Tests for taste were not made before operation. Three weeks after operation the patient could promptly taste sweet, salt, acid and bitter on both sides. The time of recognition of the taste was not noted, as this was our first test of this function. Six months later, he wrote: "The taste is perfect, so I can't understand why I am not gaining faster the sense of feeling or touch inside the mouth."

After the operation, both sides of the face were completely anesthetic to all forms of sensation.

CASE 8. A sparely nourished woman, aged sixty-two, was referred for typical right-sided neuralgia of three years' duration. For over a year, the pains were only occasional and of very short duration; gradually they became more frequent, of longer duration and more intense. Finally, each paroxysm of pain lasted about three minutes. They were induced by eating, drinking, cold air or touching the face. They began over the right eye and did not spread.

Physical and neurologic examinations gave entirely negative results.

The sensory root of the right trigeminal nerve was sectioned at the pons on Dec. 21, 1928. There was complete loss of all forms of sensation in the domain of the right trigeminal nerve after the operation.

Examination for taste was not made before or immediately after operation.

Seven months after the operation, the following results were obtained in tests for taste by one of us (W.E.D.):

TABLE I

(GROUP I), RESULTS OF EXAMINATION FOR TASTE, OVER THE ANTERIOR TWO THIRDS OF THE TONGUE, AFTER SECTION OF THE SENSORY ROOT OF TRIGEMINAL NERVE AT THE PONS; IN EVERY INSTANCE TOTAL ANESTHESIA FOR ALL FORMS OF SENSATION HAS FOLLOWED IN THE AFFECTED TRIGEMINAL DOMAIN; THESE CASES ARE THEREFORE CASES OF PURE FIFTH NERVE LESIONS

Patient	Age	Diagnosis	Operation	Time of Test	Results of Sensory Examination Over Trigeminal Area	Taste	Time of Taste Perception — Affected Side	Time of Taste Perception — Normal Side	Control Tests — Affected Side	Control Tests — (Before Operation) Normal Side
F (Case 1)	63	Trigeminal neuralgia	Section of sensory root (cerebellar route)	5 months after operation	Total anesthesia to all forms of sensation	Sugar	0	0	No tests before operation	No tests before operation
						Salt	0	40 seconds		
						Acid	15 seconds	Instantly		
						Bitter	10 seconds	5 seconds		
F (Case 2)	70	Trigeminal neuralgia	Section of sensory root (cerebellar route)	8 days after operation	Total anesthesia to all forms of sensation	Sugar	15 seconds	Instantly	No tests before operation	No tests before operation
						Salt	50 seconds	Instantly		
						Acid	20 seconds	Instantly		
						Bitter	60 seconds	Instantly		
				11 days after operation		Sugar	0	Instantly		
						Salt	0	Instantly		
						Acid	20 seconds	Instantly		
						Bitter	3 seconds	Instantly		
				9 months after operation		Sugar	0	0		
						Salt	0	0		
						Acid	0	0		
						Bitter	0	0		
				2½ years after operation		Sugar	2 seconds	2 seconds		
						Salt	2 seconds	2 seconds		
						Acid	2 seconds	30 seconds		
						Bitter	2 seconds	1 second		
F (Case 3)	51	Trigeminal neuralgia	Section of sensory root (cerebellar route)	3 days after operation	Total anesthesia to all forms of sensation	Sugar	10 seconds	10 seconds	7 seconds	Not tested
						Salt	10 seconds	2 seconds	15 seconds	
						Acid	10 seconds	2 seconds	8 seconds	
						Bitter	5 seconds	5 seconds	0	
				10 days after operation		Sugar	20 seconds	10 seconds		
						Salt	18 seconds	10 seconds		
						Acid	15 seconds	12 seconds		
						Bitter	30 seconds	20 seconds		
M (Case 4)	42	Trigeminal neuralgia	Section of sensory root (cerebellar route)	7 days after operation	Total anesthesia to all forms of sensation	Sugar	2 seconds	5 seconds	10 seconds	Not tested
						Salt	2 seconds	2 seconds	12 seconds	
						Acid	25 seconds	15 seconds	20 seconds	
						Bitter	12 seconds	5 seconds	15 seconds	
				10 days after operation		Sugar	5 seconds	7 seconds		
						Salt	20 seconds	10 seconds		
						Acid	2 seconds	2 seconds		
						Bitter	2 seconds	2 seconds		
F (Case 5)	59	Trigeminal neuralgia	Section of sensory root (cerebellar route)	7 days after operation	Total anesthesia to all forms of sensation	Sugar	20 seconds	10 seconds	Instantly	Instantly
						Salt	2 seconds	2 seconds	Instantly	Instantly
						Acid	2 seconds	Instantly	Instantly	Instantly
						Bitter	Instantly	Instantly	Recorded as normal	Recorded as normal
F (Case 6)	48	Migraine-like pain in right eye	Section of sensory root (cerebellar route)	8 days after operation	Total anesthesia to all forms of sensation	Sugar	3 seconds	2 seconds	Not tested	
						Salt	2 seconds	2 seconds		
						Acid	Instantly	2 seconds		
						Bitter	2 seconds	2 seconds		
M (Case 7)	58	Bilateral trigeminal neuralgia	Section of both sensory roots (cerebellar route)	21 days after operation	Total anesthesia to all forms of sensation, on both sides	Sugar	Promptly recognized	Promptly recognized	Not tested	
						Salt				
						Acid				
						Bitter				
F (Case 8)	62	Trigeminal neuralgia	Section of sensory root (cerebellar route)	7 months after operation	Total anesthesia to all forms of sensation	Sugar	1 second	4 seconds	Not tested	
						Salt	1 second	40 seconds		
						Acid	1 second	40 seconds		
						Bitter	12 seconds	45 seconds		

	Right (Affected Side), Seconds	Left, Seconds
Sugar	1	4
Salt	1	40
Acid	1	40
Bitter	12	45

All forms of taste were much less intense on the left (normal) side.

Summary.—In this group are included only those patients in whom total anesthesia for all forms of sensation except taste followed section of the sensory root of the trigeminus. There was essentially no difference in the acuity of taste after division of the sensory root. It may well be asked why these results should be different from those obtained by section of the sensory root by the temporal route as performed by Krause, Cushing and others. By the temporal route the petrosal nerves are torn and at times the geniculate ganglion is injured in stripping the dura from the temporal bone. Since the petrosal nerves have been included in the pathways of taste, their injury adds a complication and prevents the results from being accepted as pure fifth nerve lesions. By the subcerebellar route, which we have used exclusively, the lesion is strictly that of the fifth nerve, for no other nerves cross the line of approach.

Twenty-five additional cases of presumably total trigeminal section by this route are not included in this group because sensation in varying degrees has been retained. The preservation of sensation is not due, as might well be reasoned, to subtotal section of the sensory root but to variable adjacent accessory fibers which retain the sensory function. In none of these additional cases has taste been lost after partial or total section of the sensory root. Nor is a still greater number of cases of deliberate partial section of the sensory root included, although the results obtained are precisely similar.

Partial section of the nerve is now used exclusively instead of total division, for pain fibers have been found to be located solely in the posterior border of the sensory root and sensation to the face can be left almost intact by preservation of the anterior half of the root.

Perhaps the most impressive test of the series (group 1) that taste is not carried by the trigeminal nerve is offered in case 7, in which the sensory roots of both trigeminal nerves were totally divided at the same operation. Although all sensation of both trigeminal nerves was totally abolished, all forms of taste to the anterior two thirds of the tongue were promptly recognized.

GROUP II: PURE NINTH NERVE LESIONS

CASE 1. A robust man, aged forty-five, sought relief for agonizing, paroxysmal pains beginning in the tonsil region. These pains were brought on by swallowing and talking, and even occurred spontaneously. The pain was so terrific that he sat in terror, afraid to eat or drink, and held his head inclined at an angle so that the saliva could drool from his mouth on the unaffected side. These pains had been present for three years, though there were periods lasting for months in which the same stimuli would not produce the attacks. He said the pain felt as though a red hot poker were being thrust into the back of the tongue. He had learned that relief could be obtained by the application of cocaine to the affected jaw.

Physical and neurologic examinations gave entirely negative results. The history was typical of glossopharyngeal neuralgia.

On April 6, 1927, the glossopharyngeal nerve was divided intracranially under local anesthesia. Following the operation there was loss of sensation in the back of the tongue and the mouth on the affected side; this extended to the epiglottis below and to the roof of the pharynx above. There was also loss of taste in the posterior third of the tongue. The functions of normal. A pure ninth nerve lesion was thus produced.

Test for taste by one of us (W.E.D.) on the anterior two thirds of the tongue, ten days after the operation, gave the following results:

	Left (Affected Side), Seconds	Right
Sugar	Instantly	Instantly
Salt	Instantly	Instantly
Acid	Instantly	Instantly
Bitter	Instantly	Instantly

CASE 2. A well nourished man, aged fifty-six, pale and sallow from lack of recent nourishment, was referred by our associate, Dr. S. J. Crowe, for relief from pain that was characteristic of glossopharyngeal tic douloureux. Fifteen years before he was seen by us, while he was talking with a friend, there suddenly appeared an excruciating pain in a well localized spot in the back of the tongue and near the tonsils; it lasted only a few seconds. During the succeeding years, similar momentary pains struck him from time to time; they were so infrequent as not to be a severe handicap. The pain felt as though a red hot iron were being jabbed into the tongue. At first he was unable to discover any inciting cause, but later at certain times the attacks were brought on by eating, drinking and talking. For two weeks before entering the hospital the attacks had been almost continuous, and the patient did not dare to eat, drink or talk, sneezing or coughing also brought on the paroxysms.

Neurologic and physical examinations gave entirely negative results.

On May 11, 1927, under local anesthesia, the glossopharyngeal nerve was divided intracranially. There was loss of sensation over the same area as in the preceding case, and the same loss of taste in the posterior third of the tongue.

One week after the operation, the following results were obtained by one of us (W. E. D.)

	Left (Affected Side), Seconds	Right
Sugar	1	Instantly
Acid	1	Instantly
Bitter	1	Instantly
Salt	1	Instantly

At recent examination there was just an appreciable difference between the time of perception of taste, and to the patient there was also a slight difference in intensity of taste perception. Sensation over the domain of the fifth nerve was entirely normal.

CASE 3. A large, strong, colored man, aged thirty-two, complained of a constant severe pain in the left side of the neck and ear. Four years before this examination a peculiar sensation developed in the left ear; at first it felt as if it were a bug and then a trigger zone in the external audiutory canal. He was treated in the Johns Hopkins Dispensary for two years, at which

time a swelling was found in the auditory canal.

During the first few months there was some discharge of pus, but later, although the swelling was incised on several occasions, it did not continue to drain pus. The canal became occluded by a hard growth which was tender. From this, deafness and ringing in the ear developed. Two and one-half years ago a mastoid operation was performed, but no infection was found. A mass of fibrous and fatty tissue covered with epithelium was removed from the cartilaginous canal. Following this operation, hearing returned and there was relief from pain for over a year. One year ago, the present type of pain began; it gradually became worse so that he was unable to sleep at night without taking sedatives. The pain was continuous. It began in front of the ear, ran back of the ear and down the neck to the angle of the jaw. It was aggravated by swallowing cold air and by moving the jaw.

Physical and neurologic examinations showed nothing other than a localized lesion in the ear. The distribution of pain made us feel that the glossopharynegeal nerve was affected.

On Feb. 18, 1928, the left glossopharyngeal nerve was divided intracranially. No other nerves were injured. Before operation the following results were obtained by an associate in an examination for taste:

	Left (Affected Side), Seconds	Right, Seconds
Sugar	10	10
Salt	12	10
Acid	5	7
Bitter	5	5

Eight days after the operation, the following results were obtained by the same associate:

	Left (Affected Side), Seconds	Right, Seconds
Sugar	3	3
Salt	7	8
Acid	10	5
Bitter	4	3

Summary—In these three cases of total section of the glossopharyngeal nerve, taste remained normal over the anterior two thirds of the tongue on the affected side. There can bo no purer nerve lesions than those produced by intracranial section of the glossopharyngeal nerve, for no other nerves are touched during exposure and

TABLE II

(GROUP II). RESULTS OF EXAMINATION FOR TASTE OVER THE ANTERIOR TWO THIRDS OF TONGUE AFTER TOTAL SECTION OF THE GLOSSOPHARYNGEAL (IX) NERVE INTRACRANIALLY

Patient	Age	Diagnosis	Operation	Time of Test	Results of Sensory Examination Over Trigeminal (V) Area		Time of Taste Perception		Control Tests (Before Operation)	Remarks
							Affected Side	Normal Side	Affected Side / Normal Side	
M (Case 1)	45	Glosso-pharyngeal neuralgia	Section of ninth nerve	10 days after operation	Normal	Sugar Salt Acid Bitter	Instantly Instantly Instantly Instantly	Instantly Instantly Instantly Instantly	Not tested / Not tested	Complete loss of taste over the posterior third of the tongue
M (Case 2)	56	Glosso-pharyngeal neuralgia	Section of ninth nerve	7 days after operation	Normal	Sugar Salt Acid Bitter	1 second 1 second 1 second 1 second	Instantly Instantly Instantly Instantly	Not tested / Not tested	Complete loss of taste over the posterior third of the tongue
M (Case 3)	32	Glosso-pharyngeal neuralgia	Section of ninth nerve	8 days after operation	Normal	Sugar Salt Acid Bitter	3 seconds 7 seconds 10 seconds 4 seconds	3 seconds 8 seconds 5 seconds 3 seconds	10 seconds 12 seconds 5 seconds 5 seconds / 10 seconds 10 seconds 7 seconds 5 seconds	Complete loss of taste over the posterior third of the tongue

TABLE III

(GROUP III). RESULTS IN EXAMINATIONS FOR TASTE OVER THE ANTERIOR TWO THIRDS OF THE TONGUE AFTER TOTAL SECTION, INTRACRANIALLY, OF BOTH THE GLOSSOPHARYNGEAL (IX) AND THE TRIGEMINAL (V) NERVES

Patient	Age	Diagnosis	Operation	Time of Test	Results of Sensory Examination Over Trigeminal (V) Area		Time of Taste Perception		Control Tests (Before Operation)	Remarks
							Affected Side	Normal Side	Affected Side / Normal Side	
M (Case 1)	69	Carcinoma of the face and throat	Section of ninth and fifth nerves intracranially	7 days after operation	Complete anesthesia for all forms of sensation over the trigeminal domain	Sugar Salt Acid Bitter	30 seconds 35 seconds 10 seconds 20 seconds	Not tested	40 seconds 20 seconds 20 seconds 20 seconds / 25 seconds 25 seconds 25 seconds 15 seconds	Complete loss of taste over the posterior third of the tongue

section of the nerve. The results of this group should, therefore, dispose of the ninth nerve as a conductor of taste from the anterior two thirds of the tongue.

GROUP III: COMBINED PURE FIFTH AND NINTH NERVE LESIONS

A large, somewhat undernourished man, aged sixty-nine, complained of severe facial pain caused by carcinoma of the left side of the face. The growth, which was of eleven years' duration, was first observed just within the left auditory canal. It had been treated with radium for the past eight years. It had healed and reopened on several occasions. The pain began two weeks after treatment with "radium seeds" at another clinic two years before. It had steadily become worse. At times the whole side of the face pained. Associated with the carcinoma there was necrosis of the neck of the mandible, from which the open sinus persisted.

Section of the left fifth and ninth nerves intracranially and of the great auricular nerve superficially was performed on Feb. 21, 1928.

Before operation, the following results for taste were obtained by an associate:

	Left (Affected Side), Seconds	Right, Seconds
Sugar	40	25
Salt	20	25
Acid	20	25
Bitter	20	15

Seven days after operation, the same associate obtained the following results for taste were obtained by an associate: on the affected side only:

	Left (Affected Side), Seconds
Sugar	30
Salt	35
Acid	10
Bitter	20

There was total anesthesia for all forms of sensation over the affected trigeminal area.

Summary.—This single instance of pure experimental lesions of the fifth and ninth nerves combined merely adds emphasis to the results of the two foregoing groups; namely, that the intracranial portion of neither the trigeminal nor the glossopharyngeal nerve conducts taste sensations from the anterior two thirds of the tongue.

GROUP IV: PURE SEVENTH NERVE LESION (INTRACRANIAL)

CASE 1. A young woman, aged twenty-five, of normal appearance, was referred with the diagnosis of an unlocalized tumor of the brain. Eight months before admission, headaches began. This was one month before her baby was born. Staggering occurred from time to time and made her fearful of crossing the street. Deafness began in the right ear and soon became total. During the last months of pregnancy, she had three attacks of projectile vomiting associated with severe headache. Two months after the birth of her baby, she consulted an opthalmologist because of blurred vision; he found bilateral papilledema and advised her to consult a neurologist. Shortly afterward a cerebellar exploration was made in another clinic, but nothing was found. Five months later, symptoms having steadily progressed, she entered the Johns Hopkins Hospital.

The following positive observations indicated a right cerebellopontile tumor: (1) bilateral papilledema; (2) bulging, tight, bilateral cerebellar decompression; (3) deafness (total) in the right ear; (4) diminished sensation over the right trigeminal area; (5) slight right facial weakness of the peripheral type; (6) staggering gait; (7) a positive Romberg sign, falling to the right, and (8) ataxia on the right side.

In view of the negative cerebellar exploration at which the cerebellopontile angle had presumably been exposed, an injection of air was made. There was bilateral hydrocephalus, establishing the diagnosis of a subtentorial tumor.

On May 23, 1921, a right-sided cerebellopontile tumor was totally removed. The right facial nerve was necessarily sacrificed. A spinofacial anastomosis was refused.

Tests for taste were made on Dec. 20, 1928, or seven and one-half years after removal of the tumor. There had been no preoperative gustatory examination. All forms of sensation were normal over the domains of the trigeminal and glossopharyngeal nerves on the affected side.

	Right (Affected Side), Seconds	Left, Seconds
Sugar	0	5
Salt	0	Instantly
Acid	0	Instantly
Bitter	0	Instantly

CASE 2. A rather obese woman, aged

forty-nine, was referred by Dr. Hugh Morgan, of Nashville, Tenn., with the diagnosis of a cerebellopontile tumor. Twelve years before he consulted us, tinnitus began in the left ear; there was some associated dizziness. Six years before, deafness began in the left ear and steadily progressed. Three years before, unsteadiness of gait was first noticed. It was present only at times. There had been spells of unconsciousness with subsequent weakness of the lower limbs, but no convulsions. Headaches began in the suboccipital region four months before we saw him. There had also been left occipital pains and stiffness of the neck.

On neurologic examination, the patient showed the positive signs of a left cerebellopontile tumor; i. e., (1) complete deafness of the left ear; (2) a staggering gait; (3) a positive Romberg sign, falling backward and to the left; (4) ataxia on the left side, and (5) bilateral papilledema.

The diagnosis was a left cerebellopontile tumor.

On Nov. 3, 1923, the tumor was totally removed. The facial nerve was sacrificed. Spinofacial anastomosis gave excellent return of function.

Complete recovery followed. The patient was living and well on Aug. 1, 1929.

No tests for taste were made before operation. The sensation over the domain of the left (affected side) trigeminal and glossopharyngeal nerve was unimpaired.

In December, 1928, five years after the tumor had been removed, an examination for taste by one of us (W. E. D.) showed:

	Left (Affected Side), Seconds	Right, Seconds
Sugar	0	5
Salt	0	Instantly
Acid	0	Instantly
Bitter	0	Instantly

CASE 3. A sparely nourished woman, aged thirty-three, was referred by Dr. Louis Hamman, of Baltimore, with a diagnosis of tumor of the brain. Her symptoms began five years before we saw her with pain and stiffness in the back of the neck. These pains had grown worse and more frequent during the past two years, and they had been accompanied by dizziness and ringing in both ears. On three occasions she had lost consciousness. For about one year, she had had increasing dimness of vision and transient diplopia.

There had also been violent vomiting every few days for the past six months. This was not associated with the intake of fluid but rather with a sudden change of position. For three months, she had been unable to walk without support. For the past year, she had been much more irritable, unreasonable and irresponsible. For several months, there had been urgency and hesitancy in urination. Deafness was first noticed in the right ear two years before she consulted us.

Neurologic examinations disclosed a characteristic right cerebellopontile tumor, as revealed by the following symptoms: (1) total deafness of the right ear; (2) bilateral papilledema; (3) a staggering gait; (4) a positive Romberg sign; (5) ataxia on the right side, and (6) suggestive hyperesthesia over the right trigeminal area.

Operation: A right-sided cerebellopontile tumor was completely removed on Aug. 5, 1927. The facial nerve was sacrificed; this loss of function was repaired by a spinofacial anastomosis two weeks later.

A test for taste was made by one of us (W. E. D.) at the time of discharge from the hospital, eighteen days after operation, with the following results:

	Right (Affected Side), Seconds	Left, Seconds
Sugar	0	10
Salt	0	15
Acid	0	7
Bitter	0	10

Sensation on the affected side of the face was unimpaired.

CASE 4. A well nourished woman, aged twenty-nine, was referred by Dr. John Barron, of York, S. C. She complained of staggering and drawing of her face. Five years before we saw her, deafness was first noticed in her left ear. About a year before, the deafness became more pronounced and other symptoms developed about the same time; there were headaches, attacks of dizziness and staggering, particularly when turning. Six months before examination, her gait became unsteady; she became worried and irritable and had frequent attacks of crying. The headaches became more frequent and more severe, especially during the menstrual periods. The headaches at first were frontal, and later became general. Vision was blurred and the patient had frequent attacks of diplopia. Four months before we saw her, numbness developed in the left side of the face, and at the same time her face drew to the right side and she was unable to close her left eye.

The following positive signs were disclosed on neurologic examination: (1) bilateral papilledema; (2) deafness in the right ear; (3) paralysis of the left side of the face; (4) a staggering gait; (5) a positive Romberg sign with falling toward the left; (6) nystagmus, and (7) bilateral ankle clonus and bilateral Babinski reflex.

On Sept. 13, 1927, a large left-sided cerebellopontile tumor was completely removed. The seventh nerve was sacrificed; two weeks later a spinofacial anastomosis was performed to correct the facial deformity.

Examination for taste made by one of us (W. E. D.) at the time of discharge, seventeen days after operation, showed the following results:

	Left (Affected Side), Seconds	Right
Sugar	0	Instantly
Salt	0	Instantly
Acid	0	Instantly
Bitter	0	Instantly

Sensation on the affected side of the face was unimpaired.

CASE 5. The patient was a normal appearing woman, aged forty-two, referred by Dr. N. G. Wilson, of Norfolk, Va., with a diagnosis of tumor of the brain. The patient dated the onset of her present trouble to five years before we saw her, when she noticed a clicking, buzzing noise in her right ear. A month or two later she had had staggering gait, with falling had very few symptoms, however, until a year before examination, when a tonsillectomy was done; immediately afterward she noticed numbness and loss of sensation in the right side of the face and the side of the cheek. At the same time pains which she considered sciatica appeared in both legs time to time. For the past six months she had had staggering gait, with falling to the right. She had had some headache which concentrated in the right mastoid region and which was much intensified by straining at the stool.

The following positive neurologic observations indicated a right cerebellopontile tumor: (1) bilateral papilledema; (2) deafness in the right ear; (3) absence of corneal reflex on the right side, some loss of sensation in the right trigeminal area;

(4) a positive Romberg sign, falling to the right; (5) a staggering gait, and (6) a positive Babinski reflex.

On May 5, 1925, a right-sided cerebellopontile tumor was completely removed. The right facial nerve was sacrificed; a spinofacial anastomosis was performed three weeks later. The patient has been well to the time of writing, Aug. 1, 1929.

Tests for taste were made on July 20, 1928, over three years after the tumor was removed. There had been no preoperative tests for taste. All forms of sensation over the domain of the trigeminal and glossopharyngeal nerves on the affected side were normal. The results of the tests for taste made by one of us (W. E. D.) were as follows:

	Right (Affected Side), Seconds	Left, Seconds
Sugar	0	5
Salt	0	Instantly
Acid	0	Instantly
Bitter	0	Instantly

CASE 6 A slender woman, aged thirty-five, was referred by Dr. Sidney Miller, of Baltimore, with the diagnosis of a tumor of the brain. Illness began two years before we saw her, with severe headaches in the frontal region on both sides. The headaches were usually associated with vomiting, which sometimes was suggestive of the projectile type. They had rather diminished in severity and frequency though they were still very disturbing. Spells of dizziness began soon after the headaches; this persisted and was more marked when the patient moved about or turned the head suddenly. Impairment of hearing in the right ear was noticed about the same time; this had gradually progressed. The patient had felt weak in the knees. Her feet had seemed heavy. She had had the sensation of staggering.

Neurologic examination indicated a typical right-sided cerebellopontile tumor, as revealed by the following signs: (1) deafness of the right ear; (2) bilateral papilledema; (3) staggering gait; (4) a positive Romberg sign, with falling to the right; (5) ataxia on the right side; (6) nystagmus; (7) less active corneal reflex, and (8) diminution in sensation over the trigeminal area.

A right-sided cerebellopontile tumor was completely removed on Dec. 14, 1927. The seventh nerve was routinely sacrificed in the removal of the capsule. A spinofacial anastomosis was done two weeks later to correct this deformity.

A test for taste made by one of us (W. E. D.) at the time of discharge, twenty-seven days after the operation, gave the following results:

	Right (Affected Side), Seconds	Left, Seconds
Sugar	0	15
Salt	0	3
Acid	0	3
Bitter	0	5

Some diminution of all forms of sensation over the right trigeminal area remained.

CASE 7. A well nourished man, aged thirty-seven, was referred by Dr. R. A. King, of Pittsburgh, with the diagnosis of a tumor of the brain. The symptoms began three years before our observation, with severe pains in the vertex. At the same time dizziness began to occur several times a day. He would stagger like a drunken man during these attacks. About two years before we saw him, weakness of the facial muscles on the right side was noticed. One year before, transient attacks of blindness appeared, lasting from a few seconds to a minute. Deafness antedated all of the symptoms mentioned; it began four years before examination and became complete two and one-half years ago.

Neurologic examination showed all the signs of a right cerebellopontile tumor, as follows: (1) bilateral papilledema; (2) weakness of the right rectus muscle; (3) nystagmus; (4) absence of the corneal reflex; (5) diminished sensation over that side of the face; (6) partial right facial paralysis; (7) complete deafness in the right ear; (8) a staggering gait; (9) a positive Romberg sign, and (10) ataxia on the right side.

Operation: On May 5, 1927, a large cerebellopontile tumor on the right side was completely removed. Two weeks later a spinofacial anastomosis was done because of the facial paralysis resulting from the sacrifice of the seventh nerve.

At the time of discharge there still persisted a loss of the corneal reflex on this side and diminution of sensation over the right trigeminal area; this was less pronounced than before operation.

The following results were obtained in a test for taste made by one of us (W. E. D.) at the time of discharge, three weeks after operation:

	Right (Affected Side), Seconds	Left
Sugar	0	Instantly
Salt	0	Instantly
Acid	0	Instantly
Bitter	0	Instantly

CASE 8. A feeble, emaciated, woman, aged fifty-eight, was referred by Dr. A. E. Fink, of Newark, N. J., with the diagnosis of a cerebellopontile tumor. Three years before, she had influenza, followed by otitis media on the left side. The hearing in the left ear had since been impaired. For a year she had been totally deaf in the left ear and for the past six months she had noticed an instability of balance, with a tendency to fall to the left when the eyes were closed; she had, however, never fallen. In the left ear there had been a noise like an engine.

Neurologic examination showed the following positive observations: (1) complete deafness in the left ear; (2) slight facial weakness on the left side; (3) diminished corneal reflex and impaired sensation on the left side; (4) a positive Romberg sign and staggering gait; (5) nystagmus, and (6) ataxia on the left side.

On April 24, 1926, a left cerebellopontile tumor was completely removed. The left facial nerve was sacrificed in removing the tumor.

An examination for taste, made by one of us (W. E. D.) two and one-half years after the operation, gave the following results:

	Left (Affected Side), Seconds	Right
Sugar	0	Instantly
Salt	0	Instantly
Acid	0	Instantly
Bitter	0	Instantly

There was a slightly diminished acuity for heat, cold and sharp over the left trigeminal area. There was no loss of sensation over the glossopharyngeal domain.

CASE 9. A normal appearing woman, aged twenty-eight, entered the Johns Hopkins Hospital to be treated for a tumor of the brain. Her first symptoms began two years before with beginning deafness in the right ear. Six months before admission to the hospital she became totally deaf in this ear, and the hearing on the left side had begun to diminish. For the past six months she had had a staggering gait. Three months before examination this

TABLE IV

(GROUP IV). RESULTS OF EXAMINATIONS FOR TASTE OVER THE ANTERIOR TWO THIRDS OF THE TONGUE AFTER TOTAL SECTION OF THE FACIAL (VII) NERVE INTRACRANIALLY (IN REMOVAL OF CEREBELLOPONTINE TUMOR) SENSATION OVER THE TRIGEMINAL DOMAIN WAS SUBSEQUENTLY INTACT IN FIVE CASES, AND SOMEWHAT IMPAIRED IN FOUR CASES

Patient	Age	Diagnosis	Operation	Time of Test	Results of Sensory Examination Over Trigeminal (V) Area	Time of Taste Perception		Control Tests (Before Operation)	
						Affected Side	Normal Side	Affected Side	Normal Side
F (Case 1)	25	Cerebellopontine tumor	Total removal of tumor	7½ years after extirpation of tumor	Normal	Sugar....0 Salt....0 Acid....0 Bitter....0	5 seconds Instantly Instantly Instantly	Not tested	Not tested
F (Case 2)	49	Cerebellopontine tumor	Total removal of tumor	5 years after extirpation of tumor	Normal	Sugar....0 Salt....0 Acid....0 Bitter....0	5 seconds Instantly Instantly Instantly	Not tested	Not tested
F (Case 3)	33	Cerebellopontine tumor	Total removal of tumor	18 days after extirpation of tumor	Normal	Sugar....0 Salt....0 Acid....0 Bitter....0	10 seconds 15 seconds 7 seconds 10 seconds	Not tested	Not tested
F (Case 4)	29	Cerebellopontine tumor	Total removal of tumor	17 days after extirpation of tumor	Normal	Sugar....0 Salt....0 Acid....0 Bitter....0	Instantly Instantly Instantly Instantly	Not tested	Not tested
F (Case 6)	42	Cerebellopontine tumor	Total removal of tumor	3 years after extirpation of tumor	Normal	Sugar....0 Salt....0 Acid....0 Bitter....0	5 seconds Instantly Instantly Instantly	Not tested	Not tested
F (Case 5)	35	Cerebellopontine tumor	Total removal of tumor	27 days after extirpation of tumor	Some diminution of all forms of sensation	Sugar....0 Salt....0 Acid....0 Bitter....0	15 seconds 3 seconds 3 seconds 3 seconds	Not tested	Not tested
M (Case 7)	37	Cerebellopontine tumor	Total removal of tumor	21 days after extirpation of tumor	Some diminution of all forms of sensation	Sugar....0 Salt....0 Acid....0 Bitter....0	Instantly Instantly Instantly Instantly	Not tested	Not tested
F (Caes 8)	58	Cerebellopontine tumor	Total removal of tumor	2½ years after extirpation of tumor	Slightly diminished perception of heat, cold and sharp	Sugar....0 Salt....0 Acid....0 Bitter....0	Instantly Instantly Instantly Instantly	Not tested	Not tested
F (Case 9)	28	Cerebellopontine tumor	Total removal of tumor	14 months after extirpation of tumor	Perception of sharp dimished; sensation otherwise unaffected	Sugar....0 Salt....0 Acid....0 Bitter....0	3 seconds Instantly Instantly Instantly	Not tested	Not tested

became so severe that she fell on several occasions, always to the right side. At the same time her speech became thick and slurred, and difficulty in swallowing developed. Recently her right arm and right leg had been useless. She had had severe general headaches with intensification in the supra-orgital region, and more on the right side.

Neurologic examination indicated a right cerebellopontile tumor, as revealed by the following signs: (1) bilateral papilledema; (2) deafness in the right ear; (3) some diminution in sensation in the left side of the face; (4) slight facial weakness on the right side, peripheral in type; (5) staggering gait; (6) a positive Romberg sign, falling backward and to the right; (7) nystagmus; (8) ataxia and adiadokokinesia, and (9) bilateral Babinski reflex and bilateral ankle clonus.

A right cerebellopontile tumor was completely removed on July 16, 1926. The facial nerve was sacrificed. Fourteen months later an examination for taste made by one of us (W. E. D.) showed:

	Right (Affected Side), Seconds	Left, Seconds
Sugar	0	3
Salt	0	Instantly
Acid	0	Instantly
Bitter	0	Instantly

Sensory examination of the fifth nerve showed slightly diminished acuity for pin prick. Sensation for heat and cold was normal and equal on the two sides. There was no evidence of disturbance of the glossopharyngeal nerve.

Summary.—This group offers the positive side of the taste problem. In every instance all forms of taste were immediately and permanently abolished when the facial nerve was divided intracranially. Taste therefore is conveyed to the brain stem from the geniculate ganglion by the intracranial portion of the facial nerve (the nerve of Wrisberg). So far as is known, these are the only pure experimental lesions of the intracranial portion of the facial nerve.

In the last four cases of this group the lesions were not pure, for some impairment of trigeminal sensation persisted. This was due to stripping the tumor from the sensory root of the trigeminus. The results, however, were identical with those for the pure lesions of the nerve as represented by the first five cases of the group.

GROUP V: PURE SEVENTH NERVE LESIONS (PERIPHERAL)

CASE 1. A young girl aged seventeen, was operated on for mastoid at another clinic eighteen months before we saw her. Since the operation there had been complete facial paralysis on the corresponding side. No other cranial nerves were affected. Sensation over the trigeminal and glossopharyngeal area was normal.

A test for taste, made by one of us (W. E. D.) eighteen months after section of the facial nerve gave the following results:

	Right (Affected Side), Seconds	Left
Sugar	0	Instantly
Salt	0	Instantly
Acid	0	Instantly
Bitter	0	Instantly

CASE 2. A well nourished man, aged twenty-four, was operated on for chronic mastoid infection at another hospital ten months before we saw him. Since the operation the facial nerve has been totally paralyzed. There has been no loss of function in the trgeminal or glossopharyngeal areas. Hearing is still intact.

An examination for taste made by one of us (W. E. D.) gave the following results.

	Left (Affected Side), Seconds	Right
Sugar	0	Instantly
Salt	0	Instantly
Acid	0	Instantly
Bitter	0	Instantly

CASE 3. In a woman, aged thirty, ten days before she came under our observation there was sudden complete paralysis of the facial muscles on the left side during the night. There had been a prodrome of pain in the mastoid region for thirty-six hours before paralysis developed. No other cranial nerves were affected. Hearing was normal. The trigeminal and glossopharyngeal sensory domains were normal.

An examination for taste made by one of us (W. E. D.) ten days after the paralysis gave the following results:

	Left (Affected Side), Seconds	Right
Sugar	0	Instantly
Salt	0	Instantly

	Left (Affected Side), Seconds	Right, Seconds
Acid		0 Instantly
Bitter		0 Instantly

CASE 4. A man, aged fifty-four, had an injury to the head fifteen months before we saw him. He was unconscious for twelve hours, after which consciousness gradually returned. There was no weakness of either arm or leg after the accident, and no disturbance of speech; his hearing was normal in both ears. Sensation over the trigeminal and glossopharyngeal areas was normal. There had been complete paralysis of the left side of the face since the accident.

An examination for taste, made by one of us fifteen months after the accident, gave the following results:

	Left (Affected Side), Seconds	Right, Seconds
Sugar	0	20
Salt	0	0
Acid	0	5
Bitter	0	30

CASE 5. A young girl, aged 15, was operated on at another clinic for chronic mastoid infection of six years' duration. Following the operation, twelve months before we saw her, she had complete paralysis of the right side of the face. No other cranial nerves were affected.

A test for taste made by one of us (W. E. D.) at this time gave the following results:

	Right (Affected Side), Seconds	Left
Sugar	0	Instantly
Salt	0	Instantly
Acid	0	Instantly
Bitter	0	Instantly

CASE 6. A youth, aged eighteen, was operated on at another clinic for a chronic mastoid infection of ten years' duration. The operation was performed seven months before the patient came under our observation.

Tests for taste made by one of us (W. E. D.) at this time gave the following results.

	Right (Affected Side), Seconds	Left, Seconds
Sugar	0	5
Salt	0	20
Acid	0	3
Bitter	0	7

CASE 7. A youth, aged sixteen, was operated on at another clinic for chronic mastoid infection of two years' duration.

An operation was performed three months before we saw the patient.

A test for taste made by one of us (W. E. D.) at that time gave the following results:

	Right (Affected Side), Seconds	Left
Sugar	0	Instantly
Salt	0	5 seconds
Acid	0	Instantly
Bitter	0	Instantly

CASE 8. A large, robust, well nourished man, aged forty-seven, was referred by Dr. F. C. Schreiber, of Washington, D. C., for treatment for Meniere's disease. One year before examination, when he awoke and raised his head to get out of bed he felt dizzy and vomited, but had no nausea. For three days this dizziness persisted and prevented him from getting out of bed. Every time he moved, the dizziness was intensified and frequently caused vomiting. After the third day he was able to get out of bed, but still remained more or less dizzy for three weeks, at which time the attack had entirely cleared. Four months later he had another attack, almost exactly similar to the previous one. This attack lasted one week. Six months after the first attack, partial deafness appeared in the left ear and, at the same time, tinnitus; both the deafness and the tinnitus came on suddenly during an attack of dizziness.

The neurologic examination showed partial deafness of the left ear, staggering gait and a positive Babinski reflex on the left side. The diagnosis was Meniere's disease.

On April 12, 1927, section of the eighth nerve, left, was performed. The facial nerve was accidentally injured, producing complete facial paralysis, for which a spinofacial anastomosis was done later.

The results of an examination for taste made by one of us (W. E. D.) after the operation were as follows:

	Left (Affected Side), Seconds	Right, Seconds
Sugar	0	0
Salt	0	5
Acid	0	5
Bitter	0	10

Summary.—The results of these cases will clear any doubt which may yet remain that the facial nerve conducts sensations of taste from the point of union with the chorda tympani nerve with the

TABLE V

(GROUP V). RESULTS OF EXAMINATIONS FOR TASTE, FOLLOWING COMPLETE (PERIPHERAL) FACIAL (VII) PARALYSIS, RESULTING FROM VARIOUS CAUSES, PRINCIPALLY MASTOID OPERATIONS; SENSATION OVER THE TRIGEMINAL AREA IS NORMAL IN EVERY CASE

Patient	Age	Diagnosis	Operation	Time of Test	Sensory Examination	Time of Taste Perception		Control Tests (Before Operation)	
						Affected Side	Normal Side	Affected Side	Normal Side
F (Case 1)	17	Facial paralysis	Mastoid	18 months after injury to nerve	Normal	Sugar........ 0 Salt........ 0 Acid........ 0 Bitter........ 0	Instantly Instantly Instantly Instantly	Not tested	Not tested
M (Case 2)	24	Facial paralysis	Mastoid	10 months after facial paralysis	Normal	Sugar........ 0 Salt........ 0 Acid........ 0 Bitter........ 0	Instantly Instantly Instantly Instantly	Not tested	Not tested
F (Case 3)	30	Bell's palsy	None	10 days after paralysis	Normal	Sugar........ 0 Salt........ 0 Acid........ 0 Bitter........ 0	Instantly Instantly Instantly Instantly	Not tested	Not tested
M (Case 4)	54	Fractured skull	None	15 months after paralysis	Normal	Sugar........ 0 Salt........ 0 Acid........ 0 Bitter........ 0	20 seconds 0 5 seconds 30 seconds	Not tested	Not tested
F (Case 5)	15	Facial paralysis	Mastoid	12 months after paralysis	Normal	Sugar........ 0 Salt........ 0 Acid........ 0 Bitter........ 0	Instantly Instantly Instantly Instantly	Not tested	Not tested
M (Case 6)	18	Facial paralysis	Mastoid	7 months after paralysis	Normal	Sugar........ 0 Salt........ 0 Acid........ 0 Bitter........ 0	5 seconds 20 seconds 3 seconds 7 seconds	Not tested	Not tested
M (Case 7)	16	Facial paralysis	Mastoid	2 years after paralysis	Normal	Sugar........ 0 Salt........ 0 Acid........ 0 Bitter........ 0	Instantly 5 seconds Instantly Instantly	Not tested	Not tested
M (Case 8)	47	Meniere's disease	Section of auditory nerve	3 weeks after injury of facial nerve	Normal	Sugar........ 0 Salt........ 0 Acid........ 0 Bitter........ 0	0 5 seconds 5 seconds 10 seconds	Not tested	Not tested

geniculate ganglion. The results shown in group 4 indicate that the sensations of taste are conducted by the chorda tympani through the nervus intermedias, which represents the sensory portion of the seventh nerve of the gustatory nucleus in the pons.

SUMMARY OF RESULTS IN THE ENTIRE SERIES OF EXPERIMENTS

In this series of experiments on man, made after intracranial division of the different nerves presumably concerned with taste, several facts have been determined. Intracranial division at the brain stem of the glossopharyngeal nerve or of the sensory root of the fifth nerve or of both nerves is not accompanied by permanent loss of taste to the anterior two thirds of the tongue. Total loss of taste on the anterior two thirds of the tongue invariably follows intracranial division of the seventh nerve (at the pons) or of the peripheral portion at any point between its exit from the pons and the geniculate ganglion, from which point the fibers pursue a separate course.

At times there may be a temporary loss or diminution in acuity of taste following operations on the gasserian ganglion or the sensory root of the fifth nerve, but later taste returns to normal. Initial loss of taste, with subsequent return, has been noted by Koster and Cushing after operations on the gasserian ganglion. They assumed that another nerve had taken over the function of conducting sensations of taste in these cases. It seems improbable in the present cases that another nerve will assume the function of conducting the sensation of taste. We have no experimental or clinical observations which will warrant such an assumption.

STUDIES ON A PATIENT WITH MULTIPLE, SMALL METASTATIC TUMORS OF THE CRANIAL NERVES

Despite the untrustworthiness of the gustatory changes produced by primary or secondary tumors involving nerves conduc-ting sensations of taste, the case about to be recorded is different from those which have been reported. It is included in this paper only because the changes in taste were so closely and definitely associated with loss of function of the seventh nerve occurring first on one and then on the other side. At autopsy many tiny, discrete, secondary melanotic sarcomas were found in and along the nerves of the cauda equina, and a few nodules in the cranial nerves on both sides.

Each nodule was so small that the tumor could cause only local destruction of the nerve involved, and could not press on adjacent cranial nerves. Moreover, the loss of taste occurred during the stay of the patient in the hospital and coincided exactly with the loss of function of the facial nerves.

A young man, aged twenty-five, was under observation in the hospital over a period of three months. When first seen, his main complaint was referable to the cauda equina, but a peripheral facial paralysis was also noted on one side. In the early stages, the right facial paralysis was the only sign of intracranial disturbance. Taste was entirely lost over the anterior two thirds of the tongue on the right side. It was unaffected on the left side. Sensation, including the corneal reflex, was normal over the area of distribution of both fifth nerves. The action of the masseter, temporal and pteygoid muscles was unaffected. After a few weeks, paralysis of the left facial muscles began to develop. Within ten days this became complete, the typical mask appearance of bilateral facial paralysis developing. Coincidently, taste was lost on the left side. Loss of taste was noted over the anterior two thirds of the tongue on both sides, though neither trigeminal nerve was as yet affected. Some time later, some involvement of the right trigeminus was noted. Although this gradually progressed, it never became complete. The left trigeminus was unaffected. Toward the end, the auditory, glossopharyngeal and vagus nerves were gradually affected. Total deafness finally ensued. Dysphagia was soon followed by total inability to swallow.

CONCLUSIONS

We find no evidence to support the the-

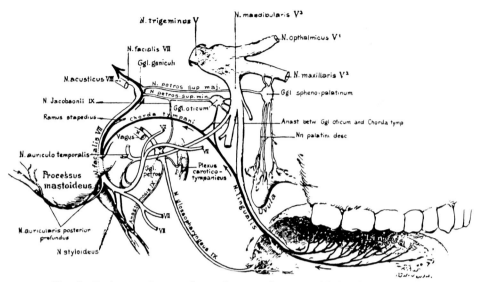

Fig. 5.—Pathway of taste from the anterior two thirds of the tongue as determined by our observations after intracranial division of the fifth and seventh nerves (Lewis and Dandy). This pathway was first suggested by Lussana.

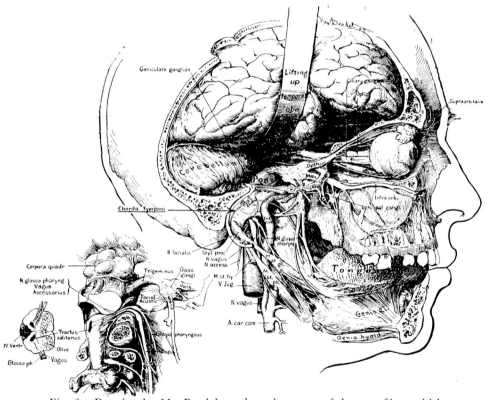

Fig. 6. Drawing by Mr. Brodel to show the course of the taste fibers which we believe to be from the tongue through the chorda tympani to the facial nerve, thence directly through the geniculate ganglion and nerve of Wrisberg to the tractus solitarius in the pons.

ory that a variable nerve supply conducts the sensations of taste, as first advanced by Krause and more recently sponsored by Harris who accepted Nageotte's anatomic demonstration that the fifth, seventh and ninth nerves have a common gustatory nucleus in the pons.

Our observations indicate that but one nerve conducts sensations of taste from the anterior two thirds of the tongue. This is the nervus intermedius (Wrisberg) or the glossopalatinus (Hardesty), which represents the sensory portion of the seventh nerve.

The course of the pathway of taste is direct. Stimuli pass from the taste buds through the chorda tympani by way of the geniculate ganglion and the nervus intermedius into the pons.

These conclusions are based on the results of intracranial division of the isolated cranial nerves in patients.

The following are the observations on which the conclusions are drawn: 1. Section of the sensory root of the fifth nerve is not followed by any permanent changes in taste, although in each instance all forms of sensation except taste over the trigeminal domain are totally absent. 2. After intracranial division of the seventh nerve, including the sensory portion (nervus intermedius of Wrisberg, the N. glossopalatinus of Hardesty), taste to the anterior two thirds of the tongue is completely and permanently lost. 3. Division of the facial nerve, between the geniculate ganglion and the point at which the chorda tympani leaves the facial nerve to pass through the middle ear, is invariably followed by total and permanent loss of taste. 4. Intracranial division of the glossopharyngeal nerve is followed by complete and permanent loss of taste to the posterior one third of the tongue, but there is no effect on taste in the anterior two thirds of the tongue.

REFERENCES

[1]Bellingeri: Claude Bernard, quoted by Frankl Hochwart, stated that Bellingeri as a result of animal experimentation and clinical observations was the first to associate conduction of

sensations of taste with the chorda tympani.

[2]Bernard, Claude: On the Alteration of the Taste in Paralysis of the Facial Nerve, 1843, trans. by Howell L. Thomas, Richmond, 1853.

[3]Bernard, Claude: *Lecons du systeme nerveux*, Paris, 1858, p. 192.

[4]Bernard, Claude: Recherches anatomiques et physiologiques sur la corde du tympanium. *Ann. med.-psychol., 1:* 408, 1843.

[5]Bernhardt, M.: Ueber die Function des Nervus trigeminus als Geschmacksnerv. *Arch. Psychiat., 6:* 541, 1876.

[6]Bigelow, H. R.: Anatomy and Physiology of the Chorda Tympani. *Brain, 3:* 43, 1880–1881.

[7]Blau, Louis: Ein Beitrag zur Lehre von der Function der Chorda tympani. *Berl. klin. Wchnschr., 16:* 671, 1879.

[8]Bruns, L.: Multiple Hirnnervenlasion nach Basisfractur: Ein Beitrag zur Frage des Verlaufs der Geschmacksnerven. *Arch. Psychiat., 20:* 495, 1889.

[9]Cassirer, R.: Ein Fall von multipler Hirnnervenlahmung: Zugleich als Beitrag zur Lehre von der Geschmacksinnervation. *Arch. Physiol.,* 1899, supplement, p. 36.

[10]Cushing, H.: The Taste Fibers and Their Independence of the Nerve Trigeminus: Deductions from Thirteen Cases of Gasserian Ganglion Extirpation. *Bull. Johns Hopkins Hosp., 14:* 71, 1903.

[10]Dana, C. L.: Case of Paralysis of Trigeminus Followed by Alternate Hemiplegia: Its Relation to Nerve of Taste. *J. Nerv. & Ment. Dis., 13:* 65, 1886.

[12]Dandy, W. E.: An Operation for the Total Removal of Cerebellopontile (Acoustic) Tumors. *Surg., Gynec. & Obst., 41:* 129 (Aug.) 1925.

[13]Dandy, W. E.: An Operation for the Cure of Tic Douloureux. *Arch. Surg., 18:* 687 (Feb.) 1929; Section of the Sensory Root of the Trigeminal Nerve at the Pons: Preliminary Report of the Operative Procedure. *Bull Johns Hopkins Hosp., 36:* 2, 1925.

[14]Dandy, W. E.: Glossopharyngeal Neuralgia (Tic Douloureux): Its Diagnosis and Treatment. *Arch. Surg., 15:* 198 (Aug.) 1927.

[15]Davidson, A.: On the Sense of Taste and its Relation to Facial Paralysis and Anesthesia. *Liverpool & Manchester M. & S. Rep., 3:* 198, 1875, reprinted from Surgeon General's Library.

[16]Davies, M.: The Function of the Trigeminal Nerve. *Brain, 30:* 219, 1907.

[17]Davis, L. E.: The Deep Sensibility of the Face. *Arch. Neurol. & Psychiat., 9:*283 (March) 1923.

[18]Dixon, A. F.: On the Course of the Taste Fibers. *Edinburgh M. J., 1:* 395, 1897.

[19]Dixon, A. F.: Further Note on the Course of the Taste Fibers *Edinburgh M. J., 1:* 628, 1897.

[20]Dixon, A. F.: On the Development of the Branches of the Fifth Cranial Nerve in Man. *Roy. Dublin Soc., Scient. Tr. (series 2), 4:* 1888-1892.

[21]Dixon, A. F.: On the Development of the Branches of the Fifth Cranial Nerve in Man. *Roy. Dublin Soc., Scient. Tr. (series 2) 6:* 19, 1896-1897.

[22]Doyle, J. B.: A Study of Four Cases of Glossopharyngeal Neuralgia. *Arch. Neurol. & Psychiat. 9:* 34 (Jan.) 1923.

[23]Duchenne: Duchenne first paralyzed the chorda in the ear and obtained a metallic taste in the anterior two thirds of the tongue.

[24]Duchenne: Recherches electrophysiologiques et pathologiques sur les proprietes et le usages deo la corde des tympani. *Arch. gen. de med., 1:* 385, 1850.

[25]Eckhard, C.: Altere Geschichte der Physiologie des Trigeminus und die ersten bie . . . experimenteller A uber disen Nerven. *Bietr. Anat. u. Physiologie Nerven, 12:*111, 1888.

[26]Erb, W.: Ueber rheumatische Facialislahmung. *Arch klin. Med., 15:*6, 1875.

[27]Eulenburg, A.: Lehrbuch der functionellen Nervenkrankheiten, Berlin, 1871, p. 292.

[28]Ferguson, J.: The Nerve Supply of the Sense of Taste. *M. News, 57:*395, 1890.

[29]Ferrier, D.: On Paralysis of the Fifth Cranial Nerve. *Lancet, 1:*1, 1888.

[30]Finney and Thomas: Three Cases of Removal of Gasserian Ganglion. *Bull. Johns Hopkins Hosp., 4:*91, 1893.

[31]Frankl-Hochwart: Die den Geshmack vermittelnden Nerven, in Northnagel: *Spezielle Pathologie und Therapie,* Wien, 1897, vol. 2.

[32]Gowers, W. R.: A Case of Paralysis of the Fifth Nerve. *Edinburgh M. J. 1:*37, 1897.

[33]Gowers: *Diesease of the Brain.* Philadelphia, P. Blakiston's Son & Company, 1885.

[34]Hagen, R.: Ueber das Verhalten der Schliemhaut der Pankenhohle nach Durch-Schneidung des Nervus trigeminus in der Schadelhohle. *Arch. exper. Path. u. Pharmakol., 11:*39, 1879.

[35]Harris, W.: Neuritis and Neuralgia. *Lancet, 1:* 218, 1912.

[36]Harris, W., and Newcomb, W. D.: A Case of Pontine Glioma with Special Reference of the Paths of Gustatory Sensation. *Proc. Roy. Soc. Med., 19:*1, 1926.

[37]Heusner, L.: Eine Beobachtung uber der Verlauf der Geschmachsnerven. *Berl. klin. Wchnschr., 23:*758, 1886.

[38]Kander: Die Storungen der Geshmacksempfindung bei chronischen Mittelohreitungen insbesondere nach Operation. *Arch. f. Ohrendh. 68:*69, 1906.

[39]Keen, C. W., and Mitchell, J. K.: Removal of the Gasserian Ganglion as the Last of Fourteen Operations in Thirteen Years for Tic Douloureux. *Proc. Philadelphia Co. M. Soc.,* 1894.

[40]Koster, G.: Klinischer und experimenteller Bietrag zur Lehre von der Lahmung des Nervus facialis, zugleich ein Beitrag zur Physiologie der Geschmackes der Schweiss-Speichel- und Thranenabsonderung. *Deutsche Arch. f. klin. Med., 68:*343, 505, 1900.

[41]Koster, G.: Eine merkwurdige zentrale Storung der Geschmacksempfindung. *Munchen. med. Wchnschr., 51:*333 and 392, 1904.

[42]Krause, F.: *Die Neuralgie der Trigeminus.* Leipzig, F. C. W. Vogel, 1896, p. 103.

[43]Krause, F.: Resection des Trigeminus innerhalb der Schadelhohle. *Verhandl. deutsch. Gesellsch. f. Chir., 21:*199, 1892; also, *Arch. klin. Chir. 44:* 821, 1892.

[44]Krause, F.: Physiologie de Trigeminus nach Untersuchungen an Menschen bei denen das Ganglion entferent worden ist. *Muchen. med. Wchnschr., 42:*577, 602 and 628, 1895.

[45]Landois, L.: *Lehrbuch der Physiologie des Menschen,* Vienna, Urban & Schwarzenberg, 1880, p. 678.

[46]Lehmann, K. B.: Ein Beitrag zur Lehre von Geschmacksinn, *Pflugers Arch Physiol., 30:*194, 1884.

[47]Luciani, L.: *Human Physiology.* London, Macmillian Company, 1915, p. 401.

[48]Lussana: Observations pathologiques sur les nerves du gout. *Arch. de physiol. norm. et path., 2:*20, 197, 1869; 4: 150, 334, 1872.

[49]Lussana and Renzi: *Arch. de physiol. norm. et path., 2:*25, 1869.

[50]Magendie, F.: *Precis elementaire de physiologie.* Translated from the French by John Revere, Baltimore, E. J. Coale & Co., 1822.

[51]Mills, C. K.: The Sensory Functions Attributed to the Seventh Nerve. *J. Nerv. & Ment. Dis., 37:*273 and 354, 1910.

[52]Montault, J.: Dissertation sur l'hemiplegie faciale: collection des theses souteneus a la faculte de medicine, Paris, 1831, p. 15.

[53]Muller, C. W.: Zwei Falle von Trigeminus-Lahmung. *Arch. Phychiat., 4:*263, 1883.

[54]Nageotte, J.: The Pons Intermedia or Nervous Intermedium of Wrisbarg, and the Bulbo-Pontine Gustatory Nucleus in Man. *Rev. Neurol. & Psychiat., 4:*473, 1906.

[55]Oppenheim, H.: Zur Brown-Sequard'schen Lahmung, *Arch Anat u. Physiol.,* 1899, supplement.

[56]Quix, F. H.: Die Storungen des Geschmacks-Sinnes. *Handbuch des Neurologie, 1:*959, 1910.

[57]Romberg, M. A.: *Nervenkrankheiten,* Berlin, 1857, part 2, p. 774.

[58]Salomonshon: Ueber den Weg der Geschmacksfoserus zum Gehirn, Diss., Berlin, 1888, p. 10.

[59]Scheier: Beitrag zur Kenntnis der Geschmacksinnervation. *Ztchr. klin. Med., 28:*441, 1895.

[60]Schiff: Origine et parcours des nerfs gustatifs de

la partie anterieure de la langue. *Ges. Beitr. z. Physiol.* 3:183, 1896; Vortrag aus dem Jahre, 1886.

[61]Schlichting, H.: Klinische Studien uber die Geschmackslahmung durch Zer-Storung der Chorda tympani und des Plexus Tymanicus. *Ztschr. Ohrenh.,* 32:388, 1898.

[62]Seeligmuller, A.: *Lehrbuch der Krankheiten der peripheren Nerven.* Braunschweig, F. Wreden, 1882, p. 122.

[63]Senator: Ein Fall von Trigeminus Affection. *Arch. Psychiat.,* 13:590, 1882; Berl. klin. Wchnschr., 1881, vol. 6, 1883, vol. 14.

[64]Spiller, W. G.: *A Physiological, Anatomical and Pathological Study of Glossopharyngeus and Vagus Nerves in Case of Fracture of Base of Skull.* Philadephia, Univ. Penn., Contrib. William Pepper Lab., 1903.

[65]Tiffany: Intracranial Operations for the Cure of Facial Neuralgia. *Ann. Surg.,* 24:575, 1896.

[66]Turner, W. A.: Facial Paralysis and the Sense of Taste. *Edinburgh Hosp. Rep.,* 4:326, 1896.

[67]Turner: Note on the course of the fibers of taste. *Edinburgh M. J.,* 2:261, 1897.

[68]Urbanschitsch, V.: Betrachtung eines Falles von Anasthesie der peripheren chorda tympani— Auslosung von Geschmacks und Gefuhlsempfindung durch Reizung des chorda tympani— Staunners. *Arch f. Ohrenh.* 19:135, 1883.

[69]Vintschan: *Arch. f. d. ges. Physiol.,* 19 and 20; *Virchow-Hirsch Jahresbericht, 1:188,* 1878.

[70]Vulpian, A.: Gaz. med. de Paris, 1878; Remarques sur la distribution anatomique de la corde du tympan. *Arch. physiol. norm. et path.,* 2:209, 1869.

[71]Vulpian, A.: De la corde du tympan. *Arch Ohrenh.,* 14:147, 1878.

[72]Weigner, K.: Ueber den Verlauf des Nervus Intermedius. *Anat. Hefte, 129:*101, 1905.

[73]Zenner, P.: Ein klinischer Beitrag uber den Verlauf des Geschmacksnerven. *Neurol Centralbl.,* 7:457, 1888.

[74]Ziehl F.: Ein Fall von isolierter Lahmung des ganzen Trigeminus asters nebst einigen Betrachtungen uber den Verlauf der Geschmacksfasern der Chorda tympani und die Innervation des Geschmackes uberhaupt. *Virchows Arch. path. Anat. 117:*52, 1889.

XL

CONGENITAL CEREBRAL CYSTS OF THE CAVUM SEPTI PELLUCIDI (FIFTH VENTRICLE) AND CAVUM VERGAE (SIXTH VENTRICLE) *

DIAGNOSIS AND TREATMENT

In the midline of the brain and within the confines of the corpus callosum either or both of the cavum septi pellucidi and cavum vergae are not infrequently found. Neither cavity has excited much interest either anatomically or clinically. The two cases here reported are, I believe, the first instances in which a diagnosis of these spaces, dilated in abnormal degree, has been made during life, the first in which the lesion has been found at or treated by operation and the first in which clinical symptoms are shown to be related to the lesions. But there is reason to believe that these cavities may not be uncommon and may not be unimportant in clinical neurology. Moreover, the diagnosis of the lesion is easy and unequivocal. The operative treatment is not difficult, though not unassociated with great danger if certain well defined precautions are not recognized. A permanent cure of the lesion can probably be expected.

In most, but not all, textbooks of anatomy there is a brief but accurate description of these two cavities. The nomenclature, however, is not uniform. For example, the cavum septi pellucidi is perhaps better known as the fifth ventricle, and the cavum vergae is called Verga's ventricle, the sixth ventricle, the ventricle of Strambio, ventriculus fornicis, ventriculus triangularis and the canal aqueduct.

The cavum septi pellucidi, the much better recognized of the two, has been known at least since the time of Sylvius and probably much longer. The cavum vergae is named for Andrea Verga, an Italian anatomist, whose observations were reported in a brief note (1851) written in response to the report by a fellow anatomist, Ferrario, of a necropsy in a case showing the cavity that bears Verga's name. Apparently, Verga's claim to priority is based on his anatomic notes rather than on priority of publication. The following excerpts from Verga's[1] letter to Ferrario show the exact status of Verga's claim to priority, which according to present tenets based on prior publication and not the date of actual observations, should go to Ferrario:

Your gracious letter, directed to our esteemed teacher, C. Panizza, and inserted in the January number of the *Gazetta medica,* comes at a most opportune time. Your interesting publication of "an unusual finding in the brain of a man who had never presented signs of mental alienation" made me resolve to publish an old note of mine about a new cerebral ventricle which receives from your observation a great impetus and a great importance. And to you—an unknowing illustrator of my discovery (let me call it mine until proven otherwise)—I first communicate this note. When I was assistant to the chair of anatomy in Pavia, examining one day the brain of a child dead of hydrocephalus, I was surprised to find . . . this cavity. I repeated the observation upon other brains . . . and always found the said cavity more or less evident, . . . but in this age of the microscope, I made nothing of the observation, for I thought there was nothing that could be seen by the naked eye that was not already known to all. Perhaps with time I might have forgotten it, had not your observation come to revive the memory of it. Now that you, learned in so many things, and especially anatomy, appear not to know that others had spoken of the cavity, I suspect that none really has ever described it.

Reprinted from the *Archives of Neurology and Psychiatry* 25: 44–66, January, 1931.

Read at the Fifty-Sixth Annual Meeting of the American Neurological Association, Atlantic City, N. J., June 9, 1930.

Verga then proceeded to describe the cavity and gave directions how to find it:

Not knowing that this ventricle was something really new . . . I refrained from giving it a name. It is therefore, an innominate ventricle. But a numerical number could be given to it—sixth ventricle—or from its shape it might be called the triangular ventricle, or from its relations, the ventricle of the vault.

He then discussed Ferrario's contention that the ventricle is an abnormality and not a uniform anatomic observation.

Before finishing I should like to remove a doubt which, it seems to me, exists in your mind. If this cavity, you say, really exists and is a normal structure it would be found in all cadavers. I have found practically the same thing in all children and neither did I have to work hard nor employ artifices of any sort. I must, therefore, conclude that it is a natural and normal finding like that of the septum pellucidum; but whether because of age or other circumstances, which are beside the question here, it is very often perfectly obliterated in the adult.

Concerning his claim to priority, he added in conclusion:

The most serious objection that can be made to my findings is, therefore, that which I myself made long ago, and I because of which I delayed so in publishing it. In truth, at this very moment, I am afraid of appearing guilty of a scientific theft and of having to suffer the brutal consequences. But I declare that I have never had such habits and I have done all this prattling only to explain the unusual lesion which you have observed and reconnected.

In the same publication, Verga mentioned the comment of Tenchini[2] that the ventricle was discovered by Verga and should be called Verga's ventricle.

POSITION AND BOUNDARIES OF THE CAVITIES

The corpus callosum defines the anterior, superior and posterior limits of the two cavities which, when not continuous, are separated from each other by the anterior limit of the fornix as it courses obliquely backward and upward from the anterior commissure to the body of the corpus callosum. Being of congenital origin, the two cavities are doubtless dependent on the development of the corpus callosum

and the fornix. They may coexist and be isolated from each other when the fornix is intact (Fig. 1.) ; they may coexist and be in communication through a defect in the fornix, or they may form a single large cavity when the fornix is not attached to the corpus callosum, as in case 1 of this report (Figs. 2 and 3). The cavum septi pellucidi is frequently present when the cavum vergae is absent, and Verga's cavity may be present when the cavum septi pellucidi is absent. Kauffmann stated that the cavum vergae may exist in one side of the midline and be absent on the other.

The cavum septi pellucidi has the following boundaries: anteriorly, the genu of the corpus callosum; superiorly, the body of the corpus callosum; posteriorly, the anterior limb and pillars of the fornix; inferiorly, the rostrum of the corpus callosum and the anterior commissure; laterally, the layers of the septum pellucidum. Viewed laterally, the cavum septi pellucidi is roughly triangular with the base at the corpus callosum. Viewed in cross-section the cavity is also triangular with the base at the corpus callosum.

The cavum vergae has the following boundaries: anteriorly, the anterior limb of the fronix; superiorly, the body of the corpus callosum; posteriorly, the spleniun of the corpus callosum; inferiorly, the psalterium (lyra davidis) and hippocampal commissure, the fibers of which bridge the space between the diverging posterior pillars of the fornix. This cavity is also triangular when viewed from the side. The cavum vergae flares out laterally on both sides with the curve of the fornix and pushes under the lateral ventricles at its extreme lateral extensions. Although the floor of Verga's cavity rests on the tela choroidea which contains the choroid plexus, evidence of choroid plexus has not been found within, but there is no available report of careful studies of the entire wall.

COMMUNICATIONS WITH THE VENTRICULAR SYSTEM

In most adult brains both spaces are absent or are at most potential, but in every

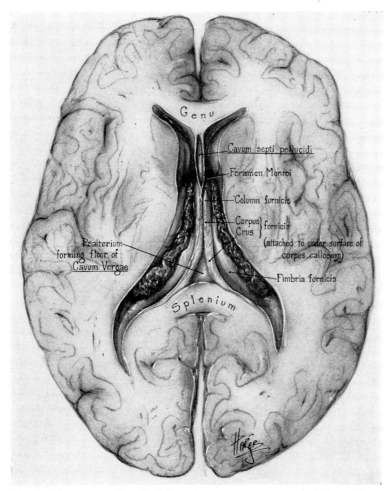

Fig. 1. Cavum septi pellucidi and cavum vergae, each independent.

one hundred necropsies actual cavities of varying size will be seen. Neither cavity can be regarded as part of the great ventricular system in which cerebrospinal fluid forms and through which it circulates. They contain no gross evidence of choroid plexus, and their development in the embryo is entirely different; any connection with the ventricular system is purely accidental and is due to contiguity. It is therefore inadvisable to retain the term "ventricle" with the numerical designations. In most necropsy specimens both of these cavities, when of unusual size, are found to communicate with the ventricular system by one or even more openings of varying size (Figs. 3 and 4). The openings are into the third and lateral ventricles. In some

textbooks of anatomy, names have been awarded to these openings, i. e., the foramen or valve of Vieussens, the foramen of Mihalkowski, etc. Verga stated that Petit (1710), and in more recent times Wenzel, Tiedemann, Meckel and Valenin, considered the openings between the cavity of the septum pellucidum and the ventricular system to be normal. Vicq d'Azyr and Santorini thought that they were artificial, a view which Verga also held.

That these openings are artificial and not performed like the interventricular foramina is evident by their inconstant position, size and number (Figs. 3 and 4), and especially by the fact that their borders are ragged and uneven, shreds of tissue usually hanging therefrom. The location of the openings is doubtless dependent on the points of greatest thinness of the walls.

Verga stated that the cavity of the septum pellucidum and the cavity that bears his name are found only in the human species.

CASES COLLECTED FROM THE LITERATURE

Verga reported five cases in which this cavity was found at necropsy. All were from psychopathic wards, the patients showing varying grades of mental disturbance. There was nothing characteristic in the assembly of symptoms. In every instance the cavity was small. He also referred to a specimen shown by his friend, Dr. Sangalli. The cyst was as large as an almond. The patient was a girl, aged seventeen, afflicted with epilepsy. He also noted that Ferrario's case, previously mentioned, was the best one that he had seen. Other cases were shown to him by his confreres, Palermo, Dubini, Biffi and De-Vincenti (1882), Inzani di Parma, Strambio and Tenchini. He quoted Tenchini as saying that the length may be as much as 13 cm.; this extreme length probably includes the cavity of the septum pellucidum in addition to the cavum vergae. Tenchini also found the cavity in 4 per cent of males and 9 per cent of females, and constantly in fetuses and the new-born.

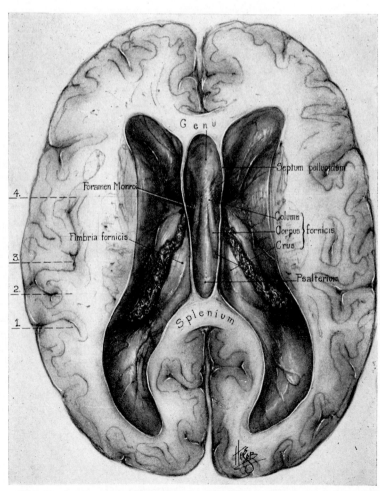

Fig. 2. Large cavity formed by union of the cavum septi pellucidi and the cavum vergae.

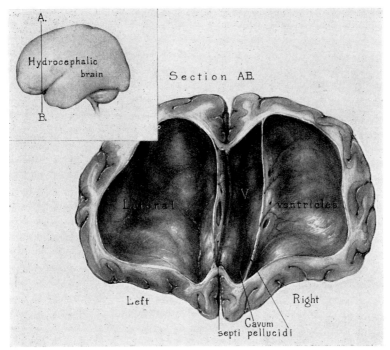

Fig. 3. A hydrocephalic brain showing a congenital malformation. The cavum septi pellucidi is formed by two distinct layers, one attached far to the right of the midline. There are numerous artificial openings between this cavity and the lateral ventricles.

It will be noted that all of the aforementioned cases were reported by Verga from the observations of his own acquaintances or at least from a restricted territory. There is every reason to believe, therefore, that the occurrence of the cavity is fairly frequent.

Examples of a dilated cavum septi pellucidi are probably even more common, though they are not easily accessible in the literature and so far as I know no effort has been made to assemble them. Kauffmann reported a necropsy showing both cavities moderately distended.

WHERE DOES THE INTRACYSTIC FLUID ARISE?

In their textbooks, Dejerine and Poirier and Charpy stated that microscopic examinations of the walls of the cavum septi lucidi have been made, and that the epithelial cells of the ependyma and choroid plexus are uniformly absent. The evidence, however, is not sufficient to accept without

further proof. One now knows that cerebrospinal fluid forms from choroid plexus and also that these cavities lie on the tela choroidea (though normally separated from it) which forms the roof of the third ventricle. Since these cavities in dilated form are uncommon, it is open to question, until disproved by more extensive microscopic studies, whether minute remnants of such cells may not be included occasionally.

Testut and Reichert have explained the existence of fluid in these cavities on the basis of transudation from the lateral ventricle, but proof of this theory is lacking. It seems much more probable that the fluid originates within the cavity, though from a source unknown. There cannot be sufficient evidence to eliminate this source until the entire ventricular wall has been subjected to microscopic study. Certainly in my two cases the walls of the cavity were far thicker than the normal thin transparent septum pellucidum, and I believe this

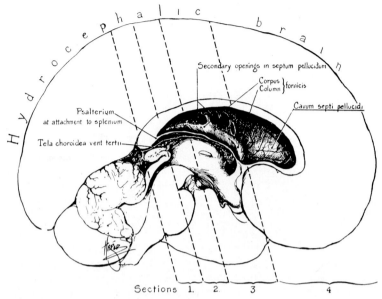

Fig. 4. Sketch of another hydrocephalic brain showing a large combined cavum septi pellucidi and cavum vergae. There are artificial openings between this cavity and the lateral ventricles, the position varying markedly from that in the two preceding cases. The presence of either or both of these cavities is not an uncommon observation in hydrocephalic brains.

to be an important reason for the isolation and growth of the "cyst," at least until by pressure absorption, erosion of the wall results at its thinnest point. The source of all fluids is not known, but there must be some unusual anatomic basis for the occasional unusual cysts that develop.

REPORT OF CASES

CASE 1. *History.*—A sparsely nourished woman, aged fifty, was referred by Dr. I. Abrahamson of New York with a probable diagnosis of tumor of the brain. Eleven years before, she began to have severe, recurring, generalized headaches, which, however, disappeared five years before the present examination and did not recur. Nine years before, she had a period of unconsciousness which lasted for only a few minutes. There were no later spells of this kind and on convulsions. Three years before, her memory began to fail. She had difficulty in understanding, and she did things incorrectly. She became slovenly in dress and personal habits. Two years before, periods of vomiting began, and in a short time she lost 40 pounds (18.1 Kg.) in weight. No satisfactory explanation

could be found for the vomiting, which later disappeared. Pain in the right arm began about two years before and had since been present at times; for this also no cause was found. Two months before, she was struck by an automobile, but sustained only bruises and was unconscious for only a few minutes. Soon thereafter she had difficulty in naming things correctly. She would put a shoe on the wrong foot. Her memory steadily became worse.

Examination.—The patient was much under weight. She was disoriented as to time, place and person. She thought that she was in a New York hotel. However, she talked fairly rationally at times. She said that her memory was poor, but that this was due to nervousness. She obeyed many commands correctly, but it was usually difficult for her to understand even simple objects; for example, when asked to in articulation. She could not name simple objects; for example, when asked to name a pencil she described its use. After some groping she frequently found the correct word. At times her speech was fairly coherent and intelligent, although she quickly wandered off the subject and frequently repeated. Cooperation was poor because of lack of understanding.

The neurologic signs were surprisingly few. There was some unsteadiness of gait. The Romberg test was positive, with falling consistently backward and not to either side. There was no ataxia or nystagmus. A positive Babinski sign on the right and hyperactive knee jerks, greater on the right, were the only other positive observations. There was no papilledema. Roentgen examination of the head gave entirely negative results. The blood pressure was 160 systolic and 100 diastolic; the pulse rate was from 70 to 80. The Wassermann reaction of the blood was negative. Ventricular fluid obtained at the time of operation was normal in every respect; there were 3 cells, no globulin and a negative Wassermann reaction.

Impression.—It was my belief that the patient had a tumor of the brain, probably situated deeply in the left hemisphere. The reasons for this diagnosis were the long period of headaches, the mental changes and the positive Babinski sign on the right side. What type of tumor could cause five years of headache and then freedom from headaches for five years was difficult to imagine. An angioma seemed the most likely possibility.

Ventriculography.—On Jan. 13, 1928, a ventricular puncture was made in the posterior horn of the lateral ventricle. The fluid was under no apparent increased pressure. Twenty cubic centimeters of fluid was removed, and the same amount of air was injected. The roentgenographic observations were as follows: In the anteroposterior view the lateral ventricles (in cross-section) were separated about 3 cm. instead of being in apposition. Moreover, the mesial margin of each ventricle was indented; i. e., there was a filling defect in each ventricle. The filling defect was much greater in the left than in the right ventricle. The third ventricle was upright but shortened in the vertical direction and wider than normal. The lateral ventricles were larger than normal; i. e., there was a low grade of hydrocephalus. The body of the lateral ventricle was smaller than the anterior and posterior parts of the ventricle. The diagnosis made on the basis of the ventriculograms was tumor in the region of the corpus callosum.

Operation.—On January 13, a small bone flap was turned down on the left side of the head just in front of the line of the rolandic area. My plan was to slide down the falx and determine the character of the tumor. If it proved to be inoperable, the small bone flap would doubtless be adequate. If there were possibilities of removing the tumor, extension of the bony defect could be made in the desired direction. Three veins were tied in the crossing from the hemisphere to the longitudinal sinus; they were doubly ligated with silk and divided. The anterior horn of the left lateral ventricle was tapped to give additional room. The mesial surface of the hemisphere was then easily retracted and the corpus callosum quickly brought into view and divided longitudinally in its anterior half. This brought me into a large smoothly lined cavity from which a clear fluid escaped. The exact color of the fluid was masked by a little oozing. The cavity looked like a lateral ventricle, but as there was no choroid plexus it was concluded that it must be a cyst. It was of tremendous size, especially in the anteroposterior direction. It extended in the midline to the anterior limit of the corpus callosum and posteriorly further than I could see or reach with an instrument, even after the corpus callosum had been divided almost as far back as the great vein of Galen. Anteriorly, the cyst was perhaps 3 cm. wide, and a smooth rounded bulge could be seen running into it longitudinally on each side. Puncture with a small aspirating needle yielded cerebrospinal fluid; they were the lateral ventricles. Posteriorly, the cyst was much wider, certainly not less than 6 or 7 cm., and on each side there was a posterior extension which went far back and under the lateral ventricle. The tip could not be seen. The posterior extension was doubtless limited by the splenium of the corpus callosum which it seemed to parallel (Figs. 5 and 6).

The nature of this tremendous cyst, which I estimated to be not less than 12 cm. long, was not clear at the time. The possibility of an enlarged cavum septi pellucidi first occurred to me, but this cavity extended much farther backward and laterally than was possible for a fifth ventricle. I clung to the view that it was probably a cyst, and that there must therefore be an underlying papilloma somewhere in the wall to cause the cyst. It was this erroneous assumption that led me to attempt a careful and thorough inspection of the whole cavity. For this purpose the corpus callosum was split to the great vein of Galen. (On several occasions when tumors of the third ventricle were remov-

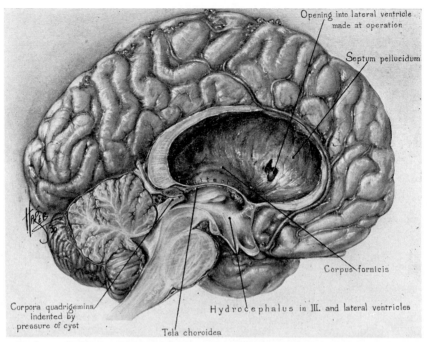

Fig. 5. (Case 1) Midsagittal view of necropsy specimen showing large cyst formed by union of the cavum septi pellucidi and the cavum vergae. The only opening in the lateral wall on either side is the one produced at operation. The absence of communication is also shown by the absence of air between the two ventricles.

ed, I had divided the body of the corpus callosum in its entire anteroposterior extent without any untoward results.) With the exception of the posterior lateral extensions of the cavity under the lateral ventricle, the entire cavity could be explored. It was everywhere smooth and glistening, but without choroid plexus and without the larger vessels which line the lateral ventricles. At no point was there an opening into either lateral ventricle or the third ventricle. There was no evidence of a tumor at any part of the wall. The conclusion was therefore forced on me that it must be, after all, an enlarged cavum septi pellucidi. If this was true, or even if a small tumor existed, opening of the cavity into the lateral ventricle should produce a cure. Openings were then made into each lateral ventricle with forceps. On puncturing the left ventricle some bleeding followed, presumably from the choroid plexus. Both ventricles filled with blood, which, however, was removed. Before closure was begun, all bleeding had stopped, and there was no particular apprehension of this postoperative complication. A decompression was performed as

an extra precaution.

Subsequent Course.—The patient died three weeks later, without regaining consciousness was due to thombosis of the left of the area of decompression. Loss of consciousness was due to thrombosis of the left anterior cerebral artery, which was doubtless injured during the exposure. This is one of the striking cases from which it has been determined that consciousness lies at some point in the left cerebral hemisphere and within the blood supply of that part of the middle cerebral artery lying above the anterior third of the corpus callosum.

Necropsy showed no other gross changes in the brain.

CASE 2. *History.*—A boy, aged four and one half years, referred by the department of pediatrics, had been born slightly prematurely at 8½ months and his weight at birth was only two and one half pounds. (1.12 Kg.). He was blue for one day, after which his color was normal. At birth the head seemed to be abnormally large. The first tooth appeared at 1 year; he sat alone at one year, walked at two years and talked at two years. The mother did not think that the head had grown faster than the body. The father said that the patient had always been mentally backward. Until six hours before admission to the hospital, the patient had been physically well though mentally backward. He had gone to bed as well as usual. At three a. m., he awoke screaming. He did not complain of any pain, but had an attack of vomiting (this was said to have been projectile). He was soon quieted, but awoke crying several more times. During the night he voided in bed, an unusual incident for

him. The following morning he was drowsy. Prior to this time he had frequently had nocturnal crying spells, but had always seemed normal in the morning.

Because of the marked drowsiness he was brought to the hospital. At that time he was comatose and was having repeated left-sided convulsions, involving the face, arm and leg.

Examination.—The patient was comatose. He had a very large head, measuring 56 cm. in circumference; it was definitely out of proportion to the rest of his body. Left-sided convulsions were frequent, but without the jacksonian "march." In fact, the convulsions were of variable character. Occasionally both legs and one (either) arm would jerk. There was at times flaccid paralysis of the entire left side; at other times only the left arm was said to have been paralyzed. The ankle jerk was absent on the left side; the biceps and triceps reflexes were equally active on both sides. A positive Babinski sign was present on both sides, but was greater on the right. Rectal and vesical sphincter control was lost. The abdominal and cremasteric reflexes were not obtainable. The eyegrounds were normal. The temperature was 103.5 F. Aside from a large head the

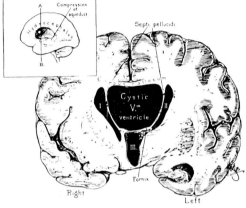

6. Position of congenital cyst in relationship to the ventricular system.

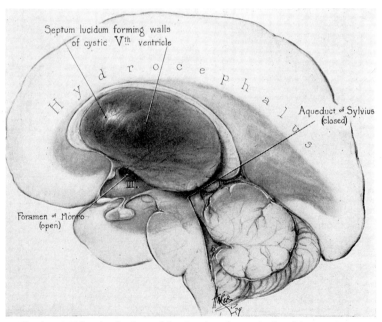

Fig. 7. Midsagittal view of brain showing relationship to the ventricular system in this place. The mild grade of hydrocephalus which resulted in this case was probably by the pressure on the aqueduct of Sylvius.

roentgen examination gave negative results.

Course.—On the afternoon of the day of admission, he was sitting up and again moving the left side apparently normally. The spinal fluid was normal. The Wassermann reaction of the blood and spinal fluid was normal.

Dr. Hodge, the resident on pediatrics, made the following note. "The striking things about the history and physical examination are: (1) questionable enlargement of the head at birth and definite enlargement at present; (2) marked mental retardation which has always been present; (3) some dilatation of the viens over the forehead and otherwise negative physical examination. The paralysis has now entirely cleared. He now runs about aimlessly, laughing in a silly, meaningless fashion. He can say few words but cannot repeat many simple words and does not know his name."

Clinical Diagnosis.—Because of the unilateral convulsions, followed by paralysis of the left side of the body, I thought of a cerebral tumor of congenital origin, perhaps an angioma. In support of this diagnosis was a rather large head. Ventriculography was suggested and was employed a few days later.

Ventriculography.—The right ventricle was reached at the posterior horn and found to be large. Thirty cubic centimeters of fluid was aspirated and an equal amount of air injected.

A positive diagnosis of an enlarged fifth ventricle was made on the basis of the precisely similar ventriculographic changes in the preceding case. There seemed no other possible lesion that could cause this ventricular deformation at this early period of life.

In the anteroposterior view the two lateral ventricles (in cross-section) were about 2 cm. apart instead of being in apposition. Moreover, the mesial aspect of each venticle was concave, and the right ventricle was rounded on its superior aspect, a positive sign of a hydrocephalic ventricle.

In the lateral view the posterior horn and a small adjoining part of the body of the ventricle were much enlarged, but anterior to this point the body of each ventricle was reduced in size. At the tip of the anterior horn the ventricles again became larger, the right more so than the left.

From these observations it was concluded that there must be a space-occupying lesion (i. e., a tumor) of some kind which separated the lateral ventricles, indented them locally and caused a mild grade of hydrocephalus by blocking the aqueduct of Sylvius.

Operation.—On May 28, 1929, a small bone flap was turned down on the right side of the head, slightly anterior to the rolandic area. The mesial side of the flap was directly over the longitudinal sinus. The dura was reflected toward the midline, and right frontoparietal part of the brain was retracted from the falx. The corpus callosum was exposed and was found to be pushed upward; it was paler and thinner than normal, owing to the underlying pressure. An anteroposterior opening, about 2 cm. in lengtn, was made in the anterior half of the corpus callosum. About an ounce of clear colorless fluid escaped as soon as the corpus callosum had been incised. The cavity from which the fluid was evacuated was everywhere smooth and glistening. Its color was essentially the same as that of the normal ventricular wall, but no blood vessels could be seen. There was no visible choroid plexus. No openings of communication could be observed, and there was no sign of papillomatous tumor. The cavity was oval. The following measurements were estimated: length (anteroposterior), 7 cm.; depth, 5 cm., and width, 5 cm. Symmetrical, smooth, longitudinally directed, rounded, bulging projections were present in each side. Each congenital projection was probably 0.75 cm. in depth and 1.5 cm. around the surface. These were the right and left lateral ventricles. With forceps an opening about 0.75 cm. long was made into lateral ventricle. Cerebrospinal fluid then escaped from each lateral ventricle. The walls were opaque and about 3 or 3 mm. in thickness—much thicker than the normal transparent wall of the septum pellucidum. The exposed surface of the brain showed a marked deformation of the cortical veins, and, doubtless, therefore, of the convolutions. There was no sylvian vein. The rolandic vein was formed just mesial to the sylvian fissure by confluence of five tributaries draining the frontal, temporal, parietal and occipital lobes. Soon after the rolandic trunk was formed, at a point about midway between the sylvian fissure and the longitudinal sinus, the vien curved sharply backward, then mesially again to

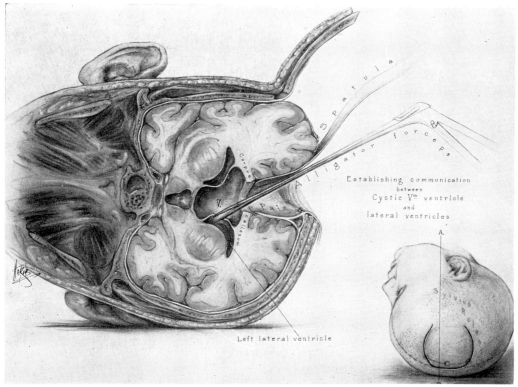

Fig. 8. The method of producing an opening between the lateral ventricle and the cystic cavum septi pellucidi. Through this approach an opening can be made into each lateral ventricle.

enter the longitudinal sinus in approximately the normal position. In its course over the hemsiphere the rolandic vein therefore formed roughly a semicircle with a radius of about 5 cm. instead of the normal direct oblique course across the brain. The rolandic vein was much larger than normal, large enough, in fact, to suggest an arteriovenous aneurysm, but this possibility was excluded by the small tributary veins and by the absence of arterial blood in the vein.

There was no evident intracranial pressure. Room for the operative exposure along the corpus callosum was obtained by releasing the fluid by a ventricular tap (right ventricle). In view of my distressing experience in the preceding case the left anterior cerebral artery was carefully avoided.

The postoperative course was uneventful, the patient returning home two weeks later.

Subsequent Course.—The patient returned for observation eight months later. He had been perfectly well in every way.

There had been no convulsions or attacks of paralysis. The Babinski reflexes were no longer positive. He appeared much brighter. His mother said that he was entirely well and much different than at any time preceding the operation. He was much more active and played with other children, whereas he had always been listless. The mental transformation seemed even greater to the mother. He was eager to learn, constantly repeating what he heard and talked of what he saw; previously he had been unconcerned. His memory was also greatly improved.

CRITICAL REVIEW OF CASE 2.—It is difficult to evaluate the clinical manifestations of this lesion except by postoperative changes, particularly as the patient had another congenital lesion, the vascular and convolutional deformations. The latter alone might cause convulsions, even unilateral convulsions, but not the convulsions of the variable character manifest in his case. He had some unilateral attacks, but others in which both legs and only one arm jerked. To produce these there must have been a mesially placed lesion in the brain. Moreover, they would not cause paralysis following the convulsions, nor a positive Babinski sign on both sides. Because of the recurring hemiplegia, the bilateral Babinski sign after the attacks, and the attacks affecting both legs but not the rest of the body, I had made a probable clinical diagnosis of an angioma near the midline of the brain, or possibly a cyst with an intracystic tumor. There had to be a gross tumor-like lesion to produce the signs of intracranial pressure, i. e., headache, vomiting, stupor and unconsciousness long after the convulsions were over. The recovery of consciousness and the relief from hemiplegia suggested a lesion that varied in size over short periods of time, as for example a cyst. The exact type of lesion was not suspected until ventriculograms were made. The diagnosis was inescapable.

How far the mental and physical improvement was due to the cure of the lesion can only be conjectured. Mental impairment may indeed be due to malformation of the left cerebral hemisphere, such as that seen at operation in the right hemisphere. The patient was righthanded, however, and the actual malformation of the right hemisphere was of no concern in the mental make-up. Explanation of the mental backwardness on the basis of a cerebral deformation could therefore be possible only by assuming another malformation of the left cerebral hemisphere. The mental improvement that resulted following the permanent opening in the septum lucidum appears to be too prompt and too great to be unrelated to the dilated cavity, particularly since during the preceding years there had been no such spontaneous improvement, even for a brief interval. I am led to believe that much, if not all, of the mental deficiency may have been dependent on the large tumor. As the lesion lay on the aqueduct of Sylvius (and third ventricle), occlusion (of the ball-valve type) of the ventricular outlet from the third ventricle led to enlargement of both lateral ventricles and probably to enlargement of the head. The lesion was, of course, of congenital origin and the enlargement of the head was noticed soon after birth. This leads me to believe that the obstruction was only partial for several years, after an initial more complete blockage.

CLINICAL FEATURES

The only symptoms that stand out in these cases were headaches and mental aberration, and neither of these symptoms was characteristic of any condition. One could only think that there must be an organic lesion of some kind and that the trouble was sufficiently serious to demand the application of every possible diagnostic aid. That an organic lesion must exist was evident from the positive Babinski sign in each case and by the motor paralysis in case 2. The intermittency of the symptoms is also doubtless significant and can surely be explained by ball-valve action of the tumor and also because of its cystic character, which denotes variability of volume. That a congenital lesion should exist for forty years before giving trouble is surprising, but scarcely more so than the fact that once headaches developed they should disappear entirely after five years and not reappear after another five years. Moreover, experience with other large congenital space-occupying lesions of the brain, such as angiomas and arteriovenous aneurysms, is not dissimilar. They may exist for many —even forty or fifty—years without causing any or many disturbances of function. As the mental disturbance in case 1 could not be due to syphilis, and as there was no reason to suspect arteriosclerosis as a cause, the diagnosis or exclusion of a new growth was demanded the more. In case 2 the mental retardation might well have been considered to be due to a congenitally malformed brain, as the patient had never been normal, but the period of coma could hardly be explained on any basis except intracranial pressure.

In neither of these cases was the location

or the character of the lesion suspected until the ventriculograms were made. In case 2 the diagnosis was made before operation solely because of the experience derived from the ventriculograms and operation in the case 1. The only other lesion that could give a similar ventriculographic picture is a neoplasm in the region of the corpus callosum; in this instance the symptoms would be more progressive, less fluctuating and doubtless most fulminating.

Whether the incidence of these cavities in normal persons is as high as in the mentally deranged cannot be answered. There is no reason to believe that the psychopathic changes evident in most of the cases reported in the literature are at all dependent on the presence of these cavities. It seems probable that they denote a general trend toward cerebral malformations (there was evidence of this in one of my cases), and that the mental disturbance is the effect of these. As the cyst grows sufficiently large to cause signs and symptoms of local pressure, mental symptoms are then inevitable, because the part of the brain compressed is most concerned in mentality. If my single case of improved mentality after operation can be accepted as evidence, it would indicate that the cyst still remaining but collapsed, was without effect.

Ferrario's original case, which Verga confessed to be the best he had seen, presented no mental symptoms. Recently I noticed both of these cavities in several postmortem examinations of patients who appeared to be normal mentally.

SUMMARY AND CONCLUSIONS

1. Two cases of cysts of the cavum septi pellucidi and cavum vergae are reported. In each case the two cavities were continuous.

2. The cysts acted as tumors and caused compression of the motor tracts on both sides. Mental symptoms were decided in both cases. One patient had peculiar epileptic attacks of varying character but indicating bilateral involvement of the motor tracts. Suggestive evidence of intermittent intracranial pressure existed in both instances.

3. The diagnosis of cysts of this type cannot as yet be made by clinical signs and symptoms.

4. The diagnosis is easily made by ventriculography. The ventriculographic picture appears to be pathognomonic.

5. An operation is offered for cysts of this character. One patient was well and apparently normal eight months after operation. His physical and mental status was entirely changed by correction of the underlying cause.

REFERENCES

[1]Verga: Dell' apparato ventricolare del setto lucido e della volta a tre pilastri, Mm. r. ist. lomb. di sc., Aug. 2, 1855; Gior. r. Isituto lomb. di sc., nos. 43 and 44, p. 89; Sul ventriculo della volta a tre pilastri. *Gass. med. lomb.*, 7, July 7, 1851.

[2]Tenchini, L.: Contributo alla storia dei progressi dell' anatomia e della fisiologia del cervello, Naples, 1880, p. 174.

XLI

EFFECTS OF TOTAL REMOVAL OF LEFT TEMPORAL LOBE IN A RIGHT-HANDED PERSON: LOCALIZATION OF AREAS OF BRAIN CONCERNED WITH SPEECH*†

In the first case reported, that of a man, aged twenty-one, the entire left temporal lobe was removed. The amount of tissue, including a tumor, was 130 Gm. Four months after the operation, there was no defect of speech that could be attributed to the extirpation of cerebral tissue. At no time did the patient have auditory aphasia. There was a profound anomia immediately after the operation. This is still present in some degree, but is steadily disappearing. We have been taught that the center for auditory aphasia is in the posterior part of the first and second left temporal convolutions. From this case it is evident that auditory speech is not located in the left temporal lobe. The anomia was doubtless due to the trauma to that part of the brain mesial to the sylvian vessel, that is, in the parietal lobe. Otherwise there would have been no return of this speech function. Unquestionably there is, as a sequel to the operative trauma, a permanent defect of some degree in the part of the parietal lobe that is contiguous to the temporal lobe.

In the second case the entire left occipital lobe in which there was a tumor, was resected; the supramarginal and supra-angular gyri were included. The plane of the cerebral incision was vertical and slightly behind the postcentral gyrus. A month after the operative precedure, the patient shows an absolute visual aphasia. He is

unable to read a letter; he can write perfectly from dictation, but cannot read anything he has written. He has no auditory aphasia. He had a slight anomia, which has disappeared. He had an almost complete apraxia after the operation; this has also disappeared. The results in this case show that the center for auditory speech is entirely independent of that for visual speech; also that the area of the brain concerned in apraxia is immediately contiguous to the tissue that was removed, and doubtless occupies the postrolandic region.

Another case is cited of a patient who had a constant series of Jacksonian convulsions beginning in the right side of the face. A small tumor was excised, together with a small zone of tissue surrounding the tumor. Unfortunately, that patient never recovered speech, so that he had a total motor aphasia, but no sensory aphasia. This case is mentioned to show that the motor speech center is in the region of Broca's area. The only reason to mention this case is that from time to time doubts have been cast on Broca's original localization of a motor speech center.

An extensive resection of the left frontal lobe is shown because it passes through the so-called Broca's area and does not cause motor aphasia. From several cases of pure motor aphasia it is my impression that the area concerned in motor speech is somewhat farther posterior than that shown in textbooks.

Slides were shown of the amount of the left hemisphere that may be removed without disturbance of speech.

Summarizing, the results of cerebral extirpations in human beings show that aud-

*Reprinted from the *Archives of Neurology and Psychiatry, 27:* 221–224, January, 1932.

†Read by invitation before, and reprinted from the proceedings of, the Joint Meeting of the New York Academy of Medicine, Section of Neurology and Psychiatry, and the New York Neurological Society held May 12, 1931.

itory speech is located in the parietal lobe, that visual speech is entirely distinct and separate anatomically from auditory speech, and that Broca's area occupies essentially the area described by Broca, except that it is possibly a little more posterior.

DISCUSSION

DR FOSTER KENNEDY: It is not easy to know what part of this presentation to approach first. Dr. Dandy has demonstrated some facts that we already know, and has demonstrated them in an extremely competent manner.

I am in entire agreement with Dr. Dandy's position that the speech areas, that is to say, the functions of integration that have to be achieved in order to effect perfect speech, live in segregated areas. It is as though in certain areas of the brain there are cells that have a certain ability of function: a general function such as vision, out of which can be educated a distinct attribute, and that attribute is highly localized and can be destroyed. Similarly, a difficulty with the motor tract may not injure a man's ability in the least to lift a heavy bucket of water, but may entirely destroy his ability to play billiards.

For a considerable time I have thought, with Dr. Dandy, that Broca's area was farther back, and I think that it is just in front of the rolandic area. I think that the reason why Dr. Dandy's patient recovered was because the lesion was behind the rolandic area. There was a motor aphasia, and I think that it was really a kind of agnosia for speech; a loss of the proper feeling of the tongue, lips and teeth that resulted in an inability to form the proper sound.

I was much interested, and it was a new idea to me, that what we have always called temporosphenoidal aphasia was really parietal. One sees such agnosias, anomias and perseverations resulting from lesions of the temporosphenoidal lobe. I have been sure for a long time that the term auditory aphasia is not a good one. It is extremely rare for any one to be so aphasic that he cannot understand heard speech. It is easy to wipe out a man's ability to know written speech. It takes a much larger lesion, or perhaps a more discrete lesion, to wipe out his heard speech. In severe temporosphenoidal lesions, the patient cannot write the symbols of speech easily, but I shall have to revise my former opinion as regards the place from which such a condition is produced.

Dr. Dandy mentioned a paper of mine in which I was able to give an explanation for the so-called crossed aphasias, that is, those occurring in people who, being right-handed and having a right hemiplegia, had no aphasia. I was able to show that many cases of the series collected occurred in persons of left-handed stock; that their right-handedness was really a sport of the stock, and that the brainedness was a stock brainedness and did not follow the handedness. I think that many of us have left-handed strains in our ancestry, and I should not be surprised to find that that left-handed strain in right-handed persons produced a condition in the brain by which the opposite side of the brain (from the usual speech area) was able to sustain the function of speech. Possibly some of the recovery of the boy whose case Dr. Dandy has reported may not be due to the parietal lobe undertaking functions regularly sustained by the temporsphenoidal lobe, but to the education of the opposite side which contains elements that are ordinarily dormant in function.

DR. ISRAEL STRAUSS: In my mind there is no question but that for clinical purposes we shall still have to adhere to the localizing symptoms that we are accustomed to attribute to certain localities of the brain. There is no doubt that we will still have to regard auditory aphasia as being in the temporosphenoidal lobe, or at least in close proximity to it, and that we will have to regard Broca's area as a center having an influence on motor speech. It was Marie who took exception to the localization of Broca's area in the left third frontal convolution, but we have all found lesions definitely placed in that part of the brain affecting motor speech. All of us have found lesions in the temporosphenoidal lobe when we have postulated them because of the presence of the so-called auditory aphasia. Dr. Dandy, however, may be correct in stating that the lower part of the parietal lobe is the seat of this disturbance in function. When a lesion exists in the temporosphenoidal lobe we would have to regard that symptom as due to pressure or edema. However, it must be borne in mind that occasionally temporosphenoidal lobe symptoms are found in cases of small abscesses in the temporal lobe, and it is hard to conceive that edema from a small abscess would cross the sylvian fissure and cause an edema in the lower part of the parietal lobe.

DR. MICHAEL OSNATO: Were serial sections made, and were studies made of the association pathways, particularly those of the inferior longitudinal fasciculus, which connects the occipital with the temporal lobes, and the long association pathway which connects the occipital pole of the brain with the island of Reil and, of course, the temporosphenoidal lobe, namely, the occipitofrontal fasciculus?

DR. JOSEPH E. J. KING: I have had no experience with complete resection of the frontal or the occipital lobe, but I have been rather impressed with the amount of destruction of the temporal lobe occurring in cases of abscess of the temporosphenoidal lobe in which no permanent aphasia remains. In some of these cases there were rather large abscesses, and one was large and not encapsulated. There is no question about the destruction of the brain substances in this region from abscess. It is not a displacing lesion but a replacing one, and it destroys that which it replaces, i. e., brain substance. I can conceive of an encapsulated tumor in this area that might displace or push some of the temporosphenoidal lobe out of position, but such is not the case in abscess of the brain.

I had one case in which an abscess of enormous size developed in the temporo-

sphenoidal lobe following an operation, with the herniation of the abscess cavity, in which a complete hemianopia developed. When the hernia receded, the hemianopia cleared up. The patient has no permanent aphasia of any kind. This patient was operated on in 1922.

DR. GEORGE VAN NESS DEARBORN: It struck me at once that more should be said about the possible "education" of substitute parts of the brain. It seems to be taken as a matter of course, at least by implication, that no education of substitute regions of the brain can occur. However, I observe in reading the latest research literature that such education may take place to a very considerable extent.

DR. W. E. DANDY: There is another important point that I neglected to mention. We are taught that there is an auditory center for hearing in each temporal lobe. The total excision of the left temporal lobe shows that there is no auditory center in the left temporal lobe. Moreover, similar negative results for hearing have been repeatedly demonstarted from total extirpation of the right temporal lobe. Unquestionably, there is a relationship between the tracts for hearing and the auditory center, but the connection must be in the parietal lobe. It has long been taught that other parts of the brain, even the opposite side of the brain, may assume the lost functions of speech, motor power, etc. I think that it was Broadbent, of England, who first proposed this theory. Victor Horsley strongly opposed such a view. I think positively that there can be no restoration of function by education of the opposite side of the brain. For example, after the total removal of a right hemisphere there will never be restoration of motor function in the left side of the body. Moreover, after resection of the left occipital lobe with hemianopia, there is no restoration of visual speech or of the hemianopia. It is true that many cases of motor aphasia and hemiplegia clear up in part or entirely. That is due to the fact that the actual destruction of these parts of the brain has been only partial, or, as in cases of edema, there may be no permanent loss of the areas controlling these functions.

XLII

PHYSIOLOGICAL STUDIES FOLLOWING EXTIRPATION OF THE RIGHT CEREBRAL HEMISPHERE IN MAN *

Attempts to localize cerebral functions based upon the effects of cerebral tumors or degenerative processes—until recently the only sources for such information—have led to the most contradictory results, and for very good reasons. The disturbances caused by a brain tumor are not restricted to the region of brain tissue that it occupies. Indeed tumors very frequently induce symptoms in far distant parts of the brain either from contiguous cerebral oedema or from the transfer of intracranial pressure. Nor can the absence of signs or symptoms be taken as evidence of the absence of function of a given part of the brain when this region is occupied by a tumor, for encapsulated or well circumscribed tumors may merely push the brain aside without altering its function; and infiltrating tumors may surround, without destroying, cerebral tracts even though the gross appearance of the tumor would give every reason to believe that non-interference with functions was impossible. The net results of tumor analyses furnishes a seeming paradox, for some tumors in a given region produce no obvious loss of function, whereas others of the same size and in precisely the same location cause the most widespread and profound alterations in their workings.

Degenerative processes, even when sharply defined and dormant, are of little more help because such processes are always multiple. This objection still clings to Broca's demonstration of the sharply defined area of the brain responsible for motor speech. And it was the capricious effects of tumors and degenerative processes that led the famous Brown-Sequard so far astray in

denying cerebral localization. How, he insisted, could such results be explained except by assuming that the brain worked as a whole?

The results of animal experimentation are of little value in determining cerebral functions and their localization because the advent in human beings of the higher intellectual faculties, including the speech mechanisms, has brought about an entirely different set-up of the tracts in the central nervous system, particularly in their transfer, in part or in whole, to the cerebral hemispheres.

It is only necessary to mention the well known cerebral extirpations of Goltz's dogs to appreciate the dangers of attempting to transfer the results of canine experiments to the human brain.

The only accurate and safe data concerning most cerebral functions can come from extirpations of parts of the human brain. From accurately defined and well performed removals of this type the functional results, if positive, must be regarded as specific and, if negative, must exclude the part of the brain concerned from participation in the functions tested. Nor can Broadbent's old theory that the corresponding part of the opposite hemisphere assumes these functions be given even remote consideration. The arm, leg and visual areas receive no such relief, and losses of function due to injuries of the left hemisphere are not aided in the least by any participation of the right hemisphere. Before drawing conclusions of the positive type from local excisions of brain tissue it is necessary to be sure that an artery that supplies a distant part of the brain has not been included. It is clear that one could remove a small region of brain and include

*Reprinted from the *Bulletin of the Johns Hopkins Hospital*, *LIII: 1:* 31–51, July, 1933.

a middle cerebral artery, or one of its larger branches, and draw entirely erroneous conclusions from the disturbed functions. Then, too, a small zone of brain contiguous to the area removed in all probability will subsequently be destroyed by the operative trauma and will add somewhat to the total volume of tissue removed.

From the following three cases the physiological results following extirpation of the entire right cerebral hemisphere, i. e., external to the basal ganglia, have been studied. One of these patients lived two years and two months, and the other six months.

CASE *I*. R. F., a preacher, aged thirty-two, was referred by Dr. John Booth of Rochester, N. Y., April 13, 1923. At the time of his admission to the Johns Hopkins Hospital he was in a state of semicoma; pulse 48; respirations 12 to 13, and irregular depth. He voided involuntarily in bed. Stimulation of the supra-orbital nerve produced movement of both arms and legs. The reflexes were normal. There was a suggestive but not definite papilloedema. The margins of the discs were hazy but the veins were neither full nor tortuous. As he had myopia of high grade, it was not certain whether these changes were due to this local condition or to intracranial pressure.

From a fellow clergyman and friend who accompanied him it was learned that the patient had been a very brilliant student; in fact, he had been an honor man at the University of Virginia. He had always worked hard and was deeply interested in his studies. He was always eccentric and egotistical and was regarded as a queer person. He was seclusive, shunned society and took no interest in social matters. His friend had not seen him for a number of years until the previous summer. At this time he noticed a pronounced change. The patient talked continuously about sexual matters and was wont to stress this subject in his sermons. He harried his congregation a great deal and gradually they ceased attendance. He then became very nervous and agitated and complained bitterly of their unfairness. About this time he began to complain of headaches, principally in the right temporal region. There was a drawl in his speech but no aphasia. He had been more or less depressed for several

months, probably because of the loss of attendance at his church. Three weeks before admission he had what was called a nervous breakdown, began to talk queerly and mumble to himself, and at other times would be depressed and unresponsive. But again there would be a flow of wit. Three months before he came to the hospital, he had stolen a communion set, but when the source of the theft was discovered he had maintained that it was his own property.

Ventricular estimation was performed April 13, 1923. The right ventricle could not be reached. The left was easily tapped and 25 cc. of fluid escaped under some pressure. From these findings a right-sided cerebral tumor was diagnosed.

Operation April 13, 1923. A fairly large bone flap was turned down on the right side. A subcortical tumor was found involving the frontal, parietal and temporal lobes. The tumor was clearly inoperable. The intracranial pressure was so great that it was necessary to remove the entire bone flap and in addition take away with the rongeur much of the remaining bone in the temporal region. The wound was then closed.

Post-operative course. Recovery was uneventful. The patient quickly regained consciousness. Four days after the operation a left hemiplegia developed progressively but quite rapidly. It was soon complete. There was a tremendous hernia at the site of decompression. Following the relief of pressure by the large decompression the patient gradually became clearer mentally. At first he wrote short notes to express what he wanted to say, then he began to talk but at times his speech was thick. He frequently joked and confabulated. He was fairly well oriented but had difficulty in maintaining intellectual contact. Occasionally he would refuse food. However, during the two weeks before the cerebral extirpation he had come to a high mental level and was in full grasp of his surroundings. He recognized old acquaintances even by their voices. He began to plan for the future and his confabulations became rarer and practically ceased. The patient and his relatives were very insistent that the tumor be removed even though they realized that the hemiplegia which was now complete would be permanent. Accordingly, at their request, the operation was undertaken.

Second operation June 4, 1923 (seven

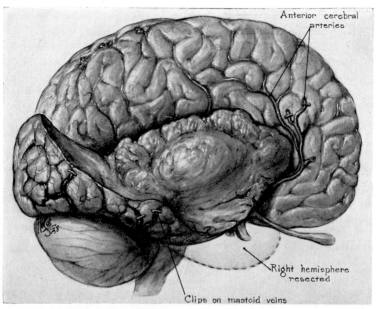

Fig. 1.　Drawing showing extent of subtotal resection of hemisphere
in Case I.

weeks after the exposure of the tumor and decompression). The right cerebral hemisphere was subtotally resected, an area of occipital lobe remaining. The tumor had now reached the surface of the brain in the parietal and frontal regions. Two small cysts opened spontaneously. The anterior, middle and posterior cerebral arteries were separately clipped and divided. The tension in the brain was much diminished by the exclusion of the arterial blood. The veins passing between the hemisphere and the longitudinal sinus were then doubly clipped and divided as they crossed in the subdural space. The hemisphere was separated from the falx. The corpus callosum was exposed and a lateral incision just above it opened the body of the lateral ventricle. The frontal, parietal and temporal lobes were removed, only a small portion of the occipital pole remaining (Fig. 1). There was everywhere so much tumor tissue that the brain ruptured in several places, exposing the growth. The total amount of extirpated brain tissue was 250 grams. In addition, there was the content of several cysts which were evacuated during the extirpation. It required 260 cc. of fluid to fill the cranial defect, and since there was a huge hernia before operation, it is clear that the actual volume of tumor and brain removed was much greater than these figures would indicate.

The basal ganglia were left intact (Fig. 2). No tumor could be seen remaining in the hemisphere but the new growth had attached itself to the dura of the middle fossa. This portion was removed as thoroughly as possible by excising the dura.

Postoperative course. Recovery was uneventful. The right third nerve had evidently been traumatized during the operation, for ptosis and external squint were present immediately after it. This palsy gradually disappeared. Immediately following the operation his mental state was essentially the same as before the cerebral excision.

He was at all times perfectly oriented as to time, place and person. He was quite quick and accurate in repartee. On June 27, 1923, three days after the removal of the hemisphere, the following statement was recorded: "That's the sickest day I had since I have been here. I have headache and my stomach aches and my heel is sore. But I ought not to complain there are others who are sick too. If you will give me an enema and get rid of this stuff in my stomach I will be better."

June 9, 1923. "How are you this morning?" "Better doctor."

"Any pain?" "In my head, heel, stomach, shoulder. I got enough to keep me busy."

"Date?" "9th of June, 1923."

"Who am I?" Dr. D."

"Who is your surgeon?" "Dr. D."

"I am Dr. H., did you see me before?" "Yes, several times."

"Which day of the week is this?" "Friday, unlucky day."

"Why unlucky? Everybody says Friday is an unlucky day. I don't know why. Old folk-lore or from the old witchcraft days, perhaps."

"How was the sherry wine you got yesterday?" "That was fine."

On July 13, 1923, five weeks after extirpation of the hemisphere he dictated the following letter:

"Dear Father and Mother:

Mr. Mason read your last letter to me, and it gave me much joy and comfort. There isn't much to write about that is new. I am perfectly well as far as my head is concerned, the only thing that is holding me back is my paralyzed leg and arm. I asked the doctor the other day when I could go home and he couldn't give me any definite answer, of course, nor can I imagine when it will be. It will be within a month I am sure. I told the doctor that I wanted to eat Thanksgiving dinner with you all at home, and he said that he thought that this could be possible. Everyone is very kind to me here. I have made many dear friends. My love and God's blessing upon all the dear ones at home. I think of you continually every day.

Your loving son,
Roy."

"P.S. The nurses in the offices have bought me several little things for which I am indebted. Please send me five one dollar bills again. This will probably be all the money I shall need.
Roy."

Following is a list of puns with which he

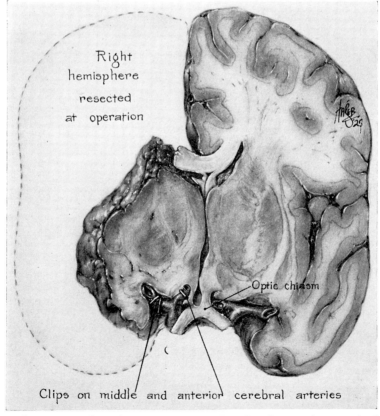

Fig. 2. Drawing of coronal section of brain after total removal of the right cerebral hemisphere above the basal ganglia.

entertained his friends both before and after the time his hemisphere was excised:

Why does a duck go under water? For diverse reasons.

Why does he come up again? For sundry purposes.

Why is the heat around the furnace like a circus? It is intense.

Why does a crow? Caws.

If you saw a Ford automobile driving down the street, and another passing it, what time of day would be represented by the scene? Ten after ten.

Why is it that next year all Fords have to be painted red? Because it is the fire law that all gasoline cans must be painted red.

Why didn't Eve have the measles? She had Adam.

After man came woman and she has been after him ever since.

I am getting worried about my hand. I want to play music for you in the hospital, and need the use of this hand for music. I play the guitar. One of the boys out there made me laugh. He said he was a musician. I said, "What music do you play?" and he said, "The victrola."

The extirpation of the hemisphere had no effect upon the facility and accuracy with which they were rattled off. Although showing no high mental level, they at least indicated a retentive memory.

On July 24, 1923, at the time of discharge, the following observations are recorded by Dr. Ford:

Cranial nerves. II. Complete homonymous hemianopsia for form and color.

V. Muscles of mastication contract strongly on the left (the paralyzed) side. Sensation is not grossly diminished in the face. Point of a pin recognized. Cotton well felt. Corneal reflex equal on both sides.

VII. The left side of the mouth does not move with voluntary efforts. When the patient smiles there is some slight movement. Eyelid closes tightly on the left. The forehead wrinkles on the left, though less strongly than the right.

VIII. Patient hears watch equally well on both sides.

XI. Sternomastoids move equally on the two sides. The left shoulder can be elevated.

XII. Tongue protrudes in the midline.

Motor and sensory changes. There is complete paralysis of the left arm. The left leg can be flexed at the knee but can-

not be extended. No movement of the toes or ankles. The muscles are all flabby. There is no spasticity. There is loss of all cutaneous sensations on the left side, except as noted in the face. Vibration of the tuning-fork is perceived on the left but not so strongly as on the right. There is complete loss of sense of position and of passive movements. Movements of the joints and compression of the muscles cause intense pain on the left. The tendon reflexes are greatly increased on the left. There is an ankle clonus, and active Hoffmann on the left. Abdominal reflexes equal. One month ago the abdominal reflex was absent on the left. Plantar stimulation on the left causes flexion of the leg but no movement of the toes. The patient retains complete sphincter control.

The patient left the hospital July 24, 1923. On June 25, 1925, I visited him at an institution maintained by the church for invalids. His mental faculties appeared to be quite normal and had so impressed his friends. He was interested in the radio, conducted vesper services on Sundays and read scripture lessons. His articulation and memory were good. He enjoyed the radio and listened with the greatest interest and late into the night to the proceedings of the Democratic National Convention which was in session in New York City during the summer. He also read the newspapers. The following month he began to become irritable and signs of weakness of the other side developed. It was evident that the tumor was recurring. He died August 16, 1925—two years and two months after extirpation of the cerebral hemisphere.

CASE II. Mrs. A. S., aged 24, entered the Johns Hopkins Hospital October 13, 1927. Complaint: Weakness of the left side of the body. Family and past histories, negative. Five weeks ago numbness of the left arm, particularly of the hand, was first observed; ten days later the weakness had extended into the arm. A few days afterward left facial weakness was evident. The arm became progressively weaker. Two weeks ago, or three weeks after the first symptom, the left foot began to drag and it too has become progressively worse. There have been no headaches, no mental changes or other disturbances.

Physical and neurological examinations. A well nourished, well developed woman, intelligent and alert. The eyegrounds are entirely negative. There is a partial paralysis of the left hand and wrist. The biceps and triceps are weak, but not entirely paralyzed. The left leg is partially paralyzed; she can drag it in walking but it is of little service. There is perhaps slight diminution of the left corneal reflex and slight loss of sensation over the left hand and forearm, but no demonstrable changes in sensation elsewhere on the left side are noted. The reflexes in the left arm are markedly exaggerated; and the arm is spastic. The knee-kicks are greatly increased on the left. The Babinski is positive on the left—negative on the right. There is no ankle-clonus. X-ray of the head negative. Blood pressure 125/80.

Diagnosis. The gradually progressive weakness of the entire left side could scarcely be due to any lesion except a tumor, and because of the rapid progress it was thought to be around the internal capsule. However, an air injection was considered in order to eliminate possible lesions of other type, particularly since removal of the hemisphere was considered in treatment. The absence of headache and papilloedema suggested a small tumor that was producing only local disturbances and not those of intracranial pressure.

Ventriculography. The right lateral ventricle could not be reached; the left ventricle was small. There was no evidence of intracranial pressure, the fluid dripping from the needle. About 15 cc. of air were injected. The air failed to pass into the right ventricle. The third ventricle was definitely though only slightly oblique. There appeared to be no dislocation of the anterior horn of the left lateral ventricle. These findings made it certain that patient had a small tumor in the right cerebral hemisphere.

Operation, October 25, 1927, three days after the air injection. Under ether anesthesia a bone flap was turned down over the right hemisphere. The dura was under no evident pressure. The surface of the brain at first appeared to be normal, but on closer inspection a slight change in the convolutions of the face and arm center in both the prerolandic and postrolandic areas was seen. The whole area involved was roughly circular and about 2.5 cm. in diameter. To make absolutely certain of the character of the lesion a nasal dilator was passed through this area and at a depth of 4 cm. a reddish-brown, semigelatinous tumor was encountered. The nasal dilator was then withdrawn. It was evident

that the only chance of successful extirpation of this tumor, which was clearly of the infiltrating type, was by an extensive resection. One could perhaps have resected the territory immediately surrounding the tumor, but this would have produced precisely the same disturbances as resection of the hemisphere, and the chances of a successful extirpation would have been very much reduced. An extension of the bone-flap was then made anteriorly. The frontal lobe was elevated, the carotid artery was doubly clipped alongside the optic nerve, and immediately following this the anterior cerebral, middle cerebral and the posterior communicating arteries were doubly clipped and divided. At once the volume of the cerebral hemisphere was markedly reduced. The veins passing to the mesial border of the hemisphere were then ligated with silk sutures just before they left the brain tissue to cross the longitudinal sinus. It was easier and safer to ligate the vessels in the brain substance than in the free subdural space, *i.e.,* between the hemispheres and sinuses. An incision was then made through the cortex from the frontal to the occipital region, leaving a small, triangular rim of brain substance lining the entire longitudinal sinus and carrying the venous stubs. The hemisphere was then separated from the falx. The corpus callosum was brought into full view. A lateral incision in the mesial surface of the hemisphere, just above the corpus callosum, brought us into the lateral ventricle. The hemisphere was then elevated with the finger in the lateral ventricle, and excised at the basal ganglia. To facilitate the extirpation the frontal lobe was resected separately, the remainder of the hemisphere, including the temporal, parietal and occipital lobes, being removed in a single mass. The lateral ventricle was now wide open. The choroid plexus and the body of the ventricle were in full view. In extirpating the mass the posterior cerebral artery was encountered and ligated. There was very little bleeding. Inspection of the mass failed to show any sign of tumor on the cut surface. The tumor was disclosed only after a later sectioning of the mass of brain tissue (Fig. 3). The weight of the brain tissue removed was 375 grams. The dura was closed tightly, the bone-flap wired in place, and the muscle, galea and skin were closed with interrupted sutures of silk.

Postoperative course. When the patient

left the operating room her pulse was 95, respirations 32, temperature 101.4°F. In the afternoon she talked and moved her right arm and leg. During the evening and night she talked quite readily and apparently normally. There was then perhaps slight spasticity of the left arm and leg and the Babinski was suggestive. At nine o'clock her pulse changed, was difficult to count but was running around 130 to 140, and she was quite restless. Temperature 102.4°, respirations 36. For the next two days her condition remained very much the same except that she responded poorly. She was in fact difficult to arouse. Respirations remained rapid, pulse around 100, temperature 100 to 102°. In the interim she had had several ventricular punctures but with no marked effect. At no time was there bleeding within the great cerebral cavity, the fluid always returning clear but under some pressure. On the third day a flanged needle was inserted into the frontal region to provide continuous drainage; it was left in place for two days. Her condition seemed to improve somewhat though I question whether this procedure produced the change. At any rate it unquestionably was the source of an infection which soon developed, and which, though of an indolent type, nevertheless was ultimately responsible for her death. In the course of the next two weeks the infection became highly purulent and required drainage through an incision and removal of the bone flap. The huge cerebral cavity filled with pus although the foramen of Monro became sealed and prevented meningitis. Her temperature gradually returned to normal. She left the hospital two months after her operation. The infection could never be eradicated nor satisfactorily handled, and she died six months after operation.

Mentality. The extensive infection is a complication which I feel must be taken into account when testing her mentality. Her brother, who is a doctor, thought that for several weeks after the operation her mind was perfectly normal. However, there were little disturbances, as evidenced by the following note by Dr. Diethelm on December 19, 1927, seven weeks after the operation: "I saw Mrs. S. on two occasions—December 15 and 17. During the first interview she was irritable and did not want to talk at all. She had many complaints, physical complaints as well as about the nurses and the hospital, all said

in a very peevish manner. Her stream of talk was always coherent. She was not depressed and her sensorium seemed to be more or less clear. She was oriented as to place, time, situation and person, but she did not remember events of the last twenty-four hours and gave an inaccurate account of her past life. Her judgment was rather poor. She did not seem to understand her treatment and showed a very poor understanding of her own peevishness and also of her poor memory for recent events.

"Last Saturday (17th) the patient was quite different. She was more alert, talked freely and joked, but the jokes were about trivial things and in a silly way. She was less irritable but still impatient. She smiled and felt more or less at ease. She still has difficulty in understanding orders, *i.e.,* she wants to get up although she knows that she cannot do it. These reactions are probably more the determination of a stubborn personality. Her sensorium is perfectly clear and her memory intact for recent and remote events as far as I was able to test it. The mistakes which she made were due more to fatigue and to a lack of being able to concentrate on certain topics for any length of time.

"I explain the difference in the two examinations by a certain cloudiness which was present the first time and which I would explain with her present organic condition. The second examination argued against an organic deficit."

In estimating her mentality it is necessary to state that she had had very little education, only going through the primary grades.

On the 20th of December, 1927 (two months after operation) the following mathematical tests were made:

9 × 7—Answered 63 promptly.

12 × 12—Answered 144 promptly.

When asked to divide 144 by 12 said "I cannot do that without a pencil."

25/5—Answered 5 fairly promptly.

30/3—Answered 10 promptly.

When asked to substract 3 from 30, said "What are you, a teacher or a doctor?" and then said "27" promptly.

Asked to add 30 and 3—Answered promptly.

She reads quickly and correctly. Can spell various names that are suggested and does so promptly without error. She learns words that she has never heard before and remembers them on subsequent days. She writes correctly and makes correct punctuations. She is facetious, suspicious and easily bored, but her brother says that she has always been so. She cooperates only when she desires to do so.

Neurological Tests for Function

Cranial nerves. I. Her sense of smell is very keen—she detects various odors promptly.

II. There is complete left homonymous hemianopsia for forms and colors.

III, IV, VI. All of the extraocular movements are normally performed without restriction. There is no nystagmus.

V. There is marked preservation of sensation over the left side of the face and corresponding exactly with the trigeminal domain. Light touch is not perceived, but when touch is slightly intensified, as by rubbing loose cotton over the face, it is accurately recognized and located. The point of a pin is registered as a painful stimulus. Sharp and dull are easily differentiated but both are considerably less acute than on the right side of the face. Heat and cold are accurately defined, though here again a somewhat greater degree of temperature is required than on the other side. The masseter muscles contact on both sides, but with somewhat less force on the left. However, the jaw is not deflected from the midline when the mouth opens. The corneal reflex is very acute and essentially the same on both sides. It will be observed that a diminution of the corneal reflex was observed in the preoperative examination.

VII. There is definite asymmetry of the face, greater contraction being, of course, toward the right, but much movement is retained. The forehead wrinkles on both sides about equally well. There is a deep nasolabial groove on the left side and the eyelids close together and completely, and almost with equal force. There is only a little less wringling of the corner of the eyes on forceful closing of the lids.

Taste tested on the 20th of December, 1927—two months after operation:

	Right	Left
Sugar	Promptly	0 (?)
Salt	Promptly	0 (?)
Acid	Promptly	Promptly
Bitter	Promptly	Five seconds

There is, therefore, definitely some taste. Unfortunately examination for taste was not made before operation. It cannot, therefore, be known whether there has actually been a postoperative loss of taste, or whether this might perhaps be the normal for this side.

VIII. Patient's hearing has been perfectly normal since the operation. There has been not the slightest sign of unilateral deafness and there has been no tinnitus. An audiometer test was made by Dr. Bunch on February 27, 1928, or four months after the operation. The hearing was essentially the same on both sides (Fig. 3).

XI. The left sternomastoid and trapezius muscles function but are weaker than on the other side.

XII. Tongue is protruded in the midline.

Motor and sensory changes in arm and

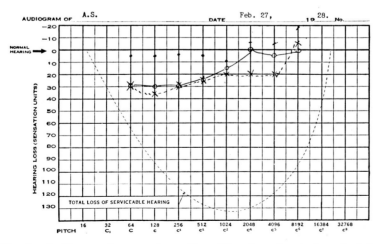

Fig. 3. Audiogram from patient (Case II) whose hemisphere had been removed four months previously.

leg. No movement whatever is possible in the left arm. There is slight movement in the muscles of the foot but they are very feeble and she cannot bend the toes or elevate the foot from the bed. No movement is possible at the knee or thigh. Cutaneous sensation is abolished over the entire left side except over the trigeminal domain, as described above. However, a deep sensation of a certain kind is present on the whole left side. When the muscles of the leg or arm are squeezed, the patient complains of severe pain and, moreover, is able to localize with fair accuracy the area that is squeezed. When the toes are manipulated, she can identify the one moved but cannot tell whether it is elevated or lowered. When the sole of the foot is scratched, the whole left leg draws up. She can tell when the leg is elevated or lowered. (Deep sensation is unchanged on the right side.) There is also severe pain on manipulation of all the joints on the left side. There is no spasticity of the left leg. Although the left hand tends to a claw formation, it is quite easy to open the fingers. There is no contracture of the forearm or the upper arm, nor is there contracture of the leg. Except for the slight claw formation of the hand one would consider the leg and hand to be in a flaccid state. There is no resistance to passive manipulation of the arm at the elbow or the leg at the knee. There are ankle and patellar clonus on the left. The biceps and knee-kicks on the left are slightly greater than on the right. There is at times an equivocal Babinski on the left; at other times it is negative. Superficial reflexes on the left side of the body are absent. Oppenheim and Gordon tests on the left are positive. Abdominal reflexes are active on the right, absent on the left. Vibrant sense is lost over the entire left arm and leg.

CASE *III.* The following is a record of the conversation—necessarily limited—beginning twenty-four hours after extirpation of a right cerebral hemisphere and contained tumor (total weight 584 grams) in a colored man, and continued at intervals during two days, after which meningitis ensued and caused his death ten days later. At the end of the reported conversation he began to become incoherent and irrational from the effects of the high fever. It is, I think, evident that immediately after the operation and before complications developed his mind functioned

quite normally.

Operation concluded March 16, 1927, 12 noon.

March 17, 1927:

2:00 p.m. "My left wrist pains." Holding wrist with right hand.

2:10 p.m. Q. "Can you straighten left leg?" No answer, but pushed it down straight by using right leg.

2:30 p.m. Q. "Can you raise your knees while I put this pillow under?" Raised right leg.
Q. "Does your wrist still hurt?"
A. "Yes mam—right here" —pointing to wrist.

3:00 p.m. Q. "Are you trying to sleep?"
A. "Yes, I'm trying, but its pretty hard."
Q. "When are you going to stop hiccoughing?"
A. "I don't know, but I'd like to."
Asked by orderly if he needed attention, answered "No."

3:20 p.m. Q. "Does your side hurt?"
A. "No miss."
Q. "Not at all?"
A. "Just a little."

3:45 p.m. Q. "Perhaps if you talk a bit the hiccoughing will stop."
A. "It might."
Q. "Did you work before coming into the hospital?"
A. "I worked until the 15th of December, then I had to quit, I couldn't work any longer and I came into the hospital."
Q. "Is that when you had your first operation?"
A. "No, I had that in 1924."
Q. "What work were you doing?"
A. "I worked for Baltimore Steel Company."

5:00 p.m. Answer a l l questions promptly, no hesitation, apparently no lack of memory. Speech not impaired at all. Voided involuntarily. When asked if he knew when he must void, answered "Yes," but offered no answer when asked why he didn't ask for some one to take care of him.

6:00 p.m.   Asked during dressing if head hurt more than before puncture was started.

A. "Yes, it hurts more now."

Q. Would you like to have some milk?"

A. "Yes, I would."

7:00 p.m.   Q. "Did you enjoy the milk?"

A. "Yes, it was very good."

9:00 p.m.   "I want the orderly, please."

9:30 p.m.   Q. "Does the light hurt your eyes?"

A. "No, Miss."

Q. "Does your chest hurt?"

A. "It's not so sore."

10:00 p.m.   Q. "Does your right hand hurt?"

A. "No, just feels numb."

10:45 p.m.   Q. "Do you know where you are?"

A. "Yes sir."

Q. "Where?"

A. "In Johns Hopkins Hospital."

Q. "Do you know who I am?"

A. "Yes sir."

Q. "Who?"

A. "Let's see. Who are you?" After a pause.

Q. "Who did you come here to see?"

A. "Mr. Dandy."

11:45 p.m.   Q. "What month is this?"

A. "March."

Q. "What day of the month?"

A. "Let's see" answered after longer pause than usual.

Q. "How do you feel?"

A. "I feel fairly good."

March 18, 1927:

1:45 a.m.

(48 hours after operation)

Q. "Would you like some orange juice?

A. "Yes Miss."

4:00 a.m.   Q. "Do you want some more water?"

A. "Yes Ma'm."

6:00 a.m.   Q. "How do you feel?

A. "All right."

8:00 a.m.   Q. "How do you feel this morning?"

A. "I feel right good, but I've got a pretty heavy fever." Pulling a t clamps on infusion.

9:30 a.m.   Q. "What do you want, Raymond?"

A. "I don't want anything."

Q. "Can you see that?"

A. "Yes Ma'm" Pulling at dressing.

10:00 a.m.   Q. "Why are you doing that?"

A. "It feels like its coming off"

10:30 a.m.   Playing with clamp on infusion.

Q. "What are you doing with that?"

A. "I'm going to play some music."

Q. "How?"

A. "Just turn it and it plays."

Q. "What is it, a Victrola?"

10:45 a.m.   A. "No'm, it's a radio."

Q. "How do you feel now?"

A. "Oh, I can't say I feel so good and I can't say I feel so bad, just about the same, I guess."

12 noon.   Visited by head nurse of ward; Recognized her immediately. Told her he felt quite well and would enjoy coming back to ward.

12:20 p.m.   Seen by Dr. Dandy.

Q. "Where are you?"

A. "At Walter Young's."

Q. "Who did you come to see here?"

A. "Dr. Dandy"—slight hesitation."

Q. "Now can you tell me where you are?"

A. "Johns Hopkins Hospital."

Q. "What month is it?"
A. "March."
Q. "What year?"
A. "1927."

12:30 p.m.   Cold sponge (begun to reduce temperature).
"It's too cold to take a bath with that water, it's almost like ice."
Asked for orderly. Voided voluntarily.

3:30 p.m.   Began talking of his own accord.
"They could get a lot of things around here to build."
Q. "What things?"
A. "Grass and things."
Q. "What is this place?"
A. "Johns Hopkins Hospital."
Q. "What would they use the grass for?"
A. "To build a nest for the young ones."
Q. "Who would?"
A. "The mice."
Q. "I didn't know that mice used grass for nests."
A. "Yes Ma'm, and feathers and cord a n d things."
Q. "What made you think of mice?
A. "I don't know, I just thought of them."

5:15 p.m.   Q. (By patient) "Is there ether in that?" Referring to alcohol.
A. (By nurse) "No, does it smell like ether?"
A. (By patient) "Seems like everything smells like ether now."

6:10 p.m. $3.00 mentioned without any provocation.
Q. "What do you want $3.00 for?"
A. "To go to Cambridge."
Q. "Why do you want to go there?"
A. "My wife wants to go."
Q. "Why?"
A. "Because her mother's there."
Q. "Does it take $3.00 to go there?"
A. "No, $1.65."

Q. "Don't you have that much?"
A. "Oh, yes'm."
Q. "If it's only $1.65, why do you need $3.00?"
A. "You see my wife's got to go and I've got to go."

SUMMARY AND CONCLUSIONS

The presentation of these three cases with extirpation of such vast areas of brain tissue without the disclosure of any resulting defect in mental functioning is most disappointing. It is still difficult to believe that some functions of the mind are not stored or at least are not activated there. Needless to say one would experience much greater elation in finding some well defined facts of positive type than in making the sweeping negative deduction that is suggested here. I am still not willing to say that the mentality of the patients was normal; but rather that abnormalities have not been disclosed. And it need scarcely be added that I have sought evidence of positive functions by referring these patients to the best available talent. I realize too that the best proof of a normal mind is the ability to carry on in the competitive world, and this opportunity was denied these unfortunates because of the hemiplegia. Then, too, little peculiarities of mental origin, such as those in the famous crow-bar case, may escape mental tests but be obvious to those who are thrown in frequent intimate contact. But such defects, if any, escaped us during the postoperative period and subsequently did not become apparent to the friends of the first patient who were associated with him in the sanitarium for over a year and a half. It is realized too that the opinion (in Case II) of a brother that his sister showed no mental abnormalities may be accepted with reservations.

It is interesting that the first patient had pronounced the progressive mental changes before his operation. These gradually cleared after the relief of intracranial pressure and remained absent after excision of the cerebral hemisphere—a splendid example of the referred effects of the tumor to that part of the brain.

Both patients were always perfectly oriented as to time, place and person. Their memory for immediate and remote events was unimpaired. They could read, write and compute without error. Moreover, the first patient (the infection reduced the period of activity in the second case) was always quick, alert and keen, as evidenced in his style of humor, but he was also interested in serious conversation, in reading and in following the world's events. His originally defective and now additionally impaired vision (hemianopsia), however, curtailed extended reading. His concentration was, I think, quite normal. Both patients were always coherent; at no time were there abnormal fears, delusions, hallucinations, confabulations, expansive ideas or obsessions. Neither was there undue melancholy nor euphoria. Both seemed emotionally quite stable, although the second patient was irritable and peevish at times. Both were normally concerned about the loss of power in the left side but knew that the handicap must be accepted and learned to do so. The habits of both were normal so far as one could judge. The habits of both were always cleanly. There was no tendency to coprolalia.

OTHER NEUROLOGICAL FUNCTIONS

One of the most interesting findings is the preservation of function in the domain of the cranial nerves, *i.e.,* evidence of autonomy of these nerves. *Hemianopsia* is, of course, complete. *Smell* is unaffected. *Taste* is preserved at least in part; the evidence is not sufficient to say whether or not it is modified.

Hearing is not altered. In an earlier paper this finding was used as proof of the absence of an acoustic center in the right temporal lobe as has long been hypothecated. And as neither patient was ever dizzy, it is fair to assume that no essential vestibular connections are present. Unfortunately a Barany test was not made.

None of the extraocular movements were altered or impaired in the slightest, nor was there nystagmus at any time in either case.

Of the greatest interest was the preservation of function in the trigeminal and facial nerves, both of which are known to have cortical representation. In one case there was a very definite but slight diminution of all forms of sensation, corresponding exactly with the trigeminal domain. In the other case it was noted that there was no sign of diminished sensation. Over the remainder of the left side of the body cutaneous sensation was abolished. The motor function of the trigeminal nerve, as evidenced by the degree of contraction of the masseter, temporal and pterygoid muscles, was possibly slightly but certainly not much depreciated. The corneal reflex was equally active on both sides in both patients.

The motor power of the facial nerve was definitely diminished but was nevertheless remarkably well preserved. Both patients could close the eyes well and move the corner of the mouth through the nasolabial groove was much shallower than on the normal side. Apparently the degree of preservation and loss of this function varies in different individuals, for in other extirpations (with shorter survival periods) there was marked difference in the degrees of facial function.

The motor power in nerves X, XI and XII is also little, if at all affected. The tongue protruded in the exact midline in both cases; and the sternomastoid and trapezius muscles appeared equally strong on the two sides. The absence of hoarseness and of difficulty in swallowing would also surely indicate preservation of the function of the vagus. Unfortunately the sensory domain of the glossopharyngeal nerve was not tested.

Another point of interest is the preservation of some (though very slight) movement in the leg of both cases. It was of no practical value in either instance. The flaccidity of the extremities was most surprising. There were no contractures, such as one sees in the many clinical examples of hemiplegia. Indeed there was very little, if any, resistance to passive movements at any time of either the arm or leg. However, the deep reflexes—biceps and knee-kicks—were greatly increased on the left in one case and but slightly in the other. An ankle and a patellar clonus were present in both cases. A positive Babinski was not present in either case.

These findings are quite different from those obtained in dogs or cats, in which the removal of a hemisphere causes no disturbance of gait and no spasticity. The great rigidity from injury to the motor tracts in dogs and cats (decerebrate rigidity) is in evidence at the midbrain. In human beings the rigidity follows lesions in the cerebral cortex and subcortex and is entirely lost or essentially so at the outer border of the basal ganglia, below which control over motor function is lost. The slight preservation of motor power in the legs of our patients is doubtless evidence that a slight residue of function is mediated by lower centers, probably like that in the dog.

The preservation of sensation in the joints, the acute pain when the deep muscles are compressed demonstrates the existence of sensations that are mediated at a lower level than the cortex. Whether or not these sensations arise from sympathetic nerves (or in part at least) is not known. In one case (Case II) there was accurate recognition of the location of the muscles that were squeezed and the joints moved. Even the toes that were flexed or extended could be accurately identified although the direction of movement was not known. These observations were checked many times. On the other hand, it is noted in Case I that there was complete loss of sense of position and of passive movements. Vibratory sense is recorded as being absent in Case II and present in Case I.

The abdominal and corneal reflexes were unchanged in both cases.

REFERENCE

[1]Dandy, W. E.: Removal of Right Cerebral Hemisphere for Certain Tumors with Hemiplegia. Preliminary Report. J.A.M.A., 90: 923, 1928.

XLIII

TREATMENT OF MENIERE'S DISEASE BY SECTION OF ONLY THE VESTIBULAR PORTION OF THE ACOUSTIC NERVE *

The cure of Meniere's disease by section of the auditory nerve intracranially is now established. Following this operative procedure, which has now been employed in thirty-five cases,[1] there have been no subsequent attack of dizziness, no loss of life and no disturbance of function, except in two of the early cases when the facial nerve was injured—a danger which is now scarcely possible. The only loss from the operation has been permanent deafness in one ear, but since there is always subtotal deafness at the time of operation, the actual loss caused by section of the eighth nerve has been of no practical concern. However, there are times when, from a number of irrelevant causes, the contralateral hearing is also diminished. In such instances preservation of hearing on the affected side, particularly if magnified by electrical instruments, might at the present or even at some future time be of important service. And again there are times when the actual loss of hearing in the affected ear—especially in the early stages of the disease—may be relatively slight.

After the cure of Meniere's disease had been established, there naturally suggested itself the possibility of a further refinement by which the remaining hearing on the defective side would be preserved. Since the disturbing symptoms of Meniere's attacks are due to explosions of function in the vestibular component of the nerve, it is reasonable to expect that section of only the vestibular division of the nerve would cure the attacks, while hearing might be left intact. Since there is no gross demarcation between the auditory and vestibular divisions of the acoustic nerve where it is attacked surgically, the exact limits of the vestibular branch can only be estimated. It was assumed that the vestibular division made up one-half of the volume of the nerve. But to be certain that all vestibular fibers were included it would even be advisable to divide some of the anterior fibers of the auditory division of the nerve. From experiences with the sensory root of the trigeminal nerve, and perhaps of the optic nerve also, there was reason to believe that loss of some auditory fibers might not be followed by reduction in hearing. The experiment at least seemed worthy of a trial and it succeeded.

CASE REPORT

Male, age fifty-one; some deafness in the right ear for twenty-six years; increased deafness in the past eight months. Humming in the right ear six months. During this time there have been frequent attacks of dizziness, lasting one-half to one hour. They have averaged about two a week. During attacks there is sound like that of church bells ringing in the right ear. He is nauseated and vomits. Dizziness is worse when lying down and when the eyes are closed. During attacks objects turn clockwise and the patient staggers to the right. Between attacks he is free from all symptoms, except tinnitus, the intensity of which, however, is greatly reduced.

Examination is negative except for the audiometer and vestibular reports. Vestibular reports. Vestibular (Barany) test: Normal response to hot and cold on the left; reduced but fairly active response on the right.

Audiometer test. The audiometer curves

*Reprinted from *Bulletin of the Johns Hopkins Hospital, LIII: 1:* 52–55, July, 1933.

are shown in Figure 2. A marked loss of hearing in the good ear made it necessary to preserve the hearing in the defective side for possible future service.

Operation, March 10, 1933. Partial section of the eighth nerve was performed under avertin anesthesia. The nerve was cocainized before division. Approximately the anterior five eighths of the nerve in cross section was divided; the posterior three eighths of the nerve (the auditory part) was preserved (Fig. 1). Assuming that the eighth nerve is equally divided (in cross section) between the auditory and vestibular divisions, the total vestibular branch should have been divided, and approximately an additional one eighth of the nerve, *i.e.,* about one fourth of the to-

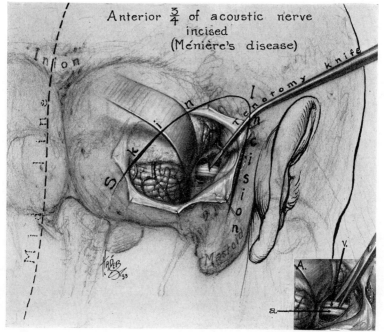

Fig. 1. Drawing showing operative approach and manner of dividing the vestibular branch of the auditory nerve leaving the acoustic division intact.

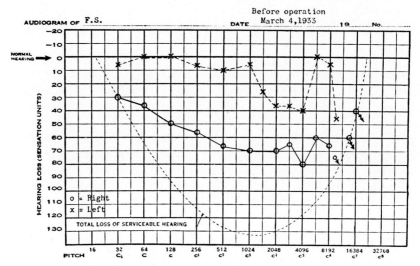

Fig. 2. Audiometer curves before operation.

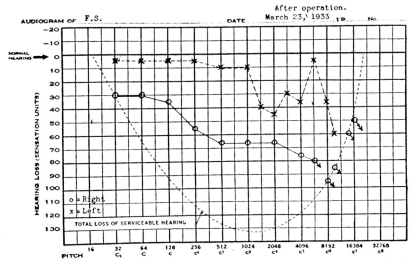

Fig. 3. Audiometer curves thirteen days after section of the vestibular
division of the nerve.

tal volume of the acoustic branch, was added in order to be reassured that no vestibular fibers could be retained in the acoustic nerve.

The postoperative course was uneventful.

Postoperative caloric test (13 days after section of the nerve): Total loss of all reactions on the right; normal on the left.

Audiometer curve. The only change from the preoperative audiometer test was a loss of the octave above 4096 (Fig. 3). Whether this slight change is actual or significant, I am not prepared to say.

The time (April 18, 1933—five weeks after operation) is as yet much too short to claim a permanent cure of the Meniere's syndrome by section of only the vestibular division of the auditory nerve, but the total absence of the caloric response indicates total absence of function in this division of the nerve and leads us to believe that a successful outcome, and with practically no loss of hearing, may be expected.

REFERENCE

[1]Dandy, W. E.: Meniere's Disease: Diagnosis and Treatment. Report of Thirty Cases. *A. J. of Surg.,* xx: 693, 1933.

XLIV

BENIGN ENCAPSULATED TUMORS IN THE LATERAL VENTRICLES OF THE BRAIN: DIAGNOSIS AND TREATMENT*

In this communication thirteen benign encapsulated tumors in the lateral ventricles of the brain are reported. There are no signs or symptoms by which enucleable tumors can be differentiated from the invasive gliomata or other malignant types of tumor which protrude into or obliterate the ventricles.

From the literature twenty-five additional cases have been found; all of these have been post-mortem findings. None has been diagnosed during life or removed at operation. From an analysis of the signs and symptoms of the tumors in the literature, together with those in my series there is no clinical syndrome by which these tumors can be localized with sufficient accuracy to be found at operation. It is true that some of them have hemiplegia, but this by no means permits accurate localization of the growth. All of these tumors can, however, be localized with absolute precision by means of ventriculography. When used correctly there is no danger whatever in this procedure. In our series all have been found at operation. Ten have been removed and the patients are well; three died from the effects of the operation. In the last nine cases there has been but one death. The longest survival period has been fourteen years. This chanced to be the first tumor that was localized by ventriculography.

Primary benign ventricular tumors occur in about 0.75 per cent. of all brain tumors. They occur in any part of the lateral ventricles. The youngest patient was twelve, the oldest forty; they, therefore, occur during the period of youth. The dur-

*Reprinted from the *Annals of Surgery*, November, 1933.

ation of symptoms varied from five months to nine years, the average being one to two years. The only constant symptom is headache. There may be nausea, vomiting, diplopia, dizziness and papilloedema, all of which are purely indications of intracranial pressure. A positive Romberg or a history of staggering gait may mislead the operator into a diagnosis of a cerebellar tumor. Some degree of sensory or motor unilateral paralysis was present in about one-half of the cases.

Character of the Tumors. The tumors are of various types, most of them ependymal gliomata, but they are entirely different from the gliomata that arise in the cerebral tissue. They are well encapsulated, except at the small point of origin in the ependyma, and this is easily removable with the tumor. In none has there been recurrence. There have been two pure fibromata; these were the largest in the series, weighing 95 and 124 grams, respectively, and both grew out of the glomus of the choroid plexus. One tumor was an adenoma of the choroid plexus, and another was a venous aneurism in the wall of the body of the ventricle (Fig. 1). This was completely extirpated following a second intracranial haemorrhage with hemiplegia.

Ventriculographic Findings. These are of various types, depending upon the size and position of the tumor; always they are pathognomonic. A sharp line indicating the termination of the air shadow accurately marks one pole of the tumor. A sharp straight or curved line suggests a benign type of tumor, but one cannot always be certain from the ventriculographical evidence alone that the tumor is of the encapsulated type. Always, there is hydrocephal-

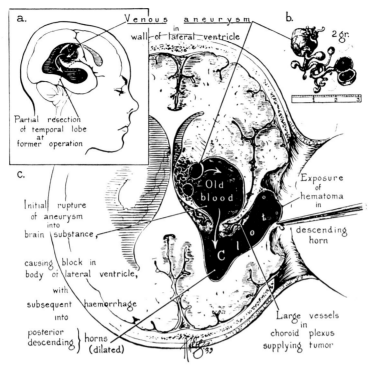

Fig. 1. Venous aneurism incorporated in the right ventricular wall.
It had bled on two occasions producing hemiplegia. After removal of
the hematoma the aneurism was disclosed and removed.

us distal to the tumor and caused by the obstruction of the ventricular system. A tumor may also block the ventricular system at a distance from the tumor, *i.e.,* by lateral compression of the aqueduct of Sylvius or the third ventricle.

TREATMENT. A cure, of course, can be accomplished only by the removal of the tumor, and the earlier the diagnosis the better the patient's chances. It is always necessary to remove an area of cortex (Fig. 2) either directly overlying the tumor, if that part of the brain is silent, or if the tumor lies in the motor or another important area of the brain, the cortical defect must be made anterior or posterior to the tumor and enucleation may be made through this defect.

DISCUSSION. Dr. George J. Heurer (New York City) remarked upon the enormous contribution which ventriculography had made to the diagnosis of certain brain tumors. He recalled in his own experience how impossible it was to make a diagnosis of an intraventricular tumor and that these cases were operated upon sometimes when the tumor was not found. They eventually came to autopsy and at that time the tumor was discovered. It is an illustration, he thought, of the advances that are being made in neurosurgery.

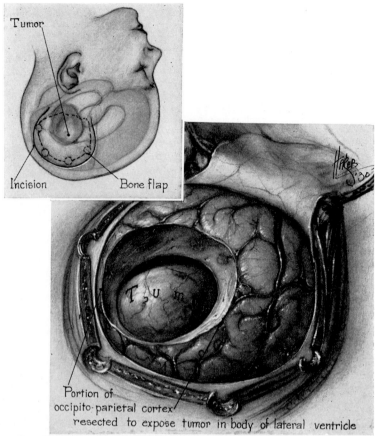

Fig. 2. Operative approach to tumor; an area of cerebral cortex is
resected in order to permit access to the growth.

XLV

CEREBRAL (VENTRICULAR) HYDRODYNAMIC TEST FOR THROMBOSIS OF THE LATERAL SINUS*

That thrombosis of the lateral or sigmoid sinuses, or the sequelae, may at times be responsible for the clinical signs and symptoms that suggest an intracranial tumor or abscess, especially the latter, is well recognized. When the character or position of the presumed intracranial lesion is not known, it is usually necessary to employ ventriculography in order to clarify both the diagnosis and the localization of the lesion. In practically all of these doubtful cases bilateral papilledema is the outstanding objective finding. Although papilledema is by no means a positive proof, it is a strong presumptive evidence of intracranial pressure.

It is of course possible, with recognized exceptions, to determine by a lumbar puncture whether or not the papilledema is due to increased intracranial pressure. But neurosurgeons have learned by unfortunate experiences that lumbar puncture is fraught with far too much danger to life and function to be used for this purpose. When a tumor or abscess is suspected, the only safe method of obtaining the necessary information is by ventricular puncture, which, in addition to the determination of the presence or absence of intracranial pressure, also permits—by the introduction of air (ventriculography)—the precise localization of the lesion, if one exists, or the elimination of this diagnosis if no lesion is present.

Heretofore in order to make a positive diagnosis of thrombosis of the lateral or sigmoid sinuses after negative results from ventricular puncture (with or without ventriculography) it has been necessary to perform lumbar puncture with the Quecken-stedt test at a later time. This test (first applied by Tobey and Ayer), though open to error, is an important advance in the recognition of thrombosis or at least of occlusion of these sinuses.

It recently occurred to me to wonder why precisely the same results could not be obtained by ventricular puncture. The hydrodynamic principles are exactly the same. Compressing one or both jugular veins causes venous congestion in the cerebral veins, and this in turn causes a rise of intracranial pressure which should register by a ventricular manometer equally and not less accurately than by the lumbar route. Occlusion or patency of a lateral sinus should, therefore, be disclosed as readily as by the Tobey-Ayer test. In the following five cases the ventricular test was checked with the Tobey-Ayer test in three instances and by necropsy in the remaining two.

REPORT OF CASES

CASE 1. C. C., a well nourished woman, aged forty, was drowsy and unresponsive though not comatose; she complained of right-sided headaches. The illness began four weeks before admission with earache on the right side; a thin yellow discharge appeared two days later. Two weeks later she was nauseated, but did not vomit. There were many hot and chilly sensations during this time and a dull, throbbing, temporal and occipital headache on the right. Shortly afterward the vision declined in the right eye, and the right eyelid drooped. She had since been bedfast and unresponsive. The discharge from the ear remained practically unchanged.

Examination. The face was flushed; the lips were dry and cracked, and the skin moist and hot. The temperature was 102 F., the pulse rate, 120. During the night the temperature and pulse remained unchanged. The respiratory rate was 20; the

*Reprinted from the *Archives of Otolaryngology,* 19: 297–302, March, 1934.

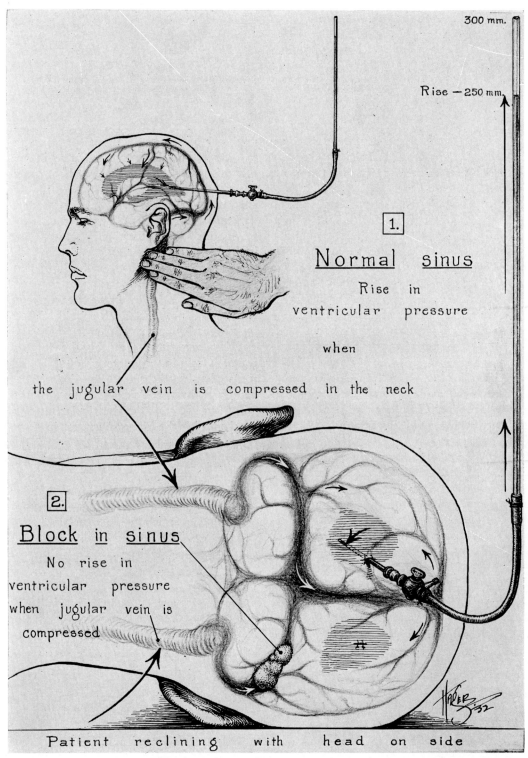

Underlying mechanical principles of the cerebral test for thrombosis of the lateral or sigmoid sinuses.

blood pressure, 180 systolic and 110 diastolic. The leukocyte count was 15,000, with 80 percent polymorphonuclears.

The neurologic examination showed papilledema of four diopters in both eyegrounds and punctate hemorrhages alongside the disks. The visual acuity in the right eye was much reduced; on rough test there was no hemianopia. The right pupil was smaller than the left. There was a definite paralysis of the abducens muscle on each side. Although there was ptosis of the right eyelid, the extraocular muscles supplied by the third nerve were not affected. A slight facial weakness of the peripheral type was evident on the right side. The hearing was markedly diminished in the right ear. On the left side there was a positive Babinski sign, and the corresponding knee jerk was increased. The Kernig sign was positive on both sides, and there was marked rigidity of the neck.

Diagnosis. There were four possibilities: (1) abscess or abscesses of the brain, (2) meningitis, (3) thrombosis of the sinus and (4) encephalitis.

Ventriculography and Subsequent Course. Ventriculography (by ventricular puncture) was necessary for the differential diagnosis and for determination of the line of treatment. On Jan. 9, 1932, the ventricular fluid was under no increased pressure; ventriculograms were normal; the ventricular fluid contained only 10 cells, 3 of which were of the polymorphonuclear type. It was therefore clear that the patient had neither meningitis nor an abscess of the brain. At once a Queckenstedt test was made by means of the spinal puncture, and it was found that jugular compression produced no rise of the fluid on the right side. However, a prompt and rapid rise resulted when the left jugular vein was compressed, and when compression of the vein was withdrawn the fluid fell rapidly to its previous level. It was clear, therefore, that the patient had thrombosis of the right lateral or sigmoid sinus. The numerous neurologic findings were, of course, not directly due to the thrombosis of the sinus, but doubtless to systemic invasion by the infection of the mastoid and perhaps of the lateral sinus.

The patient was later treated by Dr. Crowe who opened the mastoid and found a thrombosis of the lateral and sigmoid sinuses; he ligated the jugular vein in the neck. She has since remained well.

The hemolytic streptococcus was isolated from the ear and also from the lateral sinus, which was opened and cleared of its contents. The same organism grew from the blood that was taken when she was admitted to the hospital.

Ventricular Test for Thrombosis of the Lateral or Sigmoid Sinus: During her stay in the hospital it occurred to me to wonder why it might not have been possible to make a positive diagnosis of thrombosis of the lateral sinus at the time the ventricular puncture was first done. The patient would then have been spared the additional lumbar puncture for the Tobey-Ayer test.

A ventricular puncture was again made on Jan. 27, 1932. The initial height of the fluid was 19 cm. Pressure on the left jugular vein caused the fluid to rise to 33 cm., and it descended promptly when the pressure was released. Pressure on the right jugular vein produced no change in the height of the ventricular fluid at any time.

The results of the ventricular test were, therefore, identical with those of the spinal test.

CASE 2. M. C., aged thirty-five, was referred by Dr. Ralph Greene of Jacksonville, Fla., on May 7, 1932, with the probable diagnosis of an abscess of the brain.

Illness dated back to Dec. 30, 1930 (eighteen months before), when bilateral otitis media developed during a severe cold; both drums were lanced and drained for about ten days. A few weeks later an abscess of the right upper lid was opened, and shortly thereafter furuncles developed in both external auditory canals. In January, 1931, an operation on the left mastoid was followed by chills, a temperature of 105 F. and erysipelas of the face. In three weeks recovery was complete. In October, 1931, a boil developed in the right nostril, and during the following month one on the right arm. The patient was soon well again. In February, 1932, three months before admission to the Johns Hopkins Hospital, bilateral otitis media again developed, and again both drums were incised and drained about ten days. At this time the patient had a chill, a temperature of 104 F. and pains in the left side of the chest; it was said that she had some pulmonary congestion but not pneumonia; three days later this pain had disappeared. For over a month a rise in temperature of a few degrees persisted; both mastoids were again opened on March 4, 1932. The low fever continued, and two weeks later chills and high fever (from 104 to 105 F.) again developed. Altogether there were about twenty chills; these sometimes appeared on two consecutive days; at other times they were three or four days apart.

On April 3, 1932, the right mastoid was again opened and an epidural abscess evacuated. For the next month the patient continued to have right-sided headaches, which were most pronounced above the mastoid; these were of a dull character and radiated to the frontal region. Shortly afterward the same headaches developed on the left side. One week before admission there was a severe sharp pain in the left occipital region and at the same time a whistling noise in the right ear. In the last five days this had become a dull, steady roar. The patient had frequent attacks of vomiting. One month previously she complained of numbness in both legs from the ankles to the knees, but there were no objective changes. She had not had a chill for over a week before admission to the Johns Hopkins Hospital, although her temperature reached 101 F. nearly every day. There had been a pain below the left shoulder blade for the past week. About a week before admission a lumbar puncture was made by Dr. Greene, at which time greatly increased intracranial pressure was said to have been found. She had lost 31 pounds (14.06 Kg.) during the past three months.

Examination. The patient was a normal appearing young woman, slightly fatigued. There was some evidence of loss of weight, but general condition was good. The temperature was 100 F.; the pulse rate, 110, and the respiratory rate, 120; the blood pressure was 124 systolic and 78 diastolic. There was some tenderness along both mastoid wounds, which were not entirely closed, there being a small area of granulation tissue in both retracted scars.

The neurologic examination gave negative results except for a low grade of papilledema, which was perhaps more marked in the right eye.

Impression. Although a cerebral abscess was considered because of the low grade papilledema, headache, vomiting and Dr. Greene's report of increased intracranial pressure, it was doubtful that an abscess explained the condition, particularly in view of the long continued fever and chills, neither of which should have been present

had an abscess of the brain existed at the beginning of the trouble over two months before.

Roentgen Examination. Roentgenograms of the mastoid region were taken, and on the right side there appeared to be evidence of occlusion of the lateral sinus in that the curve of the lateral sinus tapered to a point midway between the torcular herophili and the mastoid. This was thought to be evidence of thrombosis of the lateral sinus, but I was entirely unfamiliar with such a positive finding.

Ventriculography and Subsequent Course. Ventriculography was needed for differential diagnosis. There was no increased intracranial pressure. The fluid barely rolled out of the needle and attained a height of only 10 cc.

Pressure on the left jugular vein produced a rapid rise to 35 cm.; on release the fluid returned to the original level. Compression of the right jugular vein produced no rise whatever in the column of ventricular fluid. Pressure on both jugular vein produced exactly the same rise that obtained when the left jugular vein alone was compressed. Thrombosis of the right lateral sinus was therefore evident.

The ventriculograms were normal, thereby excluding a cerebral abscess; moreover, the fluid contained only 8 cells.

Operation on the mastoid was later performed by Dr. Henry R. Slack, Jr., who found infected granulation tissue extending into the attic; there was no free pus. The lateral sinus was not opened. Following the operation signs of meningitis developed from which the patient died.

Autopsy. In addition to meningitis the autopsy showed an old healed thrombosis of the right lateral sinus. There were no cerebral abscesses. A small pocket of pus occupied a badly eroded anterior tip of the petrous portion of the right temporal bone, and was responsible for the chills, fever and other symptoms of recent months.

CASE 3. D. B., a well nourished girl, aged eleven years, was referred with the diagnosis of a probable tumor of the brain.

She complained of headache and vomiting. The patient had been perfectly well until the advent of severe frontal headaches six weeks before admission. These were aggravated by exercise and helped by rest. Spells of vomiting were frequent and relieved the headaches. At times there was vertigo. The mother thought that an infection in the paranasal sinus preceded the onset of the trouble, but of this she was not certain. The patient believed that she had been improving in the past week.

The physical and neurologic examinations gave entirely negative results, except for papilledema of moderate degree (two diopters) in both disks; the retinal veins were full. There was an old retinal hemorrhage on the left. The temperature was 100 F.; the pulse rate, 100, and the white cell count, 10,500.

Impression. The patient probably had a tumor, or possibly an abscess without signs of localization.

Ventriculography; Queckenstedt Test. Ventriculography was necessary for the differential diagnosis; it showed that fluid from the right ventricle reached a height of 140 mm. of water. On compression of either the right or the left jugular vein alone there was no rise. On compression of both jugular veins together the fluid immediately ascended to 300 mm. Fifteen cubic centimeters of air was injected into the right ventricle. The ventricular system was entirely normal, thereby excluding the possibility of both a tumor and an abscess. The ventricular fluid showed only 2 cells.

Three days later a spinal puncture was performed in order to inject phenolsulphonphthalein to test absorption. A Queckenstedt test was made at this time and gave precisely the same results as those obtained with the ventricular puncture.

Diagnosis. The papilledema was due to an unknown cause but not to a tumor or cerebral abscess. There was no thrombosis of the lateral sinus.

CASE 4. R. C., a well nourished young man, aged twenty-one, was referred with the diagnosis of a tumor of the brain. He complained of headache and paralysis. The family and past histories were negative. The present illness began four months before admission with a complaint of mild headaches without localization and occasional vomiting. For the past two months he had vomited several times a week; recently the vomiting had been projectile. A gradually progressive hemiplegia on the left and diplopia had begun two months previously. Recently the right side of the face had felt "dead". Clonic movements of the left arm and leg had recently appeared, without convulsions or loss of consciousness.

Physical and Neurologic Examinations. The patient was bedfast but in good general condition. There were optic atrophy in the right disk and a mild grade of papilledema with loss of visual acuity in both eyes; the vision of the left eye was 4/20; that of the right, 4/70. Paralysis of the right abducens muscle, absence of the right corneal reflex, hypo-esthesia on the right side of the face, spastic paralysis of the left arm and leg and loss of sensation; hyperactive reflexes on the left side, absence of the abdominal reflex on the left, a positive Babinski sign on the left, ankle clonus on the left and a 50 per cent reduction in hearing in the right ear were also noted.

Provisional Diagnosis. Tumor of the brain, probably in the brain stem, but possibly in the right cerebral hemisphere, was considered.

Trephination and Injection of Air; Cerebral and Spinal Queckenstedt Test. The right ventricle was tapped; the fluid registered 160 mm. of water. On compression of either the right or the left jugular vein the level of the fluid remained unchanged, but following compression of both jugular veins the fluid slowly rose to 330 mm. Additional pressure in the region of the occiput produced a further rise of 480 mm. This finding was repeated several times with similar results. Air was injected, and the lateral ventricles were found to be normal.

In order to check the interesting findings of the cerebral Queckenstedt test a spinal puncture was performed; the results were exactly the same.

Final Diagnosis and Subsequent Course. The diagnosis was that of an infiltrating tumor of the brain stem, an inoperable lesion.

The patient's signs and symptoms steadily progressed. At necropsy, three weeks later, the clinical diagnosis was substantiated. The occipital sinus was larger than either lateral sinus. It emptied into the jugular bulb on the left side.

CONCLUSIONS

A ventricular hydrodynamic test is proposed by which the diagnosis of thrombosis of the lateral sinus can be made or excluded with the same degree of accuracy as that obtained with the spinal Tobey-Ayer test.

Unilateral jugular compression (each side is tested separately) will cause the pressure of ventricular fluid to rise (with exceptions) if the lateral sinus is patent, and the level of the fluid will promptly fall when the venous compression is released. If a rise of the ventricular pressure does not follow jugular compression on one side but follows compression on the other, the lateral sinus is probably occluded or absent on the former side.

The use of this procedure instead of the spinal test is suggested only when a ventricular puncture is required to diagnose or eliminate the possibility of a tumor or an abscess of the brain by ventriculography. Under such circumstances it merely makes an additional spinal puncture unnecessary.

XLVl

THE EFFECT OF HEMISECTION OF THE COCHLEAR BRANCH OF THE HUMAN AUDITORY NERVE. PRELIMINARY REPORT*

In earlier publications it has been observed that after hemisection of the sensory root of the fifth nerve, practically no disturbance of sensation resulted. At a later date a patient whose optic nerve had been divided in more than half of its cross section the vision returned to normal following the removal of an hypophyseal tumor; in fact no difference could be determined between the vision of the intact and of the partially severed optic nerve.

This note is concerned with further evidence of much the same character after partial section of the auditory nerve. The patient, F., aged forty-four years, was operated upon for Meniere's disease, the left auditory nerve being divided in three-fourths to four-fifths of its extent. From an earlier experience in which five-eighths of the acoustic nerve—all of the vestibular

*Reprinted from *Bulletin of the Johns Hopkins Hospital, LIV: 3:* 208–210, 1934.

branch and one-eighth of the cochlear—had been sectioned, there was no post-operative loss of hearing whatever. When section of the vestibular and part of the cochlear branches of the nerve had been completed (there being no dividing lines between the component divisions of the nerve), it was my impression that about four-fifths of the total volume of the nerve had been sectioned; my assistant was asked for his opinion, and he volunteered that three-fourths of it had been divided; certainly it was not less than this amount. From this interpretation it is evident that all of the vestibular branch and one-half of the cochlear branch were divided, provided, of course, that the auditory nerve is equally divided by volume into the two branches.

Thirteen days after the operation the audiogram showed that all of the tones up to 6144 were almost exactly the same as be-

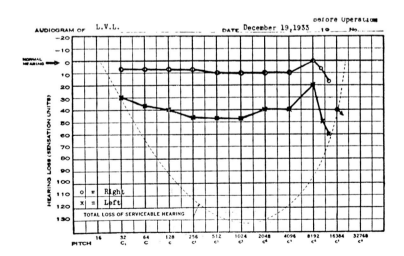

Fig. 1. Audiogram before hemisection of the cochlear division of the auditory nerve.

509

fore the operation; only the higher tones, 8192 and 12286, were lost. The highest tone, 16384, was absent both before and after the operation. On the following day another audiogram was made in order to check these findings and with identical results. The immediate result, therefore, following section of one-half, at least, of the cochlear branch of the acoustic nerve is loss of only two of the very high tones. This finding is seemingly in complete harmony with the results of partial division of the trigeminal and optic nerves.

I have no desire to speculate in general-izations concerning the significance of data of this character. It is evident, however, that there is a redundant supply of fibers in the sensory root of his as well as in that of other cranial nerves. It is also obvious that the ganglia mediate important functions and that the sensory roots lack the detailed service that obtains in the peripheral nerves. I also feel that it is difficult to harmonize such physiological facts with the neurone theory.

REFERENCES

[1]Dandy, W. E.: An operation for the cure of tic douloureux. *Arch. Surg.*, XVIII: 687, 1929.

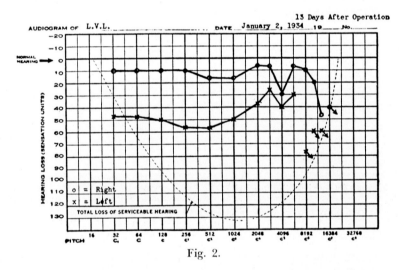

Fig. 2.

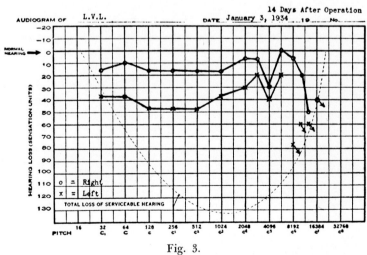

Fig. 3.

Fig. 2 and 3. Audiograms thirteen and fourteen days respectively, after hemisection of the cochlear division of the auditory nerve.

[2]*Idem*: Certain functions of the roots and ganglia of the cranial sensory nerves. *Arch. Neurol.,* *XXVII;* 22, 1932.

[3]*Idem*: Treatment of Meniere's Disease by section of only the vestibular portion of the acoustic nerve. *Bull. Johns Hopkins Hosp.,* liii; 52, 1933.

XLVII

REMOVAL OF CEREBELLOPONTILE (ACOUSTIC) TUMORS THROUGH A UNILATERAL APPROACH*

For the attack on the well recognized encapsulated tumors of the cerebellopontile angle (erroneously, I think, called acoustic tumors) the bilateral cerebellar approach has been adopted by all neurosurgeons. I know of no exception to this rule. The purpose of this communication is to present a radical departure from this standardized approach, namely, to offer in its stead, a unilateral exposure, essentially similar to that now used when the fifth, eighth and ninth nerves are divided for various symptoms referable to these nerves.

Originally a unilateral approach was proposed by Krause; it was used by others and subsequently given up because it was entirely inadequate. A pertinent query is, therefore, why again propose a seemingly similar approach which has been proved to have disastrous consequences? The answer is that new developments, particularly methods of space reduction, then not known or not properly appreciated, now offer all of the advantages obtained by the more extensive exposure. It is well known to those who have had much experience with these tumors that the patient's resources may be so severely taxed by the bilateral approach alone, particularly with the bloody midline, that the additional attack on the tumor at the same operation may be inadvisable. For many years surgeons, at least those in this country, have used the tremendous exposure provided by the so-called cross-bow incision of Cushing. Perhaps a decade ago, I gave this up for the more simple, less bloody and less arduous transverse incision, which is curved downward at the mastoid processes.

This provides the same exposure and makes the approach to the angle easier, because the big nuchal muscles fall away from, rather than toward, the line of vision. Moreover, the cerebrospinal fistulas that developed all too frequently in the vertical part of the cross-bow incision, with many disastrous sequelae, were automatically avoided. The transverse incision which I[1] employed was much like that proposed by Cotterill[2] in 1899, but it was modified by enlarging the cutaneous incision and bony defect upward and outward on the side of the tumor. Gradually the conclusion was forced on me that, after the other items in space compensation had been put into effect, the bilateral bony defect was really contributed little, if anything, to the relief of pressure in the posterior cranial fossa. In further simplification, therefore, the unilateral cerebellar approach is now proposed. It has been used in the last four tumors of this character and with no less satisfactory exposure of the tumor than with the bilateral approach. Unquestionably nothing can be worse than attempting to remove a tumor of the brain without providing adequate room not only for the existing intracranial pressure and the approach to the tumor but for all postoperative edema that develops. But it is also clear that all superfluous room is obtained at the cost of the patient's none too great physical reserve. If it is necessary to choose between too little and too much room, there can be no argument concerning the choice of the latter, but the best results are always obtainable by making the smallest approach that satisfies all needs. It will therefore be understood that, in suggesting the unilateral

*Reprinted from the *Archives of Surgery*, 29: 337–344, September, 1934.

approach for cerebellopontile tumors, it is done with the full realization that inadequate provision for room is disastrous.

I might also add that obtaining room in the standardized fashion through a bilateral cerebellar decompression is in itself frequently most injurious to the contents of the posterior cranial fossa, i.e., the cerebellum and brain stem. I have in mind the great thrust backward of the cerebellum and brain stem when the dura is widely opened. The result of this is seen in the cerebellum, which is swollen from edema and internal hemorrhages and, symptomatically, from the patient's altered pulse and respirations. It is my feeling that many postoperative deaths are due to this injury inflicted early in the operation. By the unilateral approach only the outer part of the cerebellum on the operative side can be extruded, and this part is excised in preparation for the exposure of the tumor.

REDUCTION OF PRESSURE WITHIN POSTERIOR CRANIAL FOSSA

How, then, is the increased pressure within the posterior cranial fossa reduced to the point of safety?

AVERTIN ANESTHESIA. First and perhaps most important is avertin anesthesia. Although the contents of the posterior cranial fossa are always under high pressure from three factors— (a) the tumor itself, (b) the internal hydrocephalus and (c) contiguous edema of the cerebellum and brain stem—an additional amount of pressure of variable but always important degree resulted when ether was used as an anesthetic. The absence of this effect with avertin has been commented on elsewhere. It has greatly reduced the hazards of all operations for tumors of the brain and has also permitted the exposure of tumors by such smaller cranial defects. In hypophyseal tumors, for example, the opening in the bone is now one third or less than was required when ether was in use. The proposal to reduce the cerebellar approach to

approximately one third of the former amount is only in keeping with the improvement made possible in hypophyseal operations. Without avertin as an anesthetic, the methods of space reduction that follow would doubtless be insufficient.

Tapping of a Lateral Ventricle. When a lateral ventricle is tapped until the ventricular fluid ceases to flow, the supratentorial pressure is reduced to that of the atmosphere. This procedure, probably first introduced by Krause of Berlin, greatly relieves the pressure in the posterior cranial fossa. It is now quite generally used by surgeons in all operations for tumors below the tentorium. Without it all cerebellar operations would be dangerous when a high degree of pressure obtains. By gentle and steady pressure on the exposed dura an additional amount of fluid is obtained from the lateral ventricle, and in exactly this amount the subtentorial pressure is still further reduced. The latter method of relief must be used with great caution, for the pressure is likewise on the medulla, which above all else must not suffer. It might be added that in the unilateral approach the pressure is exerted more directly on the tentorium and less directly on the medulla than when all of the bone is removed in the bilateral exposure. Rather than incorporate the ventricular openings in a high occipital incision, as many operators prefer, I make two independent horizontal incisions, exactly as for ventriculography. By so doing the transverse incision can be made very low, i.e., below the inion, and a big, overhanging cutaneous flap can thus be avoided.

Evacuation of Fluid from the Cisterna Magna and Spinal Canal. In nature's efforts toward space compensation for tumors in the posterior cranial fossa, the cerebellar tonsils are usually forced into the spinal canal, thus obliterating the cisterna magna entirely or in large degree. It might appear that this source of room, i.e., obtained by evacuating the fluid in the cisterna magna, which is of such great service in attacking the cranial nerves, would

then be denied the operator on cerebellopontile tumors. The membranous roof of
the cisterna is more difficult to reach, and
the evacuation of the cisterna is not so
spontaneous after it has been opened, but
by gentle retraction on this part of the
cerebellum the arachnoidal covering can
be pricked and the tonsil elevated sufficiently to permit the release of a large
amount of fluid with proportionate covering of the pressure below the tentorium.

*Excision of the Outer Cap of the Cere-
bellum.* This procedure is important in
two ways: (*a*) It still further reduces any
excess pressure within the posterior cranial
fossa, and (*b*) the tumor is exposed so that
it may be attacked directly, i.e., without
elevation of the cerebellum. Additional
items of importance are (*c*) that postoperative edema of the cerebellar lobe from
traction is avoided, and (*d*) that ample
room is provided for any degree of postoperative edema that may ensue.

Apparently there are no permanent effects from removal of this part of the cerebellum, the weight of which averages
about 15 Gm. First suggested by Frazier[3]
(1905), this method was rather harshly
criticized at the time and until recently
gained only a few adherents. It is an essential part of the unilateral operation.
Cerebellopontile tumors can be removed
by the bilateral operation without excision
of the outer cap of the cerebellum, but
even then to remove it makes the operation
easier and the risk to life and function less.
With the unilateral approach, removal of
the tumor could hardly be attempted without this expedient. For its success the unilateral approach is indeed dependent on
all of the methods of space reduction. It
has been used in the last four cases, in each
of which the tumor was totally removed
according to the method of attack described elsewhere. For the past ten years I have
strictly adhered to the policy of totally removing all tumors of this kind when seemingly possible, being firmly convinced that
the operative mortality is not greater than
by the partial removal and that the post-

operative course is smoother and more secure; never have I seen recurrence of such
a growth as must always obtain when the
interior of the tumor is removed. Three
of the patients operated on by the unilateral approach are living and well. One of
these was a decrepit woman, aged sixty-
two. Had a bilateral operation been performed, complete extirpation of the tumor
would hardly have been possible. The last
patient, who died, had the largest tumor
of this type that I have seen (66 Gm.).
She was comatose and badly dehydrated
and had long been blind. Earlier experiences were sufficient to prove that she
could not survive a bilateral operation
with complete removal or only partial extirpation. Up to the present comatose patients with cerebellopontile tumors have
presented an insuperable problem. Perhaps with smaller tumors the unilateral
approach may offer a degree of hope. Even
with a tumor of this size the operative attack was at no time handicapped by lack
of room or by intracranial pressure.

It cannot be claimed from this small
series that a bilateral approach may never
be indicated; certainly the need for it
would appear to be exceptional. If the
dural pressure is excessive after the release
of ventricular fluid, one can continue the
incision into the bilateral form without
loss. The only difference between the unilateral approach used in trigeminal neuralgia or Meniere's disease and that in tumors of the cerebellopontile angles is that
the bony defect is increased somewhat toward the foramen magnum in order to expose the restricted cisterna magna more
easily, and toward the tentorium so that
any tentorial vein may be safely thrombosed and divided when the cap of the cerebellum is being excised.

REFERENCES

[1]Dandy, W. E.: An Operation for the Total Re-
moval of Cerebellopontile (Acoustic) Tumors.
Surg., Gynec. & Obst., 41: 129, 1925. Cerebell-
opontine (Acoustic) Tumors, in Lewis, Dean:
Practice of Surgery. Hagerstown, Md., W. F.
Prior Company, Inc., 1933, vol. 12, chap. 1, p.

534.

²Cotterill, J. M.: Remarks on the Surgical Aspects of a Case of Cerebellopontine Tumor by Bruce. *Tr. Med.-Chir. Soc., Edinburgh, 18:* 215, 1898-

1899.

³Frazier, C. H.: Remarks upon the Surgical Aspects of Tumors of the Cerebellum. *New York M. J., 81:* 272 and 332, 1905.

XLVIII

THE TREATMENT OF SO-CALLED PSEUDO-MENIERE'S DISEASE*

The difference between the classical syndrome of Meniere's disease and so-called pseudo-Meniere's disease lies solely in the tests for hearing. In the former there is always an unilateral subtotal loss of hearing without which the diagnosis of Meniere's disease cannot be made: In pseudo-Meniere's disease the attacks of dizziness and the character of the dizziness are precisely similar, but there is no unilateral symptom or objective change in hearing by which the dizziness can be localized to one side.[1] From the standpoint of treatment this localizing distinction is all important, for Meniere's disease can be cured by sectioning the auditory nerve on the side known to be affected; whereas, in pseudo-Meniere's disease there is no indication by any objective test (or by subjective sensations) which auditory nerve is at fault, if indeed the fault lies in the nerve. In dividing the auditory nerve for Meniere's disease the loss of the remaining hearing was of relatively little importance, but one would never be willing to destroy normal hearing on one side (in pseudo-Meniere's disease) unless there was positive assurance that the attacks could be cured; and this, of course, is impossible. The recent substitution of hemisection of the auditory nerve in Meniere's disease, i.e., total section of the vestibular branch with preservation of the auditory branch and its function of hearing, has appeared to offer a solution of this difficulty. At the present time the latter procedure appears to abolish the attacks with equal certainty. Moreover, the fact that a large part of the cochlear branch of the nerve (nine-tenths in one case and more in another) can be sec-

tioned without any appreciable (to the patient) loss of hearing has offered an additional margin of safety in proposing section of the vestibular branch of both auditory nerves[2] as a rational treatment for the cure of so-called pseudo-Meniere's attacks. The following case report, at least, shows that the operative procedure is possible and the immediate results in terms of dizziness suggest the probability of a cure. However, the latter hope cannot be claimed until time has passed final judgment. The physiological effects, or rather their absence in large part, are, at least, now determinable and are of interest. The following case is presented largely because it is essentially a human experiment in which the effects of sudden total ablation of the vestibular function of both sides can be studied.

CASE. J. B., male, aged forty-four years. Occupation, structural steel worker.

Complaint. Constant dizziness and dizzy attacks.

Family history is negative.

Past history. Despite the fact that ten months and a half before admission to the Johns Hopkins Hospital patient had been rejected for life insurance by three companies because he was found to have hypertension, there had been no symptoms of any kind.

Present illness. On December 6, 1933, seven and a half months before admission, patient had gone to bed after a day's work feeling as well as usual. Upon turning quickly from the right to the left side there immediately following a very severe attack of vertigo in which objects whirled and ran together. Fifteen minutes later he began to vomit and this continued for twelve hours. He had a violent left-sided headache during the next day. During the next four weeks there was constant vertigo, but at a lower level and without acute exacerbations. During this time he remain-

*Reprinted from *Bulletin of the Johns Hopkins Hospital*, LV: 3: 232–239, September, 1934.

ed in bed. His blood pressure which had been running around 180 dropped to 140 during this period. To him there seemed no relationship between his blood pressure and his vertigo. There was some buzzing in both ears; this was increased when the vertigo was more intense. When walking on the street he says he has a tendency to deviate toward the left, but at times it is to the right also. When turning the head sharply to the left the vertigo, which has been constant, is at once increased. He has since had several acute attacks of dizziness superimposed upon the more or less constant state of dizziness and always intensified by turning the head to the left. He says that tinnitus has been present off and on for a year and a half, but it caused no concern. He also complained of some blurring of vision.

Physical and neurological examinations. Patient is a sparely nourished man, aged forty-four years. He appears depressed and admits that his situation seems hopeless. He says he always worked hard and is eager to do so now, but he sees no possibility of taking care of his family in the future. The physical examination reveals but one positive finding, namely, a hypertension which varies between 138/100 and 180/120.

The positive findings on neurological examination are: slight nystagmus on looking to either side; a suggestive Romberg; perhaps a slight tendency to stagger, although neither of the two latter findings is constant. At one time a slight ataxia was noted when the finger-to-nose test was

made, but at another time this test was negative. All the deep reflexes were normal. X-ray of the head was negative. Wassermann reaction from the blood was negative. The audiometer test (Fig. 1) showed 3 per cent loss of hearing on the right and 9 per cent loss on the left. From the caloric test patient became quite dizzy when either ear was irrigated with cold water; there was intensification of nystagmus of both sides.

Diagnosis. One could only make a diagnosis of pseudo-Meniere's disease because there was no marked loss of hearing on either side, and because tinnitus was not referred to either ear. Nor was there any discomfort in the region of either ear, such as so frequently obtained in Meniere's disease.

Operation. On July 2, 1934 a unilateral cerebellar approach was made first on the right, then on the left side. The anterior five-eighths of each anditory nerve was divided. Section of this degree was expected to insure the loss of all vestibular fibers on each side and to leave three-eighths of the auditory nerve to retain unimpaired hearing. No bleeding or other difficulties were encountered throughout the operation.

Postoperative. July 2, 1934 (day of operation), 8:00 p.m. Patient says he has no dizziness whatever but has a new and unpleasant sensation. He doesn't know the exact position of his head and feels as though it is shaking from side to side when he attempts to move it. He is surprised when told that the head is perfect-

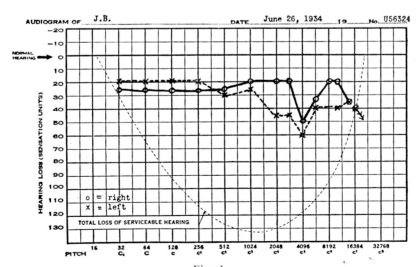

Fig. 1

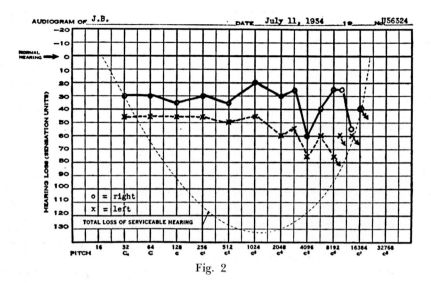

Fig. 2

ly steady. There is no rotation of objects. Diplopia is noted but there is no extra-ocular palsy. Nystagmus is present in both directions. His hearing appears to be unaffected. Nausea and vomiting are rather severe and are induced or intensi-fied by moving the head.

July 3, 1934—day following operation. Symptoms are practically unchanged. No dizziness. He still feels as though his head was turning when he moved and even when at rest. Nausea, vomiting and dip-lopia persist.

July 6, 1934—five days after operation. There has not been the slightest sugges-tion of the old dizziness at any time. Nau-sea and vomiting have ceased. Feeling of wobbling of head continues. There is no ataxia, nor has there been at any time since the operation.

July 8, 1934—seven days after operation. The "wobbling feeling" of the head is much improved.

July 11, 1934—nine days after operation. Sitting up in a chair. Says the wobbling sensation is improved, but he is uncertain about the exact position of the head and even more of the feet. Has the sensation that the feet continue turning after he moves them. Diplopia and nystagmus persist. The tinnitus has ceased. *Audio-meter test* made today; hearing is not greatly changed (see chart (Fig. 2)). The *caloric test* shows no effect whatever of irrigations of hot and cold water.

July 12, 1934—eleven days after opera-tion. Walking. Takes short steps with a rather wide base. Walks a straight line

and is quite steady. He says his feet feel as though they were whirling around, but the "wobbling sensation" of the head is nearly gone. Romberg test is negative. Still a little diplopia and nystagmus; no ataxia.

Another audiometer test was made today. (Fig. 3).

Turning tests were made to both sides with the head erect and bent forward. Not the slightest suggestion of dizziness result-ed.

July 19, 1934—seventeen days after oper-ation. Discharged.

Discharge note. When asked if he had had any trace of dizziness, says "positively not." His gait is steady, along a straight line and with no uncertainty or swerving to either side. The postoperative sensa-tion that the head was turning after move-ment has almost disappeared; the sensation of the feet turning is now present only when he walks fast.

There has been no *tinnitus* since the op-eration.

On standing with the feet together and eyes closed (Romberg) there is a little un-steadiness but he does not fall. The Rom-berg test was positive before operation, but the slight degree of unsteadiness now exist-ing is probably about that obtaining at that time. Slight nystagmus persists when the eyes are turned to either side. (It was present before the operation.) There is no ataxia. Diplopia has ceased. He has noticed no decrease from the preoperative level of hearing.

Patient was seen again July 27, 1934. He

was still annoyed by the sensation that the position of his head and feet could not be accurately estimated and appeared to continue turning after movement. He says his gait is still uncertain, although, when tested, it does not appear abnormal, unless perhaps it may be a little cautious.

SUMMARY AND CONCLUSIONS

That the vestibular nerves are totally severed by the operation is shown by the following facts: (1) Irrigation of each ear with hot and cold water (Barany test) provoked no nystagmus and induced no subjective dizziness. (2) Whirling tests with the head bent forward produced no sign of dizziness, nor did the whirling cause any symptoms whatever. It would be interesting, indeed, to know whether this patient would be subject to seasickness.

That the hearing is practically unaffected is disclosed by comparing the postoperative and preoperative audiometer curves.

It is difficult to interpret the function of the semicircular canals from this deprivative experiment. One is amazed that almost no symptoms are induced by the abrupt loss of both semicircular canals in man. Objectively, absolutely nothing could be observed at any time. Subjectively the patient complained of a "wobbling" or turning feeling of the head upon movement and to some extent of the feet. This has, he says, no similarity whatever to

dizziness with whirling objects. It appears to be more an inability to determine the exact position of his head and feet in space. It will be interesting to compare these symptoms with those of subsequent experiments of similar character. Nausea and vomiting were quite severe for a few days and perhaps are not unexpected, though it is difficult to interpret any particular relationship to the semicircular canals—perhaps no more than the diplopia which existed for ten days.

It is interesting that there was no effect whatever upon the so-called cerebellar signs, i.e., staggering gait, Romberg and ataxia.

That the state of constant dizziness which had persisted for nearly eight months, should have ceased immediately after the operation and have remained entirely absent for almost a month, at least, strongly suggests (one case over so short a time can hardly be accepted as proof) that dizziness is not possible after both vestibular nerves have been divided. In this connection it is interesting to compare the transient state of dizziness of varying degree that usually (but not always) obtains after section of one auditory nerve for Meniere's disease. On the other hand, when the function of a *normal* auditory nerve is suddenly destroyed there appears to be no post-operative dizziness.

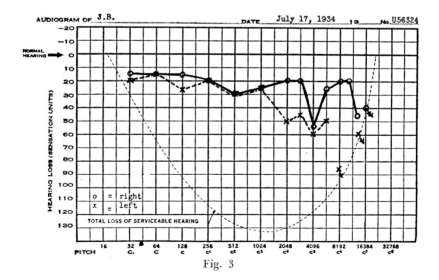

Fig. 3

If the above statements hold, the logical deductions would appear to be that: (1) Dizziness is due to a lesion (irritative or destructive) of some (doubtless any) part of the vestibular apparatus (nerve fibers and end organs). (2) That the sudden loss of one set of normal semi-circular canals does not cause symptoms of abnormal function in the contralateral intact canals, i.e., does not cause dizziness. In other words, one set of normal semicircular canals is seemingly just as effective as two. The numerous acoustic tumors without dizziness also demonstrate this point. (3) That the transient postoperative dizziness that usually follows section of one auditory nerve for Meniere's disease is due to some (unknown) underlying pathological process responsible for Meniere's disease, and located in the central nervous pathways. It is obvious that all dizziness would instantly cease after the section of the auditory nerve, if the lesion were in the semicircular canals. (4) If the results in the case presented in this communication are obtained in others, and there is every reason to believe they will be, it would be possible to stop the rare instances of protracted postoperative dizziness that obtains after sectioning the auditory nerve for Meniere's disease.

REFERENCES

[1]In a recent communication (*Archives of Otolaryngology*, July, 1934) I have expressed the belief and some evidence in support, that Meniere's disease and pseudo-Meniere's disease were really the same. At least, in many instances the unilateral alteration in hearing came months or years after the patient had been prostrated by the attacks, which in the beginning would have been classified under pseudo-Meniere's disease.

[2]Both vestibular nerves have just been sectioned in a case of bilateral Meniere's disease.

[1]Dandy, W. E.: Meniere's disease. Its Diagnosis and a Method of Treatment. *Arch. Surg., xvi:* 1127, 1928.

[2]Dandy, W. E.: An analysis of 42 cases of Meniere's disease, Symptoms, Objective Findings and Treatment. *Arch. of Otolaryng.,* July, 1934.

XLVIX

THE TREATMENT OF CAROTID CAVERNOUS ARTERIOVENOUS ANEURYSMS*

This report is based upon eight cases of carotid cavernous arteriovenous aneurysms treated surgically. Perhaps this condition is better known as pulsating exophthalmos, a term, however, that is less correct because it connotes a symptom rather than the underlying cause; pulsating exophthalmos results from other causes.

Arteriovenous aneurysms of this type are more common than arteriovenous aneurysms in any other part of the body. In fact, I think they occur with greater frequency than all arteriovenous aneurysms combined. There are now reports of over 800 in the literature. When one considers the anatomy of this region, it is not difficult to understand. There are vascular factors that are entirely different from those in any other part of the body. It is, I think, the only location in which an artery actually passes through a venous channel and that accounts, as does also the situation of the lesion, for the high frequency of these aneurysms.

For the production of an arteriovenous fistula in the arm, leg or neck, it is, of course, necessary to have a perforating wound, if the aneurysm is of traumatic origin, which penetrates the walls of both the artery and the contiguous vein. That is not necessary in the case of a carotid cavernous fistula because the arterial wall forms in large part the wall of the venous sinus so that only a tear in the carotid artery, where it traverses the cavernous sinus, is necessary for the production of a fistula.

About three fourths of these fistulae are of traumatic origin, and as so many of the lines of fissure traverse the middle fossa of the skull, it is easy to understand why tra-

uma has such an important bearing on the production of this lesion.

In the other or spontaneous group, the aneurysms, though fundamentally the same anatomically, are due to rupture of latent congenital or acquired aneurysms of the carotid artery or to arteriosclerotic patches in its wall.

Little need be said about the clinical syndrome which is sharply defined and unmistakable. There is (1) exophtalmos, (2) pulsation of the protruding eye, and in the temporal region, (3) a subjective roar which to the observer is a systolic murmur on auscultation.

The treatment of these aneurysms has been most varied. In general it has been along two lines, either from the arterial side, or from the venous side. I have had no experience with the venous side, although good results have been reported.

On the arterial side, the favorite treatment has been total occlusion of either the common or internal carotid artery on the side of the lesion. However, just as good results have now been obtained by partial ligation of either of these vessels. In fact, when one analyzes the after-effects of either partial or total ligations, the results are found to be most capricious. The aneurysms may be cured very easily, or there may be no benefit whatever. In five of our cases a cure resulted soon after ligation of the internal carotid artery (one partial and four total occlusions). In three cases there was no improvement, but in one of these a spontaneous cure resulted five years later—too late for preservation of vision.

When one analyzes the results, it is quite clear that neither the cures nor failures are dependent upon isolation of the aneurysm by occlusion of the carotid, but up-

*Reprinted from the *Annals of Surgery*, November, 1935.

on the development of a thrombus in some part of the vascular apparatus, *i.e.,* in the fistula itself, the carotid artery or venous tributaries which, of course, are principally those of the ophthalmic vein.

When the internal carotid is tied in the neck there is always immediate improvement including cessation of the roar, but in twenty-four hours or less all signs and symptoms have usually returned, though in modified degree, later gradually increasing. Whether or not there is some permanent improvement or no change depends upon whether or not thrombosis begins during the period of reduced intracranial pressure.

I am mainly concerned with the treatment of those patients who have not been cured by the arterial ligations, whether partial or total. The procedure that I wish to present is the placement of a silver clip upon the intracranial portion of the internal carotid artery just before it divides. It has been employed in two cases. The object of this attack is to isolate the aneurysm. This is not strictly correct because there is one sizable branch, namely, the ophthalmic artery between the point of the earlier ligation in the neck and the one intracranially. In one case this branch has had no effect upon maintaining the fistula which was cured immediately. In the other case it was almost a complete cure with complete return of the eyeball to normal, but a slight murmur persisted. It was necessary to excise most of the collateral branches entering the ophthalmic artery (*i.e.,* the branches of the external carotid artery) to complete the cure. In desperation these cases have not infrequently been treated by ligation of the internal or common carotid arteries bilaterally and with a very high incidence of disastrous results.

The exact treatment which one should use depends, of course, upon whether or not the carotid artery can be sacrificed without cerebral disturbances. The physiologic test—compression of this artery with the thumb—should always be made beforehand in order to determine the exact type of ligation to be used. This test has long been emphasized as a necessary prerequisite by Doctor Matas. Roughly the age of the individual is a fairly reliable guide in determining the safety or danger of total ligation, but there are too many exceptions to permit ligation without the compression test. In an elderly person one could only partially ligate the internal or common carotid artery. When partial occlusion is advisable, I perfer the internal carotid and with a band of fascia. To reduce its size one half is safe in elderly persons, and in one of our bilateral cases this was immediately and completely effective. Total arterial occlusion is permissible only when the collateral circulation is known to be adequate. Intracranial ligation of the internal carotid artery is advocated only when all the other arterial ligations have failed to cure.

L

THE TREATMENT OF BILATERAL MENIERE'S DISEASE AND PSEUDO-MENIERE'S DISEASE*

Although I have long suspected that Meniere's disease might, at times, be bilateral, and several years ago advised against operation in a patient whose signs and symptoms suggested attacks originating first on one side, then the other, it was only about a year ago that recurrence of attacks after section of one auditory nerve made the existence of bilateral Meniere's disease certain. Three additional cases have since appeared. From a series of 105 patients operated upon for Meniere's disease the bilateral syndrome has, therefore, been present in 4.1 per cent—a slightly higher frequency than obtains in trigeminal neuralgia. And if the experiences with bilateral neuralgia may be accepted as a guide, doubtless additional cases of bilateral Meniere's disease will develop from this group for the two sides may develop independently.

That the Meniere's disease is actually bilateral can only be established when the attacks continue after one auditory nerve or its vestibular division has been divided. It may be suspected when the hearing is reduced and the tinnitus is present on both sides. However, in several cases in which both of these disturbances were bilateral there have been no further attacks of dizziness following section of only one auditory nerve. And in at least one case the signs and symptoms were so nearly similar on the two sides that one could scarcely do more than guess which auditory nerve to divide.

From a series of thirty-five cases in which only the vestibular division of the nerve has been divided, unilateral Meniere's disease has, I think, been cured just as effec-

tively as by including the cochlear branch in the total division. The substitution of selective section of the vestibular branch has made it possible to propose division of both vestibular nerves; for with preservation of both cochlear branches hearing would remain unchanged. Moreover, the ability to preserve hearing makes it possible to consider treatment for pseudo-Meniere's disease in which the recurring attacks are precisely like and no less severe than those of Meniere's disease but in which there are no recognizable subjective stigmata referable to one side.

In four patients—three with bilateral Meniere's disease (i.e., recurring attacks after division or hemidivision of one auditory nerve) and one with pseudo-Meniere's disease—the vestibular nerve has been divided on both sides. In the patient with pseudo-Meniere's disease both nerves were divided at the same operation; in the other cases there were two operations.

In two of the bilateral Meniere's patients the clinical and positive story is so straight forward that little comment is necessary. In one of the two there are reasons—because of subsequent rapidly progressive deafness and the appearance of tinnitus on the unoperated side—to believe that the lesion responsible for the dizzy attacks developed on the second side after the first operation, though probably from the same underlying cause. In the other case bilateral Meniere's disease was suspected at the time of the first operation. The third case was unusual in our experience; and in the light of the subsequent events it was especially instructive. This patient was a young girl aged fifteen, the only patient in the entire series under twenty-five years of age; moreover, her at-

*From the *Acta Neuropathologica* in honorem Ludovici Puusepp LX, 1935.

tacks began at the age of four; they were identical with those of Meniere's disease, and on the whole were very frequent and devastating. Since birth she was thought to have been totally deaf in the right ear; and objectively no cochlear or vestibular response had been elicited in numerous examinations. But just before and during the attacks she always became subtotally deaf in the left (good) ear, which was essentially normal. Tinnitus was referred to both ears. After the attacks subsided the hearing returned, and although the transient loss occurred so many times, the hearing still remained unaffected between seizures.

Since the right auditory nerve was seemingly dead to all vestibular and auditory functions, there appeared no reason to believe that it could be responsible for the induction of these attacks; and since the gradual loss of hearing and the tinnitus in the left (good) ear always indicated impending attacks, the conclusion was reached that the left auditory nerve was responsible for the attacks. However, section of the vestibular nerve on this side did not prevent the attacks nor change their character. Less than a week after the operation, the right, apparently dead auditory nerve was totally divided, and at the time of this writing, eight months later, there has been no suggestion whatever of dizziness, either spontaneously or on turning the head. It is, therefore, entirely possible that this may not really be a case of bilateral Meniere's disease, and quite probable that section of the right (functionless) nerve would have stopped the attacks and without the need of sectioning the vestibular branch of the left (good) ear. If this is really strictly a case of unilateral Meniere's disease, the transient loss of hearing in the contralateral ear must be evidence that the two auditory nerves are not strictly independent. This thought has occurred before for the percentage of cases with bilateral loss of hearing and tinnitus is quite high.

In a single patient with pseudo-Me-

niere's disease (Case IV) both vestibular nerves were divided at the same operation. This patient—the first in the series to have bilateral section of these nerves—has now gone eighteen months since the operation. The indications for sectioning both vestibular nerves for pseudo-Meniere's disease are essentially the same as for Meniere's disease. Since there is no indication of the side involved there can scarcely be any alternative to section of both nerves.

After section of both vestibular nerves (four cases) the following observations have been made:

(1) There has not been a suggestion of dizziness, either in spontaneous attacks or on turning the head.

(2) Two patients were turned in whirling chairs without provoking the slightest sensation of dizziness.

(3) All of these patients complain of
   (a) Staggering in the dark or when the eyes are shut;
   (b) Inability to focus sharply when walking or riding; one patient was unable to saw a board along a straight line because he could not see the line clearly when moving the saw.

(4) Examination of these patients shows:
   (a) Romberg is negative;
   (b) Gait is a little uncertain at first, but gradually becomes steady;
   (c) No ataxia;
   (d) No nystagmus;
   (e) Hearing remains unipaired;
   (f) All caloric responses are abolished.

It is interesting that following section of one vestibular nerve, equilibrium is perfectly maintained by the vestibular apparatus of the other side. Although the errors in gait and vision that persist after loss of both vestibular nerves are cheerfully borne and considered a small price to pay for the loss of terrific attacks of dizziness, they are nevertheless sufficiently disturbing to withhold division of the second vestibular nerve until it is known that the unilateral division has not been effective.

LI

POLYURIA AND POLYDIPSIA (DIABETES INSIPIDUS) AND GLYCOSURIA RESULTING FROM ANIMAL EXPERIMENTS ON THE HYPOPHYSIS AND ITS ENVIRONS*

FREDERICK LEET REICHERT AND WALTER E. DANDY

Two decades of intensive clinical, pathological and experimental studies have failed to solve the mystery of diabetes insipidus, *i.e.,* either the manner or the exact site of its production. Although there are those who still regard this disturbance as one of primary renal origin, there can now remain little doubt that the causative lesion is in the brain and that any changes that may occur in the kidney are secondary. The great number of necropsies revealing lesions in the brain makes this statement indisputable. The leading theories at the present time may be summed up as follows:

(1) The disturbance is of hormonal origin and the hormone arises in the hypophysis.

(2) The disease is of neurogenic origin.

(A) A center for water control is located in

    (1) the hypophysis,

    (2) the diencephalon

        (a) the region of the tuber cinereum,

        (b) the supra-optic and paraventricular nuclei.

The lines of attack intended to solve this problem have been

(1) By injection of hypophyseal extracts into patients with diabetes insipidus,

(2) By injection of extracts from tumors and other lesions (human material),

(3) By animal experimentation,

(4) By human operative procedures that serve as experiments.

Although at first glance these methods might appear to supplement each other, actually they fail to do so, and the reasons for this failure are doubtless significant. From lack of adequate control, attempts to correlate the end results of these methods have been misleading.

The principal reason for assuming that the hypophyseal secretion plays an important role in the production of diabetes insipidus is that when extracts of the posterior lobe (including, of course, the pars intermedia) are applied to the nasal mucous membrane, or injected hypodermically, the urinary output and the intake of fluids are reduced. Although there are many cases of diabetes insipidus that are scarcely, if at all, improved by the administration of pituitary extract, those with decided benefit are too numerous to allow us to deny the effect, when it does occur. Nevertheless, if hypophyseal extract is the all important factor in the control of water balances, it should be unfailing and not capricious in its action. And unless a satisfactory explanation of this deficit is forthcoming—and this appears improbable—a deficiency of hypophyseal hormone as the explanation of diabetes insipidus must be untenable. Moreover, if the hypophyseal hormone is the basis for the control of water balance in the body, why does the complete removal of this structure have no effect upon this function?

A second reason for the assumption of a hypophyseal factor in diabetes inspidus has

*Reprinted from *Bulletin of the Johns Hopkins Hospital,* LVIII: 6: 418–427, June, 1936.

been deduced from a number of cases in which a tumor has been found in the region of the hypophysis. The large size of most of these tumors makes it impossible to draw any conclusions concerning a precise point of attack in the production of diabetes insipidus. On the other hand, there are occasional small and sharply defined tumors from which fairly definite impressions are obtainable, but these must be carefully separated from the general mass of material of this type.

Since we are principally concerned in this paper with the results of animal experimentation, our impressions derived from the assets and liabilities of this method will follow the presentation of material. The experiments have been conducted exclusively on dogs. The intracranial operative attack developed by the writers and reported elsewhere[1] has been used. This approach, with a shrunken brain, affords ample room for clear observations and for any desired operative procedure, without inflicting cerebral trauma—the cause of so many mis-interpretations of hypophyseal function. The animals were constantly in cages; all were studied during the fall, winter and spring; with few exceptions the ages of the puppies ranged from three weeks to three months.

In mechanically irritating the base of the brain the bent end of a probe is passed at right angles into the severed stalk of the hypophysis to a depth of 2 to 3 mm. and a longitudinal slit made by moving the probe forward to the optic chiasm and backward to the tuber cinereum. Such an incision causes injury to the so-called supra-optic and paraventricular nuclei of both sides. With the application of the cautery the entire region surrounding the hypophyseal stalk is destroyed superficially.

In order to establish controls for subsequent experiments, the intake of fluids and the output of urine were carefully measured over a period of several days before operation. The intake of fluid ranged between 100 and 1000 cc., and the output of urine between 50 and 500 cc. (Section I). We feel safe in regarding an intake of over 1000 cc. of fluid and an output of over 500 cc. of urine as evidence of polydipsia and polyuria, respectively. In a single dog, however, the intake reached 1500 and 2900 cc. and the output was proportionately high—1300 and 1450 cc. over a period of two days preceding an operation. The figures from this animal are so unusual that they should doubtless be excluded from the series of controls. The exception, however, indicates the risk of drawing conclusions from uncontrolled experiments. It, moreover provokes the thought that perhaps the occasional instance of *permanent* polyuria and polydipsia presumably produced by an operative experiment, might in reality have given the same findings before operation.

To control still further the experimental results, four (4) dogs were anaesthetized with ether over a period of time approximating that consumed in the subsequent operative procedures; they were also given the same medicaments (morphine 64 mgm. and hypertonic salt 0.5 mgm. per kilo of body weight) that were used in the experiments. There were no appreciable effects upon the quantity of fluid and urine (Section II). Among the four controls of this group was the dog with spontaneous polyuria and polydipsia; for the following three days the measurements of fluid and urine were somewhat reduced but still remained well above the levels that we consider the outside limits of normal.

Further controls were established in two instances, *i.e.*, following the usual preliminary drugs and anaesthetization, the regular hypophyseal approach was carried out but no contact was made with the hypophyseal region. The subsequent results were entirely negative (Section III). In another group (Section IV) the region of the hypophysis was explored and the rather remote environs (not including the hypothalamus) were irritated mechanically in one instance and punctured with needles in another. There was little if any effect.

The results in terms of polydipsia and polyuria of the various experiments are most inconsistent. In almost every set of experiments the results are both positive and negative. We have analyzed these seemingly capricious results from the standpoints of age of the animals, time of the year (*i.e.,* hot or cold), difference in traumatic insults, or other factors incident to the operation, but can find no satisfactory explanation. There was always ample operative room because of shrinkage of the brain with hypertonic salt solution, and controls definitely show that the preoperative treatment plays no role. The animals recovered promptly from the effects of the operation, thus further disclosing the absence of cerebral pressure from traumatic oedema. It is quite obvious that, without a large series of results, experimenters might well come to diametrically opposite conclusions.

A glance at the series of charts may perhaps suggest that the experiment in which only the anterior lobe was removed (Section VII), and in which the grade of polyuria and polydipsia was much the highest, would point to a clue concerning the hidden secret; but two (one-half) of the group failed to repeat the results, although, so far as we can determine, the experiments were duplicated precisely. We have been particularly interested to know whether polyuria and polydipsia could be induced by stimulating or destroying the base after first removing the hypophysis and allowing an interval of time to elapse before the secondary procedure. From a total of eleven cases (Sections XII, XIII, XIV and XV), in only one was there an outspoken increase in the intake and output of fluids; in two there were mild increases. But although these positive results are distinctly in the minority, they nevertheless indicate that the hypophysis is not necessary for the production of polyuria and polydipsia. Camus and Roussy, Bailey and Bremer and also Houssey have long since reached this conclusion from experi-

ments of similar character.

Following total removal of the hypophysis, polyuria and polydipsia developed in 50 per cent of the cases (six of twelve); with the additional cauterization of the base at the time of removal in 70 per cent (five of seven), but the volumetric change was decidedly less. When the hypophyseal stalk or the body of the entire hypophysis is compressed by a tightly applied silver clip (Section X), or the stalk of the hypophysis is severed from the brain (but not removed) (Section XI), or when needles are introduced into and left in the hypophysis to stimulate it mechanically, the results are essentially the same in each set of experiments; in only three of nine tests ($33\frac{1}{3}$ per cent) did a moderate grade of polyuria and polydipsia result.

Disappointing also has been our inability to induce a permanent polyuria and polydipsia such as one sees in human beings. The condition has in our experiments always been transient, lasting only two to four days in the milder grades and a maximum of seven to ten days in the more advanced grades. We are aware of the polyuria of long standing occasionally following experiments by Camus and Roussy, Bailey and Bremer, Towne and others, but so rarely that one is led to wonder if other factors may not be responsible—at times perhaps an unusual animal in which this condition occurs without the operation. Moreover, in some cases reported in the literature the polyuria and polydipsia began again weeks or months after the experiment—so late that the causal relationship is none too securely established.

CONCLUSIONS

1. Polyuria and Polydipsia

In considering the application of canine experiments to diabetes insipidus in human beings one must bear in mind that the topographical relations of this region are entirely different—so different in fact that one may well doubt that the experimental results may be transferred with any degree of safety. And further doubt may be entertained because the polyuria induced in animals compares neither in degree nor in duration with the same symptom in human beings. In dogs the hypophysis lies snugly against the base of the brain without a distinct stalk and cells of the intermediate lobe are spread over the brain. In man the hypophysis is well isolated within a dural compartment and is connected with the brain by a long stalk (2-3 cm.) that is devoid of hypophyseal tissue. In human beings operative attacks upon this region are very apt to induce permanent polyuria and polydipsia, although the temporary type also follows minor injuries.

Doubtless there is some similarity in the functions of water control dominated by this region in dogs and man, but we doubt that there is the same profound control in dogs that obtains in man. In other words, the canine experiments give us a lead but are not adequate to explain the mechanism involved in human beings. We can only conclude that there appears to be a neurogenic mechanism which can be set off by mechanical and thermal stimulation of the base of the brain and of the hypophysis as well, but that the hypophysis is not an indispensable part of it. Since polyuria and polydipsia follow injuries to the hypothalamus after the hypophysis has been removed, the conclusion is inescapable that diabetes insipidus is not due to the absence of a hypophyseal hormone. Since the paraventricular and supra-optic nuclei have unquestionably been traumatized by our mechanical and thermal injuries to the hypothalamus and with no greater effect than without such injury, we cannot believe that the center of water control is represented by these nuclei. It is our belief that only the human experiments will solve this problem.

2. GLYCOSURIA

From the foregoing table it will be seen that both the incidence and degree of glycosuria are essentially the same in the control animals in which no attack was made upon the hypophysis or upon the base of the brain as when various operative procedures were carried on these structures. Always the urinary sugar is transient and usually it occurs only in the first specimen; occasionally it persists for 24 to 48 hours. Even in dogs without anaesthesia or medication of any kind, glycosuria will be demonstrable at times. In another somewhat larger series of dogs not included in this report, glycosuria was found in four. From these observations we see no reason to infer that the hypophysis, the hypothalamus, or any part of the base of the brain in this region, has any particular bearing on the production of glycosuria in dogs.

GUIDE FOR THE INTERPRETATION OF CHARTS

Base line indicates time (each square = a day).

Abscissa indicates maximum measurements of urine and fluid (in cc.).

Solid black = urinary output.

Enclosed clear area above solid black = fluid intake.

Cross-hatched lines = output of urine and parallel oblique lines above = intake of fluids in control animals (Charts I, II, III, IV, V and IX); after the *first* of two operations in Charts XII, XIII and XIV, and after the *second* of three operations in Chart XV. (Control readings are entered only when they may modify the interpretation of the experiment).

The *normal* intake and output is charted over a period of several days in order to insure adequate control. In subsequent experiments the readings are continued only as long as an abnormal intake or output remains. When below the normal limits only the maximum figure is charted.

This number of animals showing sugar and no sugar postoperatively is noted in the square above the fluid and urine columns in each section.

The experiments recorded in the charts are grouped as follows (Roman number on the charts):

Controls:

> I. Intake or output of unoperated normal controls; 9 dogs.
>
> II. Animals given morphia (64 mgm.) hypertonic salt solution 0.5 mgm. per kilo of body weight and ether for an

hour (*i.e.,* controls without the actual operation) —4 dogs.

III. Operative exposure of hypophyseal region but nothing further done—2 dogs.

IV. Stimulation of base of brain around the hypophysis without trauma to the hypophysis or its stalk—3 dogs.

V. Total hypophysectomy — 13 dogs.

VI. Total hypophysectomy a n d cauterization of base—7 dogs.

VII. Removal of anterior lobe only —4 dogs.

VIII. Removal of posterior lobe only—3 dogs.

IX. Introduction of needles (permanent) into the hypophysis (through both lobes) —4 dogs.

X. Compression of silver clip on hypophyseal stalk—2 dogs; and across the body of the hypophysis—1 dog.

XI. Hypophyseal stalk severed— 2 dogs.

XII. (1) Total hypophysectomy and later (2) mechanical stimulation of base—3 dogs.

XIII. (1) Total hypophysectomy and later (2) application of cautery to base—3 dogs.

XIV. (1) Partial anterior and total posterior hypophysectomy, and later (2) stimulation of base—2 dogs.

XV. (1) Stalk cut; later (2) total hypophysectomy, and later (3) mechanical stimulation of base—2 dogs.

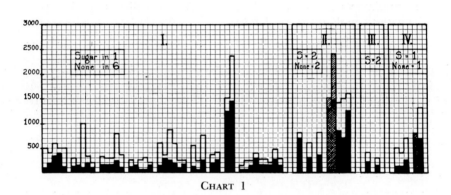

CHART 1

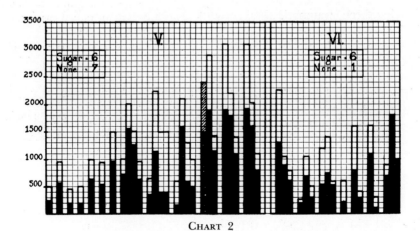

CHART 2

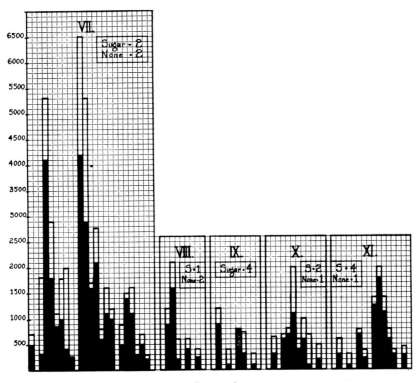

CHART 3

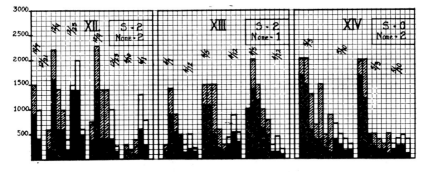

CHART 4

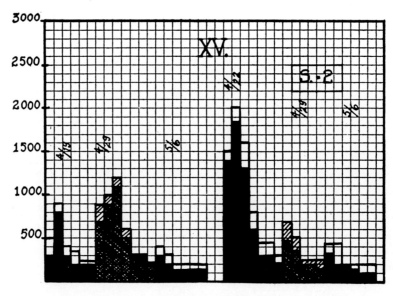

CHART 5

REFERENCE

[1]Dandy, W. E., and Reichert, F. L.: Studies on Experimental Hypophysectomy. I. Effect on the Maintenance of Life. *Bull. Johns Hopkins Hosp.,* *xxxvii:* 1, 1925.

LII

OPERATIVE EXPERIENCE IN CASES OF PINEAL TUMOR*

Although an operative approach to the pineal region was proposed by me in 1921,[1] it was not until a decade later (1931) that the first pineal tumor was successfully extirpated.[2] A disastrous toll of seven fatal issues during this long period seemed almost to indicate the futility of further efforts. Yet the same approach was used successfully in a number of cases of tumor of the third ventricle in which, though the lesion was in the same general region, less serious difficulties were offered. In addition to the aforementioned case, successful extirpation has since been performed in two others, thus indicating that the lesion is not entirely hopeless, although it remains one of the most dangerous of all intracranial growths. This seeming success, however, is still further tempered by the fact that in two of these cases the tumor has since recurred, in one after two and one-half years and in the other after three months. Only the last of the three patients remains well, and the period after operation has been only four months. Since the growth in the first case was solid and encapsulated and was extirpated intact, I expected a permanent cure. However, the growth was teratomatous, containing, in addition to the pineal element, ciliated columnar cells of ependymal origin, cartilage and tissue resembling the salivary gland. The tumor in the second case was much larger; it was so soft and cellular and its capsule so thin that it could not be shelled out intact but had to be removed in fragments. The patient died at her home three months later, but permission for necropsy was not obtained. It is, perhaps, more conceivable that cica-

*Reprinted from the *Archives of Surgery, 33:* 19–46, July, 1936.

trization at the mouth of the aqueduct caused her death than that such rapid recurrence was responsible. The tumor of the third patient was a pure pinealoma and was perfectly encapsulated. It is unbelievable that it can recur, although I felt equally secure in such a prediction for the first case. In that instance, however, the tumor was a teratoma, whereas in this case the growth was a pure pinealoma.

Reports of three cases of pineal tumor in which the patient survived the operation are appended. Particularly of interest are the remarkable transient postoperative sequelae and the absence of recognizable effects arising from the removal of part or all of the main trunks of the internal venous system of the brain.

REPORT OF CASES

CASE 1 *History.—*J. C., a boy aged ten years, was first admitted to the hospital on Nov. 24, 1931, with the complaint of headache and vomiting.

The family and the past history were not significant.

The present trouble began five weeks prior to admission, with moderately severe bilateral frontal headache and double vision. The patient slept all afternoon and remained in bed two days, during which time he vomited once. He returned to school, but two days later headache, nausea and vomiting returned. During the first week of his illness the mother noticed that he staggered and "did not seem to go where he wished."

For some time he was improved and played with other children. Good days alternated with bad. Then double vision returned, and there were spells of dizziness. A diagnosis of intracranial tumor was made by Dr. George Wright of Pittsburgh.

Physical and Neurologic Examination. The patient was slender and of normal size. The pupils were large and did not

533

react. There was paresis of both the right and the left external rectus muscles. No ptosis was present. A rough test of the visual fields and the perimetric examination, which had been made at Pittsburgh, revealed nothing abnormal. There was papilledema of four diopters in each fundus, and fresh hemorrhages covered each disk and the surrounding fundus. The patient was too ill for an audiometer test, but a watch could be heard when placed against either ear. He walked with a wide base and had a suggestion of but not a positive Romberg sign. There was no ataxia. The deep reflexes were exaggerated but equal on the two sides. A slight ankle clonus was detected on the left but was absent when the test was repeated. The Babinski and Kernig signs were absent. Bradycardia (with a pulse rate between 50 and 60) was present throughout the day prior to operation.

Roentgenographic Examination.—A roentgenogram of the head showed a large calcified shadow (Fig. 1 *B*) in the region of the pineal body, a probable pathologic finding in a person of the age of the patient and one that should suggest pineal tumor.

Ventriculography (Nov. 25, 1931).—The left ventricle, which was uppermost, was tapped, and fluid spurted under tremendous pressure 75 cc. of fluid was aspirated and an equal amount of air injected. Both lateral ventricles were much enlarged, and enlargement of the third ventricle showed in the anteroposterior but not in the lateral view. It was suspected that the absence of air in the third ventricle (lateral view) was due to the injection of an insufficient amount of air, and because of the history of staggering gait it was decided to explore the cerebellum first and proceed to the pineal region at the same operation if the result of the first exploration was without significance.

The ventricular fluid contained 6 cells, all of which were mononuclears. The Wassermann reaction was negative.

Operation (Nov. 25, 1931).—Immediately after the ventriculograms had been interpreted, the patient underwent operation under anesthesia induced with tribromethanol in amylene hydrate. Exploration of the cerebellum revealed nothing of significance. The fourth ventricle was inspected to the iter. The wound was closed, and a pineal flap was at once made in the right occipital region. The dura was reflected mesially over the longitudinal sinus. It was not necessary to dispose of any veins crossing from the hemisphere to the longitudinal sinus. After the lateral ventricle was tapped and additional fluid released by gentle compression of the brain, the hemisphere was easily retracted. The corpus callosum was split perhaps three fourths of its horizontal extent. At first, no tumor was visible. The great vein and the two small veins of Galen were in full view. A small circumscribed part of the tumor was then detected just lateral to the small vein of Galen on the left and at a point near its junction with the great vein of Galen. With the forceps the left vein of Galen was gently stripped from the sur-

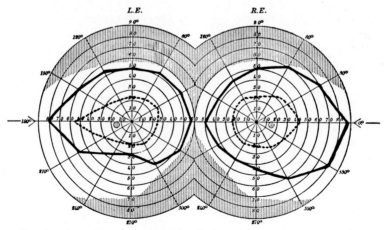

Fig. 1. (case 1). Visual fields of the patient taken two and one-half years after removal of a pineal tumor. It will be seen that hemianopia did not follow removal of the tumor.

face of the tumor, which was then seen to extend far anteriorly. Fortunately, the attachment of the small vein of Galen to the tumor was slight, so that it could be gently pushed aside. It is worthy of note that the two small veins of Galen were close together in their parallel course; i. e., they were not separated as usually obtains when a tumor lies immediately beneath and is thrust between these vessels.

The tumor appeared to be well encapsulated. It was picked up with the forceps and gently withdrawn between the small veins of Galen, which had been separated by cleaving the thin fibrous tissues between them—the roof of the third ventricle. As the tumor was gently elevated, a transparent area came into view and was tapped; a few drops of fluid escaped, but the amount was too small to permit impression of its character or color. The capsule of the tumor was again grasped, and with steady traction the tumor was soon delivered from its bed. There remained a slight attachment posteriorly, which for the moment was left undisturbed. As the tumor was delivered up to this point, the third ventricle was opened, and more air and fluid escaped. It could then be seen that the tumor was attached posteriorly to the great vein of Galen by a small fibrous band; a small knife divided this bloodlessly. At no time during the removal of the tumor was there any bleeding.

Roentgenograms then showed that the calcified shadow was absent in the pineal region and present in the specimen.

Macroscopic Description of the Tumor.— The tumor weighed 3 Gm. It was roughly oval and well encapsulated, with a smooth but somewhat irregular surface. From the posterior and upper surface of the tumor a small, pear-shaped nodule (about as large as a pea) projected, which strongly suggested an enlarged pineal body. At the time the tumor was removed it was looked on as having arisen from the pineal body, largely because of this isolated protuberance. Roentgenograms showed the area of calcification to be in this part of the tumor.

*Microscopic Description.—*In places an ependymal lining could be seen on the outside of the tumor, but usually it was not evident. A heavy external layer of fibrous tissue indicated the capsule. The tumor contained numerous large and small cysts lined with low cubical epithelium, but no basement membrane. Cilia were visible in many places; they were clearly derived from ependymal cells. The basic tissue of the tumor was of loose areolar type (doubtless glia), with few cells; in many places it looked almost like myxomatous tissue. Throughout this fibrous tissue were clusters of large cells with deeply staining nuclei; the cytoplasm was ill defined and sent strands from cell to cell. These were characteristic pineal cells. Clusters of smaller and more deeply staining nuclei like those of lymphocytes were scattered throughout (second type of pineal tumor cell), though they were far less numerous than the large cells.

In places were acini of high columnar cells, with basal nuclei and much cytoplasm, which was sometimes vacuolated; such acini suggested the salivary gland. At one point there was a small island of cartilage. Many areas af calcification were present.

*Microscopic Diagnosis.—*The diagnosis was teratoma, with pineal and ependymal cells predominating.

*Further Course of the Illness.—*After the operation the patient was quite ill for ten days; he was listless and voided in bed frequently. Ventricular punctures were necessary for relief of the increased pressure. As the pressure began to diminish, the general condition improved. He then complained that he was unable to see. For the first time, he could see a little on the thirteenth day. At the time of his discharge from the hospital, on December 14, a rough test revealed that the visual fields were still constricted but that there was no hemianopia (Fig. 1). At the time of admission to the hospital vision was known to be greatly reduced, but the patient had been too ill for taking of the visual fields. At the time of his discharge the palsy of the left abducens nerve had entirely cleared, and that of the right was much improved. An audiometer test six days after the operation showed loss on both sides of the upper tones (from 3,000 to 16,000 vibrations) —a finding that made us wonder whether it carried significance as a localizing sign.

Subsequent Admission to the Hospital (March 15, 1934).—The patient had grown at a normal rate and appeared normal. He had no extra-ocular palsy, and vision was said to have been normal. He had been playing football and engaged in other sports at school. He stated that he could throw a ball accurately but was unable to catch it.

Two weeks prior to his admission head-ache and vomiting reappeared; they then disappeared for a week and returned in much the same position as before the first operation. Again, diplopia, stiffness of the neck, unsteadiness on the feet and stagger-ing appeared. The cerebellar region had begun to bulge.

Neurologic Examination.—The following findings were of significance: bilateral fix-ation of the pupils; bilateral paresis of the sixth nerve, probably more marked on the right, and bilateral ptosis. Vision and the visual fields were practically normal. Visual acuity was 20/30+ in the right eye and 20/30— in the left. The audiometer curve, which was of interest during the first stay in the hospital, was unchanged.

Operation (March 16, 1934).—A recur-rent tumor was removed. Since recurrence of the tumor had been regarded as improb-able, the possibility of stricture of the aqueduct was entertained. In order to differentiate between the two conditions, an injection of air was made. One hun-dred and twenty-five cubic centimeters of air replaced an equal amount of fluid. The fluid was under marked pressure. Ven-triculograms showed a large filling defect in the posterior part of the third ventricle, thus demonstrating recurrence of the tumor. The bone, which had healed well, was cut anew. A vein tore at the longitud-inal sinus and had to be packed during the operative procedure. Subsequently, when the pack was removed the bleeding was difficult to control, and a fair amount of blood was lost. The falx was tightly ad-herent to the mesial surface of the hemis-phere. Everywhere, oozing followed sep-aration of the adhesions. A dense mass of adhesions filled the split in the corpus call-osum; when these were divided the recur-rent tumor came into view. The tumor was smooth and round and, though firmly embedded, could be dislodged without great difficulty or trauma. Again, a small cyst with white gelatinous fluid (indica-tive of ependymal lining) was evacuated during the delivery of the tumor, which was accomplished by traction on the firm capsule. The tumor was firmly adherent to the great vein of Galen, which tore during the liberation of the mass. It was necessary to thrombose the entire trunk, but this was accomplished without difficul-ty or much loss of blood. The tumor weighed 6.9 Gm.—more than twice as much

as the original tumor.

As the patient had lost a fair amount of blood during the operation and the blood pressure was low, he was given a transfus-ion of his citrated blood that had been col-lected during the operation. This was an unfortunate procedure, however, for soon after its administration the blood oozed from all points, owing to the effect of the citrate. It was then impossible to com-bat the bleeding, and the patient died on the operating table.

The microscopic appearance of the tum-or was similar to that of the first specimen, but with much more fibrous tissue. Mitoses were abundant.

CASE 2. *History.*—H. S., a white woman aged twenty-eight, was admitted to the hos-pital on Aug. 29, 1935, with the complaint of headache and failing vision.

The family and the past history were not significant.

Present Illness.—Beginning seven months prior to the patient's admission to the hos-pital, generalized headache occurred first periodically and then more or less con-stantly. In the last three months the head-ache had been much improved, there being constant dull ache in the frontal region. Three months prior to admission a whir-ring noise, like that of a motor, developed in the right ear, and this persisted till the time of examination. The patient express-ed the belief that there had been some loss of hearing in this ear. Diplopia developed two months before, and for the last two months vision became progressively worse. On two occasions the left upper eyelid drooped for a period of half an hour or more. There were staggering gait and difficulty in control of the finer movements of the hands and arms during the past two months. The patient was generally weak but had no paralysis.

Physical Examination.—The patient was well nourished and well developed. The blood pressure was 128 systolic and 80 diastolic.

Neurologic Examination.—There were papilledema of 5 diopters in each eye-ground and numerous flame-shaped hem-orrhages in the right. The visual fields were normal for form, but no colors were distinguished except with central vision. Visual acuity was 20/40 in the left eye and 20/200 in the right. The pupils were dilated and reacted feebly to light. There was slight, quick lateral nystagmus to either side, but no extra-ocular palsy. The corneal reflexes, though still present, were diminished on both sides. Hearing was somewhat lost in the right ear and was normal in the left. Knee kicks were exaggerated on both sides, more so on the right. The patient staggered somewhat when walking, but the Romberg sign was absent.

Diagnosis.—The diagnosis was tumor of the brain of undetermined location.

Trephine and Injection of Air (Aug. 31, 1935).—One hundred and twenty-five cubic centimeters of fluid was removed from the ventricular system and an equal amount of air injected. The fluid was under tremendous pressure. Ventriculograms showed a filling defect in the posterior part of the third ventricle; both lateral ventricles and the anterior part of the third ventricle were greatly dilated.

Operation (Aug. 31, 1935).—A pineal approach was made in the right parieto-occipital region. The right hemisphere was retracted from the falx without difficulty. The corpus callosum was exposed and divided. The third ventricle was reached anteriorly; its roof was at once perforated, and a large amount of fluid and air escaped, thus reducing the intracranial pressure. Even then there was inadequate room, so that in exposing the region of the tumor undue pressure had to be made on the cerebral hemisphere. One could then see the bulging tumor in the region of the great vein of Galen. The small vein of Galen on the right was torn in the attempt to dissect it from the tumor; bleeding from this tear was finally controlled by electrocautery, though with some difficulty. A little later during the dissection the great vein of Galen, which was densely adherent to the tumor, was torn, and was even more difficult to isolate and thrombose this vessel. Finally, because there was inadequate room, it was necessary to resect quickly the right occipital lobe. Extirpation included part of the parietal lobe, for the transverse plane of the cerebral section was on a level with the great vein of Galen and passed through the anterior part of the posterior horn, exposing the glomus of the choroid plexus. Little bleeding attended this extirpation. The tumor projected so far posteriorly that it was necessary to resect the tentorium. It could then be seen that the great vein of Galen actually traversed the tumor, and since it had already been thrombosed and divided and additional room was required because the tumor was so large,

the incision was made in the falx and carried backward to the straight sinus, which was closed by a transfixion suture of silk and divided. The incision was then carried forward into the left side of the tentorium, thus removing a large section of dura overlying the tumor. The tumor was then in full view. The posterior part was dissected away from the cerebellum, into which it protruded but did not infiltrate. The tumor was soft and had a thin capsule which permitted no pull. However, by traction with the spatula it was possible to dissect the tumor from its bed in the quadrigeminal plate and to enucleate it completely. It extended far forward and projected deep into the third ventricle, which it filled completely. During its removal the mass broke into many fragments, but no gross tumor remained. Several small bleeding vessels were thrombosed in the neighborhood of the left vein of Galen.

Since the third ventricle was widely open and had been subjected to sponging, subsequent cicatrization was thought to be a distinct possibility. In removing the tumor, much of it was aspirated through the suction tube. Its soft, cellular nature made it possible to remove much of the interior in this way. The weight of the tumor that was collected, which was but a small fragment of the whole, was 2 Gm. I estimate that the weight of the tumor was about 15 Gm.

Postoperative Course.—The patient was drowsy and listless for a number of days after the operation. Intracranial pressure continued to be high and was relieved by ventricular punctures during the next three weeks. The patient was blind for several days after operation. Vision gradually returned, and at the time of her discharge from the hospital, on September 28, one month after operation, visual acuity in each eye was the same as that at the time of admission. There was, in addition, left homonymous hemianopia. Colors were not recognized. All the extra-ocular movements were restricted but not completely lost; they had steadily improved during the last week. The patient was disoriented for three weeks but became normal in this respect before her discharge from the hospital. Improvement was rapid in every way during the last week.

On Nov. 15, 1935, the following letter was received from her husband: "Until last Friday we had much hope for my wife.

On that day Dr. ——, of this city, told me that it was only a matter of time until she died. Doctor, it is tough to see and hear her talking and laughing and know that she has to die. Isn't there something we can do for her?"

A letter was sent in reply in what way she was troubled, and I was advised that she died on Dec. 1, 1935. Permission for autopsy was not obtained.

Microscopic Diagnosis.—The diagnosis was pure pinealoma.

CASE 3 *History.*—R. P., a youth aged fifteen, was admitted to the hospital on Sept. 28, 1935, with the complaint of headache, vomiting and diplopia.

The family and the past history were not significant.

Present Illness.—When the patient was 8 or 9 years old (six years prior to his admission) he had periods of severe headache, lasting for several hours and occurring at irregular intervals, but never more frequent than once or twice a week; they were accompanied by vomiting. Four years before he had a fainting spell, but no more information could be elicited; apparently it was not a clonic convulsion. During the past year he was almost free from headache, until two months prior to admission, when the attacks became severe, occurred almost daily and were associated with vomiting; they were generalized but were worse in the occipital region. At about the same time diplopia appeared, and this had remained since. It was notic-

ed that the patient held his head tilted backward and at times complained of pain and stiffness in the neck. He was also said to have walked stiff-legged, but apparently he did not stagger. Photophobia was present during the last two months. At first, he carried on a more or less normal life and was able to play golf. The symptoms gradually became more severe, and a month before his admission he entered another hospital, where he remained for three weeks, at the end of which time he was discharged. Immediately on reaching home, he became much worse and was irritable and drowsy. He was readmitted to the hospital. Lumbar puncture was performed, but no improvement resulted. He then came to Baltimore. On the way he became disoriented, screamed with pain, was extremely listless and talked incoherently.

Physical Examination.—The patient was well nourished and of normal development. He was acutely ill.

Neurologic Examination.—The neurologic examination was difficult because of the patient's condition. Any attempt at examination made him combative. He saw fingers with either eye. The pupils reacted to light. There was probably slight weakness of the left side of the face of the central type. An audiometer test could not be made. There was marked gross tremor when the hands were used, and the left arm and leg appeared to be somewhat weaker than the right. The

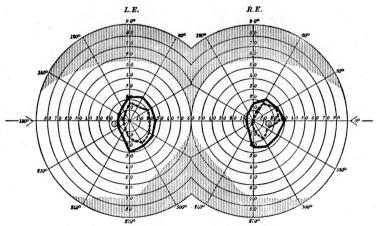

Fig. 2. (case 3). Visual fields for form and color, taken with a 1 degree test object, showing homonymous hemianopia, which not infrequently follows removal of a tumor in the region of the pineal body and third ventricle. It is doubtless due to traction on the cuneus and is permanent.

biceps and triceps reflexes and the knee and ankle jerks were extremely hyperactive, but more on the left than on the right. Abdominal reflexes were not obtained. There was a definite Babinski sign on the left and an equivocal one on the right; no ankle clonus was present. The eyegrounds could not be examined until the patient was under anesthesia, when high grade papilledema (5 diopters) was found on both sides; there were no hemorrhages.

Trephine and Injection of Air (Sept. 28, 1935).—One hundred and fifty cubic centimeters of fluid was removed from the right ventricle, which was lowermost, and 130 cc. of air was injected. The ventricular system was enlarged; this included the anterior half of the third ventricle. There was a filling defect in the posterior half of the third ventricle, indicating the location of the tumor to be in the pineal body. The ventricular fluid was clear and contained no cells or globulin. A small area of calcification showed in the region of the pineal body.

Operation (Sept. 28, 1935).—A pineal tumor was removed. Immediately after the ventriculograms had been read, the patient was placed under anesthesia with tribromethanol in amylene hydrate, and a pineal approach was made on the right side. The corpus callosum was split practically its entire length. Fluid oozed from the subarachnoid spaces surrounding the corpus callosum in large amounts. Finally, the third ventricle was exposed anteriorly and was punctured. An abundance of fluid escaped, providing ample room for the attack on the tumor, which was immediately beneath the corpus callosum. The tumor was white, slightly pink, hard and perfectly encapsulated. The small vein of Galen could be seen skirting the right side of the tumor and, of course, running in a longitudinal direction; it could be observed as it entered the great vein of Galen and for about 3 cm., where it turned to the region of the foramen of Monro. The small vein of Galen on the left could be seen near the great vein. It arched around the tumor and was lost to view. An attempt was made to strip the small vein of Galen on the right, but it was bound too tightly to the tumor and finally had to be thrombosed with the cautery and divided at the anterior and posterior pole of the tumor. The capsule of the tumor was then incised, and an attempt was made to extirpate its con-

tents with the curet. The tumor was much too hard, however, and nothing could be accomplished by this attempt. The small area of calcification that showed in the roentgenogram was soon encountered, in the posterior part of the tumor. The cutting loop of the cautery was not used, because the application of heat to the brain stem was feared. The firmness of the capsule, however, made it possible to dislocate the tumor by exerting traction on it, and gradually the tumor was elevated and, after much blunt and sharp dissection, was lifted from its bed. It was firmly embedded in the underlying quadrigeminal plate. Gradually, the left vein of Galen came into view, and it was possible to withdraw the tumor from it without injury. The entire growth lay on the roof of the third ventricle, which was not opened, except anteriorly, where a puncture was deliberately made in order to relieve the excess of cerebrospinal fluid. The part of the tumor attached to the roof of the third ventricle was much less firmly fixed than the portion attached posteriorly. The dense attachment to the quadrigemenial plate required numerous applications of fine-pointed scissors and the scalpel before the delivery of the tumor was accomplished. The great vein of Galen was at no time injured. The tumor bulged a little more to the left than to the right. There was almost no bleeding during the removal of the tumor, for its attachments were bloodless. A tiny oozing at the end was traced to a small artery, which was thrombosed with the cautery. The wound was closed with drainage, and the dura and bone were accurately restored.

The tumor weighed 4 Gm. It was solid everywhere and had slight nodulations on its surface. Histologically, it was a typical pinealoma.

Postoperative Course.—The general condition of the patient steadily improved. Ventricular punctures were required for seven days. On the second day the patient was thought to be blind, but the pupils reacted slightly to light. There appeared to be weakness in the left arm and leg, although both were used; this seemed a little more evident than before operation. The patient remained totally blind until the seventh day after the operation, when he recognized light and movements of the hand. He sat up on the twelfth day. Vision steadily improved. The mental condition was clear. He was discharged from the hospital on Oct. 12, 1935. Extensive impairment of the extra-ocular muscles and the state of vision were described by Dr. Alan Woods as follows:

"There was conjugate deviation of the eyes to the right. They could be brought back to the midline independently or together, but no lateral motion was possible to the left side. Elevation of the eyeballs and the upper lids was poorly performed; immediately, conjugate deviation of the eyes to the right recurred. The pupils were dilated and showed only the faintest suggestion of reaction to light. Visual acuity on the right was 20/70, and on the left only movements of the hand were perceived. There was complete homonymous hemianopia (Fig. 2)."

I next saw the patient on Dec. 2, 1935, at which time the accompanying photograph was taken. The Romberg sign was absent. He could walk without staggering. He had no headache and was cheerful and normal mentally. The following report on vision and the extra-ocular muscles was made by Dr. Alan Woods:

"The eyes were normal externally, except for rather widely dilated pupils, which reacted sluggishly to light. Extra-ocular movements showed failure of the left eye to converge, but adduction was normal and lateral movements were normal in every direction, except for the almost abolished upper gaze. Left homonymous hemianopia still persisted.

"Ophthalmoscopic examination showed clear media in both eyes. The disks were flat and of good color, without manifest atrophy, but above and below each disk was residual indication of 'shot-silk' retinitis.

"The manifest refraction of each eye was −0.37 sph., with which correction vision was 20/20.

"Tests for muscle balance revealed exophoria of approximately 1 degree for distant vision and of 9 degrees for near vision.

"Diagnosis: At the time of writing the boy presented a rather typical picture of pineal lesion, with involvement of the quadrigeminal plate below, resulting in limitation of upward gaze and disturbances in motility of the pupillary sphincter, due to interruption of fibers to the superior colliculus. The lesion was undoubtedly on the right side, for it probably involved the middle branch of the optic tract to the external geniculate body. All evidence of choking of the disk had disappeared, as had conjugate deviation of the eyes."

DIAGNOSIS OF PINEAL TUMOR

The diagnosis of a pineal tumor by neurologic signs and symptoms is only occasionally possible. The most significant disturbance is limitation of the upward gaze, the objective evidence of which is ptosis, usually bilateral but at times unilateral; it may be inconstant, particularly in the beginning. Although not a pathognomonic sign, for in some instances a tumor placed anteriorly in the posterior cranial fossa also causes ptosis, it places the burden of proof on tumor other than that of the pineal body. Since in most cases a pineal tumor causes staggering gait, the differential diagnosis of this type and a tumor of the cerebellum is always one of great difficulty, and since cerebellar tumor is very common and pineal tumor relatively infrequent, the law of probability has often led to cerebellar exploration, which yielded negative results. The most common clinical story in this series of cases was headache, nausea, vomiting, diplopia and bilateral papilledema—in other words, the signs and symptoms of tumor of the brain, without signs of localization. Fixation and dilation of the pupils were noted in two patients; this condition is probably one of the most important localizing signs; it is also found in cases of tumor of the third ventricle. Three of the patients complained of unilateral tinnitus (one with partial deafness). The incidence of this symptom is too great to be dismissed as a coincidence.

The ages of the ten patients in this series were 10, 11, 12, 13, 15, 17, 28, 28, 30 and 36 years; in nearly two thirds of the cases, therefore, operation was performed during the period of youth. The earliest symptoms of the existence of a tumor developed in one patient at the age of 9 years; in this case the tumor did not cause dangerous symptoms until six years later. Seven of the patients were males, and three were females. All of the six tumors occurring before the twentieth year were in males. A larger series of cases will be necessary to determine whether these striking figures in relation to age and sex are significant.

Perhaps the most noteworthy localizing sign is an area of calcification in the pineal region of children. After the age of twenty, calcification of the pineal body is an expected and nonsignificant finding, unless it is of unusual size or intensity. But during youth calcification of the pineal body, while not entirely trustworthy, strongly suggests a tumor and the larger and more dense the shadow the greater the reason for assuming that there is a neoplasm. In four of six children in the present series there was a striking shadow in the pineal region. Curiously, in none of the four adults was the shadow greater than one finds in the normal condition. The area of calcification is therefore significant only in children. The most extreme shadow that I have seen in this region was one in a case of tumor of the choroid plexus lying in the third ventricle. Tumor in the third ventricle casts a shadow in over two thirds of the cases and in practically the same position, so that the differential diagnosis of tumor of the pineal body and tumor in the third ventricle cannot be made on the basis of the roentgenographic findings. For practical purposes, however, this is not important, for the two require identically the same operative attack.

A precise diagnosis of pineal tumor is probably always possible by ventriculography, but to accomplish this end perfect visualization of the third ventricle is necessary. This is never difficult, because the ventricular system is always greatly enlarged. That one may be assured that the third ventricle will be clearly shown, the fluid in the entire ventricular system must be exhausted and replaced by air; otherwise, the air takes the course of least resistance and passes into the larger cavity, the lateral ventricle. Two ventriculographic changes are probably always in evidence—a filling defect in the posterior part of the third ventricle and absence of the

suprapineal recess—always a striking space when present. I am not prepared to state that every pineal tumor encroaches on the third ventricle and thus produces a filling defect, but in all the cases that I have observed, it has done so. Every pineal tumor must obliterate the suprapineal recess.

Since the suprapineal recess is not always normally present, one cannot be certain that the absence of this space means the presence of a tumor in this region. But given a suprapineal recess in the ventriculogram, one can be certain that a pineal tumor is not present and that there is either a cerebellar tumor or a stricture of the aqueduct of Sylvius—a lesion by no means uncommon. Therefore, while the absence of the suprapineal recess is significant in a positive way, its presence is pathognomonic in a negative way in excluding the possibility of a pineal tumor. However, since in all the cases of pineal tumor that I have observed a filling defect has been shown in the third ventricle, the obliteration of the pineal recess is of secondary importance.

To obtain perfect filling of the ventricular system, it is necessary only to exhaust the fluid from the lowermost ventricle. It has been stated by enthusiasts for the use of liquids producing opaque shadows (such as thorium dioxide and iodized poppy-seed oil) that the employment of these solutions is especially advisable in the differentiation of tumors in this region because ventriculography (with air) is frequently ineffective. Such a statement is only an admission that the injection of air was not properly made. There is no tumor of the brain causing intracranial pressure, and this includes tumor of the pineal body and tumor of the third ventricle, that cannot be accurately localized by ventriculography. There is never, therefore, in my opinion, justification for the use of opaque material as a means of diagnosis or localization of any tumor of the brain. It need scarcely be added that spinal injections of air contribute little or nothing to the localization of such a tumor. Always dangerous when intracranial pressure exists, spinal injections of air are particularly so when the brain stem is contiguous to the tumor.

OPERATIVE PROCEDURE

The operative attack on pineal tumor is, with minor improvements, essentially the same as that described in the earlier publication. The size of the bone flap is smaller and is situated perhaps a little more posteriorly. The anterior margin of the cerebral exposure is situated well back of the rolandic vein, and the posterior margin is from about 4 to 5 cm. anterior to the transverse sinus; the usual posterior perforator opening used in ventriculography forms the posterior limit of the cranial defect. The mesial border of the incision in the skin is in the exact midline, and the mesial incision in the bone is made at the outer edge of the longitudinal sinus. Fortunately, this part of the sinus rarely bleeds when uncovered, and with the reduction in the size of the bone flap one can approach the midline directly and without the need of subsequent use of the rongeur. Veins from the cerebral hemisphere to the longitudinal sinus are now much more easily handled by coagulation with the electrocautery. Frequently, there are no such veins, but there may be as many as four or five in the field. If a fairly large vein should be situated well anteriorly and should be placed on a stretch when the hemisphere is separated from the falx, it is usually safer to coagulate it and divide it in the beginning than to run the risk of subsequent tear that would be more difficult to control and, in addition, might well interrupt the extirpation of the tumor at a critical time.

The corpus callosum is split longitudinally from its posterior extremity to a point anteriorly where the third or the lateral ventricle comes into view; this incision is bloodless. Usually this incision takes most, and sometimes all, of this structure to its downward bend. No symptoms follow its division. This simple experiment at once disposes of the extravagant claims to function of the corpus callosum.

The so-called cerebellar position with the patient recumbent and the face toward the floor is best, because there is need for less retraction of the cerebral hemisphere. The amount of room available for the direct attack on the tumor is in proportion to the size of the lateral ventricles, which, of course, are always greatly enlarged, owing to the obstruction by the tumor at the aqueduct of Sylvius.

Evacuation of fluid from the ventricular system is perhaps the most essential part of the operative precedure. Fortunately, both enlarged lateral ventricles may be emptied through a single puncture which may be made into the anterior horn of either lateral ventricle (usually the left) or into the anterior part of the third ventricle. It makes little difference at what point the puncture is made. However, a large opening in the roof of the third ventricle should be avoided because of the danger of sponging and injuring the iter. One of the differential points between tumor of the pineal body and tumor of the third ventricle may be that the former (at times only) grows forward over the roof of the third ventricle and the latter, of course, is always under it. Preservation of the roof of the third ventricle greatly facilitates the subsequent flow of fluid through the sylvian aqueduct and therefore shortens the period of convalescence. After the ventricular fluid is released to the utmost, the opening is packed loosely with cotton to preclude the entrance of blood, for a hematoma extending to the remote recesses of the lateral ventricle could not be retrieved. Hydrocephalus, although always present, varies considerably in degree. The ventricles are always larger in young persons and in patients with a long-standing tumor that has acted as a ball-valve for a time, i.e., in patients with periodic headache and vomiting. The tumors in this series ranged from 3 to 18 Gm. The size of the operative field at the site of the tumor may be greatly reduced by the large tumor; usually, too, a larger tumor develops more

rapidly, blocks the aqueduct more promptly and therefore is associated with smaller
lateral ventricles at the time of operation.
Under such circumstances, there is only
one possible way of producing more room
—excision of the occipital and part of the
parietal lobe, as in case 2. This we were
forced to do in four of the series of cases.
Removal of the occipital lobe is the easiest
of all lobe resections, because there are
usually no large veins (the veins entering
the lateral sinus at the mastoid are avoided) and only the posterior cerebral artery
requires ligation. Without this expedient
there is no possibility of carefully extirpating a tumor, for each forceful retraction
of the cerebral hemisphere produces trauma that quickly swells the brain and reduces the field of operation. Needless to
say, the infliction of cerebral trauma by
operative approach, when the injury is
superimposed on trauma at the site of the
tumor, leaves little hope that the patient
will survive. Sacrifice of the right occipital
lobe (because of the possible need of sacrificing an occipital lobe of the brain the
operative exposure is always made on the
right side) adds more than the necessary
room and brings the major part of the tumor directly into view, permitting the
operator to use both hands to extirpate
the growth.

The need at times of splitting the tentorium longitudinally or the falx vertically
and retracting the flaps with sutures of silk
has been stressed in the earlier publication.
Resection of part of either structure, or of
both, may even be necessary, as in case 2.

Two factors make the removal of a pineal tumor much more hazardous than that
of a tumor of the third ventricle: the tight
adherence to the quadrigeminal plate and
the much greater intimacy with the veins
of Galen. Tumor of the third ventricle is
usually only marginally attached at the
lateral and posterior borders to the roof of
the ventricle and below this merely lies
loose in the ventricle, thus making it unnecessary to injure the midbrain or quadrigeminal bodies in the removal. But the
entire inferior surface of a pineal tumor is
firmly embedded in and tightly adherent
to the quadrigeminal plate. Moreover,
such a tumor is usually oval, with the long
diameter in a longitudinal direction, thus
increasing the area of the adherent surface.

The great vein and the small veins of
Galen always lie on a tumor of the third
ventricle, but usually the attachment is not
difficult to separate and at least one of the
veins can be spared. But these veins are
usually firmly bound to a pineal tumor
and frequently grow into it. In fact, the
great vein of Galen had penetrated and
was inseparable from the pineal growth in
most of the specimens that I exposed at
operation.

Liberation of the great vein of Galen
and the small vein of Galen on the right
(that on the left is not visible at first because it lies beyond the curvation of the
tumor) is necessary before enucleation of
the tumor can be attempted. This may or
may not be possible. When the great vein
or its smaller divisions actually traverse
the tumor, the operator has no choice
other than ligation or thrombosis and division of the great vein of Galen as it leaves
the tumor to enter the straight sinus and
of the small veins of Galen as they enter
the anterior pole of the tumor. But every
effort should be made to spare these vessels
before resorting to their destruction. Since
it was realized that the entire internal venous system of the brain has its outlet through the great vein of Galen, its sacrifice
was at first thought to be incompatible
with life, although there was no precedent
on which such a belief could be established. That none of the first patients who
had undergone removal of a pineal tumor
survived was not proof that the loss of the
veins of Galen was the cause, for other factors may have been and actually were responsible. However, the burden of proof
rests strongly on one who denies that this
venous system is necessary to life, or at
least, to the anatomic and functional preservation of the brain. Instances of thrombi of the straight sinus or the great vein of

Galen have, indeed, been reported, but the complete eradication of the major part of these venous trunks is different from the formation of a cicatrix which may allow some restoration of function by collateral channels. Gradually, from the removal of tumors of the third ventricle it was learned that one small vein of Galen could be sacrificed without apparent functional loss. Indeed, it is no simple task to avoid injury to and consequent loss of one small vein of Galen. Although there is less danger of injury to the more distant (left) small vein, its preservation is no mean accomplishment. When intracapsular enucleation of much of the tumor is possible, the loosened capsule can be withdrawn and dissected from the vein, after which the vein remains fairly distant from the field of operation. The near (right) small vein, on the contrary, continues to lie in the line of operative attack and, though protected by moist cotton, is susceptible to operative trauma. The second case in this series of cases of pineal tumor is proof that both the small veins of Galen, the great vein of Galen and at least a third of the straight sinus can be removed without apparent loss of cerebral functions.

After the veins of Galen were disposed of, no large vessels were seen to enter any pineal tumor that has come under my observation. A few tiny arteries and veins enter from the pia covering the quadrigeminal bodies, but one easily disposes of them by packing with moist cotton or by electrocoagulation. However, in some instances the tumor is quite vascular, and the suppression of blood within the tumor —when intracapsular enucleation is employed—may be tedious and difficult.

The most serious problem in disposing of pineal tumor is freeing the tumor from its bed in the quadrigeminal plate. Too deeply situated to be reached with the fingers, the growth must be liberated with instruments. This is just as well, for enucleation with the finger would cause trauma incompatible with the preservation of life or function. The dangers would be pre-cisely the same as those attending the removal of a tumor of the acoustic nerve. Slow, painstaking extirpation of the tumor from its bed is facilitated greatly if intracapsular enucleation is possible and the capsule is strong enough to support traction with forceps. If one or both of these contributions are possible, traction is made upward from the under-surface of the anterior pole of the tumor with the left hand, and the underlying attachments are liberated by cautious blunt dissection or are divided by the knife and scissors with the right hand. The field must, of course, be constantly dry so that no step is made in the dark. Usually the tumor extends so far posteriorly that additional exposure is required. This is provided by cutting the right side of the tentorium for some distance in a posterior direction and reflecting the mesial cut border over the straight sinus by a traction suture.

Three important sequelae are usual after the successful operative removal of such tumor: intracranial pressure, blindness and extraocular palsy. All these complications are due to edema of the tissues from which the tumor has been liberated, and, if actual injury has not been inflicted, are transient. Although at the time these disturbances are terrifying to the surgeon and patient, they all begin to disappear at about the same time, i. e., a week or ten days after the operation.

The acute intracranial pressure is, of course, due to the edematous closure of the aqueduct of Sylvius. Treatment with ventricular puncture is repeated as often as the condition demands—usually three or four times a day.

Blindness results from edema of the centers of vision in the superior colliculi and the external geniculate bodies. In the early stages of visual return, vision may be present one moment and gone the next, but soon thereafter it is as good as it was before the operation.

It is also of interest that in two of the three instances reported in this paper (cases 2 and 3) a sharply defined homonymous hemianopia to the contralateral side remained permanently (Fig. 2). In case 1 the perimetric fields were subsequently normal for both form and color. This sequel of the operation has also been observed in two cases in which tumor of the third ventricle was removed. Although it is conceivable that injury of the external geniculate body may be responsible, this explanation seems hardly probable, for blindness of this origin resulting from traumatic edema clears a few days after operation. Moreover, there is scarcely less trauma to one external geniculate body than to the other. It appears much more probable that the hemianopia results from retraction of the cuneus during the operation.

Disturbance of the function of the extra-ocular muscles is doubtless due to edema of the nuclei of their nerves and the central pathways in the midbrain. Usually the extra-ocular palsy is unequal on the two sides. As a result, the position of the two eyes is markedly different, and their actions may not be correlated. Conjugate deviation resulted in one case. Restriction of the upward movements of the eyeball—an important diagnostic sign of pineal tumor—was apparently not present in case 3 at the time of admission but has persisted to date, so that the return of extra-ocular muscular function may not be complete. Perhaps this represents the degree of permanent injury resulting from the extirpation of the tumor. It has never been clear how this limitation of movement could be effected alone, i. e., without similar loss in the remaining extra-ocular movements referable to the oculomotor nerve.

SUMMARY AND CONCLUSIONS

Three patients with tumor of the pineal body survived extirpation—seemingly total. One patient died three months later (cause undetermined); in the second patient the tumor recurred in two and one-half years, and the third patient is living and apparently well four months later.

In most cases a pineal tumor causes only signs and symptoms of intracranial pressure, due to occlusion of the aqueduct of Sylvius.

Important localizing signs occurring at times are ptosis, usually bilateral, limitation of the upward movements of the eyes and fixation and dilatation of the pupils.

In none of the ten cases were there any disturbances of endocrine character.

Perhaps the most important objective evidence of a pineal tumor in young children—but not in adults—is calcified shadow.

Precise localization in all cases of pineal tumor can be made by ventriculography. The pathognomonic changes are a filling defect in the posterior part of the third ventricle and obliteration of the suprapineal recess.

Six (60 per cent) of the ten tumors in this series were in children between 10 and 17 years of age.

The weights of the tumors ranged from 3 to 18 Gm.

A pineal tumor is exposed by an occipital approach, separation of the right cerebral hemisphere from the falx and splitting of the corpus callosum.

In cases of large tumor in which the ventricles are smaller, resection of the posterior part of the right cerebral hemisphere is necessary. This method was used in four cases (in three of which the outcome was fatal and in one, successful).

Transient blindness and subtotal paralysis of all the extra-ocular muscles followed operation in each of the three cases in which the intervention was successful. These disturbances disappeared a week or ten days later. They were doubtless due to edema resulting from trauma to the quadrigeminal plate, in which the tumor is always firmly embedded, and to the underlying brain stem.

Left homonymous hemianopia may or may not follow and be permanent. It is probably due to compression of the cuneus during the separation of the hemisphere at operation.

REFERENCES

[1]Dandy, W. E.: An Operation for the Removal of Pineal Tumors. *Surg., Gynec. & Obst., 33:* 113, 1921.

[2]Dandy, W. E.: *Benign Tumors in the Third Ventricle of the Brain.* Springfield, Ill., Charles C Thomas, Publisher, 1933, p. 88.

LIII

ETIOLOGICAL AND CLINICAL TYPES OF SO-CALLED NERVE DEAFNESS*

NERVE DEAFNESS OF KNOWN PATHOLOGY OR ETIOLOGY FROM CENTRAL OR CORTICAL LESIONS PARTIAL SECTION OF THE VIIITH NERVE†

From a series of human intracranial operations, which serve as experiments, I wish to bring you certain facts concerning the effects upon hearing in two different lines in the pathways of hearing.

This sketch is that which you will see in any textbook, with the exception of the central pathways for hearing; *i.e.,* those in the cerebral hemispheres.

It is, I think, universally claimed that the centre for hearing lies in each temporal lobe. How this conception has arisen is difficult to understand, but it is certainly a mistake, for one can remove either the entire right or left temporal lobe with no effects whatsoever upon hearing. Audiometer tests have, of course, been used in checking these experiments.

Another more extensive experiment is perhaps even more impressive when the entire right cerebral hemisphere is removed—this has been done seven or eight times —there is not the slightest effect upon hearing.

After removing the occipital, frontal and temporal lobes on the left side (in different individuals), there is no effect upon hearing; therefore, the only possible location for a centre of hearing is in the left parietal lobe. It is unquestionably connected with the auditory speech centre, which is located in the parietal lobe, and not in the temporal lobe, as most textbooks

state.

In this connection, two interesting points from a negative standpoint are: 1. that between the mesial geniculate body and the inferior colliculus anteriorly, and the point of entrance of the VIIIth nerve into the brain stem posteriorly, I have never seen a brain tumor that has produced deafness; and, 2. I have never seen a tumor in the cerebral hemispheres, right or left, that has produced deafness unless there has been an associated deficiency of auditory speech. These facts must carry significance, although I am not prepared to make a positive explanation. Possibly there may be one central region in which defects of hearing may carry diagnostic significance; *i.e.,* at the inferior colliculus or the medial geniculate body. I have had three cases in which tumors in this region (pineal or adjacent tumors) have shown an abrupt bilateral drop in the high tones. These may have been purely coincidental findings, but I believe they are significant. In one case where an auditometer test had not been made, the tumor was found in this location, a subsequent check-up disclosed this same suspected finding.

Other than this, when deafness results from an intracranial tumor the lesion is always located along the VIIIth nerve itself. It is, therefore, of the greatest and most certain diagnostic import.

Why the absence of defects of hearing from tumors throughout the brain stem? My only explanation is that the fibres scatter after the arrival in the brain stem.

My next point of experimental attack is

*Reprinted from *The Laryngoscope,* August, 1937.
†Read as part of the Symposium, *The Neural Mechanism of Hearing,* at the Seventieth Annual Meeting of the American Otological Society, Long Beach, N. Y., May 27, 1937.

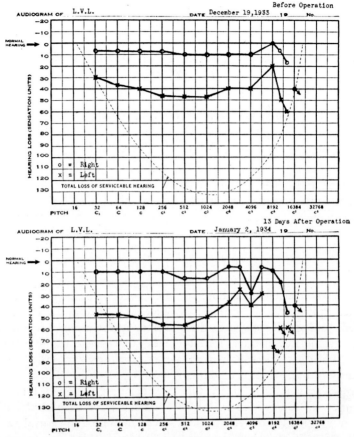

Fig. 1. Audiograms before and after division of three-fourths of the auditory nerve, or one-half of the hearing division of the nerve. The only loss of function is in the very high tones.

in the VIIIth nerve itself; *i.e.,* in the intracranial portion between the spiral ganglion and the brain stem. From a large series of operations for Meniere's disease, we have found this one very interesting observation; namely, that one can divide one-half to two-thirds, at least, of the auditory division of the VIIIth nerve and lose practically nothing in hearing (Fig. 1). When slight losses do occur they are restricted to the very high tones.

In Meniere's disease, where deafness is always associated with the attacks, the lesion must be in the nerve itself. In several specimens removed at operation there has been fibrosis of the nerve. This is, I think, the explanation of the syndrome. It is the only intrinsic change I have been able to find. In about 20 per cent of the cases a large artery (one of the branches of the superior-inferior cerebellar artery) lies against the nerve, and is, I think, one of the causes of the deafness and dizziness of this disease.

LIV

INTRACRANIAL PRESSURE WITHOUT BRAIN TUMOR*

DIAGNOSIS AND TREATMENT

During the past seven years there have gradually accumulated 22 cases in each of which the signs and symptoms of intracranial pressure have been indubitable, and yet in none has there been an intracranial tumor or a space occupying lesion of any kind. Almost without exception a clinical diagnosis of an unlocalized brain tumor has been made; but by ventriculography a brain tumor has been excluded. All of these patients have complained of headache, most of them of nausea, vomiting, diplopia, dizziness, many of loss of vision, and objectively in every instance there have been bilateral papilledema and usually hemorrhages in one or both eyegrounds to indicate, or at least strongly suggest, that intracranial pressure of advanced degree was present. And in each case the intracranial pressure has been objectively demonstrated and usually actually measured by ventricular or lumbar punctures; and finally the subsequent demonstration of pressure over a period of months or years is merely a matter of inspecting the site of the subtemporal decompression to which most of these patients were subjected for treatment. The increased intracranial pressure may last only a few months, but it at times persists five to seven years, and doubtless longer. Curiously, the decompression is almost never consistently at its maximum fulness but is intermittent, and the pressure may come and go with surprising rapidity—from one extreme to the other in a few minutes. The cause of the sudden changes

—indeed the cause of the increased pressure at all—is unknown.

HISTORIES OF THE CASES CONSIDERED

CASE I Unit 11820: B. O. F. Age twenty-one. April 27 to May 14, 1927.

Complaints.—Headache and failing vision.

Present Illness.—Three months ago patient awoke from her sleep smelling illuminating gas. She tried to get up, but fell and struck the back of her head. She vomited that day and the following day. There has been headache in the occipital region since that time and she ascribed it to the injury of the head. The headache is worse in the morning. Since the original episode her vision has been failing; objects are indistinct and there are spots before her eyes. When she tries to read she becomes dizzy and the print melts away. Two weeks ago she thought she staggered, but this lasted only for a day.

Examination.—Patient is a normal appearing young woman of 21. There is papilledema of both eyegrounds, measuring two and one-half diopters on each side. There are several large hemorrhages along both disks. Vision acuity is 20/15 in each eye. Visual fields are normal.

Trephine and Air Injection.—April 30, 1927. Fluid spurted under pressure. The ventriculograms, however, were entirely normal. Wassermann of the cerebrospinal fluid was negative.

Operation.—Right subtemporal decompression, May 6, 1927. The dura was quite tight and the brain bulged markedly through the bony defect. No note was made concerning the amount of fluid obtained at the operation.

Subsequent Course.—Patient was not seen again until November, 1936, at which time the decompression was soft and not bulging; however, it was not sunken. She

*Reprinted from the *Annals of Surgery*, 106: 4, October, 1937.

549

says it has always varied, occasionally being prominent and fairly tense, and at other times sunken. The difference was particularly noticeable in the first two or three years following the operation, but recently the site of the decompression has not become full or tense.

CASE 2 Unit 27949: V. R. F. Age twenty-seven. November 12 to November 22, 1929.

Complaints.—Headaches a n d failing vision.

Present Illness.—Patient was perfectly well in every way until two years ago when she awakened one morning with a severe occipital headache, nausea and vomiting varying from once a month to two or three times a week. For the past 18 months the associated nausea and vomiting have disappeared entirely. Seven months ago an ophthalmologist found bilateral choked disks. For the past six months there have been progressive visual disturbances; at times there are spells of momentary blindness which she thinks are more likely to develop when she has been exposed to a bright light. At times she has noticed a narrowing of the field of vision to such an extent that it appeared to her as though she were looking through a key hole. This has been more progressive in the right eye. Between attacks of disturbed vision the eyesight is clear. Her eyes ache at times and there may be flashes of light when she closes her eyes, particularly when she is facing a bright light. There has been a buzzing in the ears at times, also noise like escaping steam. Her friends have told her that she staggers when she walks. There have been three or four spells of numbness in the right side of the face, sharply down the midline; these last for an hour or more, after which the normal sensation returns.

Examination.—Bilateral papilledema of three diopters in the right eye and two diopters in the left. There are numerous large hemorrhages in and about the left disk. The visual acuity is 20/20 in the right eye and 20/30+ in the left. The blind spot is about four times its normal size in each field of vision. At one time a little hypo-esthesia was disclosed in the right trigeminal area; at other times this could not be found. There are no other positive neurologic findings. Her Romberg is negative, despite her history of staggering gait. The blood Wassermann was negative.

Trephine and Air Injection.—November 15, 1929. The left ventricle was tapped. Fluid spurted under great pressure and stopped abruptly when about 10 cc. had escaped. An equal amount of air was replaced. It was necessary to use pressure to force the air into the ventricle. The ventricular system was small and perfectly normal in every way. The third ventricle was upright and in the midline.

Operation.—A right subtemporal decompression was performed, under avertin anesthesia, immediately after the ventriculograms had been interpreted. The dura was exceedingly tense, so much so that we were fearful of the cortical rupturing in opening it. The descending horn of the ventricle was tapped and some air and fluid escaped, reducing the pressure to a point where the dura could be opened safely. The brain bulged almost to the maximum degree. There was very little fluid on the surface of the brain. Because of the great tension of the brain it was not possible to close the temporal fascia.

Examination of the Cerebrospinal Fluid.—Eight cells, all lymphocytes; globulin negative; Wassermann negative.

Postoperative Course.—Uneventful. Decompression remained full and fairly tense during her stay in the hospital. She has not been seen since. The following report was contained in a letter received December 14, 1934, five years after the operation: "It was about a year and a half after the operation before I could walk without staggering, although this is the first time I have ever admitted it, and from that time on I got much better. The lump on my head remained about the same until last winter when it went down to almost normal and has since remained unchanged. I get very few headaches and usually know the reason. I cannot stoop over much, or keep going too long without paying with a headache. However, I am really just fine and feel great. My eyes do not bother me at all. Have gained in weight—present weight 150 lbs."

CASE 3. Unit 29509: M. C. M. Age forty-five. February 13 to March 1, 1930.

Complaints.—Dizzy spells and drowsiness.

Present Illness.—Ten months ago patient noticed a tendency to become drowsy. He would fall asleep when reading or sitting quietly; had a tendency to mix his words when he was talking, and he had many spells in which both arms and legs would drop limp at his sides and he would be unable to talk. This would last from one to five minutes. Consciousness was not lost. There were no convulsions. He had no headaches. Diplopia has been present at times.

Examination.—Patient is a well developed, strong looking man. Blood pressure 120/80. The neurologic examination is negative except for a low grade papilledema in each disk; there are no hemorrhages.

Trephine and Air Injection.—February 18, 1930. Fifteen cubic centimeters of fluid were removed under great pressure. An equal amount of air was injected. The ventricular system was normal. The ventricular fluid showed no cells; no Pandy; negative Wassermann. Patient had a bradycardia at the time of his admission. During the next 48 hours he was somewhat stuperous, with a pulse running around 38 and 40.

Operation.—February 18, 1930. The left hemisphere was explored because of the history of weakness on the right side and difficulty in speech. There was moderately increased pressure, but the surface of the brain everywhere looked normal. The bone flap was removed for a decompression. The decompression bulged markedly at the time of his discharge from the hospital.

CASE 4. Unit 42619: A. C. F. Age forty-two. April 5 to May 12, 1932.

Complaints.—Dizziness, headache and double vision.

Past History.—Patient has always been extremely constipated. Because her basal metabolism was inconsistently low, ranging between —10 and —30, for the past nine years she has been taking 1 to 3 gr. of thyroid extract daily.

Present Illness.—Eight months ago she began getting dizzy when changing from a sitting to a recumbent position, or vice versa; also when turning the head from side to side, and more especially when she leaned forward. This was during a very hot summer. At times when leaning forward there was momentary blurring of vision. A month later a terrific right side hemicrania lasted for an hour. During this time the vision was quite blurred and she was very dizzy; this attack began when she suddenly changed her position in bed. A month later, or five months ago, diplopia developed and the dizzy spells became so severe on changing position that she became frightened and was unwilling to lean forward to pick up anything. This condition remained essentially unchanged

until a month ago when several more severe right sided headaches developed; the pain was more in the occipital region. There was a little nausea but no vomiting. Curiously, when the dizziness is on, it and the blurred vision can frequently be made to disappear instantly by throwing the head backward.

During the past two weeks there have been flushing spells, so severe that she feels that her face is burning up. She never had a keen sense of smell, but it has been worse in the past few years, and more so in the past few months.

Examination.—Patient is a brilliant, normal looking woman, without nervous tendencies. Blood pressure 112/76. Basal metabolism —17. Both disks are swollen about four diopters. There are small hemorrhages about both disks. The visual fields and visual acuity are normal. Except for diminution of the sense of smell there are no other positive neurologic findings.

Cerebral Pneumography.—A ventricular air injection was attempted but neither lateral ventricle could be reached. A spinal air injection was then performed under gas anesthesia. Fluid spurted under pressure. In view of the type of anesthesia one could not be certain that the pressure was not due to the anesthetic. Seventy-five cubic centimeters of fluid were removed; this exhausted the cerebrospinal fluid. An equal amount of air was injected. The ventricular system was small but normal in every way.

Five days later, without an anesthetic, a lumbar puncture was performed. The pressure was 300 Mm. of water. The fluid was clear, contained four cells; negative globulin and negative Wassermann.

Since the ventriculograms showed a normal ventricular system, a tumor could be excluded. The interpretation, therefore, was that there was intracranial pressure of undetermined cause.

Operation.—April 18, 1932. Under avertin anesthesia a second spinal air injection was done because we were still apprehensive that there might possibly be metastatic nodules which could so easily escape detection by an air injection, or perhaps even a tumor of the olfactory groove. Again the ventricular system was well filled and perfectly normal.

A right subtemporal decompression was then performed. Much to our surprise the brain was sunken beneath the dura. It was quite clear, therefore, that we were dealing with a condition in which there were marked variations in the intracranial pressure. It is also worthy of note that there was no excess of fluid on the surface of the brain.

The postoperative course was uneventful. During her subsequent stay of three weeks in the hospital, the decompression remained, for the most part, full and tense, although there were times when it was quite flat and soft. Her diplopia and dizziness gradually diminished and had practically disappeared at this time. Up to the present time, five years later, neither the diplopia nor dizziness has ever reappeared. Her eyegrounds were found to be normal when examined a few months after her return home, and they have remained normal to date. The vision has been entirely normal. The decompression is still tense at times and it may be just as hard and tense as it was at the time of her operation five years ago. Perhaps more than half of the time it is soft and flat. She is well in every way and leads a very active life with many social activities (May 1, 1937).

I have been particularly eager to determine what may cause the rise and fall of the decompression, but on the whole have been quite unsuccessful. The pressure does appear to rise with any excitement, although this is not always true. A relationship with her obstinate constipation cannot be established, nor does the intake or restriction of fluid materially change it. She suffers no inconvenience whatever. There have been four or five convulsions during the past five years; none were present before. Since there is nothing connected with the air injections or decompression that could cause the convulsions, it has been assumed that they are in no way related to the intracranial condition that is responsible for the increased pressure. On the other hand, she is the only patient in the series who has had a convulsion subsequent to operation.

CASE 5. Unit 37125: B. P. F. Age twenty-three. May 16 to 22, 1931, and again May 9 to 18, 1932.

Complaint.—Impairment of vision.

Present Illness.—Eight months ago patient became totally blind when changing from a recumbent to a sitting position. For the following six weeks the visual loss recurred several times a day. She is quite certain that shifting to other positions did not produce the same effect. Six months

ago there were attacks suggesting right homonymous hemianopia. Objects would disappear in the right half of her field. She had 100 or more such attacks during a day. Her eyes were then examined but nothing abnormal was found. Owing to the continuance of the same symptoms, a lumbar puncture was performed six weeks ago by Doctor Colella of Johnson City, N. Y. Fluid was said not to have been under pressure, although it was not measured. There was one cell and no globulin.

Five weeks ago headaches appeared in both frontal regions; these would last for two or three hours and disappear during sleep; they were throbbing and pounding in character. There had been nausea with the headaches, but no vomiting. In recent weeks the attacks of momentary blindness have come only in the right eye.

At the age of fourteen or fifteen (eight or nine years ago) she had some spells in which she could not get her breath. There is said to have been stertorous breathing. She could not talk, but understood what was said to her. These spells lasted about one-half hour and occurred once or twice a month. There were severe bifrontal headaches for about two hours after each attack.

Examination.—She is considerably over weight, weighing 150 pounds. At the age of sixteen she weighed 192 pounds and two months ago, 170 pounds. The present reduction in weight has occurred without dieting. The neurologic examination reveals only one finding, namely, papilledema measuring three diopters in the right eye, and one diopter in the left. The veins are full and slightly tortuous. There are no hemorrhages in either eyeground. The visual acuity is 20/20 in the right eye and 20/15 in the left. The visual fields are normal. The blind spot in the right eye is enlarged to about three times its normal size; on the left it is normal.

Trephine and Air Injection.—May 19, 1931. Both ventricles were tapped. Fluid spurted under great pressure, then stopped abruptly. About 7 cc of air were injected into each ventricle. Pressure was required to inject the air. The ventriculograms were entirely normal.

Subsequent Course.—Since she could be carefully followed at home she returned, hoping the condition might clear spontaneously. Her blind spells decreased in number but still remained. Her headaches were improved for some time, but again reappeared. She was again having attacks similar to those she had had at the age of fourteen or fifteen, and which she now recognized as being hysterical. Four months later a spinal puncture was performed; the pressure was 250 Mm.

She was again admitted to the hospital, May 9, 1932. Her papilledema now measured only one and one-half diopters in the right eye and one diopter in the left. The visual acuity was 20/20 in each eye; the disks were definitely paler than before. Lumbar puncture on two successive days registered 300 and then 400 Mm. of water.

On May 10, 1932, air was again injected into the lateral ventricles, which were, as previously determined, small and apparently normal. This time there were 16 mononuclear cells in the spinal fluid.

Operation.—May 10, 1932. A right subtemporal decompression was performed. The brain was very tense and bulged greatly but did not rupture when the dura was opened. There was no excess of fluid on the surface.

She returned for observation June 2, 1932, and stated that her headaches were less frequent and less severe. Two days after returning home her right arm and leg began to jerk occasionally and she could not control them so well. She says it caused her to break many dishes. She had another blind spell three days ago; on this occasion only the right eye was affected. The decompression was soft most of the time while at home, but has again become quite bulging and tense. Three days ago both legs became weak and she developed a stumbling gait. There still appears to be some slight motor weakness in the right hand and the finer movements are less well performed. There is no tremor; no ataxia and no astereognosis. She walks with a rather broad base, but there is no definite staggering, and her Romberg is negative.

She was again seen March 19, 1937. The decompression still protruded slightly, but it was quite soft. She says it does get more tense at times. Her vision is normal. Her blind spells have ceased. The disturbances with the legs, and particularly the right leg, and also the right arm, have cleared. She is quite nervous and has become addicted to drugs.

CASE 6. Unit 43567: C. B. F. Age forty-six. May 28 to June 11, 1932.

Complaints.—Headaches and buzzing in the right ear.

Present Illness.—Began four months ago when she developed inconstant, dull, aching pain in the region of the right mastoid. There was also pain in the right frontal region, and a little tinnitus in the right ear. Dizziness has been present at times.

Examination.—Patient looks well, though somewhat overweight. Blood pressure 128/80. The neurologic examination is negative, except for papilledema of four diopters in each disk; there are numerous hemorrhages on both sides. Vision and visual fields are normal. Roentgenologic examination of the head is negative.

Trephine and Air Injection.—May 31, 1932. Fifteen cubic centimeters of fluid were removed from the right ventricle and an equal amount of air injected. The ventricular system was normal. The cerebrospinal fluid contained two cells and no globulin; Wassermann was negative. A spinal puncture was performed three days later; pressure was 550 Mm. of water.

Operation.—June 3, 1932. A right subtemporal decompression was performed. The brain was under great pressure and bulged almost to the maximum degree. The decompression was full and tense at the time of her discharge from the hospital.

CASE 7. Unit 45653: A. R. F. Age thirty-four. October 3 to 25, 1932.

Complaint.—Headaches.

Present Illness.—Eight months ago patient had an attack of headache lasting three days; it was continuous day and night and was accompanied by nausea and vomiting. The headache was more in the right frontal region than elsewhere, but it was also generalized. At the same time there was marked photophobia. A month later there was a similar attack lasting for five days. In the interim she had been well. Two months later a third attack lasted three weeks. She vomited three or four times a day. Two weeks later a fourth attack was accompanied by stiffness and soreness in the neck and a sensation of pins and needles along the inner sides of both arms. The attacks since recurred about once a month. On her visit to the Johns Hopkins Dispensary during the past month, bilateral papilledema was discovered.

Examination.—A large, obese woman, age thirty-four. Blood pressure 110/80; pulse 82; blood Wassermann negative. The neurologic examination reveals but one finding, namely, papilledema of about two diopters in each eye. The veins are full and tortuous but there are no hemorrhages. Visual acuity and visual fields are normal.

Trephine and Air Injection.—October 5, 1932. Twelve cubic centimeters of air were injected into the right ventricle. Fluid spurted under pressure. The ventriculograms showed a normal ventricular system. The fluid contained four mononuclear cells, no globulin. Four days later a lumbar puncture was performed. The pressure was 330 Mm. of water. The Queckenstedt test was normal. There was a response of over 20 Mm. on compression of each jugular, and 40 Mm. on compression of both.

Operation.—October 15, 1932. A right subtemporal decompression was performed. The dura was quite tense. A large amount of fluid escaped under pressure when the dura was opened; the fluid was in the subarachnoid space. After the fluid had escaped, the brain still bulged through the bony defect.

Subsequent Course.—The decompression was usually full and tense, but on many occasions was soft and sunken. When I saw her four months after the operation the decompression was soft, but protruding; she said that on the day preceding it had been so tight and hard that she could not lie upon it.

Her headaches continued, but with much less severity and are practically confined to the right side. These headaches come on an average of once a week and last for two or three days; they are sharp, like a knife thrust. There has been some dizziness during these attacks and some ringing in the right ear. She is quite sure that the headaches have no relationship to the tight decompression. She says they come just as much when the decompression is soft. Both disks are normal in outline and color, and the veins are of normal size.

Hoping to relieve the headaches, I removed the stellate ganglion. She went for three months without a headache, but they again recurred and were of the same type. She is quite nervous, cannot sleep at night and has bad dreams. How much her headaches are genuine and how much functional is difficult to determine.

At the time of my examination a year ago (May, 1936), the decompression was full and very tense.

CASE 8. Unit 46919: S. H. F. Age thirty-two. December 15, 1932, to January 2, 1933.

Complaints.—Headaches; blurring of vision; colored spots before the eyes; double vision.

Past History.—Ovarian tumor was removed three years ago. Prior to this operation she had lost 40 pounds in weight; this has been regained. Her periods again became regular after the operation and have since been normal.

Present Illness.—Soon after her ovarian operation three years ago, occasional dull headaches began; they were more in the frontal and occipital regions, were not especially severe and occurred quite irregularly; at times they might come every two or three days, and again would not reappear for two or three months. Four months ago she began to tire easily, felt badly, and found it difficult to do her house work. Her condition was worse at the menstrual period, at which time there was a dull ache in the right side of her abdomen.

Five weeks ago a sudden, sharp pain developed in the back of the head, perhaps more severe on the left side; this pain has been continuous to date and is worse at night. There have been diplopia and black spots in front of her eyes. Three weeks ago her vision was found to be failing, particularly in the right eye, and a week later she was unable to see anything with this eye. There was vomiting on one occasion, three weeks ago. There was also a transient numbness in the left arm at that time. She staggered for a time and had ringing in the right ear. Four days ago, for no apparent reason, the vision returned in the right eye so that she had a definite field of vision, including colors.

Examination.—Patient is a large woman, considerably overweight (present weight 190 pounds). There is swelling of four diopters in each disk. There are numerous hemorrhages in both eyegrounds; the veins are full and tortuous. The visual acuity is 20/50+ in the right and 20/20 in the left eye; the field of vision is normal in the left and about one-fifth of the normal in the right. The neurologic examination otherwise is entirely negative. Vaginal examination reveals no signs of a tumor recurring from her operation of three years ago.

Tentative Diagnosis.—It was clear that patient had severe grade of intracranial pressure. The possibility of metastases from a malignant abdominal lesion was strongly considered.

Trephine and Air Injection.—December 20, 1932. Twenty cubic centimeters of fluid were removed from the right ventricle and 10 cc. of air injected. There were two cells in the fluid. I could not be sure about the degree of pressure. A lumbar puncture was performed four days later and the pressure registered 320 Mm. of water. The Queckenstedt test was normal; there was no globulin; Wassermann negative.

Operation.—December 24, 1932. A right subtemporal decompression was performed. A fair amount of fluid on the surface of the brain, which was very tense, but when the fluid had been evacuated the brain bulged but slightly.

Subsequent Course.—Letter received June 4, 1936 (three and one-half years after operation): Patient is well and does housework for family of six. Her vision is good in the left eye, still defective in the right. She has no headaches. The decompression swells at times, especially when tired, and goes down quickly when she rests.

Case 9. Unit 60526: E. V. F. Age nine and one-half. February 8 to 25, 1935.

Complaints.—Headaches and vomiting.

Present Illness.—Five months ago generalized headaches appeared, which occurred in spells and quite frequently. Two and one-half months ago she fell off her horse, struck her left jaw, was not unconscious, but was somewhat dizzy. She rode the horse home; vomited that night after dinner but seemed her usual self the next day. Her parents thought the headaches became frequent following this injury. Two months ago one of the episodes of headache and vomiting lasted five days, but following this she was well for nearly a month, when the headaches again returned, accompanied by vomiting. At this time she had an attack that lasted eight days. Her urine was said to have contained acetone and her NPN. was elevated to 68 mg. Four days later the blood chemistry was within its normal limits. About this time diplopia was first noted and an examination of the fundi revealed bilateral papilledema. Ten days ago a lumbar puncture was performed at her home in Mexico City; xanthochromic fluid was said to have been recovered; Pandy was positive, four cells. Her physician also noted paralysis of the left external rectus muscle.

During this time the headaches continued. There was numbness of the hands at times, during the past month. The headaches have never been localized. Appetite has been rather poor during the past month. There has been no disturbance in

gait; no convulsions and no change in personality.

Examination.—An undernourished girl is in bed because she feels ill. Blood pressure 120/70; pulse 90 to 100. Tuberculin test (0.1 mg.) was markedly positive.

The neurologic examination is negative, except for papilledema of three diopters in each eye. There are several hemorrhages in the right disk; the veins are full and tortuous. The appearance of the left disk is essentially similar, except that there are no hemorrhages. The visual acuity is 20/50 in each eye. Visual fields are normal. There are no scotomata. The abducens palsy has disappeared.

Operation.—An air injection was performed February 8, 1935. The ventricular system was perhaps a trifle enlarged, although within the limits of normal. There did not appear to be any pressure, although this could not be definitely determined. The ventricular fluid contained no cells and no globulin. A guinea-pig which was injected with this fluid later died of tuberculosis.

One week later a spinal puncture was made without anesthesia. The pressure registered 500 Mm. of water. There were two cells in the spinal fluid; Pandy was negative. A guinea-pig was also injected with this fluid and eventually died of tuberculosis.

A right subtemporal decompression was performed February 15, 1935. The dura was very tense; when opened the fluid poured out in tremendous quantities, much as obtains in fractures of the skull. We looked carefully for evidence of tuberculosis, but none could be found. Even with the escape of the tremendous amount of fluid, and the loss of 85 cc. of fluid from the lumbar puncture immediately preceding the anesthetic, the brain was now only flush with the dura. After operation the decompression was never tense. She left the hospital February 25, 1935, quite free from symptoms.

Subsequent Course.—A letter received from the father March 12, 1937, two years after operation, stated that the patient had been entirely free from symptoms up to that date and was well in every way. Her physician reported normal eyegrounds and normal vision. We had been apprehensive because two guinea-pigs had died of tuberculosis.

Case 10. Unit 66287: A. M. M. Age forty-four. November 22 to December 9,

1935.

Complaints.—Headaches and dizzy spells.

Present Illness.—Dull headaches have been present in the right frontal region for the past eight months; they come in spells lasting several hours and occur almost daily. They have not become more severe nor more frequent. On two occasions he has had a feeling of giddiness; once so severe that he fell.

Examination.—Patient is a large, well nourished man, seemingly in good health. The physical examination is negative. Blood pressure 118/64. The neurologic examination is negative except for papilledema of three diopters in each eye. There are numerous small hemorrhages on both sides. Vision is normal. Roentgenologic examination of the head is normal.

Trephine and Air Injection.—November 26, 1935. Fluid spurted under high pressure but only 55 cc. of fluid were obtainable. Ten cubic centimeters of air were injected. The ventricular system was normal. The cerebrospinal fluid was not examined.

Operation.—November 26, 1935. Immediately after the ventriculograms were read, a right subtemporal decompression was performed. The brain was under tremendous pressure. Despite the release of a considerable quantity of fluid, the brain still protruded markedly.

Subsequent Course.—The decompression was full and tense at the time of his discharge from the hospital.

I examined the patient again March 17, 1937, 16 months after the operation. He was quite well and played golf. The decompression was full and tense. He says it is that way very much of the time but is also frequently flat. When the decompression is very tense there is a little headache and the eyes feel as though they were being pushed out; at these times there are colored rings about both eyes. The vision and visual fields are normal; the disks are sharply defined and the veins of normal appearance. He says reading, talking and nervousness quickly cause the decompression to become tense and full— the time required for it to change from one extreme to the other is less than two minutes. He also thinks the decompression becomes more tense when he is constipated.

CASE 11. Unit 66817: R.H. F. Age forty-one. December 20 to 30, 1935.

Complaint.—Blurring of vision in the left eye.

Present Illness.—One and one-half years ago an intermittent blowing sound developed in the right ear. This was synchronous with the heart beat. She found by lying in certain positions or by holding the upper right side of her neck with her hand the noise would stop. The noise occurred irregularly, and was not sufficiently disturbing to keep her awake. Three months ago blurring of vision was noted in the left eye. This was not associated with any other symptoms. She is quite certain that she has had no headache, and aside from loss of vision there have been no other disturbances.

Examination.—Patient is a well nourished, normal looking woman, a little overweight. Blood Wassermann negative. Blood pressure 140/76. Roentgenologic examinations of the head are negative. In each fundus there is papilledema of three diopters, large hemorrhages cover both eyegrounds. Visual acuity is 20/20 in the right eye; 20/40 in the left. Visual fields are normal. The blind spots are slightly enlarged.

Trephine and Air Injection.—December 21, 1935. Fluid spurted under great pressure; only a few cubic centimeters of ventricular fluid escaped. Ten cubic centimeters of air were injected. The ventricular system was normal in every way, but both lateral ventricles were markedly undersized.

Operation.—A right subtemporal decompression was performed the same day. The dura was exceedingly tense and the brain bulged greatly when it was opened. However, there was quite a free flow of fluid from the subarachnoid space and before the operation was concluded the brain was flush with the level of the dura, but not beneath it. There were no signs of abnormalities in the brain. The patient was discharged December 30, 1935; the decompression was full and tense.

Subsequent Course.—A letter from her husband February 4, 1937 (fifteen months after operation), states: "Mrs. H. feels fine. She doesn't sleep very well at night. The bump on her head where she was operated seems swollen quite a bit, but otherwise she is in fine health." Visual acuity and visual fields taken by Dr. Walter R. Parker, of Detroit, were normal.

CASE 12. Unit 67385: S.W. F. Age thirteen. January 21 to February 16, 1936.

Complaints.—Failing vision, diplopia

and headache.

Present Illness.—Seven months ago pain developed in her left hip causing her to limp. The pain progressed steadily for three months when she was no longer able to walk. Roentgenograms were taken and were said to have been negative. A month later a second roentgenologic examination revealed an abnormality about the epiphysis at the head of the femur and atrophy of its neck. The leg was placed in a plaster spica. The pain immediately disappeared. She felt better, ate heartily and gained some weight. A month later, *i.e.,* two months ago, she had an attack of vomiting. One month later, *i.e.,* one month ago, she complained of dizziness and headache over both eyes. Within a week her eyesight became blurred, there was double vision and the headache had become much more severe. It was then located in the occipital as well as the frontal region. There were pain and stiffness in the neck. Vomiting became more severe, occurring several times a day. Three weeks ago the plaster spica was removed and an appendectomy performed because of the vomiting. There was no upset following the operation, and although her headache continued, the vomiting ceased. One week ago her vision had become so poor that she could only recognize light with the left eye. She was still able to read with the right eye. For the past three or four weeks there have been attacks of numbness in the right leg (not the leg in the spica).

Examination.—Patient is a sallow, fairly well nourished, young girl suffering severely with headache. Temperature normal; pulse 110; respirations 24; blood pressure 120; W.B.C. 7,800. There is a definite cracked-pot sound (Macewen's sign) on tapping the frontoparietal suture line. Moreover, roentgenologic examination showed separation of sutures—unusual at the age of 13, and indicative of an extreme degree of intracranial pressure. There is only light perception in the left eye. She can read ordinary print with the right eye. Being bedfast and in a plaster spica, a more detailed eye examination is not possible. There is papilledema of five to six diopters in the right eye; two to three diopters in the left (the blind eye). The disk and surrounding retina are filled with large flame-like hemorrhages; these are more pronounced on the right side. There is weakness of the external rectus muscle on the left, but the parents say this has always

been present. The knee jerks on the right could not be elicited; the left leg is in a plaster spica. Babinski is negative; no clonus.

Diagnosis.—Although I had suspected a tuberculous hip and a metastatic infection of the brain, Dr. George Bennett, who saw her with me, excluded tuberculosis from the study of the roentgenograms. The co-existence of the two lesions made us suspect a relationship between the two, but the only positive finding in the hip was the epiphyseal separation and atrophy of the neck and upper part of the shaft. There was no positive infective process.

Trephine and Air Injection.—January 22, 1936. The right ventricle was tapped. Fluid spurted out under tremendous pressure—at least at a distance of three feet. About 15 cc. of fluid escaped and then the flow shut down abruptly. Ten cubic centimeters of air were injected under pressure to replace the fluid. The ventriculograms showed a perfectly normal ventricular system. The fluid showed four cells, all lymphocytes. A guinea-pig was inoculated with the fluid, because of the suspicion of tuberculosis; it had no effect upon the animal.

A right subtemporal decompression was performed immediately after the ventriculograms had been interpreted. The dura was exceedingly tense. A small nick was made in the dura, hoping that fluid might be encountered and thus reduce the terrific tension. A large amount of fluid did escape, but it seemed to make little, of any, impression upon the tension of the dura. The dura was rapidly opened but the pressure was still so extreme that the cortex ruptured inferiorly. The intracranial pressure had just about reached its limit.

Following the operation the decompression was exceedingly tense. A spinal puncture on the third day after operation registered 460 Mm. of water; this, in spite of the decompression. With this great pressure it looked as though the decompression would be futile. A lumbar puncture was performed on each of the following seven days; about 30 cc. of fluid being removed each time. On the eighth day after operation the spinal fluid pressure registered 350 Mm. The tension of the decompression gradually decreased during the next five days. On the fourteenth day the decompression was flat and the spinal fluid pressure measured 160 Mm. Patient remained in the hospital a week longer.

The decompression remained perfectly flat throughout that time.

For a few days after operation patient was unable to see with either eye. As the pressure became less her vision returned and at the time of her discharge she was able to read fine print with the right eye, but the left eye still remained blind. Her general condition had changed entirely, her color was better, and she was very much more alert and active mentally.

Subsequent Course.—When examined by me three months later, she was totally blind, had severe headaches, and the decompression was as full and as tense as it could possibly be. The left optic disk showed extreme optic atrophy with sharply defined disk and normal sized veins. The right had much the same appearance but slightly less advanced. It did not look as though vision could ever return. Within two weeks the decompression was again flat, and vision returned in the right eye. February 12, 1937, 13 months after operation, she was well; had had no more evidences of increased pressure, the decompression had remained soft; her vision was 20/70 in the right eye and there was a fairly normal field of vision. Her femur has healed and gives no trouble; there is no limp.

CASE 13. Unit 69343: R.W. F. Age thirty-one. July 8 to 20, 1936.

Complaints.—Headache and blurred vision.

Past History.—Aside from a chronic discharging ear on the left side since the age of nine, the past history is negative.

Present Illness.—This is dated, by the patient, to an automobile accident five years ago. Since this time she has had occipital headaches; more recently they have become generalized. At times there is a feeling of giddiness and unsteadiness on her feet, but no true vertigo. At times there are spots before her eyes and the vision is blurred. There has been no diplopia.

Examination.—Patient is a rather obese, well developed, healthy looking but highly nervous woman. She does not appear ill. Blood pressure is 124/76; blood Wassermann negative. There is papilledema measuring two diopters in each disk. There are a few small hemorrhages about each disk. The visual fields and visual acuity are normal.

Trephine and Air Injection.—June 13, 1936. Both ventricles were small. Ten cubic centimeters of fluid were removed from each ventricle and an equal amount

of air injected. The ventriculograms were negative. The ventricular pressure could not be determined because the ventricles were too small. The ventricular fluid showed three cells and a negative Pandy.

Spinal Puncture.—July 8, 1936. Pressure measured 430 Mm. of water. Fluid was clear; four cells; negative Pandy. Wassermann negative.

Operation.—July 11, 1936: Decompression. The dura was under high tension. Fluid poured out in large amounts when the dura was opened. Fluid was everywhere through the subarachnoid spaces. When the fluid had ceased to flow the brain still bulged markedly.

Subsequent Course.—January 4, 1937, patient states swelling has disappeared.

CASE 14. Unit 71733: V.D. F. Age twenty. August 10 to 22, 1936.

Complaint.—Headache.

Present Illness.—Three years ago (April, 1933) severe generalized headaches developed. An examination of her eyegrounds at that time revealed choking of the right disk. She had no visual symptoms at that time; in fact no symptoms except headache. Two months later air was injected into her spine by her physician. A year later she was seen by a neurologic surgeon who performed a ventricular air injection. The ventricles were apparently normal. She was blind for twenty-four hours following this procedure. Since then she says her vision has not been as good as it was before. She says there has been fever off and on during her illness of the past three years. At one time she kept a record and found that her temperature rose to 100° or 101° F. nearly every afternoon. She has been examined for various infections, but nothing has ever been found. Headache still remains the only symptom. It remains essentially unchanged and is not localized.

Examination.—Patient is a normal appearing female, age twenty. Her physical examination reveals no abnormalities. Blood Wassermann negative. Blood pressure normal. Roentgenologic examination of the head is normal. Neurologic examination reveals only bilateral papilledema. This is of low grade in the left eye but there is an elevation of four diopters in the right. There are no hemorrhages in the eyegrounds. Her vision and visual fields are normal.

Spinal Air Injection.—August 14, 1936. Since a tumor was not regarded as a very strong probability, a spinal air injection was made. The spinal pressure was 330 Mm. of water. One hundred cubic centimeters of fluid were removed and an equal amount of air injected. The lateral ventricles were imperfectly filled and were very small but normally placed.

Operation.—August 14, 1936. A right subtemporal decompression was performed. The brain was very tense and bulged through the dural defect, but there was no fluid on the surface of the brain.

CASE 15. Unit 74033: P.W. F. Age nineteen. November 3 to 11, 1936.

Complaints.—Blurring of vision; double vision; headaches.

Present Illness.—Three months ago vision became blurred and distant objects were seen double. Headaches began at the same time; they were generalized and appeared to begin and end in no particular region; they were somewhat worse at night. There was no vomiting or vertigo.

Examination.—Blood pressure, 124/70. Wassermann negative. Neurologic examination is entirely negative except for bilateral papilledema of two diopters and some diminution in visual acuity. There are numerous hemorrhages about both disks. The visual fields are normal. The visual acuity is 20/40 in each eye. The blind spots are perhaps very slightly enlarged. *Tentative Diagnosis:* Brain tumor.

A lumbar puncture was performed immediately before the air injection. The pressure registered 530 Mm. of water. On account of the severe pressure, air was not injected by the spinal route.

Trephine and Air Injection.—November 4, 1936. Intracranial pressure was very high, the fluid spurting. The ventricular system was entirely normal.

Operation.—A right subtemporal decompression was performed the same day. The brain was very tense, and great quantities of fluid poured from the arachnoid when it was punctured. At the time of closure the cortex bulged slightly.

Subsequent Course.—June 10, 1937. Patient states that the operative area swells when she lies down; at other times it is flat. Her vision is good.

CASE 16. Unit 74464: B.F.S. M. Age twenty-nine. December 8 to 18, 1936.

Complaints.—Headaches and loss of vision.

Family and Past Histories.—History of syphilis. Patient lost the left eye in an accident during childhood.

Present Illness.—Three years ago headaches began; they were in the occiput and behind both ears. For six months the neck was stiff. He then began vomiting and the headaches became intensified, subsequently subsiding. During the past three months more or less constant dull frontal headaches have occurred. For the past two months the vision in his left eye (only) has been impaired. He also thinks he has staggered during this time; some dizziness, frequent vomiting; loss of 34 pounds in weight.

Examination.—Patient is a very much undernourished, ill looking man with sallow complexion. He clearly shows the loss of 34 pounds in weight. Blood Wassermann four plus. Papilledema of two diopters in the left eye—the right has been removed. There are no other positive neurologic findings.

Trephine and Air Injection.—December 9, 1936. The ventricular system was entirely normal. Later the pressure of the spinal fluid measured 250 Mm. of water; there was no cells; Pandy was positive and the Wassermann four plus.

Right Subtemporal Decompression.—December 11, 1936. Since patient had only one eye a decompression was made, even though the intracranial pressure was not greatly increased. The brain bulged moderately, with a fair amount of fluid, after the evacuation of which the brain became flush with the dura. The patient was discharged December 18, 1936.

Letter May 18, 1937: Condition is essentially unchanged.

CASE 17. Unit 104829: A.S. M. Age forty-four. April 19 to 29, 1937.

Complaints.—Pain in the back of the head and blurring of vision.

Present Illness.—Began three months ago when a severe pain developed in the lumbar region and radiated to the back of the head where a severe headache developed which persisted for two days. During the time of the severe headache there was a numbness and tingling in his right foot and hand, but there was no loss of motor power. One week ago he vomited on several occasions. Nine days after the first attack a similar lumbar pain again developed which radiated to the head; this persisted for only one day but the back pain lasted for ten days; only during the past week has he been free of it. Ten days ago diplopia developed but soon disappeared; it recurred several times during the following three days. His vision has been blurred to such an extent that he has been unable to read fine print. At the present time there is very little headache and this is not at all localized. It is not intensified by change of position.

Examination.—Patient is a well developed, well nourished man. Blood pressure 126/84; blood Wassermann negative. There is bilateral papilledema of three diopters and numerous hemorrhages in both eyegrounds; the veins are full and tortuous. The visual fields are normal, but the visual acuity is reduced to 20/30 in each eye following correction by glasses. Possibly there may be slight weakness of both external recti. Roentgenologic examination of the head is negative.

Ventricular Air Injection.—April 20, 1937. Fluid spurted under marked pressure. Fifteen cubic centimeters of fluid were removed and an equal amount of air injected. The ventricular system was normal.

A spinal puncture was performed immediately and registered 480 Mm. of water. The fluid showed four cells, no globulin and negative Wassermann.

Operation.—A decompression was performed on the same day. The brain was exceedingly tense. There was quite a little fluid on the surface, enough to reduce the pressure so that finally the brain bulged but slightly beyond the cranial vault. Patient was discharged from the hospital nine days later. At the time of his discharge the decompression area bulged but slightly.

Subsequent Course.—Three weeks later the site of the decompression had suddenly become very full and tense. He said before this it had not protruded. This fulness and increased tension had been present for the preceding 48 hours.

CASE 18. Unit 103973: H.B. Colored F. Age twenty-nine. April 28 to May 10, 1937.

Complaint.—Pain in the head.

Present Illness.—One year ago bifrontal headaches began; they also extended into the temporal region and were especially pronounced just back of the eyes. They were intensified by bending over and on returning to the upright position. For the past three weeks the headache has been very severe. There has been slight diminution in visual acuity, but no diplopia. There have been no other symptoms.

Examination.—Patient is a rather obese, but healthy looking colored woman. The physical examination is entirely negative except for a slight increased blood pressure which registered 150/90; three weeks previously, when taken in the dispensary, it was 170/100. Blood Wassermann negative Urine two plus albumin. There is papilledema of two diopters in each fundus. There are no hemorrhages. The visual fields are normal; visual acuity 20/15 in each eye. Roentgenograms of the head are negative.

Ventricular Air Injection.—April 28, 1937. Entirely negative. The ventricles were rather small.

Spinal Puncture, May 3, 1937, registered 250 Mm. of water. The Queckenstedt test was negative on both sides. The spinal fluid contained no cells and no globulin; Wassermann was negative.

Operation.—A right subtemporal decompression was performed May 5, 1937. The brain was very full and tense. There was almost no fluid on the surface of the brain so that it bulged markedly at the time the temporal muscles were approximated.

CASE 19. Unit 27262: M.G. F. Age twenty-four. October 4 to 25, 1929.

Complaint.—Headache.

Present Illness.—Began two years ago with terrific headaches lasting a few hours and occurring every five or six days; they were mainly in the right frontal region. Four months ago they became more severe and were present almost every day. During the past month the headaches had been almost constant, but worse at night. On two occasions the patient had vomited when the headache was especially severe. There had been a little dizziness at times, particularly when the patient moved abruptly or stooped over.

Examination.—Patient is a large well nourished colored girl, age 24. Blood pressure 110/82; pulse 70. Blood Wassermann negative. There is bilateral papilledema of four diopters, a little more marked on the left, and a few small hemorrhages at the disk margin on the left. Her vision is normal.

Trephine and Air Injection.—October 5, 1929. Fluid spurted under high pressure, but only a few cubic centimeters were obtained. Ten cubic centimeters of air were injected under pressure. Ventriculograms showed the ventricular system to be entirely normal. There were three cells and no globulin in the ventricular fluid. Wassermann negative.

Operation.—October 5, 1929. As the right ventricle was not as well filled as the left, and her headaches were definitely unilateral, we felt that if it were a tumor it would be on the right side. Accordingly an exploration of the right hemisphere was made. The brain was very tense, but there was fluid everywhere in the sulci, and when this was evacuated and the ventricle tapped it was not difficult to close the dura. A decompression was not performed.

Subsequent Course.—On October 22, 1929, seventeen days after operation, another air injection was performed. Again the ventricular fluid was under high pressure and the ventriculograms again showed the ventricular system to be entirely normal. The patient was seen two months later, at which time the papilledema was still present, but less than when she was in the hospital. She was then free of headaches entirely. A letter April 1, 1936, says patient is normal in every way and vision is unaffected.

CASE 20. Unit 65474: S.M. M. Age forty-eight. October 14 to November 23, 1935.

Complaints.—Headache and drowsiness.

Past History.—Negative, except that patient is said to have had attacks of kidney stone without hematuria.

Present Illness.—Patient was first seen when he was comatose. He had right sided headaches for the past three weeks. When the headaches began he had suddenly become irrational. A spinal puncture was done at his home and a pressure of 300 Mm. of water was reported. Following this he was somewhat improved. He was brought to a hospital in Baltimore where he again suddenly became drowsy, then unconscious. A lumbar puncture was done in another hospital; it measured 200 Mm. and the fluid was said to have been xanthochromic.

A careful neurologic examination was made by Dr. Irving Spear and was entirely negative. I saw him when he again passed into coma; at this time his pulse ranged between 60 and 70. I thought he had a brain tumor and advised ventriculography.

Trephine and Air Injection.—October 14, 1935. Air injection showed definitely increased pressure, though it was not excessive and was not measured. Twenty-five cubic centimeters of fluid were removed and an equal amount of air injected. The ventricular system was entirely normal. As the fluid was somewhat bloody, a cell count and globulin examination were not made. During the next few days the patient became gradually more responsive, but was disoriented and had hallucinations. He had some pain in the right side. of his head. Gradually he became quite normal again.

Nine days after the operation for ventriculography, he still complained of a little headache. A lumbar puncture was done and registered 160 Mm. of water. The fluid was perfectly clear and there were no cells and no increased globulin.

On October 29, 1935, there suddenly developed a severe attack of auricular fibrillation with pulse deficit of 64; the heart beat was 114. Under treatment improvement began at once and the heart rate was soon normal, and remained so up to the time of his discharge. His wife then recalled that he had had a seemingly similar attack at the beginning of his present illness. Following this last attack his general condition was improved and he was seemingly quite normal in every way.

On October 31, 1935, another lumbar puncture was done. He was then having increased headaches and the ventricular pressure registered 230 Mm. of water. The fluid showed 48 cells and a positive Pandy, but the fluid was blood tinged. The Wassermann reaction was normal. He had no more attacks of arrhythmia or hallucinations, and his headache disappeared. He left the hospital November 23, 1935.

It should be noted that although his eyegrounds were negative on admission, there was a definite papilledema of two diopters in each eye. and a single hemorrhage in the left eye, when examined on November 11, 1935.

In view of the fact that he was symtomatically so well, that his vision could be watched, and that his spinal pressure had not been high, it was not thought advisable to perform a decompression.

Subsequent Course.—Five months later he wrote that he was quite well, except for some dizziness and pains in the head when active.

CASE 21. Unit 67255: M.D. F. Age twenty-seven. January 14 to 21, 1936.

Complaint.—Headache.

Present Illness.—Twelve days before admission patient was delivered of a full term baby. Throughout pregnancy and delivery nothing unusual happened. Three days after confinement a sudden severe right frontal headache developed, which soon became generalized, although it remained more intense on the right side. On the following day she vomited many times, and on the next day there was intense nausea but no vomiting. The headaches persisted, though they were less severe. On the seventh day there was numbness of the left arm; this spread to the left leg and to the left side of the face. There were a number of attacks of numbness of this character during the following day, each attack lasting for about twenty minutes. There was transient diplopia. Her appetite became poor. A lumbar puncture was performed, the fluid registered 400 Mm. of water. There were four cells in the fluid.

Examination.—Patient is a well developed, large woman. She was very drowsy. At the time of her admission to the hospital her pulse, temperature, respirations and blood pressure were normal, but there was a slight trace of sugar and albumin in the urine. There was bilateral papilledema of four diopters in each eyeground and one large flame shaped hemorrhage just below the left disk. The left external rectus was paralyzed.

Trephine and Air Injection.—January 13, 1936. The right ventricle was tapped; the fluid did not appear to be under increased pressure. Fifteen cubic centimeters of fluid were removed and 10 cc. of air injected. The ventricular system was entirely normal. Patient remained in the hospital only five days. Her general condition improved rapidly. Since the attack of intracranial pressure was so acute, the vision was unimpaired, and since her vision could be carefully watched, a decompression was not considered necessary. It was hoped that the condition would clear spontaneously. At the time of her discharge there was no apparent difference in the eyegrounds and the abducens palsies remained.

Subsequent Course.—Letter May 15, 1936 (four months after admission to the hospital) : Patient reports that she is perfectly well in every way. Her double vision has cleared. Ophthalmoscopic examination is entirely negative.

CASE 22. Unit 74786: A. K. M. Age twenty-one. January 4 to 13, 1937.

Complaints.—Headache and dimness of vision when reading.

Present Illness.—Began eight months ago with headaches which were generalized. There has been some dimness of vision

during the past eight months. He has had no other symptoms. A lumbar puncture had been performed a week before admission, which registered 250 Mm. of water. Subsequently, when tested by us, it was 300 Mm.

Examination.—Patient is a well nourished, normal appearing young man, age 21. Blood pressure 130/75. Blood Wasserman and roentgenologic examination of the head are negative. The neurologic examination is entirely negative, except for bilateral papilledema of one and two diopters in each eye. There are no hemorrhages in the eyegrounds. Vision is 20/30 in the right eye, and 20/40 in the left. Visual fields are normal. Blind spots are not enlarged.

Trephine and Air Injection.—January 8, 1937. Only about 5cc. of fluid were obtainable. Ten cubic centimeters of air were injected, each ventricle being filled independently. The ventricular system was very small, but of normal shape. A tumor could be definitely excluded.

A lumbar puncture was made three days later in order to check the previous findings of increased pressure. It now registered 300 Mm. of water, and contained three cells, globulin negative; Wasserman negative. A decompression is held in abeyance awaiting visual examination a month hence.

Subsequent Course.—Patient was well and had normal vision on May 1, 1937 (four months) .

Age and Sex Incidence.—The youngest patient was nine and one-half, the next thirteen years of age; the latter had much the more rapid and severe intracranial pressure in the series. One other case was under twenty, and a fourth just twenty. Seven occurred in the second decade. Half of the patients were, therefore, in the first two decades and the remaining in the third and fourth decades. The oldest patient in the series was forty-eight.

Sixteen of the patients were females and only six were males. Two (females) were colored.

Symptoms.—Headache or pain was the first symptom in seventeen cases; blurring of vision was the first symptom in four cases, although in two it was practically synchronous with the headache. Dizziness, drowsiness and vomiting were the other three initial symptoms.

Dizziness—a sensation of swooning or uncertainty in the head, not a sensation of whirling objects—was a fairly common disturbance and was doubtless a symptom of intracranial pressure and not of localizing import. It occurred in twelve of the twenty-two cases.

Nausea was present in seven; vomiting in eleven, and diplopia in eleven of the twenty-two cases. These symptoms occurring in about half of the cases are also due to intracranial pressure.

Duration of Symptoms.—In 13 of the 22 cases the symptoms had been present less than a year when the patient applied for treatment. The shortest duration of symptoms was twelve days; another was three weeks; in neither of these were the symptoms severe and in neither was an operation performed. In several cases the symptoms were of only three months' duration. The most fulminating case in the series had had symptoms only ten weeks and was then permanently blind in one eye. Symptoms were present for a year or more (five years in one) in six cases (22 per cent).

The Eyegrounds.—In every case papilledema was present and was the outstanding objective finding. In every instance (excepting one patient who had only one eye) the papilledema was bilateral and usually it was symmetrical; occasionally it was slightly greater in one eye. The papilledema varied from one to four diopters. Hemorrhages were very common (15 of the 22 cases). In 11 cases the hemorrhages were bilateral, in four unilateral. Usually they were multiple and scattered over or beyond the disks; in two cases only a single hemorrhage was found in the eyegrounds.

Vision.—Blurring of vision was one of the most common complaints. Reduction in visual acuity, enlarged blind spots, scotomata and blindness were found in 11 cases (50 per cent).

Other Symptoms.—Numerous other complaints have been assembled but with few exceptions there is no semblance of uniformity. The most common complaint, except those enumerated above, was staggering gait in four cases, though in one instance it lasted for only one day. In six cases there was numbness of some part of parts of the body. There were episodes of numbness in both hands (two cases), a leg, an arm, one side of the face and half of the body (each one case); weakness of both arms and legs (one case) and transient hemiplegia (one case). Buzzing of one or both ears was a symptom in three cases. Other complaints were drowsiness in spells (one), nycturia (one), hallucinations (one), anosmia (one), stiffness of neck (one), pain in lumbar region (one) and loss of weight (one).

Findings from Various Examinations.—The neurologic examinations were practically negative in every case. A positive Romberg was disclosed only once, hyperactive knee jerks, once, abducens palsy, twice. In only a single instance did the roentgenologic examination disclose a positive finding; the frontoparietal sutures were separated in a girl of 13 who had the extreme intracranial pressure over a short period of time.

The blood pressure was elevated in only one instance; it was 150/90 in a woman age twenty-nine. At an earlier examination it was said to have been 170/100. Her urine also contained two plus albumin.

In only one case was the Wassermann reaction positive in the blood and spinal fluid. He gave a definite history of syphilis.

The Cerebrospinal Fluid.—With two exceptions the cell count and globulin were well within normal limits. In one case a lymphocyte count of 36 was recorded. A year later on reexamination there were 16 cells. She also had 50 mg. of albumin. She is still living and well six years later, so there can be no serious significance to the increases. In only one other case in the series was there globulin in the cerebrospinal fluid (the patient with syphilis).

Intracranial Pressure.—The pressure of the spinal fluid varied from 250 to 550 Mm. of water. In Case 12, a girl, age 13, the frontoparietal sutures were separated by the intracranial pressure. This was evident by percussion of the head (MacEwen's sign) and in the roentgenograms. In no other case in the series was the roentgenologic examination of any value.

Ventriculography.—In every instance the ventricles have been small—usually markedly undersized—and symmetrical. An intracranial tumor causing the grade of intracranial pressure that is indicated by the papilledema, hemorrhages and measured pressure could not exist with such small symmetrical ventricles.

Treatment.—The treatment of these cases is purely upon a mechanical basis. A right subtemporal decompression is performed if the symptoms and objective signs (eyegrounds and vision) indicate its need. It is necessary in most, but not all, cases because the intracranial pressure frequently persists for months, and frequently years. In four cases in this series there was every indication of a mild degree of intracranial pressure but since the vision and eyegrounds could be periodically observed they were not operated upon. So far, in every case there has been every indication of a complete, spontaneous cure. When operation is indicated the maximum opening in the subtemporal region should be provided. Although the pressure is always high, the cortex has never ruptured in the bony defect. The latter complication is avoided because sufficient fluid escapes from the subarachnoid space to reduce the pressure. Nor has the decompression—although very full and tense—suggested the need of further temporary relief by puncture of the spinal canal. There was one exception to this statement, the little girl previously mentioned with the extreme pressure (Case 12). Following a spinal puncture with collapse of the decompression, the pressure returned to its maximum within an hour.

SUMMARY AND CONCLUSIONS

The facts concerning this condition may be summed up from the 22 cases reported,

as follows: There is intracranial pressure of varying duration and intensity. Frequently it persists over several years, though it may be of only a few months' duration. Usually in each individual there are marked variations in the degree of intracranial pressure from time to time and the changes from one extreme to the other and in either direction may occur, at times at least, very rapidly, *i.e.,* over a period of a few minutes. The subjective disturbances are those of intracranial pressure alone, though at times vague neurologic symptoms may appear; the latter, when present, are fleeting, inconstant, and too ill defined to be of localizing significance. This condition is both immediately and permanently controlled (possibly with rare exceptions) by a subtemporal decompression. To this extent, therefore, it is a self limited disease. Without operative relief, vision, at least, is lost. On the other hand, spontaneous recovery may result before vision is seriously affected. The effect upon life is difficult to estimate, but it is quite probable that in only the most severe grades would life be lost.

The cause of this condition is not known. It can be reasoned with safety that the increased intracranial pressure is dependent upon the intracranial fluid content, *i.e.,* either blood or cerebrospinal fluid, otherwise the very rapid changes could not occur. But whether blood or cerebrospinal fluid is chiefly or entirely responsible can only be conjectured. Moreover, the variable fluid content must be in the brain itself and not in the meningeal spaces. Proof of this statement is demonstrated by two observations: (1) The protruding brain at the time of operation is usually only partially, and at times scarcely at all, relieved by evacuating the fluid from the subarachnoid spaces over the temporal lobe; and (2) because the ventricular system is always small, and usually much smaller than normal. If the fluid in the meninges were increased the ventricular system would naturally participate and, therefore, be correspondingly enlarged from the backlog. Since fluid is never in the subdural space the only other place where it could form in excess and cause intracranial pressure would be in the substance of the brain. Fluid in this position would maintain the fulness of the brain after evacuating the subarachnoid space and would also diminish rather than increase the size of the lateral ventricle. Whether or not such a condition actually obtains, or could obtain, I do not know. Disturbances of this kind are not known, nor is there sufficient information concerning the circulation of fluid within the brain to advance a hypothesis of this kind.

The only other possible explanation of the increased pressure is by variations in the intracranial vascular bed probably by vasomotor control. It is, I think, more amply demonstrated that such influences are at work. There are at least two reasons for thinking that this may be the most satisfactory explanation. The very rapid increase and decrease of the decompression—in two or three minutes from one extreme to the other—could hardly occur except from variations in the vascular bed; certainly the change is much too rapid for an increase or decrease of cerebrospinal fluid. And secondly, fright, fatigue, mental or physical, and sudden nervousness may cause the decompression to become more tense very rapidly. However, an abnormal psychogenic background in three patients is certainly the exception rather than the rule. In not more than one, or at most two instances, was the patient highly emotional. On the other hand, these sudden changes may be merely effects that are superimposed upon the underlying condition with another explanation. Nor is there any reason to believe from a study of these patients that the underlying condition can be dependent upon any obstruction in the big venous sinuses, for the Queckenstedt test is usually made routinely and has never been positive. Other etiologic factors are entirely unknown.

That all of these cases have, or have not, the same underlying cause I do not know.

We may well be dealing with a condition that has more than one underlying anatomic or etiologic basis. The facts do not permit discussion of this thought. They behave in much the same way, except in degree and duration. Four cases with signs and symptoms of lesser degree were observed without operation and recovered in a few months. One was so fulminating that blindness of one eye resulted in two months; and three months after a seemingly complete recovery, with a collapsed decompression, the pressure again suddenly became extreme and vision was abolished in the remaining eye; within another month the pressure again returned to, and has since remained, normal, with partial return of vision in this eye. Despite every search no cause of the original or subsequent increased pressure could be suggested. She was a very placid girl and only thirteen years old (Case 12).

One patient feels that "after reading or talking to people the decompression may get as tight as a drum, and within two minutes it may be perfectly soft." He also thinks that nervousness (he is not of nervous temperament), or getting in or out of a car, will cause a sudden increase in the pressure. He also thinks the decompression is more tense when he is constipated. Another patient who is chronically constipated does not think there is any relationship between the degree of pressure and her constipation, nor is there any appreciable difference.

In only one case is there reason to consider an inflammatory lesion, such as an encephalitic process, as a possible factor in this condition. In Case 5 the cell count (36) and globulin were increased, and a year later the cell count was still 16. It may well be that this case differs from the others, although the end-result is essentially the same. Certainly there have been numerous neurologic complaints in this case, although no objective findings. Indeed the history in the case is not unlike that of multiple sclerosis; but after five years she is again without neurologic symptoms. It is worthy of note also that this patient went a year with her intermittent pressure and without diminution of vision. On the whole, the periods of increased pressure may well have been of short duration.

Nor can it be denied that syphilis is a factor in Case 16, in which the Wassermann reaction from both blood and cerebrospinal fluid was positive. In none of the remaining cases, however, do the examinations of the spinal fluid suggest an underlying inflammatory lesion of any type.

That the increased pressure usually sets its limit within the bounds of relief afforded by a subtemporal decompression is indeed surprising. In one case this was certainly not true, for the vision was lost when the decompression became more tense than any I have ever seen; recovery of vision followed the spontaneous relief of the underlying condition. It is quite certain that vision and probably even life itself were spared by the decompression that had been made.

The significance of papilledema in these and other cases of suspected intracranial pressure should be emphasized. Needless to say there is no difference between the ophthalmoscopic picture in these cases and those due to tumors, for both are due to intracranial pressure. There is another ophthalmoscopic picture, however, where a differential diagnosis is all important, *i.e.*, optic neuritis. Although it is, at times, possible by the ophthalmoscopic studies to differentiate between a mechanical papilledema due to pressure and the local one of optic neuritis, this is usually not true. In fact in a condition so serious, I should rarely feel safe in depending exclusively upon an ophthalmoscopic examination for the differentiation of these two lesions. But the differential diagnosis can be, and always should be, made by directly ascertaining the intracranial pressure.

The diagnosis of this condition is made by the ventriculograms and by measurement of the pressure of the cerebrospinal fluid. It may be reasoned that a tumor is really present and has been overlooked. If ventriculograms are properly made and carefully interpreted, no single brain tumor can fail to escape diagnosis and localization. It is possible for multiple metastatic tumors to exist throughout the brain and not appreciably deform the ventricular system. Moreover, most of the cases in this group have stood the test of time. It is not conceivable that tumors would be disclosed after several years.

Visualization of the lateral cerebral ventricles should be made by injecting air into them (directly not by lumbar puncture). If the ventricular system is normal a tumor can be excluded with absolute certainty. If there then remains any doubt whether the intracranial pressure is increased, a lumbar puncture can then be safely performed and the pressure measured. To inject air in the presence, or suspected presence, of intracranial pressure is far too dangerous to be justifiable. The secondary spinal puncture for pressure readings can be made immediately or a few days later—I usually prefer the latter though the severity of the symptoms may dictate its prompt performance. When the lateral cerebral ventricles are small the indications of increased intracranial pressure from the ventricular puncture may be absent or equivocal; it is for this reason that so many of these cases have had the spinal in addition to the ventricular puncture. Given increased pressure plus papilledema the diagnosis and indications for mechanical treatment are clear. Without increased pressure it is equally evident that the ophthalmoscopic picture is one of optic neuritis and operative treatment is contraindicated.

The periodic nature of the attacks, and also the permanency of cure in four cases known to have remained well without treatment, lead one to suspect that this condition may be a very common one and that only the most severe grades fall into our hands; and that many of the transient, unexplainable headaches may really be instances of this condition, though in lesser degree.

DISCUSSION. DR. WILDER G. PENFIELD (Montreal) : I should like to ask Doctor Dandy if he feels that there may not be an increase in subdural fluid in those cases. Occasionally it does happen secondary to an inflammatory process in the mastoid or one of the sinuses, or secondary to trauma, that there is definite increase of subdural fluid. The subdural fluid has a higher protein content which is unable to pass through into the subarachnoid space because of the presence of that protein. Such fluid escapes at decompression and the pressure is relieved. It is difficult to be sure, in any surgical approach, where fluid comes from.

DR. ALFRED ADSON (Rochester, Minn.) : There is no question but that this group does exist. In addition, I think probably we also have had the experience of examining patients who have come with the symptoms of intracranial pressure and even localizing evidence, and have used ventriculography in connection with exploration, at which time no tumor was found. A biopsy made in conjunction with exploration resulted in the report of inflammatory tissue, and I have had the same patients return several years later seeking medical release in order that they might be accepted for life insurance. It is very evident that these patients did not have brain tumors and that some of these undoubtedly had localized encephalitis. We have encountered a number of cases of retrobulbar neuritis in which there were choked disk and evidence of intracranial pressure. It was our impression that probably we were dealing with some type of leptomeningitis.

DR. WALTER E. DANDY (Baltimore) closing: I can answer Doctor Penfield's suggestion very positively. When a temporal lobe is exposed, one can, of course, see where the fluid is coming from, and it is always from the subarachnoid space. You can clearly see it coming through the arachnoid membrane.

I do not think Doctor Adson's suggestion of encephalitis probably belongs in this group. Certainly the effects of an encephalitis would not exist over as long a period as five, six or seven years. I think that is a different lesion. But neither would it account for the very sudden fluctuations in the size of the decompression for which the only explanation I can offer is that it probably has some relationship to the intracranial vascular bed. How could a decompression rise in two or three minutes and then fall in the same length of time, except from a sudden change in the vascular bed? There could scarcely be a rise and fall in the amount of cerebrospinal fluid so rapidly.

LV

STUDIES ON EXPERIMENTAL HYPOPHYSECTOMY IN DOGS*

III. SOMATIC, MENTAL AND GLANDULAR EFFECTS

Walter E. Dandy, M. D., and Frederick Leet Reichart, M. D.

Our first report (1925) (1) on the total removal of the hypophysis in dogs went to show that the hypophysis was not essential to the maintenance of life.[1] This, our third and greatly delayed publication on this subject, is concerned with the somatic, mental and sexual changes induced by the removal of this gland during the various periods of life. Some of these results have been published in Volume I of *Engelbach's Endocrine Medicine* (2) and in Volume II of the *Memoirs of the University of California* (3). When our studies were begun there were two diametrically opposite conclusions concerning the relationship of the hypophysis to the maintenance of life: (1) Aschner (4) had shown that it was not essential, while (2) Paulesco, Cushing and his coworkers had concluded that animals could not survive its total extirpation.

To Cushing (12) the explanation of Aschner's survivals lay in incomplete extirpations. He was further convinced that a definite train of symptoms marked the few remaining hours or days of life in a totally hypophysectomized dog. These—loss of weight, subnormal temperature, increasing lethargy—he chose to group as a syndrome—cachexia hypophyseopriva. Aschner was never able to understand the differences. It was in the hope of finding the cause of these discordant results that our experiments were undertaken. That the one (Cushing) used an intracranial, the other (Aschner) a transbuccal route did

not then appear to be of any particular importance. To one with a surgical bent a clean temporal route was always superior to one through the roof of the mouth teeming with organisms. However, infections could not be said to have caused any of Aschner's results. Nor could it be claimed that total extirpation of the hypophysis should be any more difficult or uncertain by the buccal approach: on the contrary, the reverse was more probably true. It was not long before we found that the animals did survive total removal of the hypophysis by the intracranial route; it was next learned that the number of survivals was in direct proportion to the ease and rapidity with which the hypophysis could be extirpated, *i.e.*, the avoidance of trauma to the brain during retraction of the temporal lobe to expose the hypophysis. To better attain these ends two operative improvements were developed: (1) the brain was shrunken by injecting hypertonic salt intracranially, and (2) by inverting the head so that the brain gravitated from the bone of the skull and required almost no retraction. Only by the use of these expedients was it possible to carry out the operation successfully on young puppies (three to four weeks old.) When adept, the operator should be able to complete the operation in twenty minutes or less and to require less than two minutes for actual retraction of the temporal lobe. Our results, therefore, were in absolute accord with those of Aschner. The so-called "cachexia hypophyseopriva" syndrome (in animals) proved to be nothing more than the mani-

*Reprinted from the *Bulletin of the Johns Hopkins Hospital*, LXII: 2: 122–155, February, 1938.

festations of approaching death from intracranial pressure, pneumonia or other causes.

In this report are included the ultimate somatic and sexual changes from a series of dogs subjected to partial and total hypophysectomy by this method. To insure, when desired, the elimination of cellular remnants, the infundibular attachment to the base of the brain was cauterized with the red hot bulbous tip of a metal probe. At least it can be said that the removal of the hypophysis and its cellular prolongations along the stalk have been even more complete than was possible by mechanical means used exclusively up to that time.

After reviewing our results, we find nothing to detract from and little to add to the admirable contributions of Aschner. There are few experimental studies that can rank higher in accuracy and thoroughness, and few will better stand the test of time. He antedated the excellent experimental results of Smith (1916) (6) and Allen (1916 (13) in tadpoles, and his findings for the higher animals were essentially the same as those attained in the lower forms.[2]

EXPERIMENTS

Most of the puppies were operated upon when three, four, or at the most, six or eight weeks old. The younger the animal the more profound is the disturbance of development. The operative risks are much greater (by the intracranial route) in very young puppies because the brain is much softer and consequently more easily traumatized. Moreover, there is less intracranial room because the amount of cerebrospinal fluid is relatively less and sufficient traction to expose the hypophysis is impossible without great injury to the brain. By a preliminary injection of hypertonic salt solution, intravenously, the volume of the brain is reduced to such a degree that undue trauma to it is avoided. The procedure of rotating the head nearly 180° is also important in that it permits the brain to fall away and thus reduces the

retraction to a minimum. When cauterization of the infundibular region is employed to destroy all hypophyseal cells, the operator must be careful not to apply it too severely, for too much heat will quickly cause death from cerebral oedema.

Because of the excessive mortality when dogs are kept in the laboratory the puppies were either returned immediately after the operation to the original litter and put on a roof garden in pleasant weather, or kept by interested friends in more ideal surroundings in the city. Puppies from the same litter were always used as controls and were kept with the hypophysectomized puppies as long as possible. Similar feeding conditions were maintained. Most of the puppies were mongrels, but only litter mates and of approximately the same size were selected as controls. They were photographed, weighed and x-rayed at frequent intervals. When one of the hypophysectomized animals died, a control, when possible, was sacrificed in order that accurate comparative gross and microscopic studies could be made of all the organs. The hypothalamus of the hypophysectomized animals was serially sectioned in order to permit search for hypophyseal cells.

The protocols with charts and illustrations that have been selected for this report concern eight puppies with their controls. Each, except two (H[32] and H[33]), on study of serial sections of the base of the brain, was found to have undergone a total hypophysectomy, that is, complete removal of anterior and posterior lobes, but minute bits of pars tuberalis were found attached to the base of the brain in H[16], H[76], H[92] and H[99]. In puppies H[23] and H[33] there were small macroscopic remnants of anterior lobe cells, so that these animals will serve as examples of subtotal hypophysectomy.

The rate of growth was determined by roentgenograms at frequent intervals of the skull, and the right hind limb in particular. The tube was uniformly placed six feet from the animal and by measuring on the roentgenogram the distance from inion to nasion, and the length of the femur and the tibia, a fairly accurate index of the skeletal growth was obtained. From the roentgenograms it was also possible to determine the condition of the epiphyseal lines and their time of closure; the x-rays of the skull showed the time of appearance of second dentition. In the tables, growth is recorded by the length of the skull and by the sum of the lengths of the femur and tibia.

PROCTOCOLS OF EXPERIMENTS

I. TOTAL HYPOPHYSECTOMY. H¹ (TOTAL

HYPOPHYSECTOMY) AND H² (CONTROL). A male, fox terrier puppy (H¹) was totally hypophysectomized June 29, 1924, when exactly three weeks old. The operation was performed under ether anesthesia and before the adoption of intravenous hypertonic salt solution to shrink the brain. The traumatized temporal lobe was partially resected. The puppy's weight at the time of the operation was 1.2 kgs., while the male litter mate control (H²) weighed 1.0 kg.

First series of x-rays of H¹ was taken August 24, 1924 (eight weeks after the hypophysectomy). Measurements of the control are in parentheses.

H¹ and control
2 mos.

Humerus	4.5 (8.2)	Small epiphyses at both ends (larger epihyses in control).
Ulna	4.7 (8.2)	
Radius	4.5 (7.8)	
Femur	4.4 (9.2)	Small epiphyses. (Larger epiphyses in control).
Tibia		
Fibula	4.8 (8.2)	
Pelvis	4.4 (7)	Ischium still divided on each side (United in crontrol).
Metacarpal	1.7 (3.5)	Tiny epiphyses. (Large in control) no union.
Metatarsal	1.5 (3.8)	Only two bones—astragalus and another (all well developed big bones in control).
Skull (Nasion Inion)	6.6 (9)	
Teeth		Baby teeth in operated puppy (second teeth formed in control, but not erupted).
Vertebrae		Thin epiphyseal plates (traces of fissure still present in control).
Tarsals		Only two small tarsal bones in operated puppy (well developed in control).
Carpals		Five tiny carpals in operated puppy (well developed in control).
Penis		No bone in penis of operated puppy (but slight calcification in control). No signs of union of any epiphyses in either operated or control puppy.

Second series of x-rays was taken October 30, 1924 (18 weeks after hypophysectomy). The following measurements were made (control measurements are in parentheses).

Humerus	4.7 + epiphyses = 5.7 (11.00)	
Ulna	5.8 (12.5)	Fairly large epiphyses in hypo-
Radius	5 (11.0)	physectomized animal, but
Femur	5.8 (12.4)	shapeless. (Much larger and
Tibia		well formed in control.)
Fibula	5.4 (11.5)	
Pelvis	Still united (well united).	
Metacarpal	2.0 (4.4)	
Metatarsal	2.2 (5.3)	
Skull (Nasion Inion)	6.6 (12.7)	
Teeth	Second teeth beginning to form (many permanent teeth erupted in control).	
Vertebrae	Epiphyseal lines not visible (closed in control).	

Control..............	All epiphyseal lines are still open in the control puppy. Only lower ends of humerus and tibia are united.
Tarsals and Carpals......	Much more developed than at 5 months; carpals have little shape, tarsals are taking form. (In control all are well developed.)
Penis.................	No bone in penis. (Well developed bone in penis of control.)

Third series of x-rays was taken March 1, 1925, 39 weeks after operation.

Hypophysectomized
puppy H^1 Control H^2

Length of femur...	6.0 cm.	15.1 cm.
Length of tibia.....	6.0 cm.	16.1 cm.

In the hypophysectomized dog the proximal epiphysis of the femur is closed and the distal one is closing. No calcification in bone of penis. Permanent teeth are just erupting.

In control dog all epiphyses (of tibia and femur) are closed. Bone of penis is calcified. Permanent teeth have been present (*cf.* table above at 18 weeks postoperative).

Weights
Hypophysectomized
H^1 Control H^2

Time of operation.....	1.2 kilos	1.0 kilo
18 weeks after operation	1.7 kilos	7.4 kilos
39 weeks after operation	1.8 kilos	7.7 kilos
41 weeks after operation (at death)	1.4 kilos	

The chart (Fig. 1) shows the weights and the lengths of tibia and femur during the life of these animals. The hypophysectomized animal gained 600 grams (mostly fat) during the 39 weeks after operation compared to a gain of 6700 grams in the control. During this period the operated animal showed only 4 cms. increase in the combined length of femur and tibia, while in the control the increase was 23 cms.

The hypophysectomized puppy always retained the long lanugo hair; at least the hair was soft and downy at the skin, but many of the hairs became coarse distally. Curiously enough, the tail soon lost nearly all the hair and until death had the appearance of a rat's tail. This was also noticed in other operated puppies. The skin became a little thicker in the later months.

The testicles could never be seen or palpated, possibly owing to large pads of abdominal fat in the groins. The scrotum never developed.

Eight months after operation (when nearly nine months old) this puppy and the control were placed with a bitch in heat. The hypophysectomized puppy was entirely indifferent; the control behaved normally.

Although playful and fairly active the hypophysectomized animal always tired easily, much more so than a normal puppy of six weeks. It soon took on the general appearance of a senile animal (progeria) in spite of its puppy size. It was always snappy and cranky. Its bark was shrill and high pitched. It ran in a little trot but never jumped about in joyous play like a normal dog. In the later months of life it waddled as though tired and took little interest in anything except eating and resting. It knew its friends, wagging its tail in recognition; it barked in anger when strangers appeared. It died March 26, 1925, of pneumonia, when eleven months old and forty-one weeks after operation. Autopsy showed very small organs, although all were well formed. Their size was roughly that belonging to a puppy of one month. No trace of thymus could be found. The left kidney and ureter were absent.

Unfortunately the weights and photographs of some of the organs have since been lost, but the following weights and measurements after formalin fixation were found: Adrenals, 1.5 gms.; right kidney (no left), 9.9 gms.; testicles, 0.85 gm.; lungs, 18.6 gms.; left femur, 6.35 gms.; left tibia, 5.0 gms.; length of large bowel, 9.0 cms.; of oesophagus, 12 cms.; total length of gastrointestinal tract, 87.0 gms. Serial sections were made of the base of the brain and no hypophyseal cells could be found.

Since permission could not be obtained to sacrifice the control at the time of death of the operated animal, sections of a three weeks' old puppy of approximately the same weight will be used for control. The histological appearance of the testes of the hypophysectomized puppy is that of immaturity. There are no spermatozoa, spermatocytes and only spermatogonia. There appears to be an almost total absence of the interstitial cells. In the adrenal which is smaller than that of a six weeks' puppy no histological abnormalities can be detected. Nor do the histological appearances of the pancreas, liver, heart, kidney or spleen seem abnormal.

The chart (Fig. 1) showing the growth illustrates the profound changes resulting from total hypophysectomy in the early weeks (third week) of canine life.

II. H[16] (TOTAL HYPOPHYSECTOMY) AND H[17] CONTROL. H[16] was a female fox terrier puppy; she was hypophysectomized September 1, 1927, when six weeks old. During the first six months after operation the puppy remained infantile, failed to grow, retain-

ed the puppy face and hair, failed to erupt permanent teeth (which occurred in the litter mate control H[17] between the third and fifth months), and exhibited infantile genitalia. Six months after hypophysectomy (when seven and one-half months old) she showed an increase in weight of 1300 gms., whereas the control had increased 6700 gms. The growth in the length of femur and tibia of H[16] for the same period was 1.5 cms., while in H[17] the increase was 9.0 cms. The increase in the length of the skull in H[16] was 0.7 cm., and in H[17], 3.4 cms.

During the next four months pituitary replacement therapy (reported by Reichert) was given to the operated animal, her weight increased 800 gms., the same amount as in the control. The increase in length of femur and tibia of H[16] during this treatment was 2.4 cms., and in the control (now nearly grown), 0.5 cm., and the resultant growth of skull of H[16] was 0.7

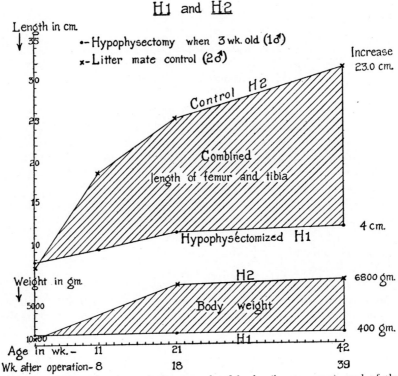

Fig 1. Curves showing relative growth of body (lower curve) and of the hind leg (upper curve) in Hypophysectomized puppy H[1] and its litter-mate Control H[2]

cm., while in H[17] it was 0.2 cm. Besides causing some growth until the epiphyses became closed in the treated dog, the replacement therapy erupted the permanent teeth and changed the hair to a coarser and longer coat. Portions of the thyroid, adrenal and ovary were removed by operation in both H[16] and H[17] at the end of the period of replacement therapy. The histological picture of these organs in H[16] is of interest, although the adrenals were not remarkable. The thyroid showed definite parenchymatous hyperplasia with several layers of cuboidal cells, the ovary (since the puppy was in a state of oestrus throughout the period of treatment) was larger and contained a large cystic corpus luteum, while the uterine endometrium was thicker and showed an excessive increase in number, size and tortuosity of the glands.

Subsequently the hypophysectomized animal lived to be 2⅓ years old. There was no further growth; recession of the swollen genitalia occurred with the ending of replacement therapy. A growth and weight chart of H[16] and H[17] will not be reproduced here, since it is found in Chart VII, page 90 in Volume I of *Engelbach's Endocrinology*. The animal died of pneumonia and the control was sacrificed at the same time. Serial sections were made through the base of the brain; there was no trace of anterior or posterior lobe cells, but there was a small remnant of cells of the pars tuberalis.

The weights of the organs were as follows:

	H[16]	H[17]
Right thyroids ...	0.4 gm .	0.8 gm.
Adrenals	1.3 gms.	4.0 gms.
Pancreas	8.9 gms.	16.5 gms.
Spleen	10.5 gms.	21.6 gms.
Kidneys	29.5 gms.	64.5 gms.
Liver	150.5 gms.	369.0 gms.
Heart	54.0 gms.	73.5 gms.
Length of gastro-intestinal tract..	233 cms.	369 cms.
Sex, ovary and uterus, developed from previous replacement therapy	10.4 gms.	7.0 gms.

The organs, excepting those of sex, were all smaller than in the control, but histologically only the thyroid, ovaries and uterus differed noticeably from the normal. The thyroid was atrophic, showed small acini with flattened epithelium and much less colloid than the control. The breast tissue unfortunately was not saved for histological study.

The ovary, which had been affected for a short period a year and a half before death by replacement therapy, was now atrophied with only a few ova and follicles in the periphery surrounded by dense stroma—the control ovary had many ova and follicles and a fairly large cystic corpus luteum. The uterus was small and markedly fibrosed; there was a sparsity of glandu-

TABLE I

MEASUREMENTS FROM X-RAYS AT VARYING INTERVALS AFTER HYPOPHYSECTOMY.

DATE AND WEEKS AFTER OPERATION	NO. H[30]					NO. H[31] (CONTROL)				
	Weight	Length of skull	Length of femur	Length of tibia	Length of femur and tibia	Weight	Length of skull	Length of femur	Length of tibia	Length of femur and tibia
	kilos.	cm.	cm.	cm.	cm.	kilos.	cm.	cm.	cm.	cm.
Operation, 4/26/28	1.19	8.3	5.3	4.7	9.0	1.98	9.7	6.6	5.5	12.1
5/ 4/28—1 week	1.42					2.5				
5/11/28—2 weeks	1.5	8.6	6.0	5.4	11.4	3.12	10.5	8.1	7.4	15.4
5/18/28—3 weeks	1.55					3.3				
5/24/28—4 weeks	1.5	9.0	6.4	5.8	12.2	3.18	11.0	9.1	8.1	17.2
5/31/28—5 weeks	1.56	Distemper				3.18	Distemper			
6/ 7/28—6 weeks	1.56					3.22				
6/15/28—7 weeks	1.24	9.0	6.6	6.2	12.8	3.12	11.3	10.1	9.3	19.4
Maximum gain since operation	0.37	0.7	1.3	1.5	3.8	1.24	1.6	3.5	3.8	7.2

lar elements.

III. H[30] (TOTAL HYPOPHYSECTOMY) AND H[31] CONTROL. Both were female litter mate puppies; H[30] was totally hypophysectomized April 26, 1928, when four weeks old and died of pneumonia seven weeks later. Although the period of survival was short, this experiment, together with that on H[76] will demonstrate the comparative differences in growth, weights of organs and in the endocrine glands. Weekly measurements of skeletal growth were made from the roentgenograms; the table at the end of this section shows that growth was greatly inhibited two weeks postoperatively and was stopped by the fourth week. The growth of hair in a shaved area was almost twice as fast in the control as in the operated puppy. The weight of the control failed to increase at a normal rate because of the presence of intestinal worms. Histologically, marked differences can be seen in the thyroid and sex organs.

Serial sections through the base of the brain of H[30] showed total absence of cells of the anterior and posterior lobes and the pars tuberalis. Histologically, the thyroid of H[30] showed marked atrophy with diminution in the amount of colloid and in the size of the acini. The epithelium is flattened. The ovary of H[30] showed atrophy, especially in the center, with a scant number of ova and follicles in the periphery in contrast to the sections of the control H[31]. The uterus of H[30] was smaller, with a thinning endometrium and only a few glands. The adrenals, although of smaller size, showed no discernible histological change; the relation of cortex and medulla, as well as the relative thickness of the three cortical zones, appeared to be he same. (See table I).

IV. H[76] (TOTAL HYPOPHYSECTOMY) AND H[77] (CONTROL). These were litter mate female puppies of the collie type. When six weeks old H[76] was totally hypophysectomized and the cautery applied to the base (July 25, 1929). The operated animal was sacrificed because of distemper thirteen weeks after operation, when nineteen weeks old. Here again the profound inhibition of growth is found.

Serial sections of the base of the brain of H[76] revealed no cells of the anterior or posterior lobe, but there was a small cluster of pars tuberalis cells found.

As in H[30], the histological changes that were most marked were found in the thyroid and sex glands. The thyroid of H[76] was quite different from that of the control; it showed marked atrophy of the gland, smaller acini and a sparsity of colloid; the epithelial cells were smaller and flattened. The endometrium of the operated puppy was definitely more fibrotic and less cellular than the control. The pancreas seemed to have about the usual number of normal appearing islets and the adrenal, though smaller, showed the normal differences in thickness of the three zones; possibly there was a suggestion of a thinner cortex in relation to the medulla. No difference could be noted in the histological appearance of the spleen and liver. (See Table II.)

V. H[99] (TOTAL HYPOPHYSECTOMY) AND H[100] (CONTROL). A long-haired breed female puppy (H[99]) was totally hypophysectomized and the cautery applied to the base when six weeks old (June 20, 1930). Eleven and a quarter months after hypophysectomy (May 5, 1931) H[99] was used for another experiment showing the effect of daily injections of prolan and growth hormone in conjunction with Dr. H. M. Evans and his co-workers, and that experiment was reported in Section 12, in Volume II, *Memoirs of the University of California*, 1933 (3).

Forty-five weeks after hypophysectomy H[99] was still infantile, with puppy teeth and hair (the teeth in the control had changed at the age of three and one-half months); the epiphyseal lines were still open, though in the control they had closed at nine months.

Because of the subsequent experiment with the hormones the organ weights and the histological changes may possibly have been influenced by the therapy and are not

TABLE II
WEIGHTS AND MEASUREMENTS OF BONE FROM X-RAYS TAKEN AT INTERVALS OF ABOUT ONE WEEK

DATE AND WEEKS AFTER OPERATION	NO. H[76] (HYPOPHYSECTOMIZED)			NO. H[77] (CONTROL)		
	Weight	Length of skull	Length of femur and tibia	Weight	Length of skull	Length of femur and tibia
	kilos	cm.	cm.	kilos	cm.	cm.
Operated 7/25/29, 6 weeks old	1.8	9.0	12.0	1.68	9.1	11.8
8/ 1/29— 1 week	1.9			2.0		
8/ 8/29— 2 weeks	2.1	9.8	13.5	2.3	10.4	15.4
8/13/29— 3 weeks	2.1			2.8		
8/22/29— 4 weeks	2.3			3.4		
8/29/29— 5 weeks	2.5			4.1		
9/ 6/29— 6 weeks	2.6			4.7		
9/12/29— 7 weeks	2.6			5.4		
9/19/29— 8 weeks	2.7			5.9		
9/26/29— 9 weeks	2.6			6.6		
10/ 4/29—10 weeks	2.6	9.8	15.0	7.1	13.6	24.5
10/10/29—11 weeks	2.5			7.0		
10/17/29—12 weeks	2.5			8.2		
10/24/29—13 weeks	2.3	9.9	15.0	8.2	14.5	26.5
Maximum gain since operation	0.9	0.9	3.0	6.52	5.4	14.7

used in this present report.

The photographs of these litter mate puppies at various intervals of time taken at the standard distance from the camera revealed the cessation of growth following hypophysectomy. The roentgenograms show the failure of skeletal growth. The puppy teeth and the open epiphyses persisted nearly a year after operation. This cessation of growth is expressed graphically in the weight and growth chart.

Serial section of the base of the brain of the operated animal, H[99], showed a total absence of anterior and posterior lobe cells, but there was a small remnant of pars tuberalis cells at the base.

VI. H[92] (TOTAL HYPOPHYSECTOMY.) AND H[93] (CONTROL). A female litter mate collie breed puppy (H[92]) was totally hypophysectomized and the cautery applied to the base when seven weeks old (April 28, 1930). It died of distemper forty-seven and one-half weeks after operation: the baby teeth, baby hair and high-pitched voice were still present; the epiphyseal lines had remained open. The teeth in the litter mate control (H[93]) changed at four and one-half months and the epiphyseal lines were closed at nine and one-half months.

The photographs of the animals taken at the same distance from the camera, showed the marked change with a striking senile appearance in the operated animal similar to that revealed in H[1] and H[99]. She was playful, combative and learned to follow tortuous and intricate passageways almost as quickly as her litter mate. But as she grew older she became deliberate in her gait and tired easily.

The photographs of the roentgenograms of the two animals, taken at the time of the hypophysectomy and ten and one-quarter months after operation, show the retention in the operated animal of the puppy shape of the skull, the first denture and the open epiphyseal lines. The curves of weight and growth (Fig. 2) are similar to those of the others with total hypophysectomy.

Serial sections of the base of the brain in H[92] showed a complete removal of the anterior and posterior lobes; a tiny remnant of pars tuberalis remained.

A study of the sections of the organs showed a small atrophied thyroid, with small acini and flattened cells. No difference could be seen in the parathyroids of the two animals. The ovary of the operated animal was very small, hard and almost entirely fibrotic; a few small ova could be seen in the periphery. The adrenal was small but showed no definite histological differences from the normal; the relative thickness of the three zones was essentially the same as the normal. The ovary contained no ripening follicles or corpora lutea. The breast tissue was small, atrophic and only occasional acini and ducts were visible.

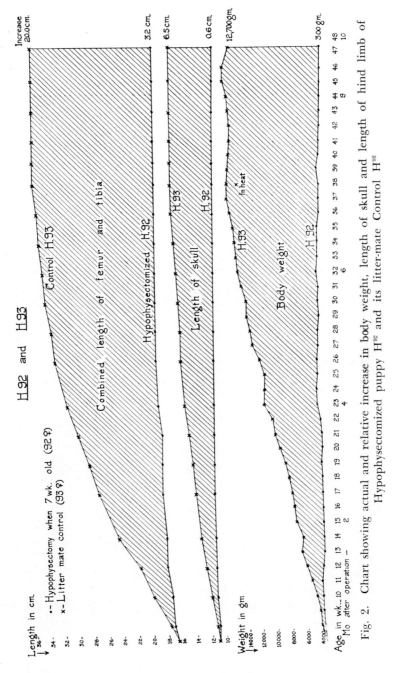

Fig. 2. Chart showing actual and relative increase in body weight, length of skull and length of hind limb of Hypophysectomized puppy H⁹² and its litter-mate Control H⁹³

WEIGHT OF ORGANS	H⁹²	H⁹³
Ovary, right (1.4 x 0.5 x 0.4 cm.)	0.225 gm. (both)	
Control (2.0 x 1.1 x 0.9 cm.)		0.92 gm.
Thyroids (1.7 x 0.6 x 0.4 cm.)	0.225 gm.	2.70 gm.

Adrenals (2)	0.705 gm.	3.6 gm.
Thymus	9.960 gm.	
Pancreas	10.850 gm.	35.4 gm.
Spleen	12.500 gm.	62.0 gm.
Kidneys (2)	43.4 gm	127.5 gm.
Heart	49.8 gm.	158.5 gm.
Lungs (right lower lobe pneumonia)	103.0 gm.	Pneumonia
Liver and gall bladder	220.5 gm.	680.0 gm.
Gastrointestinal tract, weight	360.0 gm.	
Gastrointestinal tract, length	316 cm.	515 cm.
Brain (skull bone brittle)	70.2 gm.	98.5 gm.

VII AND VIII. H³² AND H³³ (SUBTOTAL HYPOPHYSECTOMY) AND H³²ᴬ AND H³³ᴬ (CONTROLS). These were *subtotally* hypophysectomized puppies and had as their litter mate controls H³²ᴬ and H³³ᴬ.

Puppy H³² was a male, bred from an Esquimo bitch, which was hypophysectomized April 26, 1926, when five weeks old. The cautery was not applied to the base of the brain. At the time of the operation H³² weighed 1.8 kilos and the male litter mate control (H³²ᴬ) weighed 1.75 kilos.

Puppy H³³ was a female of the same litter as the H³² puppy; it was hypophysectomized on the same day as H³², when five weeks old. She weighed 1.85 kilos and her female litter mate control (H³³ᴬ) weighed 1.85 kilos. All of the puppies were kept in the country by an interested friend.

The first roentgenograms were taken August 14, 1926, fourteen weeks after operation and showed:

	Hypophysectomized		Controls	
	H³²ᴬ, male		*H³³ᴬ, female*	
Length of femur	8.2 cm.	8.5 cm.	11.6 cm.	10.2 cm.
Length of tibia	8.3 cm.	8.1 cm.	11.2 cm.	10.4 cm.

The second roetgenograms were made October 10, 1927, seventy-six weeks after operation, when the puppies were eighty-one weeks old, and the following measurements were recorded:

	Hypophysectomized		Controls	
	H³²ᴬ, male		*H³³ᴬ, female*	
Length of head	7.0 cm.		10.5 cm.	
Length of femur	9.0 cm.	9.6 cm.	11.2 cm.	
Length of tibia	8.9 cm.	9.7 cm.	10.9 cm.	

Fourteen weeks after operation all the epiphyses were open in the hypophysectomized puppies; in the controls the proximal epiphyses of the femur were closed, and the remaining epiphyses of femur and tibia were open. At the age of eighty-one weeks (seventy-six weeks after operation) all epiphyses of both operated and control animals were united. The permanent den-

ture had erupted in all animals at that time. Penile bone calcification occurred in the control when nineteen weeks old, but not in the operated puppy. It was calcified in the latter nineteen months after operation.

The recorded weights of the animals were as follows:

	Operated		Controls	
	H³²	*H³³*	*H³²ᴬ*	*H³³ᴬ*
At time of operation (5 weeks old) ..	1.8 kilos	1.85 kilos	1.75 kilos	1.85 kilos
19 weeks old (14 weeks p.o.)	2.3 kilos	3.3 kilos	4.0 kilos	2.0 kilos
1½ years old.....................	4.21 kilos	4.3 kilos	5.0 kilos	4.3 kilos
		6.0 kilos		

H[32] died of pneumonia October 27, 1927, when one and one-half years old, and H[33] died of pneumonia, August 22, 1928, when two and one-half years old.

Serial sections of the base of the brain in both operated animals, H[32] and H[33] showed small nubbins of anterior lobe, just visible to the naked eye.

The two operated puppies were very playful and alert, in marked contrast to the exhibition of premature senility exhibited in H[1]. They became house pets and were bright, although they lacked the virility and extreme vivacity of the control puppies. At no time before the last illness had either animal shown any signs of advancing senility and both would probably have lived much longer if intercurrent disease had not caused death. Their stature actually increased considerably, though falling far short of the controls.

Unfortunately it was not possible to obtain the control animals to sacrifice at the time of the death of the operated puppies, but comparative studies by photography and by weights of the organs were therefore, made from (1) a normal six weeks old puppy, (2) a six months old puppy, and (3) an adult dog, all of fox terrier breed. It was felt that these animals essentially served the purpose of controls, since the ultimate size of the animals was almost the same as shown in table III.

Although not weighed, the photographs of the ovaries, thyroids and adrenals of H[33] showed marked atrophy of the ovaries and thyroid when compared with a normal six weeks puppy, but the adrenals were about equal in size to that of a six weeks animal. The ovaries were small, hard and fibrous, but with quite a few immature ova in the periphery. The thyroids showed a marked

atrophy with smaller acini and a diminished amount of colloid. The adrenals showed on definite histological differences from the normal.

HISTOLOGICAL STUDIES

Under the microscope it is not possible to detect any abnormality in the heart, lungs, liver, spleen, pancreas, kidney or thymus. Histological deviations from the normal are found only in certain glands of internal secretion, *i.e.*, the thyroid and sex glands. The adrenals certainly are grossly changed as much as the thyroid but we can detect no histological difference from the normal. No positive change could be seen in the parathyroids.

The ovaries and testes show all signs of immaturity. In the female subtotal hypophysectomies there are graafian follicles in varying degrees of development, but the number of such functioning follicles is tremendously reduced. However, from a microscopic inspection of the ovary alone one could predict that the hypophysectomy had not been total. None of the developing follicles were present in the totally hypophysectomized animals. It was difficult to find any glandular tissue in the breast.

In order to reach a purely objective and unbiased view concerning any possible histological changes in the adrenals and thyroids a test was made as follows: Six unlabeled sections of thyroid— (1) from total hypophysectomy, (2) and (3) from subtotal hypophysectomy, (4) from a normal dog of six weeks, (5) from a normal of six months, (6) from a normal adult dog— were given to Drs. Arnold R. Rich, Henry M. Thomas, Jr., and William F. Rienhoff, Jr. (all specialists on this gland), and each was able to pick out the total and subtotal

TABLE III

ORGANS	HYPOPHYSECTOMIZED		CONTROLS		ADULT
	H[32]	H[33]	At 6 weeks	At 6 months	
Body weight	3.0 kilos	1.5 kilos	1.4 kilos	3.2 kilos	5.7 kilos
Brain	52.5 gms.	49.5 gms.	49.0 gms.	67.5 gms.	63.5 gms.
Spleen	5.0 gms.	4.0 gms.	5.0 gms.	10.2 gms.	17.0 gms.
Liver	86.7 gms.	89.5 gms.	88.5 gms.	206.0 gms.	300.0 gms.
Kidneys (2)	14.8 gms.	16.5 gms.	15.0 gms.	50.5 gms.	46.0 gms.

specimens and in addition could tell which was from the subtotal hypophysectomy. Similarly sections of adrenals— (1) and (2) from total, and (3) subtotal, and (4), (5) and (6) from normals, six weeks, six months and adult respectively—were given to Drs. George A. Harrop and Arnold R. Rich, who have been especially interested in this gland, and neither was able to see any difference between the normal and hypophysectomized specimens.

SUMMARY AND CONCLUSIONS

The longest life span in our series of total hypophysectomies was two years and seven months, another two years and five months. The longest period of survival of any hypophysectomized dog in the literature was three years (Brown). Distemper and pneumonia were the usual causes of death. That they were more susceptible to the contraction and less resistant to the effects of disease than normal dogs is, we think, quite definite.

Dogs without a hypophysis definitely show signs of senility much sooner; indeed they very closely suggest the well known human state of progeria. Although playful, they are much less active and far less rough in their play. They appear to be bright, and they learn and make good household pets. However, their mentality is unquestionably far lower than that of normal dogs.

These hypophysectomized puppies, besides remaining infantile in growth, retain their soft puppy hair, their shrill puppy bark, their first denture, their infantile external sexual apparatus, their playful investigative, combative and destructive puppy attitude. Growth of hair on the shaved head is delayed fully twice as long as on the control.

The almost total cessation of skeletal growth soon after total hypophysectomy is the most astounding of all changes. It appears quite probable that, from some unknown cause, there is a very slight skeletal growth for two to three weeks after the removal of the gland; after this the growth

ceases entirely. This is in contrast to the immediate cessation of growth that has been shown to occur in rats (Smith). The younger the age of the animal at the time of hypophysectomy, the more striking the skeletal deficiency, probably because the relative growth is so much greater in the early weeks of life. Our case 1 (H[1]) is probably the youngest successful hypophysectomy. It exhibits a much more striking "midget" than H[92] which was operated on when seven weeks old, or Aschner's beautiful pioneer result (his figure 85) from the eighth week.

The closure of the epiphyseal lines was delayed to nineteen months in the subtotal hypophysectomized animals H[32] and H[33], whereas in the other animals they remained open for over a year without any evidence of closure; in the controls the epiphyseal lines closed and growth ceased between the seventh and ninth months. When the control had reached adult life the epiphyses of the hypophysectomized dogs could be closed in from two to four months by anterior lobe replacement therapy as reported elsewhere (Reichert). The penile bone never calcified in totally hypophysectomized puppies and calcification was greatly delayed (nineteen months) in the subtotally hypophysectomized puppy H[32]. Penile calcification in the normal dog begins at the fourth to fifth month.

Along with the cessation of skeletal development is a similar cessation of growth, perhaps in some glands an actual recession in size, of all organs of the body. In the table of organ weights of H[30] and H[31], and H[76] and H[77] the brain, lungs and liver show relatively less difference in weight than other organs, probably because in the early weeks of life they already have attained a proportionately larger size; the heart, spleen, kidneys, long bones and length of gastrointestinal tract show a greater disproportion, and the endocrine group of glands, *i.e.*, the thyroids, adrenals, sex glands and pancreas, show the greatest disproportion in weight and size.

REFERENCES

[1]Dandy, W. E., and Reichert, F. L.: Studies on Experimental Hypophysectomy. I. Effect on the Maintenance of Life. *Bull. Johns Hopkins Hosp., 37:* 1, July, 1925.

[2]Engelbach, William: *Endocrine Medicine,* Vol. I, 1932, pp. 67–73, 90–93 and 100. Springfield, Ill., Charles C. Thomas, 1932.

[3]Evans, H. M., Meyer, K., Simpson, M. E., and Reichert, F. L.: The Effect of Combinations of Prolan and Hypophyseal Extract on the Atrophic Genital System of an Hypophysectomized Dog. Section XII of The Growth and Gonad-Stimulating Hormones of the Anterior Hypophysis. Vol. II, *Memoirs of the University of California.* University of California Press, Berkeley, Calif., 1933.

[4]Aschner, B.: Ueber die Funktion der Hypophyse. *Pfluger's Arch., ges. Physiol., 146:* 1, 1912.

[5]Chaikoff, I. L., Reichert, F. L., Larson, P. S., and Mathes, M. E.: The Effect of Hypophysectomy and Cerebral Manipulation in the Dog upon the Response of the Blood Sugar and Inorganic Phosphorus to Insulin. *Amer. J. Physiol., Vol, 112:* 493–503, July, 1935.

[6]Smith, P. E.: Hypophysectomy and a Replacement Therapy in the Rat. *Amer. Journ. Anat.,* Vol. 45, p. 205, March 15, 1930.

[7]Grollman, A., and Firor, W. M.: The Role of the Hypophysis in Experimental Chronic Adrenal Insufficiency. *Am. J. Physiol., 112:* 310–319, June, 1935.

[8]Brown, C. G.: The Effects of Complete Extirpation of the Hypophysis in the Dog. (Preliminary Report.) *Proc. Soc. Exper. Biol. & Med., 20:* 275, 1923.

[9]Reichert, F. L.: The Results of Replacement Therapy in an Hypophysectomized Puppy: Four Months of Treatment with Daily Pituitary Heterotransplants. *Endocrinology, 12:* 451, July–Aug., 1928.

[10]Reichert, F. L., and Dandy, W. E.: Polyuria and Polydipsia (Diabetes Insipidus) and Glycosuria Resulting from Animal Experiments on the Hypophysis and Its Environs. *Bull. Johns Hopkins Hosp., LVIII:* 418–427, June, 1936.

[11]Smith, P. E.: The Disabilities Caused by Hypophysectomy and Their Repairs. *J.A.M.A.,* 1927; Jan. 15, p. 158.

[12]Cushing, H.: *The Pituitary Body and Its Disorders.* Philadelphia, 1912.

[13]Allen, B. M.: The Results of Extirpation of the Anterior Lobe of the Hypophysis and of the Thyroid of Rana Pipiens. *Science, 44:* 755, 1916.

[1]We wish to take this opportunity of correcting our mistake in stating that Houssay had found the hypophysis to be essential to life. He—using the buccal route—had clearly stated that animals survived its total extirpation.

[2]For a more complete review of experimental studies of the hypophysis especially in lower animals, the reader is referred to the splendid publications of Evans (3) , and of Van Dyke, *The Physiology and Pharmacology of the Pituitary Body,* The University of Chicago Press, 1936.

LVI

INTRACRANIAL ANEURYSM OF THE INTERNAL CAROTID ARTERY*

CURED BY OPERATION

CASE REPORT. A rather frail, small, sallow, man, age forty-three, applied at the Johns Hopkins Dispensary February 16, 1937, because of complete paralysis in the distribution of the right oculomotor (third) nerve. The family history was negative. His general health was good until last year when his stomach "went bad" from drinking. He was hospitalized from July to September, 1936, for this gastic disorder which was pronounced "ulcer". He has been a very heavy drinker for the past 18 months.

Present History.—Six days ago he was awakened by a severe pain in the right frontal region. During the afternoon there was a very severe shooting pain in the right eye, but it lasted only a moment. He slept poorly that night because of the pain. On the following morning diplopia was first noted and in the evening the right eyelid drooped. The eye was completely closed the next morning. The pain became less severe but two days later became greatly intensified and prevented his sleeping. Since then the pain has been present but less severe. Examination at that time showed a complete paralysis of the right, third cranial nerve. There were no other positive findings. The eyegrounds, visual fields and reflexes were normal. A diagnosis of aneurysm along the circle of Willis was made. A roentgenologic examination of the head revealed no abnormality. The patient returned to the dispensary from time to time until March 19, 1937—nearly five weeks after the onset of his trouble—when Dr. Frank Ford referred him to me with the thought that a surgical effort might be worth while. There had been no improvement in the local condition in the interim.

The following findings were reported by Dr. Frank Walsh, of the Ophthalmological Department, March 12, 1937:

"The upper lid is completely closed and can only be moved slightly by the frontalis muscle. The globe is abducted to 45° and only moves laterally and slightly down when it rotates inward. The pupil is 4½ Mm. in diameter and one-fourth larger than the left. It reacts slightly to light, directly and consensually. Visual acuity 20/40 right and 20/25 left. Visual fields normal. Fourth and sixth nerves are functioning." The Wassermann reaction was negative.

Operation.—March 23, 1937: A small hypophyseal approach was made on the right side, using the concealed incision. There was marked cortical atrophy, evidenced by the pools of fluid in the subarachnoid spaces (doubtless the result of his heavy drinking). The removal of this fluid and that from the cisterna chiasmatis gave ample room for exposure of the chiasmal region upon retraction of the frontal and temporal lobes. A pea-sized aneurysm projected from the outer wall of the internal carotid artery and adjacent to the entry of the posterior communicating artery. The aneurysm, however, did not involve this vessel, but arose from the internal carotid by a narrow neck beyond which it expanded to the size of a pea; therefore, it was quite a small aneurysm. Laterally it bridged the adjacent cerebral space and firmly attached itself to the free border of the dura which projects mesially from the middle cranial fossa; it spread out beneath the dura forming quite a broad attachment. At this site the covering of the aneurysm changed from the normal grayish-white, shiny covering, similar to that of the carotid artery, to a deep red color. Moreover, the surface was irregular, three or four tiny nodules projecting along the margin of the cavernous sinus. This change represented the false aneurysmal sac resulting from rupture of the aneurys-

*Reprinted from the *Annals of Surgery, 107:* 5, May, 1938.

mal sac. The third nerve passed obliquely backward in its normal course and was attached to the aneurysm at only one point —where it entered the carvernous sinus. Since it was quite evident that the red color of the aneurysmal wall indicated a reduction in its thickness, no attempt was made to dissect the attachment to the wall of the carvernous sinus. There was no evidence of subarachnoid bleeding; doubtless the growth into the wall of the carvernous sinus prevented this. Forceps placed upon the thick aneurysmal wall pulsating forcibly.

The small neck of the aneurysm afforded an easy surgical attack. An ordinary flat silver clip was placed over the neck of the sac and tightly compressed, obliterating it completely. The clip was flush with the wall of the carotid artery. The sac, lateral to the silver clip, was then picked up with the forceps and thrombosed by the electrocautery. It shriveled to a thin shred of tissue. It is worthy of note that the aneurysm became much softer after the silver clip had been applied; it also ceased to pulsate.

Postoperative Course.—Aside from an attack of delirium tremens which lasted three days, patient made an uneventful recovery and left the hospital April 5, 1937— two weeks after the operation. At that time there was a definite improvement in the function of the extra-ocular muscles.

On April 8, 1937, (three days later), Doctor Walsh reports: (1) Improvement in the ptosis; (2) slight upward movement; and (3) the lateral movements of the eyeball are close to normal. The pupillary reaction is still a little less than the left. Seven months later there was complete return of all functions referable to the third nerve.

Perhaps ten years ago I saw, with Dr. Fuller Albright, an aneurysm situated in a somewhat similar position, localized because of the paralysis of the third nerve and pain in the eye. An attempt was made to cure it by ligation of the internal carotid artery in the neck, but the patient died of cerebral softening as a result, probably from an extending thrombus. Such an indirect attack surely had little chance of curing the aneurysm but there then seemed no other rational effort indicated. The present case in a sequel to this unsuccessful attempt. The precise point of origin of this aneurysm could not be predetermined; it might have arisen from the carotid or the posterior communicating artery; the latter was our impression at the time of operation. If it had arisen from the posterior communicating artery it was hoped that a silver clip could be placed upon the artery on each side of the aneurysm if there was not a satisfactory neck by which the aneurysm could be attached directly.

A number of publications have appeared in recent years indicating that aneurysms of the circle of Willis are quite common. It is from them that most of the subarachnoid hemorrhages arise. Unfortunately, in most instances there are no localizing signs by which the position of the aneurysm or, indeed, the size of the aneurysm can be estimated. Those with paralysis of the third nerve, as in our case, are exceptional. Sands[4] makes the statement that 47 per cent of those along the posterior communicating artery produce signs referable to the third nerve. Certainly those with palsies of the third nerve may be given the chance of surgical cure. On the other hand, there is no assurance that the aneurysm after its disclosure may be amenable to surgical attack—the aneurysm may be too large, or it may be placed too far posteriorly on the posterior communicating artery. Under the latter condition perhaps a single clip anterior to the aneurysm might be effective; or the aneurysm, if arising from the carotid, may be less favored by a narrow neck by which it can be isolated and cured by the application of a silver clip. The present effort is but a beginning or a suggestion that an aneurysm at the circle of Willis is not entirely hopeless. A word may be added concerning the cauterization of the aneurysm by which it is shriveled to a small shred. The silver clip, of course, added the same sense of security against an extending thrombus, which, I should think, would be quite likely if the cautery were used alone, but perhaps no more probable than by a spontaneous thrombosis, which may conceivably occur.

At least I should be fearful of such an outcome without the intervening clip to prevent its spread. Should the outlook be hopeless one would, of course, be justified in this attempt, and it is not inconceivable that even then a cure might result from thrombosis of the aneurysm without extension into the main arterial trunk.

In general, the indications for operation on aneurysms at the circle of Willis and causing only subarachnoid hemorrhage, are none too clear. Certainly without a knowledge of the side of the circle of Willis upon which the aneurysm is located there would be no justification in exploring either side in search of the lesion. When a patient has had a subdural hemorrhage and has recovered, one is loath to suggest an operation, which certainly would be classed as hazardous, because another hemorrhage may never occur; at least many go for years with no further trouble, although this is not the usual story. During a subarachnoid hemorrhage and the immediate period thereafter one would not dare operate because the intracranial room needed for operation would be occupied by blood —and one needs all the room obtainable for the operation. For cases with a third nerve palsy the indications are clear enough. And where subarachnoid hemorrhages are recurring and the eventual outlook seems hopeless I should feel inclined to advise operative attack of there is even a suggestion that the aneurysm may be on one side. Arteriography may here become an important means of locating one of these aneurysms around the circle of Willis. Then, too, the frequency of multiple aneurysms, and under such circumstances the difficulty of locating the one that is at fault, make the problem of therapy an even more difficult one.

So far as I know, this is the first attempt to cure an aneurysm at the circle of Willis by direct attack upon the aneurysm.

REFERENCES

[1]Albright, Fuller: The Syndrome Produced by Aneurysm at or Near the Junction of the Internal Carotid Artery and the Circle of Willis. *Bull. Johns Hopkins Hosp., 44:* 215, 1929.

[2]Dandy, Walter E.: Carotid-Cavernous Aneurysm (Pulsating Exophthalmos). *Zentralbl. Neurochir., 2:* 77, 1937. Also *Annals of Surgery, 102:* 916, 1935.

[3]Forbus, on Wiley D.: Ueber den Ursprung Gewisser Aneurysmen der basalen Hirnarterien. *Centralbl. Allg. Pathologie u. Pathologische*

[4]Sands, I. J.: Aneurysms of Cerebral Vessels. *Arch. Anatomie, 44:* 243, 1928–1929.

[5]Symonds, C. P.: Contributions to the Clinical Study of Intracranial Aneurysms. *Guy's Hosp. Rep., 73:* 39, 1923.

LVII

THE OPERATIVE TREATMENT OF COMMU-
NICATING HYDROCEPHALUS*

There can, I think, no longer be any doubt concerning the underlying causes of hydrocephalus, nor can there be any instances where the cause of the hydrocephalus cannot be unequivocally demonstrated. The underlying lesions vary greatly in character, but with those rare exceptions where fluid is overproduced, all cause the same effect: namely, an *obstruction* to some part of the system through which the cerebrospinal fluid circulates. The obstruction prevents the fluid from reaching that part of the system where most of the absorption occurs: namely, the subarachnoid spaces over both cerebral hemispheres. Fundamentally, hydrocephalus is not at all different from hydro-ureter and hydronephrosis, or from the effect upon the biliary tracts of stones and other obstructions, which, too, may be quite variable in character; but the effects of the obstructions are the same.

In hydrocephalus, as in other conditions, the obstructions occur in many different locations. When the obstruction closes all or part of the cisternae at the base of the brain, the hydrocephalus is known as *communicating* because the ventricles communicate freely with the spinal canal. When the obstruction closes any part or all of the ventricular system the type of hydrocephalus is called *noncommunicating* because the ventricular system, or the affected part, does not communicate with the spinal canal. The differentiation between these two major types of hydrocephalus is all important from the standpoint of surgical therapy because two fundamentally different anatomic set-ups exist. When the ventricles do not communicate with the

spinal canal (and the obstruction is in the ventricular system), it may be assumed that the cisternae are open and that it is only necessary to sidetrack the fluid which may then enter the cisternae and thence be passed along to the subarachnoid space for absorption. (This presumption is by no means always correct, for not infrequently more than one congenital obstruction exists.) But when the *cisternae* are blocked there is no way by which fluid can be made to enter the subarachnoid spaces to be absorbed. There are indeed many instances of communicating hydrocephalus in which the crucial part of the cisternae—the cisternae interpeduncularis and chiasmatis from which all the subarachnoid spaces radiate—are beyond the obstruction; but whether, since they have never contained fluid, they are still potentially patent and could receive fluid from an opening in the floor of the third ventricle is difficult to determine. At any rate there is no safe way of separating this group from those in which the entire length of the cisternae or at least the important anterior half (the cisternae interpeduncularis and chiasmatis) is included. This being true, for the present, at least, all cases of communicating hydrocephalus are considered alike. The cure of this type of hydrocephalus cannot (except perhaps in some of the isolated exceptions noted above) be accomplished by sidetracking the fluid to any location where great absorption can occur. This being true, the only hope must be in reducing the amount of cerebrospinal fluid that is formed.

Twenty years ago the writer[1] proposed a procedure by which the large glomus of the choroid plexus was removed from both lateral ventricles. It was hoped that the

*Reprinted from the *Annals of Surgery, 108:* 2, August, 1938.

absorption of fluid that occurs in the spinal and cerebellar subarachnoid spaces might take care of the fluid that formed from the remaining choroid plexuses. I have had several undoubted cures resulting from this procedure. It has been my impression that the cures have been principally, though not entirely, in the older infants, where the size of the head was somewhat fixed and the hydrocephalus was, therefore, progressing at a slower pace. That the rate of growth of the head in hydrocephalics is very variable is well known. It has also been my impression that those with the larger choroid plexuses and those with more histologic evidence of obliterations of the vessels in the choroid plexus did better following the removal of the plexuses. It has also seemed that there is a relationship between the histologic degenerative changes in the choroid plexus—which are often profound—and the rate at which the hydrocephalus grows. In effect, the latter changes are the equivalent of partial removal of the plexus.

The purpose of this communication is to show the effect of further operative removal of the choroid plexus from the brain when removal of the glomus from both sides has been found to be inadequate. Since the brain is so rapidly destroyed by advancing hydrocephalus, it is important that delay be avoided when further surgical efforts are to be instituted. One cannot, therefore, wait very long to determine that the earlier operation has been inadequate. In this connection it should be emphasized that unless hydrocephalics are brought very early for treatment, attempted cures are not worth-while. There is no point in curing or attempting to cure a baby that is certainly going to be subnormal mentally. For the rapidly growing hydrocephalics, three months is the outside limit for surgical intervention; for those that are growing less rapidly, the limit may vary from six months to a year, all depending, of course, on the actual size and rapidity of the growth of the head. But the earlier the treatment the better the results, both in terms of life and of subsequent mentality.

The surgical procedures that are herewith suggested, and which were carried out with apparent success in one patient, are: (1) The cauterization with or without removal of the choroid plexus lying in the posterior cranial fossa: namely, that in the fourth ventricle and along both flocculi; and, (2) cauterization of the plexus in the bodies of both lateral ventricles. These procedures are in addition to the routine removal of the glomus and the plexus in the descending horn of both lateral ventricles.

CASE REPORTS

CASE 1. P. G., female, age one year, was admitted to the Johns Hopkins Hospital April 8, 1936, with the history that four days before birth the mother had been operated upon for appendicitis. Mother and baby remained in the hospital for nearly three months. At the age of five or six weeks the head was definitely oversize and had since continued to grow, though the rate of growth has not been even. At times it would appear to grow very rapidly and again the increase would be much less. At the age of three months she could hold up the head and even despite its great enlargement she was able to sit up. The head was fairly symmetrically enlarged and measured 54 cm. in circumference. The anterior fontanelle was very large, measuring 9x8 cm. The posterior fontanelle was closed. The veins of the scalp stood out prominently. The baby weighed 9,700 Gm.

The phenolsulphonephthalein test showed free communication between the spinal canal, into which the dye was injected, and the ventricular system. The cerebral cortex was perhaps $3/4$ cm. thick.

Operations.—April 11, 1936: *Removal of glomus from the right lateral ventricles.* It was first thoroughly coagulated, then removed.

April 17, 1936: *Coagulation and removal of glomus of left lateral ventricle.*

April 28, 1936: *Coagulation of choroid plexus on under surface of vermis at the foramen of Magendie and the prolongation of the choroid into each lateral recess.* There was quite a mass of plexus at each terminus; this was similarly destroyed with the cautery.

June 30, 1936: Patient returned because of vomiting. The circumference of the head was unchanged but the fontanelle was somewhat tense. Through a small opening in the right side of the anterior fontanelle the ventriculoscope was introduced into the anterior horn of the large right ventricle and *the choroid plexus was quickly cauterized from the foramen of Monro to the scar marking the removal of the glomus.* The septum pellucidum, curiously, was everywhere intact. An opening was cut through this structure by the cautery, and the *plexus of the left lateral ventricle was destroyed with the cautery precisely as on the right side.*

The baby was discharged from the hospital July 19, 1936.

Subsequent Course.—The baby was next seen one year later (July 8, 1937). At that time it was holding up its head, and appeared bright. The mother says it understands much that she says to it.

The circumference of the head was 57 cm. The anterior fontanelle was reduced to 4:5 cm. in the anteroposterior diameter and 7 cm. in the lateral.

The last visit was January 15, 1938, one and one-half years after the operation. The head measured 57 cm. in circumference; the anterior fontanelle 5.5x2 cm. The baby looks bright, sees and is beginning to talk. Both arms and legs are used freely. When lying on her stomach she raises her head and looks from side to side. She plays with her toys all day long; she loves to listen to the radio. She has made no effort to get on her feet.

This series of operative procedures had been carried out in another child, age five months, a year previously; the patient died, however, six weeks following the final operation, too soon to estimate upon the effects of it on the hydrocephalus.

In this connection the results on a third little patient are of interest because pathologic considerations prevented the attempted removal of the choroid plexus from the posterior fossa, and cauterization of that in the bodies of the lateral ventricles has so far been withheld; but the little baby is, at the end of eight months, seemingly well and apparently cured.

CASE 2. R. H., male, age three months, was admitted to the Johns Hopkins Hospital, with the history of having had a difficult birth. The head was thought to have been large at that time; the mother, however, was reported to have had a contracted pelvis. The baby was delivered with instruments. It cried feebly but took its feeding by the breast immediately after birth. It was not until the end of the ninth week that Dr. C. Rosenberg of Newark, N. J., observed the first evidence of hydrocephalus.

Examination.—Except for the enlarged head the baby was well developed, well nourished and looked healthy. The head was markedly enlarged, measuring 50 cm. in circumference; the anterior fontanelle measured 6x6 cm. The veins of the scalp were dilated.

Operations.—June 12, 1937: The glomus of the choroid was removed from both lateral ventricles at one operation. The cauterization was continued down both descending horns and for some distance along the body of the ventricles. The cerebral hemispheres were not more than 1 cm. thick at the site of the ventricular openings. The ventricular fluid was strongly colored with phenolsulphonephthalein that had been introduced into the spinal canal on the preceding day.

June 25, 1937: Assuming that further operative treatment would be necessary, a bilateral cerebellar exploration was made. Cauterization of the plexus in the posterior cranial fossa was intended. However, there was a very dense scar at the foramen of Magendie which was tightly sealed and the cerebellar tonsils projected slightly into the spinal canal. Hoping to reach and remove the choroid plexus within the fourth ventricle, the vermis was split and an opening that would admit the index finder was made into the large fourth ventricle. The incision was carried posteriorly to the medulla in the midline. The choroid plexus could not be seen; it was all incorporated within the scarred mass and was beyond reach. Since the hydrocephalus was clearly of the communicating type, the opening into the fourth ventricle could play no part in the subsequent cure of the hydrocephalus.

Subsequent Course.—This little patient was last seen November 15, 1937—five months after the first operation. It was a very normal looking baby with bright eyes; it was cooing and playful. Its head had increased only 1 cm. since the admission to the hospital—a normal rate of growth. The anterior fontanelle now measured 5x2 cm., a reduction of 1x4 cm.; it was neither tight nor bulging. A letter received February 1, 1938, stated that the baby continued to thrive, was seemingly normal and measurement of the head showed no increase.

Cauterization and Removal of the Glomus.—Preparatory to this and all the other operative precedures upon hydrocephalic children whose sutures have not united, it is necessary to fix the head in a plaster encasement. If this is not done, the head will collapse as the fluid escapes, and collapse of the head is almost necessarily fatal.

I always prefer to attack the choroid plexus through an air medium because it is much more simple; the plexus is so much better seen and so much easier of cauterization and removal. I have tried the various water cystoscopes used by Dr. Hugh Young, and with special improvements for the local situation, but have never been able to get results as satisfactorily as with the air medium. Working in an air medium, one has a far sharper, clearer view, never obscured, as in a water medium, by any little bleeding; moreover, any bleeding points can be promptly controlled either with cotton pledgets or the electrocautery.

The cutaneous incision is straight and vertical (about 2 cm. in length) in the occipital region of each side and about 2½ to 3 cm. from the midline. The bone is ronguered away until its opening is almost exactly the size of the small ventriculoscope. After opening the dura and cauterizing any cortical vessels, the underlying cortex is incised and the ventriculoscope is introduced into the posterior horn of the ventricle. The ventricular fluid is collected, kept warm and replaced at the end of the operation. After much experimentation the Cameron light has been found to be much the most satisfactory. The illumination of the ventricle is almost perfect and without sacrificing room in the tube. In order to prevent the effects of the electrocautery from spreading, an insulated German bakelite tube is used. Prior to the use of this ventriculoscope I used a

headlight of German make and from which parallel rays of light passed down the narrow tube; although very satisfactory, it was not so simple, in that frequent adjustments of the head mirror were necessary to attain the exact angle for passage of light down the ventriculoscope.

In recent years I have usually, but not invariably, removed the glomus of only one ventricle at a time (Case 2 is an exception). It is so easy to remove both at a single operation that it is tempting to do so, but there is no doubt that it carries a higher mortality. Usually an interval of a week between the right and left sides is sufficient. It is worthy of note that when the head is in a plaster encasement, rapid removal of the ventricular fluid has no effect upon the baby's pulse, respirations or color. Such changes are very promptly induced by even a slight loss of blood. The best method of attack upon this mass of dangling choroid plexus—the glomus—has also been determined only after much experimentation. It can be aspirated (only in young babies) into a continuous suction tube very easily and with scarcely any bleeding because the vessels of this age are small and contract promptly. However, it is probably preferable to cauterize the mass by applying a metal probe to its surface until it is greatly shrunken. This mass can then be removed with long slender bladed forceps, or sucked through the tube, or even left in place. Every effort is made to cauterize that portion of the choroid plexus that passes to the tip of the descending horn and also that in the body of the lateral ventricle; from this point of attack one can rarely cauterize the plexus far beyond the bend into the body of the ventricle.

Before withdrawing the ventriculoscope, the ventricular fluid is replaced and any deficit is supplied by Ringer's solution. Since the ventriculoscope is accurately applied to the dural defect and the opening in the cortex, air cannot pass outside the cortex and cause it to collapse. It might be supposed that fluid would subsequently pass through the cortical opening and collect outside the cerebral cortex, causing it to collapse, but this does not happen when the cortical opening is small. In fact, this opening soon heals over and in the course of time can scarcely be found. It is, of course, obvious that these openings are made in a silent part of the cerebral cortex. Conceivably the visual cortex might be injured, but I have not seen this happen.

Removal of the Choroid Plexus in the Posterior Cranial Fossa.—There is quite a volume of choroid plexus in the posterior cranial fossa. Usually the cisterna magna, the foramen of Magendie and the fourth ventricle are all exceedingly large in communicating hydrocephalus. Exposure of the posterior cranial fossa by a small bilateral suboccipital craniotomy brings all of the choroid plexus in this region immediately into view. Even the extension of the choroid plexus laterally into each lateral recess is directly visible because the large cisterna magna extends laterally around the brain stem and lifts the cerebellum upwards as far as the inferior peduncles, under which the choroidal extensions pass to the foramina of Luschka where they form a mass comparable to, but smaller in size than, the glomi of the lateral ventricles. It requires only a few minutes to completely cauterize all of the choroid plexus in the posterior cranial fossa. As the choroid passes along the vagus nerve the cauterization must be cautiously performed to avoid dysphagia. This actually resulted in this little patient but cleared after several days.

There are exceptions to the above topographic relations. At times the foramen of Magendie is closed and the fluid must then escape through the ventricles through the lateral foramina of Luschka. Under these conditions the cisterna magna may be very small and the cerebellum snugly applied to the brain stem, thus completely hiding and making difficult or impossible of exposure the entire mass of choroid plexus in the posterior fossa. In the second case of this report this situation was encountered. The cerebellum was tightly bound to the me-

dulla everywhere and the foramen of Magendie was closed by a dense scar so that neither the lateral extensions of the choroid nor that in the fourth ventricle could be safely reached. I am not prepared to say that many cases of hydrocephalus cannot be cured without including this portion of the choroid plexus in the sum total that is extirpated or necrosed, but the evidence at hand appears to indicate that it is essential in many.

Cauterization of the Choroid Plexus in the Body of Each Lateral Ventricle.—Extirpation of the choroid plexus from the bodies of the lateral ventricle is not possible because the plexus is but slightly elevated. However, it is only necessary to lightly draw the coagulating needle of the electrocautery (or better a probe which is touched by the cautery) along it from the scar at which the glomus has been previously removed posteriorly to the foramen of Monro, to see it shrivel to a white streak. It has seemed better to coagulate this part of the plexus on both sides at a single sitting, first because it is necessary to remove only about two-thirds of the ventricular fluid; second, because the amount of cauterization is less than elsewhere; third, because of the desire to avoid entry through the more important left hemisphere; and finally, because both sides can be reached almost as easily as one. To accomplish this end the same sized Cameron ventriculoscope is passed through the right side of the anterior fontanelle, which is always large. The air medium is also used in the attack upon this part of the plexus. Usually the septum pellucidum is already perforated, or even largely destroyed by the pressure of the hydrocephalic fluid. It is then only necessary to shift the ventriculoscope through the openings to expose the choroid plexus on the left side. But if no perforation exists, as in the above case, one of adequate size can easily be incised with the cautery.

SUMMARY AND CONCLUSIONS

In the treatment of communicating hydrocephalus the removal of the glomus from each lateral ventricle may or may not be sufficient to produce a cure. If not adequate, additional choroid plexus may be removed or destroyed by the cautery: (1) From the posterior cranial fossa (fourth ventricle and lateral recesses); and/or, (2) from the bodies of both lateral ventricles. Only experience and careful study of the effects of each attack can tell when the added removal is necessary. There is so much individual variation in the rate of growth of hydrocephalus that no set rule can indicate beforehand whether additional removal is necessary, and if so, how much. Since most cases do require more than the removal of the glomi, I am inclined to destroy the plexus in the posterior cranial fossa (when this is possible) without waiting to see the effects of removal of the glomi. By so doing the extensive destruction of brain tissue in the unsuccessful cases may be avoided.

The test of success or failure of these operations is, to a very large extent, dependent upon measurements of the head; and by the time it is known that the operation has not been successful extensive destructive of the brain tissue has resulted; which may well mean the difference between a subsequent normal and impaired mentality. Nothing should be left undone to insure, when possible, the minimum of cerebral damage. By the large, the destruction of brain tissue is far more serious than the risk of the added operation.

The final suggested attack, namely, cauterization of the plexus along the bodies of both lateral ventricles, should, I feel, be left until it is definitely demonstrated that both of the other procedures have been inadequate.

Admittedly each of the above operative procedures is one of magnitude and is fraught with danger, but when the hydrocephalus of the communicating type continues to progress, there appears to be no alternative. It seems impossible that this type of hydrocephalus can be cured except by the removal of a sufficient amount of choroid plexus. In the case here reported and the one that died subsequently, it was only the continuation of pressure, as indicated by a tense fontanelle and vomiting, that made the need of the last choroid plexus removal necessary (from the bodies of the lateral ventricle), if this line of attack were going to be successful. Only the choroid plexus in the roof of the third ventricle remains, and even the beginning of this at the foramina of Munro has been included in the cauterization. Even this could be removed very simply by splitting the corpus callosum, but it is difficult to believe that this small remaining amount of plexus could maintain a progressive hydrocephalus of this type.

REFERENCE

[1]Dandy, Walter E.: Extirpation of the Choroid Plexus of the Lateral Ventricles in Communicating Hydrocephalus. *Ann. Surg., 68:* 569, 1918.

LVIII

SUBDURAL HEMATOMA*

DIAGNOSIS AND TREATMENT

Paul A. Kunkel, M.D. and Walter E. Dandy M.D.

In 1925 Cushing and Putnam [1] published reports of 11 cases of subdural hematoma in which the condition apparently arose as the result of trauma to the head. At the same time they summarized the theories regarding the nature of this lesion and discussed its relation to the pachymeningitis haemorrhagica interna described by Virchow.[2] They expressed the opinion that the only pathologic difference between the two is in the microscopic appearance of the membranes of the hematoma, the traumatic form possessing large mesothelial-lined spaces and smaller capillaries. They also concluded that late hemorrhages into the sac are of common occurrence. In 1927 Griswold and Jelsma,[3] in a similar study, concluded that the microscopic appearance of the membranes was the same in both forms. Whatever the relation between the two forms of subdural hematoma, these papers served to emphasize the importance of trauma as a cause, if not the only cause, of the lesion considered in this paper. Such causation is in contradistinction to that of Virchow's pachymeningitis, a condition which occurs in decrepit persons and probably results from systemic causes. Although the microscopic appearance of the membranes is essentially the same with the two types of lesion, the gross lesions are entirely different; with Virchow's pachymeningitis there is solid, thick membrane with little or no blood, and with subdural hematoma these membranes are very thin and the blood is in great volume. As early as 1804, Bell [4] in

his "A System of Surgery" wrote of the importance of incising the dura after trephining the skull, for the possible release of subdural blood, in cases of head injuries in which an extradural hemorrhage is not encountered. (There is no record of a case in which the lesion was cured in this way by Bell.) He further stated that subdural hemorrhages may not give rise to symptoms for several weeks after the injury. The frequency with which cases of traumatic subdural hematoma were reported in surgical papers during the nineteenth century is indicated by the article of Bowen,[5] who in 1905 was able to collect seventy-two cases (presenting both acute and chronic conditions) from the literature. He divided them into two groups. In the first were those in which the hematomas were unassociated with severe cerebral injury, the hemorrhages apparently having arisen from a tear in a pial vein or a vein running to the longitudinal sinus, and in the second group were those in which the hematomas were associated with severe cerebral lacerations or contusions and produced immediate symptoms. He pointed out that in the first group a period of freedom from symptoms after the injury frequently occurred. Henschen [6] in 1912 also reviewed a series of cases in which the condition was of traumatic origin, and Trotter [7] in 1914 called attention to the fact that the causative injury may be trivial. Subsequently, Rand [8] in 1926 demonstrated that the pial vessels were the source of the hemorrhage in several of his cases. The traumatic origin of this lesion is now widely accepted, as is indicated by the recent

*Reprinted from the *Archives of Surgery*, 38: 24–54, January, 1939.

papers of Kaplan,[9] Fleming and Jones,[10] McKenzie,[11] Gardner,[12] Fischer and de Morsier,[13] Keegan,[14] Frazier,[15] Coleman,[18] and Furlow.[17] A full discussion of its occurrence in infants is given in a paper of Sherwood's [18] in 1930, although in none of his cases was there a history of trauma. Peet and Kahn [19] in 1932 pointed out the importance of operative intervention in cases in which the patients are infants and children. Jelsma [20] in 1930 summarized the symptoms and clinical findings in forty-two surgical cases previously reported in the literature and added two cases of his own. It is apparent that subdural hematoma is recognized more frequently than formerly, although the number of surgical cases reported is still rather small.

In the neurosurgical service of the Johns Hopkins Hospital between 1914 and 1935 there have been forty-eight cases of subdural hematoma in which the lesions at operation were found to have the characteristics of the traumatic hematomas described by others.[21] The first case was described by Heuer and Dandy [22] in 1916. That there may have been others in which the condition was unrecognized is likely only before the introduction of ventriculography by one of us (W. E. D.) in 1918. Prior to that time a right subtemporal decompression was frequently performed on patients suspected of having a tumor of the brain but not having localizing signs. The lesions in cases 2, 3 and 4 were apparently discovered during such an operation, and had the hematomas occurred on the left side it is readily seen that they would have escaped recognition. With the aid of ventriculography the diagnosis and localization of such a lesion has been greatly simplified.

AGE. Of the forty-eight patients forty were adults, six were minors and two were infants each nine months of age. The largest number of hematomas (11) occurred in the sixth decade of life, and the smallest number (3) occurred in the first decade. Five occurred in the second decade. That the lesion occurs occasionally in young persons has been recognized before. The average age for the entire group was 41.2 years. Jelsma in his analysis of forty-two cases found an average age of 39.2 years and a fairly similar age distribution.

SEX. There were forty-three male and five female patients, a disproportion encountered in all other case reports and doubtless correctly attributed to the accepted cause, that is, trauma.

COLOR. Forty-four patients were white, and four were Negroes.

SIDE OF OCCURRENCE OF THE HEMATOMA. In thirty cases, or 61.7 per cent, the hematoma was on the left side, and in fifteen, or 32.1 per cent, it was on the right. In two cases, or 4.2 per cent, the lesion was bilateral. We can think of no reason for assuming that the much greater incidence of this lesion on the left side has any anatomic significance. In one case it lay about the sella turcica.

CAUSE. That an injury to the head is generally regarded as the cause of this lesion has already been mentioned. Futhermore, the frequency with which subdural hemorrhages accompany severe injuries to the head has recently been emphasized by Leary [23] and Munro.[24] These authors and Coleman [16] included the "acute" lesions in their analysis of the subject. In this series, however, patients with fresh subdural clots, showing immediate symptoms of severe injury requiring prompt operative intervention, have been excluded because from a clinical standpoint they fall under the classification of patients suffering from the immediate effects of acute injury to the head.

The incidence of trauma in this series was found to be lower than that recorded in most reports; a definite history of injury was obtained either before or after operation in thirty-one cases, or 65.9 per cent. In the other seventeen cases, or 36.1 per cent, no history of even a trivial injury could be elicited despite our constant interest in this phase of the lesion. Futhermore, in the group of patients with a history of injury, the trauma was minor for

TABLE I. SUMMARY REPORT OF FORTY-

Patient and Date of Admission	Age, Sex, Race	Chief Symptoms	Type of Trauma Time Before Admission	Duration of Symptoms	Latent Interval	Headache	Nausea or Vomiting	Drowsiness	Diplopia	Vertigo	Convulsions	Coma	Mental Confusion	Papilledema Retinal Hemorrhages	Involvement of Other Cranial Nerves	Motor and Sensory Changes
1 C. C. 2/28/14	26 M W	Headache; vertigo; failing vision; failing hearing; tinnitus	No history of trauma	14 mo.	0	+	+	0	0	+	0	0	0	Bilateral 5 to 6 D; nearly blind	Hearing impaired both ears	0
2 G. B. 4/22/16	38 M W	Headache	Fall; unconscious; 8 weeks	8 wk.	0	+	+	+	0	0	0	0	0	Bilateral 6 D with hemorrhages	0	0
3 L. D. 10/22/16	55 M W	Headache; drowsiness	Auto accident; not unconscious; 7 weeks	6 wk.	1 wk.	+	+	+	0	+	0	0	0	Bilateral 3 D	0	0
4 T. V. 12/11/16	24 M W	Headache; drowsiness; earache	Fall with unconsciousness; 4 weeks	4 wk.	0	+	0	0	0	0	0	6	0	Bilateral 2 D	0	0
5 B. C. 12/27/16	47 M W	Headache; vomiting	Kicked on head by horse; unconsciousness; 3 years?	2 yr.?	1 yr.?	+	+	0	0	0	0	0	0	Bilateral	0	0
6 J. T. 9/13/20	18 M W	Headache; vomiting	No history of trauma	10 wk.	0	+	+	0	0	+	0	0	0	Bilateral	0	Slight weakness of right side
7 I. H. 12/19/22	26 M W	Headaches; drowsiness	Struck on left side of head boxing; 6 months	6 mo.	0	+	0	+	0	0	0	0	0	0	0	0
8 L. B. 6/19/23	44 M W	Headache; drowsiness; paralysis right side	Struck head on auto fender; 3 weeks	2 wk.	1 wk.	+	0	+	0	+	0	+ 24 hr.	0	Bilateral papilledema	0	Flaccid paralysis right arm and leg
9 D. L. 5/5/34	9 mo. F W	Enlargement of head; convulsions	Birth injury?	5 mo.	0	0	0	+	0	0	+	0	0	0	0	Slight weakness left arm and leg
10 W. S. 2/15/25	64 M W	Headache; mental confusion; drowsiness	Struck by auto; dazed; 8 weeks	8 wk.	0	+	+	+	+	+	0	+	+	0	0	0
11 V. C. 5/27/25	30 M W	Headache; drowsiness	Struck by "knucks"; unconscious; 5 weeks	5 wk.	0	+	+	+	0	0	0	+	0	Bilateral	0	0
12 T. G. 7/7/25	40 M N	Headache; weakness of legs	Struck by auto; unconscious; 9 weeks	3 wk.	6 wk.	+	0	0	0	0	0	0	0	0	0	Marked muscular weakness, unable to walk
13 L. B. 11/13/25	37 M W	Headache; drowsiness	Struck head in fall; 6 months	6 mo.	0	+	+	+	0	+	0	+	+	Bilateral 1 D	0	0
14 L. S. 11/21/25	47 M W	Headache; weakness right side; unable to talk	Struck head in fall; unconscious; 5 weeks	4 wk.	1 wk.	+	0	+	0	0	0	0	0	0	0	Spastic paralysis right arm and leg; unable to talk
15 J. A. 3/30/26	53 M W	Headache; drowsiness	0	8 wk.	0	+	+	+	+	+	0	0	+	Bilateral papilledema	0	Marked muscular weakness, unable to stand or walk
16 J. S. 7/10/26	43 M W	Headache;	0	6 mo.	0	+	+	+	0	0	0	0	0	0	0	0
17 J. H. 8/31/26	32 M W	Drowsiness	Auto accident; unconscious 10 hours; 9 weeks	4 wk.	5 wk.	+	+	+	0	0	0	0	0	Bilateral papilledema	0	Left facial weakness (central)

EIGHT CASES OF SUBDURAL HEMATOMA

Reflex Changes	Temperature, Pulse, Blood Pressure, W.B.C.	Other Positive Findings	Roentgen Findings	Clinical Impression	Trephine Ventriculography	Side of Lesion, Type of Operation and Date	Recurrence After Operation	Result	Comment
Dp reflexes, hyperactive both sides	T 98.6 F. P 60 WBC 6,400	Bulging right subtemporal decompression; operated on elsewhere 4 months previously	Erosion posterior clinoids	Tumor of the brain	0	Right craniotomy Mar. 14, 1914; drains used	0	Discharged well Apr. 9, 1914	Died one year later; cause unknown
Dp reflexes more active left	T 98 F. P 60	0	Normal	Tumor of the brain	0	Right subtemporal decompression; drains used; Apr. 23, 1916	0	Discharged well May 16, 1916	Well in 1937
Dp reflexes more active left; Babinski sign left	T 101.8 F. P 60 BP 130/80 WBC 15,000	0	0	Tumor of the brain	0	Right subtemporal decompression; drains used; Oct. 22, 1916	0	Discharged well Nov. 23, 1916	Died in 1932 of cardiac disease
Dp reflexes hyperactive	T 98.6 F. P 66 BP 100/70	0	Fracture at base	None given	0	Right subtemporal decompression; drains used; Dec. 16, 1916	0	Discharged well Dec. 30, 1916	0
Dp reflexes more active left	BP 145/105 WBC 8,400	0	Normal	Tumor of the brain	0	Right craniotomy; drains; Dec. 27, 1916	0	Discharged well Jan. 11, 1917	History confusing as to when present illness began; well in 1937
Dp reflexes more active left; Babinski sign right	T 98.6 F. P 90	0	0	Tumor of the brain	+	Right craniotomy; drains; Sept. 20, 1920	0	Discharged well Oct. 8, 1920	Homolateral signs; well in 1937
Babinski on left	T 98.6 F. P 60 BP 95/50 WBC 11,200	Head is described as being very large	0	Tumor of the brain	+ Dec. 22, 1922	Left craniotomy; drains; Dec. 26, 1922	+ Subdural clot evacuated Dec. 26, 1922	Discharged well Jan. 13, 1923	Homolateral signs
Dp reflexes more active right; Babinski sign right;	T 103.6 F. P 70 WBC 15,000	0	0	Cerebral tumor	0	Left craniotomy; drains; June 20, 1923	0	Died June 21, 1923	Autopsy showed no recurrence of hematoma; brain edematous
0	T 98.6 F.	Enlargement of head; right side larger than left; separation sutures	Hydrocephalus	Hydrocephalus	+	Right tap subdural space; 80 cc. obtained; May 6, 1924	0	Discharged well June 4, 1924	Well in 1933
Romberg	T 98.6 F. P 58	0	0	Brain abscess or cerebral tumor	Trephine revealed hematoma,	Right subtemporal decompression; drains; Feb. 15, 1925	Right craniotomy Feb. 25, 1925; removal bone flap Feb. 27, 1925	Discharged well Apr. 4, 1925	Subtemporal decompression insufficient for complete evacuation
0	T 99.2 F. P 60	0	0	Subdural hematoma	Trephine revealed hematoma frontal	Left craniotomy May 27, 1925	+ Evacuation extradural hematoma May 29, 1925	Discharged well June 22, 1925	Well in 1937 save for focal epilepsy
Lateral Babinski	T 98.6 F. P 60 BP 170/100	0	Normal	Tumor of the brain	+	Left craniotomy July 30, 1925	0	Discharged well Aug. 7, 1925	
0	T 98.6 F. P 46	0	Normal	Subdural hematoma	+	Left craniotomy, Nov. 13, 1926 120 cc. old blood	0	Discharged well Nov. 26, 1925	Well in 1937
Dp reflexes more active right; Babinski positive on right; stiff neck	T 98.6 F. P 80 WBC 20,000	0	Normal	Brain abscess	Trephine revealed hematoma frontal	Left craniotomy Nov. 25, 1925	Explored Dec. 1, 1925; extra-and subdural clots	Discharged well Feb. 2, 1926	Well in 1937
Lateral Babinski	T 99 F. P 46 BP 105/80 WBC 15,000	0	Normal	Tumor of the brain	+	Left craniotomy Mar. 21, 1926	0	Discharged well Apr. 15, 1926	Patient epileptic before hematoma; no convulsions during present illness; well in 1937
Lateral Babinski	T 98.6 F. P 56 BP 117/70	0	Normal	Tumor of the brain	Trephine disclosed hematoma frontal	Left craniotomy July 12, 1926	Evacuation extra- and subdural hemorrhage July 13, 1926	Discharged well July 26, 1926	Well in 1937
Dp reflexes more active left	T 98.6 F. P 60 BP 106/70	0	0	Subdural hematoma	Trephine disclosed hematoma	Bilateral craniotomy Sept. 15, 1926		Discharged well Oct. 29, 1926	Bilateral hematoma

TABLE I. Summary Report of For[

Patient and Date of Admission	Age, Sex, Race	Chief Symptoms	Type of Trauma Time Before Admission	Duration of Symptoms	Latent Interval	Headache	Nausea or Vomiting	Drowsiness	Diplopia	Vertigo	Convulsions	Coma	Mental Confusion	Papilledema Retinal Hemorrhages	Involvement of Other Cranial Nerves	Motor and Sensory Change
18 W. W. 11/15/26	57 M W	Headache; drowsiness	0	4 mo.	0	+	+	+	+	0	0	+ 12 hr.	0	0	0	0
19 F. W. 12/27/26	20 M W	Headache	Struck on head in football game; 3 months	3 mo.	0	+	+	0	+	0	0	0	0	Bilateral 2 D	0	0
20 J. E. 11/24/27	59 M W	Headache; vomiting	0	4 mo.	0	+	+	0	0	+	0	0	+	0	0	0
21 F. F. 5/18/28	43 M W	Headache; drowsiness	0	6 wk.	0	+	0	+	0	0	0	Periods of coma	0	Bilateral less than 1 D	Left ptosis (iii)	Left facial weakness (central)
22 C. A. 11/28/28	26 M W	Headache; vomiting	Struck on head with bare fists; 8 weeks	5 wk.	3 wk.	+	+	0	0	+	0	0	0	Bilateral 1 D	0	0
23 C. B. 3/15/29	52 M N	Headache; vertigo	0	5 wk.	0	+	0	0	0	+	0	0	0	Bilateral with hemorrhages	0	0
24 J. O. 3/16/29	29 M W	Headache; loss of vision	Auto accident; unconscious; 1 year	1 yr.	0	+	0	+	+	+	0	0	0	Optic atrophy; blind	Anisocoria; right pupil larger than left	0
25 W W. 4/16/29	24 M N	Headache; vomiting	Punched about head in boxing; 6 weeks	6 wk.	0	+	+	0	0	0	0	0	0	Bilateral 1 D	0	0
26 R. G. 9/24/29	18 M W	Headache; diplopia	0	3 wk.	0	+	+	0	+	+	0	0	0	Bilateral 1 D	Right facial (vii); absent corneal, left; motor V left; nystagmus	0
27 F. P. 12/20/29	61 M W	Headache; vomiting	0	4 wk.	0	+	+	+	0	0	0	0	0	0	Nystagmus	0
28 W. M. 6/11/30	70 M W	Weakness and numbness of left extremity	0	6 mo.	0	0	0	+	0	0	0	0	0	0	0	Motor weakness of entire left side
29 L. F. 6/11/30	38 F W	Headache; vomiting; tinnitus	0	6 mo.	0	+	+	0	+	0	+ Right focal	0	0	Bilateral 1 D; hemorrhages	0	Slight weakness right arm
30 M. R. 5/15/31	53 F W	Headache; vomiting; drowsiness	Struck head during paroxysm of sneezing; 3 weeks	2 wk.	1 wk.	+	+	+	+	0	0	0	0	0	Bilateral ptosis; inability to look up; sluggish pupils (iii)	0
31 H. P. 6/15/31	53 M W	Headache	Struck by auto; unconscious; 4 months	4 mo.	0	+	0	+	0	0	0	0	0	0	0	Hypesthesia left extremities; pa[ ] entire left side
32 S. H. 7/18/31	19 M W	Headache; staggering	0	8 mo.	0	+	+	0	0	+	0	0	+	Bilateral 2 D	0	General muscular weakness
33 J. W. 1/23/32	67 M N	Headache; drowsiness	Struck head in fall; unconscious; 5 weeks	5 wk.	0	+	0	+	0	0	0	0	0	0	0	General muscular weakness
34 E. H. 6/28/32	51 M W	Headache; fainting spells	Struck head in fall; unconscious; 3 months	3 mo.	0	+	0	0	+	+	Focal right extremity	0	0	Bilateral 3 D; hemorrhages	Nystagmus; right pupil larger than left	0

GHT CASES OF SUBDURAL HEMATOMA *(Continued)*

Reflex Changes	Temperature, Pulse, Blood Pressure, W.B.C.	Other Positive Findings	Roentgen Findings	Clinical Impression	Trephine Ventriculography	Side of Lesion Type of Operation and Date	Recurrence After Operation	Result	Comment
p reflexes e active left; teral inski sign	T 99.8 F. P 52 BP 120/75 WBC 9,000	Arteriosclerosis of peripheral vessels	Normal	Tumor of the brain	+	Right craniotomy Nov. 16, 1926	Nov. 18 evacuation extradural hemorrhage; Nov. 19 decompression	Discharged well Jan. 11, 1927	Small; removed intact with membrane
0	T 99 F. P 60 BP 110/60 WBC 5,400	0	0	Tumor of the brain	+	Left craniotomy Dec. 28, 1926	0	Discharged well Jan. 11, 1927	Well in 1937
0	T 98.6 F. P 58 BP 105/70 WBC 16,000	Arteriosclerosis of peripheral vessels	0	Tumor of the brain	+	Right craniotomy Nov. 26, 1927	Evacuation extra- and subdural hemorrhage Nov. 29, 1927; same Dec. 2,1927	Discharged well Dec. 14, 1927	Well in 1937
o reflexes e active left	T 98.6 F. P 60 BP 180/120	Arteriosclerosis of peripheral vessels	Normal	Tumor of the brain	Trephine disclosed hematoma	Left craniotomy May 21, 1928	0	Discharged well June 14, 1928	
0	T 98.6 F. P 62 BP 100/60 WBC 8,400	0	Normal	Tumor of the brain	+	Right craniotomy Nov. 30, 1928	Evacuation extra- and subdural hemorrhage Dec. 2, 1928	Discharged well Dec. 22, 1928	
0	T 98.6 F. P 60 BP 115/70 WBC 5,300	0	Normal	Tumor of the brain	+	Left craniotomy Mar. 19, 1928	Evacuation extra- and subdural hemorrhage Mar. 21, 1929	Discharged well Apr. 1, 1929	Well in 1937
0	T 98.6 F. P 74 BP 90/60	0	0	Pituitary tumor	+ Cisternal air injection	Left craniotomy Mar. 24, 1929 (hematoma about sella)	0	Discharged improved Apr. 10, 1929	
0	T 98.2 F. P 58 BP 115/70 WBC 7,300	0	0	Subdural hematoma	Trephine disclosed hemorrhage, occipital	Left subtemporal decompression Apr. 19, 1929	0	Discharged well May 15, 1929	
0	T 99 F. P 100 BP 120/80 WBC 6,800	0	Normal	Tumor of the brain	+	Left craniotomy Sept. 25, 1929	0	Discharged well Oct. 7, 1929	5,000,000 R.B.C. bloody cerebrospinal fluid; hydroma associated with hematoma;
0	T 97 F. P 66 BP 190/100	0	Normal	Tumor of the brain	+	Left craniotomy Dec. 20, 1929	Evacuation extra- and subdural hemorrhage Dec. 21, 1929; also twice more with removal bone flap	Discharged well Jan. 24, 1930	Died in 1935 angina pectoris
o reflexes e active eft; inski posi- on left	T 98.6 F. P 60 BP 140/100 WBC 7,300	Arteriosclerosis of peripheral vessels	0	Cerebral hemorrhage	+	Right craniotomy June 14, 1930	Exploration; evacuation bloody fluid June 17	Died June 25, 1930; staphylococcus wound infection; meningitis	Autopsy; no abnormality noted save meningitis and membrane of hematoma; no recurrence
o reflexes e active ight	T 98.6 F. P 90 BP 100/65 WBC 7,400	0	Normal	Tumor of the brain	+	Left craniotomy June 1930	0	Discharged well June 28, 1930	
o reflexes eractive; eral inski	T 99 F. P 60 BP 140/90	0	Normal	Tumor of the brain	+	Left craniotomy May 16, 1931	Evacuation extra- and subdural hemorrhage May 17; same and removal bone flap May 19	Discharged well June 4, 1930	Bleeding and clotting time normal; well in 1937
o reflexes e active eft side; eral nski	T 99 F. P 60 BP 98/62 WBC 7,900	Tenderness right frontal region	0	Subdural hematoma	0	Right craniotomy June 15, 1931	0	Discharged well June 30, 1931	Well in 1937
0	T 99.6 F. P 62 BP 90/50 WBC 8,000	0	Normal	Tumor of the brain	+	Right craniotomy July 21, 1931	0	Discharged well Aug. 4, 1931	Well in 1937
o reflexes eractive; eral inski	T 100 F. P 60 WBC 10,400	Arteriosclerosis of peripheral vessels	Normal	Cerebral hemorrhage	+	Left craniotomy Jan. 26, 1932	0	Discharged well Feb. 2, 1932	Died 3½ years later of intestinal obstruction; no autopsy on head
0	T 99.6 F. P 80 WBC 6,000	0	0	Subdural hematoma	0	Left craniotomy June 29, 1932	0	Discharged well July 6, 1932	Well in 1937

TABLE I. SUMMARY REPORT OF FOR

Patient and Date of Admission	Age, Sex, Race	Chief Symptoms	Type of Trauma Time Before Admission	Duration of Symptoms	Latent Interval	Headache	Nausea or Vomiting	Drowsiness	Diplopia	Vertigo	Convulsions	Coma	Mental Confusion	Papilledema Retinal Hemorrhages	Involvement of Other Cranial Nerves	Motor and Sensory Change
35 J. D. 7/25/32	65 M W	Headache; unconscious spells	Fall from a horse; unconscious; 3 months	3 mo.	0	+	+	+	0	+	+	0	+	0	0	0
36 J. H. 8/13/32	59 M W	Unconsciousness	Struck head in fall; unconscious; 1 week	1 wk.	0	0	+	0	+	0	0	+12 hr.	0	0	0	Deep reflexes bilaterally hyperactive
37 P. F. 5/1/33	36 M W	Headache; drowsiness; tinnitus	In auto accident; unconscious; 6 weeks	6 wk.	0	0	+	+	+	0	0	0	0	Bilateral 2 D; hemorrhages	Absent corneal reflex left (v)	Hpyesthesia all extremities; loss of sense of position of toes bilateral
38 J. P. 5/2/34	67 M W	Headache; drowsiness; mental confusion	0	5 mo.	0	+	0	+	0	0	0	0	+	0	0	Slight weakness of left side
39 E. B. 5/12/34	53 F W	Headache	Struck head on bureau; 2 months	5 wk.	3 wk.	+	0	0	0	0	0	0	0	0	0	General muscular weakness; unable to stand
40 R. B. 6/23/34	62 M W	Headache; drowsiness; mental confusion	0	2 mo.	0	+	0	+	0	0	0	0	+	0	0	General muscular weakness; unable to stand
41 E. A. 9/15/34	64 F W	Headache; drowsiness	Struck head on wall; 3 weeks	2 wk.	1 wk.	+	+	+	0	0	0	+24 hr.	0	0	0	0
42 C. W. 10/31/34	47 M W	Headache; vomiting	In auto accident; unconscious; 3 months	5 mo.	0	+	+	+	+	0	0	0	0	0	Right vi nerve palsy	General weakness; unable to stand
43 R. C. 11/20/34	8 M W	Headache; vomiting; photophobia	In auto accident; left eye discolored; 3 months	11 days	7 wk.	+	+	+	0	0	0	0	0	Bilateral loss 1 D; hemorrhages	0	0
44 A. H. 11/28/34	9 mo. M N	Drowsiness; convulsions	Fall from bed; 1 week	3 days	4 days	0	0	+	0	0	+	+24 hr.	0	Bilateral with hemorrhages	0	Right facial weakness (central type)
45 H. K. 2/9/36	17 M W	Headache; drowsiness	0	1 wk.	0	+	+	+	+	0	0	0	0	Bilateral 4 D with hemorrhages	0	General muscular weakness; unable to stand
46 W. R. 3/3/36	55 M W	Headache; drowsiness	Fall on sidewalk; 6 weeks	6 wk.	2 days	+	+	+	+	0	0	0	+	0	Pupils sluggish	0
47 R. W. 9/5/36	38 M W	Headache, left and general; blurred vision; vertigo	Struck on head with brick; unconscious; 4 weeks	4 wk.	0	+	+	+	0	+	+	0	0	Bilateral 7-8 D	0	0
48 H. R. 7/9/37	59 M W	Headache; convulsion	Fall 8 weeks before admission; not unconscious	3½ wk.	2½ wk.	0	0	0	0	0	0	0	0	0	0	0

GHT CASES OF SUBDURAL HEMATOMA

Reflex Changes	Tempera-ture, Pulse, Blood Pressure, W.B.C.	Other Positive Findings	Roentgen Findings	Clinical Impres-sion	Trephine Ventricu-lography	Side of Lesion Type of Operation and Date	Recurrence After Operation	Result	Comment
binski on ht	T 99.2 F. P 50 BP 90/50	Arterio-sclerosis of peripheral and retinal vessels	Normal	Cerebral arterio-sclerosis	+	Left craniot-omy Aug. 2, 1932	0	Discharged well Aug. 14, 1932	Well in 1937
binski on right; le clonus right	T 100.6 F. P 80 BP 150/80	Arterio-sclerosis of peripheral vessels	0	Subdural hematoma	Trephine disclosed hema-toma	Left craniot-omy Aug. 13, 1932 (men-branes very thin)	0	Discharged well Aug. 23, 1932	Alcoholic; died in 1933 of stricture of esophagus
ep reflexes eractive aterally; vical dity	T 99 F. P 54 BP 130/90 WBC 8,000	0	Normal	Subdural hematoma	Puncture	Left craniot-omy; right subtemporal decompression; May 6, 1933	0	Discharged well May 23, 1933	Bilateral hematoma; well in 1937 save for slight degree of optic atrophy
ep reflexes eractive; ateral binski	T 99 F. P 54 BP 130/90 WBC 7,900	Arterio-sclerosis of peripheral and retinal vessels	Normal	Tumor of the brain	Trephine disclosed hema-toma occipital	Left craniot-omy May 3, 1934	Evacua-tion extra- and sub-dural hem-orrhage; decompres-sion May 4, 1934	Discharged well May 21, 1934	Well in 1937
ep reflexes eractive aterally; ateral Ba-ski sign	T 99 F. P 58 BP 130/80 WBC 6,600	0	Normal	Tumor of the brain	+	Left craniot-omy May 15, 1934	Evacua-tion extra- and sub-dural hem-orrhage; decompres-sion May 16, 1934	Discharged well June 3, 1934	Well in 1937
ep reflexes eractive	T 98.6 F P 56 BP 140/90 WBC 6,600	Arterio-sclerosis of peripheral vessels	Normal	Tumor of the brain	+	Left craniot-omy June 25, 1934	Evacua-tion extra- and sub-dural hem-orrhage; decompres-sion July 3, 1934	Discharged well July 9, 1934	Well in 1937
binski on t	Not re-corded	Arterio-sclerosis of peripheral vessels	0	Tumor of the brain	+	Left craniot-omy Sept. 15, 1934	Evacua-tion extra- and sub-dural hem-orrhage; decompres-sion; Sept. 16, 1934	Discharged well Sept. 28, 1934	
p reflexes re active left	T 99 F. P 66 BP 140/90 WBC 10,400	0	Normal	Tumor of the brain	+	Right crani-otomy Nov. 2, 1934	0	Discharged well Nov. 12, 1934	History of some headache preceding auto accident by 2 months; well in 1937
0	T 299 F. P 72 BP 90/60 WBC 8,800	Tenderness to pressure left side of skull; cervical rigidity	0	Tumor of the brain	+	Left craniot-omy Nov. 21, 1934	0	Discharged well Nov. 28, 1934	175 cc. fluid blood; few clots; hgb. 103%; RBC 4,100,000; WBC 6,100; NPN 28 mg.; NaCl 552 mg.; sugar 40 mg.; total pro-tein 5.6; albu-min-globulin ratio 65/35; well in 1937
ateral binski	T 101 F. WBC 12,000	0	0	Subdural hematoma	Puncture of sub-dural space	Left craniot-omy decom-pression; Nov. 30, 1934	0	Discharged well Jan. 3, 1935	Died in fire 2 months later
0	T 100 F. P 48 BP 120/80 WBC 14,500	0	Normal	Tumor of the brain	+	Left craniot-omy Feb. 11, 1935	0	Discharged well Feb. 20, 1935	Well in 1937
ep reflexes re active right; teral Ba-ski sign	T 98.6 F. P 60 BP 170/100	Arterio-sclerosis	Normal	Subdural hematoma	+	Left craniot-omy Mar. 4, 1936; 12 hours later decom-pression	0	Discharged well Mar. 13, 1936	Small hema-toma, 40 cc. blood laked; sugar 25 mg; NPN 38 mg.
0	T 98.6 F. P 70-90 BP 120/80	0	0	Subdural hematoma	+	Left craniot-omy Sept. 8, 1936	0	Discharged well Sept. 16, 1936	Small hema-toma, 40 cc. blood laked; NPN 28 mg. per 100 cc.
0	T 98.6 F. P 90 BP 150/100 WBC 8,000	0	Normal	Subdural hematoma	+	Left craniot-omy July 9, 1937	0	Discharged well July 21, 1937	Small hema-toma, 40 cc. or less; no RBC in fluid

TABLE II
Age Incident in Decades

Age, Years	Number of Cases	Percentage
0-10	3	6.3
10-20	5	10.6
20-30	6	12.7
30-40	7	15
40-50	7	15
50-60	12	23.4
60-70	8	17

Average age, 41.2 years

exactly half of this number and might be considered major, in that consciousness was lost at the time, for the other half. Almost every type of accident has been described as giving rise to this lesion, particularly blows on the front and back of the head (Gardner [25]). It is of interest that eleven patients were injured in falls, ten in automobile accidents and four in boxing; three accidentally bumped their heads on stationary objects, one was struck by a brick, one was kicked by a horse and one was injured playing football. In only two instances was it doubtful that the trauma recorded could have been the cause of the hematoma. One patient (the patient in case 5) was injured three years before admission and at least one year before symptoms arose. In contrast, the patient in case 42 had a history of headaches and diplopia two months before he was rendered unconscious by an automobile accident. Among the seventeen patients without a history of trauma, other possible predisposing factors, such as arteriosclerosis or alcoholism, were not of frequent occurrence. Only two patients had a history of alcoholism; both also had injuries. Of the eleven patients with clinical arteriosclerosis, seven had injuries and four did not. It has been assumed by others that in such cases trauma has invariably occurred, although it may have been trivial and therefore forgotten by the patient. Whether or not this assumption is justified is open to question, but it would seem to be upheld by the fact that the clinical and operative findings in such cases are identical with those in cases in which there is a definite history of trauma.

Duration of Present Illness. The present illness was of comparatively short duration in all but two cases. The patient in case 1 had been ill for fourteen months and was practically blind on admission. He also had been operated on elsewhere, a right subtemporal decompression having been done four months before. The patient in case 5 had a history of sick headaches for years, which were stated to have been worse for two years before admission; the time at which his other symptoms arose is not recorded. None of the other patients had symptoms of more than a year's duration. The shortest illness among the adults and minors was one week (case 36) and among the infants three days (case 44). The other infant, the child in case 9, was ill for five months. The average duration of the present illness for the entire group was thirteen weeks.

Latent Interval. Of the 30 cases in which there was a history of trauma, a latent interval was present in only fourteen, or 43.3 per cent, the patients in the remaining sixteen cases dating their symptoms from the time of the accident. In case 5 this period was a year (further evidence that the recorded injury was not the cause of the hematoma in this case), while in case 44 it was but four days. If these two extremes are excluded, the average length of this period was only three weeks.

Symptoms. As noted by others, for the majority of patients with subdural hematomas the principal symptoms are those of intracranial pressure. Of the 46 adults and minors, 45, or 93.6 per cent, complained of headache, the patient in case 28 being the only exception. In but five cases was headache more pronounced on the side on which the hematoma occurred, while in three the opposite side was more affected. Headache, therefore, is of no value as a sign of localization. The next most common complaint was drowsiness, occurring in thirty-one patients, or 66 per cent. Nearly the same number, twenty-nine, or 61.7 per cent, had diplopia, and ten, or 21.2 Vertigo, apparently arising with changes in position, was recorded for sixteen, or 34 per cent. Only thirteen patients, or 27.6 per cent, had diplopia, and ten, or 21.2 per cent, had periods of mental confusion. Weakness of one side of the body was a principal symptom for only three patients, or 6.3 per cent, and the same number complained of tinnitus. Convulsions occurred in 7, or 12.7 per cent. Both infants, the patients in cases 9 and 44, had generalized convulsions. Of the five adults, the patients in cases 29 and 34 had focal seizures and those in cases 35 and 47 and 48 had generalized convulsions. The patient in case 15 was epileptic but had no attacks during the present illness. Visual failure was complained of in two instances. The patient in case 1 was nearly blind with a high grade of papilledema. This was the only patient with a history of progressive deafness. The patient in case 24 was totally blind. The case of this patient was the most unusual in the series and has previously been reported by one of us (W. E. D.[26]). The visual failure and associated atrophy of the optic nerve were due to direct pressure on the optic chiasm by a hematoma surrounding the sella turcica (Fig. 1). In summary, a history of symptoms possessing localizing value was obtained in but five cases, or 10.6 per cent (cases 8, 14, 28, 29 and 34).

OBJECTIVE FINDINGS. For most of the patients the clinical findings were indicative of intracranial pressure only. Papilledema was present in twenty-five, or 53.2 per cent, and absent in twenty-one, or 44.7 per cent. Associated retinal hemorrhages occurred in seven, or 14.8 per cent. The degree of papilledema varied from less than one diopter to six diopters, with little difference on the two sides. No significant abnormalities of the visual fields were recorded. In no instance was there hemianopia. The patient in case 24, who has been mentioned, was the only patient with atrophy of the optic nerve. Central facial weakness was present in eight cases (17 per cent), being an isolated finding in four. Three patients (6.3 per cent) had nystagmus, and

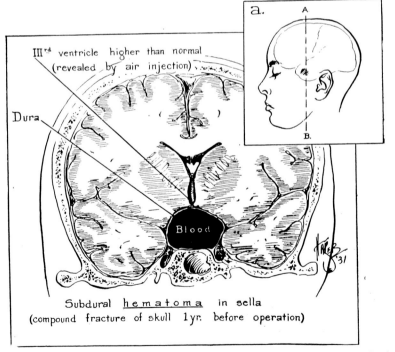

Fig. 1 Post-traumatic subdural hematoma about the pituitary body in case 29. This patient had signs of a hypophysial tumor, including destruction of the sella turcica.

two (4.4 per cent) had ptosis. The patient in case 30 had bilateral ptosis, sluggish pupils and inability to look upward, while the patient in case 21 had unilateral ptosis corresponding to the side on which the hematoma was present. Anisocoria was noted in a single case (33), the larger pupil being on the same side as the hematoma. The corneal reflex was absent in two cases (4.4 per cent). In case 25 it corresponded to the side on which the hematoma occurred, whereas in case 37 it was also unilateral although the hematoma was bilateral. Cases 1 and 24 were the only instances of marked reduction in vision, the patient in case 24 being blind. Of the remaining cranial nerves, none except the sixth was recorded as abnormal.

General muscular weakness was a rather frequent observation, eight patients, or 17 per cent, being unable to stand unassisted. Weakness of the extremities on one side also occurred in 8 cases, being marked in only two, cases 8 and 14. Interestingly, this hemiparesis occurred on the same side as the hematoma in two cases (cases 6 and 38). Case 31 was the only instance of hemihypesthesia. Astereognosis was not noted in a single case.

The reflexes were more frequently disturbed. The deep reflexes were bilaterally hyperactive in 9 cases, or 19.2 per cent, and unilaterally more active in 14 cases, or 30 per cent. In case 21 this hyperactivity occurred on the same side as the hematoma, while in case 17, with unilateral activity, there were bilateral hematomas. The Babinski sign was recorded in 20 cases, 44.6 per cent; it was bilaterally present in 12 cases, or 27.6 per cent, and unilaterally present in 8 cases, or 17 per cent. In cases 6 and 7 the Babinski sign occurred only on the side on which the hematoma was present. It is significant that Fleming and Jones,[10] Frazier[15] and Kaplan[9] have noted the presence of homolateral neurologic findings, the last-named author having observed them in 5 of 8 cases. Another reflex which occurs occasionally in the presence of a tumor of the brain, namely, cervical

rigidity, was observed in 3 cases (6.4 per cent).

The frequency with which a history of drowsiness was obtained has already been recorded, but it is worthy of note that eight patients, or 17 per cent, were in coma at the time of admission and required immediate operation. Although mental confusion was recorded for 10 patients, and although a majority of the hematomas were on the left side, the patient in case 14 was the only one showing motor aphasia.

In summary, then, if one considers the reflex changes having value in the localization of the cerebral lesion and the presence of motor weakness, sensory loss and aphasia, one finds that twenty-five patients, or 53.2 per cent, were without positive findings, nineteen patients, or 40.3 per cent, possessed them in part, and three patients, or 6.7 per cent, showed neurologic findings referable to the uninvolved hemisphere.

TABLE III
Symptoms in Order of Occurrence

Symptom	Number of Cases	Percentage
Headache	44	93.6
Drowsiness	31	66
Nausea and vomiting	29	61.7
Vertigo	16	34
Diplopia	13	27.6
Mental confusion	10	21.2
Convulsions	7	12.7
Weakness on 1 side of body	3	6.3
Tinnitus	3	6.3
Failing vision	2	4.2
Failing hearing	1	2.1
Numbness of 1 side of body	1	2.1

Elevation of temperature above 101 F. occurred in but two instances (cases 3 and 8). On the other hand, in seven cases, or 15.5 per cent, there were leukocyte counts of more than 12,000; in cases 3, 9, 15 and 20 there was leukocytosis, the leukocyte count ranging between 15,000 and 20,000. Such a high leukocyte count is fairly common in association with subdural hydroma. Of greater significance was the pulse rate before operation. Twenty-six patients, or 55.3 per cent, had bradycardia, the pulse rate being 60 or below; nine, or 19.1 per cent, had a pulse rate between 60 and 70; and only eight, or 17 per cent, had a pulse rate above 70. In four cases, or 8.8 per cent, the rate was not recorded prior to operation. The only other positive physical findings of note were also in the cardiovascular system. Arteriosclerosis of the peripheral or retinal vessels was noted in ten cases (21.2 per cent), and ten patients had a blood pressure of 140 systolic and 90 diastolic (or higher). It is interesting that the patient in case 9, an infant, had an enlarged head and separation of the sutures suggesting hydrocephalus. The other infant (case 43) had a head of normal size with bulging fontanels and was in coma. Both had generalized convulsions.

Most of the laboratory studies gave negative results. The Wassermann reaction of the blood was negative in every case. Lumbar punctures were done on the two infants, one of whom (case 9) had normal fluid and the other (case 43) xanthochromic fluid, apparently the most common abnormality occurring in association with this lesion. Only in case 4 did the roentgenograms show a fracture of the skull.

CLINICAL DIAGNOSIS. From what has been recorded concerning the histories of this group of patients it is not surprising that a presumptive diagnosis of subdural hematoma was made in only twelve cases, or 23.3 per cent. Twenty-nine patients, or 61.7 per cent, were thought to have a tumor of the brain; two patients, or 4.2 per cent, were thought to have abscesses of the brain, and for a similar number the condition was diagnosed as cerebral hemorrhage. The condition of one patient (2.1 per cent) was diagnosed as hydrocephalus and that of 1 as arteriosclerosis of the brain. Because of the presence of blindness and atrophy of the optic nerve the patient in case 24 was believed before operation to have a tumor of the pituitary gland. Clinical differentiation between the manifestations of subdural hematoma and those of tumor of the brain is especially difficult because of the common tendency of patients to attribute their symptoms to injuries.

TABLE IV
NEUROLOGIC FINDINGS

	Number of Cases	Percentage
Papilledema	25	53.2
Retinal hemorrhages	7	14.8
Atrophy of the optic nerve	1	2.2
Facial weakness (central)	8	17.0
Nystagmus	3	6.6
Ptosis	2	4.4
Anisocoria	1	2.2
Absence of corneal reflex	2	4.4
General weakness	8	17.0
Hemiparesis	8	17.0
Hemihypesthesia	1	2.2
Hyperactive deep reflexes (bilateral)	9	19.2
Unilaterally hyperactive deep reflexes	14	30.0
Bilateral Babinski sign	12	27.6
Unilateral Babinski sign	8	17.0
Cervical rigidity	3	6.4
Coma	8	17.0
Aphasia	1	2.2

VENTRICULOGRAPHY

Since an unlocalized tumor of the brain is suspected in a high percentage of cases of subdural hematoma, the localization of the lesion is ultimately dependent on ventriculographic examination or its equivalent, direct puncture of the hematoma. A subdural hematoma cannot escape detection by ventriculographic study and not infrequently the exact character of the lesion can be determined from the ventriculograms alone.

In our series of cases only the ventricular injection of air has been used. This is certain and safe, and the results are absolute. Unless there are undoubted signs of localization (and in few of these cases was this true a surgeon will no longer take chances in finding the lesion through an operative exposure of the brain. Subdural hematomas are therefore (with only rare exceptions) localized by ventriculographic study. The spinal route for injection of air has not been used because it entails unnecessary danger and the results are capricious. In approximately one third of all spinal injections the air injected into the spinal canal will not reach the ventricular system, because the foramen of Magendie is not patent and air cannot pass through the foramens of Luschka. It is interesting in this connection that Van Dyke[27] has localized a hematoma by the subarachnoid picture of the air and regards the findings as pathognomonic.

When there is a history of recent trauma and the diagnosis of subdural hematoma is a probability or even a possibility, the openings for the ventricular puncture are regularly made anteriorly, i.e., over the anterior horns of the lateral ventricle instead of at the usual posterior site. In addition, the bony opening, instead of being made solely by a perforator, is enlarged by a burr in order that the color of the dura may be better seen and the dura may be carefully inspected as it is opened in search of a hematoma. If the dura is punctured blindly through a conical perforator opening in the bone, one may easily mistake the blood of a punctured superficial cerebral vein for that of a subdural hematoma; with a perforator opening enlarged by means of a burr, this mistake is not possible, for with such an opening one can actually see the outer membrane lining the inner surface of the dura, and if a hematoma does not exist the cortex will present. The reason for making the bony openings anteriorly is that the hematoma will usually be encountered at that point, for with occasional exceptions it extends to the midline. Frequently the hematoma ends slightly anterior to the usual site of the posterior openings, and it would be missed if the puncture were made in the occiput. There are cases in which the anterior opening also just misses a subdural hematoma. The mesial border of this lesion may be irregular, reaching the falx only in part of its course, and in one of its outward bends the dural puncture may just miss the hematoma. The only advantage in reaching a hematoma directly is the avoidance of an injection of air. If a hematoma is not encountered the wounds are closed, and ventriculographic examination is completed in the usual fashion.

Another advantage of the anterior openings is that the occasional bilateral hematoma may be disclosed without the necessity of ventriculographic study. Moreover, in such cases it is highly probable that both lateral ventricles will be nearly or entirely obliterated by the space-occupying lesions, so that ventricular puncture is difficult or even impossible. In both of our cases in which the condition was bilateral the double lesions were disclosed solely by anterior puncture.

In twenty-seven cases, or 57.7 per cent of the series, ventriculographic studies were made prior to operation. In seven others, or 15.5 per cent, preparations were made

TABLE V. SUMMARY OF FINDINGS IN VENTRICULOGRAMS FROM CASES OF SUBDURAL HEMATOMA

Do Both Ventricles Contain Air?	Is There Contralateral Hydrocephalus	Anteroposterior View		Contralateral Ventricle Compressed	Lateral View	
		Sharp Upper Cut in Ventricle	Concavity of Outer Border		Homolateral Ventricle Reduced in Size	Filling Noted in Contralateral Ventricle
+	+ Small rounded	+	+	Slight	Entire ventricle but more in anterior horn and body	None
+	+ Slight	+ Slight	+ Slight	No	Anterior half reduced; posterior absent	+
Only contralateral	+ Slight	Not filled	Not filled	+	Ventricle obliterated	None
Only contralateral	+ Big	Not filled	Not filled	..	Ventricle obliterated	+
+	No	+	+	No	Only shred of posterior half; anterior reduced	None
+	No	+	+	No	Only slight remains	+
Only contralateral	+ Posteriorly; small anteriorly from compression	Not filled	Not filled	+	Ventricle obliterated	None

for ventriculographic examination but the hematoma was encountered when the dura was punctured enroute to the ventricle. Of the total number of cases, therefore, ventriculographic examination or its equivalent was required in 75 per cent. These figures, however, do not portray the actual facts in this regard, for five of the cases were observed before the introduction of ventriculography in 1918. Since this time the occasion is rare indeed when ventriculographic study or its equivalent is not deemed necessary. Since 1918 these tests have been used in 64.3 per cent of cases. In 18 air was present in the third ventricle and in both lateral ventricles. In nine cases the lateral ventricle on the side on which the hematoma was present did not contain air. In every case air reached the third ventricle, which was markedly oblique.

VENTRICULOGRAPHIC FINDINGS

For several years it has been evident that the ventriculographic plates will frequently disclose a change in the ventricular system that is pathognomonic. From the ventriculograms alone, therefore, one can frequently make the diagnosis of subdural hematoma even though the history may have offered no suggestion of this lesion. To know that the intracranial lesion is a subdural hematoma and not a tumor is of the greatest importance to the operator and the patient, for the extent of the cranioplastic procedure is reduced by half and the position of the bone flap is changed.

In general it may be said that the changes demonstrable by ventriculography in cases of subdural hematoma closely resemble those in cases of dural endothelioma, which are almost but not quite pathognomonic. A dural tumor is recognized by the sharp, straight line that represents the border of the growth in the deformed ventricle. This is particularly evident in the anteroposterior view, which shows the lateral ventricle in cross section. A subdural hematoma produces a precisely similar ventricular change, i.e., a sharp, straight ventricular defect which is always on the superior surface of the affected ventricle (in cross section); and, in addition, it usually but not invariably induces a concave indentation on the outer surface of the lateral ventricle (in cross section). That both the superior and the outer surface of the ventricle are affected is due to the extensive distribution of the hematoma; i.e., it is both superior and lateral to the ventricle. Such a bilateral effect on the ventricle is occasionally seen with a large dural tumor, but this is infrequent. The third important ventriculographic change is seen in the lateral view. Since the hematoma usually extends from the frontal to the occipital pole, the lateral ventricle is correspondingly compressed so that the resultant ventriculographic picture shows a lateral ventricle greatly reduced in size throughout most of its horizontal extent, i.e., from the anterior horn through the body to and not infrequently including the posterior and descending horns. This again is a picture that is occasionally but uncommonly reproduced by a cerebral tumor. We have occasionally seen the aforementioned ventriculographic deformations caused by cerebral tumors surrounded by extensive cerebral edema; the findings are therefore not absolute.

The ventriculographic changes in both lateral and anteroposterior views taken in our last nine cases are shown in the accompanying sketch (Fig. 2). The pneumographic shadows have been traced from the roentgen plates. All of our earlier ventriculograms were destroyed when the inflammable roentgen plates were superseded by the modern ones that do not burn.

Ventricular changes on the side on which the lesion was present were as follows:

1. Anteroposterior view.

(*a*.) In all instances there was dislocation of the ventricular system to the contralateral side.

(*b*.) With one exception (G) the anterior horn in cross section was smaller on the side on which the lesion is present. In this instance it was about twice as large on the affected side. Why this exception occurred

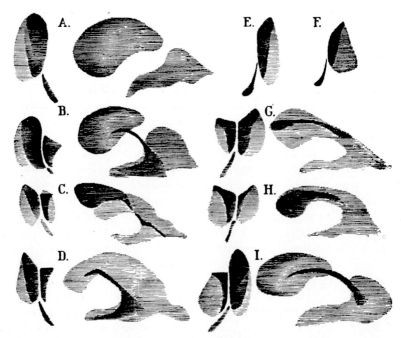

Fig 2.　Shadows traced from ventriculograms taken in 9 cases of subdural hematoma. See text for explanation.

we do not know. In the remaining cases the ventricle on the side on which the lesion was present varied in size from slightly smaller than the other to complete absence in three cases (*C, F,* and *I*).

(*c*) The telltale sharp upper border was present in four and absent in two of the affected ventricles that filled.

(*d*) The equally telltale concave lateral border was also present in four and absent in two of the affected ventricles that filled. The absence of these nearly pathognomonic changes in the ventricles is doubtless due to the lesser volume of the hematoma over the frontal region in these cases.

(*e*) The all-important obliquity of the ventricle was well defined in every instance.

(*f*) In two plates the shadow of the third ventricle was strikingly club shaped (and in two others the change was present but less pronounced), rounded inferiorly and gradually flattening to an acute angle superiorly. This effect was due to the varying degree of pressure from the hematoma in the upper (greater) and the lower (lesser) end of the ventricle. It is hardly probable that this deformation has any relation to subdural hematoma.

2. Lateral view.

(*a*) Without exception the lateral ventricle in all cases was tremendously reduced in size throughout its longitudinal extent. The reduction in the ventricular volume may be greater in front, greater behind or essentially equal throughout. The character and extent of the reduction may be seen in Fig. 2. In three cases (33.3 per cent) the ventricle was entirely collapsed on the affected side.

Ventricular changes on the contralateral side were as follows:

1. Hydrocephalus of varying degree was present in six of the nine cases. It was advanced in three cases, slight in three and absent in three. The cause of hydrocephalus was compression of the aqueduct of Sylvius. The lesser degree of hydrocephalus was diagnosed from the anteroposterior view when the corners of the ventricle were rounded; this is always the earliest objective evidence of ventricular dilatation. The moderate degree of hydrocephalus leads us

to believe that in these cases occlusion of the aqueduct was partial and was of the ball valve type.

2. A partial filling defect about the middle of the contralateral ventricle was present in two cases (lateral view). This was due to the fact that the maximum volume of the hematoma compressed the opposite ventricle in this region. The greater obliquity of the third ventricle is also evidence of the great compression effect in this transverse plane.

3. Flattening of the anterior horn was definite in two cases (Figs. 2C and 2I) and probably present in slight degree in a third (Fig. 2A, anteroposterior view).

PATHOLOGIC PICTURE

The stricking pathologic findings in cases of subdural hematoma are:

1. A large collection of dark fluid is present, with a few soft brownish yellow clots dangling from the outer membrane but sometimes extending across and attached to both membranes.

2. The fluid blood when left standing in a test tube will never clot, even when normal blood is added to it; i.e., the clotting element has been completely eliminated.

3. The blood is hermetically sealed in membranes that cannot extend; the hematoma is therefore not progressive.

4. The outer membrane is always thick (1 to 4 mm.); it is snugly attached to the dura but can be stripped from it; it is opaque and fairly vascular. Its vascularity is derived from the dura, from which new vascular channels connect with newly formed blood spaces in the membrane.

5. The inner membrane is thin, transparent and avascular. It lies loosely on the pia-arachnoid, but there is no attachment except at the margins of the hematoma, where the inner and the outer membrane are confluent; in this region there may be a firm line of attachment to the brain.

In this series the volume of the hematoma was estimated to have varied from 1.3 ounces (40 cc.) to 8 ounces (240 cc.). In case 9,80 cc. of old blood was aspirated; in case 43, 175 cc. of fluid blood was removed from the sac, and in addition there were several fair-sized clots; in cases 46 and 47 the contents of the sac were entirely fluid and measured but 40 cc. Except for the lesions in cases 16 and 24, the hematomas were described as lying on the frontal and parietal lobes and frequently on the occipital lobe; they extended from the longitudinal sinus to the region of the sylvian vein. In one instance the hematoma was exclusively in the temporal region; it was directly over the site of a blow, and beneath it the brain was excavated from absorption of the contused area. In another case the hematoma was in the sella turcica, causing the sellar contents to bulge and act like a tumor. In one case (case 26), associated with the hematoma but separate from it was a subdural hydroma (Fig. 3). In no instance have we been able to determine the source of the blood. In case 16 it seemed probable that a large thrombosed vein crossing from the atrophic defect in the temporal lobe to the dura may have been the source of the original bleeding, but there is, of course, no proof.

The condition of the blood within the membranes is of interest. That such blood no longer has power to clot is doubtless due to the extraction of the clotting substance in the formation of the outer membrane. That there remain a few small and seemingly degenerative clots within the hematoma indicates that there has originally been clot formation; it would be difficult to believe that the blood had not quickly clotted in the beginning. But why should the new tissue representing the outer membrane develop exclusively along the dura and not form throughout the volume of blood, as in Virchow's pachymeningitis interna? And why, too, should it never form on the arachnoid membrane? The fact that the dura is vascular unquestionably accounts for the growth of vascular channels within the outer membrane, but hardly for its thickness, which is fairly uniform, or for its intrinsic character. That the inner membrane is not caused by any

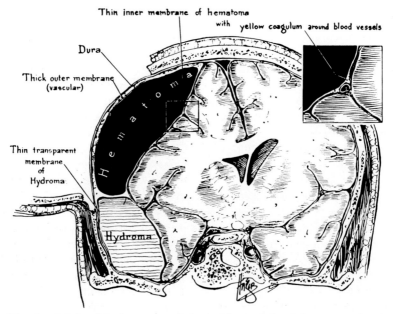

Fig. 3. Subdural hydroma coexisting with a subdural hematoma in case 26. Both resulted from the same injury.

derivative of the blood is shown by the fact that precisely the same membrane forms in cases of subdural hydroma, in which, of course, no blood is present. One can therefore only conclude that the membrane is a product of reaction of the pia-arachnoid. It is also worthy of interest that exactly the same thin, transparent membrane is present on the dural side of a subdural hydroma, although as time advances it becomes somewhat thicker and more opaque than the inner membrane, and it too adheres tightly to the dura.

Can a subdural hematoma disappear spontaneously? This hardly seems possible, because the limiting membranes can scarcely absorb blood. Although vascularized, the inner surface of the outer membrane is smooth and glistening from pressure alone. We have never seen, either at operation or at necropsy, a hematoma as late as a year after its origin (except one solid clot, in case 18). This fact, together with our clinical experience, leads us to doubt that survival is possible after this time. Most of the patients that come for operation appear at a time when an ac-

count of advanced intracranial pressure the tenure of life is unquestionably short. These statements naturally lead us to doubt, and even to deny, that Virchow's pachymeningitis is the same lesion as the subdural hematoma, even though the end result of Virchow's lesion as seen at necropsy might well lead one to assume that a large hematoma has become absorbed and replaced by fibrous tissue.

One of the most surprising findings in cases of subdural hematoma is the gross and microscopic appearance of the blood. The blood when viewed in bulk is black, but venous blood is also dark, and when the specimen is small and unless specimens of the blood from the different sources are side by side it may be difficult to tell from inspection alone that the blood is unquestionably that of a hematoma. Even when a small amount of blood from a subdural hematoma is placed on a white towel at operation and its color compared with the color of venous and arterial blood from the scalp and the dura it may be difficult to be certain that the blood from the hematoma is actually different. Usually, however, the hematomatous blood when spread on a white background is rusty brown, in contrast to the red of fresh blood. The difficulty in being absolutely certain led us to inspect the dura and the outer membranes directly through a burr opening rather than through the smaller perforator opening used for a ventricular or cerebral puncture. On one occasion a specimen of blood had been obtained through a smaller bony opening through which the dura could not be inspected. The appearance of the specimen and its color on the towel were such that a competent physician insisted that the blood was from a punctured vein; and even when the specimen was examined under a microscope most of the corpuscles were found to be well rounded or only slightly crenated—and this after being free for a period of several weeks in the cranial chamber!

Other amazing features of subdural hematoma are that it is nearly always located in the same region and that the brain almost never shows any signs of injury. Only in case 16 was the brain injured; this case presented also one of the two exceptions to the usual location, the lesion being in the temporal region. In this instance the brain was lacerated and excavated, and bridging vascular trunks crossed the defect. Except for these features the resultant hematoma was precisely similar to the remaining ones in the series. Since the hematoma almost invariably begins at the midline of the cranial chamber and spreads outward, since the outer membrane is thickest along the midline, since there are no torn veins over the surface of the brain and since the large cerebral veins are most exposed where they "jump" across from the cerebral hemisphere to the longitudinal sinus, the only conceivable explanation for a hematoma is rupture of one of these crossing veins. The bleeding would almost necessarily be into a potential cavity, and this does exist along the falx. Venous bleeding elsewhere would, with rare exceptions, be quickly stopped spontaneously by the apposition of tissues. Moreover,

arterial bleeding could scarcely be responsible, for the only arteries in this region are in the substance of the brain, and the brain is practically always uninjured. Then, too, spontaneous cessation of arterial bleeding just short of severe intracranial pressure at the time would be far less probable as a consistent outcome. It might happen occasionally, but not repeatedly. One other exception to the almost uniform picture of this lesion should be noted. In one case (case 18) the hematoma was entirely solid and could be shelled out like a tumor and there were no membranes. In case 43 the hematoma was in large part solid.

Why this difference exists we do not know. Whether subdural hematoma uncomplicated by other factors ever causes death at once is not certain. Certainly in a high percentage of cases the danger has been little at the time and symptoms have developed a few weeks or months later. It is the progressive nature of the symptoms that has led to the widespread belief that the hematoma itself is progressive. This is, of course, precluded by the rigid and unchanging walls of the hematoma. What, then, causes the progressive symptoms and eventually death? That intracranial pressure is the cause cannot be questioned, because its relief brings immediate preservation of life. It is hardly believeable that the volume of fluid blood in the hermetically sealed capsule which precludes absorption can become greater. Nor is it conceivable that new hemorrhages can occur within the rigid walls, because there are no exposed vessels that can bleed. The answer we believe to be in the reaction of the brain to the hematoma as a foreign body. We know that tremendous areas of cerebral edema surround tumors of the brain and that this occurs in variable degrees with different tumors. We also know that patients with tumors of the brain and other lesions causing intracranial pressure may be physically entirely well one minute and unconscious or dead the next from sudden strain or from a cough or even with no recognizable predisposing cause. The sudden change is due to increased cerebral edema and not to hemorrhage into the tumor. Precisely the same factors, we believe, are responsible for the gradual progression of subdural hematoma and the eventual death of the patient, i.e., the reaction in the brain from a lesion that already occupies a volume so great that the margin of security at any time is slight.

In only three cases was any study made of the cellular and chemical constituents of the blood. In case 26 a red blood cell count showed 5,000,000 cells per cubic centimeter. In case 43 the hemoglobin percentage (Sahli) was 103, the red blood cell count 4,100,000 per cubic centimeter and the white blood cell count 6,100 per cubic centimeter. A smear stained by the method of Wright showed the cells to be normal in appearance but with an apparent absence of platelets. Chemical analysis showed a nonprotein nitrogen content of 28 mg. per hundred cubic centimeters, a sodium chloride content of 552 mg. and a sugar content of 40 mg. The total protein content was 5.6 mg. per hundred cubic centimeters, and the albumin-globulin ratio, 65:35. The hematomas that occurred in cases 46, 47 and 48, which were relatively small, measuring approximately 40 cc. each in contrast to the hematoma in case 42 measuring 175 cc., contained blood which was entirely laked, as no red blood cells could be demonstrated in preparations. The nonprotein nitrogen content was 38 mg., and the sugar content, 25 mg., per hundred cubic centimeters. From this evidence alone the theory of gradual enlargement of the hematoma from repeated hemorrhages from the membranes, first proposed by Virchow,[2] and the more recent theory of Gardner,[12] McKenzie [11] and Zollinger,[28] that the hematoma enlarges by the acquisition of fluid from the subarachnoid spaces by osmosis, are both seen to be impossible. What is more probable is that, whereas the patient's symptoms are progressive, the hematoma is actually regressive after the initial period of hemorrhage. The absence

of severe symptoms accompanying the original hemorrhage is probably due to the fact that it is venous and not arterial in origin. Furthermore, microscopic sections from the inner and outer membranes of the sac in all cases in which operation was done [6] showed them to be composed of granulation tissue containing numerous capillaries, especially in the outer membrane. Both membranes were infiltrated with leukocytes, particularly the outer membrane. There were also occasional interstitial hemorrhages. In no case was there evidence of any mesothelial-lined spaces as described by Cushing and Putnam.[1]

TREATMENT

Obviously the only treatment is surgical. Although repeated aspirations of a subdural hematoma have been advocated, our experience with 1 hematoma so treated was the least satisfactory of the series; the patient recovered completely but required repeated tappings for three months. A decompression had been made, and its fulness indicated the need for the repeated relief of pressure. Our plan of attack in recent years has consistently been to turn down a very small bone flap (Fig. 4), excise with the electrocautery the outer membrane flush with the dural incision and strip the thin, avascular and unattached inner membrane as far as possible from the surface of the brain. We irrigate the hematoma from the cranial chamber by flushing with Ringer's solution. Not infrequently one or more isolated pockets of blood exist in the subdural space. Careful inspection of this space will disclose them bulging into the large primary cavity. They are punctured, evacuated and irrigated; it has not been necessary to remove any of their covering membranes.

Whether or not removal of the inner and outer membranes is necessary cannot be stated. Since only a fraction of the entire surface area is removed and cures are unequivocal and prompt, we have gradually lessened the size of the cranial exposure and have seen no difference in the immediate or ultimate results. It is largely for this reason that the preoperative defferential diagnosis of a subdural hematoma is important. If a hematoma is still questioned after ventriculographic studies have been made, a burr opening in the line of the proposed cranial approach is inspected before the incision is made. If a hematoma is discovered in incising the dura an osteoplastic flap of approximately half the size of that necessary for a tumor will answer every purpose and correspondingly reduce the severity of the operation.

In this series the chief postoperative complication was hemorrhage, subdural or extradural or both; this occurred in sixteen cases, or 34.2 per cent. In fifteen of these an osteoplastic flap had been employed, and it was necessary in two instances to evacuate the hematoma a second time. It is interesting that on this second exposure the blood was always clotted. In case 10, in which operation was done by the subtemporal route, evacuation of the hematoma through a superimposed craniotomy opening was required. Also, the patient in case 46, with a very small hematoma, showed signs of intracranial pressure in twelve hours, owing to cerebral edema alone; he was rescued by a decompression.

The principal source of subdural postoperative bleeding is the raw edge of the outer membrane of the sac, which is fairly vascular. Bleeding from this source can now be prevented by incising the membrane by the cutting current of the electrocautery. Because of the great vascularity of the outer membrane it is important that it be not stripped from the dura beyond the dural defect, where oozing would be

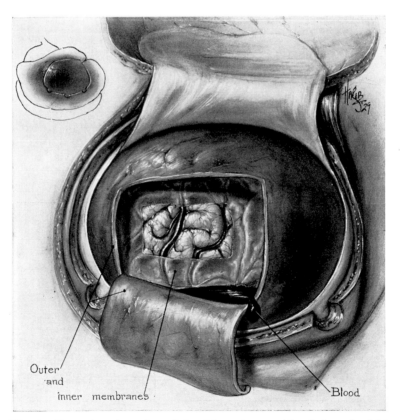

Fig. 4. Operative view of a subdural hematoma, with windows in thicker outer membrane and thinner inner membrane. The intact brain lies beneath. Blood fills the space between the membranes. The hematoma usually covers most of the outer surface of the cerebral hemisphere.

out of reach. Extradural bleeding is the source of greater concern than is bleeding beneath the dura. With meticulous care this can now be avoided; at least the incidence will be very low if the dura is completely incised parallel to and near the bony margins, the dura drawn tightly to the skull by several sutures and the bone largely stripped of its blood supply. Failure of the affected hemisphere to expand after operation in the absence of hemorrhage occurred in one case; it was overcome by placing the patient in the head-down position for twenty-four hours and by adding fluids to the circulation. Important in the postoperative care was the release of fluid and air from the subdural space by occasional tapping with a ventricular needle during the first forty-eight hours.

The danger of postoperative bleeding is scarcely less and may be even greater than that of the original hematoma; it would usually quickly end in death if not immediately recognized and promptly treated by reopening of the wound and evacuation of the clot. The detection of a postoperative hematoma requires constant and careful observation of the patient, the state of consciousness being by far the most important item. If the lesion is detected early the reopening of the wound entails no risk; if the discovery is delayed the risk increases rapidly. As most patients are very drowsy and even comatose at the time of operation, a few hours' delay in recognizing a postoperative hematoma may well cause the death of the patient. The low mortality rate in the series is evidence of the careful study of patients by the resident surgeons. Failure to discover a postoperative hematoma is a fault scarcely to be forgiven.

The unusually high incidence of postoperative bleeding with this lesion has often led us to wonder if there may be some predisposing tendency to bleed. This probably is not so. With anesthesia induced by means of avertin with amylene hydrate there is unquestionably less bleeding, but on the other hand quite a number of these patients were operated on with the region under local anesthesia. The reduction in the size of the bone flap has unquestionably reduced both the number and the size of hematomas.

When patients are very ill from the effects of intracranial pressure there is always the thought that it would be safer to remove the bone flap—now a small one—and play safe with life. Moreover, a postoperative hematoma would rarely form after removal of a flap. However, for cosmetic reasons, we have never done this at the primary operation because of a feeling of security as to the prompt detection of a hematoma. However, it has been necessary in several instances to remove the flap at the subsequent operation when a further risk of life was unjustifiable.

That postoperative bleeding is a serious argument against a cranioplastic operation and in favor of tapping and irrigating a hematoma cannot be denied. However, with the very low mortality in the series the argument loses most of its force. If the patient is carefully watched there is scarcely any justification for loss of life. Then, too, when one considers the fact that the primary lesion is frequently multiple, it is clear that unless operation is performed the remaining pocket or pockets of blood may be missed, and in such circumstances a cure is scarcely to be expected. And of course tapping and irrigation offer no benefit for a patient with a solid hematoma.

Extradural drains were employed in nine of the earlier cases (20 per cent) but were given up because of the risk of infection and because they contributed nothing to the prevention of hematoma.

When a subdural hematoma is present on both sides, the patient is placed in the so-called cerebellar position and the same procedure carried out on each side. Since the reduced size of the bone flap has cut the operative risk proportionately, both sides can be operated on with a single procedure.

RESULTS

Among the forty-eight patients there were fifty hematomas, the lesions of two patients being bilateral. Forty-six patients recovered and two died. The patient mortality therefore is 4.1 per cent; the case mortality, 4 per cent. The patient in case 27 had a wound infection and died of staphylococcic meningitis on the tenth day after the operation. Autopsy showed no other pathologic change. The patient in case 7 was in coma, with a temperature of 103.6 F., at the time of operation and died two days later. Autopsy in this case revealed nothing except edema of the brain. At the time of discharge from the hospital all the other patients were well. Subsequent reports from this group of patients have been gratifying. Twenty-eight are known to be in normal health in 1937, and among these are two who were operated on twenty years ago. No replies were received from twelve patients, and six are known to have died from causes unrelated to the hematoma a considerable time after their discharge from the hospital.

In summary, then, from this review of forty-eight cases one may conclude:

1. Subdural hematoma occurs with almost equal frequency in every decade of life.

2. Whereas trauma is probably the immediate cause of the hemorrhage, there may be some additional but unrecognized factor.

3. After the initial hemorrhage there can scarcely be any increase in size of the hematoma.

4. The diagnosis is difficult because unless the history of trauma is acceptable the clinical symptoms and findings do not differ from those produced by any intracranial space-occupying lesion.

5. In the cases in which trephining does not disclose the hematoma, adequate and at times precise localization can be made by ventriculographic study.

6. When a hematoma is suspected but not proved, a burr opening is made over the parietal region. Incision of the dura will establish or eliminate the diagnosis and determine the size and position of the bone flap.

7. A small craniotomy opening with evacuation of the hematoma is the operation of choice.

8. Postoperative bleeding has been of frequent occurrence. For very ill patients a decompression may occasionally be essential to recovery.

REFERENCES

[1] Putnam, T. J., and Cushing, H.: Chronic Subdural Hematoma. *Arch. Surg. 11:* 329 (Sept.) 1925.

[2] Virchow, R.: Hematoma durae matris, *Verhandl. d. phys.-med. Gesellsch.,* 7: 134, 1857.

[3] Griswold, R. A., and Jelsma, F.: Chronic Subdural Hematoma. *Arch. Surg., 15:* 45 (July) 1927.

[4] Bell, B.: *A System of Surgery,* Ed. 3, Philadelphia, T. Dobson, 1806, vol. 2, chap. 10.

[5] Bowen, W. H.: Traumatic Subdural Hematomas. *Guy's Hosp. Rep.,* 59: 21, 1905.

[6] Henschen, K.: Diganostik und Operation der traumatischen Subduralblutung. *Arch. klin. Chir.,* 99: 67, 1912.

[7] Trotter, W.: Chronic Subdural Hemorrhage of Traumatic Origin and Its Relation to Pachymeningitis Hemorrhagica Interna. *Brit. J. Surg.,* 2: 271, 1914.

[8] Rand, C. W.: Chronic Subdural Hematoma. *Arch. Surg., 14:* 1136 (June) 1927.

[9] Kaplan, A.: Chronic Subdural Hematoma. *Brain,* 45: 430, 1931.

[10] Fleming, H. W., and Jones, O. W., Jr.: Chronic Subdural Hematoma. *Surg., Gynec. & Obst., 54:* 81, 1932.

[11] McKenzie, K. G.: Surgical and Clinical Study of Nine Cases of Chronic Subdural Hematoma. *Canad. M. A. J.,* 26: 534, 1932.

[12] Gardner, W. J.: Traumatic Subdural Hematoma with Particular Reference to the Latent Interval. *Arch. Neurol. & Psychiat.,* 27: 847 (April) 1932.

[13] Fischer, R., and de Morsier, G.: Chronic Subdural Hematoma Following Cranial Trauma. *Presse med., 41:* 1517, 1933.

[14] Keegan, J. J.: Chronic Subdural Hematoma. *Arch. Surg., 27:* 629 (Oct.) 1933.

[15] Frazier, C. H.: Surgical Management of Chronic Subdural Hematoma. *Ann. Surg., 101:* 671, 1935.

[16] Coleman, C. C.: Chronic Subdural Hematoma. *Am. J. Surg., 28:* 341, 1935.

[17] Furlow, L. T.: Chronic Subdural Hematoma. *Arch. Surg., 32:* 688 (April) 1936.

[18] Sherwood, D.: Chronic Subdural Hematoma in Infants. *Am. J. Dis. Child., 39:* 980 (May) 1930.

[19]Peet, M. M., and Kahn, E. A.: Subdural Hematoma in Infants. *J.A.M.A., 98:* 1851 (May 28) 1932.

[20]Jelsma, F.: Chronic Subdural Hematoma: Summary and Analysis of Forty-Two Cases. *Arch. Surg., 21:* 128 (July) 1930.

[21]Putnam, T. J., and Putnam, I. K.: The Experimental Study of Pachymeningitis Hemorrhagica. *J. Nerv. & Ment. Dis., 65:* 260, 1927.

[22]Heuer, G., and Dandy, W. E.: A Report of Seventy Cases of Brain Tumor. *Bull. Johns Hopkins Hosp., 27:* 224, 1916.

[23]Leary, T.: Subdural Hemorrhages. *J.A.M.A., 103:* 897 (Sept. 22) 1934.

[24]Munro, D.: The Diagnosis and Treatment of Subdural Hematomata. *New England J. Med., 210:* 1145, 1934.

[25]Gardner, W. J.: Traumatic Subdural Hematoma. *Ohio State M. J., 31:* 9, 1935.

[26]Dandy, W. E.: The Brain: Subdural Hematoma, in Lewis, D.: *Practice of Surgery.* Hagerstown, Md., W. F. Prior Company, Inc., 1932, Vol. 12, Chap. 1, p. 299.

[27]Van Dyke, C. H.: A Pathognomonic Encephalographic Sign of Subdural Hematoma. *Bull. Neurol. Inst. New York, 5:* 135, 1936.

[28]Zollinger, R., and Gross, R.: Traumatic Subdural Tematoma. *J.A.M.A., 103:* 245 (July 28) 1934.

LIX

THE TREATMENT OF INTERNAL CAROTID ANEURYSMS WITHIN THE CAVERNOUS SINUS AND THE CRANIAL CHAMBER*

REPORT OF THREE CASES

The surgical attack upon intracranial aneurysms is just beginning. Nor is it the insuperable problem that the desperate nature of the lesions might lead one to believe. Indeed, a few have unquestionably been cured. Within the past few years several aneurysms have been disclosed at operation, others demonstrated just as unequivocally by Moniz's arteriography, and procedures of different types have been directed toward their cure. In general, the surgical attack has been of two kinds—(1) direct, and (2) indirect. The former attempts to deal with the aneurysm directly, the latter indirectly by inducing thrombosis: (1) Through ligation of the internal carotid artery—Hunter's method of proximal ligation; or (2) by trapping the aneurysm between ligatures. The three aneurysms included in this report have been treated by the latter method. The type of operation will always be dictated by the position and to some degree by the size of the aneurysm.

Although the direct attack upon aneurysms would appear to be the more logical and more certain of permanent results, it is only certain aneurysms that are amenable to such treatment and, at best, the procedure must be regarded as one carrying definite hazards. Two successful direct attacks upon intracranial aneurysms have been recorded, both appearing during 1937, and each was operated upon by a different method. McConnell[11] (1937) incised an aneurysm (probably from the internal carotid artery) and despite a furious

*Reprinted from the *Annals of Surgery, 109:* 5, May, 1939.

hemorrhage plugged the sac with muscle. The visual defects resulting from the aneurysm have since disappeared, and the patient is free of symptoms and is back at work.

The writer[4] (1937) closed a silver clip upon the neck of an aneurysm of the internal carotid artery and shriveled the aneurysm distal to the clip with the electrocautery. The clip was flush with the wall of the carotid. The third nerve palsy cleared completely in six weeks and the patient is perfectly well and free of all symptoms, 21 months later (December, 1938).

Dott[5] (1937) placed silver clips upon both sides of an aneurysm of the anterior communicating artery but an unfortunate postoperative accident deprived him of a beautiful result—the patient died from an intrathoracic puncture of an infusion needle.

Tonnis[20] (1936) by splitting the corpus callosum, made a most difficult exposure of a cherry-sized aneurysm of the anterior communicating artery (shown by arteriography), found the aneurysm surrounded by a "walnut-sized" hematoma. Fearing injury to the arterial trunk from which the aneurysm arose, he merely covered its surface with a piece of muscle. The patient made an uneventful recovery. However, one cannot believe that muscle applied to the outer surface of the aneurysmal sac could play any part in curing the aneurysm; possibly it might, as the operator hoped, seal the leak and prevent further bleeding. Dott[5] (1933) wrapped a sheath of muscle around an intracranial aneurysm of the carotid at the junction with the posterior cerebral artery and later [5] (1937) reported the patient well after four years. Here again, one cannot believe the application of muscle could have had any curative, effect upon the aneurysm. Trevani[21] (1932) evacuated an intracranial carotid aneurysm, suspecting it to be a tumor, when aspiration was negative; the internal carotid artery was ligated in the neck to control bleeding, but the patient died five hours later. Sosman and Vogt [18] (1926) included in their paper on the roentgenologic examinations of aneurysms of the circle of Willis, a case operated upon by Cushing; an aneurysmal sac on the intracranial portion of the carotid had been deliberately opened and was packed with muscle. The patient, age fifty-eight recovered with hemiplegia, doubtless due to closure of the carotid artery. There was partial return of motor function but she died six months later. A note from Doctor Sosman related that at necropsy the aneurysm was found to be thrombosed.

By the indirect attack, there is reason to believe that several intracranial aneurysms have been cured. Dott, who has just presented a most interesting series of intracranial aneurysms, is probably entitled to the credit of the first successful surgical treatment by simply ligating the internal carotid artery. His first cure was reported in 1933, and is doubtless the one that was reported well four years later (1937). In his later report (1937) there is good reason to believe that three of his verified aneurysms have been cured by simply ligating the internal carotid artery in the neck. The remaining four of his seven verified cases died, although two were unconscious when the operation was performed. Walsh and Love[22] (1937) reported another almost certain cure by the same method of ligating the internal carotid in the neck. Subsequent photographs showed the oculomotor palsy to have disappeared and the patient was back at work three months after the operation. In Jefferson's [10] series of carotid-cavernous aneurysms (1938) is one (Case 5) demonstrated by angiography

and probably cured by this method. Another (Case 15) developed transient contralateral motor numbness thirty-six hours after ligation of the internal carotid, but at the time of his publication was reported to be improving.

In the accompanying report three additional cases of intracranial aneurysms are added. All arose in the intracavernous portion of the internal carotid artery or just as the carotid enters the cranial chamber. All projected into the cranial chamber alongside the carotid artery. In each there is every reason to believe that the aneurysm is cured. The method of treatment has consisted of trapping the aneurysms between two occlusions of the internal carotid artery (1) intracranially; and (2) in the neck. This method is similar to that carried out by the writer in the treatment of carotid-cavernous-arteriovenous aneurysms.

CASE REPORTS

CASE 1. History No. U-73513: L. B., white, female, age twenty-eight. Admitted September 25, 1936, discharged October 15, 1936. Referred by Dr. Roger G. Doughty and Dr. J. Heyward Gibbes, Columbia, S. C.

Complaints.—Headache and drooping of the left eye.

Family and Past Histories were negative.

Present Illness.—Four or five months ago generalized headaches appeared, became periodic, but were not severe. Six weeks ago, sudden, intense headache appeared over the left side of the head and continued for twenty-four hours. After the headache had subsided the vision was impaired, but she did not then see double. Objects seemed a little less clear than previously, but she could not say definitely that only the left eye was affected. Four days later there was another similar, equally severe attack that lasted for two days and again the pain was mainly over the left side of the head. She was not exactly unconscious but she could remember very little that happened during that period. For two or three days before this attack there was mental haziness. Patient was taken to a hospital and repeated lumbar punctures done; blood was obtained from these punctures. These, she thought, gave her temporary relief.

A third and similar attack of pain occurred three weeks ago. At this time the left eyelid drooped and the eyeball pulled outward. Since that time she has been unable to open the left eye. There has since been a constant dull headache with exacerbations on three different occasions.

Physical Examination.—Patient is somewhat undernourished; Blood pressure, 130/70; Wassermann, negative.

Neurologic Examination showed complete paralysis of all motor functions referable to the left third nerve. Patient was unable to elevate the eyelid even slightly. The pupil was widely dilated and did not react to light or accommodation. There was also complete paralysis of the left fourth nerve; the sixth was intact. The following negative findings are perhaps worthy of note: Both visual fields were normal; the visual acuity was not recorded. The eyegrounds were normal on both sides. No murmur was audible over the head. Compression of the left carotid artery over a period of five minutes produced no symptoms. Roentgenologic examination of the head was negative.

Clinical Diagnosis.—Aneurysm of the left carotid artery or the posterior communicating artery.

Operation.—October 6, 1936: A hypophyseal flap was turned down on the left side, using the concealed incision. Behind the left carotid artery was a small, rounded, reddish mass, about the size of a pea, bulging from the inner margin of the dura lining the middle fossa of the skull, *i.e.*, covering the cavernous sinus. When this little mass was touched with the forceps it pulsated strongly. It appeared to be part of the carotid as it passed through the dura. When the carotid artery was gently separated from the aneurysm with forceps there was a small spurt of arterial blood. This ceased as soon as the carotid fell back upon the arterial wall; this gentle separation was repeated three times and with each there was a spurt of arterial blood. In other words, the posterior wall of the carotid artery was blocking the small opening in the aneurysm and this was doubtless the source of bleeding on former occasions. The third nerve could be seen pushed backward and outward by the aneurysm.

A silver clip was placed upon the internal carotid artery and compressed, completely occluding it. After closing the cranial wound, the internal carotid artery was then exposed in the neck. This vessel was elevated upon a tape and compressed with the finger. An opening was made into the carotid cephalad to the point of compression; a strong spurt of blood indicated the rapidity with which a return circulation develops from the ophthalmic artery (its principal source of collateral). A small piece of muscle was introduced into the opening of the carotid artery (Brooks' method) and a clip placed upon it for subsequent identification roentgenologically. The artery was then ligated above and below the opening. Roentgenograms subsequently showed the position of the clip on the piece of muscle to have remained at the site at which it was introduced into the artery.

The patient made an uneventful recovery and was discharged October 15, 1936, nine days after the operation.

Subsequent Course.—Patient returned for observation April 6, 1938, eighteen months after the operation. She had been perfectly well; had had no headaches and had been doing all of her own house work. She had gained thirty-two pounds in weight. A later note, November 15, 1938 (twenty-five months after the operation), says that she still remains well and free of symptoms.

When examined April 6, 1938, the left pupil did not react either to light or accommodation, nor did it react consensually. There was a normal movement inward of the left eyeball, but an almost complete inability to look up or down. The left palpebral fissure was only 2 Mm. narrower than the right, and she could elevate the lid. There was no vision in the left eye, normal in the right. Unfortunately, visual acuity was not recorded before the operation, but the visul fields were normal. There must, therefore, have been a very pronounced loss of vision in the left eye as a result of the arterial ligation, or, more probably, as a result of thrombus formation that included the ophthalmic artery. The left disk showed marked primary optic atrophy and the arteries were greatly narrowed.

COMMENT. The headaches in this patient have been entirely relieved over a period of twenty-five months. There has been improvement in the extra-ocular movements, principally the inner movement of the eye, and a marked improvement in the ptosis, but the functions of the extra-ocular muscles have not been completely restored. One is curious to know the cause of the loss of vision in the left eye. The natural assumption is that it is due to the ligature of the carotid, of which the ophthalmic artery is the only accessible branch. However, the same ligatures have been placed on the internal carotid artery in the other two cases, and in several other cases for carotid-cavernous aneurysms, and without loss of vision. It is conceivable, indeed it is my belief, that the small piece of muscle that was introduced into the artery may have led to the formation of a propagating thrombus that occluded the mouth of the ophthalmic artery and perhaps extended along it to the retinal artery. Unfortunately, our records are not sufficiently clear on the preoperative state of vision to warrant any conclusion, though I think there cannot be any doubt that her vision was quite good, although perhaps not perfect, before the operation was performed; certainly her visual field was normal in this eye.

CASE 2   History No. U-137770: C. L. S., white, male, age thirty-six. Admitted April 20, 1938; discharged May 7, 1938. Referred by Dr. Edward F. Milan, of Baltimore, Md.

Complaints.—Headache and trouble with left eye.

Family and Past Histories were negative.

Present Illness.—This began eight months ago with headaches localized to the left orbit and the left frontal region; and associated with these was a tickling sensation in the nose. There was some nasal discharge and he thought he had a fresh cold. Headaches were not constant; they occurred almost every morning and frequently awakened him from a sound sleep. The attacks came on suddenly and without warning, "like a flash," and lasted about one hour; he had one or two every day. If an attack did not come in the morning, it would be certain to come in the afternoon and usually around four o'clock. Since the onset there had never been a day without an attack. They left him exhausted and he had found nothing to give relief.

Five months ago the left eye began to close and draw. This progressed so that he could no longer keep the eye open. Vision in the left eye has been blurred dur-

ing the last month. At times the ptosis came on in spells lasting from 30 to 60 minutes, and then in large part cleared, but always with a little residual droop. Generally he has felt "tired and droopy," but there has been no generalized weakness. He has had no convulsions, and has never been comatose. The eye has never protruded. There has been no noise in the ear or head.

Physical Examination was entirely negative. Patient is a well nourished, average-sized man of thirty-six years. Blood pressure was 120/70, and the Wassermann reaction from the blood was negative.

Neurologic Examination. — Incomplete ptosis of the left upper lid. Some swelling of both upper and lower lids. Exophthalmometer measured 16 Mm. on the left and 14 Mm. on the right. Exophthalmos, if real, could not be detected on inspection. There was limitation in adduction and downward and upward movements of the left eye. The left pupil was larger than the right but reacted well. Vision in the left eye was 20/30, and the right 20/20; the left could not be improved by lenses. The visual fields were normal; the blind spots were normal in both eyes. No murmur could be heard with a stethoscope. Roentgenologic examination of the head was negative.

Clinical Impressions.—This patient was first seen in the Diagnostic Clinic, where Doctor Ford made a diagnosis of a tumor, or more probably an aneurysm of the carotid or posterior communication arteries. My own diagnosis was the same; I thought it was almost certainly an aneurysm.

Operation.—April 22, 1938: A hypophyseal approach was made on the left side, using the concealed incision. This exposure provided ample room for inspection of the carotid artery. A branch of the sylvian vein crossing to the dura along the lesser wing of the sphenoid was thrombosed and divided, and this permitted inspection of the floor of the middle fossa of the skull. The third nerve was seen to be elevated by a lesion beneath, *i.e.,* from the region of the cavernous sinus. When the optic nerves and the carotid artery were separated one could see a small reddish-brown mass projecting between them on the mesial side (Fig. 1). The region of the cavernous sinus was much fuller than normal and pulsated when the forceps pushed upon it. The branches of the caro-

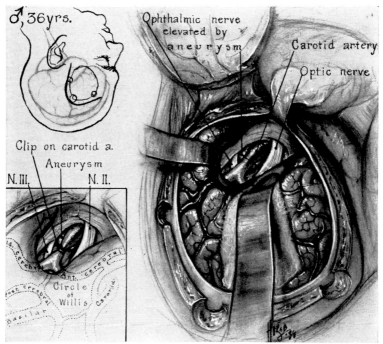

Fig. 1. Drawing of aneurysm (Case 2), which lies just behind the carotid artery and pushes the oculomotor nerve backward. The difference in color of the carotid artery at the point of entrance into the skull and that farther along on the artery is noted and probably carries some significance. The artery is also larger at the point of entrance into the skull than where it approaches the brain. The lower inset shows the clip placed upon the carotid artery.

tid along the base of the brain were visible and the lesion was not attached to any of these. One point was perhaps noteworthy, *i.e.,* in the first half of the carotid intracranially the wall of the artery was pink (Fig. 1), but beginning with a very sharp line about its midpoint the normally white thickened wall continued onward to the base of the brain; it was assumed that the whiter coating meant a greater thickness of the artery. A flat silver clip was clamped upon the internal carotid artery completely obliterating it. (Fig. 1, inset.) This was accomplished without difficulty and without bleeding. Five days later the internal carotid artery was ligated in the neck. The artery was distinctly smaller than usual.

Subsequent Course.—Patient returned June 4, 1938, one month after discharge, and six weeks after the first operation. He was perfectly well in every way. His ptosis and all of the extra-ocular palsies had entirely cleared. He had no pain, no headache and the tickling sensation in the left side of the nose had disappeared. There

was no sign of atrophy of the disk. His visual fields were normal on rough test. He said the vision in that eye was perfectly normal. He was seen again August 1, 1938; was perfectly well and was back at his work—a clerical position. He remained well, November 15, 1938.

Case 3 History No. U-135470: D. R., white, female, age thirty-seven. Admitted April 4, 1938, discharged April 30, 1938. Referred by Dr. John F. Daly, Teaneck, N. J.

Complaints.—Drooping of the right eyelid and headaches.

Family and Past Histories were negative.

Present Illness.—For the past five years, patient has been having brief, mild headaches about once a week and readily relieved by aspirin. Four months ago she had a peculiar pain about the right eye; this lasted three days when it became suddenly very much more severe and remained concentrated in the right eye. She described the sensation as though the eye was being torn out. During this attack she fell unconscious. After two or three minutes she was able to get up and went to bed unassisted. A terrific headache and pain over the entire right side of the face persisted. She was nauseated and vomited frequently. At that time drooping of the right upper eyelid and double vision developed. A week later there was a similar attack, following which the right eyelid was completely closed and she was unable to elevate it. A week later she had a third attack. She was then taken to a hospital where she remained 12 weeks. The physicians said they could hear a "swishing" noise in the head, but the patient has never heard it. When she had obtained no relief during a months stay in the hospital, the right internal carotid artery was ligated. The physicians told her that the bruit had disappeared, but patient recognized no subjective improvement.

During the past month she has had a noise in the right ear like escaping steam from a locomotive. She thinks there may have been some protusion of the right eye which has since disappeared; she was, however, not certain of this. Her right pupil has been persistently dilated.

Physical Examination. — Patient is a large, obese woman, seemingly normal, except for her local deformity. Blood pressure 138/96; Blood Wassermann reaction, negative.

Neurologic Examination showed the right eye to be strongly abducted. The pupil was dilated to 6 Mm. and did not react to light either directly or consensually, or to accommodation. All movements of the muscles supplied by the third nerve

were completely paralyzed. Slight rotary movement of the eyeball was possible, doubtless due to an intact fourth nerve. The external rectus muscle functioned normally. Ptosis was complete.

Vision in the right eye was 20/50, in the left 20/15. It was impossible to chart the visual field in the right eye because of the very strong abduction of the eyeball. The eyegrounds were normal. The tension of the eyeball was normal on both sides. There was no exophthalmos and no murmur could be heard with the stethoscope. Compression of the right internal carotid artery for five minutes caused no cerebral disturbance. Roentgenologic examination of the head was negative.

Operation.—April 13, 1938: A right hypophyseal approach was made, using the concealed incision. The brain was quite tight and surprisingly little room could be obtained by evacuating the cisterna chiasmatis. The lateral ventricle was tapped and 25 cc of fluid obtained; even then it was difficult to get sufficient room to expose the carotid artery. In order to gain access to the anterior part of the middle fossa, it was necessary to thrombose and divide two branches of the sylvian vein crossing to the lesser wing of the sphenoid; finally, an adequate exposure of the carotid region was obtained. There was a small piece of fibrin over the outer surface of the carotid artery as it passed through the base of the skull. (Fig. 2). This was cautiously divided and one could see beneath it a bulging pulsating mass, about the size of a pea, extending from the cavernous sinus, which

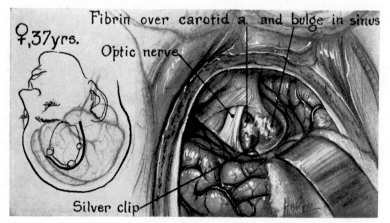

Fig. 2. Case III: Operative findings: A clip has been placed upon the carotid artery. The layer of fibrin, which was so conspicuous in this case, is undoubtedly an indication of the weakness of the aneurysm.

bulged markedly and pulsated (Fig. 2). The small intracranial protrusion was everywhere smooth and glistening and had no relationship to the posterior communicating artery. The third nerve could not be seen because the bulging mass covered its course. The carotid artery was isolated from the optic nerve, a silver clip placed upon it and compressed. There was no difficulty in doing this and no bleeding resulted.

Second Operation.—April 22, 1938: Ligation of the Right Internal Carotid Artery in the Neck:

In another hospital, ligation of the internal carotid artery was said to have been done. The wound had become infected and drained for several weeks, so that there was now an exceedingly dense scar throughout the depth of the old incision. Cautiously the scar tissue was cut away until the carotid artery was located. The common carotid artery was finally exposed, then the internal and external carotids for a short distance. Both the internal and external carotid arteries were essentially normal in size and both pulsated normally. We could find no ligatures or fascia or foreign material of any type that had been placed around the carotid. The internal carotid artery was then ligated with a double ligature of medium silk; a second ligature was placed just above the first one. On palpating the vessel, cephalad to the ligature, no pulsation could be detected. The patient made an uninterrupted recovery and was discharged April 30, 1938.

*Subsequent Course.—*Patient wrote, July 10, 1938, that the ptosis was improving; she could elevate it slightly. She returned for observation, August 27, 1938; she could then elevate the lid almost to the normal, though when at rest it lagged markedly. There was just a beginning abduction of the eyeball; the upward and downward movements were unimproved and the pupil though less dilated than formerly did not react to light. Oblique rotation of the eyeball was present. The vision fields on the affected side were normal. The vision in the affected eye was 20/20; before operation it was 20/50. Her general health was perfect. She had had no headaches and the noise in the head had disappeared. In a later photograph, taken in December, 1938, eight months after the operation, a still further improvement was noticeable.

Diagnosis of Intracranial Aneurysms.— The intensive cultivation of any field usually discloses the lesion to be of far greater frequency than we have been wont to believe. This has already been found to be true with intracranial aneurysms. Sporadically, cases have been reported for over half a century. Blane (1800) and Adams [1] (1869) reported specimens at necropsy. Hutchinson [9] (1875) presented a postmortem report of one that had been diagnosed correctly 11 years earlier. A spontaneous cure had resulted from thrombosis. During the past decade the number of cases has increased quite rapidly; in most instances there are several from a single clinic. Jefferson [10] has just reported seventeen aneurysms in the cavernous sinus alone, and in his experience has had fifty-five arterial aneurysms of the brain; many of these, however, have not been verified either by operation or necropsy.

The diagnosis of an intracranial aneurysm may be made with the greatest of ease or with great difficulty. Similarly, the localization of the aneurysm, which, of course, is all essential for surgical treatment, may be simple or difficult. Unfortunately, the easy localizations from clinical signs and symptoms are in the minority. However, arteriography, introduced a decade ago by Moniz,[16] frequently makes the diagnosis and localization with precision, when the signs and symptoms fail completely, or are at least uncertain.

Intracranial aneurysms may be divided into two general groups: (1) Those within the substance of the brain; and (2) those on the surface of the base of the brain. The latter arise from the circle of Willis, or from the carotid in its intracranial course or within the carotid canal (and project into the cranial chamber). The former are frequently larger, because a tissue wall withstands their progress; they are usually encountered during operations for brain tumors. The aneurysms at the base of the brain are usually relatively or actually small, are frequently multiple and their presence is known or suspected from five disturbances: (1) Recurring, sudden, severe pain and headache back of an eye; (2) subarachnoid hemorrhage; (3) palsies of the nerves to the extra-ocular muscles, particularly the third; (4) involvement of the trigeminal and sympathetic nerves; and (5) unilateral loss of vision with primary optic atrophy. One must always suspect an intracranial aneurysm when there are sudden, severe pains or headaches confined to one side and in the general region of the eye or temple. And the diagnosis becomes highly probable when one of the nerves entering the cavernous sinus is affected. The sudden severe pains or headaches will usually recur at relatively short intervals. The syndrome of recurring, sudden, severe pains in one eye, side of the head, or side of the face (frequently all are combined), plus ptosis and other evidence of disturbed function of the nerve, are almost pathognomonic of an aneurysm of the internal carotid artery or the posterior communicating artery. In each of the three aneurysms reported and in a fourth reported elsewhere, this syndrome was the sole basis for the diagnosis, and was regarded with sufficient certainty to warrant exploration of the aneurysm. This was also true in the case of Walsh and Love.[22] Although this syndrome has long been known and emphasized (Hutchinson, [9] Beadles, [3] Symonds,[19] Sands,[17] etc.), it has been only during the last few years that surgeons could feel sufficiently secure of its pathognomonic significance and at the same time of the surgical possibilities to permit exploration of the lesion.

Subarachnoid bleeding is with almost equal certainty an indication of an aneurysm on the circle of Willis, but rarely is there any indication of the location of the aneurysm, even to the right or left side of this vascular circle. The eyegrounds may give an indication. Not infrequently a huge round hemorrhage develops in the disk or retina in addition to many other smaller ones. This picture is pathognomonis of a subarachnoid hemorrhage, and in two recent cases the major hemorrhages were on the side of the aneurysm. A rapidly developing choked disk is usually also present and this, too, is more advanced on the side of the aneurysm. However, these indications are usually in the very severe hemorrhages, or are usually late manifestations. Ophthalmic migraine is often due to aneurysms of the carotid artery and should always be borne in mind as the probable cause.

Roentgenologic examination of the head is at times helpful in the differential diagnosis of intracranial aneurysms. Linear, curved shadows always suggest an aneurysm, and several examples of this have been demonstrated. Erosions of the landmarks of the sella and middle fossa of the skull, have resulted from large aneurysms of the carotid, usually arising within the cavernous sinus. Heuer and writer [8] described such a case in 1916; Schuller another, in 1918; both were substantiated by necropsy. Sosman and Vogt (1926) added three more. Other writers contributing on this subject are McKinney, Acree and Soltz [13] (1936), and Jefferson (1938). In one of Jefferson's cases the shadow appeared seven years after her first symptom and seven years before death.

Arteriography, introduced by Moniz, in 1937, gives every promise of the greatest help in precisely diagnosing and localizing intracranial aneurysms. Already, quite a number have been so graphically demonstrated by the intra-arterial (intrenal or common carotid) injections of thorotrast that one cannot be skeptical of its importance. A glance at the beautiful roentgenograms, with the sharply defined and unmistakable aneurysms, shown by Dott, Tonnis and Jefferson, after these injections, is absolutely convincing. So graphic are they, that nothing is left to the imagination. And yet one wonders whether the absence of an aneurysmal shadow can be accepted as positive evidence that an aneurysm does not exist, *i.e.*, whether one can exclude an aneurysm on negative evidence. Also, is a bilateral internal carotid injection indicated after negative single injections, and even then would bilateral negative injections be absolute evidence in excluding an aneurysm? I must confess a great reluctance to use arteriography, fearing thrombosis of the big arterial trunk, or some cerebral complication from thrombosis of one of the smaller trunks, possibly even the induction of hemorrhages from the aneurysm. This may well be a prejudice of one who withholds all accessory methods in diagnosis, even lumbar punctures and ventriculography, unless there are very necessary indications for their employment. It is always my feeling that the least done to a patient, the better. Complications are bound to arise from time to time as a result of seemingly trivial accessory examinations (lumbar punctures and air injections, intravenous injections, *etc.*, for example) and the patient may lose his life as a result. I realize full well that no bad results have been reported from the use of arteriography, but when deaths have occurred in patients who have previously had injections of thorotrast, one wonders whether this method can be excluded as a factor, or at least whether in the very ill state of the patients they would not have been better off without the additional insult, even though reportedly a harmless one. There can be no quarrels in its employment when the silent aneurysms causing subarachnoid hemorrhages are sought, but I can see little, if any, reason for its employment when the history and localizing neurologic evidence is so convincing. Even in the group associated with subarachnoid hemorrhages, without any indication of the side of the lesion, there is room for disagreement. So many of these patients recover from the immediate effects of the hemorrhage, and go for many years without further trouble, that one is reluctant to add to the immediate risk. I have seen many such cases. On the other hand, only recently, I advised against a vascular injection of thorotrast when the patient was recovering and was seemingly well after a subarachnoid injection. A week later she had another hemorrhage, and death re-

sulted promptly. Unquestionably, precision and elimination of guesswork will eventually be the better course with lesions so grave and at the same time so capricious in their course. And the attainment of this end can, from the present outlook, be only through arteriography. Doubtless, with time, the writer will use it more, but only when there is no indication whatever of the side of the lesion. At present, however, if by headache, pains or other subjective sensation there is indication of the side of the circle on which the aneurysm is located, I should prefer (in cases with subarachnoid hemorrhage) operative exposure of the base of the brain on that side, rather than arterial injections. However, it is only fair to add that since the type of operation to be employed in the treatment of intracranial aneurysms differs with the surgeon, the reaction to the use of angiography may differ accordingly. Those who feel that ligation of the carotid in the neck is safer, and on the whole preferable to direct inspection of the aneurysm, may feel more justification in viewing the aneurysm roentgenologically.

Treatment of Arterial Aneurysms.—Since the treatment of arterial aneurysms is still in its infancy, one cannot be dogmatic concerning any method of handling them, or indeed, in many instances, that surgery should be undertaken. That a certain number of aneurysms have been cured spontaneously from thrombosis is perhaps true, although one cannot be too certain of this. The long absence of symptoms leads us to suspect a cure, but subsequently, much of the false aneurysmal sac is largely filled by a laminated clot when the mouth of the aneurysm and a small portion of the sac adjoining the mouth remain patent; and the aneurysm is not only actually still active but may be of tremendous size. Although further bleeding may not occur and the patient may be symptomless for a long period of time, the silence may well be only deceptive. I have seen several such examples within the brain substance and the aneurysm has gained considerable

size—even to the proportion of a large tumor—gradually and doubtlessly paroxys-
mally, and yet without external bleeding
or other symptoms. In this state of apparent rest, the aneurysm is merely bleeding
into the false sac and behind a thrombotic
wall which is slowly extending; under such
circumstances the aneurysmal cavity may
be very small. This is probably more true
of aneurysms within the brain substance
than those on the exterior. Such findings
lead one to suspect that in many instances
the reputed cure of the aneurysm may be
more apparent than real. However this
may be, one is reluctant to advise surgical
treatment for aneurysms on the circle of
Willis unless the subarachnoid hemorrhages are sufficiently severe to endanger
life and are known to recur.

For aneurysms of the producing oculomotor palsies and severe recurring pains
there can be no doubt concerning the need
for surgical intervention. Nor is there, in
safe hands, such a formidable risk as the
subject of aneurysms might suggest. However, for aneurysms elsewhere along the
circle of Willis one must assume at the present time, in the absence of surgical tests,
that the risk is greater and the possibilities
of aneurysms favorable for treatment are
undoubtedly less. Many of them involve
both the carotid and anterior or posterior
communicating or the middle cerebral arteries, making the eradication or the trapping of the aneurysm seemingly impossible.
Then, too, these aneurysms must be localized, at least, to the side of the circle of
Willis. In most instances this determination can be arrived at only by arteriography. The risk attending surgical efforts
must, therefore, depend upon the exact site
and the size of the aneurysm. There is no
reason to believe that the surgical treatment of aneurysms of the anterior cerebral
artery, or even the anterior communicating
artery, should be attended by any more risk
than one of the carotid, and probably not
so much, but aneurysms of the posterior
communicating or posterior cerebral or
basilar arteries would be much more diffi-

cult to expose sufficiently to "clip" the
trunk of the artery on both sides of the
aneurysm. However, if nothing more
could be done, it is not impossible that
clipping of the arterial trunk on one side
of the aneurysm may be adequate.

For aneurysms of the internal carotid
artery, either within the carotid canal or
within the cranium, the best type of surgical treatment can only be evolved from experience. Unquestionably, the best treatment for such aneurysms within the cranial chamber is "clipping" the neck of the
aneurysm with or without coagulation of
the sac beyond the clip. The great advantages of this method are, of course, that the
treatment is a direct one with an absolute
assurance of cure, and that the internal
carotid artery is not sacrificed. But from a
pathologic study of quite a number of
these aneurysms, it is hardly conceivable
that many of them are so favorably situated and constructed that closure of the
neck will be possible. It is not impossible
that the application of a silver clip to the
body of a small aneurysm, that exhibits no
appreciable neck, may not suffice, or even
the application of the cautery to the aneurysm, without an intermediary clip, may
prove to cure an aneurysm that otherwise
would appear hopeless. Opening and packing an aneurysm such as was done by Ter-
vani and Cushing is far more hazardous
and more difficult. Certainly this method
of attack would be a last resort.

For those aneurysms of this vessel that
are within the cranial chamber and below
the main branches, or are within the carotid canal, two lines of attack may be used:
(1) Ligation of the internal carotid in
the neck—Hunter's operation of ligation
in continuity; and (2) ligation of the internal carotid, both within the cranial
chamber and in the neck, *i.e.,* trapping the
aneurysm between two ligatures (Fig. 3).
It is assumed that the diagnosis can be
established in these cases solely by the
history and the neurologic examination.
The three cases included in this report
have been operated upon by the later

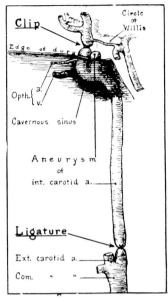

Fig. 3. Diagrammatic representation indicating the position of the aneurysm and the method of surgical attack upon it, by trapping the aneurysm between the carotid, intracranially, and the ligature of the internal carotid artery in the neck.

method. Five of Dott's carotid aneurysms have been operated upon by the first method, three surviving and two ending fatally; however, since his deaths were in very ill patients, the ligation of the carotid may or may not have been contributory. However, both of his deaths were in patients whose ages, 49 and 50, were beyond the safe limit for total ligation of the internal carotid. My reasons for the intracranial approach first and ligation of the carotid at that site, have been that one could see the aneurysm and perhaps treat it by ligating the sac alone without sacrificing the internal carotid artery. And at least one can be certain of the character of the lesion, for tumors not infrequently must be considered in the differential diagnosis. Ligation of the neck of the sac has been possible in one of four cases. On the other hand, it may well be preferable to define the exact position and size of the aneurysm by arteriography and be guided

in the subsequent method of surgical treatment by these results. Doubtless, to many, perhaps most surgeons, such a precise test will be preferable to a cranial exposure which, if ligation of the carotid in the neck should prove to be sufficient in producing a cure, may in the end be unnecessary. One's reaction to these alternative views will eventually depend upon: (1) Whether or not arteriography carries more or less danger than the cranial exposure; and (2) whether the degree of assurance of simple cervical ligation is sufficiently great.

The cure of an aneurysm by ligation of the internal carotid in the neck (in continuity) is thought to be dependent upon the development of a thrombus due to lowered blood pressure. The thrombus is presumed to be formed in the aneurysmal sac and either solely there or as a secondary extension of a thrombus extending from the site of the ligature in the internal carotid to and including the aneurysm. Our knowledge of thrombus formation in vessels with normal walls and without infection is none too secure. That such a progressive thrombus does form in the presence of infection or a ruptured intima is well recognized, but neither in experiments upon animals nor in clean human ligations, is there any certain evidence that a thrombus develops and spreads from the point of the ligature. Recently, I have seen at necropsy, two internal carotid arteries that have been ligated with silk, one three months, the other six weeks, and there was no gross thrombus formation in one and a tiny one, just visible to the eye, in the other. And in another case, I explored and opened an internal carotid artery in the neck just above a total ligature of this vessel, that had been placed several months earlier, and it not only bled freely but had no thrombus at that point. On the other hand, I have seen a thrombus develop spontaneously from a defective calcified wall in the cavernous portion of the internal carotid with a break in the intima and spread far down the neck and upward into the three intracranial branches of this vessel. In one of Dott's cases, a thrombus was said to have extended from the site of a cervical ligature on the internal carotid almost to the intracranial division of the carotid and including the aneurysm. However, since death resulted only eighteen hours after the ligature was placed, one wonders whether, after such a short interval, it is possible to differentiate with any degree of certainty between a postoperative and a postmortem thrombus.

In a recent publication, the writer [4] has shown that, in an analysis of many cases of carotid-cavernous arteriovenous aneurysms treated by ligation of the internal carotid artery in the neck, only about one-third are cured either immediately or within a short period thereafter. The cure of these aneurysms, when it occurs, is by advent of thrombosis, just as in arterial aneurysms. But in every reported case of arterial aneurysm that has survived ligation of the internal carotid artery in the neck (three by Dott, one by Walsh and Love, and one by Jefferson) a seeming cure has resulted, and promptly. These results are far superior to those obtained by proximal ligation for aneurysms affecting other large arteries, where indeed the resultant cure is unusual. Certainly this difference in results cannot be due to a lesser collateral blood supply because the return of blood from the circle of Willis is very prompt and great. If these results hold even approximately, arterial aneurysms are decidedly easier to cure by ligation of the internal carotid than the arteriovenous type. And if subsequent tests prove this to be true intracranial ligation of the internal carotid artery would be unnecessary. At least, it can be withheld until the cervical ligation has proved to be ineffective. Possibly one should be prepared to believe that the cure of arterial aneurysms following this line of treatment would be more frequent than in the arteriovenous variety because they are blind-end sacs; whereas, in the latter there is only a thin-walled fistula in a continuous vascular channel, and through this the continuity of blood flow would be

more probable. This alone will answer the question of the permanency of cures by simple ligation. For the moment, the cures appear to be no less perfect than by the double ligation.

Moreover, cervical ligations of the carotid can be effective only when the aneurysms are in certain locations. When situated in certain other positions, it may be very dangerous, *i.e.,* where the collateral circulation through the circle of Willis may be compromised or congenitally inadequate. In the case reported by Albright,[2] in 1929, I had tried this method of tying the internal carotid in the neck, using, however, the seemingly safer partial closure with a fascial band instead of a total occlusion with a ligature. This was done because the total occlusion test (by finger compression) indicated that complete closure of the internal carotid artery would not be tolerated. About eight hours after the operation (which was performed under local anesthesia), cerebral signs began to appear and steadily progressed. Death resulted three and one-half days after the operation, despite the removal of the fascial band within two hours after the first cerebral sign. There was no suggestion of a thrombus within the carotid artery or its branches. Cerebral softening resulted in the part of the brain supplied by the middle cerebral artery. Cerebral anemia was found at necropsy to be due to pressure of the aneurysm, which was a fairly large one, on both the middle cerebral and the posterior communicating arteries, thus precluding adequate collateral blood supply to the brain.

When an aneurysm is located along the circle of Willis and is so situated and is large enough to compromise or destroy by compression the circulation in the posterior communicating or middle cerebral or anterior communicating arteries, it is quite probable that the middle cerebral artery will receive an insufficient blood flow and the result will be cerebral softening. The above case is an example and is probably not exceptional. Dott came to a similar conclusion from his arteriographic studies. Then, too, one of these collateral trunks may be congenitally too small to play its part in maintaining the collateral circulation. It is doubtful how dependable the preoperative test of occluding the carotid artery with the finger may be, especially when it is negative, for in the above case the test was negative and it was eight hours before the effects of cerebral anemia were manifest. The importance of this test lies in detecting those cases in which an immediate effect is produced by closing the carotid.

Another reason for preferring exploration of the lesion, is that tumors at times may be disclosed when an aneurysm is suspected. Frequently the differential diagnosis between an aneurysm and tumor must be considered unless, of course, arteriography is used. And finally in reviewing the fatal case reported by Albright, I wonder if a direct attack upon the aneurysm might not now offer hope of success.

The age of a patient will always be an important determining factor in the line of treatment. After the age of 40 or 45 total ligation of the internal carotid artery unquestionably carries an increasing hazard from cerebral complications, due to inadequate blood supply. Before the of 40 or 45 ligation of this important trunk is usually without adverse effect, though this is not always true, as our cerebral anemia from partial ligation demonstrates; this patient was only thirty-three.

To protect patients over forty—indeed, all ages— the carotid compression is indispensable; it should be carried out for ten minutes without interrupton. The importance of this test has been repeatedly emphasized by Matas.[15] It does not insure against eventual trouble, such as has been noted above, but when positive it does pick out individuals in whom ligation of the carotid would certainly be followed by hemiplegia and probably death. If, therefore, an aneurysm of the brain is suspected, the primary exposure of the aneurysm would not be attempted unless this test were neg-

ative. And, therefore, if the test were positive one would be forced to forego the intracranial exposure. But total ligation of the carotid in the neck would be equally contraindicated. The only safe surgical attack would then be, first a partial occlusion of the carotid in the neck, with a band of some type; I prefer a band of fascia lata. Four to six weeks later this artery can with safety be totally occluded. Finally, if there remains evidence of the patency of the aneurysm the intracranial exposure and attack can be carried out without risk of inadequate cerebral blood supply. That the age at which the carotid can be ligated with impunity varies with different individuals is shown by the fact that Magnus[14] ligated the internal carotid artery in a patient sixty-nine years old, and McKendree and Doshay[12] report another ligation by Elsberg in a patient age fifty-eight; Jefferson's case was fifty-seven. The end-result, of course, depends entirely upon the amount of collateral circulation through the anterior cerebral and posterior communicating arteries, and this will always be a variable factor regardless of age.

RESULTS.—In Case 2, the return of all functions and the disappearance of all symptoms were prompt and complete. Within six weeks the eyelid and all of the movements of the extra-ocular muscles were perfectly normal. In Case 1, the symptomic cure was just as prompt and complete but the return of the muscular function in the lids and eyeballs has been slow and two years after the operation is still incomplete. In Case 3, all symptoms disappeared immediately. It was nearly three months before the eyelid began to elevate and at the end of four and one-half months the first return of movement in abduction of the eyeball had begun; other movements were as yet unchanged. The great difference in the rapidity with which the ptosis and extra-ocular palsies have cleared is noteworthy. The explanation can only be conjectured. It is noteworthy that the two cases in which the beginning and rate of improvement has been slower, had absolutely complete loss of all functions referable to the third nerve before operation; whereas, the patient whose oculomotor functions cleared so quickly and so rapidly had only weakness and not total paralysis of these functions. Our conclusion is that in the latter case the aneurysm had only pressed upon the nerve, whereas, in the other two, more slowly improving cases, the third nerve was probably incorporated in the wall of the aneurysm within the cavernous sinus.

The visual changes following the operations have also been interesting. In the paper on the treatment of carotid-cavernous arteriovenous aneurysms it was shown that the same two ligations of the internal carotid artery, *i.e.*, in the neck and intracranially, did not affect the vision on the affected side. Since the ophthalmic artery arises from the carotid between the two ligatures, the effect upon vision was anxiously awaited and fortunately proved to be unaffected. Doubtless because there was adequate collateral circulation from the branches of the external carotid within the orbit. From the three cases in this series, the vision remained normal in two; in fact it was greatly improved in one, *i.e.*, from 20/50 to 20/20. In the remaining case, Case 1, however, the vision was totally lost. In this case a plug of muscle was introduced into the carotid (Brooks' method) in the neck. It would seem reasonable to believe that from this a propagating thrombus had developed and incorporated the lumen of the ophthalmic artery and perhaps even of the retinal artery. Proof of this is, of course, not obtainable, but in none of the six other patients with the same double ligation was vision made worse.

SUMMARY AND CONCLUSIONS

(1) Three cases of arterial aneurysms of the intracranial portion of the internal carotid artery are presented. In each the aneurysm was alongside the carotid as it came through the cavernous sinus.

(2) Each was treated by ligating the in-

ternal artery, both intracranially (with a clip) and in the neck (with a ligature of silk). All are symptomatically well.

(3) The use of arteriography to disclose the aneurysm is discussed. It is a valuable diagnostic abjunct in silent aneurysms with subarachnoid bleeding. At the present time its use would appear to be indicated only when a diagnosis is impossible by other means. Perhaps its more frequent employment in precise localization and size of the aneurysm when its diagnosis is clear may be in the offing.

REFERENCES

[1]Adams, J.: Aneurysm of Internal Carotid in the Cavenous Sinus. *Lancet, 2:* 768, 1869.

[2]Albright, F.: The Syndrome Produced by Aneurysm At or Near the Junction of the Internal Carotid Artery and the Circle of Willis. Bull., *Johns Hopkins Hosp., 44:* 215, 1929.

[3]Beadles, C. F.: Aneurysms of the Large Cerebral Arteries. *Brain, 30:* 20, 1907.

[4]Dandy, W. E.: Intracranial Aneurysm of the Internal Carotid Artery. *Ann. Surg., 107:* 654, 1938. *Idem:* Carotid-Cavernous Aneurysms (Pulsating Exophthalmos). *Zentralbl. Neurochir., 2:* 77, 1937; *Ann. Surg., 102:* 916, 1935.

[5]Dott, N. M.: Intracranial Aneurysms: Cerebral Arterio-Radiography: Surgical Treatments. *Edindurgh M.J., 40:* 219, 1933. *Idem:* Intracranial Aneurysms and Allied Clinical Syndromes: Cerebral Arteriography in Their Management. *Lisboa med., 14:* 782, 1937.

[6]Fearnsides, E. S.: Intracranial Aneurysms. *Brain, 39:* 224, 1916.

[7]Forbus, W. D.: Uber den Ursprung gewisser Aneurysmen der basalen Hirnarterien. *Centralbl. f. Allge. Path. und Pathol. Anat., 44:* 243, 1928–1929.

[8]Heuer, G. J., and Dandy, W. E.: Roentgenography in the Localization of Brain Tumors, Based Upon a Series of One Hundred Consecutive Cases. *Bull. Johns Hopkins Hosp., 26:* 311, 1916.

[9]Hutchinson, J.: Aneurysm of the Internal Carotid Within the Skull; Diagnosed Eleven Years Before Patient's Death; Spontaneous Cure. *Trans. Clin. Soc. London, 8:* 127, 1875.

[10]Jefferson, G.: On the Saccular Aneurysms of the Internal Carotid Artery in the Cavernous Sinus. *Brit. J. Surg., 26:* 267, 1938.

[11]McConnell, A. A.: Subchiasmal Aneurysm Treated by Implantation of Muscle. *Zentralbl. Neurochir., 5–6:* 269, 1937.

[12]McKendree, C. A., and Doshay, L. J.: Visual Disturbances of Obscure Etiology, Produced by

Focal Intracranial Lesions Implicating the Optic Nerves. *Bull. New York Neurol. Inst.*, *5:* 223, 1936.

[13]McKinney, J. M., Acree, T., and Soltz, S. E.: The Syndrome of the Unruptured Aneurysm of the Intracranial Portion of the Internal Carotid Artery. *Bull. New York Neurol. Inst.*, *5:* 247, 1936.

[14]Magnus, V.: Aneurysm of the Internal Carotid Artery. *J.A.M.A.*, *88:* 1712–1713, 1927.

[15]Matas, R.: Aneurysms of the Circle of Willis. *Ann. Surg.*, *107:* 660, 1938.

[16]Moniz, E.: *L'Angiographie Cerebrales.* Masson, Paris, 1934.

[17]Sands, I. J.: Aneurysms of Cerebral Vessels. *Arch. Neurol. & Psychiat.*, *21:* 37, 1929.

[18]Sosman, M. C., and Vogt, E. C.: Aneurysms of the Internal Carotid Artery and the Circle of Willis from a Roentgenological Viewpoint. *Am. J. Roentgenol.*, *15:* 122, 1926.

[19]Symonds, C. P.: Contributions to the Clinical Study of Intracranial Aneurysms. *Guy's Hosp. Rep.*, *73:* 139, 1923.

[20]Tonnis, W.: Traumatischer Aneurysma der linken Art. carotis int., *etc. Zentralbl. Chir.*, *61:* 844, 1934.

[21]Trevani, E.: Ein als para-sellar Tumor operiertes Aneurysma der carotis interna. *Deutsch. Ztschr. f. Chir.*, *237:* 534, 1932.

[22]Walsh, M. N., and Love, J. S.: Intracranial Carotid Aneurysm—Successful Surgical Treatment. *Proc. Staff Meeting, Mayo Clin.*, *12:* 81–88, 1937.

LX

PAPILLEDEMA WITHOUT INTRACRANIAL PRESSURE (OPTIC NEURITIS)*

Although papilledema is the most significant objective finding in brain tumors, it is by no means pathognomonic of this lesion. In 1937, the writer[1] reported a series of cases in which there was bilateral papilledema with intracranial pressure and yet no brain tumor. This condition, whatever the unknown cause or causes may be, could be safely differentiated from the tumor group by ventriculography. The ventricles were uniformly small, but showed no displacement. In the course of a most variable period of time, the intracranial pressure subsided and the patients remained permanently well. They were spared major operative procedures which would otherwise have been indicated, only a subtemporal decompression was necessary to preserve life and vision pending subsidence of the intracranial pressure.

The present report is concerned with another, even larger, group of cases having papilledema, usually bilateral, at times unilateral, frequently with hemorrhages in the eyegrounds, and usually with a mild degree of headache and with varying degrees of visual loss. This group differs from the foregoing one in the absence of intracranial pressure. The underlying pathologic process causing the papilledema, whatever its character or the underlying cause, is, therefore, largely of local origin and may be classified as "optic neuritis," "papillitis," or "retrobulbar neuritis," if it is understood that these designations do not connote an inflammatory process, which it may or may not be. There can be little doubt that the pathologic process is, in many instances at least, not strictly confined to the optic nerve or

nerves because of the frequent coexistence of other signs and symptoms, such as headaches, diplopia, dizziness and perhaps nausea and vomiting. But the intracranial involvement beyond the optic nerves is rarely great or severe. There can also, I think, be no doubt that this is not strictly a pathologic or clinical entity, for in a few cases at least, the ophthalmologic picture is an initial manifestation of multiple sclerosis, and in one patient who died 14 months later the microscopic sections of the brain showed diffuse chronic encephalitis involving the cerebral cortex. However, the number of such cases, studied over a long period of time, is so small that one can be equally certain that multiple sclerosis or encephalitis is the exception rather than the rule. From the evidence at hand it is not possible to say that the pathologic process is one of demyelinization in the optic nerves, or an inflammatory or perhaps some other process.

On the whole, the pathologic process and its signs and symptoms are acute or relatively so; it subsides spontaneously with or without a permanent visual defect and has almost no tendency to recur (a single exception). In most of these cases the differential diagnosis from a brain tumor has been made by ventriculography, and the absence of intracranial pressure has been determined by manometric readings of the spinal fluid by spinal puncture. In some of the later cases the clinical picture has seemed adequate to make the diagnosis without either ventriculography or spinal puncture. The principal differential diagnostic test of this condition is a rather precipitate loss of vision—much too rapid to be possible from the effects of intracranial pressure. One also considers, though with

*Reprinted from the *Annals of Surgery*, 110: 2, August, 1939.

628

less assurance, the relatively slight headache accompanying such a high grade of papilledema with retinal hemorrhages.

Since there is no intracranial pressure, operations upon the brain are not indicated. It is cases of this kind that have been subjected to exploratory craniotomies with negative findings, to decompressions and to operations upon the paranasal sinuses. The latter operations have been performed on the assumption that an inflammatory process has extended through the bone of the skull and into the optic nerves. And many teeth have been pulled in the search for an inflammatory focus.

Since the pathologic process is one of relatively short duration and clears spontaneously, it is not surprising that excellent results have been claimed following any therapeutic efforts, whether surgical or medical, but the results are, of course, *post hoc, propter hoc.*

Forty-four cases of this condition are included in this report, and the end-results presented in thirty-one. From the remaining thirteen, no answer has been received to inquiries by letter. The cases are spread over the past 15 years. The results of the study are presented in the accompanying table and are summarized in the ensuing resume.

SEX AND AGE INCIDENCE. Curiously enough, females are almost three times as frequently affected as are males—the exact number of each being thirty-two and twelve. Such a great difference in the sexes must carry some significance but I know of no explanation.

This condition occurs in every decade of life up to the seventieth year, and with surprising regularity except in the second decade where the number was more than double. The actual numbers by decades were six, fifteen, six, six, seven and four.

RESUME OF SIGNS AND SYMPTOMS: DURATION. To the time of admission to the hospital, the condition has existed less than one month in twenty-one, or nearly half of the cases; less than three months in thirty-one, 70 per cent of the cases. It was less than six months in thirty-eight cases, or 86 per cent; less than one year in the remaining six. In one case, under observation almost from the beginning of the illness, the patient was practically blind within five days; three days later the visual fields and visual acuity were normal, and one year later the vision was still perfect. There can be no doubt that many patients who appear months or years after an initial attack of visual loss have had edema at the onset, and at this late date there remains only some evidence of pallor in the optic disks.

HEADACHE. In thirty-seven cases from the series, headache was a conspicuous symptom; in five it was absent, and in two not mentioned. In most instances the headache appeared almost simultaneously with loss of vision. It was never as severe as in brain tumors, although instances of the latter without headache are by no means uncommon. At times the headache was bilateral, and at other times unilateral. Often it was in the frontal region, or behind the eye, and not infrequently more of a stinging, boring pain rather than an ache.

As noted above, the relatively slight degree of headache was in such marked contrast to the severe grade of papilledema that the diagnosis of an intracranial neoplasm was considered unlikely.

DIPLOPIA, NAUSEA, VOMITING, DIZZINESS AND CONVULSIONS. Double vision was present in thirteen cases and absent in twenty-five, *i.e.,* it was present in roughly one-third of the cases. Only in three cases was there an extra-ocular palsy and in one of these it was bilateral. One of the unilateral palsies was the case of encephalitis; the bilateral palsy was in a particularly severe illness with total blindness which has persisted through the patient is otherwise well, eleven years later; the third case has not responded to our letter of inquiry. The appearance of diplopia means, of course, that the pathologic process has extended beyond the optic nerves. Except in the cases where an extra-ocular palsy has followed, the diplopia has always been of short duration—in one instance only thirty minutes.

In nine cases there was nausea, and in twelve vomiting, but in two of the latter it was said to have followed medicine by mouth. In no instance was either the nausea or vomiting prolonged or severe, and in many vomiting occurred only once.

Dizziness occurred in ten cases and was never severe.

Convulsions were present in none. This negative note is recorded because it is fairly important evidence against any degree of cerebral involvement.

OTHER SIGNS AND SYMPTOMS. One patient had numbness of the face; she has since been followed (two and three-fourths years) and has had no return of it. Another had weakness of the right arm, polydipsia and palsy of the right sixth nerve; her subsequent course is unknown; it may be a case of multiple sclerosis. Another patient subsequently developed characteristic signs and symptoms of multiple sclerosis, *i.e.,* ataxia, Romberg, staggering gait and urinary incontinence. A bilateral Babinski sign was elicited in one patient; it has since disappeared and she remains perfectly well. Bilateral ataxia was noted in another patient, who probably had an acute encephalitis following pneumonia (Streptococcus); except for a severe loss of vision she recovered completely. Buzzing in one ear was noted by one patient whose subsequent course is not known, and by another who recovered with total blindness but with no return of the buzzing; bilateral exophthalmos of low grade developed during the present illness and subsequently disappeared.

In three patients adiposity was excessive. In two, the menses had disappeared, and in the third, they subsequently disappeared but returned following injections of hypophyseal extract. In each of the above three adipose individuals the increased weight had long antedated (one, three and twelve years) the visual disturbance and could, therefore, have had no bearing upon it. Since this abnormal grade of adiposity is so commonly associated with menstrual irregularity and loss, it is probable that this disturbed function was also not related to the papilledema. However, in one patient the amenorrhea developed only one month before her visual loss and she dated the present illness from it.

Polydipsia was a symptom in one case and was perhaps a manifestation of encephalitis.

Three patients in this series had hypertension—two of moderate (170, 168) and one of severe grade (220). The frequent association of papilledema with hypertension of severe grade is well known. I have excluded from this series those cases in which the papilledema appeared to be directly related to the hypertension. In the three cases included in this report, there can scarcely be a doubt that the hypertension was entirely independent and unrelated. One patient with a blood pressure of one hundred and seventy eight died eight years later following an abdominal operation, the findings of which are unknown. Her vision had remained unchanged in the interim. The most surprising case was that of a colored woman, age forty-four, blood pressure 220/110. Following an acute visual disturbance, with 4 D. of papilledema and hemorrhages in both eyegrounds, the patient's vision returned almost to normal and has remained so for six and one-half years, and despite continuous hard work she is symptomless and her blood pressure remains 220/110. Her blood pressure surely has nothing to do with her acute visual episode. The third patient, whose pressure was 180, cannot be traced.

In only a single patient was there a positive Wassermann reaction; this was positive both in the blood and spinal fluid. Whether or not it was related to the papilledema cannot be determined. The eyegrounds rapidly became normal during vigorous antisyphilitic treatment. The story is so similar to that of so many other cases—all without syphilis—that I doubt the relationship.

ETIOLOGY.—That this series of cases contains not a single pathologic entity is shown by the fact that there is certainly one and probably a second case of multiple sclerosis, and one and perhaps two more cases of encephalitis. The association of papilledema with both of these lesions is well known. But I do not believe any of the remaining cases could fall under either multiple sclerosis or encephalitis.

A nonspecific inflammatory origin is suggested in three cases. In one instance there was tenderness and swelling of one eyelid at the onset of symptoms, and the papilledema developed only in the corresponding eyeground which contained numerous small hemorrhages. Five and one-half years later the center of the disk was filled with a scar that entirely concealed the entering blood vessels; the visual acuity was 20/20 in each eye but a temporal defect remained in the affected eye. In another case, the left eyelid was swollen and painful and there was lacrimation at the time of onset of the visual change. The other eye had been blind from birth. She had had unilateral retinal hemorrhages, but her subsequent course is not known. The third patient had redness of the eyeball for two months before vision was affected. Although the eyesight was badly affected and there were numerous hemorrhages in the eyegrounds, he reports normal vision 11 years later.

A fourth patient had just returned from a ride on horseback, three weeks after recovery from pneumonia (Streptococcus and influenza organisms were grown from cultures), when she suddenly became confused, semicomatose and delirious. She is said to have had fever, vomiting, ataxia of both hands, in addition to papilledema and loss of vision. There must have been a very diffuse encephalopathy, and occurring so soon after the attack of pneumonia it would appear probable that this was the same source of the inflammatory process in the brain—though without pus formation.

A fifth patient had stinging eyes and photophobia—both suggestive, but not indicative of mild inflammatory origin.

It is worthy of note and perhaps significant that cases with the probable evidence of slight inflammatory character have all been severe, in that they have had hemorrhages and visual defects. However, if these findings are evidences of inflammatory origin, none of them have been pyogenic and none have shown alterations of the cerebrospinal fluid. In none of the remaining cases—excepting the single case of syphilis—has there been any evidence to suggest that the process may be of inflammatory nature.

From six of the forty-four cases (13 per cent), therefore, there is evidence of an underlying inflammatory process of some peculiar type. There were pain, redness and swelling of the eyelids—cardinal signs of infection—but in none was there the slightest indication of the character of the infection.

Although a demyelinizing process is conceivable (perhaps like that of multiple sclerosis), there is no proof. Moreover, with one exception, there has been but a single insult to the optic nerves, and after this has passed the cure has appeared to be permanent. One would expect repeated and long continued attacks if a demyelinization process were the cause.

THE CEREBROSPINAL FLUID: PRESSURE. The pressure of spinal fluid was measured in nine cases, in only two of which were the readings in the higher reaches of normal—250 and 280. The actual readings were 80, 120, 120, 130, 170, 170, 250 and 280.

In twenty-four cases, the flow of fluid from the ventricular fluid (tapped for ventriculography) was such as to indicate the absence of intracranial pressure. In two instances it was reported to have been slightly increased.

CELL COUNT. Cells were counted in twenty-two cases. The highest count was twelve; in the remaining it was 10 (one case) or less.

GLOBULIN CONTENT. The fluid was examined for excess globulin, but in no instance, even the case of syphilis, was there an increased amount.

ROENTGENOGRAMS AND VENTRICULOGRAPHY. Roentgenograms of the head were made in nearly all cases, and in none was there a positive or even a suggestive finding. Ventriculograms were made in thirty-seven cases, and since tumors were suspected, all injections of air were made through ventricular punctures. All showed normal, symmetrical ventricles, thereby unequivocally excluding intracranial tumors. In two instances, the ventricles were fairly large (both in older persons) and representing, we thought, the normal for those individuals. The ventricles, though small, were, on the whole, somewhat larger than in the group with papilledema and intracranial pressure but without brain tumor.

VISION. Of the forty-four cases, forty-one complained of disturbance of vision. The most common complaint was dimness or blurring of vision. The degree of visual loss varied from a purely subjective disturbance without actual objective loss in any form to complete blindness. In fourteen or approximately one-third of the cases, the visual acuity and visual fields were normal. In eight, there was unilateral loss of vision in some degree, and in twenty-two, or 50 per cent, there was bilateral loss of some degree. In two-thirds of the total number there was visual loss.

In nineteen cases, blind spots were enlarged on one or both sides, and in ten the blind spots were normal. In thirteen, there were scotomata or field defects of varying size.

EYEGROUNDS. In every case there was papilledema in one or both eyes—forty-two bilateral and two unilateral. Hemorrhages were present in the eyegrounds in nineteen cases (43 per cent); in five, the hemorrhages were unilateral and in fourteen bilateral. The hemorrhages were usually petechial, but in two cases they were large and flame-shaped.

ULTIMATE RESULTS. Thirty-one cases have been traced, some by letters; others

have returned for examination. Two are dead, one, eighteen months later of chronic encephalitis, which was doubtless the lesion at the time of our examination; the other patient died eight years later following an abdominal operation. Only two of these patients are reported in less than a year after the initial study; seven have gone two years or less; four between two and three years; two between three and five years; nine between five and ten years; and seven more than ten years; the longest 14½ years.

In seeking the ultimate effects upon vision, the original cases have been divided into four groups: Those with (1) papilledema only; (2) hemorrhages in the eyegrounds; (3) scotomata and enlarged blind spots; and (4) field defects.

PAPILLEDEMA ONLY. There were nine cases in this group, and in all the vision has remained normal both subjectively according to the patients' report and objectively in those who have come for examination in the check-up. Five of these are over ten years, the remaining between one and one-half and three and one-half years.

HEMORRHAGES IN EYEGROUNDS. Of the thirteen cases with hemorrhages in the eyegrounds, one is blind and was blind at the time of our first study nine years earlier; a field defect remains in three; and in nine the vision is said to be normal.

The return of visual acuity in several of these patients is most striking. One patient's visual acuity returned from 12/200 to 20/70 (six and one-half years); another from 3/200 and 12/200 to 20/30 in each eye (three years); and another from 10/200 and 80/200 to 20/20 in each eye (six years).

SCOTOMATA AND BLIND SPOTS. Of thirteen patients who have been followed, nine are now normal, and in four the vision has remained unchanged.

FIELD DEFECTS. This is the group with the most severe visual changes and with the poorest prognosis. Of eleven cases, the vision in seven has remained unchanged; in one, the vision returned to normal in one eye and is only useful in the other (one and one-half years later). At the time of the original study in the latter patient both eyes were essentially the same, he being practically blind. In the three remaining cases of this group the vision has returned to normal in both eyes. In one of these patients, blind when first seen, the visual acuity and visual fields are normal six years later. In another who was blind in one eye, the visual acuity and fields are again normal two years later.

SUMMARY AND CONCLUSIONS

(1) Forty-four cases of papilledema without intracranial pressure are presented. The underlying etiologic or pathologic basis is unknown, except that two cases of multiple sclerosis and two of encephalitis are included. No evidence of either of these lesions can be found in the remaining cases. A few of the cases appear to follow a mild nonspecific inflammatory process in the eye or lids, but these cases are distinctly in the minority.

(2) Although there is evidence of some intracranial involvement in some cases, in others there is none. Moreover, the papilledema may be unilateral, although it is much more commonly bilateral. On the whole, the pathologic process is decidedly local and any intracranial extension and its effects are usually mild and of little concern. Exceptions to this statement are, of course, the examples of encephalitis and multiple sclerosis.

(3) The condition carries no danger to life, and heals spontaneously in the course of a few weeks or months. No form of treatment is known to be effective. Certainly, all forms of operative intervention are contraindicated.

(4) Women are affected nearly three times as frequently as men. It occurs in all decades of life in about equal frequency, except the second, where it is two and one-half times as common.

(5) The ontstanding symptom is loss of vision—usually a blurring at first. Scotomata, field defects and blindness may develop with great rapidity, and may or may not remain. Great defects of vision and visual acuity, even blindness, may disappear and even normal vision may return. Permanent blindness resulted in one case. Hemorrhages in the eyegrounds occur with great frequency.

(6) There are no changes in the cerebrospinal fluid; the pressure is not increased. Ventriculograms are always normal.

(7) In only one case did the papilledema recur. This was three years after the initial attack and three years ago. On each occasion the vision was seriously defective, but returned almost to normal. The eyegrounds show only slight pallor of the disks. In another case, a dense scar fills the disk and obliterates all of its landmarks.

REFERENCES

[1]Dandy, W. E.: Intracranial Pressure Without Brain Tumor. Diagnosis and Treatment. *Ann. Surg., 106:* 492, 1937.

[2]Bordley, James, Jr.: Ocular Manifestations of the Paranasal Sinuses. *Arch. Ophth., 1:* 137, 1921.

[3]Cushing, H.: Accessory Sinus Disease and Choked Disk. *J.A.M.A., 75:* 236, 1920.

[4]Fuchs: Case of Eye Disturbance in Accessory Sinus Disease. *Lehrbuch der Augenheikunde, 10:* 766, 1905.

[5]Hajek, H.: Kritik des rhinogenen Ursprunges der retrobulbaren neuritis. *Wien. klin. Wchnschr., 33:* 267, 1920.

[6]Marburg, O.: Retrobulbar Optic Neuritis and Multiple Sclerosis (Bibl.). *Zeitschr. Augenh., 44:* 125, 1920.

[7]Oliver, K. S., and Crowe, S. J.: Retrobulbar Neuritis and Infection of Accessory Nasal Sinuses. *Arch. Otolaryngol., 6:* 503, 1927.

[8]Richardson, S. A.: Optic Neuritis: Resulting from Hyperplastic Ethmoiditis and Sphenoiditis. *J. Florida M.A., 9:* 22, 1922.

[9]Stark, H. H.: Retrobulbar Neuritis, Secondary to Disease of the Nasal Sinuses. *J.A.M.A., 77:* 678, 1921.

[10]Stough, J. T.: Choking of Optic Disks in Diseases Other Than Tumor of Brain. *Arch. Ophth., 8:* 821, 1932.

[11]Walker, C. B.: Retrobulbar Neuritis and Multiple Sclerosis. *California and Western Med., 34:* 1, 5; 2, 83, 1931.

[12]Weill, G.: Relationship Between Inflammation of Posterior Sinuses and Disease of Nervus Opticus. *Arch. Ophth., 1:* 307, 1929.

[13]White, L. E.: Blindness from Teeth, Tonsils and Accessory Sinuses. *Boston Med. & Surg. J., 192:* 64, 1925.

LXI

THE CENTRAL CONNECTIONS OF THE VESTIBULAR PATHWAYS*

AN EXPERIMENTAL STUDY

WALTER E. DANDY AND PAUL A. KUNKEL

Our interest in the unsolved problems of Meniere's disease prompted this experimental investigation on the auditory nerves and cerebellum. The results following section of the vestibular nerves in animals are so different from those obtained in human beings that their transfer to man is impossible. Indeed had the devastating effects of dividing the auditory nerve in dogs and cats antedated the operation on human beings [1a,b,c,d] the cure of Meniere's disease by this operative attack might well have been delayed.

Apparently there is no difference in the effects produced in dogs and cats except in degree, the cats reacting more severely. The operative attack upon the auditory nerves and the cerebellum was found to be much more difficult in both dogs and cats than upon human beings, largely because of the excessive vascularity about the dural sinuses in the posterior cranial fossa. Bleeding from this source is difficult to avoid, because the dura is so thin and so closely attached to the bone. By "rongeuring" the bone very cautiously and in very small amounts at each step, it is possible to separate the dura and stop effectively the bleeding by application of wax. The attack upon either the auditory nerves or the cerebellum is merely a matter of painstaking care. Without a bony defect of adequate size the soft cerebellum quickly becomes edematous from the effects of trauma and thereby the interpretation of the

results may be vitiated by the complications. This warning applies both to section of the auditory nerve and to the removal of the cerebellum. In hemisection the remaining half of the cerebellum may be damaged so severely as to be in large part necrotic. In partial or total section the brain stem may be injured. With either complication the experiment may be so defective that the results will be worthless.

In cutting the auditory nerve the bony defect must be made so far laterally that the cerebellum may be retracted without trauma. Hemisection of the cerebellum is done by splitting the vermis from the tentorium anteriorly to the membranous covering of the apex of the fourth ventricle; this is practically bloodless. The hemisphere then is turned outward and upward until the large peduncle is isolated. This is transected with a scalpel; the cerebellar lobe has only minor attachments along the upper margin of the fourth ventricle. Midsection of the vermis makes either unilateral or total removal of the cerebellum much simpler and practically devoid of trauma to the remaining structures.

Section of the restiform body (middle peduncle) in animals dates back nearly a century. Vulpian [8] (1866) refers to Magendie's experiments in sectioning the middle peduncle of the cerebellum in cats; rotation of the animal with incredible rapidity followed and to the same side. His results were confirmed by Vulpian, Schiff, Hitzig [6] and other great physiologists working about the middle of the nineteenth century. The results were the exact equi-

*Reprinted from the *American Journal of Medical Scienes, 198*:149–155, August, 1939.

valent of destruction of the semicircular canals (Flourens' experiments). Ferrier[3] (1880) and Ferrier and Turner[4] (1898) divided the auditory nerve in rabbits and monkeys; their results were similar to those following section of the restiform body. They refer to earlier experiments of this type by Brown-Sequard. In the course of time the rolling movements subsided and the animals walked again, but in a sprawling, unsteady fashion. Ferrier[3] comments upon the great mortality attending his attempts to expose the cerebellum in dogs and cats: he "succeeded in comparatively few," but the results were the same as in rabbits.

In recent years, Fulton, Liddell and Rioch[5] (1930) sectioned the auditory nerve in cats with greater ease and with more assurance that contiguous structures have not been injured. Their results, however, are not different and were identical with libyrinthectomies. They stress the advantage of "dial" (a barbiturate) anesthesia in facilitating the operative procedure, and doubtless the prolonged anesthesia (36 hours or longer) is responsible for the fact that their animals usually survived and after a period of nine to thirteen days walked again, at first in a very poor sprawling fashion, but gradually improving. Owing to the short duration of ether anesthesia all our animals succumbed within forty-eight hours, the period in which the severity of the whirling movements is at its maximum. After 36 hours it was found that these movements steadily diminished. This was the experience of Ferrier and Turner and later of Northington and Barrera[7] (1934) and of Dow[2] (1938) in monkeys. This also corresponds fairly well with the subjective rotary effects in man following the sectioin of the vestibular nerves. Dow has emphasized the fact that the severity of this disturbance decreases as one ascends the phylogenetic scales. He even found that the effects produced by destruction of the labyrinth in anthropoids (baboons and chimpanzees) were less than in monkeys. Ferrier[3] dwells at some length on the shift from the actual rotation of the body in animals, including monkeys, to the purely subjective visual disturbance that attends lesions of the auditory nerve in human beings. At that time the auditory nerve had, of course, not been sectioned in man.

Our results following section of the auditory nerves in animals are in complete accord with those of all other experimentalists on this line. We are, however, less concerned with these effects than with the central pathways of vestibular function which we believe are concentrated almost entirely in the cerebellum. This view was expressed by Meynert (see Ferrier[3]), but he apparently also believed that the same was true of the auditory pathways, an utterly untenable concept, according to Ferrier, because his experiments had led him to the conclusion that a center for hearing was located in each temporal lobe—a view,

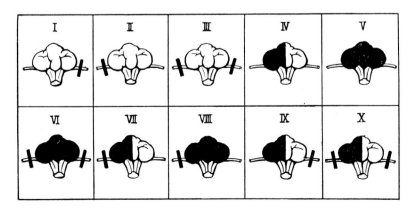

Fɪɢ. 1. Tabulation of experiments.

by the way, that modern cerebral excisions have rendered impossible, at least in human beings.

Experiments

In order to avoid repetition only one protocol has been entered for each experiment, although each has been repeated at least once.

I. ADULT CAT. Section of right eighth nerve (N VIII) (cerebellar approach); ether, November 15, 1934. The animal stood the operation well; 6 hours later it was awake and nervous. There was facial paralysis on the right. It lay against the side of the cage on the right side. Placed on the floor it rolled violently to the right, spinning until it finished exhausted against the wall. If placed on the left side, it immediately rolled over and over, but always to the the the right. It could not stand or walk. Nov. 16: Same reactions. Unable to eat or drink and is fed by tube. Nov. 17: Died. Autopsy showed total section of the right seventh and eighth nerves.

II. ADULT CAT. Total section of eighth nerve left; ether, November 15, 1934. Exactly the same reactions, except whirling to the left. Unable to stand or walk.

III. ADULT CAT. Bilateral section of eighth nerve (cerebellar approach); ether, December 3, 1935. Cat in good condition at end of operation. Six hours later it was awake and lying against the side of the cage. Both sides of the face were paralyzed. It did not respond to noises. Placed on the floor it rolled violently to the right, at other times to the left. It was unable to sit, stand or walk and would not take water or food. Dec. 4: Same reaction as before. Dec. 6: Died. Autopsy showed

total section of both seventh and both eighth nerves.

III. (A) ADULT DOG. Section of nerves VIII, bilateral (cerebellar approach); ether, February 14, 1935. Animal stood operation well. Five hours later marked nystagmus; rolled and spun violently to either side, but not as violently as the cat. Unable to stand, sit or walk. Died following day. Necropsy showed both auditory nerves totally divided.

IV. ADULT CAT. Removed of left half of cerebellum; ether, January 21, 1935. Six hours later cat awake and quite. No turning movements and no rolling at any time. Lay on left side; could not sit up or stand.

V. ADULT CAT. Removal entire cerebellum, January 10, 1935. Cat remained quite, did not whirl at any time. Could maintain sitting position, but could not stand or walk.

VI. ADULT CAT. Removal entire cerebellum and section of both nerves VIII; ether, January 14, 1935. Animal stood the operation well. Six hours later it was awake, lying on right side. Gave no evidence of hearing noises. For most part animal was limp and unable to stand; it remained on either side or back when so placed. When picked up by hind quarters with head and front of body hanging, it executed normal movements (coordinated) of forelegs and turned head from side to side. Jan. 15: Same reactions as yesterday. Will not eat or drink. Jan. 17: Died. Autopsy showed complete extirpation of cerebellum and both eighth nerves were totally divided.

VII. ADULT CAT. Removal left half cerebellum and section nerve VIII *left;* ether, January 17, 1935. Six hours later animal in good condition. Placed on floor it turned and rolled violently *to the left,* coming to rest on

TABLE I
RESULTS OF EXPERIMENTS.

Operation	*Result*
I. Total section *right* N VIII	Violent whirling to right; cannot stand or walk.
II. Total section *left* N VIII	Violent whirling to left; cannot stand or walk.
III. Total section *both right and left* N's VIII	Violent whirling to both sides; cannot stand or walk.
IV. Removal *left* half of cerebellum	No whirling; cannot stand or walk.
V. Removal entire cerebellum	No whirling; cannot stand or walk.
VI. Removal *entire* cerebellum and total section of both N's VIII	No whirling; cannot stand or walk.
VII. Removal *left* half of cerebellum and total section *left* N VIII	Violent whirling to *left;* cannot stand or walk.
VIII. Removal *entire* cerebellum and total section *left* N VIII	*No* whirling; cannot stand or walk.
IX. Removal *left* half of cerebellum and total section right N VIII	No. whirling.
X. Removal *left* half of cerebellum and total section both N's VIII	Violent whirling to left.

the left side. Movements began with turning of head to *left* and then body was rapidly turned. Died following day. Remaining half of cerebellum showed no necrosis; eighth nerve had been totally divided.

VIII. Adult Cat. Section left nerve VIII and left half of cerebellum removed; ether, January 17, 1935. It has since been whirling to the left. Jan. 18: Removed the remaining right half of the cerebellum. Six hours later the cat was awake, quiet and without turning movements. Lay quietly on either side. Picked up by hind quarters, it turned normally either to right or left; moved both forelegs in normal manner. Died the following day. Autopsy showed all cerebellum removed; left auditory nerve was totally divided. Brain stem showed no softening.

IX. Adult Cat. Section right nerve VIII and removal of left half of cerebellum, ether, January 30, 1935. Five hours later it was wide awake. Nystagmus present. It lay on the left side in the cage, tried to push itself about but *did not spin*. Regardless of position and movements induced, no whirling movements could be provoked. When picked up and put on right side it lay quietly. There was a striking contrast to the cats with the cerebellum intact, or with half of cerebellum removed and the ipsolateral nerve VIII sectioned. Movements of all extremities were good. Jan. 31: Same reactions as yesterday. No spinning movements. Feb. 1: Reactions unchanged; it died during the night. Autopsy showed nerve VIII sectioned on right. Right half of cerebellum was in good condition.

X. Adult Cat. Section under ether of both nerves VIII and removal left cerebellar lobe, October 18, 1936. Awake three hours later, had nystagmus. Rolled violently to the *left* until exhausted. Lay on the right side. Oct. 19: similar violent whirling to *left* only. Died during night. Autopsy showed total division of both eighth nerves and an intact right cerebellar lobe.

Summary and Conclusions

A summary of the above experiments in terms of whirling indicates the following:

1. Section of either N VIII results in frequent spells of violent whirling—always rolls to the side of the lesion (Experiments I and II).

2. Section of both N's VIII results in violent whirling—turns to either side (Experiment III).

3. After removal of one-half of the cerebellum there are no rotary movements (Experiment IV).

4. After removal of the entire cerebellum there is no whirling (Experiment V).

5. After section of N VIII and removal of the cerebellar lobe of the same side, violent rotation follows; and the whirling is to the same side (Experiment VII).

6. After secton of one N VIII and removal of the opposite cerebellar hemisphere no whirling results (Experiments IX and X).

From these experiments it will be seen that the ability to sit or stand or walk is completely lost immediately after section of either or both auditory nerves, and as far as we can tell the result is, in this respect, exactly the same as removing either half or all of the cerebellum. The great difference following these two procedures is that after removal of half or all of the cerebellum the animal lies quietly, whereas after section of one or both auditory nerves a terrific whirling of the body results and continues until death results from exhaustion. Fulton, Liddell and Rioch [5] have shown that after section of one or both auditory nerves under prolonged "dial" anesthetic the severe period may be passed under the anesthetic. When the animal responds after thirty-six to forty-eight hours, the rotation is so much less severe that the animal will recover.

The profound effects produced by sectioning one or both auditory nerves are entirely different from those in man.[1a,b,c,d] The body itself is set in motion in a series of violent whirling movements that are precipitated by any slight movement of the body and always occur to the side of the sectioned nerve, or to either side when both nerves are cut. These violent whirling attacks are immediately abolished when the entire cerebellum is removed.

In man, the body itself does not rotate following section of a vestibular nerve, but the effect is one of rotation of objects in the room, or when the eyes are closed of rotation of the body. In man, therefore, the aberrations of vestibular function are transferred to, and translated by, the visual tracts so that the effect produced is subjective and visual; in animals, the untoward effect is somatic and objective. Doubtless the transfer of the vestibular function from the cerebellum in dogs and cats to the visual tracts in human beings is related to a lessened importance of the semicircular canals in man as compared to animals.

In keeping with this change in the functional setup of the vestibular pathways, it is interesting that section of both eighth nerves in man has little, if any, effect upon the equilibrium of the body, but rather the effect is one of jumbling the appearance of objects when the body is in motion, *i.e.,* the effects are upon ocular coordination. These physiologic effects, therefore, indicate the probability that when the vestibular pathways can be accurately charted, those in dogs and cats will predominantly pass to the cerebellum, whereas those in human beings will pass up the brain stem to the centers controlling the extraocular movements.

The fact that the violent rotary movements of the body are instantly and permanently abolished (in dogs and cats) when both cerebellar lobes are removed doubt-less indicates that the central apparatus concerned with equilibrium is very largely, if not entirely concentrated there.

Another striking and perhaps surprising feature of the experiments is the contralateral relationship between the cerebellum and the peripheral vestibular tracts, *i.e.,* bodily rotation after section of an eighth nerve is unaffected by removal of the ipsolateral half of the cerebellum, but is abolished by removal of the contralateral half. This can only mean that the vestibular pathways decussate like the pyramidal tracts.

REFERENCES

[1]Dandy, W. E.: (a) *Arch. Surg., 16:* 1125, 1928; (b) *Bull. Johns Hopkins Hosp., 55:* 232, 1934; (c) *Arch. Otalaryng., 20:* 1, 1934; (d) *Laryngoscope, 47:* 594, 1937.

[2]Dow, R. S.: *Am. J. Physiol., 121:*392, 1938.

[3]Ferrier, D.: *The Functions of the Brain.* New York, G. P. Putnam's Sons, 1880.

[4]Ferrier, D., and Turner, W. A.: *Phil. Trans., 190:*1, 1898.

[5]Fulton, J. F., Liddell, E. S. T., and Rioch, D. McK.: *Brain, 53:*327, 1930.

[6]Hitzig, E.: *Untersuchungen uber das Gehirn,* Berlin, August Hirschwald, 1874.

[7]Northington, P., and Barrera, S. E.: *Arch. Neurol. & Psychiat., 32:*51, 1934.

[8]Vulpian, A.: *Lecons sur la Physiologie du Systeme Nerveux.* Paris, German Bailliere, 1866.

LXII

INTRACRANIAL ANEURYSMS*

There are three types of intracranial aneurysms, venous, arteriovenous and arterial. Venous aneurysms are less common; they arise in the dura or as congenital anlage in the brain. I shall not dwell upon these because they are less difficult to handle surgically.

Arteriovenous aneurysms are of two types, congenital and acquired. All arteriovenous aneurysms that occur in the brain substance are of congenital type. The acquired type are located exclusively in the cavernous sinus in the base of the skull. Acquired arteriovenous aneurysms cannot arise in the brain substance because there are no generalized large arteries and veins, so that when they occur in the brain substance they are due to coils of vessels arising congenitally and failing to develop into the usual capillary system and, therefore, maintaining direct communication between the arteries and veins. They are usually productive of epilepsy and are diagnosed either by calcifications that occur in the arterial walls, or by an air injection or exploration. There is very little that can be done for most of them. There are many of these aneurysms that extend directly through the skull into the scalp, and these can be treated by removing a portion of the aneurysm in the scalp and bone, but unless the intracranial aneurysm is in the silent part of the brain it does not lend itself to extirpation.

The arteriovenous aneurysms arising in the cavernous sinus may be congenital or acquired. They arise between lines of fracture that extend through the middle fossa of the base of the skull. The carotid artery is torn and its blood then passes directly into the cavernous sinus and the main channels from the cavernous sinus pass into the orbit largely through the orbital veins. These become of enormous size, contain pulsating arterial blood, they push the eyeball forward causing exophthalmos and cause greatly dilated channels over the forehead, nose and face. Eventually they lead to blindness with or without a glaucoma. This is the only place in the body where a large artery passes through a large venous channel. Usually for the development of an arteriovenous aneurysm it is necessary to have a perforation of a contiguous artery and vein, but in the cavernous sinus it is only necessary to rupture the wall of the artery to produce an aneurysm because the aneurysm lies in the vein.

About one-third of these aneurysms are cured by ligating the internal carotid artery in the neck. These are cured only because of stasis resulting from the lowered blood pressure. In two-thirds of the cases this does not occur and no material benefit is obtained. When ligation of the internal carotid in the neck does not effect a cure, it is then necessary to ligate the internal carotid artery intracranially. This is done by placing a silver clip upon the carotid where it enters the cranial chamber along the optic nerve. It is not a difficult procedure and is attended with very little risk in skilled hands.

This will cure the aneurysm because there is only one sizable branch between the ligation in the neck and that in the cranial chamber, namely the ophthalmic artery and this is not enough to maintain the aneurysm.

We have had eight such aneurysms which have been cured in this way.

The remaining aneurysms that I wish to consider are arterial; they arise within the carotid canal and bulge into the cranial chamber, or they arise along the carotid artery where its dividing branches are

639

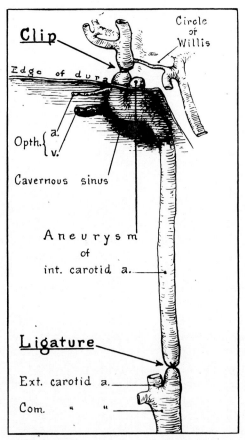

Fig. 1 Diagrammatic representation of position of arterial and arteriovenous aneurysms in the carotid canal. The drawing indicates the method of trapping the aneurysm between ligatures.

reached at the base of the brain. The diagnosis of these aneurysms is made upon the third nerve palsy and sudden pain in the left side of the head and back of the eye. This pain is due to an extensive rupture of the aneurysm and may be repeated several times before a large hemorrhage results in death.

The treatment of these aneurysms is of two types: If the aneurysm comes off the carotid artery intracranially the neck of the sac can at times be closed by a silver clip and the sac itself shrivelled with the electrocautery. This we have done once for an aneurysm that broke through from the cavernous sinus. We have had six of these. The carotid artery is ligated intracranially with a silver clip and the internal carotid artery is ligated with silk in the neck. The aneurysm is then trapped between these ligatures exactly in the same fashion as with the arteriovenous aneurysms. These double ligations will cure the aneurysm because the collateral is inadequate to maintain it.

Another type of aneurysm is a small miliary dilitation at any point along the circle of Willis. This gives rise to a subarachnoid hemorrhage and does not give localizing signs. The only way to localize this aneurysm is by the injection of thorotrast into the internal carotid. I have never been willing to use this very extensively because of the danger of cerebral thrombi which have been reported in a very high percentage of the cases. It may be that the seriousness of the lesion may warrant its use, even with such handicaps in the future.

The treatment of intracranial aneurysms is just beginning, but the cure of eight arteriovenous and seven arterial aneurysms is evidence that the lesion is not of the hopeless type that one might suspect from their vicious character.

LXIII

SECTION OF THE HUMAN HYPOPHYSIAL STALK*

ITS RELATION TO DIABETES INSIPIDUS AND HYPOPHYSIAL FUNCTIONS

That diabetes insipidus in man is caused by lesions in the environs of the hypothalamus is well established by human clinical and pathologic material. It is indeed pathognomonic of a lesion of some type in this general region. However, the precise limits of the neurogenic center have not been established. For example, the relationship of the stalk of the hypophysis (infundibulum), the supra-optic and paraventricular nuclei, the tuber cinereum and the component parts of the hypophysis itself still remain in dispute. Human pathologic material, particularly tumors, although the safest source of interpretation as applied to man, has nevertheless been of little value in sharply localizing this center because, with few exceptions, the lesions have been so large that more than one of the disputed areas have been involved.

The animal experiments on this problem are open to even more criticism, because the component parts of the so-called hypothalamic-hypophysial ensemble are so closely related that it is virtually impossible to attack one part without affecting others. In dogs and cats the hypophysis lies in such direct contact with the base of the brain that the hypophysial stalk is little more than a name. It is impossible to divide or place a clip on the infundibulum without at the same time traumatizing both the hypophysis and the hypothalamus. Moreover, in these animals hypophysial cells are spread along the pars tuberalis and always the microscopic presence or absence of these cells constitutes support or objection to any particular theory. Reich-

ert and I[1] inspected this region directly and produced lesions with the greatest possible precision but concluded from the capricious results that the experimental attack could not, in its present form at least, offer a solution of the problem. Camus and Roussy[2] and soon thereafter Bailey and Bremer[3] concluded from their canine experiments that the center was at the base of the brain and that the hypophysis had nothing to do with diabetes insipidus. We were inclined to agree with them. On the other hand, Biggart and Alexander[4] and Fisher, Ingram and Ranson,[5] who have concentrated on the experimental attack, are quite dogmatic in concluding from results which appear to be no less capricious than our own that the hypophysis is a necessary part of the anatomic setup for water control and therefore for the induction of diabetes insipidus. Both Biggart and the Northwestern University investigators have probably done the best experimental work that is possible and their work is quite generally accepted, and yet their conclusions are not satisfying to one who has been intimately associated with the clinical side of diabetes insipidus. It is their opinion that polyuria and polydipsia are due to the loss of an antidiuretic hormone which is secreted by the posterior lobe of the hypophysis and that the loss of this hormone is due to the deprivation of its nerve supply which passes from the supraoptic nuclei down the infundibulum to the posterior lobe. They also agree that the intact, or at least partially functioning, anterior lobe is an indispensable part of the mechanism—a conception first advanced by von Hann[6] based on a group of human

*Reprinted from *The Journal of the American Medical Association, 114*:312–314, January 27, 1940.

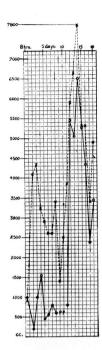

Chart 1. Degree of polyuria and polydipsia immediately after section of the hypophysial stalk, Jan. 24, 1928. Fluid intake is indicated in these charts by dashes and the urine output by the solid line.

hypophysial material—which was poorly chosen, however, for such a hypothesis.

Their conclusions, however, do not answer the following clinical facts: (1) Hypophysial tumors confined to the sella turcica (i.e., not affecting the hypophysial stalk or the hypothalamus) never induce diabetes insipidus regardless of the amount of destruction of the hypophysis; (2) operations on the human hypophysis for hypophysial tumors are never followed by diabetes insipidus unless the stalk or base of the brain is traumatized.

Recently the supra-optic and paraventricular nuclei have been postulated as part of the neurogenic mechanism. They may well be part or even an essential part of a center for water control, but the evidence is not convincing. In this connection it is worthy of note that in a recent assembly of six cases of colloid cysts filling the third ventricle I did not find a history of diabetes insipidus in one before operation, and in none did it follow their removal.

Of nineteen other solid tumors filling the third ventricle and producing greater pressure on the hypothalamus, there was a history of polyuria and polydipsia in only three. These facts only make one wonder why compression of the supra-optic and paraventricular nuclei, if they are parts of the center, produces diabetes insipidus so infrequently.

Two quite contradictory facts at once confuse the picture when an attempt is made to draw final deductions concerning a possible hormone from the posterior lobe: (1) Injections of the posterior lobe usually, but not always, markedly diminish the output of urine and intake of fluids in diabetes insipidus, and yet (2) the posterior lobe is excessively a nervous structure and does not contain glandular cells unless one accepts the occasional acini of the pars intermedia that intrude or unless the pars intermedia is included as part of the posterior lobe.

The transfer of results obtained on experimental animals to man is never too certain. The solution of this problem will doubtless be from well selected cases of human material. In man there is complete anatomic separation of the hypophalamus and hypophysis by a hypophysial stalk that is a centimeter or more in length, and hypophysial cells are not scattered along its course. In due time small tumors, or perhaps other lesions, will be found involving

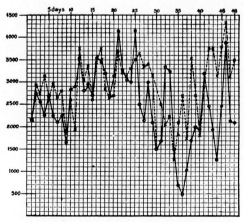

Chart 2. Fluid intake and urine output on second admission, Feb. 6, 1933.

only one part of the ensemble. Indeed one perfect specimen of this type has been described by Futcher.[7] It was a small metastatic tumor at the base of the brain beginning at the cerebral side of the infundibulum and extending intracerebrally. The hypophysis itself was far removed from any direct effect of the growth. A precise surgical experiment is added in the present communication—sharp transverse section of the hypophysial stalk at its middle and without trauma to either the base of the brain or the hypophysis; a permanent polyuria and polydipsia followed. This case is presented not only for its effect on the production of diabetes insipidus but also for the effects on the hypophysis—all essentially negative.

REPORT OF A CASE

A girl aged seventeen years was admitted to the Johns Hopkins Hospital Jan. 21, 1928, because of loss of vision. Before admission she had been studied in the neurologic dispensary, where no definite diagnosis was made. At this time she had been totally blind in the left eye for ten weeks, and, although there was no well defined hemianopia in the right eye, I thought there was a very definite difference in the intensity for color in the nasal and temporal field, the color being more clearly recognized in the nasal field. Moreover, she had volunteered that she could see things more plainly to her left than to her right with the right eye. This led me to suspect a tumor in the region of the optic tracts. Visual acuity was 15/200 in the right eye. There were no other subjective complaints or objective signs.

The hypophysial region was explored on the left (blind) side January 24. The optic nerves looked quite normal from the superior view. Since she was totally blind in the left eye, this optic nerve was divided in order to make a further search beneath the optic tracts. The hypophysial stalk was then in full view. To obtain a better view, the hypophysial stalk was divided with scissors midway between the base of the brain and the diaphragm of the sella. This was done without the slightest bleeding and without sponging either to the cut side of the stalk or to the contiguous region. The stalk was about 1 cm. long. The

operation, therefore, serves as an example of a precise experiment in which the sharply defined transection at the middle of the stalk is responsible for the subsequent effects. It also excludes from consideration and direct participation of the base of the brain or of the hypophysis itself.

On the evening of the operation, soon after consciousness appeared, there was marked thirst, and this was quickly followed by a very high output of colorless urine with a very low specific gravity. Chart 1 shows the course of the polyuria and polydipsia during her subsequent stay in the hospital, a period of nineteen days. A postoperative specimen of urine examined for sugar was normal.

The patient returned to the hospital Dec. 5, 1930, nearly three years after the operation, therefore, serves as an example changed until eight days previously, when she became totally blind in the remaining eye. In 1928 she had had numbness and weakness of the right leg lasting a month and clearing completely. Another similar attack occurred in May 1930 but involved both sides of the body. She was pregnant at the time. The sensory and motor changes disappeared almost completely in six weeks. It was now evident that the correct diagnosis was multiple sclerosis. She said that ever since the operation she had been troubled with severe thirst and frequency of urination—it was necessary for her to get up several times every night to void. Vision returned to the previous level soon after she left the hospital.

Feb. 6, 1933, the patient again entered the hospital because of advanced sensory and motor changes over the entire body. A fluid and urine chart was kept during her stay of eight days (chart 2).

In August 1933 she again entered the hospital. She now appeared to be in the terminal stages of the disseminated disease and was practically helpless. The polyuria and polydipsia still persisted unchanged (chart 3).

She was again seen during October 1937. Her general recovery had been remarkable. She was doing her own housework and walked without support, although with a difficulty of gait. The vision in the right eye (4/200) was good enough to permit reading. However, there was only a small central field. The urinary output and intake of water were essentially unchanged; voluntary control over the urine had

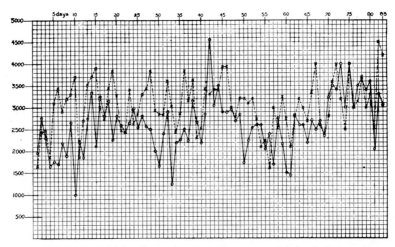

Chart 3. Fluid intake and urine output on third admission, June 3, 1933. The three charts cover a period of five and one half years. The polyuria and polydipsia remain practically unchanged after eleven years.

returned. She looked well.

The last word from her was received by letter May 1, 1939, more than eleven years after the operation. She said "My general condition remains about the same as when I last saw you, except that I cannot walk quite so well. My weight remains the same. The thirst and increased urination are unchanged. I get up two and three times every night to urinate."

SUMMARY

From a very sharply defined lesion, i.e., division of the stalk of the hypophysis without trauma to the contiguous parts of the brain, a permanent (eleven years) polyuria and polydipsia ensued. It is therefore evident that division of the stalk of the hypophysis is solely responsible for polyuria and polydipsia. This, of course, does not mean that injury to, or a lesion on, the base of the brain would not also produce the same disturbances. In fact there is every reason to believe that it would do so. Futcher's case is ample evidence. Clinical experience has shown that trauma to the hypophysis does not produce polyuria and polydipsia.

NOTES ON HYPOPHYSIAL FUNCTIONS

The patient subsequently married. A baby was born Sept. 1, 1930 (two years and nine months after section of the hypophysial stalk). Pregnancy and labor were normal. She nursed the baby for three months and had ample milk.

In 1933 she had a second child at full term and by normal delivery. This baby was nursed four months; supplementary feedings became necessary when the amount of milk became less abundant.

The menstrual periods were regular following the operation and for several years thereafter. In 1934 some irregularity first appeared; at times a period would be passed.

There have been many blood pressure readings. Before operation the pressure was 140/90, 136/80 and 135/90. Two years after the operation it was 120/76. Five years later it was 140/90, 130/90, 138/80, 105/75, 118/68 and 110/70.

Her weight was 122 pounds (55.3 Kg.) at the time of the operation and 140 pounds (63.5 Kg.) in 1933, five years after the operation.

The skin has retained its normal color; there has been no loss of hair on the head, axillae or pubic region.

Numerous examinations of the urine have been made. There was no sugar in the urine in the first postoperative specimen and none in three subsequent specimens. On her subsequent admissions twenty-seven examinations were recorded and a trace of sugar was found on two occasions. Seven times a trace of albumin was found.

CONCLUSIONS

1. A sharply defined lesion transection of the hypophysial stalk in man, without trauma to the base of the brain or to the hypophysis, produced a permanent (eleven years) polyuria and polydipsia.

2. This failed to disturb the known hypophysial functions, such as (*a*) menstruation, (*b*) pregnancy, (*c*) lactation, (*d*) weight, (*e*) blood pressure, (*f*) sugar content of urine (there was no glycosuria immediately after the operation or subsequently except for a trace on two occasions).

REFERENCES

[1]Dandy, W. E., and Reichert, F. L.: Studies on Experimental Hypophysectomy: I. Effect on the Maintenance of Life. *Bull., Johns Hopkins Hosp. 37:* 1 (July) 1925. Dandy, W. E.: *Benign Tumors of the Third Ventricle: Their Diagnosis and Treatment.* Springfield, Ill., Charles C. Thomas, Publisher, 1933.

[2]Camus, J., and Roussy, M. C.: Presentation de sept chiens hypophysectomisés depuis quelques mois. *Soc. de biol., 74:* 1386, 1913.

[3]Bailey, Percival, and Bremer, Frederic: Experimental Diabetes Insipidus. *Arch. Int. Med., 28:* 773 (Dec.) 1921.

[4]Biggart, J. H., and Alexander, G. L.: Experimental Diabetes Insipidus. *J. Path. & Bact., 48:* 405 (March) 1939.

[5]Fisher, Charles; Ingram, W. R., and Ranson, S. W.: *Diabetes Insipidus and the Neurohormonal Control of Water Balance: A Contribution to the Structure and Function of the Hypothalamic Hypophysial System.* Ann Arbor, Mich., Edward Brothers, Inc., 1938.

[6]von Hann, F.: Ueber die Bedeutung der Hypophysenveranderungen bei Diabetes insipidus. *Frankfurt. Ztschr. Path., 21:* 337, 1918.

[7]Futcher, T. B.: Diabetes Insipidus and Lesions of the Midbrain. *Am. J. M. Sc., 178:* 837 (Dec.) 1929.

LXIV

REMOVAL OF LONGITUDINAL SINUS INVOLVED IN TUMORS*

There is occasionally presented to the neurosurgeon the problem of dealing with dural meningiomas that have invaded the longitudinal sinus and especially with bilateral dural tumors in which the longitudinal sinus is incorporated in the mass. Unless the affected part of the longitudinal sinus is resected there is no possibility of curing the tumor, and, in most instances, so extensively has the tumor grown to the falx and sinus that even removal of the mass with the full expectation of recurrence is well nigh impossible. When the great size of the longitudinal sinus and the numerous large tributary cortical veins entering it from both sides are considered, it is not difficult to realize that surgeons have hesitated to resect the longitudinal sinus both from fear of producing irreparable harm to such a seemingly all-important venous trunk and from the technical difficulties involved. There has been scant evidence indeed to support the thought that resection of this sinus might be tolerated, particularly in its posterior portion. Many patients with thrombosis of the longitudinal sinus have come to necropsy. But in the case of such a patient there is frequently an acute inflammatory basis, and many of the contiguous cerebral veins are also included in the process. Moreover, in many an acute septicemia coexists. It is doubtful whether experimental evidence would be pertinent, except perhaps in monkeys. In dogs there is only one cluster of cerebral veins on either side that enters the sinus, whereas in man there are many.

It is, of course, clear that in dealing with bilateral tumors and frequently even with unilateral dural tumors the longitudinal sinus is frequently occluded by the tumor either by compression or by direct invasion, so that removal of a section of the longitudinal sinus really adds little or nothing to the demand for collateral venous circulation. In these cases the venous obstruction has doubtless been gradually progressive, and because of this there has been time for the collateral circulation to develop. This condition was true in both of my cases in which the longitudinal sinus was resected posterior to the rolandic vein, and doubtless it was also true in nearly all of the cases reported in the literature. Whether a patient sinus could be similarly resected can only be conjectured; there is no evidence from the literature to support or deny such a claim.

Gradually a small number of cases of resection of the longitudinal sinus in the course of tumor extirpations have been assembled from the literature. Kenyon (1915) reported the first case in which the longitudinal sinus was doubly ligated in the frontal region, the ligatures being 2½ inches (6.3 cm.) apart. Rand (1923) was apparently the first deliberately to resect about 10 cm. of the sinus with a large bilateral dural meningioma with massive hyperostosis over it. The resected sinus was well in front of the rolandic vein. The patient made a splendid recovery with no loss of motor function, and a note from Dr. Rand on March 19, 1940, stated that the patient is well eighteen years later, an occasional epileptic attack being the only residual disturbance. In 1926 Towne removed a similar tumor weighing 428 Gm. and a section of the longitudinal sinus (length not stated), but his patient died two months later. The longitudinal sinus was filled with tumor.

*Reprinted from the *Archives of Surgery*, 41: 244–256, August, 1940.

David, Bissery and Brun (1935) reported a case in which operation was done by
Vincent of Paris, France. A bilateral tumor—12 Gm. on the left and 18 Gm. on
the right—was removed with 5 or 6 cm. of
longitudinal sinus just in front of the rolandic vein. The result was excellent, with
no motor loss. No note was made of the
patency or occlusion of the longitudinal
sinus. Horrax has successfully removed
sections of the longtiudinal sinus in two
cases, one (1931) included in Cushing's
book on meningiomas (6 cm. of sinus in
front of the rolandic vein was resected)
and another, reported by Maltby (1939),
in which 4 cm. of the sinus posterior to the
rolandic vein was excised. The patients in
both cases made excellent recoveries, with
slight but gradually diminishing spasticity
of the extremity. In Horrax' second case
resection was done in a single operation,
doubtless because his earlier experience
had given him a greater sense of security
concerning removal of a section of longitudinal sinus. In all the preceding cases the
sinus had been resected after recurrence or
in stages for tumors of excessive size and
vascularity. In Horrax' second case (Maltby) a prolongation of the tumor was drawn
out of and doubtless occluded the longitudinal sinus. Rowe (1939) reported another splendid result, with a large bilateral
dural tumor with hyperostosis, together
with which 6 cm. of the longitudinal sinus
was resected. A letter from Dr. Rowe stated that he has since been unable to locate
the patient and that the patency or occlusion of the sinus was not investigated.

Two remarkable cases (Davidoff [1937]
and Tonnis [1935]) complete the series of
cases of resection of the longitudinal sinus
that I have been able to assemble from the
literature—a total, therefore, of 9 (in Kenyon's case ligation, not resection, was
done). The operation in all except
Towne's case was successful, without any
disturbances attributable to resection of
the sinus, and Towne's patient lived over
two months. Most of these patients had
some degree of temporary spasticity of the
lower extremities after operation, but this
was clearly due to trauma of the motor
cortex incident to extirpation of the growth and not to any effects of removal of the
longitudinal sinus.

Davidoff's case and also that of Tonnis
give evidence of the very highest surgical
skill, as indeed do all the others, for such
operations are no mean feats. Davidoff's
tumor, removed in three stages, weighed
835 Gm. and was perhaps the largest cranial tumor to have been successfully removed. The hyperostosis and contained tumor weighed 270 Gm., and the intracranial
portion, 565 Gm.! The length of sinus removed is not stated. A letter from Dr.
Davidoff (Jan. 22, 1940) states that, although the patient has some slight spasticity on the right and a slightly hesitant
speech, she is quite well and does her own
housework.

Tonnis removed not only a section of
the longitudinal sinus (length not stated)
but part of one transverse sinus and the
tentorium, through which the tumor had
penetrated into the posterior cranial fossa.
And his patient recovered with no defects
except homonymous hemianopia.

To the aforementioned group of cases
four of my own are added. In two resection was done in the anteriormost part of
the sinus, and in two, posterior to the rolandic vein. In two of the cases the sinus
was excised when the tumor had recurred,
and in two the sinus was removed at the
first operation, when the tumor was known
to be bilateral.

REPORT OF CASES

Case 1. C. W. L., a white man aged
forty-nine, was admitted to the hospital
because of headache and a "change of disposition." A cerebral injection of air was
performed May 7, 1927. This showed a
tumor in the left frontal lobe. An exploration was made May 8, and a small dural
tumor, weighing 27 Gm., was removed
from the anterior portion of the falx. The
tumor was thought to be a dural meningioma. The patient made a complete recovery, and his headache and mental symptoms entirely disappeared.

Four months later he reentered the hospital because his original symptoms had returned. The wound was reopened, and a recurrent tumor weighing 20.6 Gm. was shelled out with the finger. It was realized that this could not be a permanent cure, and two and one-half weeks later (September 20) the wound was reopened and the bone removed over the longitudinal sinus and to some distance on the right side. There were no veins entering the longitudinal sinus on the right side. Clamps were placed across the longitudinal sinus anteriorly, and the sinus was divided. The incision was carried through the longitudinal sinus, and the inferior longitudinal sinus was clipped and divided. The longitudinal sinus was then divided and transfixed even with the posterior margin of the bony defect, and the entire intervening part of the longitudinal sinus and the falx were removed. The remaining ends of the longitudinal sinus were then transfixed with medium silk. The amount of longitudinal sinus removed was 8 cm.; this was well in front of the rolandic area, the posterior ligature in the sinus being about 4 cm. anterior to the rolandic vein.

The patient had no after-effects from ligation of the sinus. He recovered completely but returned again seven months later because of recurrence, which was evident from the protrusion at the site of the removal of bone. There was such an extensive return of the tumor that no attempt was made to remove it. The patient died three months later, June 27, 1928.

Autopsy showed massive recurrence of the tumor. No note was made concerning thrombosis of the remaining part of the longitudinal sinus. It was noted that 3 cm. of the longitudinal sinus remained anterior to the ligature in the longitudinal sinus.

CASE 2. F. R., a white woman aged forty, had observed a swelling of the forehead for the past twenty-three years; it had been steadily progressing (Fig 1). There had been headache and pain over both frontal regions for the past two years and exophthalmos of the right eye over the same period; this, too, had been steadily progressing. Roentgenograms showed tremendous hyperostosis of the frontal bones (Fig. 2).

Operation.—On Nov. 21, 1936, a large sweeping curved incision was made across the frontal region, just under the hair line; it was directed posteriorly and extended from one temporal region to the other. A flap of galea and skin was thrown forward to the supraorbital ridges. The tumor had eroded through the bone on the right side over a considerable area, but the surface was intact. The bone was so thick that several burr openings were made, and the intervening bone was cut with large biting forceps. When the bone was turned back and broken across at the supraorbital region the tumor came out with it. It was a large bilateral dural growth (Fig. 3). The sinus tore across at the posterior margin of the bone, but it bled very little. The mass in the orbit had broken off from the main growth and was shelled out separately. Several veins crossing from the anterior lobe to the longitudinal sinus were coagulated with the electrocautery. The tumor mass with the overlying bone weighed 296 Gm.

The patient made an uneventful recovery and has been well to date (March 10, 1940). She is constantly employed at full time (Fig. 1).

The length of sinus removed was about 8 cm.

CASE 3. J. W., a man twenty-two years of age, consulted me May 21, 1939, because of a prominent swelling over the vertex of the skull. He had had headaches for three or four years, and for the past five months these had become more persistent and more severe, occurring almost daily and lasting from a few minutes to a few hours; they were bilateral and biparietal. The lump on the head was steadily increasing but was not tender. His work in college had gradually declined, and during the past year he had barely made passing grades. Concentration was difficult; his memory was poor, and there had been some difficulty in getting out words and phrases, although he knew them well. On some occasions there had been transitory attacks of blurred vision. On a few occasions he had had cramps in the right leg but not a convulsion.

Neurologic examination showed slight but definite papilledema, with fulness and tortuosity of the retinal veins. The grip of the right hand was slightly weaker than that of the left. During the examination he had a cramp which drew up the right leg severely, and it was very painful. There was slight hypoesthesia in the right arm and leg; the station and gait were not af-

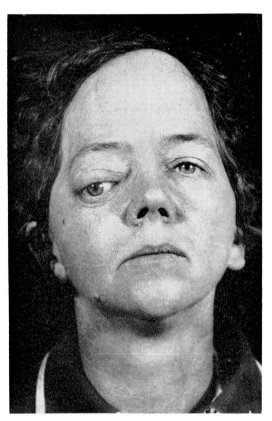

Fig. 1 (case 2).—Preoperative photograph of the patient. The tumor was a bilateral dural endothelioma with tremendous hyperostosis The tumor had broken through the roof of the orbit on the right side.

fected. The patient's speech was halting; reading was stumbling but correctly done, but it seemed difficult to get the context of what he was reading. The Wassermann reaction of the blood was negative. Roentgen examination showed marked hyperotosis at the vertex, about equal on both sides of the midline. The protrusion was about 1 inch (2.5 cm.) above the normal level of the scalp; it was diffuse and even.

Operation.—On May 23 a long midline incision was made over the tumor and extending well beyond it anteriorly and posteriorly. The galea and skin were then retracted; this exposed the hyperostosis, which was not very vascular. Several burr openings were made in a circle just beyond the hyperostosis, where the bone was nearly normal. With the Gigli saw these openings were connected, and the mass of bone was lifted off the dura and longitudinal sinus. As the bone was being ele-

vated, the tumor could be seen projecting into a deep concavity in the inferior surface of the bone; it was firmly attached to it. By gradually elevating the bone flap and inserting the finger beneath it the tumor was stripped from the concavity in the bone. There was very little bleeding from the exposed dura and tumor; application of the electrocautery controlled this. The concavity in the bone was about 2 inches (5 cm.) long and 1¼ inches (3.1 cm.) wide. The tumor was entirely on the left side of the longitudinal sinus, which was pushed in a curve to the right. The wound was closed without drainage.

The weight of the bone was 159.1 Gm.

The second stage operation was performed on June 3, ten days after the first operation. The wound was reopened; there was some necrosis on the surface of the exposed tumor. The dura was first opened in a semicircle on the right side, the termini being at the border of the longitudinal sinus. The tumor was then seen pushing the cerebral hemisphere to the right. It was a large, hard growth and was clearly a dural meningioma. It extended deeply along the falx. The dura was then opened on the left side in a similar fashion, and the incision extended to the longitudinal sinus. The longitudinal sinus was then doubly clamped at both ends and just at the margins of the large defect in the skull. The sinus was then cut between the clamps, and the ends were transfixed with sutures of medium silk. Several veins entering the longitudinal sinus from the hemispheres were thrombosed with the electrocautery and divided. These veins included the rolandic veins on both sides. About eight veins were thrombosed on the two sides; all of them were very tortuous. The falx was then divided through its entire length, including the inferior longitudinal sinus at both ends. The clips shown in the roentgenograms were on the posterior part of the longitudinal sinus. After the falx had been cut through at both ends the tumor was gently shelled away from both hemispheres; it protruded far out on both sides, undermining the hemispheres, but much more on the left. On the right side it was necessary to cut away a small slice of the attached leg center to the depth of about 2 cm. and about 1 cm. in thickness. This was necessary because the tumor was adherent to the brain at this point. The tumor was bulging far

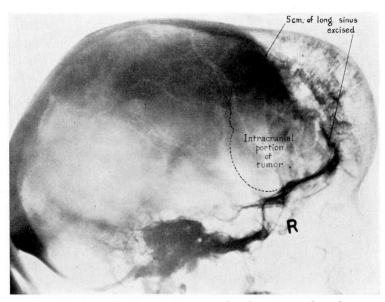

FIG. 2. (case 2). Roentgenogram showing tremendous hyperostosis over a bilateral dural tumor.

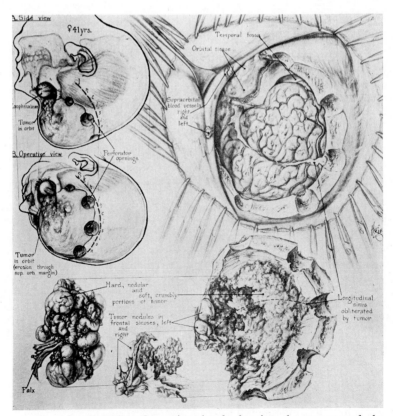

FIG. 3. (case 2). Operative sketch showing the tumor and the amount of longitudinal sinus resected.

out on both sides in the depths of the brain, but it was easily separated from it, with very slight trauma; the bulge was greater to the left. Little bleeding attended extirpation of this mass. A piece of fascia lata was removed from the right leg and carefully sutured to the dural margins, completely covering the entire dural defect. The wound was closed without drainage.

The tumor weighed 170.3 Gm. The total weight of the bony growth and the bilateral tumor was 329.4 Gm.

The patient was conscious soon after the operation and moved both legs and arms freely. Later in the afternoon he was unable to move either leg. The first movement in the left began six days later, and slight movement in the right leg began on the following day. There was also diminished sensation in the legs during this period, but on the day before the motor function began to return he noticed increased feeling in both legs.

Microscopic section of the bone showed typical dural meningioma cells, and sections of the tumor showed typical dural meningioma with whorls of fibrous tissue. The longitudinal sinus was totally occluded over about three-fourths of the removed portion. The length of the longitudinal sinus was determined at the time of operation and was 12.5 cm.

Subsequent Course.—The patient's motor function steadily improved. He left the hospital June 18, thirteen days after the last operation. At that time the power was not sufficient to support him, but during the summer months he improved rapidly, and when I last saw him (Jan. 20, 1940) he was walking with very slight disturbance of gait; the two legs were equally good. He had just returned to college for the second semester; he was keen and alert and said he felt that he had completely returned to his normal mental state. The wound was soft and sunken, and there was no evidence of recurrence.

Case 4. L. P., a white man aged fifty-six, was operated on May 6, 1933. A dural endothelioma was removed from the falx on the left side, in the postrolandic area. The symptoms of the tumor were convulsions beginning in the right leg and weakness of the right leg. The tumor removed at this time weighed 63 Gm.

Four and one-half years later (Jan. 7, 1938) a recurrent tumor was removed from the same side; it weighed 12 Gm. The patient had slight motor disturbance in the right leg following this operation, but he walked well.

On Jan. 17, 1940, he returned because of a similar weakness in the left leg. It was clear that he had a similar tumor on the right side of the falx. He was again operated on (January 23), and a tumor weighing 35 Gm. was removed from the right side, together with the intervening longitudinal sinus and falx. There was no recurrence on the left side. The length of resected longitudinal sinus was 6.5 cm. and extended backward from a point about 3 cm. posterior to the rolandic vein. Five centimeters of this had been completely obliterated by the tumor, which had grown directly through it.

The patient had no increase in motor weakness following removal of the sinus and tumor. On the day after the operation his general condition was as good as before the operation. There were no noticeable effects from extirpation of the longitudinal sinus, and none could be expected, because the sinus had been completely obliterated by the tumor. He left the hospital two weeks later.

The postoperative course was uneventful.

SUMMARY

In none of the four cases was there any motor, sensory or other loss that could be attributed to removal of the longitudinal sinus.

The length of the longitudinal sinus removed was 5 cm. and 8 cm., respectively, in the two cases in which resection was anterior to the rolandic vein and 6.5 cm. and 10 cm., respectively, in the two cases in which resection was posterior to the rolandic vein.

In three cases and probably in the fourth the longitudinal sinus was already obliterated over much of the excised portion owing to compression or actual invasion by the tumor. There is as yet no available evidence by which it can be known whether the longitudinal sinus can be removed in part before gradually progressive occlusion has occurred.

REFERENCES

[1]Cushing, H., and Eisenhardt, L.: *Meningiomas.*

Springfield, Ill., Charles C. Thomas, Publisher, 1938, p. 463.

[2]David, M.; Bissery, M., and Brun, M.: Sur un cas de meningiome de la faux opere avec succes. Absence de troubles paralytiques apres resection du sinus longitudinal au nivean de l'abouchement des veines rolandiques. *Rev. neurol., 1:* 725, 1934.

[3]Davidoff, L. M.: Meningioma: Report of an Unusual Case. *Bull. Neurol. Inst. New York, 6:* 300, 1937.

[4]Frazier, C. H., and Alpers, B. J.: Meningeal Fibroblastomas of the Cerebrum. *Arch. Neurol. & Psychiat., 29:* 935 (May) 1933.

[5]Holmes, G., and Sargent, P.: Injuries of the Superior Longitudinal Sinus. *Brit. M. J., 2:* 493, 1915.

[6]Kenyon, J. H.: Endothelioma of the Brain, Three Years After Operation. *Ann. Surg., 61:* 106, 1915.

[7]Maltby, G. L.: Resection of Longitudinal Sinus Posterior to the Rolandic Area for Complete Removal of Meningioma. *Arch. Neurol. & Psychiat., 42:* 1135 (Dec.) 1939.

[8]Olivercrona, H.: *Die parasagittal Meningeome.* Leipzig, Georg Thieme, 1934.

[9]Rand, C. W.: Osteoma of the Skull: Report of Two Cases, One Being Associated with a Large Intracranial Endothelioma. *Arch. Surg., 6:* 573 (March) 1923.

[10]Rowe, S. N.: Parasagittal Meningiomas. *Am. J. Surg., 43:* 138, 1939.

[11]Tonnis, W.: Die Zulassigheit der Resektion des Langs-blutleiters des Gehirns. *Deutsche Ztschr. Nervenh., 136:* 186, 1935.

[12]Towne, E. B.: Invasion of the Intracranial Venous Sinuses by Meningioma (Dural Endothelioma). *Ann. Surg., 83:* 321, 1926.

LXV

RESULTS FOLLOWING THE TRANSCRANIAL OPER-ATIVE ATTACK ON ORBITAL TUMORS*†

Two excellent papers on the pathologic aspects of intraorbital tumors by Byers[1] (1901) and Hudson[2] (1912) emphasized the high percentage of these growths that passed into the cranial chamber. Removal of such a tumor by one of the usual orbital operations, therefore, meant that the patient ordinarily succumbed later to the intracranial growth that remained, and in addition there was local recurrence in the orbit. In 1921 I[3] encountered by the cranial route an intracranial tumor that had extended through the optic foramen into the orbital cavity. The orbital roof was removed in order to follow and extirpate this portion of the tumor. So simple was the operative attack and so perfectly could the intraorbital contents be exposed that this method suggested great improvement in operative attack on the great group of intraorbital tumors. No matter in which direction the intracranial portion of the tumor extends or in which part of the orbit the tumor is situated, this approach has proved far superior to the usual frontal or lateral (Kronlein) routes by which such tumors had previously been attacked. This paper presents the results that have followed the use of this operative approach. And even for the tumors that are confined to the orbit alone, this approach has been found to be preferable to those formerly used by ophthalmologists. The great advantage of this approach lies in the much fuller and safer exposure of the intraorbital contents. The optic nerve, the eyeball, three of the extraocular muscles and the ophthalmic veins and arteries can well be exposed and avoided during the dissection of the orbital tumor.

Since the original publication, the operative approach (Fig. 1), which is identical with that used for hypophysial tumors, has been greatly reduced and simplified, owing in large part to the introduction of avertin with amylene hydrate as an anesthetic. It has been found that swelling of the brain that so commonly follows ether anesthesia is avoided when avertin with amylene hydrate is used, and for that reason the size of the bone flap necessary for the exposure of the base of the brain can be greatly modified.

From the clinical examination of patients with exophthalmos it is not usually possible to tell whether or not there is an intracranial extension of the orbital tumor. And all too frequently the orbital tumor is but a small fraction of the large but silent intracranial tumor which is usually the primary growth. Since intracranial tumors are present in approximately three fourths of the orbital tumors in this series, it should be assumed on the law of probabilities that the tumor extends into the cranial chamber. And anything less than the combined transcranial and intraorbital surgical approach will offer no solution of the problem. All too frequently the orbital contents have been exenterated in a radical attempt to remove the tumor from the front of the orbit, and an infected granulating wound has resulted. Such a result would forever preclude the transcranial approach, because of the certainty that infection would follow. In safe hands the transcranial approach carries very little risk, and it offers the maximum hope of cure, unless the frontal bone is involved,

*Reprinted from the *Archives of Ophthalmology*, 25: 191–213, February 1941.

†Read before the Section on Ophthalmology at the Ninety-First Annual Session of the American Medical Association, New York, June 14, 1940.

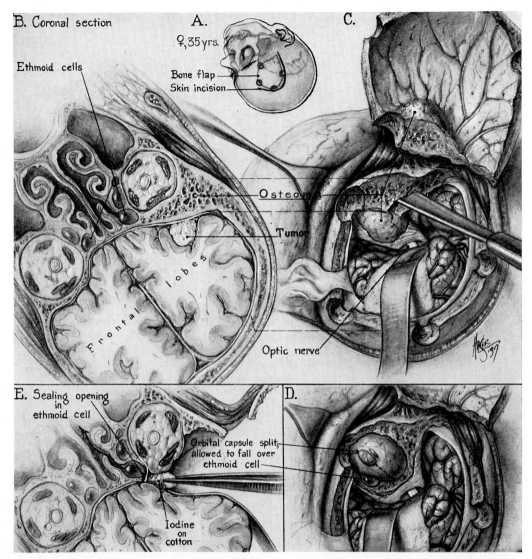

B. Coronal section   A.   C.

♀, 35 yrs.

Ethmoid cells

Bone flap
Skin incision

Osteoma

Tumor

F r o n t a l   l o b e s

Optic nerve

E. Sealing opening in ethmoid cell

Orbital capsule split, allowed to fall over ethmoid cell

D.

Iodine on cotton

Fig. 1. Steps in the operative procedure for removal of an orbital tumor by the transcranial route. This particular tumor was one of the intracranial and intraorbital dural meningiomas with marked hyperostosis of the skull and of the orbit.

and without cosmetic defects. Even when the character of the tumor prevents a permanent cure, the maximum period of relief and extension of life is afforded by subtotal removal of the extensive tumor.

Although the best available evidence of an intracranial component of the tumor is obtained from the roentgenograms, this proof is all too frequently lacking. The optic foramen is occasionally enlarged or reduced in size, but the vast majority of tumors are not continuous through this

opening. The dural tumors, which comprise almost half of the tumors in the series, usually but not always show diffuse hyperostosis of the walls of the skull and of the orbit. In cases in which this condition is present there is usually no gross defect in the orbital roof and the extension of the tumor is due to diffuse invasion of the bone. At times calcification may be detected in the intracranial part of the tumor, entirely unsuspected from the clinical data, or a bony prominence may indicate an underlying growth. In none of the cases has enlargement of the sphenoid fissure indicated intracranial participation in the tumor.

TYPES OF GROWTH STUDIED

The data on twenty-four patients with surgically treated orbital tumors and combined orbital and intracranial tumors are included in this report; in addition, data on seven other patients who have come to necropsy and have not been subjected to this operation are included for the sake of pathologic study of combined orbital and intracranial tumors. The case reports and operative results in this group will be reserved for a later and more comprehensive paper on this subject. From symptoms alone intracranial extension of the tumor would have been suspected in perhaps 2 patients; in 1 there was headache but no papilledema, and in another there were uncinate attacks.

The character, number and percentage of tumors in the entire series of thirty-one cases may be summarized as follows:

Type of Growth	No. of Cases	Percentage
Inflammatory mass	1	3.2
Pure fibroma	1	3.2
Pure osteoma (diffuse)	2	6.4
Osteomatous cyst	1	3.2
Spindle cell sarcoma	1	3.2
Round cell sarcoma	1	3.2
Schuller-Christian disease (probable)	5	16
Dural meningioma of nerve sheath (bilateral)	1	3.2
Dural tumors without hyperostosis of the skull (by roentgen examination)	2	6.4
Sarcoma with tremendous hyperostosis of the skull	1	3.2
Dural meningioma with hyperostosis of the skull	11	36
Periosteal sarcoma	1	3.2
Carcinoma	1	3.2

INFLAMMATORY NODULE. An example of this type of tumor is that in case 1. The patient is well at the time of writing, three and one-half years later. The proximity of the paranasal sinuses would suggest a much greater frequency of lesions of this type. Doubtless this is true, for it must be in the exceptional case that a persisting mass would form. Most infections would doubtless subside completely spontaneously or after evacuation of an orbital abscess. There was nothing in the histologic picture of this small mass to suggest tuberculosis or syphilis, and the subsequent history of freedom from progression over three and one-half years would be ample evidence against them.

PURE FIBROMA. The origin of the remarkable tumor in case 2 is not entirely clear. It most probably arose from the inferior surface of the dura to which it was so tightly grown that the dura had to be excised with the growth. Moreover, judging by its intracranial position, where its habitat must have been for many years before it broke through the roof of the orbit and the cribriform plate, its dural origin would appear even more probable. But it is unlike any of the other dural meningiomas in that it contains so few cells. The patient is apparently well four years later. Stokes and Bowers[4] reported a pure fibroma of the orbit; it was made up of whorls of fibrous tissue.

PURE OSTEOMA. By pure osteoma is meant a growth of bone that is not due to a soft tissue-invasive tumor that causes hypertrophy of the bone. The latter type of growth occurs with such relative frequency in this series that a degree of skepticism is justified when the diagnosis of pure osteoma is made. One patient (the first reported in this paper but not included in the series of those operated on) has been followed for twenty-one years and is known to have had the growth for forty-three years (since the age of six years). The tumor was fully exposed intracranially, as well as intraorbitally, and no sign of an additional soft tumor was found, Moreover, the duration of the tumor's life, with almost no progression in twenty-one years, would appear to exclude safely the possibility of an additional soft tumor. The second patient (case 4) has been followed only two years. It is possible to say only that no soft tumor was found when the entire roof of the orbit was removed. The roentgenologic picture of a pure osteoma differs but little from that of the larger group of secondary soft tumors. Perhaps in these two cases the growth invaded the paranasal sinuses to a greater extent, but the involvement of the roof and side of the orbit and of the walls of the skull appears to be precisely similar. The bony growth is diffuse in both cases and its complete removal therefore impossible. It can only be hoped that the results in the second case will be like those in the first.

Well defined localized pure osteomas also occur but have not been encountered in this series. So frequently associated with the frontal or ethmoid sinuses and breaking into the orbit, they have been grouped by Cushing[5] under orbitoethmoid osteomas. Another case has been reported by Pilcher.[6]

OSTEOMATOUS CYST. In case 4 an unusual tumor arose in or below the floor of the orbit and projected upward into the orbit. The cyst, with serous fluid, was perhaps as large as a bantam's egg. Lining the exposed part of the cyst wall was a thin layer of tumor tissue. Microscopically the lining of the tumor was made up of cellular connective tissue throughout which were thickly intredispersed small roughly spherical and irregularly shaped masses of bone. There were numerous osteoblasts and large multinuclear osteoclasts. In most of the bony deposits were osteocytes. The newly formed bone had none of the arrangements of true bone.

SPINDLE CELL SARCOMA. It is worthy of note that the tumor in case 5 was removed by intracapsular enucleation, a procedure that would favor local implantation at the site of removal, and yet four years later the patient is well and there has been no recurrence. At the time of the operation the tumor was thought to be malignant, and the lapse of time without recurrence has been a pleasant surprise, the more so because the patient's other eye had been removed several years previously, after an accident.

ROUND CELL SARCOMA. There was a single case of a pure round cell sarcoma (case 6), in a child two and one-half years old. Symptoms rapidly developed, and after removal of the growth recurrence quickly

followed. In the contiguous region several metastatic or transplanted nodules appeared a few weeks after the operation. This tumor was much the most malignant one in the entire series, death occurring five and one-half months after the first sign of exophthalmos.

SCHULLER-CHRISTIAN DISEASE. Case 7 furnishes a clinical example of a nodule of this type, which so characteristically perforates the bone. Histologically there were seen numerous masses of foam cells and diffuse infiltration with eosinophils and small round cells, both in great abundance. The duration of life cannot be told, because the operation was recently performed.

In the four remaining cases (8, 9, 10 and 11) the clinical and the gross pathologic appearances were entirely dissimilar. The neoplasm in case 8 behaved like any slowly growing malignant tumor, with local recurrence and localized tumor implants about the site of operation. The gross appearance of the mass was like that of a hard, slowly growing, invasive tumor. The patient is still alive six and three-fourths years after the first symptoms. In none of the sections obtained at two operations were there tumor cells. Because of the foam cells and eosinophils and considering the microscopic, gross and clinical pictures as a whole, Dr. Rich looked on the diagnosis of Schuller-Christian disease as the most probable one.

The growth in case 9 was very rapid (total duration of symptoms until death was ten months) in both orbits, within the cranial chamber and scattered throughout the body. The tumors were salmon colored. From the gross appearance, Dr. Roger Baker, of Duke University, made a diagnosis of xanthomatosis. From the microscopic study of the various masses removed at operation, Dr. Rich stated the opinion that the diagnosis lay between a xanthofibroma and Schuller-Christian disease. No tumor cells were present.

The tumors in cases 10 and 11 were similar in their gross appearance. They were single masses of tissue that grossly resembled hard tumors. Both were firmly fixed, one at the apex of the orbit and the other to the orbital capsule; both had invaded the extraocular muscles, and in both, although the mass could be extirpated, it was clear that the contiguous tissues were infiltrated and that the removal was incomplete. In neither of these, nor in the two preceding cases, were there perforations of the cranial vault, which are so typical of Schuller-Christian disease. Only in case 7 was this bony perforation present. This diagnosis in the remaining four cases has therefore been made solely on the histologic picture, which more closely resembles Schuller-Christian disease than any other known lesion.

Many cases of Schuller-Christian disease affecting the orbit have been reported, some as instances of xanthomatosis and others of lipoid granulomatosis; and since the condition is not an actual tumor, in many cases it has been classified as a pseudotumor, a designation proposed by Birch-Hirschfeld.[7] Examples of the foregoing reports are those of Ringel,[8] Rowland,[9] Chester,[10] Chiari,[11] Heath,[12] Knapp,[13] and Sautter.[14] Among seventy primary orbital tumors Schreck[15] included twelve as pseudotumors, a proportion of non-neoplastic masses not greatly different from those in this series. Six of them were reported to be chronic inflammatory tissue, a diagnosis that could easily have been made in two of my cases of Schuller-Christian disease that only Dr. Rich's expert eye would have placed in this group. In two of Schreck's twelve cases the diagnosis were lymphogranuloma and aleukemic lymphadenoma. As Schreck did not mention Schuller-Christian disease in his cases, one is led to wonder if the condition in many of them may not have been of this origin.

Voelkel[16] collected forty cases of bilateral symmetric orbital growths, most of which he thought to be of lymphomatous origin. Doubtless in some of these cases the condition was similar to that in my case 9.

PSAMMOMA (DURAL TUMOR OF THE OPTIC SHEATH). Almost identical tumors were present in both optic nerves in case 12. The point of origin of the growths was from the dura in the optic canal, from which point each projected slightly intracranially and much more intraorbitally. On the side operated on the tumor strangulated the optic nerve like a tight constricting band. Microscopically the tumor was made up of fibrous tissue and was loaded with psammoma bodies. Although the vision was not improved by the operation, the patient is still alive and well except for blindness twenty-four years after the onset of symptoms. Olivecrona and Urban[17] (1935) reported an almost identical case, in which the condition was also bilateral. Schott[18] (1877) reported bilateral symmetric bodies of psammoma of the optic nerves at the optic foramen, but they were more circumscribed than in my case.

DURAL TUMORS WITHOUT ROENTGENOLOGIC EVIDENCE OF HYPEROSTOSIS OF THE SKULL AND OF THE ORBIT. The qualification of roentgenologic evidence is added because it is exceptional in this series (cases 14 and 15) for a dural tumor to be unassociated with hyperostosis. As a matter of fact, definite thickening of the sphenoid ridge was seen at operation in both cases, although it was not demonstrable in the roentgenograms either before operation or on subsequent restudy. The highly malignant tumor in case 14 showed only occasionally the arrangement of cells so characteristic of a cellular dural meningioma. Had one not known its character from the gross picture, a diagnosis of sarcoma might well have been made. The duration of life was two years after the first symptoms. After the operation transplanted nodules developed about the operative site.

The tumor in case 15 was like others of the cellular type of dural growths. The cells in most part were grouped in round or oval columns of varying size throughout the sections. The same columns of cells were found in the marrow spaces of the bone. Histologically this growth was similar to the tumors with hyperostosis, to be described.

Tumors With Roentgenographic Evidence of Hyperostosis of the Skull and
of the Orbit. Nine tumors, or over one
third of the surgically removed tumors in
this series, were associated with such pronounced hypertrophy of the skull and walls
of the orbit that it was strikingly shown in
the roetgenograms. The cause of this relation, recognized by Spiller [19] in 1899 and
by Brissaud and Lereboullet,[20] in 1903, was
probably first demonstrated by Cushing [21]
in 1922. Under the microscope he found
the marrow spaces in the bone to be filled
with tumor cells (dural meningioma in
each instance). Phemister,[22] Penfield [23]
and Berard and Dunet [24] quickly verified
Cushing's findings. This same combination of a dural tumor and superimposed
thickening of bone occurs not only with
orbital growths but also with those located
along all parts of the vault and base of the
skull, and always there is the same explanation: The cells of the dural tumor have
invaded the overlying part of the skull.
That the hyperostosis is not absolutely, although nearly, pathognomonic of a dural
meningioma is shown by the same extensive bony proliferation in a case of a
sarcoma (spindle cell); the same sarcoma-
tous cells that made an enormous soft tumor also filled the marrow spaces of the
skull. Doubtless the bony change is similar
in its development to that of the well recognized areas of hypertrophy of the vertebral column associated with metastases
from carcinoma of the prostate.

The roentgenograms of the benign osteomas in this region and elsewhere presented
no demonstrable difference from those of
the invasive meningeal growths. Doubtless the age of the patient is an important
differential point, for in both of the benign hyperostoses the bony thickening was
present in the first decade. And none of
the dural tumors was known to be present
before the thirtieth year. Although benign
osteoma may well appear later, the burden
of proof must be on the acceptance of such
a diagnosis after this age.

The size, position and general character
of the dural tumor in relation to the size
of the hyperostosis of the orbit and of the
skull is worthy of consideration. The dural growth in case 16 is especially interesting because there was no dural meningioma on the side of the dura contiguous to
the hyperostosis. It was only because the
dura was opened that it was seen at all;
and then it was only a flat plaque, about
the thickness of paper and very loosely applied to the cerebral side of the dura. It
gave no gross appearance of having infiltrated the dura and was stripped from
the dura with the greatest ease. Sections of
the bone, which was tremendously thickened, showed the same type of tumor. In two
other cases (17 and 22, the latter studied
at necropsy) there was no gross dural tumor; but in the orbital fat of each there
was a small diffuse irregular mass looking
like firm granulation tissue, and this proved to be tumor. From the gross appearance
one would be led to wonder if this orbital
tumor might not have been a secondary
outgrowth from the tumor within the bone.
Could this dural tumor have arisen from
dural rests within the bone which in each
instance was of enormous size? In case 22
the hyperostosis was the most extensive of
the entire series. In case 23 the dural growth was hard and flat, about 1 cm. thick and
spread like a carpet over the entire orbital
roof, to which it was firmly attached; it extended posteriorly, covering the dura over
two thirds of the floor of the middle fossa;
the hyperostosis was of moderate grade. In
case 19 the dural tumor arising from the
orbital roof was about the size of a hazelnut. In case 20 a hazelnut-sized dural tumor projected from the sphenoid wing. In
case 21 a small (2 cm. in diameter) round
dural tumor projected intracranially from
the orbital roof, and the irregular mass of
grayish brown tissue like granulation tissue
projected into the posterior part of the orbit.

On the other hand, the dural tumor in
case 18 was of great size and very hard
(Fig. 2). In this case the orbital roof was
destroyed and the hyperostosis was confin-

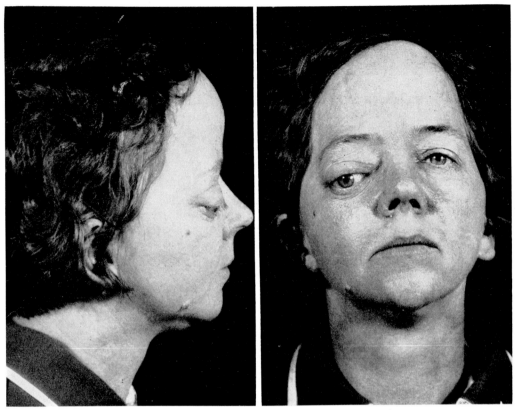

Fig. 2. Patient with bilateral frontal dural meningioma.

ed to both frontal bones.

Viewed histologically, with a single exception (case 18), the tumors were all of the very cellular type of meningioma and were lacking in the whorls and palisades of fibrous tissue. In case 18, however, the tumor was made up of whorls and palisades and was lacking in the solid masses of cells. Both types of dural tumor can, therefore, be responsible for the extensive contiguous hyperostosis. Moreover, the degree of hyperostosis is just as great with small circumscribed or thick carpet-like tumors as with the larger growths. Cushing and Eisenhardt[25] commented on the fact that a greater proportion of dural tumors "en plaque" produced hyperostosis than those of the large, hard, rounded tumors, which he termed the "global type." However, the same change in the bone is produced by both types. Surprising indeed is the extensive and widespread distribution of the hyperostosis which so frequent-

ly involves much of the orbital bones, the side and front of the skull and all too frequently the paranasal sinuses. So much are the paranasal sinuses involved that these growths have been included by Cushing under "orbitoethmoid" tumors.

Operative removal of tumors of this type has been reported by Cushing,[21] Armitage,[26] Patterson and Cairns,[27] Vorhis and Adson,[28] Love,[29] Hoover and Horrax,[30] Vincent and Mahoudeau,[31] Pilcher[6] and Cairns.[32] Knapp[33] reported two cases, in one of which an operation was performed and in the other of which roentgen therapy was given. Elsberg, Hare and Dyke[34] reported five cases of tumors of this type, in some of which the dural growth was removed, but apparently without removal of the orbital hyperostosis.

GLIOMA OF THE OPTIC TRACTS. Four cases are added for pathologic study; in all exploratory operations were performed, but in none did the operation include the orbital attack, the tumor being clearly inoperable. In two of the cases there was no exophthalmos despite the fact that the growth had continued into the orbit. All the growths were widespread, involving the chiasm and one or both optic nerves within the cranial chamber and also in the orbits, and in each the brain was also involved. In one instance the tumor extended through the third ventricle and the temporal, frontal, parietal and occipital lobes on one side. All these tumors were in young children, the ages being four, five, seven and thirteen years. This type of tumor may be suspected when hemianopia in the eye without exophthalmos is present or beginning. A case of this type was reported by Willemer[35] as early as 1879; an excellent drawing was included. Other cases have been reported by Martin and Cushing.[36]

Lundberg[37] made an extended study of this tumor, which he classified as an "oligodendrocytoma." He emphasized the early age of onset. Busch[38] suggested partial extirpation of the growth and recorded two cases in which there was improvement after two and one-half and seven and one-half years. However, very little operative trauma can be sustained without mortality, because the subsequent edema involves the hypothalamus, which tolerates trauma poorly.

OTHER TUMORS IN THE ORBIT. The foregoing pathologic report by no means exhausts the orbital tumors. They merely represent the cases that have occurred in the experience of a neurosurgeon and very probably are fairly representative of the commoner types. Coulter and Coats[39] reported an orbital teratoma and Gow[40] a large cyst that was probably of this character. Mancilla[41] and Byers[42] each reported a cavernous angioma of the orbit; Adson and Benedict,[43] a hemangio-endothelioma, Franklin and Cordes,[44] a lymphangioma; Knapp,[45] an oil cyst lined by epithelial cells and containing many sebaceous glands and a few hair follicles; Wheeler,[46] an orbital cyst with epithelial lining; Stall-

ard,[47] a cavernous angioma; de Schweinitz,[48] a myxosarcoma and a lipoma; Pinkus,[49] two cases of cholesteatoma of the orbit, and Cairns,[32] a cholesteatoma arising beneath the orbital roof. Van der Hoeve[50] reported a case of von Recklinghausen's neurofibroma and Steurer[51] two other cases of this condition; the latter also included a case of an epidermoid with slight hyperostosis of the orbital roof with six cases of dural hyperostosis causing exophthalmos. Davis[52] reported two cases of plexiform neurofibromatosis, in one of which the condition was associated with a glioma of the optic nerve. There are doubtless few tumors encountered elsewhere in the body that do not also appear in the orbit.

THE OPERATIVE PROCEDURE

The size of the cranial exposure has been greatly reduced since the earlier report. This is in large part due to the use of avertin with amylene hydrate as the routine anesthetic in operations on the brain. The great operative disadvantage of ether lies in the swelling of the brain that usually follows. It was to make allowance for this that the larger bony exposure was required. With the use of avertin with amylene hydrate the brain does not swell, and therefore a much smaller bony opening will serve just as effectively as the larger one when ether is used.

For exposure of the orbital roof the regular hypophysial approach is made. The concealed incision has for many years been employed in all operations on the brain and with no loss of room or increased difficulty of approach. The cutaneous incision begins about 2 cm. anterior to the ear, passes straight toward the midline and about 3 cm. from it makes a sharp curve forward and ends anteriorly at, or slightly in front of, the hair line. The galea and the skin are then stripped from the bone and temporal muscle and retracted anteriorly.

The bone flap is made so that the anterior border misses the frontal sinus and skirts the supraorbital ridge as far laterally as possible. When turned back and broken under the temporal muscle it is retracted laterally and is well out of the way. The dura is opened just within the bony margin, and the roughly circular incision is so complete that it becomes practically an autotransplant, thus being a factor in preventing postoperative extradural bleeding. The frontal lobe is elevated and the cisterna chiasmatis evacuated, thus reducing the volume of intracranial contents and providing room for attack on the roof of the orbit. The head is then lowered to permit the frontal lobe to fall away without the need of traction.

If the cisterna chiasmatis is not opened, the brain so completely fills the operative field that undue pressure would usually be necessary to retract the frontal lobe to a degree sufficient to permit the attack on the orbit and its contents.

From the optic foramen the dural covering of the orbital roof is incised in a curve, sweeping it laterally around the outer margin of the orbit and then curving anteriorly almost to the cribriform plate. The dural flap is stripped toward the midline with a periosteal elevator.

The initial opening in the orbital roof can frequently be made by applying slight force with the periosteal elevator at the thinnest point of the bone. The remainder of the roof is removed with rongeurs, care being taken not to extend the defect into the ethmoid cells. In 2 of my cases this happened and rhinorrhea promptly followed, necessitating reopening the wound and covering the opening with bone wax and the flap of dura. At times the bone is so thickened (by an osteoma) that the chisel is necessary to make the primary defect, and it may then be necessary to complete the removal of the roof with numerous applications of this instrument.

The capsule of the orbit then presents and is incised longitudinally and the edges retracted. Either the tumor or orbital fat presents, depending on the position of the growth. If fat presents, the growth is under pressure and extrudes and must be excised. Identification of the superior rectus muscle is usually immediate, unless the tumor is superimposed. This muscle is surrounded by a silk suture and retracted to one side, which provides inspection of the entire superior half of the orbit. From this view a tumor in any part of the orbit will be found, and its extirpation can be carried out deliberately. The optic nerve, the posterior part of the eyeball and the ophthalmic artery and vein are readily identified.

In only one case, in which evacuation of the cisterna provided much less room than normal, was there any trauma to the frontal lobe. Rather than take any chance with subsequent postoperative edema and intracranial pressure, a small part of the frontal lobe was removed. In closing, the dura is snugly resutured; the bone flap is replaced and wired, and the galea and the skin are closed without drainage.

There has been but one death in the series (case 22). With the huge mass of bone along the base of the middle and the anterior fossa, it doubtless would have been wiser to be content with a partial removal of the growth with the chisel rather than to attempt such an extensive extirpation.

The thought doubtless occurs: Does not pulsating exophthalmos follow removal of the orbital roof? I have looked carefully for such a sequel but have never found it, despite the fact that pulsating exophthalmos is known to occur when the orbital roof is congenitally absent.

Although I have never done a lateral Kronlein operation for an orbital tumor, it does not seem possible that it can provide the exposure for deliberate painstaking dissection of a tumor that is necessary to avoid injury to important structures within the orbit. And for tumors that extend beyond the orbital cavity, the Kronlein operation would, of course, be perfectly futile.

When an orbital tumor is small and protrudes anteriorly beyond the orbital ridge, the attack on the tumor by an incision under the supraorbital ridge is doubtless adequate, but when the tumor extends back of the eyeball the intracranial approach is advisable.

Before the operation is begun, the size and position of the frontal sinuses should be known. In making the anterior bony incision it is important that the frontal sinus be avoided. Entry into a frontal sinus is a potential source of infection and of subsequent rhinorrhea. If a frontal sinus is opened a flap of dura should be tightly sutured over the opening. If an ethmoid cell is opened it can be covered with wax and the dural flap replaced over it. A small opening in the frontal sinus may also be covered with wax, but the larger openings would require a dural flap. In none of the cases in this series was the frontal sinus opened. In case 18 the enormous tumor of long standing had completely obliterated the frontal sinuses, but the paranasal sinuses communicated with the wide open cerebral chamber (the whole frontal dura on both sides was removed with the attached tumor). No attempt was made to close this defect, and neither rhinorrhea nor infection followed. In two cases of this series infection followed entry into the ethmoid sinus and the bone flap had to be sacrificed.

The method of attack on the intracranial part of the tumor is dependent on the nature and position of the growth. Usually the hypophysial approach affords ample room. If the middle fossa or temporal lobe contains a large dural growth, it may be necessary to rongeur away an additional area of bone beneath the temporal muscle. This was done in two of my cases. It has not been necessary to enlarge the cutaneous incision or to turn down an additional bone flap, either of which, however, is easily possible if the situation should demand. Retraction of the temporal muscle with or without transverse division of its fibers will, after the underlying bone has been removed, expose most of the temporal lobe and even permit its resection

in large part if necessary. The removal of a large dural endothelioma is always a difficult feat and requires ample room. Since the arterial bleeding is from the middle meningeal artery, the tributaries of which cover the middle fossa to the foramen spinosum, it is essential that access to this area be unimpeded by inadequate exposure. The dural attachments should, when possible, be totally excised. As long as the dura along the floor of the middle fossa is the site of origin this is not difficult; in fact, the removal of this dura also greatly facilitates control of the severe bleeding from the middle meningeal artery. Not infrequently control of this bleeding is best accomplished by immediately following the middle meningeal artery to the foramen spinosum. Ligation or cauterization of the trunk of this vessel is usually far easier and safer than attempting to control the numerous bleeding points from its many branches.

The problems associated with the intracranial portion of these tumors are those encountered in any series of tumors of the brain. The risk involved in removing combined intraorbital and intracranial growths is confined almost exclusively to the part of the tumor within the cranial chamber, and the accompanying group of cases shows that even with enormous growths the danger is relatively slight.

Occasionally the internal carotid artery is surrounded by tumor, or at least attached to it. This complication occurred once (case 15) in this series of cases. To injure the internal carotid artery or the middle cerebral artery would mean disaster and must be avoided at all hazards. Rather than invite hemiplegia and probably death from arterial thrombosis by shaving the tumor too closely, there is no choice but deliberately to leave a nest of cells on this vessel.

When there is some exophthalmos and a dural endothelioma has been completely removed from the middle or anterior fossa, should one open the orbit? The answer is dictated by the fact that the bone about the tumor is thickened because of tumor contained within it. In 1 patient with this condition I removed the orbital roof, but since the eye was already blind (case 15) I did not incise the orbital fascia. Since the additional exposure of the orbit is simple and not time consuming and adds practically nothing to the operative risk, the surgical possibilities should be completed in one stage; moreover, a second stage is much more difficult, and the possibilities of a complete cure are reduced.

The most difficult surgical problem with this series of tumors has been in attacking the bilateral frontal tumors of enormous size. This was done in two cases. A bilateral approach was made with a long sweeping curve from one ear to the other and just under the hair line. The bone was so thick that the ordinary instruments used for making bone flaps were of little avail. Between large deep burr openings the bone was cut in a curve from the supraorbital ridge on one side to that on the other with large bone-cutting forceps. When the huge bone flap was turned back on the supraorbital ridge, the dura, which was densely attached, tore with it; this included the anterior part of the frontal sinuses, which, however, were practically obliterated by the tumor masses. This bone must, of course, be removed.

In May 1884 a remarkable extirpation of a tumor was performed by Durante,[53] of Rome, perhaps the earliest successful operation of its kind. It antedated by seven months the celebrated case of Rickman Gorlee, of England, to whom is usually accredited the first successful extirpation, although the removal was only partial. Whether or not Lister's aseptic methods were used is not stated in Durante's publication. His patient survived many years and was even apparently cured, the tumor doubtless being a dural endothelioma. The patient happened to be one with exophthalmos secondary to rupture of the orbital roof. A drain was placed from the depths of what Durante thought to be the nasal cavity, from rupture of the ethmoids,

but one is led to wonder if on account of the exophthalmos it might not have been the orbit; no infection followed. Durante's diagnosis was based on the patient's loss of smell, and the case is therefore one of the very earliest ones in which operation was performed after localization of the growth had been made from neurologic signs. The field of cerebral localization, based on the experiments of Fritsch and Hitzig and of Ferrier, was just beginning to stimulate interest and bring results. Except for the facts that the frontal bone was chiseled away and therefore sacrificed and no attempt was made to remove the orbital roof, the operative approach was strikingly similar to that presented in this paper.

In a recent publication on meningiomas (1938), Cushing and Eisenhardt[25] called attention to this approach, which they expected to use in forthcoming cases of tumor of the orbit. Adson and Benedict[43] (1934), Hoover and Horrax[30] (1935) and doubtless others have used this approach to remove orbital tumors.

PROPORTION OF (1) PURELY ORBITAL AND (2) COMBINED ORBITAL AND INTRACRANIAL TUMORS

Of all the tumors included in this report, only six, or 20 per cent, were confined solely to the orbit, and one of these was an inflammatory nodule. The combined incidence of orbital and intracranial tumors was, therefore, 80 per cent. If only the tumors in the operative series of twenty-four cases are analyzed, 25 per cent would be solely orbital and 75 per cent combined orbital and intracranial. In the entire series (both pathologic and operative observations) it is probable that all of the combined tumors arose primarily in the cranial chamber, except perhaps those which were multiple (in the four cases of glioma and the one case of Schuller-Christian disease, case 9). The earlier papers of Hudson and of Byers had prepared us for the high percentage of combined orbital and intracranial tumors, but their figures were even lower than our own. They, however, did not have the advantage of direct inspection of both cavities simultaneously but were dependent on necropsies or histories providing unmistakable evidence of subsequent intracranial lesions. If, however, the twenty-three postmortem examinations of orbital tumors reported in the combined papers of Byers and Hudson with twenty-one intracranial extensions of the growth are considered, it will be seen that the involvement of both the orbital and the cranial chambers actually exceeds the figures in this report.

MALIGNANCY OF TUMORS IN THIS SERIES

From the series of twenty-four patients operated on the outcome for only one is unknown (case 13). Five are known to be dead of the following causes and after the following intervals: (1) round cell sarcoma, three and one-half months after operation (case 6); (2) Schuller-Christian disease or xanthoma, five months after operation (case 9); (3) a malignant dural meningioma, twenty-two months after operation (case 14); (4) a dural meningioma with hyperostosis, ten years after operation (case 16), and (5) an operative death (case 22).

In three cases at least, and probably more, the condition is benign and should be permanently cured: case 1, an inflammatory nodule, three and one-quarter years; case 2, a fibroma, four years, and case 3, a spindle cell sarcoma, three years.

In the remaining cases the tumors must be looked on as malignant or as benign growths that could not be completely removed. The great group of dural tumors must be considered malignant because the orbital roof and frequently the skull over a large area were invaded by such a neoplasm and its complete extirpation was therefore impossible. The growth of a dural tumor, however, is usually very slow, and there should be relief for many years; one patient (case 16) survived ten years, and all the patients have survived a num-

ber of years. The same is doubtless true of the sarcoma with hyperostosis (case 13); this patient's subsequent course cannot be traced, but he was well when he left the hospital. Two other potentially benign tumors could not be completely removed (case 3, an osteoma, and case 12, a bilateral dural psammoma of the optic sheath). In the latter case eighteen years has passed since the operation and the tumor has made no observable progress. It is hoped that the osteoma (case 3), operated on two years ago, will grow as slowly as that in the introductory case in this paper, which has shown no recognizable progress in twenty-one years.

In the four living patients with Schuller-Christian disease the condition must be considered malignant. In the case of one of them (case 8) nearly three years has passed, but local recurrence is slowly progressive. The other three patients (cases 7, 10 and 11) have been operated on in the past few months, and although other lesions cannot be found and the orbital growth has been thoroughly removed, with contiguous tissue, a cure can hardly be expected.

SUMMARY

A series of twenty-four intraorbital tumors that have been operated on by the transcranial route is reported. Five, or 21 per cent, of these tumors were confined to the orbit; 18, 79 per cent, were combined intraorbital and intracranial growths; one of the former and two of the latter were metastatic. With an additional seven cases in which necropsy was performed but this operation had not been employed, the percentages are even more pronounced, 16 2/3 per cent and 83 1/3 per cent respectively. The pathologic features of the tumors are discussed.

The operative attack, proposed in 1921, is through a transcranial (hypophysial) approach. The roof of the orbit is removed after evacuating the cisterna chiasmatis; retraction of the frontal lobe then provides sufficient room.

The operation is offered not only for all

combined intraorbital and intracranial tumors but for growths that are restricted to the orbital cavity. As a matter of fact, it is rarely possible before operation to be certain whether or not the tumor also lies within the cranial chamber, as so many of them do (roughly 75 to 80 per cent in this series). Their coexistence should therefore be assumed on the law of probability.

For tumors confined to the orbit this operation offers a far better exposure of the tumor than is possible by any other method. Deliberate, careful dissection of the tumor is possible only by this approach. There is therefore much less chance of injury to the extraocular muscles, their nerve supply, the optic nerve and the ophthalmic vessels by this approach.

It offers the only hope of a permanent cure when the tumor is in both cavities, and when the condition is incurable it offers the maximum palliative result.

The operative risk in safe hands should be very low (41 per cent in this series) in regard to both tumors confined to the orbit and those with intracranial extensions. Prior exenteration of the orbit or removal of the eyeball will prevent the utilization of this operation, because the orbital tissues will be infected.

REFERENCES

[1]Byers, W. G. M.: Primary Intradural Tumors of the Optic Nerve. *Stud. Roy, Victoria Hosp., Montreal 1:* 3–82, 1901.

[2]Hudson, A. C.: Primary Tumours of the Optic Nerve. *Roy. London Ophth. Hosp. Rep., 18:* 317, 1910–1912.

[3]Dandy, W. E.: Prechiasmal Intracranial Tumors of the Optic Nerves. *Am. J. Ophth., 5:* 1, 1922; Prechiasmal Tumors Along the Optic Nerves, in Lewis, D.: *Practice of Surgery.* Hagerstown, Md., W. F. Prior Company, Inc., 1932, vol. 12, p. 662.

[4]Stokes, W. H., and Bowers, W. F.: Pure Fibroma of the Orbit: Report of Case and Review of Literature. *Arch. Ophth., 11:* 279 (Feb.) 1934.

[5]Cushing, H.: Experiences with Orbito-Ethmoidal Osteomata Having Intracranial Complications. *Surg., Gynec. & Obst., 44:* 721, 1927.

[6]Pilcher, C.: Bony Intracranial Tumors. *South. M. J., 31:* 613, 1938.

[7]Birch-Hirschfeld, A., in Schieck, F., and Bruckner, A.: *Kurzes Handbuch der Ophthalmologie.* Berlin, Julius Springer, 1930, vol. 3, p. 78.

[8]Ringel, T.: Ueber Tumoren, Pseudotumoren und Fremdkorper der Orbita. *Beitr. z. klin. Chir., 126:* 239, 1922.

[9]Rowland, R. S.: Xanthomatosis and Reticulo-Endothelial System. *Arch. Int. Med., 42:* 611 (Nov.) 1928; The Christian Syndrome and Lipoid Cell Hyperostosis of the Reticulo-Endothelial System. *Ann. Int. Med., 2:* 1277, 1929.

[10]Chester, W.: Ueber lipoid Granulomatose. *Virchows Arch. f. path. Anat., 279:* 561, 1930.

[11]Chiari, H.: Die generalisierte Xanthomatose vom Typus Schuller-Christian. *Ergebn. d. allg. path. u. path. Anat., 24:* 396, 1931.

[12]Heath, P.: Ocular Lipoid Histiocytosis and Allied Phenomena. *Arch. Ophth., 10:* 342 (Sept.) 1933.

[13]Knapp, A.: Xanthomatosis of the Orbit: Report of Two Cases. *Arch. Ophth., 11:* 141 (Jan.) 1934.

[14]Sautter, H.: Beitrag zur Kapitel der entzundlichen Pseudotumoren der Orbita am Hand. *Klin. Monatsbl. Augenh., 100:* 29, 1938.

[15]Schreck, E.: Zur Klinik und pathologischen Anatomie der Orbitaltumoren. *Klin. Monatsbl. Augenh., 103:* 1, 1939.

[16]Voelkel, R.: Zur Frage der symmetrischen Orbitaltumoren. *Klin. Monatsbl. Augenh., 98:* 169, 1937.

[17]Olivercrona, H., and Urban, H.: Ueber Meningeome der Siebbeinplatte. *Beitr. klin. Chir., 161:* 224, 1935.

[18]Schott: On Some Affections of the Optic Nerves. *Arch. Ophth. & Otolaryng., 6:*262, 1877.

[19]Spiller, W. S.: Hemicraniosis and Cure of Brain Tumor by Operation. *J.A.M.A., 49:*2059 (Dec. 21) 1907.

[20]Brissaud and Lerebloullet, P.: Deux cas d'hemicraniose. *Rev. neurol., 11:*537, 1903.

[21]Cushing, H.: The Cranial Hyperostoses Produced by Meningeal Endotheliomas. *Arch. Neurol. & Psychiat., 8:*139 (Aug.) 1922.

[22]Phemister, D. H.: The Nature of Cranial Hyperostosis Overlying Endothelioma of the Meninges. *Arch. Surg., 6:*554 (March) 1923.

[23]Penfield, W.: Cranial and Intracranial Endotheliomata Hemicraniosis. *Surg., Gynec. & Obst., 36:*657, 1923.

[24]Berard, L., and Dunet, C.: Hyperostosis craniennes et tumeurs meningees, *Lyon chir., 12:*502, 1924.

[25]Cushing, H., and Eisenhardt, L.: *Meningiomas.* Springfield, Ill., Charles C Thomas, Publisher, 1938.

[26]Armitage, A.: Osteoma of Frontal Sinus with Intracranial Complications, *Brit. J. Surg., 18:*565, 1931.

[27]Patterson, H., and Cairns, H.: Observations on the Treatment of Orbital Osteoma, with Report of a Case. *Brit. J. Ophth., 15:*458, 1931.

[28]Vorhis, H. C., and Adson, A. W.: Meningiomas

of the Spheniodal Ridge with Unilateral Exophthalmos. *S. Clin. North America, 14*:663, 1934.

²⁹Love, J. G.: Transcranial Removal of an Intraorbital Meningioma. *Proc. Staff Meet., Mayo Clin., 10*:213, 1935.

³⁰Hoover, W. B., and Horrax, G.: Osteomas of the Nasal Accessory Sinuses, with Report of a Case Illustrating the Transcranial Approach to Orbital Structures. *Surg., Gynec. & Obst., 61*:821, 1935.

³¹Vincent, C., and Mahoudeau, D.: Sur un cas d'osteome ethmoidoorbitaire avec pneumatocele opere par la methode de Cushing. *Rev. neurol., 68*:993, 1935.

³²Cairns, H.: Peripheral Ocular Palsies from the Neurosurgical Point of View. *Tr. Ophth. Soc. U. Kingdom, 58*:464, 1938.

³³Knapp, A.: Orbital Hyperostosis: Its Occurence in Two Cases of Meningioma of the Skull. *Arch. Ophth., 20*:996 (Dec.) 1938.

³⁴Elsberg, C. A.; Hare, C. C., and Dyke, C. G.: Unilateral Exophthalmos in Intracranial Tumors with Special Reference to Its Occurrence in the Meningiomata. *Surg., Gynec. & Obst., 55*:681, 1932.

³⁵Willemer, W.: Ueber eigentliche d. h. sich innerhalb der ausseren Scheide entwickelnde Tumoren des Sehnerven. *Arch. f. Ophth. (pt. 1), 25*:189, 1879.

³⁶Martin, P., and Cushing, H.: Primary Gliomas of the Chiasm and Optic Nerves in Their Intracranial Portion. *Arch. Ophth., 52*:209, 1923.

³⁷Lundberg, A.: Ueber die primaren Tumoren des Sehnerven und der Sehnervenkreuzung, Inaug. Dissert., Stockholm, Nordiska Bokhandeln, 1935.

³⁸Busch, E.: Surgical Treatment of Gliomas of the Optic Nerve and the Chiasma. *Zentralbl. Neurochir., 2*:364, 1938.

³⁹Coulter, R. J., and Coats, G.: Teratoma of the Orbit. *Roy. London Ophth. Hosp. Rep., 18*:64, 1910–1912.

⁴⁰Gow, W. H.: Orbital Tumor: Report of Unusual Case. *Brit. J. Ophth., 18*:520, 1934.

⁴¹Mancilla, G. A.: A Cavernous Angioma of the Orbit. *Rev. med. de Sevilla, 42*:26, 1923.

⁴²Byers, W. G. M.: Case of Encapsulated Angioma of Orbit. *Arch. Ophth. 53*:280, 1923.

⁴³Adson, A. W., and Benedict, W. L.: Hemangio-Endothelioma of the Orbit: Removal Through Transcranial Approach. *Arch. Ophth., 12*:484 (Oct.) 1934.

⁴⁴Franklin, W. S., and Cordes, F. G.: A Case of Orbital Lymphangioma. *J.A.M.A., 83*:1741 (Feb. 16) 1924.

⁴⁵Knapp, A.: Oil Cyst of Orbit. *Arch. Ophth., 52*:163, 1923.

⁴⁶Wheeler, J. M.: Orbital Cyst Without Epithelial Lining: Report of Two Cases of Blood Cyst. *Arch. Ophth., 18*:356 (Sept.) 1937.

⁴⁷Stallard, H. B.: Cavernous Hemangioma of the Orbit Successfully Removed by Kronlein's Operation. *Lancet, 1*:131, 1938.

⁴⁸de Schweinitz, G. E.: A Contribution to the Subject of Tumors of the Eyelid and Orbit. *Tr. Am. Ophth. Soc., 14*:341, 1915.

⁴⁹Pinkus, F.: Ueber "Cholesteatoma" der Orbite. *Klin. Monatsbl. Augenh., 90*:145, 1933.

⁵⁰van der Hoeve, J.: Rontgenphotographie des Foramen opticum bei Geschwulsten und Erkrankungen der Sehnerven. *Arch. Ophth., 115*:355, 1925.

⁵¹Steurer, O.: Ueber Beiteilung des inneren Ohres und des Hornerven bei multipler Neurofibromatosis Recklinghausen, mit besonderer Berucksichtigung des sekundar absteigenden Degeneration des Hornerven. *Ztschr. Hals-, Nasen- u. Ohrenh., 4*:124, 1922.

⁵²Davis, F. A.: Plexiform Neurofibromatosis (Recklinghausen's Disease) of Orbit and Globe, with Associated Glioma of Optic Nerve and Brain: Report of Case. *Arch. Ophth., 22*:761 (Nov.) 1939.

⁵³Durante, F.: Contribution to Endocranial Surgery. *Lancet, 2*:654, 1887.

LXVI

ON THE PATHOLOGY OF CAROTID-CAVERNOUS ANEURYSMS (PULSATING EXOPHTHALMOS)*

WALTER E. DANDY, M. D. AND RICHARD H. FOLLIS JR., M. D.

The last word upon the clinical features of carotid–cavernous-sinus aneurysms has probably been said by C. H. Sattler in his exhaustive publication on pulsating exophthalmos (Handbuch der gesamten Augenheilkunde, 1920). It is unlikely that more than minor variations in the clinical expressions of this lesion will be found. A method of curing these desperate lesions when they proved to be refractory to the simpler surgical efforts heretofore in vogue was recently presented by one of us (W. E. D.). The hazards of any form of surgical treatment of such cases are attested by the two pathological specimens to be described, obtained at necropsy in the only two fatal cases in the series. These dangers are in part due to the risks of the operative attack *per se* and in even greater degree to the variable and unpredictable vascular patterns of the circle of Willis, upon which the development of an adequate collateral arterial circulation to the brain is dependent. The age of the patient is always an additional risk which unquestionably increases with the years. However, because of congenital variations of the circle of Willis, youth is no assurance against this danger.

It is principally with the anatomical details of carotid–cavernous-sinus aneurysms that this publication is concerned. Two post-mortem specimens are presented: the patient in one case died from rupture of the carotid artery when a clip was placed intracranially; in the other, probably from multiple infarcts in the brain stem. The

relationship, if any, of these infarcts to the operative application of a partially occluding band on the internal carotid artery in the neck is not clear. The temporary cerebral anemia in the second case was doubtless due to a minute posterior communicating artery on the affected side and to a small anterior cerebral artery by which alone a collateral arterial blood supply was possible. At the time of Dandy's recent publication on carotid-cavernous aneurysms (1937), twenty-nine pathological specimens of carotid-cavernous arteriovenous aneurysms were recorded in the literature, most of them inadequately described, and in the great majority it was merely noted that an opening existed in the carotid artery within the cavernous sinus. It has previously been emphasized: (1) that in no other part of the body does an artery actually traverse a venous channel and thus lend itself so readily to the development of an arteriovenous fistula, and (2) that within the cranial chamber large arteries and veins are not contiguous and, therefore, (3) in no other part of the cranial chamber can a *traumatic* or otherwise *acquired* arteriovenous fistula develop. All arteriovenous aneurysms within the brain (and there are many of these) are, therefore, of congenital origin. Carotid–cavernous-sinus aneurysms may arise either as a direct or indirect result of trauma to a normal or abnormal (preexisting aneurysm) carotid artery within the cavernous sinus; or they may result from spontaneous rupture of an arteriosclerotic internal carotid artery or a preexisting aneurysm of this artery within the cavernous sinus. Of the twenty-nine postmortem specimens, six-

*Reprinted from the *American Journal of Ophthalmology*, 24:4, April, 1941.

teen were presumably of traumatic, and thirteen of spontaneous origin. It is not entirely unlikely that in some of these entered as traumatic there may well have been, as possibly in one of our cases, a preexisting aneurysm that was already on the point of rupture, and the trauma may have had little, or perhaps no, bearing upon its production. There are, in fact, reasons to believe that seriously defective walls of the internal carotid artery are more common in its intracavernous portion than in the neck or intracranially.

Case Reports

CASE 1. (U-135247). *Diagnosis.* Bilatlateral carotid-cavernous-sinus arteriovenous aneurysms—presumably postraumatic (16 years' duration).

Treatment. (1) Fascial band applied to left internal carotid artery (April 18, 1938). (2) Portion of internal, external, and common carotid arteries about band area removed 58 days later. (3) Attempted application of silver clip to internal carotid artery intracranially (death five hours later). (4) Necropsy 67 days after application of the band, and nine days after removal of portion of the arteries.

A colored male, aged 53 years, entered the Johns Hopkins Hospital on March 17, 1938, because of bilateral carotid-cavernous-sinus arteriovenous aneurysms, from the effects of which he was almost blind. He had long been a patient in the dispensary, where he was treated for syphilis of the cardiovascular system. His blood pressure was 160/105 in 1932. He had arteriosclerosis and dilation of the aorta.

The present illness began sixteen years ago (at another time he said eleven years ago) following an injury to the head. The history of trauma is none too dependable. Whether or not his pulsating exophthalmos dated from that time is not certain; he remembered very little about the injury and did not know whether he was unconscious afterwards. However, at that (indefinite) time the left eye turned outward and he became aware of a noise in the head. On further inquiry into the hospital records it was found that he did have an accident in 1932. This great disparity in dates is indicative of the patient's mental unreliability. He was very forgetful, and all his statements concerning

past history were so changeable as to be entirely uncertain.

He was first seen in the Johns Hopkins Dispensary in December, 1930, and again in 1932. At the time of the latter admission he complained of a continual roar in the head, dizziness, ringing in the left ear, and poor vision in both eyes. The objective findings were: bilateral strabismus, slight bilateral exophthalmos, ectropion of the left lower lid, paresis of both sixth nerves, and total paralysis of the left third nerve. He said he had been advised from time to time to have something done, but as long as any vision remained he was averse to surgical treatment.

He again entered the Johns Hopkins Hospital, March 17, 1938, following a drunken brawl. He was semiconscious, but his condition rapidly cleared. At that time there was marked proptosis of the right eye, none of the left. (Proptosis was not measured.) The right eyeball pulsated strongly and synchronously with the pulse; the left did not. There was marked convergent strabismus in the left eye, but none in the right; movement of the left eye was impossible. Tremendous tortuous bulging vessels stood out over the forehead on both sides, but much more on the right. There was a big bed of pulsating vessels along the bridge of the nose; all of these vessels pulsated strongly. A thrill was palpable over the vessels and a loud murmer heard over practically the entire head, but more intensely over the temporal and frontal regions. The pupils were of average size: that of the left eye barely reacted to light; that of the right reacted somewhat better. The optic discs were atrophic and pale but sharply defined, the veins engorged and tortuous. The blood pressure was then 176/100. Compression of the right carotid artery in the neck did not affect the bruit nor the size of the vessels over the forehead. Obliteration of the left carotid artery modified but did not entirely stop the loud bruit; there remained a slight humming sound. Following compression of either internal carotid for half a minute the patient became dizzy.

The patient was entirely blind in the left eye and could only count fingers with the right. Both eyes were turned inward toward the nose, the left much more than the right.

One month later the patient was squeezing a furuncle on the nose when he opened one of the large vessels. The bleeding was quite severe; he came at once to the dispensary where pressure was applied and the bleeding controlled. Frightened by the possibility of further hemorrhages he was eager for surgical intervention.

OPERATIONS. *First, April 16, 1938.* Partial occlusion of the *left* internal carotid artery by a band of fascia lata (W. E. D.).

One could only assume that the arteriovenous fistula was on the left side because (1) the bruit was markedly affected by closure of the left internal carotid artery in the neck; that of the right had no effect; and (2) the third-nerve palsy was complete on the left. On the other hand, the exophthalmos was only on the right, and the tortuous pulsating vessels were on the right. It was therefore, necessary to assume that the left ophthalmic vien was thrombosed.

Since it was clear from the compression test that total ligation of the internal carotid artery in the neck could not be tolerated, partial occlusion of the internal carotid was performed under local anesthesia. The internal carotid artery was very large and pulsated strongly; it was at least twice as large as the external carotid artery. The fascial band was placed around the internal carotid artery just above the bifurcation and sutured when it had reduced the artery to approximately one third of its original circumference. Pulsation and a thrill were still present above the band, but the difference in the degree of pulsation above and below the band was very marked. The patient was carefully watched before the band was permanently fixed, but there were no symptoms. He immediately realized the great diminution of the noise in the head, but it was still present.

The patient was discharged ten days later, after an uneventful recovery. The bruit remained, perhaps somewhat diminished, but still strongly heard over the entire head.

The patient was readmitted on June 14, 1938, two months after the partial ligation of the carotid artery in the neck. The size of the vessels in the forehead and eyes and the pulsating exophthalmos were practically unchanged from the findings at the first admission. The blood pressure was now 230/105. Compression of the artery in the neck was well borne for five minutes without cerebral symptoms.

Second operation, June 15, 1938. Excision of part of left internal carotid artery with band. Total occlusion of internal carotid.

The old wound was reopened under avertin anesthesia. The carotid artery was surrounded by a very dense scar which made the dissection difficult. The vagus nerve and the jugular vein were tightly matted to the artery and required sharp dissection for their liberation. The jugular vein was opened during this process and ligated. The internal carotid artery was totally occluded with a silk ligature just above the scarred area. After this the internal carotid artery, the external carotid artery, and the common carotid artery were closed with silk sutures and the intervening trunks (containing the old band) were removed in one piece. It is worthy of note that no change occurred in pulse, blood pressure, or respirations during this procedure. The patient's postoperative course was uneventful.

Nine days later, June 24, 1938, an attempt was made to place a silver clip on the left internal carotid artery intracranially. The artery was so large that the clip which had heretofore been used in other cases would not straddle the vessel and in an attempt to force it with a little pressure, the calcified artery tore. Although the immediate bleeding was terrific, it was quickly suppressed with the spatula and both ends were clipped without injury to the circle of Wills. But the hemorrhage into the posterior fossa had been sufficient to cause death five hours later.

PATHOLOGICAL REPORT (Autopsy No. 15915). The autopsy was performed fourteen hours after death. Aside from cardiac hypertrophy (510 grams), moderate arteriosclerosis, and pulmonary emphysema, all the important gross and microscopic pathological changes were found in the cervical and cranial vascular system. It should be noted that the partially occulding fascial band had been placed on the internal carotid artery just cephalad to the bifurcation 67 days before death, and the section of the arteries including the band had been removed nine days before death.

Arteriovenous fistulae. The entire sphenoid bone together with the anterior portion of the occipital bone was removed, and two transverse sections were made through the specimen. The first was through the stalk of the hypophysis, and the second just anterior to the posterior clinoid process, making it possible to see both carotid arteries and both cavernous sinuses.

Description of specimen. In its course through the foramen lacerum the wall of the left internal carotid artery and related structures was so greatly thickened that quite a mass had been formed; the thickness of the wall (2 mm.) was about three times the normal, but its lumen (4.5 mm.) was not affected and in size equal to that of the opposite side. There was a small, flat, partially obliterating thrombus within the artery in this region; this may possibly have been related to the greater thickness of the overlying arterial wall. After the first bend in the artery as it entered the cavernous sinus, the vessel remained unchanged in size for a distance of 1.25 cm.; at this point the anterior, posterior, and lateral walls diverged, forming a sac measuring 1.5 cm. in its greatest diameter, and 6 mm. in width; the major bulge was in the anterior wall of the sac (artery). In the lateral wall of the aneurysmal sac was a small calcified plaque. On the anterior wall of this sac and at a point 5 mm. above its origin was the first of two openings into the cavernous sinus. It was roughly oval and measured 4 by 7 mm. Its margins were slightly irregular but smooth. A second fistulous opening from the aneurysmal sac was approximately of the same size; it was 1 cm. above the first opening and on the superior wall of the sac. The margins of this opening were also somewhat irregular but smooth. The walls of the aneurysmal sac were much thinner than those of the carotid artery and eventually for this reason it became difficult to tell where the artery terminated and the thickened walls of the cavernous sinus began. The superior continuation of the carotid artery from the aneurysmal sac is shown by the entering probe. It is worthy of note that, in cross section, the continuation of the internal carotid artery above the aneurysmal dilatation was distinctly smaller than that of the opposite side and was triangular in shape, owing to the compression on all sides by an enlarged cavernous sinus and the aneurysmal sac.

Microscopically, the thickening of the left catrotid artery at its entrance into the cavernous sinus was found to be due to an increase in the size of the media. The elastica was intact as the artery entered the skull. However, at the point where the lumen began to widen, the elastic layer

completely disappeared and the wall of the dilated artery was composed for the most part of elongated muscle cells and hyaline connective tissue. There was no evidence of any inflammatory change. The wall of the left carotid above the dilatation was normal.

The cavernous sinus, left side. The cavernous sinus was a very large sac measuring 2.5 cm. (vertical) by 2.5 cm. (width) by 1.5 cm. (anteroposterior). A mesial pouch of the cavernous sinus extended beneath the internal carotid artery and pushed the hypophysis toward the opposite side; the left border of the hypophysis just reached the midline. This pouch also elevated the intracranial portion of the internal carotid artery and this in turn produced sharp angulation of the optic nerve where it was fixed at the optic foramen. The wall of the cavernous sinus on the left side was composed of dense, hyaline connective tissue. In places there were bluish staining granules of calcium. Hyaline thrombus was adherent to the wall; in the anterior portion there was a fresher thrombus undergoing organization.

A second round pouch (1 cm. by 1 cm.) of the left cavernous sinus lay just over fistula no. 2, and projected intracranially through the opening where the third nerve entered the wall of the sinus. It was sharply defined and looked like a little tumor. This venous pouch flattened the oculomotor nerve, which was spread like a fan over its anterior border. The normal trabeculae within the cavernous sinus had been entirely destroyed so that a single big smooth cavity resulted. The walls of the sinus were everywhere greatly thickened, in places to 2 or 3 mm., and in one place were definitely calcified.

The *right cavernous* sinus was roughly a third as large as the left and contained numerous trabeculae. The two pouches that were present in the left were also represented here but both were very much smaller. The places at which these pouches developed were doubtless the weak spots in the wall of the cavernous sinus.

The *intervacernous connection* is interesting. Immediately beneath the hypophysis was a roughly oval venous sac measuring 1 cm. by 8 mm. This sac communicated with each cavernous sinus by an opening about 2 mm. in diameter. This was the only direct communication between the two cavernous sinuses. A very wide patent basilar sinus afforded much greater communication, although in a slightly more indirect way; that is, downward behind the posterior clinoid process.

Venous tributaries. The superior ophthalmic vien on the *left* was completely thrombosed from its mouth in the cavernous sinus to the most anterior part of the orbital contents (5 cm.) that remained after removal at necropsy. No trace of an inferior ophthalmic vein could be found. The lumen of the thrombosed vein was only about 1 mm. wide at the cavernous sinus and about 2 to 3 mm. at its greatest diameter within the orbit. The wall of this thrombosed vessel was as thick as the normal carotid artery. Microscopically, this vein presented an interesting appearance. There was an adventitial layer a little thicker than normal. Next was found a layer of connective-tissue cells together with a few muscle cells which probably represented the media. Farther in, were numerous thinwalled vascular channels all infiltrated with lymphocytes. Between these and the lumen, there was a band of hyaline connective tissue to which organized thrombus was attached.

The right superior ophthalmic vein was enormous (diameter 1.2 cm.), elongated, and tortuous. There was no inferior ophthalmic vein on this side. The walls were not thickened, but were probably actually thinner than normal.

The *inferior petrosal* sinuses were fairly symmetrical blind pouches which did not communicate with the jugular system; apparently no communication had ever existed. The basilar sinus afforded connection between the two inferior petrosal sinuses and indirectly between the two cavernous sinuses was like an hourglass in shape, the constricting center being at the midline and only 2 mm. in diameter. Trabeculae were present in the *right* inferior petrosal and *right* half of the basilar sinus, but were absent in both of these sinuses on the *left side.*

The superior petrosal sinuses were also blind, roughly symmetrical pouches on both sides; they measured 1 cm. in length and 8 mm. in width. They did not communicate with the lateral sinuses, but ended over the dural foramina conveying the sensory root of the trigeminus. The sphenoparietal sinuses appeared to be absent; at least, extension of the cavernous sinus through either foramina ovale could not be demonstrated.

Arteries. The intracavernous portion of the left internal carotid artery has been described under the fistula. It may be added that this artery was closely applied to the sphenoid bone and the hypophysis except anteriorly, where a bulge in the cavernous sinus projected below the bone and the artery, pushing the latter laterally. On the right, the carotid artery was everywhere fixed mesially. In the other case described in this paper these arteries were closely applied to the lateral wall of the sinus and were separated from the hypophysis by the venous bed.

In the accompanying drawing the differences in size and position of the intracavernous portion of the internal carotid artery on the two sides are shown. On the *left* the lower portion of the artery was pushed to the midline of the head; on the *right* the artery was pushed laterally at one point by a projection of the cavernous sinus.

Other arterial abnormalities. The markedly abnormal circle of Willis is shown in the accompanying drawing. All of the arteries were full of sclerotic plaques. The anterior communicating artery was double and each trunk as large as the anterior cerebral artery. A small dilatation (aneurysm) bulged posteriorly along the right anterior cerebral artery.

The posterior communicating artery on the *right* was small; the one on the *left,* nearly as large as the carotid. The posterior communicating artery was practically continuous with the posterior cerebral artery—a not uncommon finding.

At the junction between the left posterior communicating and posterior cerebral arteries was a sacculated aneurysm that measured 1 cm. by 8 mm. This was unruptured and contained no thrombus. The basilar and both vertebral arteries were very large; the walls contained many calcified plaques.

Thrombi. A well-organized gray single thrombus 1.7 cm. by 1.2 cm. filled the inferior portion of the left cavernous sinus. This thrombus lay 2 or 3 mm. beyond fistula no. 1 and did not, therefore, reach the fistula. The extensive and doubtless much older thrombosis of the left ophthalmic vein has been noted. There was no connection between this thrombus and that in the pouch of the cavernous sinus. A small, fiat, partially obliterating (by about one third) thrombus in the carotid just before it entered the skull coincided with the thickened arterial wall. There was no thrombus at any point in the intracavernous portion of the carotid artery.

Brain. When the calvarium and dura were removed, a small amount of blood was found beneath the dura on the left side. The convolutions were slightly flattened but there was no marked pressure cone. A large hemorrhage was observed beneath the arachnoid at the base and especially over the cerebellar hemispheres on their inferior aspect.

The lateral cerebral ventricles were of normal size; a blood clot partially filled the posterior horns as well as the fourth ventricle. On numerous sections of the brain the only lesion found was a small area of punctate hemorrhages in the cortex about the level of the anterior limit of the caudate nucleus on the left. Microscopically, no change that might be referable to the carotid ligation could be made out on the left side. The ganglion cells had normal-appearing nuclei and their cytoplasmic contents showed no change. There were several small arteries with calcified walls in the corpus striatum, on both sides.

Eyes. There was distinct atrophy of the optic nerves. Except for a few thickened blood vessels in the choroid, the remaining portions of the posterior segments of the eyes showed nothing upon histological examination.

CASE 2. (U-143515). Admittance, June 10, 1938; death, July 18, 1938.

Diagnosis. Bilateral carotid-cavernous-sinus arteriovenous aneurysms—posttraumatic (three weeks' duration).

Treatment. (1) Partially constricting fascial band on internal carotid artery (June 11, 1938). (2) Removal of band one day later (recovery of symptoms followed). (3) Band replaced 10 days later. (4) Total ligation of internal carotid artery 24 days later (death two days later).

A quite feeble old lady, aged sixty-eight years, had been perfectly well until she had had a fall three weeks previous to admittance. She was stunned momentarily but was not unconscious. A resulting Colles fracture was reduced and a cast applied in another hospital, where she remained seven days. Her right eye was swollen immediately after the accident and there was some protrusion of the eyeball. Since the accident there had been a continuous roar in the right side of her head. Because of the noise and the protruding eye she was brought to the Johns Hopkins Dispensary, where Dr. Frank Ford made the diagnosis

of a carotid-cavernous-sinus arteriovenous aneurysm and sent her into the Johns Hopkins Hospital, on June 10, 1938.

The following positive observations were recorded: (1) Marked protrusion of the right eyeball, with (2) complete ophthalmoplegia, and (3) complete ptosis of the upper lid; (4) marked edema of the conjunctivae of both upper and lower lids and slight eversion of the lids from this cause; (5) over the right side of the skull a loud systolic bruit could be heard. It could be stopped by pressure upon the internal carotid artery, but pressure upon the artery could be tolerated only a few seconds, after which the patient swooned. The exophthalmos of the right eye measured 6 mm. No pulsation could be seen or felt at any time in the protruding eye. The visual acuity was 20/70 in the right eye and 20/30 in the left. There was a temporal quadrantal defect for form and color in the right eye; the fields for form and color in the remaining vision were markedly restricted.

At this time there was no protrusion of the left eye, nor was there any fullness nor tortuosity of the veins over the forehead on either side. On account of the subjective roar and the objective systolic murmur we believe that there must be an arteriovenous aneurysm, and that there was no enlargement of the veins of the forehead because of local venous thrombosis. The patient's blood pressure was 150/90.

OPERATIONS. *First, June 11, 1938.* Under local anesthesia, a band of fascia lata about 1 cm. wide was placed around the internal carotid artery just above the bifurcation of the common carotid (W. E. D.). Aside from the fact that the internal carotid made a complete S-shaped loop in the neck, there were no anatomical variations. Its size was quite normal. In making this loop the artery ran exactly transversely in the neck for a short distance. This same observation had been made in the case of the other patient. There was a tremendous thrill in the transverse portion of the loop, but no thrill could be felt in the arterial trunk just above the bifurcation. At first we thought the transverse portion of the artery was a big vein, as it was distinctly blue, but when the artery was dissected upwards it was found to be simply a loop which when untangled made the artery quite redundant. It was thought that the thrill was probably due to the kink in the vessel from the formation of the redundant loop, but when the artery was straightened out the thrill persisted.

When the band was drawn so as to constrict the artery and then sutured in place there was still pulsation above the constriction. Prior to this we had tied the band a little more tightly, but, as the pulse above was quite feeble, we decided that in view of the patient's age it might reduce the circulation too seriously. The sutures were removed and replaced in order to provide a larger opening in the arterial lumen. It was thought that following this the circulation should be adequate.

Subsequent course. During the night the patient was quite well, but on the following day she became slightly drowsy; the lethargy steadily deepened and at the same time a definite left-sided facial weakness was noted. Under local anesthesia the band was removed and immediately the pulse returned in the exposed artery above the band, and promptly thereafter function in the left side of the body improved; in another 24 hours it was quite normal. The drowsiness also became less marked. The patient appeared to be essentially as she had been before the operation. Immediately after the band had been placed and during the first night, the murmur that had been heard over the right side of the head was abolished, but upon removal of the band it was heard as before. It is also worthy of note that the thrill in the loop of the cervical carotid artery, which was exposed at the operation, again returned when the band was removed.

On the following day—that is, 24 hours after the band was removed—the *left eyeball became edematous and the murmur could now be heard over the left side of the head.* The patient's general condition was good; she was quite responsive, and had normal power in the left leg and arm. There was no facial weakness and no Babinski. On the following day, June 14th, the left eye was definitely more prominent; there was ptosis of the upper lid and almost complete paralysis of the third nerve, all of which came on overnight. The edema of the lids was further increased, but there was no definite pulsation in either eye. There was now definitely bilateral exophthalmos. The exophthalmos of the second side, therefore, developed 25 days after the accident. The extraocular movements were now equally limited on the two sides, there being almost complete

bilateral ophthalmoplegia.

On June 22, 1938, the wound was opened and a partially constricting band of fascia lata again placed around the vessel, care being taken not to constrict the vessel too severely. It was hoped that new tissue, building up around the band, would eventually induce occlusion. A good pulse remained above the band. The bruit was reduced but was distinctly present. On the following day the bruit had returned to the preoperative level.

On July 7th—27 days after admission—the vision had rapidly declined in both eyes to R.E. 6/100, and L.E. 6/40 (it was 6/40 right and 6/12 left on admission). The visual fields had not changed. The exophthalmometer readings were 25 left and 24 right (12 left and 18 right on admission). There was then slight blurring of both nerve heads, but no hemorrhages; the retinal veins were full and quite tortuous (examinations were made by Dr. Alan Woods).

The patient's condition remained practically unchanged until July 13th, 21 days following the replacement of the fascial band, and one month following the first application of the band. Her blood pressure was then 150/100, essentially the same as on admission. From that time on the patient began to decline rapidly; she became progressively more drowsy, but there was no return of the weakness on the left side of the body.

On July 15, 1938, under local anesthesia, the right internal carotid artery was totally ligated above the band with a double suture of medium silk. There was no immediate effect following this operation. The left side was not weak, but during the following two days the drowsiness that had already become apparent and progressive before the operation steadily deepened, and the patient died on July 18, 1938. Fever first appeared five days before her death and gradually increased until the end. Three days before her death there was early papilledema of both discs, and numerous small hemorrhages were seen scattered throughout both fundi.

PATHOLOGICAL REPORT (Autopsy No. 15959). The autopsy was performed one and a half hours after death. Permission was restricted to an examination of the head, neck, and thorax. The aorta showed only moderate arteriosclerosis. The right lung was normal. There was some fibrinous exudate over the surface of the left lung and scattered areas of lobular pneumonia. This was verified by microscopic study.

Arteriovenous fistula and related structures. The sphenoid bone together with the anterior portion of the occipital bone was removed *in toto.* A frontal section was made (a.a.') directly through the hypophyseal stalk in order to show the cavernous sinuses and the carotid arteries. A few millimeters after it passed through the foramen lacerum, the right carotid artery presented an oval opening (9 by 7 mm.) on the superior lateral wall. The edges of the opening were smooth and regular. The artery beyond was smaller than the left internal carotid. This difference in size was found within both the cavernous sinus and the cranial chamber, where this vessel was about two thirds as large as the opposite artery. The left internal carotid showed no lesion. Miscroscopic study of the wall of both intracranial portions of the carotid arteries revealed no change. A section through the fistula in the right carotid showed elastic tissue extending almost to the margin of the opening in normal fashion. At this point the elastic fibers became frayed and ceased entirely, and beyond this for a short distance the margin of the opening was made up of connective-tissue cells with very little collagen present.

Cavernous sinuses. Both cavernous sinuses were approximately the same size, each being at least twice the normal size. When the base of the skull was viewed from above one could see a distinct though not marked bulge in the region of the cavernous sinuses. The bulge would doubtless have been much increased during life when filled with blood. There was wide communication between the two cavernous sinuses through a *single* large intercavernous sinus, the width of which was 1.2 cm. at the maximum and 5 mm. at the narrowest part. This extensive intercavernous sinus (circular) extended about 3 mm. posterior to the hypophysis and ended about 3 mm. posterior to anterior border of the hypophysis. The pituitary body was elevated and compressed by it from beneath, and laterally was also compressed by the symmetrically enlarged cavernous sinuses. Trabeculae were still present in both cavernous sinuses but were more in evidence on the left. The enlargement of the cavernous sinuses had pushed both internal carotid arteries laterally, had mark-

edly compressed both oculomotor nerves, and had elevated both optic nerves at the optic foramina to such a degree that a decided angulation resulted. Both Gasserian ganglia were elevated and flattened by the lateral extension of the enlarged cavernous sinuses.

Venous tributaries. On both sides the superior and inferior ophthalmic veins entered the cavernous sinuses separately; the superior branches were about twice the normal size, and the inferior branches slightly less. The inferior petrosal sinuses were somewhat enlarged where they arose from the cavernous sinuses. Each measured about 1.2 cm. in diameter and retained this dimension for a distance of 2 cm., when they abruptly diminished to a diameter of 4 mm. The basilar sinus measured 1 cm. in width and was fairly uniformly dilated from side to side. It was at least 5 mm. in depth.

A superior petrosal sinus was present on each side, but showed no definite dilatation. Although the cavernous sinus was actually much enlarged under the mandibular branch of the trigemenus as far as the foramen ovale, one could detect no enlargement of the connections with the pterygoid plexus.

The spenoparietal sinuses were present on both sides but barely admitted a probe.

Thrombi. There were no thrombi in any part of the arterial or venous components of the arteriovenous lesion nor of the arteries or veins in the neck.

Anomalies along the circle of Willis. At three points there were curious outpouchings of the arterial wall and at

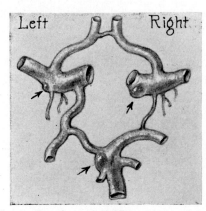

Fig. 1 (Dandy and Follis). Circle of Willis, case 2. Note small right posterior communicating branch as well as inadequate communicating artery.

these places the wall became very thin (potential aneurysms). On the posterior wall of the right internal carotid artery was a small bulging area (4 by 4 mm.) of marked thinning—so thin that a rupture seemed imminent, but the wall was intact. On the left carotid where the choroidal artery began there was a similar thin pouch like tiny aneurysm; it too, was unruptured. On the basilar artery (left side) was a similar thinning, at the point where the superior cerebellar artery began. The anterior communicating artery was tiny, not more than 1 mm. in diameter. The right posterior communicating artery was not larger. It was in marked contrast to the unusually large posterior communicating artery on the left side. A section through one of the out-pouchings on the circle of Willis showed a greatly thinned wall, with loss of elastic tissue.

Brain. Externally the brain showed nothing except a few small hemorrhages in several convolutions on the orbital surface of the right frontal lobe. There was very light sclerosis of the vessels at the base. The right carotid was about two thirds the diameter of the left carotid. The basilar and vertebral arteries were normal.

Infarct within the brain. On section through the brain there was seen an infarct with a rather curious distribution. On the right side beginning in the anterior part of the right frontal lobe a little anterior to the internal capsule the white matter showed some old softening. As one proceeded posteriorly, the white matter was found to be soft until the anterior portion of the globus pallidus was reached. Here the tissue was likewise soft, and there was an old cavity between the globus pallidus and the internal capsule. All had the appearance of an old lesion. In the cortex of the island of Reil on the left side there were small hemorrhages with some softening. Proceeding posteriorly, there was found in the midline a fresher lesion consisting of hemorrhage and necrosis of the mesencephalic tissues; the mesial margins of both cerebral peduncles were involved at this level. Still farther back the lesion continued. In the anterior part of the pons the tissue in the midline beneath the aqueduct was softened, and there was a hemorrhage in the inferior half of the left side of the pons. Farther back in the pons at its posterior extremity, the whole inferior half was

necrotic and there was a triangular area of necrosis and hemorrhage in the tissue beneath the fourth ventricle. Microscopically, at the site of the gross lesions described above, there were areas of hemorrhage and necrosis. At many such points all the ganglion and glial cells were necrotic, and the tissue was swollen and vacuolated. No completely occluded vessels could be made out in numerous sections. The areas of hemorrhage and necrosis were accompanied by another interesting change. Especially marked in the globus pallidus, though to a lesser extent in the thalamus, cerebellum, and even the cerebral cortex, were many small arteries with calcified walls. Even out in the tissues there were numerous granules which took a dark blue stain with hematoxylin, and some of these had the outlines of nerve cells. Some of the vessels were narrowed by the deposition of this material in their walls but none, as stated above, could be found which were completely occluded. There was just as much of this material on the right as on the left side.

Eyes. Microscopic study of the posterior segments of both eyes revealed very little atrophy of the optic nerve. There were a few small hemorrhages in the retina as well as edema of the choroid. The vessels in the latter seemed prominent.

Summary of Vascular Findings at and Near the Carotid—Cavernous-Sinus Arteriovenous Aneurysms

CASE 1. (1) Two separate fistulae of approximately the same size and roughly circular were found between the left internal carotid artery and the cavernous sinus. Each measured 4.7 mm. in the two directions. The edges were smooth.

(2) The first fistula was in the anterior wall of an arterial dilatation within the cavernous sinus—doubtless a preexisting arterial aneurysm. The second fistula was on the superior wall of the sac and was 1 cm. distant from the first fistula.

(3) The cavernous sinus was dilated and measured 2.5 cm. vertically, 2.5 cm. in width, and 1.5 in length. The contralateral cavernous sinus was about one third as large.

(4) A mesial pouch of the sinus dis-

located the hypophysis to the opposite side.

(5) A second mesial pouch of the sinus projected intracranially and compressed the oculomotor nerve.

(6) The walls of the cavernous sinus were thickened (in places 2 to 3 mm.), and in one place there was calcification.

(7) The walls of the ethmoid cells were eroded and the mucosa was displaced.

(8) The two cavernous sinuses were connected directly by a 2-mm. opening lying between the two dilated pouches of the cavernous sinuses. Indirectly they communicated through the basilar sinus by a 2-mm. opening that was continuous with the inferior petrosal sinuses.

(9) The inferior and superior petrosal sinuses ended laterally in blind pouches and did not connect with the jugular system.

(10) The superior ophthalmic vein on the left was completely occluded; the inferior was not present.

The superior ophthalmic vein on the right was enormous, elongated, and tortuous.

(11) The wall of the internal carotid on the affected side was thickened before it entered the aneurysm.

(12) A well-organized gray thrombus measuring 1.7 by 1.2 cm. filled the inferior portion of the left cavernous sinus. It lay 2 or 3 mm. anterior to fistula no. 1, hence did not reach the fistula. The left ophthalmic vein was totally obliterated by an older thrombus. There was no connection between this thrombus and that of the cavernous sinus. There was a thrombus in the carotid artery after it had passed through the foramen lacerum.

(13) At the junction of the left posterior communicating and posterior cerebral arteries was a small sacculated aneurysm measuring 1 cm. by 8 mm.

CASE 2. (1) A single fistula (9 by 7 mm.) was found on the posterolateral wall of the carotid artery within the cavernous sinus. The edges were smooth and regular.

(2) Both cavernous sinuses were enlarged to at least twice the normal size.

(3) There was a wide communication between the two cavernous sinuses by a single intercavernous sinus that measured 1.2 cm. at the maximum and 0.5 cm. at the minimum diameter. It was just posterior to and beneath the hypophysis, which was elevated and compressed.

(4) Both internal carotid arteries were dislocated laterally.

(5) Both Gasserian ganglia were elevated and compressed by lateral extensions of the cavernous sinuses.

(6) The superior ophthalmic veins on both sides were about twice the normal size.

(7) Both inferior petrosal sinuses were somewhat enlarged. The superior petrosal sinuses showed no definite dilatation.

(8) The internal carotid artery was distanctly smaller beyond the fistula and its size not appreciably changed below it.

(9) The elastic coat of the carotid artery was lost at the fistula.

(10) There were no thrombi in the cavernous sinus nor in the carotid artery.

(11) The anterior communicating artery was small; the right posterior communicating artery, tiny. These probably were not sufficient to maintain a collateral circulation.

Unusual Clinical Features

The clinical aspects of case 1 are of interest because of the absence of exophthalmos and pulsation on the side of the fistula, and the marked proptosis with pulsation on the contralateral side. However, the complete third-nerve palsy could leave no doubt of the marked involvement of this side also; that is, bilateral involvement of the cavernous sinuses. It could only be inferred that total thrombosis of the ophthalmic vein was present and precluded pulsating exophthalmos on the side of the fistula. This was confirmed by the necropsy specimen. Two other cases of this character have been described (Nuel and Pincus). In Nuel's case thrombosis of the ophthalmic vein was demonstrated at necropsy. Pincus probably rightly inferred that destruction of the sympathetics was responsible for an actual exophthalmos in his case, but one cannot avoid the conclusion that the ophthalmic vein was also thrombosed. His patient did not come to necropsy. In Reif's case there was greater exophthalmos on the contralateral than on the affected side. This could be due only to some factor, such as a partial venous thrombus, that made the dilated venous bed smaller.

In our case 1 there is the added information that on a previous admission to the Johns Hopkins Hospital exophthalmos of low grade was present on *both* sides and that it was equal on the two sides. If this observation is correct, it would mean that the thrombosis was of later development and had allowed the exophthalmos to recede. The thrombus, as disclosed at post-mortem examination, had stopped short of the fistula and had, therefore, merely changed the expression of the lesion.

The choice of sides upon which to ligate the internal carotid artery is dependent upon more fundamental considerations—that is, the side upon which the murmur is altered, both subjectively and objectively, by compression of the carotid artery in the neck. One cannot overestimate the importance of this test in arriving at the side of the lesion. Had the wrong side been chosen by the greater exophthalmos on the *right,* it is hardly possible that any benefit would have resulted and subsequent closure of the *left* internal carotid would have been out of question.

Another case upon which the importance of this test rested was reported by Dandy a few years ago. In a case with equal and symmetrical bilateral pulsating exophthalmos, the side of the fistula was disclosed in this way and the patient responded promptly to partial occlusion of the artery on that side.

The importance of the compression test as a preliminary to treatment also cannot be overemphasized. If compression of the carotid in the neck cannot be tolerated for a 5- or 10-minute period total occlusion of the internal carotid will surely cause disastrous results to the brain; only a partial occlusion is then in order. Two or three weeks hence the total occlusion will be safe. Matas has long emphasized the importance of this test, which would doubtless be known as the "Matas test."

There were several noteworthy features in case 2. The late appearance of the exophthalmos on the second side was 24 days after the accident, whereas the exophthalmos appeared immediately after the accident on the other side. This came suddenly four days after the patient's admission to the hospital. Sattler's beautiful study of this lesion has shown that, in the bilateral form, the exophthalmos on the two sides develops synchronously in one third of the cases and that in the remaining cases the time of appearance on the second side varies from a day to 15 months. In 19 such cases the second side developed exophthalmos in 1 to 7 days in five cases; in from 1 to 7 weeks in three; and in from 2 to 15 weeks in four. One would suppose that the arterial pressure within the small venous channels connecting the two cavernous sinuses gradually caused them to dilate. In those cases in which exophthalmos appears at once, the venous connections are already well developed; in the remaining cases the connections are only potential, or at least inadequate until the intravascular pressure causes their enlargement.

The rapid appearance of paralysis of the functions of the third nerve and of vision on the side of the first exophthalmos is also interesting. With the appearance of exophthalmos on the second side—overnight—there was an equally immediate and complete paralysis of the corresponding third nerve.

The loss of vision appears to be due to pressure upon the optic nerve through the intervening carotid artery, which was pushed forward by the enlarged cavernous sinus. In case 1 the same effect in exaggerated form was observed and commented upon at the operation. It does not seem possible that vision could be lost by the exophthalmos *per se* because orbital tumors growing with equal rapidity spare vision unless the optic nerve is directly attacked. And since there was no papilledema until the end stages, vision could not be lost from that effect. Moreover, the third nerve is similarly bent at the fixed point in the dura from the underlying pressure in the enlarged cavernous sinus, and the sudden loss of function of this nerve, with the appearance of the exophthalmos on the other side, could have no other explanation. The same explanation doubtless holds for the sixth nerve also. In case 1 there was a well-defined round herniation of the cavernous sinus beneath the third nerve, which was markedly flattened by it, as if by a tumor.

The frequency of extraocular palsies with pulsating exophthalmos has long been recognized. Keller (1898) found an immobile eye in 23 per cent and partial loss of function in an additional 37 per cent of ninety-two cases. In one hundred twenty eight cases of extraocular palsies Sattler found that the third nerve was affected in 28 per cent, the fourth nerve in 10 per cent, and the abducens in 62 per cent.

Pathological findings. One of these aneurysms was purely traumatic, the other probably arose from rupture of a pre-existing aneurysm. Whether trauma played any role in the rupture cannot be established.

In one of these specimens there was a single opening (9 by 7 mm.), in the other there were two openings about 1 cm. apart, each measuring 7 by 4 mm. Double fistulae have been reported by Usher, Nuel, and Seyfarth, and three distinct openings by Schlaefke. Reclus reported a case in which there was a single opening in each carotid artery.

The development of arteriovenous fistulae from preexisting carotid aneurysms has been demonstrated in post-mortem ex-aninations by Morax and Ducamp, Hirschfeld, Karplus, Jack, Baron, and Nunnelly. In his first excellent description of a pathological specimen—the most perfectly described specimen to date—Delens stated that Vieussens and Morgagni had described dilatations of the carotid within the cavernous sinus and that Charcot had disclosed miliary aneurysms of the brain with which he thought the intracavernous arterial dilatations were probably analogous. Following carotid injections of fluids under pressure in cadavers, Charcot also found that ruptures always occurred in this region, thereby disclosing the inherent weakness of the carotid in its intracavernous portion. In his search through the literature Charcot found a case in which a small aneurysm had developed in the carotid canal from a spicule of bone. Many unruptured arterial aneurysms of the internal carotid within the cavernous sinus and of varying size up to very large masses have since been reported. However, it is highly improbable that the large ones can form an arteriovenous fistula because they have obliterated the cavernous sinus and, therefore, eliminated the venous receptacle which is necessary for the development of an arteriovenous aneurysm.

That the intracavernous portion of the carotid is perhaps the weakest portion of the carotid in keeping with Charcot's experiment is beginning to be realized. In case 1 of this report there is a large calcified plaque in this portion of the carotid; and in a case reported by Dandy (*Zentralbl. Neurochir.,* 1937) there was diffuse calcification of the media and erosion of the intima from which a propagating thrombus developed in an otherwise healthy man of thirty-seven. In yet another of our (W. E. D.) cases there were large bilateral aneurysms of the carotid arteries arising within the carotid canal. From clinical experiences we know that there are also frequent instances in which a sudden cerebral thrombosis has unquestionably occurred with partial loss of cerebral functions and in which the ventriculograms show such a diffuse unilateral cerebral atrophy, involving the entire hemisphere, that only a carotid occlusion could be responsible for the cerebral changes. These cases do not come to necropsy, so that the proof of such a lesion is lacking. In two recent cases of this kind the carotid pulsation in the neck appeared to be less on the affected side, and total occlusion of this vessel in the neck produced no cerebral changes on the affected side, but caused swooning quickly when the other side that was presumed to be unaffected was occluded.

The size of the opening in the carotid in our two cases was 9.7 mm. (single fistula) and 4 by 7 mm. in each of the two fistulae (double fistulae). All of these are slightly larger than the measurements recorded in the literature. The fistula in Nelaton's specimen (first reported by Henry, 1856) was 6 mm. long (it contained a splinter of bone); in Nelaton's second case, reported by Delens, the fistula was nearly as long and 2 mm. wide; in that of Cantonnet and Cerise 3 mm., in Jack's 3.25 mm., and in Karplus's 3 mm. In Stuelp's case it was the size of a pea and in Sloman's the size of a hempseed.

The location of the fistula, particularly with reference to the side of the artery involved, is noted in several reports. In our first case one opening is on the anterior and inferior surface of the carotid (aneurysm), the other on the superior surface of the artery. In the second case the opening is on the superior and lateral surface of the artery. The cases reported in the literature show the openings to be in almost any position—on the superior wall in Delen's case, on the outer wall in three cases (Schleafke, Stuelp, and Gibson), and on the mesial surface in five (Usher, Cantonnet, and Cerise, Jack, Nuel, Seyfarth). The position of the fistula appears to have no bearing upon the development of unilateral or bilateral pulsating exophthalmos. Except for Sloman's case, in which the site of the fistula is not detailed, our cases are the only bilateral ones in which

the location of the fistula is described. C. H. Sattler advanced the view that the position of the fistula might be responsible for the development of the unilateral or bilateral form—that if the fistula lay well anteriorly, unilateral exophthalmos would develop, and if the opening was situated more posteriorly. bilateral involvement would occur. We, too, had entertained this view but are more dubious about it now.

The degree of exophthalmos does not appear to be dependent upon the size of the fistula alone. In our second case the fistula was larger than either of the two fistulae in the first case, but smaller than the two combined, but the degree of exophthalmos was very much less. Moreover, although the opening in the second case was larger than in any of the cases reported in the literature, the grade of exophthalmos was among the lowest. It appears more probable that the degree of exophthalmos is dependent upon the varying amount of venous collateral that can take the burden of the ophthalmic veins. This collateral would be principally the basilar sinus and the superior and inferior petrosals. The *changes in the venous system* in these two cases are, on the whole, not surprising. In both cases the cavernous sinuses are bilaterally much enlarged, and there is free communication between the two sides by an intercavernous sinus and by a larger basilar sinus. In case 1 the intercavernous connection is hourglass-shaped with a minimum diameter of 2 mm., but in case 2 the communication was very wide and not restricted in its course.

The relatively low grade of exophthalmos and the absence of large veins on the forehead in case 2, and in other cases from the literature, are, of course, dependent upon the size of the ophthalmic veins. In case 1 the right ophthalmic vein was enormous. In case 2 these veins were enlarged, but only to a moderate degree. Time unquestionably accounts for much of this difference, but in many other cases the exophthalmos had developed to an extraordinary degree in a very short time. One can only infer that the resistance of the venous walls in the orbit differs with the individual, or perhaps the stricture at the sphenoidal fissure is less distensible. In case 1 the size of the ophthalmic vein was much smaller at the sphenoidal fissure and progressively enlarged distal thereto. Then, too, the presence or absence of the varying degree of venous collateral from the cavernous sinus must make a difference in the volume of the load that is thrust upon the ophthalmic veins. For example, in case 1 both the superior and inferior petrosal sinuses were absent, only pouches remaining at the basilar sinus; all the blood, therefore, had to pass into the ophthalmic veins. In case 2 both superior and inferior petrosal sinuses were present, so that part of the blood was probably diverted to the internal jugular veins.

It is particularly interesting that the left ophthalmic vein (on the side of the fistula) was obliterated by an old thrombus that extended into the anterior part of the cavernous sinus. This finding was predicted by the absence of exophthalmos. Its absence thrust an additional large burden upon the contralateral ophthalmic vein. Had this thrombus continued backward, as happened in some cases, and included the fistula, a spontaneous cure would have resulted. This finding also demonstrates the fact that the pulsating exophthalmos may be cured without curing the fistula. The ultimate test of a cure is the disappearance of the murmur.

Another small mural thrombus only partially occluded the internal carotid as it entered the base of the skull. Both this thrombus and that in the ophthalmic vein show that the propagation or non-propagation of a thrombus is a matter of chance.

In both cases the hypophysis was displaced upward and forward by the enlarged intercavernous sinus. Whether this would interfere with hypophyseal functions would doubtless depend upon how much destruc-

tion of the hypophysis occurred with time. This structure was well preserved in both cases. Both patients were beyond the age when the symptoms of pituitary dysfunction would be obvious.

In case 2 there was no thrombus at any point in either the arterial or venous system contiguous to the fistula.

The internal carotid arteries within the cavernous sinuses were closely applied to the sphenoid bone and hypophysis in case 1 (except anteriorly on the left where an interposed pouch of the cavernous sinus dislocated it laterally), but were displaced laterally in case 2. The internal carotid artery was considerably smaller distal to the fistula in both cases than on the contralateral side—probably due to the diversion of blood through the fistula.

In case 1 there were two small aneurysms of the circle of Willis—one in the right anterior cerebral artery, the other at the junction of the left posterior communicating and posterior cerebral arteries. Doubtless the aneurysm of the carotid with rupture into an arteriovenous fistula was a similar one of congenital origin. The frequency of such aneurysms is now well recognized.

REFERENCES

[1]Baron: Report at anatomical society by M. Bell, secretary. *Bull. de la Soc. Anat., Paris,* 1835, p. 178.

[2]Cantonnet and Cerise, L.: Anevrisme arterioveineux spontane de l'orbite. *Arch. d'Opht.,* 27: 34, 1907, v. 27, p. 34.

[3]Dandy, W. E.: The treatment of carotid-cavernous aneurysms. *Ann. Surg., 102:*916, 1935.

[4]———: Carotid-cavernous aneurysms (pulsating exophthalmos). Zentralbl. f. Neurochir., 1937, 2 Jahrgang, no. 2.

[5]Delens, E.: De la communication de la carotide interne et du sinus caverneux. These de Paris, 1870.

[6]Henry, A. A.: Considerations sur l'aneurysms arterio-veineux. These de Paris, 1856.

[7]Hirschfeld, L.: Epanchement de sang dans le sinus caverneux du cote gauche; diagnostique pendant la vie. *Gaz. des Hosp.,* 32:57, 1859.

[8]Jack, E. E.: A case of pulsating exophthalmos— Ligation of the common carotid artery—Death. *Am. Ophth. Soc.,* 11:439, 1907.

[9]Karplus, P.: Anatomical preparation demonstra-

tion before Gesellschaft der Aerzte in Wien. *Wien. med. Wchuschr.*, *13*:357, 1900.

[10]Keller, E.: Beitrage zur Kasuistik des Exophthalmus pulsans. *Inaug. Dissert., Zurich,* 1898.

[11]Matas, R.: Surgery of the vascular system, *Keen's Surgery,* 5:320, 1909.

[12]————.: Occlusion of large surgical arteries with removable metallic bands to test the efficiency of the collateral circulation. *J.A.M.A., 56:*233, 1911.

[13]Morax et Ducamp: Anevrisme arteriosoveineux non traumatique consecutif a la rupture d'une poche aneurysmale de la carotide interne dans le sinus caverneux. Ann. d'Ocul., Juin, 1916. *Klin. M. f. Augenh.,* 2:443, 1916.

[14]Nelaton: Sur l'aneurisme arterioveineux. *Lancet (Holmes lecture),* 2:142, 1873. *Also see* These d'Henry, 1857.

[15]Nuel, J. P.: Externe Oculomotoriusparese als einziges Symptom einer traumatischen Verbindung der Carotis interna und der Sinus cavernosus. *Centralbl. f. Ophth.,* 1902, p. 43.

[16]Nunnelly, T.: Vascular protrusion of the eyeball. *Lancet,* 1864 (Dec.).

[17]Pincus, F.: Spontanheilung eines traumatischen pulsierenden Exophthalmus. *Ztschr. Augenh., 18*:33, 1907.

[18]Reclus, P.: Sur une observation d'exophtalmos pulsatile. *Gaz. des Hosp.,* 1908, p. 1001.

[19]Reif, E.: Ein Fall von doppelseitigen hauptsachlich gekreuzten pulsierenden Exophthalmus. *Beitr. Augenh., 38:*25, 1899.

[20]Sattler, C. H.: Beitrag zur Kenntnis des pulsierenden Exophthalmus. *Ztschr. Augenh.,* 1920.

[21]Schlaefke, W.: Die Aetiologie des pulsierenden Exophthalmus. v. Graefe's *Arch. Ophth., 25*:112, 1879.

[22]Seyfarth, C.: Arteriovenose Aneurysmen der Carotis interna mit dem Sinus cavernosus und Exophthalmus pulsans. *Munch. med. Wchuschr., 67:*1092, 1920.

[23]Sloman, H. C.: Bidrag til Laeren om d. puls. Exophth. *Dissert. Kopenhagen,* 1898.

[24]Usher, C. H.: Notes on cases of pulsating exophthalmos. *Ophth. Rev., 23:*315, 1904.

LXVII

THE SURGICAL TREATMENT OF INTRACRANIAL ANEURYSMS OF THE INTERNAL CAROTID ARTERY*†

Intracranial aneurysms arise on any part of the arterial vascular tree. Over one-half spring from the circle of Willis, the remaining are distributed throughout the brain and from the vertebral and basilar arteries. There are three types of intracranial aneurysms: (1) Congenital, comprising about 80 per cent of the entire number; (2) arteriosclerotic (about 15 per cent); and (3) mycotic (about 5 per cent). Contrary to a very prevalent opinion, syphilis plays no role, or almost none, in the formation of these aneurysms. There are no surgical possibilities in the mycotic aneurysms, which are one of the terminal phases of endocarditis, and are almost always in the brain substance and on the middle cerebral artery or one of its branches. Arteriosclerotic aneurysms offer very little returns from surgery; as yet none have been cured, though it is quite probable that the vertebral and basilar aneurysms may be benefited by ligation of one vertebral artery in the neck. It is principally with the congenital aneurysms that surgery has a place in the treatment. Usually they are small berry-like nubbins in one of the vascular trunks—not uncommonly they are multiple. Since their walls are congenitally defective, they give rise to intracranial hemmorrhage—usually the so-called subarachnoid hemorrhage—and in the early years of life, although they may rupture in later life.

Until a sudden rupture, aneurysms are usually silent. The immediate result of the hemorrhage depends in large degree upon the presence or absence of opposing tissue at the site of the rupture. If the rupture is into cerebral substance, the bleeding may be controlled, and a large progressive false aneurysmal sac form and in time, by gradual expansion, give signs and symptoms like those of a brain tumor. Should the rupture be along a structure like the third nerve or the carotid artery itself, the bleeding may be controlled temporarily, but subsequent ruptures will probably occur and usually end fatally. Should there be no opposing tissue, the bleeding would then be into the cerebrospinal fluid (the cisternae) and rapid, fatal hemorrhage is almost inevitable.

The great deterrent to operative intervention in subarachnoid hemorrhage is the inability to localize the aneurysm by symptoms or signs. At times, there are prodromal manifestations but all too frequently, the patient passes quickly into coma and then, all too frequently, there are no objective localizing signs.

If it were even possible to localize the side (right or left) of the aneurysm, the operative exposure would be adequate to disclose the aneurysm, if it were located on the circle of Willis. This is a hope for the future, for up to the present time the only aneurysms that have been operated upon successfully are those causing a third nerve palsy or paralysis—a sign that is almost but not quite pathognomonic of an aneurysm and its location.

In a search for better and earlier means of diagnosis of aneurysms and their location, I have analyzed 103 cases that have appeared in the records of the Johns Hopkins Hospital. In a very high percentage of cases, no help was elicited, but in many of them there was adequate information to

---

*Reprinted from the *Annals of Surgery, 114:3,* September, 1941.

†Read before the American Surgical Association, White Sulphur Springs, W. Va., April 28, 29, 30, 1941.

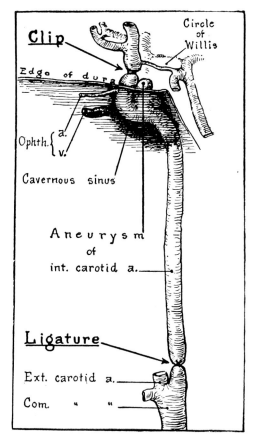

Fig. 1. Diagrammatic drawing illustrating the method of curing carotid aneurysms arising within the carotid canal. A clip is placed on the internal carotid artery intracranially, and the internal carotid artery is ligated in the neck. This traps the aneurysm between the two ligatures, and the only sizeable branch between the ligature it the ophthalmic artery. Vision is not lost as the result of the ligation.

determine the side of the lesion. In nearly all of the aneurysms of the middle cerebral artery there was hemiplegia, but it is highly improbable that more than an occasional aneurysm of this vessel can ever be cured without a permanent hemiplega, and treatment of this character would not be considered. On the other hand, some aneurysms of the anterior cerebral artery give a partial hemiplegia or Babinski, and these are amenable to treatment, although none have as yet been cured. Bilateral cerebellar and brain-stem signs of sudden onset may also indicate aneurysms of the

basilar and vertebral arteries, but here again there are little prospects of a cure by surgical means, at least none have yet been successfully treated. It is the silent aneurysms, with few or no signs or symptoms arising from the internal carotid arteries and the circle of Willis, that offer the maximum from prompt surgical treatment.

The only symptom that is useful in detecting the side of the aneurysm is an unilateral headache, or pain in one eye. This may or may not be present, either as a prodromal symptom before rupture, or as

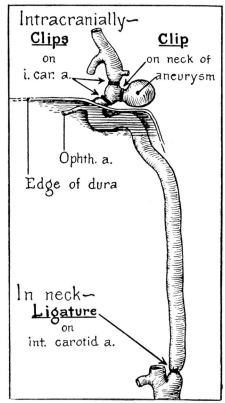

Fig. 2. Diagrammatic drawing illustrating the method of treating intracranial aneurysms arising from the internal carotid artery, before the first branch is given off. The neck of the aneurysm may be clipped and nothing done to the internal carotid, or the internal carotid may be clipped on either side of the neck of the aneurysm, thus isolating it. The aneurysm is then shrunk by the electrocautery, in order to remove its contact with the third nerve, or it may actually be removed; this was done in one case.

an excruciating pain at the time of rupture; and even occasionally it may be misleading. A positive Babinski sign may at times betray the side of the lesion; but by far the most important sign of all is weakness of a third nerve.

Intra-arterial injections of thorotrast have for some time been used to define aneurysms and with remarkable results. Against its use is the risk of cerebral emboli, the frequent necessity of injecting both internal carotid arteries, since only one side fills well with one injection; and in the acute stage of bleeding the patient is much too ill. For patients who are not in the acute stage of subarachnoid bleeding, it will doubtless be a distinct asset, but should be employed with caution and discrimination.

Thirteen intracranial aneurysms of the internal carotid artery have been operated upon; all have been diagnosed and localized by a third nerve palsy or paralysis, plus sharp, severe, sudden pains in the eye and the corresponding side of the head. Six of these arose in the carotid canal and broke through into the cranial chamber alongside the internal carotid artery. Five of these are cured, the longest for four and one-half years. The single death was due to a rupture of the carotid artery in applying to a very large arteriosclerotic vessel a silver clip that was too small. This was a case of an arteriovenous aneurysm (pulsating exophthalmos). The arterial aneurysm which had ruptured and caused this arteriovenous fistula was found at necropsy. Seven arose from the internal carotid artery intracranially, before the anterior cerebral artery is given off. Five of these are cured and two have died.

Two of the five cures were obtained by placing a silver clip on the neck of the aneurysm, leaving the carotid artery intact. The remaining three cures were obtained by clipping or coagulating with the cautery the internal carotid artery on both sides of the aneurysm. The two deaths were due to (1) an abnormally placed posterior communicating artery, which was between the two clips and prevented collateral circulation; and (2) to subsequent rupture of the electrically coagulated internal carotid artery. This occurred one month postoperative, after the patient had returned home, and was presumably cured. Ligation of the internal carotid artery in the neck would have prevented this death.

The mortality in this series is, therefore, 23 per cent—the cures 77 per cent.

LXVIII

SERIOUS COMPLICATIONS OF RUPTURED INTERVERTEBRAL DISKS*

Ruptured intervertebral disks are now known to be exceedingly common; they are, in fact, among the most frequent lesions treated surgically. Over 95 per cent of them are in the lumbar region, where they explain the overwhelming percentage of recurring pains low in the back plus scaitica in one or both legs. With rare exceptions it is now possible to diagnose and localize those in the lumbar region without spinal injections of iodized oil, air or other contrast medium or even without a lumbar puncture.[1] Up to the present time the course in all reported cases of ruptured disk except our first two has run true to form and there were no serious complications. Three serious sequelae encountered during the past month emphasize the potential dangers of this simple lesion when the diagnosis and treatment are delayed. One of the disks ruptured was in the cervical, another in the thoracic and the third in the lumbar region. The rupture of the cervical and the thoracic disk had disastrous results—total paralysis and death from pressure necrosis of the spinal cord in the former; in the latter the paralysis has partly cleared. The rupture of the lumbar disk caused permanent sensory paralysis in addition to long-continued pain and loss of bladder function with subsequent infection of the urinary system.

In addition to these three recent cases I have had two cases of ruptured disk (lumbar disk) with complete paraplegia (previously reported) and loss of bladder function and another (lumbar disk) with long-continued bladder incontinence and infection. These six cases of serious complications occurred in a series of perhaps three hundred operative cases of ruptured disk, a percentage, therefore, of about two. All the sequelae could have been prevented with early diagnosis and treatment. Although all the patients except the one with a cervical disk ruptured have survived, the paralysis of the patient with a thoracic disk ruptured will probably be permanent, and perhaps some permanent stigmas will affect the others, particularly those with infection of the urinary tract. Delay in treating a ruptured cervical or thoracic disk is disastrous because only a few hours is required to destroy the spinal cord irreparably. After paralysis due to a ruptured lumbar disk, function can be restored because the lesion involves the peripheral nerves. Moreover, spontaneous healing of a ruptured disk must be unusual.

Report of Cases

CASE 1. *Rupture of fourth lumbar intervertebral disk into spinal canal.* A laboring man aged fifty-three had had a sudden severe attack of "sciatica" on the right side and pain low in the back five years before that kept him in bed over three months. The recovery was slow, covering a period of three months.

Thirteen months before, while he was shoveling sand, a pain (not very severe) stabbed him in the lower part of the back. As he continued at work the pain became intense and was increased by movement. Two days later, while he was at work, "something gave way in his back" and the pain became excruciating. He went to bed, and in the afternoon control of his bladder became difficult and then impossible. For four days he could not pass urine and was catheterized. The pain was unbearable, and he was unable to get out of bed; morphine was given repeatedly. On the fourth day the pain was somewhat improved; he was able to get up but could

*Reprinted from *The Journal of the Americacn Medical Association Vol. 119:*474–477, June 6, 1942.

not use his right leg. The urine then began to dribble, but retention still made catheterization necessary. There was also fecal incontinence.

By degrees the pain lessened, but an infection of the bladder kept the patient in a hospital seventy-eight days. During this period he noticed numbness in the back of both legs, but the motor power in the right leg improved so that he could walk, although with difficulty. The disturbance and anesthesia of the bladder and rectum were still present when he was admitted to the Johns Hopkins Hospital one year later. The infection in the bladder had cleared despite continued intermittent use of the catheter.

Examination on Dec. 19, 1941 revealed (1) weakness of the flexor and extensor movements of the right foot, (2) bilateral anesthesia of all nerve segments on the right below the fourth lumbar vertebra, including (3) saddle anesthesia and (4) anesthesia of the penis and the scrotum, (5) loss of both achilles tendon reflexes and (6) only slight response of the rectal sphincter.

This patient was presented at ward rounds with the students, and an unequivocal diagnosis of ruptured intervertebral disk with compression of the lumbar spinal nerves was made; no other diagnosis could be considered. My assistant, Dr. Troland, whose diagnostic acumen is almost perfection, was gently chidded for having entertained the diagnosis of a tumor of the spinal cord and injected 1 cc. of iodized oil. This was our second spinal puncture and injection of iodized oil in 100 cases of ruptured intervertebral disk—a procedure that we have denounced for ruptured lumbar disks as unnecessary, misleading, painful and harmful. Roentgenograms with the iodized oil showed a complete block at the fourth lumbar disk.

We had assumed that the situation revealed at operation would be similar to that in other cases in which the protruding extradural disk was so large that the cauda equina had been compressed by the extradural mass. One exceptional objective observation, however, was noteworthy; i.e., the sensory loss was much greater than the motor, whereas the reverse would have been expected.

At operation (Fig. 1) on the following day the usual unilateral approach was made. The fifth ligamentum flavum was reflected on a hinge and replaced when the subdural space was seen to be normal. Exploration of the fourth subflaval space immediately revealed a scar so dense that exposure beneath the dura was impossible. Removal of a notch in the upper part of the fifth lamina showed the same impenetrable scar. The only safe approach then was to expose the dura by a complete laminectomy. On the dorsal surface the dura

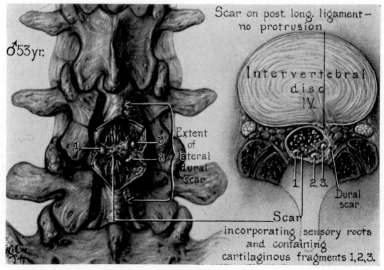

Fig. 1. (Case 1). Operative sketch showing intradural scar wrapped around the posterior roots of the cauda equina. Note the three little isolated fragments of intact cartilage (1, 2, 3). Sketch representing the cross section of the scar in the spinal canal.

became more normal and was opened. At the level of the fourth lumbar interspace a dense scar was encountered extending entirely across the spinal canal. The dura was then opened below the scar and the incision continued upward to it. The intradural scar was about 0.5 cm. wide and very dense and had two distinct components; there were three small pure white glistening nodules, each about 3 mm. in diameter, one far over to the left side of the dura on its dorsal aspect and the other two with a dumbbell formation on the right lateral aspect of the inner dura. These little white nodules were tightly bound together with the usual dense brownish red connective tissue of a scar. The mass clearly did not contain neoplastic elements. Three sensory nerve roots passed through the dense fibrous mass, and two had to be excised with it. Curiously this transverse fibrous mass was on the dorsal aspect of the spinal canal; the motor roots could be seen beneath and were intact after removal of the scar. On the right side the dura was an integral part of the scar and retained none of its normal appearance. The vertebral disk was then inspected. The posterior spinal ligament was a dense white scar but there was no localized protrusion, and when it was incised with a scalpel there was only very hard tissue beneath. The disk itself had, therefore, healed spontaneously after extrusion of the disk.

There could scarcely be a doubt that the scar throughout the interior of the spinal canal was the end product of the rupture of a disk into the spinal canal. And it was suspected that the small white glistening bodies in the scar represented actual remains of the extruded cartilage. In the strained microscopic sections cartilaginous remains were disclosed, some fairly normal and others so greatly disintegrated that only suggestions of cartilage were in evidence.

The patient left the hospital on Jan. 10, 1942, entirely relieved of pain and with some diminution in the anesthesia.

CASE 2. *Rupture of sixth cervical disk with necrosis of spinal cord.* A man aged twenty-nine entered the hospital Jan. 2, 1942 and was operated on a few hours later. He was totally paralyzed in both legs and partly paralyzed in both arms and had bladder retention and loss of rectal control. Breathing was labored and was reinforced by use of the sternocleidomas-

toid muscles. There were rales in the lungs and much mucus which could not be delivered. The temperature was 104.2 F., the leukocytes numbered 18,000 and a patch of pneumonia in the base of the right lung was suspected because of clinical signs and its presence confirmed by roentgenogram twenty-four hours later.

Forty-eight hours before the time of operation the patient was seemingly perfectly well in every way. While straining at stool he suddenly became paralyzed to the degree noted, and all sensation was lost below the neck. All this paralysis developed within a few seconds; it appeared to begin in the left foot, went to the right and passed upward like a flash. Thirty-six hours later the condition showed no improvement; the patient was then rushed by ambulance from a neighboring city.

Examination showed complete motor and sensory paralysis with a sharp sensory level at the sixth cervical segment. The patient was perfectly conscious but apprehensive and somewhat panicky because of the embarrassed respirations.

It was possible to obtain a history of pain in the neck and shoulder over a period of six or eight months, always intensified by throwing a ball or moving the neck. The pain had probably been somewhat less during the past month. I suspected an extradural or intradural encapsulated tumor (probably a meningioma) because of the past history of pain and the associated sudden paralysis following straining at stool. In a case reported several years ago[2] this sequence of events was regarded as pathognomonic of an encapsulated tumor, and it has since been found to be a trustworthy sign. A ruptured intervertebral disk was not suspected.

At operation with the patient under local anesthesia, a cervical laminectomy was performed. At the level of the sixth cervical vertebra a sharply defined lesion was encountered. For a distance of perhaps 2 cm. the cord was reddish brown, the vessels on the surface were enlarged and, for a moment, an aneurysm was considered. The cord was distinctly swollen; had iodized oil been injected (it was not) a block would probably have been shown. When the leptomeninges were stripped an area of pinhead size in the center looked almost transparent and was nicked with a knife; a large amount of the necrotic interior of the spinal cord oozed from the opening (Fig. 2). The incision was ex-

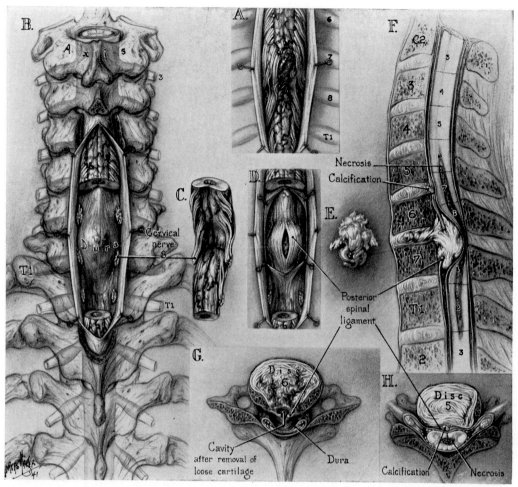

Fig. 2. (Case 2). *A*, the cord with the necrotic interior beginning to protrude at the surface. *B*, section of the cord removed to show the dura bulging because of rupture of the intervertebral disk. *C*, a drawing of the cord to show the effects of compression by the disk. *D* and *E*, cartilage removed from the bulging disk. *F*, diagram showing the effect of the lesion on the cord; note the extent of the necrosis of the interior of the cord. *G*, transverse section of the affected disk, showing the extent of the necrotic interior. *H*, cross section of a normal disk for comparison with the affected disk (*G*).

tended almost the length of the lesion, and an increasing volume of necrotic material was spontaneously extruded. It contained no blood or fluid and was not even blood tinged; it was grayish white. It should be noted that a network of vessels extended up and down for some distance in the other layer of the arachnoid membrane, indicating a vascular support to the contiguous lesion in the cord. It is known that the white matter in the brain and spinal cord is much softer than the gray matter and, therefore, far more susceptible to trauma. It being evident, therefore, that this was a traumatic lesion, the cause was

sought beneath the cord by gently retracting it. A rounded hard mass was seen bulging beneath the dura, which did not appear thickened or abnormal. An extradural search quickly revealed the protruding disk. When it was incised several pieces of cartilage extruded spontaneously; more were removed with forceps.

There appeared to be no possibility that return of function could follow so much necrosis of the interior of the cord. With administration of sulfathiazole the pneumonia cleared, but the patient died ten days later of paralysis of the respiratory tract. Examination of only the cervical portion of the cord and vertebrae was carried out.

CASE 3. *Rupture of second thoracic disk with paraplegia.* A Negro man aged forty-two was admitted to the medical service Feb. 11, 1942 complaining of pain in the neck and inability to walk. The present illness had begun two months before with severe pains in the chest; a diagnosis of pneumonia had been made (probably erroneously). Five weeks before he had had a temperature of 103 F. During a stay of three weeks in another hospital the diagnosis of sinus infection was made. He was discharged, apparently well. Shortly thereafter there were some stiffness of the neck and some difficulty in bending forward. Two weeks before admission severe pains in the chest returned and radiated to both shoulders. Any movement intensified the pains, but they were not aggravated by coughing and sneezing. About the same time both legs became weak, and he could not walk. There were also urinary infrequency and dribbling. Within twenty-four hours the paralysis of the legs became almost complete. Examinations revealed (1) some pain on pressure over the first and second thoracic vertebrae, (2) almost total paralysis of both legs, (3) sharp sensory loss at the level of the third thoracic vertebra, (4) paralysis of the abdominal and the lower intercostal muscles, (5) extreme hyperactivity of the knee kicks and ankle jerks, (6) presence of the Babinski sign bilaterally, (7) loss of the position and the vibratory sense in the legs, (8) presence of the Queckenstedt sign (complete block), (9) a count of 50 cells (lymphocytes) in the spinal fluid, (10) a complete block at the second thoracic vertebra as shown with iodized oil (roentgenograms of the spine were normal) and (11) a temperature of 100 F.

The tentative diagnosis was epidural abscess or tubercle. A ruptured disk was not considered.

At operation on February 13, perfomed by Dr. Troland, rupture of the second thoracic vertebral disk was found. One large and many small pieces of cartilage were removed.

The paralysis was unimproved on March 11, 1942, but on May 1 there was decided improvement, the patient being able to take steps.

COMMENT

Among perhaps three hundred operations for ruptured intervertebral disks these are the only instances of such complications, except our first two previously reported cases, and none, I think, have been reported in the literature. Although these complications are relatively uncommon, the quick succession of these 3 cases indicates that they are probably to be expected more frequently in the future.

Spontaneous resolution of ruptured intervertebral disks has been suspected from the history of patients whose signs and symptoms appeared to indicate clearly the existence of a ruptured disk and later disappeared. The usual history is one of recurrent attacks with intervals varying up to several months or years. However, it is my belief that a spontaneous cure is infrequent and occurs only after a period of many years. In case 1 the lesion in the disk had remained dormant for four years and then had sprung up anew from the effects of the trauma incident to heavy lifting. This is the common story. I have suspected but cannot prove that a permanent cure results only when the protruding cartilage actually ruptures through the posterior ligament, where it is gradually absorbed. The reason for such a conception is the course of events after operation. It is now known that the important part of operative treatment is the adequate opening of the retaining posterior spinal ligament, which permits the eventual extrusion of the defective cartilaginous content of both the disk and the protrusion. The actual removal of a cartilaginous sequestrum doubtless hastens the healing and cure, but rarely, if ever, can all the defective disk be removed, and frequently, particularly of the disk is concealed, few or none of the fragments are removable without the inducing of an inadvisable degree of trauma. An adequate opening of the ligamentous cover is, therefore, the indicated treatment. This is probably the reason that ruptured disks are not found after severe crushing injuries of the spine or soon after dislocation; i.e., the posterior spinal ligament is torn and permits the injured disk to extrude spontaneously.

The high percentage of permanent cures which follow operation and are without sequelae therefore suggests that the extruded cartilage eventually is absorbed and disappears. Only twice have I seen at operation actual spontaneous rupture of the posterior spinal ligament with freely lying cartilage in the extradural space. I suspected that had operation not intervened a spontaneous cure might have resulted, but it is probable that the trauma (bending the spine) incident to lifting the patient to the operating table may have induced the rupture; in both instances the rupture through the spinal ligament could not long have antedated the operation. In case 1 the acute pressure of the protruded disk eroded and overlying dura and permitted its penetration into the spinal canal—an unusual sequel and almost a cure. Had the protrusion remained extradural a cure would probably have resulted. The long preservation of cartilage in the spinal canal and its incorporation in the scar indicate the disposition of an autogenous graft of cartilage in this situation.

In case 2 a successful result with restoration of spinal functions could not have been possible after the lapse of much time—probably a few hours. Once necrosis of the interior of the cord had begun the loss of function could only be rapidly progressive and permanent. The optimum time for the diagnosis and treatment, therefore, was before the spinal cord had been compressed with such suddenness. It is true that at the time of operation rupture of a vertebral disk was not suspected, but had the patient been seen earlier and an opportunity of study been provided it would probably have been suspected. Rupture of a cervical disk is far less common than rupture of a lumbar disk (in 10 of our three hundred cases the ruptured disk has been in the cervical region), but it is sufficiently frequent to be considered seriously when a patient complains of pain in

the neck—especially in the lower part of the neck—the shoulders and the arms. In all our cases the rupture has been at the sixth or the seventh cervical disk.

A postmortem examination in case 2 revealed only the cortical shell of the spinal cord remaining at the level of the rupture. When held to the light it was transparent for a distance of about 2 cm. A large cavity extended up and down the center of the spinal cord from the top of the fifth cervical vertebra to the top of the second thoracic—a distance of four vertebrae! This cavity was due to the extension of the necrosed spinal cord along the path of least resistance: extrusion through the meningeal covering is the more resistant course. The ruptured disk, as large as a hickory nut, pushed the dura posteriorly and in the exact midline. The entire center of the disk was loose cartilage, about one third of the entire disk being grossly destroyed. The area of necrosis extended through the antero-posterior extent of the disk; a seemingly normal cushion remained on each side. The lateral position of so many disks had prepared us to believe that the nucleus pulposus has nothing to do with the development of a ruptured disk. This specimen, however, which I believe is the only one reported post mortem, suggests that the destruction of cartilage did and probably always does begin in the nucleus pulposus. The greater frequency of lateral protrusions doubtless is explained by the looser attachment of the posterior spinal ligament to the vertebral body on the sides than in the center. Moreover, the ligament is definitely thicker in the middle. The much tighter binding of the ligament in the center is easily and strikingly demonstrated by stripping it with forceps. Eventually, however, the pressure beneath the ligament may become great enough to force the central attachment also, as in this case.

CONCLUSIONS

1. Though not frequent (occurring in 6 of 300 cases, an incidence of 2 per cent),

serious sequelae resulting from rupture of an intervertebral disk produce severe loss of function referable to the spinal cord or the cauda equina (depending on their site).

2. A ruptured disk in the cervical or the thoracic region is a potential source of permanent destruction of the spinal cord. Its diagnosis and treatment before involvement of the spinal cord is of permanent importance. The diagnosis is suggested by localized and referred pain. After the spinal cord is involved operative treatment within a few hours is imperative if any function referable to the spinal cord is to be expected. Iodized oil is indicated for an early diagnosis when the spinal cord is involved, i. e. when the ruptured disk is in the cervical or the thoracic region. It is not indicated for rupture of a lumbar disk because with rare exceptions the diagnosis can be made with much more accuracy and certainty without it.

REFERENCES

[1]Dandy, W. E.: Concealed Ruptured Intervertebral Disks: A Plea for the Elimination of Contrast Mediums in Diagnosis. *J. A. M. A., 117*:821 (Sept. 6) 1941; Loose Cartilage from Intervertebral Disk Simulating Tumor of the Spinal Cord. *Arch. Surg., 19*:660 (Oct.) 1929.

[2]Dandy, W. E.: A Sign and Symptom of Spinal Cord Tumors. *Arch. Neurol. & Psychiat., 16*:435 (Oct.) 1926.

LXIX

ANEURYSM OF THE ANTERIOR CEREBRAL ARTERY*

During the past decade intracranial aneurysms have been added to the group of lesions that are curable by operation. I now have cured fifteen patients with aneurysms of the internal carotid artery arising in the cavernous sinus and along the intracranial course of this vessel. The treatment of aneurysms of the internal carotid artery is relatively simple, it being necessary only to isolate the aneurysms between ligatures or silver clips, or to clip the neck of the aneurysms when they lie within the cranial chamber.

Herewith is a report of an aneurysm of the anterior cerebral artery. As it is one of the most common aneurysms of the brain, and one with a fairly easy approach, the hope is entertained that the surgical attack will become increasingly more frequent. Up to the present aneurysms of other arteries in the brain have not been cured, but doubtless with time the list will be increased.

Report of Case

A well nourished, normal looking woman, aged forty-five was referred by Dr. Robert Sullivan of Murfreesboro, Tenn., Dec. 1, 1941, became of defective vision.

Her only complaint was loss of vision, which began two months before and had steadily increased. There had been no headaches.

Dr. Alan C. Woods examined the patient's eyes and found (1) visual acuity to be 15/200 in the right and 20/70 in the left eye; (2) loss of all color vision in the right eye; (3) central scotoma in the right eye; (4) suggestive altitudinal hemianopsia for form in the right eye; (5) some pallor of the right optic disk; (6) central scotoma for color in the left eye, and (7) only a small field for colors remaining in

*Reprinted from *The Journal of the American Medical Association*, *119*:1253–1254, August 15, 1942.

the left eye.

The blood pressure was 120 systolic and 85 diastolic, the Wassermann reaction of the blood was negative and roentgenograms of the head were negative.

The diagnosis was a tumor in the supraseller region; an aneurysm was not suspected.

An operation was performed on December 3. A right hypophysial approach was made with a concealed incision. There was no increased intracranial pressure. Less than 0.5 cm. from the optic foramen the optic nerve began to show a brownish red discoloration and was increased in size. My first thought was that this was a glioma of the optic nerve and chiasm. The internal carotid artery lay alongside for a distance of probably 3 cm., was free of any attachment and looked perfectly normal. The space between the artery and the nerve was inspected but extension of the tumor was not seen. On further withdrawal of the frontal lobe for inspection of the chiasm a large mass was seen extending upward into the base of the brain. It was smooth and well rounded and was certainly not a glioma. Suspecting that it was a tumor I incised the capsule and made an attempt to curet the interior, but the content was so hard that the curet made no impression on it. Since it was firmly attached to the right optic nerve and a line of cleveage could not be found, I cut away the upper half of this nerve, freeing the presumed tumor just before the chiasm was reached. The incised bed of the nerve was about 0.75 cm. long; approximately the upper half of the optic nerve had been exised. With very slight traction on the incised capsule the mass was lifted slowly and with no apparent point of fixation. After a little progress, however, the wound suddenly filled with blood. I suspected that the internal carotid might have been torn and promptly passed a silver clip through the blood and closed it. The blood was then aspirated and it was seen that the bleeding had completely stopped. With gentle dissection the tumor was separated from the optic chiasm and lifted out of its bed; no further bleeding resulted. The tumor was then recognized to be an aneurysm. An opening in the wall, as large as the end of a lead pencil, was the source of the sudden hemorrhage. The aneurysm could have arisen only from the right anterior cerebral artery. However, at no time was this vessel actually seen, and curiously no bleeding appeared from it subsequently, although only the internal carotid artery had been ligated.

The aneurysm was about the size of a bantam's egg. It was the shape of a dumbell and the upper part was about twice as large as the lower part. The constriction between the two parts was at the level of the optic chiasm, behind which it lay.

The upper portion protruded upward between the two frontal lobes and the lower portion passed back of the optic chiasm and must have rested on the sella turcica. There was only a small cavity in the aneurysm; this connected with the opening on the exterior, at which point the attachment to the trunk of the anterior cerebral artery had been torn off. The larger upper subdivision of the aneurysm was white and the lower half was black; the striking difference in color was due to the age of the contained thrombus, the upper part being quite old and very firm and the lower part being fresh and softer. The cavity in the aneurysm was entirely in the upper part. The weight of the aneurysm was 16 Gm.

Fortunately the Matas test had been made before the operation and was negative. This test is now routinely performed on every patient whose lesion is in the environs of the sella, because a number of aneurysms have been encountered when tumors were suspected. Without a prior knowledge of the adequacy of the collateral circulation through the circle of Willis, closure of the carotid artery would be taking a serious risk, although in this case the risk was inescapable. There can, I think, be no doubt that the cerebral circulation on the right side of the brain is now maintained solely through the posterior communicating artery.

On coming out of the anesthesia (about two hours after the operation was concluded) the patient had half a dozen convulsions on the left side, but there was no weakness of that side of the body then or at any time subsequently. The following day she was in excellent condition, quite alert, happy and apparently normal in every way. Nine days later when asleep she apparently had a convulsion and broke open the wound; this was immediately closed; no one was in the room at the time of the convulsion. There was no subsequent weakness of the left side, but she was disoriented and less alert for three or four days thereafter. I assumed that the convulsion and the after-effects were the result of necrosis of the brain from loss of the anterior cerebral artery. This may or may not be true, but it appears to resemble a similar state that at times follows the operation of Freeman and Watts in prefrontal lobotomies.

The patient left the hospital December 21, eighteen days after the operation. Mentally she was as well as before the operation. A complete third nerve paralysis has persisted since the operation, doubtless owing to an injury sustained when the internal carotid artery was closed; this was entirely unexpected, since bleeding was controlled quickly and seemingly without trauma.

Vision in the right (affected) eye was practically unchanged; the same visual field with a central scotoma and altitudinal hemianopsia remained, and visual acuity was 20/400. I was prepared to believe that vision would have been lost after excision of at least the upper half of the nerve with the firmly attached aneurysm. The vision in the left eye was definitely improved; the visual acuity was 20/20, the central scotoma had disappeared and the color fields, which were barely present alongside the central scotoma, were normal (examination of the eyes was done by Dr. Woods). On Jan. 15, 1942 (six weeks after the operation) she was reported to be in excellent health, and her vision was good.

LXX

INTRACRANIAL ARTERIAL ANEURYSMS IN THE CAROTID CANAL*

DIAGNOSIS AND TREATMENT

Aneurysms of the cranial division of the internal carotid artery may arise (1) in the carotid canal and (2) within the cranium. There may or may not be differences in the signs and the symptoms of the two types, and the surgical attack which has been developed in the past few years may or may not be the same for both. The only symptomatic difference between aneurysms in these two locations is that many of those in the cavernous sinus produce disturbances of the trigeminal nerve while those of the intracranial portion do not. Nearly all aneurysms in the carotid canal are amenable to operative treatment with minimal risk; those in the intracranial division may or may not be curable, depending on the exact relation to the branches at the circle of Willis. I am concerned in this publication only with the arterial aneurysms in the carotid canal, particularly with the large ones. This location is also a favored seat for carotid-cavernous arteriovenous aneurysms with resultant pulsating exophthalmos, but these have been considered elsewhere. Rupture of the smaller arterial aneurysms in this region is indeed one source of the arteriovenous variety, and one of my cases has been included because this finding was present at necropsy. Most of the arteriovenous aneurysms in this position are of traumatic origin and are a common result because the torn internal carotid actually traverses the cavernous sinus.

*Reprinted from the *Archives of Surgery*, 45:335–350, September, 1942.

Report of a Case of a Large Aneurysm Arising in the Carotid Canal

The patient was a rather frail woman fifty-two years of age. She was referred by Dr. Warde B. Allan, of Baltimore, on Nov. 19, 1941, with the probable diagnosis of an intracranial aneurysm. Dr. Frank Ford, the neurologist at Johns Hopkins Hospital, made the same diagnosis. The illness for which she was admitted to the hospital began three years before with diplopia which lasted a month and was said to have been corrected by glasses. However, it recurred periodically during the next three years. Four months before admission a tingling sensation in the right maxillary region and quickly thereafter numbness of the cheek and forehead appeared. At the same time severe pain struck the right eye. Three weeks later, a sudden piercing headache developed in the right frontal region; this was accompanied by nausea and vomiting. On the following morning, the pain had concentrated in the right eye, and the right upper eyelid drooped (ptosis). The pains and the headache persisted, although for the last three weeks there was gradual improvement and for the last week they were barely noticeable. A spinal puncture had been made at the Gorgas Hospital at Ancon in the Panama Canal Zone six weeks before and was entirely negative.

The following findings were elicited on examination of the eyes by Dr. Frank Walsh, who also suggested an intracranial aneurysm: (1) total paralysis of all extraocular muscles on the right side (the third, fourth and sixth nerves); (2) exophthalmos of 4 mm. of the right eye; (3) enlargement and absence of reaction in the right pupil; (4) visual acuity, 20/50 for the right eye and 20/20 for the left; (5) small central scotoma on the right and normal fundi; (6) anesthesia of the first and second branches of the right trigeminus nerve; (7) destruction of the anterior and posterior clinoid processes on the right (no calcifield shadows); (8) blood pressure, 192 systolic and 100 diastolic; negative Wassermann test.

In 1941, I reported the cases of five presumably cured patients with carotid aneurysms in the carotid canal. The cure was accomplished by trapping the aneurysm between a clip on the intracranial carotid and a total ligation in the neck. All of these patients were fairly young; the collateral circulation was adequate, and the aneurysms were small. I had feared that huge aneurysms of this type would probably be beyond hope of operative treatment, although I had not yet exposed one at operation. It was assumed that the intracranial portion of the internal carotid artery would probably be hidden from view by the large intracranial protrusion of the aneurysm and furthermore that the possible collateral circulation through the circle of Willis would be compromised by the projection of the mass on the anterior and posterior communicating arteries. As is so frequently true, this supposition proved to be unfounded, and the problem, although not as simple as that of the smaller aneurysms because of other considerations, was solved without undue difficulties.

The collateral circulation was indeed demonstrated to be entirely inadequate by the Matas test, i. e., compression of the internal carotid artery in the neck. Total occlusion of this vessel could be tolerated less than a minute, and, therefore, ligation of the vessel without disastrous cerebral sequelae was precluded. However, after partial occlusion of the internal carotid artery in the neck by a fascial band, the collateral circulation was found to be adequate, and four days later, the internal carotid was totally occluded intracranially by a silver clip and in the neck by a ligature (over the fascial band), thus trapping the aneurysm (Fig 1). Between the two ligatures there is only one sizable branch of the internal carotid artery, namely, the ophthalmic artery, and this, I believe, will not maintain the aneurysm. At least in none of the other five patients reported as cured has there been a suggestion of failure by subsequent signs or symptoms.

At the time of the final operation the internal carotid was simultaneously exposed intracranially and in the neck. When the silver clip was clamped on the internal carotid artery within the cranial chamb-

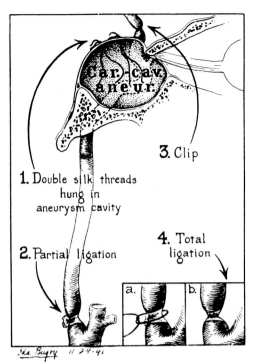

Fig. 1. The final treatment of the aneurysm is indicated in this sketch. First the internal carotid was partially closed with a fascial band. Four days later, the internal carotid was clipped intracranially and ligated in the neck. A silk ligature was tied over the fascial band.

er, there was no visible effect on the violent pulsation of the aneurysm. Perhaps five minutes later the internal carotid was ligated with silk in the neck, and all pulsation in the aneurysm immediately stopped. It is probably worthy of note that the intracranial ligation was performed first. It perhaps made no difference which ligation was placed first since the time interval between the two ligatures was so short, but with a longer interval there is reason to believe that cerebral emboli may be prevented by ligating this artery intracranially first. It may or may not be important to place both ligatures almost simultaneously, but the thought occurred that an aneurysm not receiving blood would be smaller and therefore compromise the collateral circulation through the circle of Willis to a lesser degree. Recovery from the operation was uneventful and without any trace of cerebral involvement. It also should be added that at the time of the initial exposure of the aneurysm five days before these ligations, four double silk sutures of medium size were left dangling in the interior of the aneurysm. Each of the eight sutures was about 2 cm. in length. Owing to the thick capsule of the aneurysm, long curved needles could be passed through the aneurysmal wall and pulled until one end of the suture was left dangling inside. There was no evidence from the degree of pulsation of the aneurysm that they had induced a thrombus. Perhaps in the smaller berry aneurysms they may be more effective and may possibly offer a means of curing those that cannot be extirpated or clipped at the neck of the sac.

The chronology of events in the surgical treatment of the aneurysm was: (1) exposure of the aneurysm intracranially on Nov. 24, 1941; (2) partial ligation of the internal carotid in the neck on Nov. 25, 1941; (3) clipping of the internal carotid intracranially and total ligation in the neck on Nov. 29, 1941 (Fig. 1); (4) discharge from the hospital on Dec. 22, 1941.

Subsequent Course.—The patient was examined by Dr. Walsh two months after the operation, on Jan. 28, 1942; at that time she was free from all symptoms and had been since operation. The vision in the affected eye had returned to 20/20 (from 20/50), and the central scotoma had disappeared. She could elevate the upper lid so that the entire pupil was exposed. The eye abducted 35 and adducted 7 degrees; it moved upward 2 and downward 2 degrees. Before operation the eyeball had been fixed. The exophthalmos had not diminished. She was then returning to her home in Panama.

Heretofore, an interval of three to four weeks had been allowed between the partial and the total closure of the internal carotid artery. The advent of facial weakness on the contralateral side from a small extradural hemorrhage necessitated reopening the wound, and for that reason it was reluctantly determined to close the carotid at the same time (the Matas test then indicating that the circulation was adequate).

Comment

In a recent review of one hundred and eight arterial aneurysms of the brain that came to operation or necropsy, nine (8.3 per cent) were in the carotid canal; in one case the condition was bilateral. From the literature, twenty-seven additional cases have been collected, in three of which the condition was bilateral. The total number of cases therefore is thirty-five, and the total number of aneurysms, thirty-nine. The four bilateral cases in the literature were reported by Blane (1800), Heuer and Dandy (1916), Jefferson (1938) and Bozzoli (1937). When bilateral, aneurysms may be symmetric (Blane), nearly symmetric (Bozzoli) or markedly asymmetric (Heuer and Dandy, Jefferson).

Jefferson (1938), in an excellent paper, reported seventeen cases, but only six of these (including two in one patient) were authenticated; the remainder were assumed to be cases of aneurysm in the carotid canal because of signs and symptoms. But important as are the subjective and objective disturbances, they are by no means pathognomonic either of aneurysms or of the exact location of the lesion, i. e., whether in the carotid canal or intracranial. Two of Jefferson's aneurysms diagnosed by angiograms were clearly intracranial because they extended to the circle of Willis.

There are three methods by which the aneurysm and its exact position can be determined: (1) by necropsy; (2) by operation, and (3) by angiograms. A fourth method should probably be included, viz., roentgenograms of wire inserted into the aneurysm (Werner, Blakemore and King's case). There may be occasional calcifications which are adequately demonstrated by roentgen examination, but in most cases, even with the knowledge that calcifications are present, one is still left in doubt whether the lesion is a tumor or an aneurysm. For example, it is possible that two of the aneurysms reported by McKinney, Acree and Soltz may have been in the carotid canal, but no differentiation was made between these two subdivisions of the carotid, and it is impossible to make the determination from their roentgenograms; moreover, the writers placed them in the cranial chamber. The first description of the curved linear intracranial roentgen shadows that are almost pathognomonic of the calcified walls of aneurysms was reported by Heuer and myself in 1916 (case 1). Although neither Heuer nor I was aware of their significance at the time, their import was recognized by Dr. H. M. Thomas, then professor of neurology at the Johns Hopkins University School of Medicine, and the suggestion of an aneurysm was made by him and is so recorded in the history. Shadows of similar character are shown in the plates presented by Sosman and Vogt (1926) and McKinney, Acree and Soltz (1936). In one other case (case 6) in my series, a small dense irregular calcification in the carotid canal could leave no doubt concerning the diagnosis, especially when connected with the history. In Bozzoli's case, bilateral shadows alongside the sella turcica were of similar character.

Since the advent of angiography by Egas Moniz in 1933, intraarterial injections of colloidal thorium dioxide have demonstrated many intracranial aneurysms. Beautiful examples of those in the carotid canal have been reported by Fincher (1938), Reichert (1939), Krayenbuhl (1941) and Kosic (1941). A second aneurysm of Krayenbuhl failed to show in an arteriogram and was disclosed at operation. The demonstrations of aneurysms of this type at operation have been made by Cushing (1918—reported by Viets), Magnus (1927), Jefferson (1938) —four cases—and me—six cases. There can be no uncertainty about the diagnosis at operation, for the aneurysms pulsate, and blood can be aspirated from them if there is any doubt. Magnus opened an aneurysm while operating for trigeminal neuralgia, but the patient survived after the aneurysm had been packed and the internal carotid artery ligated in the neck. Cushing exposed one through a decompression opening. In 1 of Jefferson's cases, the aneurysm was exposed during a trigeminal operation, and the patient lived fourteen years. In his other three cases, the aneurysms were found when the clinically localized lesions were explored. In all of my 6 operative cases, the pa-

tients were operated on with the impression that the lesions were aneurysms and with surgical attack in mind.

Aneurysms in the carotid canal vary in size, like those located intracranially, from the so-called small berry aneurysm to those the size of an orange. Some are localized projections from the wall of the artery; others are dilatations of the whole arterial trunk.

According to signs and symptoms, aneurysms of the carotid canal fall into three types: (1) those giving palsies of the extraocular muscles; (2) those giving trigeminal neuralgia and corresponding sensory loss, and (3) those in which types 1 and 2 are combined. By far the most important manifestations of an aneurysm in this region are palsy or paralysis of the third nerve and periodic severe pain in the affected eye or frontal region. These disturbances are equally present with intracranial aneurysms of the internal carotid or even of the posterior communicating artery. But when to this pain and paralysis is added involvement, whether subjective or both, of the first and second branches of the trigeminal nerve (eventually of all three branches), the diagnosis of an aneurysm, and that one in the carotid canal, is almost absolute. Usually paralysis of the fourth and sixth nerves coexist. In Czermak's case palsy of the abducens antedated that of the third nerve by six years (in his case anesthesia of the cornea [fifth cranial nerve] also antedated involvement of the third nerve by the same time). Dural tumors of the lesser wing of the sphenoid and neuritis of the third nerve also may give identical objective findings, but with both of these conditions the severe attacks of pain in the eye and the frontal region are absent. Pain of this character and location has been perhaps the most consistent subjective complaint in all of the recorded cases. A sudden severe pain is always suggestive of vascular expansion or rupture.

Since these aneurysms lie on the gasserian ganglion, it is expected that trigeminal

Author	Date	How Proved	Size	Unilateral or Bilateral	Patient		Duration of Symptoms	Headache	Pain	Parilysis of Third Nerve	Paralysis of Fourth and Sixth Nerves
					Age, Yr.	Sex					
Blane..........	1800	Necropsy	....	Bilateral and symmetric	..	..	......	....	....	....	....
Holmes.........	1861	Necropsy	Size of a small nut	Unilateral	16	M	3 mo.	General	Over the left eye	Complete	Complete
Adams.........	1869	Necropsy	Size of a walnut	Unilateral	56	M	5 mo.	....	Right temporal	Complete	Complete
Romberg.......	1853	Necropsy	Double normal size of carotid	Unilateral	57	M	10 yr.	....	Facial neuralgia	None	None
Hutchinson.....	1875	Necropsy	Size of a bantam's egg	Unilateral	50	F	11 yr.	Periodic	Throbbing temple	Partial; later, complete	Complete in the sixth
Bramwell.......	1886	Necropsy	3 in. (7.6 cm.)	Unilateral	31	M	6 yr.	....	....	....	....
Dempsey.......	1886	Necropsy	¾ in. (1.9 cm.) in diameter	Unilateral	22	F	......	None	+ From ophthalmic aneurysm	None	None
Czermak........	1902	Necropsy	5.5 cm.	Unilateral	..	..	8 yr.	....	....	Complete	Complete
Czermak........	1902	Necropsy	Size of a mandarin	Unilateral	61	M	8 yr.	+ Right frontal	....	Complete	Complete
Reinhardt......	1913	Necropsy,	4.5 by 4 cm.	Unilateral	41	M	9 yr.	Severe	In the left part of the forehead and the left eye	Complete	Complete
Nettleship...... (reported by Beadles)	1907 (1889)	Necropsy	4 cm.	Unilateral	61	F	10 yr.	....	In the nose	Complete	Complete
Heuer and Dand (case 1)	1916	Necropsy	3.5 by 2 by 2 cm. and 8 by 7 by 7 cm.	Bilateral	29	M	5 yr.	Violent	In the left eye and the head	Complete	Complete
Cushing........ (reported by Viets)	1918	Operation; decompression	Size of a walnut	Unilateral	26	F	7 wk.	+	Sudden in the right side of the head	Complete	Complete
Magnus........	1927	Operation	Size of a chestnut	Unilateral	69	M	3 mo.	None	Constant facial neuralgia	None	Abducens only
Bozzoli.........	1937	Necropsy	Large	Bilateral	59	M	3 mo. (following trauma ?)	None	....	None	None
Jefferson.......	1937	Operation	Very large in drawing	Unilateral	50	F	5 yr.	Dull left sided	....	Complete	Partial in the sixth
Robinson....... (reported by Beadles)	1937	Necropsy	1 inch (2.5 cm.) diameter	Unilateral	..	..	......	....	None	None	None
Fincher........	1938	Colloidal thorium dioxide	Small	Unilateral	35	M	5 mo.	+ Vertical	+	Complete	Abducens palsy
Jefferson....... (case 1)	1938	Operation for trigeminal neuralgia	Large	Unilateral	65	F	18 yr.	+	Constant trigeminal neuralgia and pain in the head	None	Complete

CAROTID CANAL REPORTED IN THE LITERATURE

Paralysis of Fifth Nerve	Visual Loss	Exophthalmos	Other Signs and Symptoms	Intracranial Pressure	Diagnosed Correctly	Treatment	Result	Rupture	Comments
....	....	.....	....	None	No	....	.....	.....	
First branch	Blind on affected side	.....	Giddiness	None	No	None	Dead	No	Partly filled with clot; center open; thought to be due to endocarditis
First and second branches	Blind on affected side	.....	Giddiness; cornea ulcerated	None	No	None	Dead	No	Partly filled with clot; center open
Neuralgia	None	.....	Giddiness	.. ..	No	None	Dead	No	Patient had only trigeminal neuralgia
All branches	None	.....	"Beating under the ears"	Probably	Yes	None, but it was proposed to ligate the carotid	Dead	No	Aneurysm removed and preserved in the museum of the Royal College of Surgeons; thought to be solid; calcified walls
....	Bitemporal hemianopia	....	....	Probably	No	None	Dead	No	Protruded into cranial cavity
None	.. ..	+ From ophthalmic aneurysm	Principal symptoms from ophthalmic aneurysm	None	No	Common carotid tied	Dead	No	Patient had intravranial carotid aneurysm and one of the ophthalmic artery also
All branches	....	.....	....	Present	No	None	Dead	Yes	
All branches	Blind on affected side from keratitis	None	Syphilis; keratitis first symptom	Probably	No	None	Dead	+	Abducens palsy 6 yr. before advent of third nerve change
All branches	Blind on affected side	+	....	Present	No tumor diagnosed	None	Dead	No	Photograph of enormous aneurysm; much of the aneurysm filled with firm clot
Probably not involved	Blind in one eye	+	Exophthalmos; bleeding from nose repeatedly	Present	No	None; ligation suggested	Dead	Yes; into the nose	Another small aneurysm was in the neck; patient died of nasal hemorrhage; specimen in museum
All branches	Blind in the left eye; temporal hemianopia on the right	+	.. ..	Marked	No; but suggested as a possibility by Dr. H. M. Thomas	None (decompression)	Dead	No	Marked long linear shadows in the brain; destruction of sella (first case with roentgen changes)
First and second branches	None	None	Discomfort in the neck; dizziness; vomiting	Present	No	None	Died 1 yr. later	?	Died suddenly; no autopsy
All branches; hypoesthesia	None	.....	....	None	At operation for trigeminal neuralgia	Internal carotid ligated in the neck	.. ...	.....	Encountered and opened during operation for tic douloureux (temporal route)
None	Visual acuity 1/10 for the left eye; 2/10 for the right eye	None	Syphilis; calcification alongside the sella	None	No	None	Dead	No	
All branches	Visual acuity, 6/60	+	Weakness on the right side of the body; erosion of the wing of the sphenoid; faint roentgen shadow; the sella not eroded	Present	No	None	Dead	No	Patient died 8 wk. later following increase in hemiplegia; "almost completely" thrombosed
None	None	.....	None	None	No	None	Dead	No	Recorded in museum; Beadles stated that there was no clinical evidence of the existence of an aneurysm
None	None	.....	....	None	Yes	Clipping carotid intracranially after tying in neck	Well	No	
Possibly (alcohol injection given)	None	None	Calcikcation developed in aneurysm; several years later there was periodic bleeding from the nose; blood pressure, 175/100	None	No	None	Died 14 yr. later	....	Began with sudden severe pain in the head; vomiting; coma for 2 or 3 days

Author	Date	How Proved	Size	Unilateral or Bilateral	Patient Age, Yr.	Sex	Duration of Symptoms	Headache	Pain	Parilysis of Third Nerve	Paraly of Four and Six Nerve
Jefferson (case 3)	1938	Operation	Large	Unilateral	61	F	20 yr. (headache)	+	....	Complete	Compl
Jefferson (case 8)	1938	Operation	Small	Unilateral	61	F	3 mo.	+ Right frontal	+ Behind the right eye	Complete	Comp
Jefferson (case 16)	1938	Necropsy	Large	Bilateral	72	F	1 mo.	+ Left	Trigeminal	Incomplete on the left	Incom on the
Sands and Hyman	1938	Necropsy	4.5 by 4 by 3.5 cm.	Unilateral	24	F	10 yr.	Present at end	....	....	Abdúc palsy
Dandy (case 2)	1939	Operation	Small	Unilateral	28	F	5 mo.	+ Left frontal	In the left eye	Complete	Comp in the fourth not in sixth
Dandy (case 3)	1939	Operation	Small	Unilateral	36	M	8 mo.	+ Left frontal	In the left eye	Partial	None
Dandy (case 4)	1939	Operation	Small	Unilateral	37	F	5 yr.	+ Right frontal	In the right eye	Complete	None
Reichert	1938	Colloidal thorium dioxide	Large	Unilateral	50	M	9 yr.	+ Present 2 to 3 yr.	+ In the right part of the forehead	Complete	Compl
Dandy (case 5)	1941	Necropsy	Size of a hazelnut	Unilateral (2 lesions)	53	M	None from arterial aneurysm until rupture	....	....	....	.....
Kosic	1941	Colloidal thorium dioxide	Small	Unilateral	42	F	3 wk.	....	....	Complete	Comp
Krayenbuhl	1941	Colloidal thorium dioxide	4 by 3.5 cm.	Unilateral	21	F	8 mo.	+	Severe in the left part of the forehead	None	Comp in the sixth
Krayenbuhl	1941	Operation (colloidal thorium dioxide negative)	Walnut size	Unilateral	44	M	18 mo.	+	+ In the left eye and the left part of the forehead	Complete	Comp
Werner, Blakemore and King	1941	By wiring (roentgenograms)	Very large	Unilateral	17	F	6 yr.	Generalized and severe	In the right eye and temple	None	Diplo withou ptosis
Dandy (case 6)	1942	Operation	Small	Unilateral	24	M	22 yr.	+ Left frontal	In the left eye	Complete	Partia
Dandy (case 7)	1942	Operation	Small	Unilateral	20	M	3 mo.	+ Right frontal	In the right eye	Complete	Comp
Dandy (case 8)	1942	Operation	Huge	Unilateral	52	F	4 yr.	+ Right frontal	In the right cheek	Complete	Comp

...ROTID CANAL REPORTED IN THE LITERATURE *(Continued)*

Paralysis of Fifth Nerve	Visual Loss	Exophthalmos	Other Signs and Symptoms	Intracranial Pressure	Diagnosed Correctly	Treatment	Result	Rupture	Comments
...l branches	None	......	Began with sudden terrific pain in the left temple; diplopia for a few days (3 yr. earlier); blood pressure, 135/90	?	Yes	None	Living 5 yr. later	No	Exposed through decompression
...rst branch	None	None	Erosion of the sella	None	Yes	None	Living 6 yr. later	No	
...poalgesia ...the whole ...t side	Loss to visual acuity of 2/24 in each eye	None		None	Yes	None	Dead	No	Patient died of coronary occlusion; the left aneurysm was five or six times as large as the right
...esthesia ...the cornea	None	......	Double vision; convulsions; attacks of mental confusion	Present	No	None	Dead	Yes	Projected into the brain
...ne	Vision reduced on the affected side	None	....	None	Yes	Internal carotid ligated intracranially in the neck	Living 5 yr.	+	Aneurysm broke through the dura; small protrusion intracranially alongside the carotid
...ckling ...sation ...the neck	Blurring in the left eye; visual acuity 20/30 for the left eye and 20/120 for the right	None	....	None	Yes	Aneurysm trapped between ligatures	Living 3½ yr.	No	Aneurysm broke through dura alongside the intracranial part of the carotid
...ne	Visual acuity 20/50 for the right eye and 20/25 for the left	None	....	None	Yes	Aneurysm trapped between ligatures	Living 3½ yr.	Probably	Aneurysm broke through dura alongside the intracranial part of the carotid
...ne	Visual acuity 5/10; small central scotoma	+	Noise in the ear on the same side; no pulsation in exophthalmus; papilledema	?	Yes	Partial ligation of the carotid with fascia	Well	No	Improvement after operation (3 weeks)
....	Not from arterial aneurysm	+ Not from arterial aneurysm	All signs of pulsating exophthalmos	None	No	Attempted closure of internal carotid	Dead	No	Operation for carotid-cavernous arteriovenous aneurysm; cause found at necropsy to be rupture of two small arterial aneurysms; artery tore, death resulting
...ne	None	None	....	None	Yes	None	Living	No	
...ne	None	+	Some erosion of the sella; double vision first symptom	None	Yes	Ligation of the carotid	Well	No	Two years later strabismus gone and the patient felt well
...t and ...nd ...ches	Blind on affected side	+	....	None	Yes	Ligation of the carotid	Well	No	Three weeks after operation extraocular palsies much improved and anesthesia of the face reduced
...eresia of all ...ches	Eventually blind	+ 5 mo.	Bruit heard; erosion of the sella, the orbit and the sphenoid: Simmonds' disease; amenorrhea	Probably	Yes	Wiring (30 ft. [914.4 cm.]); both common carotids tied	Living 22 mo.	No	
...e	Visual acuity 10/400 for the left eye and 20/15 for the right	None	Small dense calcification in the cavernous sinus	None	Yes	Aneurysm trapped between ligatures	Living 2¾ yr.	Probably	Third nerve palsy persisted since age of 2 yr.; aneurysm confined to sinus
...e	None	None	....	None	Yes	Aneurysm trapped between ligatures	Living 3¾ yr.	Probably (bloody spinal fluid)	Large nut-sized aneurysm broke through dura alongside the carotid
...branches ...tial)	Visual acuity. 20/50 for the right eye and 20/20 for the left	+ 4 mm.	The sella destroyed; central scotoma on the right	Present	Yes	Aneurysm trapped between ligatures after partial ligation in the neck	Living 2 mo.	No	One of the enormous aneurysms pushing far upward into the temporal lobe

neuralgia, probably more or less continuous, and eventually sensory loss should be present. Actually, however, in 10 cases these subjective and objective disturbances were absent or not noted. Their absence therefore does not militate against the diagnosis of an aneurysm in the carotid canal, but their presence is all important. Romberg's (1853) patient, who had 1 of the smallest aneurysms reported, had only facial neuralgia; the patients of Magnus (1927) and Jefferson (1937) had this type of neuralgia plus palsy of the abducens. Jefferson proposed subdivision of aneurysms in the carotid canal into three further types: (1) posterior; (2) middle, and (3) anterior, i.e., corresponding with the three positions of the lesion in the carotid canal. Under the posterior type of aneurysm he placed those with involvement of all three branches of the trigeminus and palsies of all the extraocular muscles. With the middle type the third branch of the trigeminus is spared, and with the anterior type only the first branch of the trigeminus is involved. However, there appears to be little point in this finer classification. The greatest involvement of nerves is more an index of the size of the aneurysm.

Loss of vsion is an important and common subjective and objective disturbance. It is of course due to direct pressure of the bulging aneurysm on the optic nerve or on the nerve through the interposed carotid artery as in one of my cases (case 8) in which there was only a central scotoma. Eventually there may be blindness in the eye on the affected side. Occasionally, as in one of my cases, the aneurysm may enlarge sufficiently to attack the optic chiasm and produce hemianopia in the other eye. When one sees the enormous size of many of these aneurysms, it is surprising that vison is retained so long. It is the tightly attached dura at the anterior part of the middle fossa that protects the actual contact with the optic nerve until the size of the aneurysm grows excessive and finally compresses it.

At times papilledema results from intracranial pressure as the aneurysm grows upward into the cranial chamber. Both eyegrounds may be similarly affected, or there may be primary optic atrophy on the affected side and papilledema on the other side.

The very nature of aneurysms, i.e., their being due to defective arterial walls, predisposes them to rupture, and since a high percentage—at least 75 per cent—are of congenital origin, frequently the rupture occurs in the early years of life. Aneurysms in the carotid canal are less susceptible to rupture than those within the cranial chamber because they are covered by the firm layer of dura which expands slowly. This accounts for the long duration of symptoms in so many instances. However, they are by no means immune to this termination. Four deaths resulted in this collected series from this cause—the rupture taking place into the cranial chamber. In three of my operative cases, the rupture had probably occurred alongside the carotid (from small intracranial extensions), and the point of rupture had healed owing to the contact with the carotid artery. In 1 of my cases (case 2) two separate small aneurysms had ruptured into the cavernous sinus and produced an arteriovenous aneurysm (pulsating exophthalmos). This is one of the important causes of this remarkable lesion; it may occur spontaneously or be induced by trauma. In this case the existence of the arterial aneurysm as the underlying cause was recognized only at necropsy. In Nettleship's case repeated ruptures had occurred into the nose, death finally resulting.

Exophthalmos was noted in nine cases, including the case reported here. This can occur only with the large aneurysms which have eroded the walls of the sphenoid fissure and have therefore broken through into the orbit. Pulsation of the eyeball was noted but rarely in spite of the violent pulsation of these aneurysms; doubtless it was missed in some instances. Dempsey's case is noteworthy because in it there was an aneurysm of the ophthalmic artery in addition to the diffuse enlargement of the internal carotid artery (¾ inch [1.9 cm.]) in the canal.

Bruit was noted only in the case reported by Werner, Blakemore and King. Hutchinson was skeptical of reports of bruits with intracranial aneurysms and concluded that a bruit was present only with the arteriovenous variety—then termed aneurysm by anastomosis. In none of my cases was a bruit detected. It does occur, but only rarely, and is hardly worthy of consideration in differential diagnosis.

That a spontaneous cure of an aneurysm of this type ever occurs is doubtful, though perhaps possible. Frequently the aneurysm is partially filled with a firm old thrombus that is laid down in layers. Hutchinson noted that the aneurysm in his case was "almost entirely" filled with thrombus; however, the specimen was not opened, and his deduction was made by probing. Jefferson stated that 1 of his large aneurysms was "almost completely" thrombosed. Many aneurysms are indeed almost completely filled with thrombus, but a central channel is usually patent and is in communication with the lumen of the artery, and they still remain active aneurysms. In 1 of Krayenbuhl's cases, the internal carotid and the middle cerebral arteries were completely thrombosed (hemiplegia resulting). It appears probable that this may have been a case of complete thrombosis and cure of the aneurysm, but the patient survived, and no pathologic report was therefore in evidence.

The ages of patients at the time of operation, death or disclosure of the aneurysm run fairly evenly according to decades. Only two were under twenty, although several of those in the succeeding decade had their origin before twenty. In one of my cases (case 6), the aneurysm ruptured at the age of two years. Eight aneurysms occurred in the third and sixth decades; six in the seventh; four, in the fourth; and three, in the fifth. The oldest patient was seventy-two (Jefferson). Sixteen patients were male and sixteen female. Twenty of the aneurysms were of the large type that protrudes upward into the cerebral chamber; many of these caused intracranial pressure.

The duration of symptoms varies considerably; eighteen patients (over 50 per cent) had symptoms over three years; nine had symptoms nine years or more; three lived eighteen, twenty and twenty-two years, and at the time of writing, one (case 6) is still living after twenty-five years. In several cases, however, the course was more fulminating, lasting a few weeks or months.

The fact that thirteen of these aneurysms were actually disclosed at operation testifies to the great progress in neurosurgery in recent years. A few were accidental disclosures, two (Magnus and Jefferson) being found during operation for trigeminal neuralgia by the temporal route. Magnus had the terrifying experience of opening the aneurysm but was able to pack the opening and tie the internal carotid artery in the neck. Despite the advanced age of the patient (sixty-nine years), the ligation caused no ill affects. The extradural approach to the gasserian ganglion of course reduces the hazards of a ruptured aneurysm in this position.

The disclosure of aneurysms by angiography has attained a great vogue since its introduction by Egas Moniz, and viewed superficially, the results appear to be remarkable. Certainly the roentgenograms depict the lesion beautifully both in diagnosis and localization, but from a practical point of view, I consider its use inadvisable. It is not a procedure without risk. Cerebral thromboses were reported by Ekstrom and Lindgren in 60 per cent of the brains examined after death. These may or may not cause symptoms at the time, but they certainly are a potential cause of epilepsy. Moreover, the colloidal thorium dioxide is a permanent deposit in the reticuloendothelial system. There is no reason to inject it when the signs and symptoms clearly indicate the site of a lesion which should be exposed at operation.

This statement holds true for all aneurysms in the carotid canal, where the localizing disturbances are so pathognomonic of the site of the lesion and clinical judgment is almost adequate to identify the character of the lesion. If it was a matter of diagnosing a hopeless type of lesion and thus avoiding an operation, it might be a procedure of merit, but all the aneurysms in this group are operable and should be operated on. In one of Karyenbuhl's cases, the angiogram did not disclose the lesion which was subsequently found at operation. Patients are certainly better without it!

Of the seven patients operated on there was one who died—a mortality rate of 14 per cent. The death occurred in a case in which operation was done for a carotid-cavernous arteriovenous aneurysm, and at necropsy the cause of the arteriovenous aneurysm was found to be rupture of two small arterial aneurysms in the carotid canal. Death was due to rupture of an oversized arteriosclerotic artery during the application of a silver clip that was too small. In over twenty closures of the carotid intracranially by this method, this was the only accident. The other six patients were cured, the longest period after operation being three and one-half years.

SUMMARY

The case of a presumably cured patient with a large aneurysm of the internal carotid artery arising in the carotid canal and extending into the cranial chamber is presented.

The differential diagnostic signs and symptoms are emphasized.

The surgical attack previously employed for the smaller aneurysms, viz., trapping the aneurysm by ligating the internal carotid artery intracranially and in the neck, was applied with equal success to one of enormous size after forcing adequate collateral circulation through the circle of Willis by preliminary partial ligation of the internal carotid in the neck.

REFERENCES

[1]Adams, J.: Aneurysm of Internal Carotid in the Cavernous Sinus. *Lancet*, 2:768, 1869.

[2]Beadles, C. F.: Aneurysms of the Larger Cerebral Arteries. *Brain*, 30:20, 1907.

[3]Blane: *Tr. Soc. Improv. M. & Chir. Knowledge*, 2:192, 1800; cited by Beadles.

[4]Bozzoli, A.: Aneurisma bilaterale della carotide interne. *Riv. oto-neuro-oftal.*, 14:304, 1937.

[5]Bramwell: Two Enormous Intracranial Aneurysms. *Edinburgh M. J.*, 32:918, 1886-1887.

[6]Cushing, H.: Contributions to the Study of Intracranial Aneurysm. *Guy's Hosp. Rep.*, 73:159, 1923.

[7]Czermak: Case Report, Verein deutscher Aerzte in Prag. *Prag. med. Wchnschr.*, 27:227, 1902.

[8]Dandy, W. E.: The Treatment of Carotid-Cavernous Arteriovenous Aneurysms. *Ann. Surk.*, 102:916, 1935.
The Treatment of Internal Carotid Aneurysms Within the Cavernous Sinuses and the Cranial Chamber, *Ann. Surg.*, 109:689, 1939.

[9]———— and Follis, R. H.: On the Pathology of Carotid Cavernous Aneurysms. *Am. J. Ophth.*, 24:365, 1941.

[10]Dempsey, A.: A Case of Oribital Aneurysm. *Brit. M. J.*, 2:541, 1886.

[11]Ekstrom, S., and Lindgren, G. H.: Gehirnschadigungen nach cerebraler Arteriographie mit Thorotrast. *Zentralbl. Neurochir.*, 4:227, 1938.

[12]Fincher, E. F.: An Aneurysm of the Intracranial Carotid Artery Treated Surgically. *Yale J. Biol. & Med.*, 11:423, 1939.

[13]Heuer, G. J., and Dandy, W. E.: Roentgenography in the Localization of Brain Tumors. *Bull. Johns Hopkins Hosp.*, 26:311, 1916.

[14]Holmes, T.: Aneurysm of the Internal Carotid Artery in the Cavernous Sinus. *Tr. Path. Soc. London*, 12:61, 1861.

[15]Hutchinson, J.: Aneurysm of the Internal Carotid Within the Skull Diagnosed Eleven Years Before the Patient's Death: Spontaneous Cure. *Tr. Clin. Soc.*, 8:127, 1875.

[16]Jefferson, G.: Compression of the Chiasma, Optic Nerve and Optic Tracts by Intracranial Aneurysms. *Brain*, 60:444, 1937.
On the Saccular Aneurysms of the Internal Carotid Artery in the Cavernous Sinus. *Brit. J. Surg.*, 26:267, 1938.

[17]Kosic, H.: Die Tumoren der Gegend der Sella turcica. *Arch. klin. Chir.*, 201:89, 1941.

[18]Krayenbuhl, H.: Das Hirnaneurysma. *Schweiz. Arch. f. Neurol. u. Psychiat.*, 47:155, 1941.

[19]McKinney, J. M.; Acree, T., and Soltz, S. E.: The Syndrome of the Unrupted Aneurysm of the Intracranial Portion of the Internal Carotid Artery. *Bull. Neurol. Inst. New York*, 5:247, 1936.

[20]Magnus, V.: Aneurysm of Internal Carotid Artery. *J.A.M.A.*, 88:1712 (May 28) 1927.

[21]Reichert, T.: Ueber Hirnaneurysmen. *Zentralbl.*

*Neurochir., 4:*111, 1939.

[22]Reinhardt, S.: Ueber Hirnarterienaneurysmen und ihre Folgen. *Mitt. Grenzgeb. d. Med. u. Chir., 26:*432, 1913.

[23]Romberg, M. H.: A Manual of the Nervous Diseases of Man, translated and edited by E. H. Sieveking, London. *New Sydenham Society, 1:* 37, 1853.

[24]Sands, I. J., and Hyman, M. A.: An Intracranial Carotid Aneurysm of Long Duration. *Ann. Int.*

*Med., 12:*708, 1938.

[25]Sosman, M. C., and Vogt, E. C.: Aneurysms of the Internal Carotid Artery and the Circle of Willis from a Roentgenological Viewpoint. *Am. J. Roentgenol., 15:*122, 1926.

[26]Viets, H.: Unilateral Ophthalmoplegia. *J. Nerv. & Ment. Dis., 47:*249, 1918.

[27]Werner, S. C.; Blakemore, A. H., and King B. G.: Aneurysm of the Internal Carotid Artery Within the Skull. *J.A.M.A., 116:*578 (Feb. 15) 1941.

LXXI

RESULTS FOLLOWING LIGATION OF THE INTERNAL CAROTID ARTERY*

It has long been known that ligation of the internal or common carotid artery is followed by (1) a high mortality rate and (2) a high percentage of cerebral complications. Some of the patients in whom cerebral complications develop survive with residual sequelae, such as varying degrees of hemiplegia, aphasia, mental changes and epilepsy. In prelisterian days the surgical mortality rate from carotid ligation approached and frequently surpassed 50 per cent. It has since been learned that the mortality rate is less when wounds are clean and that sepsis was responsible for many deaths through the intravascular spread of an infected thrombus into the cranial chamber. However, precisely the same sequence of events occurs with and without sepsis; the only difference is in the relative frequency. There are two causes of death and disability: (1) cerebral anemia from inadequate collateral circulation through the circle of Willis, the effects of which appear immediately and may be abrupt or progressive, and (2) cerebral thrombosis and embolism, the effects of which are late in appearing, i.e., develop twelve hours to several days later, and are usually abrupt, though at times a preceding small attack may warn of the impending event.

The purpose of this communication is to show that (1) by care in the preoperative tests for the adequacy of collateral circulation in the brain and (2) by the proper choice of the methods of ligation these risks can now be largely eliminated.

Pilz [1] collected six hundred cases of common carotid ligation, the mortality rate being 38.5 per cent and cerebral compli-

cations being present in 32 per cent. Lefort[2] reported a mortality rate of 54.5 per cent. Wyeth [3] and Ballance and Edmunds [4] reported seven hundred eighty-nine collected cases in each of their writings with a mortality rate of 41 per cent (they probably had reference to the same material). The writings of these authors give a fair estimate of the risks to life in the days when operations were almost always attended by sepsis.

In 1891 Zimmermann [5] collected sixty-five cases reported since 1880 with a mortality rate of 31 per cent and an incidence of cerebral complications of 26 per cent, and in 1899 Siegrist [6] reported 825 cases collected since 1880 with a mortality rate of 40 per cent. More recently, Cauchoix [7] reported one hundred fifty cases of ligation of the common carotid with a mortality rate of 10 per cent and thirteen cases of ligation of the internal carotid with a mortality rate of 16.7 per cent; Walcker [8] reported a mortality rate of 40 per cent in 601 collected cases; Matas,[9] in sixty-six cases of his own (sixty cases of ligation of the common carotid and six of ligation of the internal carotid), had eight deaths (including two reported as due to angina) —representing a death rate of 12 per cent. The report of Matas brought the risk to the lowest figure yet obtained and represented the best work of an individual investigator rather than an ensemble of results collected from the literature. I have made no effort to separate ligations of the internal and common carotid arteries. It is frequently stated that ligations of the common carotid are less dangerous than those of the internal carotid because of the collateral circulation through the external carotid in the former. Theoretical-

*Reprinted from the *Archives of Surgery,* 45:521–533, October, 1942.

ly this appears reasonable, and perhaps there may be a slight difference, but I doubt that it is much. A recent report by Watson and Silverstone [10] of a death rate of 55 per cent and of an incidence of cerebral complications of 70 per cent in their twenty cases should be noted in passing. In all of their cases, however, the ligations were done in conjunction with the removal of large carcinomatous masses (many of them ulcerated and infected) in the neck. Such statistics cannot give a fair appraisal of the risks incurred with simple ligations of the carotid arteries, but they do indicate the dangers that attend the procedures.

RESULTS IN THIS SERIES OF EIGHTY-EIGHT LIGATIONS (PARTIAL AND TOTAL)

In this series, except for three ligations of the common carotid, all have been ligations of the internal carotid. In each of the 3 exceptions, however, in addition to the common carotid the external carotid was tied, so that the equivalent of ligation of the internal carotid was done. All ligations were performed by myself or my associates, and all were "clean cases." In all but three of the cases of partial ligation, total ligation was done subsequently. In the overwhelming percentage of the cases the ligations were performed for verified arterial or arteriovenous aneurysm of the brain; in a few they were done for brain tumor. The ligations may be divided into three groups: (1) partial ligation in the neck (with fascial bands), twenty-five cases; (2) total ligation in the neck, thirty-six cases; (3) total intracranial ligation (with silver clips), twenty-seven cases. The total number of cases was eighty-eight.

PARTIAL LIGATION IN THE NECK. Partial occlusion of the internal carotid with fascial bands was done in twenty-five cases. Immediate cerebral complications developed in three cases (12 per cent); death occurred in one case (4 per cent).

The single death was due to an aneu-

rysm that was known to have ruptured at the time of the ligation. The ruptured aneurysm therefore probably did not contribute to the death but perhaps did induce the paralysis.

In the three cases in which there were immediate complications, the band was removed in each instance within a few hours with the following results: complete return of function in one; complete return of speech but not of motor power in one; no improvement in one.

In fifteen cases the lesion for which the carotid was ligated was intracranial arterial aneurysm; in nine cases it was intracranial arteriovenous aneurysm.

The ages af the patients were 33, 36, 36, 38, 38, 40, 45, 45, 48, 50, 51, 52, 53, 54, 56, 58, 60, 61, 67, 68, 68, 68, 70, 72 and 73 years.

The ages of the 3 patients with cerebral complications were 56, 58 and 70 years respectively.

TOTAL LIGATION IN THE NECK. Total ligation in the neck was done in thirty-six cases. In seven cases it was done after partial ligation in the neck; in these seven cases there were no immediate or late cerebral complications, and there was one death. In twelve cases it was done after intracranial clipping of the carotid; in these cases there were no cerebral complications or deaths. In seventeen cases it was done without any prior attack on the artery; in these cases there were no immediate cerebral complications, but in one case there were late cerebral complications followed by death.

The age of the patient with the cerebral complication (hemiplegia) was thirteen years. Hemiplegia occurred suddenly twenty-four hours after the artery had been tied. The patient died eighteen days later. Postmortem examination was not obtained. This complication and death could, I am sure, now be avoided by tying the artery over a band of fascia lata.

The death noted as following partial ligation, which was done when the patient was dying and was not in any way responsible for her death, was shown at necropsy to have been due to multiple scattered venous thrombi. In view of these observations the ligation was ill advised. Her original lesion was a carotid arteriovenous aneurysm. It was for this that the original partial ligation had been performed. The relation, if any, between this lesion and the multiple venous intracranial thrombi is not clear.

The ages of the patients in whom the internal carotid was ligated were as follows: (1) of those whose internal carotid was ligated after partial occlusion—38, 48, 50, 52, 53, 54 and 68 years; (2) of those whose internal carotid was ligated after intracranial clipping—20, 20, 23, 28, 36, 37, 38, 42, 43, 47, 48 and 54 years; (3) of those whose internal carotid was ligated without prior attack on the artery—13, 18, 23 ,23, 24, 27, 28, 32, 35, 36, 39, 43, 45, 47, 48, 48 and 55 years.

In 15 cases the lesion for which the carotid was ligated was intracranial arterial aneurysm; in twenty cases it was carotid-cavernous and cerebral arteriovenous aneurysm; in 1 case it was tumor of the gasserian ganglion.

TOTAL INTRACRANIAL LIGATION. The internal carotid was clipped intracranially in twenty-seven cases. In six cases this was done after partial ligation in the neck; in these cases there were no cerebral disturbances, but there was one death. In six cases the clipping was done after total ligation in the neck; in these cases there were no cerebral disturbances or deaths. In fifteen cases the clipping was done without prior attack on the artery in the neck; in 1 of these cases there was an immediate cerebral complication.

The single death (giving a mortality rate of 4 per cent) was due to rupture of the carotid when an undersized clip was applied to a greatly enlarged arteriosclerotic artery. The single immediate cerebral complication (hemiplegia) was due to inadequate collateral circulation in the circle of Willis. Since this was known beforehand from the positive reaction to the Matas test, it was poor judgment to take the chance involved in clipping the artery intracranially.

In sixteen cases the lesion for which the internal carotid was clipped intracranially was intracranial arterial aneurysm; in nine it was carotid cavernous arteriovenous aneurysm; in two it was tumor of the gasserian ganglion.

The ages of the patients were 18, 20, 20, 21, 23, 23, 23, 24, 27, 28, 32, 36, 38, 37, 42, 43, 45, 45, 45, 47, 48, 52, 53, 53, 54, 58 and 60 years.

SUMMARY OF RESULTS OF ALL EIGHTY-EIGHT LIGATIONS. Among all eighty-eight cases in which ligation was done there were immediate cerebral complications in four, or 4.5 per cent, late cerebral complications in one, or 1.1 per cent, and deaths in four, or 4.5 per cent.

COMMENT

It is certain that in one case of total ligation the death was in no way connected with the operation, for the patient was dying at the time ligation was done. The operation was a desperate but ill considered attempt to do something for a condition which could not be diagnosed but which was thought to be related to an arteriovenous aneurysm which had nothing to do with the patient's impending death. In another case death was due to rupture of an intracranial aneurysm which was known to have broken at the time the operation was performed. If these two cases are eliminated, the mortality rate is 2.25 per cent. With greater care in applying an intracranial silver clip another death would have been prevented, and finally, if a band of fascia had been interposed between the internal carotid and the silk ligature, there is reason to believe that the late-appearing hemiplegia and subsequent death would have been avoided. With careful preoperative care in the choice of ligations of the internal carotid and with the best of operative skill, ligations of this vessel should now be possible with little risk.

From the complications already mentioned it can be seen that partial ligations are the most hazardous. There can be no doubt that the application of the Matas test [11] used throughout this series, i. e., compression of the internal carotid with the finger for ten minutes to determine whether or not cerebral functions are disturbed, is responsible for the low figures both of mortality and cerebral complications. Without this test and the resulting operative attack, the results in this series would scarcely have been different from those of other reports. A high percentage of patients, regardless of age (but certainly increasing with age), will not tolerate total ligation of the carotid, but by partial closure of the carotid and cerebral collateral circulation becomes quickly established, and complete closure can be safely concluded later. The exact time between the partial and total closures of this vessel has been determined empirically. At first an interval of four to six weeks was thought to be advisable, but gradually this was lessened until now a week is considered ample, and in one of the most severe tests in this series (a large carotid aneurysm) the total closure was made after four days. By this means the reduced flow of blood through the internal carotid is adequate for the cerebral blood supply, but at the same time the demand is made for the anterior and posterior communicating arteries to supply the deficit that is created.

In none of the cases was there any disturbance when total ligation followed preliminary partial closure. And without the Matas test most if not all of these patients would certainly have been lost or badly crippled by the effects of inadequate cerebral circulation if the total occlusion had been done first.

Only once did preliminary partial ligation fail to establish the collateral circulation so that total occlusion could be performed. This was in the last case included in this report. Two months earlier I had done partial ligation of the carotid for post-traumatic carotid-cavernous arteriovenous aneurysm. The patient was so much improved that he was allowed to return home with the hope that the intra-arterial thrombosis would clear the lesion in time. When he subsequently returned, compression of the carotid could still not be sustained, numbness of the arm developing within a minute. The lumen of the carotid was then further reduced by another band. At the time of the operation (with the patient under local anesthesia) temporary direct occlusion of the artery with forceps produced precisely the same numbness of the arm as the Matas test. It can only be assumed that the circle of Willis was congenitally defective (the patient's age at the time of writing is 36), that probably one of the communicating branches was absent and that the other was too small to maintain the cerebral circulation. One week later the artery was totally ligated in the neck and clipped intracranially without any untoward effects.

PARTIAL CLOSURE OF THE INTERNAL CAROTID

Throughout this series of cases a band of fascia lata was used for partial closure of the internal carotid. It has the advantage of a living tissue, is soft and can therefore be removed with ease and safety if signs of vascular anemia develop. Dr. W. S. Halsted [12] performed many experiments on animals, using all types of bands, and concluded that metallic (aluminum) rolled bands were superior, even though at times the vessel was eroded by the band. His objection to fascia lata was the disintegration of the fascia due to the strong arterial pulsation. However, his experiments were performed on the abdominal aorta, which is larger and has a more violent pulsation. Even on the internal carotid the fascia does disintegrate, the fibers fragmenting, but apparently this can be entirely overcome either by doubling the fascial band or encircling the vessel twice; the fascia then does not break up. In four instances I have subsequently removed the section of the carotid covered by the double bands and subjected them to microscopic study; the fibers appeared to be intact after intervals of two to four months. One noticeable difference appears to be evident, that there is always a reaction and deposition of new tissue about a band, but it is far greater when the band is single and the fibers fragmented; the fibers are then engulfed in such a dense, bulbous, fibrous mass that the original fascia (after two months) can scarcely be found on gross dissection. When the band is double, the original band is just as distinct as when it was applied. With either the single or the double layer of fascia, however, the result is essentially the same. In addition to the constriction by the band itself, there is gradually added an increasing constriction of the lumen by the added connective tissues. In time total occlusion would probably ensue.

The first application of fascial bands to human arteries was probably made by Perthes [13] and has since been used by Freeman [14] and in improved fashion by Kerr.[15] Pearse [16] recently suggested cellophane bands because of the marked connective tissue reaction that follows and which in time gradually obliterates the lumen, but I see no advantage over the fascial bands which do precisely the same thing though perhaps more slowly. There is apparently no need for greater rapidity of progressive constriction of the lumen than that produced by fascia lata. Whether or not the lumen would be too rapidly constricted by the cellophane reaction I do not know.

The degree of initial constriction of the lumen of the carotid is all important and requires great care. At best it is a rough estimate guided by the appearance of the constricted region and by the effect on the pulsation above the band. Since in three of my earlier cases cerebral disturbances developed owing to too much constriction, I have preferred to err on the side of too little constriction rather than that of too much and to depend on the subsequent tissue reaction to increase it. Roughly a reduction of the lumen by one half is safe and has led to no cerebral symptoms in re-

cent years. This still leaves a good pulse above but one distinctly less than that below the band. It is less than the thrill stage, which is much too far. In none of the partial constrictions that have been done in the past four years have there been any adverse after-effects.

In one of the earlier cases removal of the fascial band restored the cerebral functions. Similar results have been reported by Matas (aluminum band) and Moses (fascial band).[17] In order to appraise the immediate response to partial ligation, the operation should be performed with the patient under local anesthesia, or at least one of the anesthetics from which consciousness is quickly restored should be used. It is important also that the band be removed when the first sign of cerebral failure is manifest, for progression of the disturbance is probable.

CAUSE OF LATE CEREBRAL DISTURBANCE FROM CAROTID LIGATIONS

The immediate cerebral complications, of which hemiplegia is the outspoken evidence, are clearly explained on the basis of inadequate circulation to the affected side of the brain. The late cerebral involvement is just as certainly explained on the basis of a propagating thrombus in the carotid, or possibly in some cases an embolus that has broken off from a thrombus and lodged in the cerebral arteries. Usually the onset is precipitate, but there may be premonitory cerebral attacks with recovery, followed in the succeeding twenty-four to forty-eight hours by the complete loss of function.

The pathologic reports confirming this view are not numerous but are conclusive. Zimmermann [5] collected 5 reported cases with postmortem examinations of the carotid artery following ligations; in all there were thrombi extending the length of the carotid in the neck. Two of the specimens were examined intracranially, and all three branches of the carotid (in the brain) were filled with a continuation of the thrombus

(Verneuil's case, 1871) and (Schanborn's case, 1879). In four of his own cases the entire carotid in the neck was closed by a thrombus, and in 1 of these it was continuous into the ophthalmic and middle cerebral arteries. Stierlin and Meyerburg[18] reported a specimen obtained after a bullet wound in the neck in which the internal carotid was not torn; the thrombus extended from a point 4 or 5 cm. above the carotid bifurcation into the anterior cerebral and middle cerebral arteries and their branches. In another of Zimmermann's cases (following thyroidectomy), the thrombus extended down the external carotid into and up the internal carotid artery and closed the middle cerebral artery. Cerebral symptoms appeared suddenly four days after the operation, and death occurred two days later. Perthes traced a postoperative thrombus (artery tied at the base of the skull) into all three intracranial branches of the internal carotid. Paralysis and aphasia appeared eight hours after the ligation and were complete in three hours. Death occurred six days later. The intima and the media had been cut by the ligation. In another of Perthes' cases hemiplegia developed during the night following ligation of the carotid. There were a thrombus at the site of the ligature and an embolus in the terminus of the intracranial portion of the carotid. Apparently the thrombus was not continuous, but a fragment of it was carried up the carotid.

An interesting case was recorded by Esmarch.[19] While an aneurysm of the carotid in the neck was being palpated, the patient suddenly became hemiplegic and died three days later. Necropsy showed a thrombus formation (from an embolus) in the internal carotid from the ophthalmic artery into the middle cerebral and anterior cerebral arteries and their branches.

In a personal communication Dr. Cyril Courville, of Los Angeles, has forwarded me unpublished reports of carefully studied postmortem examinations made in two cases. In one case a thrombus extended the entire length of the internal carotid and into the anterior and middle cerebral arteries. In the other the artery in the neck contained a thrombus that extended part way up the neck, and an embolus had lodged in the middle cerebral artery, the anterior cerebral artery being intact.

I[20] recently reported a necropsy specimen (nontraumatic and non-operative) from a spontaneously arising thrombus that extended continuously from the bifurcation of the carotid into the middle cerebral artery and its branches and for some distance into the anterior cerebral artery. It apparently arose from a defective calcified area in the artery within the carotid canal (see illustration).

Pettermann[21] reported four cases of sudden cerebral death after carotid ligations with postmortem studies in three. Softening in the brain was reported in one, and a thrombus of the internal carotid extending from the ligature was reported in another. Although he explained the cerebral disturbances by propagation of thrombi (and they undoubtedly are due to this), the pathologic studies were not sufficiently complete to use for evidence.

Fetterman and Pritchard[22] reported the postmortem observations in the case of a patient aged thirty-seven whose internal carotid had been ligated one and one-half years earlier; two and one-half hours after the operation aphasia and right hemiplegia resulted. The internal carotid (intracranially) was completely obliterated. No note was made concerning the extension of the thrombus into the middle cerebral artery, nor can one determine this from the excellent photographs of the exterior of the cerebral vascular tree. The posterior communicating artery was absent on that side and small on the other, but the anterior cerebral artery appears to have been of ample size to take care of the collateral circulation.

In a recent communication Schorstein[23] argued at some length to refute this explanation of the cause of cerebral complications after carotid ligations. These he explained by anoxemia and without actual occlusion of the vessels. He based his conclusions on three cases reported by others, in none of which was a thrombus seen at autopsy. However, a lesion of this kind may well have been missed. He admitted that in one of the cases the local pressure of the intracranial aneurysm may have been responsible; this compression would, of course, act precisely like an intravascular occlusion from a thrombus, and the end result would therefore be essentially the same.

Schorstein failed to differentiate between the immediate and late sequelae of carotid ligations. The former, occurring within the first six or eight hours, are unquestionably due to anoxemia, but after this period, in which the cerebral circulation has been tested and proved adequate, subsequent disturbances of the brain can be due only to intracranial occlusions from thrombi or emboli.

PREVENTION OF THROMBI AND EMBOLI IN CLEAN WOUNDS

From a long and carefully studied series of vascular occlusions, Dr. Halsted [24] concluded that injury to the intima was responsible for the development of intravascular thrombi. This view has since been amply supported by experimental and clinical data. A silk ligature applied tightly enough to obliterate a large artery always cuts the intima and the media, and this wound is the starting point for the thrombus. Doubtless the diminished pressure and flow within an occluded large artery is also an important item in thrombus formation. This was long ago stressed by Virchow and later by Senn [25] and by Perthes. A retarded circulation is doubtless also an important factor in the formation of venous thrombi and subsequent pulmonary emboli.

Realizing the importance of intimal injury from ligatures as the cause of late cerebral complication, Perthes suggested two methods of obliterating the artery by which the intima would not be injured: (1) by tying the artery with a band of fascia lata (using a knot) and (2) by tying the artery around an interposed bar of fascia lying on one side of the artery. Kerr improved this procedure by suturing the fascia (for partial occlusion). In recent cases I have placed a band of fascia around the carotid for either partial or complete occlusions; in the former the artery is subsequently tied with silk around the band of fascia, and in the latter the silk ligature is applied over the fascia to make the total ligation initially. I feel certain that had this been done in my single case of late cerebral complication and death, the disaster would not have occurred.

CLIPPING THE CAROTID INTRACRANIALLY

Clipping the carotid intracranially has become a frequently used procedure in the treatment of certain intracranial aneurysms, both arterial and arteriovenous, and is occasionally necessary with tumors in the region of the cavernous sinus and the gasserian ganglion. The clip is placed astraddle the artery and closed by light compression. Except for a death from rupture of an oversized arteriosclerotic artery when applying an undersized clip there were no fatalities. The only cerebral complication was an immediate one which occurred when the artery was closed despite a preoperative warning by the Matas test that the collateral circulation was inadequate (pressure on the carotid was tolerated only five minutes). Such developments as these would now be better handled and the sequelae avoided. I have had occasion to reexpose at operation two clips, each after a period of several months, and in neither of the cases was there any thrombus formation on the cardiac side of the clip, the carotid being normally full and compressible about the clip. And in no case was there any late cerebral complications. It therefore appears to be an ideal method of occluding the internal carotid intracranially. And because the intracranial division of the internal carotid is so much smaller than the cervical portion (perhaps five times as small), I feel more secure against thrombus formation when it is clipped intracranially than when the artery is ligated in the neck. When both intracranial and cervical ligations are indicated, I therefore prefer to do the intracranial one first. Certainly the possibility of a propagating thrombus is less with a small artery than with a large one.

SUMMARY AND CONCLUSIONS

Eighty-eight partial and total ligations of the internal carotid artery are included in this report. Death occurred in four cases (a mortality rate of 4.5 per cent); immediate cerebral complications were present in 1 case (1.1 per cent), and late complications were present in four cases (4.5 per cent). By evaluating and avoiding the causes and the sequelae the subsequent results should be improved.

The Matas test, which demonstrates the efficiency or nonefficiency of the collateral cerebral circulation, is all important in avoiding disaster following immediate total ligation of this vessel.

After partial ligation of this vessel (with fascial bands) a later total occlusion can be safely performed in one to two weeks, or even less.

The great danger in partial occlusion is in obliterating the lumen too far. If cerebral signs develop during the succeeding six or eight hours, the band can be removed, and at times the cerebral circulation will be restored.

For total ligation of this vessel an interposed fascial band is probably the best assurance against thrombosis and the resulting late cerebral complications.

Clipping the internal carotid artery intracranially is relatively safe and easy and is essential in treating many intracranial aneurysms.

REFERENCES

[1]Pilz, C.: Zur Ligatur der Arteria carotis communis, nebst einer Statistik dieser Operation. *Arch. klin., 9*:257, 1886.

[2]Lefort: A. carotis, in Archambault; Arnould, J.; Axenfeld; Baillarger, and others: *Dictionnaire encyclopedique des sciences medicales, Paris. 12*:621, 1879.

[3]Wyeth, J. A.: *Essays on the Surgery and Surgical Anatomy of the Great Vessels of the Neck.* New York, William Wood & Company, 1879.

[4]Ballance, C. A., and Edmunds, W.: *A Treatise on the Ligation of the Great Arteries in Continuity.* London, Macmillan & Co., 1891.

[5]Zimmermann, W.: Ueber rie Gehirnerweichung nach Unterbindung der Carotis communis. *Beitr. klin. Chir., 8*:364, 1891.

[6]Siegrist, A.: Die Gefahren der Ligatur der grossen Halsschlagadern fur das Auge und das Leben des Menschen. *Arch. Ophth., 1*:511, 1900.

[7]Cauchoix, cited by Niedner, F.: Ueber die Unterbindung der Arteria carotis. *Beitr. klin. Chir., 171*:524, 1941.

[8]Walcker, F.: Einige neue Wege zur Vorbestimmung der moglichen Komplikationen nach der Unterbindung der A. carotis communis. *Arch. klin. Chir., 130*:736, 1924.

[9]Matas, R.: Classified Summary of Six Hundred and Twenty Operations upon the Blood Vessels, Performed for All Causes. *Tr. Am. S. A., 58*:335, 1940.

[10]Watson, W. L., and Silverstone, S. M.: Ligature of the Common Carotid Artery in Cancer of the Head and Neck. *Ann. Surg., 109*:1, 1939.

[11]Matas, R.: Testing the Efficiency of the Collateral Circulation as a Preliminary to the Occlusion of the Great Surgical Arteries. *J.A.M.A., 63*:1441 (Oct. 24) 1914.

[12]Halsted, W. S.: Partial, Progressive and Complete Occlusion of the Aorta and Other Large Arteries in the Dog by Means of the Metal Band. *J. Exper. Med., 15*:373, 1909.

[13]Perthes: Ueber die Ursache der Hirnstorungen nach Karotisunterbindung und uber Arterienunterbindung ohne Schadigung der Intima. *Arch. klin. Chir., 114*:403, 1920.

[14]Freeman, L.: The Causation and Avoidance of Cerebral Complications in Ligation of the Common Carotid Artery. *Ann. Surg., 74*:316, 1921.

[15]Kerr, H. H.: Fractional Ligation of the Common Carotid Artery in the Treatment of Pulsating Exophthalmos. *Surg., Gynec. & Obst., 46*:565, 1925.

[16]Pearse, H. E.: Experimental Studies on the Gradual Occlusion of Large Arteries. *Tr. Am. S. A., 58*:443, 1940.

[16]Pearse, H. E.: Experimental Studies on the Gradual Occlusion of Large Arteries. *Tr. Am. S. A., 58*:443, 1940.

[17]Moses, H.: Hirnstorungen nach Carotisunterbindung. *Zentralbl. Chir., 9*:321, 1921.

[18]Stierlin and Meyerberg: Die fortschreitende Thrombose und Embolie im Gebiet der Carotis interna nach Contusion und Unterbindung.

*Deutsche Ztschr. Chir., 142:*1, 1920.

[19]Esmarch, F.: Embolische Apoplexia durch Losung von Fibringerinnseln aus einen Aneurysma der Carotis. *Virchows Arch. path. Anat., 11:*410, 1857.

[20]Dandy, W. E.: Carotid-Cavernous Aneurysms (Pulsating Exophthalmos). *Zentralbl. Neurochir., 2:*77, 1937.

[21]Pettermann: Unterbindung der A. carotis interna. *Zentralbl. Chir., 59:*3073, 1932.

[22]Fetterman, J. L., and Pritchard, W. H.: Cerebral Complications Following Ligation of the Carotid Artery. *J.A.M.A., 112:*1317 (April 8) 1939.

[23]Schorstein, J.: Carotid Ligation in Saccular Intracranial Aneurysms. *Brit. J. Surg., 28:*50, 1940.

[24]Halsted, W. S.: *The Effect on the Walls of Blood Vessels of Partially and Completely Occluding Bands.* Baltimore, Johns Hopkins Press, 1924, p. 585.

[25]Senn, N.: Cicatrization of Blood-Vessels After Ligature. *Tr. Am. S. A., 2:*249, 1885.

LXXII

NEWER ASPECTS OF RUPTURED INTERVERTEBRAL DISKS*†

Inspection of the spinal column explains the cause of defective lumbar intervertebral disks, their frequency and the fact that they are nearly always multiple or potentially multiple. The key to these disclosures lies in the lateral facets of articulation between the vertebrae. The first and second lumbar articulations parallel the spinous processes and prevent not only lateral but little forward, backward or side motion. At the third lumbar articulation the lateral articulations usually, but not always, begin to turn outward from the horizontal plane, and as far as 25°. The fourth articulation turns laterally to as much as 45°, and the fifth may reach 90°. Doubtless the purpose of the directional shift in the facets is to provide movement and flexibility of the spinal column, but at the same time it creates a potential weakness in the spinal column. There are many variations at all of these points and much asymmetry between the two sides but this tendency is always present. In addition, some of the facets are round, others oval; some concave and convex, others flat. These differences account for further weakness at these points.

The sequence of events in low back pain and sciatica is, I think, as follows: (1) A sudden, severe lift, or twist, tears the capsule at the lateral articulations, and loosens the joints. (2) These loose joints automatically throw an additional strain on the intervertebral cartilages, which is the third component in the articulations between the vertebrae. (3) The result of this sustained trauma is an injured disk which protrudes and impinges upon the emerging spinal nerve lying immediately in contact with the intervertebral disk.

Since the three articular facets of the three lower vertebrae participate in the anatomic variation, the high incidence of multiple disks is to be expected and actively obtains in practically all cases. In at least 5 per cent of the cases three disks are present at the time of operation, or will subsequently develop. Without a proper appreciation of multiple disks, any operative treatment will be ineffectual. This is one of the principal reasons for the disappointing results in the past.

TEST FOR MOBILE JOINTS

When the articular facets become loose the whole vertebral junction is similarly affected. The abnormal mobility can be determined at operation by pushing a spinous process in the horizontal direction. And, conversely, if this test shows mobility there are defective articular facets and at the same time a defective disk. This test is, I think, absolute with one exception, *i.e.*, when the roentgenogram shows a reduced interspace; a fusion or partial fusion has then occurred and this may or may not reduce or entirely eliminate the movement, the result depending upon the duration and degree of fusion. This is nature's attempt at curing a disk—the contents of the disk having gradually absorbed over a period of many years, but the protrusion may remain and compress the nerve.

TREATMENT

Nature's method of absorbing a disk is the key to the proposed surgical treatment, *i.e.*, complete or essentially complete removal of the affected disks. This is done

*Reprinted from the *Annals of Surgery*, 119:4, April, 1944.

†Read before the Southern Surgical Association, December 7–9, 1943, New Orleans, La.

by thoroughly curetting the interior of the disk, extracting its contents and at the same time removing the protruding portion. The end-result is fusion of the entire vertebral surfaces. There have now been 30 cases in which at an earlier period a single disk has been removed and return of symptoms necessitated reopening the wound for a second disk; after six months the vertebrae at the site of the first operation are absolutely fixed when the disk has been completely removed. Unless a disk is thoroughly removed (*i.e.,* if only the protruding sequestrum of cartilage is extracted) the surfaces will not fuse, the joint remains mobile and it is more than probable that a new protrusion (recurrence) will form. The end-result of a cured disk is, therefore, firm fusion of the apposing surfaces of the vertebrae. Furthermore, by this treatment, when properly done, a cure must result and if the pain returns another disk must be the cause.

IDENTIFICATION OF DISKS

There are varying degrees of protrusion of disks; the smaller ones, that would not show with contrast media in the spinal canal, I have termed "concealed" disks, and these are two-thirds to three-quarters of the total number. Some of these bulge only slightly, but they fluctuate and in most instances are bound to the surrounding epidural tissues by adhesions which indicate that they must have protruded more than appears at operation. It might well be asked whether some of these are really abnormal. I am not sure. At necropsy much the same appearance has been found but without adhesions, *i,e.,* they protrude slightly and fluctuate. Of this I am certain, if there is abnormal mobility of the joint, removal of the disk is the only method of obtaining successful treatment, and it will be successful. With periodic backaches there is always a loose joint and this is almost the only cause of such backaches. Moreover, there is no difference, except in the degree of sciatica, between the cases having protrusions and those with the concealed disks.

It is natural to ask why fusions by autogenous grafts to the lumbar spine will not accomplish the same result. The answer is that with a graft fusion the protruding disk is merely covered up and continues to cause sciatica. And in several cases that have been fused the backache persists as well as the sciatica because of the defective disk. There can be no fusion so complete and effective as that obtained by denuding the broad surfaces of the vertebrae. Moreover, fusion by removing the disks is simple and requires but a week or ten days in the hospital. A spinal graft is a big performance and requires a plaster encasement for six weeks and a prolonged stay in the hospital, and will not produce a cure.

DIAGNOSIS AND LOCALIZATION OF THE DISKS

Neither the diagnosis nor the localization of disks require intraspinal injections. They miss over two-thirds of the disks (concealed disks) and the history alone is almost pathognomonic, *i.e.,* periodic attacks of low backache plus sciatica, both usually (but not always) made worse by coughing and sneezing (because of the mobility of the joint). The *localization* of the defective disk or disks (mobile joints may be preferable) is perfectly simple and certain by the mobility test* described above. The only possibility of error in diagnosis is a spinal cord tumor. These occur in a little less than one per cent of the cases. This is, indeed, a difficult and often impossible differential diagnosis to make solely from routine examinations, but is no excuse for subjecting the 99 per cent to intraspinal injections. If the diagnosis is suspected a lumbar puncture alone is indicated—the fluid will be xanthochromic if a tumor is present; there may or may not be a positive Quecken-

---

*This test was shown to me by Dr. Ray E. Lenhard when demonstrating a congenitally defective lumbar vertebra. It was then tried on the disk cases and found to be all-important.

stedt test. I have missed five tumors in the series of 900 disks—700 patients.

Recently we have treated 15 cases of backache without sciatica, six with congenitally defective lumbar vertebrae, and ten with spondylolisthesis, by the same procedure, *i.e.,* removal of the intervertebral disks to produce vertebral fusion. The results in backache without sciatica are precisely the same as those with sciatica. Sufficient time has not elapsed to determine the results in the defective vertebrae and spondylolisthesis.

Before concluding I should like to call attention to a medical classic that I have never seen mentioned, namely, that of Goldthwaite, of Boston, published in 1911. The anatomic weakness of the spinal column to which I have alluded has long been known to orthopedists and has been considered by them to be the potential source of low back pain and sciatica. Indeed Ghormley has very aptly called it the "facet syndrome" which is probably responsible for the backache. But Goldth-waite not only described the anatomic variation of the three lumbar facets and ascribed to them the low backache, but he postulated the development of ruptured intervertebral disks upon the same basis, and this was eighteen years before the first disk was found at operation. This remarkable anticipation of ruptured disks and their cause was made from careful studies in the anatomical laboratory and was prompted by a negative surgical exploration in one of his patients whose symptoms he always maintained could only be caused by a ruptured intervertebral disk.

REFERENCES

[1]Goldthwaite, J. E.: The Lumbosacral Articulation. *Boston Med. & Surg. J., 164:*365, 1911.

[2]Ghormley, R. K.: Low Back Pain, with Special Reference to the Articular Facets: Presentation of the Operative Procedure. *J.A.M.A., 101:*1773, 1933.

[3]Dandy, W. E.: Loose Cartilage from Intervertebral Disk Simulating Tumor of the Spinal Cord. *Arch. Surg., 19:*660, 1929.

LXXIII

PATHOGENESIS OF INTERMITTENT EXOPHTHALMOS*

Frank B. Walsh, M.D., and Walter E. Dandy, M.D.

Intermittent exophthalmos is a rare, but striking and unmistakable, syndrome. It is characterized by pronounced and rapid—almost instantaneous—protrusion of one eye when venous stasis is induced by bending the head forward; by lowering the head; by turning the head forcibly; by hyperextension of the neck; by coughing; by forced expiration, with or without compression of the nostrils, and by pressure on the jugular veins. The ocular protrusion disappears immediately when the head is erect and when artificially induced venous congestion is relieved.

Usually, but not invariably, there is enophthalmos when venous congestion does not obtain. There may or apparently may not (to judge from cases reported in the literature) be pulsation of the eyeball. Vision may or may not be affected. The condition is progressive and may be productive of unbearable pain and troublesome diplopia. The appearance is unsightly, but life is not at stake.

The case here reported—the only one we have seen—is presented because the pathologic features were disclosed at operation. Most previous reports of cases are mainly clinical presentations, and the clinical study is not followed by detection of the underlying lesion. Orbital operations have been performed in a few cases, and venous beds have been described in the orbit. These may or may not represent the whole pathologic picture. No postmortem examinations have been made.

*Reprinted from the *Archives of Ophthalmology* 32:1–10, June, 1944.

Report of a Case

A white girl aged eighteen was referred by Dr. Milton Little, of Hartford, Conn., with the complaint of bulging of the left eye induced by posture and associated with pain in the head.

The family and past histories were without significance.

PRESENT ILLNESS. From the age of ten years the patient had known that her left eye was sometimes more prominent and at other times less prominent than her right eye. When she sat erect or stood, the left eye became sunken. When she lay down, it bulged. When she became excited, it protruded. For six months, every morning on awakening, there had been a throbbing pain in the eye, which disappeared soon after she got up. The pain disappeared after rest in bed for a week, but on resumption of her usual activities it soon returned. For a week there had been severe pain in the left eye and the left temple. The throbs were noted to occur at the same rate as the heart beat. From the age of ten years there had been occasional periods when diplopia was present, but strabismus or ptosis had not been observed.

EXAMINATION. When the patient stood, there was striking enophthalmos. Immediately after she lay down, the eye commenced to protrude, and pronounced exophthalmos persisted throughout the recumbent period. Moreover, the eyeball pulsated; this was visible and palpable. When she leaned forward (head down) the exophthalmos became extreme. This was also true when the jugular veins were compressed or when she blew her nose. The exophthalmos was also increased when the common carotid artery was compressed (because the internal jugular vein was then also compressed), but the pulsation ceased. There was no audible bruit.

There were weakness of the left external and inferior rectus muscles and absence of ptosis when the patient was sitting erect. When the eye was protruded as a result of change of position of the head, ptosis appeared. Measurements were made with the Hertel exophthalmometer. There was enophthalmos of 3 mm. when the head was erect (in the sitting or standing position the measurement for the right eye was 15 mm. and for the left eye 12 mm.) There was exophthalmos of the left eye: 6 mm. when she was lying recumbent; 11 mm. when the head was turned forcibly to the jugular vein was compressed; 18 mm. when expiration was forced and the nostrils were compressed (patient standing; 5 mm. when the head was tilted forward or the left, and 3 mm. when it was turned to the right. Visual acuity was 20/15 in the right eye and 20/30 in the left eye (with the patient sitting upright). The left pupil dilated slightly when the eyeball protruded. The eyegrounds were normal except for slight overfilling of the retinal veins of the left eye when that eye was maximally protruded.

Roentgenograms showed thickening of the superior margin of the left orbit, which was increased in density, as was the left wing of the sphenoid. The sphenoid fissure was widened. A small, diffuse area of calcification was visible in the outer orbit.

DIAGNOSIS. 1. The quick protrusion and sinking of the eyeball with the postural changes, and the rapid protrusion induced by coughing, sneezing and jugular compression could only mean filling of a large venous bed.

2. The pulsation of the eyeball indicated an arterial component. The lesion, therefore, had to be an arteriovenous aneurysm.

3. The absence of a murmur indicated that the communication between arteries and veins was through vascular "coils," and not through a fistula.

4. The enophthalmos (with the patient sitting or standing) was thought to be due to atrophy of the orbital fat from long-continued pressure.

5. The most puzzling point was the absence of exophthalmos when the patient was erect. Coiled vessels could be expected to produce a space-occupying mass in the orbit. The explanation of this was obtained at operation. The coils making a space-occupying mass were in the cranial chamber, and not in the orbit.

OPERATION (W.E.D.). On July 24, 1943, a frontotemporal approach to the cranial chamber was made—a typical hypophysial approach. When the dura was turned back, a finger-like projection of vascular coils was observed extending from the region of the pterion backward and mesially, and finally paralleling the sylvian vein. A few minor vascular attachments to the brain were thrombosed with the electrocautery, after which the brain was free of attachment to the dura. The cerebral vessels were unaffected and of normal size. In the region of the sphenoid fissure and the anterior part of the middle fossa was a mass of coiled vessels; this overflowed the sphenoid wing and extended a short distance over the orbital plate (about 1 cm.) as a thin, pink film (of arterial blood), which blanched with slight pressure. The mass was intimately grown into, and was inseparable from, the dura and was made up of intertwining coils of vessels, easily compressible, like a sponge, and immediately returning to the original size when pressure was released. The vascular mass was repeatedly attacked by the electrocautery, and the volume gradually shrank until the scar was flush with the sphenoid fissure.

From time to time the cautery cut through the vessels, and brisk arterial bleeding occurred. The bleeding areas were covered with pieces of muscle, and the coagulation was carried out through them. The sphenoid fissure was greatly widened and filled with the vascular coils, but no attempt was made to carry the cauterization forward into the orbit, there being no reason to believe that a mass was located therein. Because of diffuse bleeding, the middle meningeal artery was isolated and coagulated at the foramen spinosum. It was our impression that the arterial component of the arteriovenous aneurysm arose from this vessel because of its intimate relation to the coiled mass and because no other large artery was nearby. The intracranial division of the internal carotid artery was distant and was entirely normal. The optic nerve was in full view, was not implicated and was not injured at any time. The aneurysmal mass completely covered the dura over the gasserian ganglion and the cavernous sinus. It could not be determined whether or not these were communications with the latter. That there were no communications with the internal carotid artery in the cavernous sinus cannot be stated dogmatically, but this could be possible only through an anomalous branch. It was realized throughout the operation that the nerves to the extraocular muscles lying in the cavernous sinus and the sphenoid fissure were passing through the vascular mass that was being coagulated, and that their injury, or even destruction, was a distinct possibility. However, the cure of the aneurysm was thought to be advisable in view of the progressively increasing pain.

POSTOPERATIVE COURSE. Immediately after operation the eyeball was free of all the intermittent changes that previously obtained with posture, blowing the nose, jugular compression, etc. However, vision was entirely lost in the left eye, and all the extraocular muscles were paralyzed. The pupil did not respond directly or consensually to stimulation with light. Three months later the intermittent exophthalmos remained cured, but the extraocular paralyses persisted in part. The pupil exhibited a consensual reaction. There was enophthalmos of 3 mm. The upper lid could be elevated incompletely, and internal and downward rotation of the eyeball had improved to about half-normal. The price of a cure was therefore high, but the patient is happy over the end result. We have wondered whether it would have been practical and preferable to have attempted ligation of the orbital veins in the orbit (through the same transcranial approach) and to have left the aneurysm untouched. The practicability of this procedure is uncertain, but even if the operation had been successful, the pulsation of the eyeball would have persisted.

NOTE. The patient was seen again ten months after discharge from the hospital. There had been no discomfort except on one occasion, three weeks before reexamination, when she had a severe pain in the head. She stated that at this time there was some protrusion of the left eye.

Examination revealed incomplete ptosis and inward deviation of the eye of about 30 degrees. She was unable to elevate the left eye but could lower it 20 to 30 degrees. The eye was blind and the nerve atrophic. There was enophthalmos of the left eye, which was not influenced by such factors as position and pressure on the jugular vein.

Symptomatology and Brief Review of Literature

Intermittent exophthalmos has been re-cognized as a clinical entity since 1805, when it was first described in an infant. In a classic paper, Birch-Hirschfeld reviewed the literature up to 1906 and presented observations of prime importance concerning not only the intermittent exophthalmos but the anteroposterior position of the normal eye in relation to various positions of the head. He described the syndrome in a physician, Dr. Minor, who also wrote regarding it. Wissmann and Schulz (1922) added a single case and collected the cases appearing between 1906 and 1922, a total of seventy-four. Kraupa and Mendl (1936) described a case and brought the number reported in the literature to ninety-six cases. They rejected two cases included by Wissmann and Schulz.

The following reports of cases of intermittent exophthalmos have been found since Kraupa and Mendl's publication, and the list also includes two cases not mentioned by them: Bartok (1931), Chapman (1931), de-Petri (1935), Marchesini (1935), Hippert (1936), Muirhead (1936), Lipovich (1936), Petrov (1939), Spektor (1939), Giqueaux (1942), Poole (1942), Dunphy (1942) and Rones (1942). The cases reported by the two last-named authors were mentioned in the discussion on Poole's paper. Rychener (1942) and Ellett (1940) made subsequent reports on Chapman's case. These, with our case, bring the total number of cases to one hundred and eleven.

From the clinical viewpoint little has been added since Birch-Hirschfeld's comprehensive review.

OCCURRENCE. As the foregoing figures indicate, true intermittent exophthalmos is rare. Birch-Hirschfeld saw a single case among 150,000 patients with ophthalmic disease, and de Schweinitz, one case among 100,000 such patients; the case described here is the only one of the condition recorded at the Johns Hopkins Hospital. Krauss, Hippert and Weisner each encountered two cases. In the United States and Canada, the condition has been described by Sattler, de Schweinitz, Byers,

Chapman, Ellett, Poole, Dunphy, Rychener and Rones.

SEX. Possibly more men than women are victims of this condition. Birch-Hirschfeld's series contained thirty-five men and fifteen women. In Kraupa and Mendl's series ten patients were males and eight females.

TRAUMA. Trauma has been suggested as a factor in the development of intermittent exophthalmos, but it is difficult to believe it can play more than a precipitating role. The patient described by Rumjanzewa was first observed to exhibit the syndrome during childbirth.

AGE OF ONSET. Since persons with intermittent exophthalmos may be wholly unaware of its existence until it has been pointed out to them, it is impossible to obtain accurate information regarding the age of onset. The condition has been seen in infants, and it has been observed for the first time during the sixth decade of life (Birch-Hirschfeld). Sattler expressed the opinion that it occurred in young persons almost, or quite, exclusively, but there is ample evidence that this concept is erroneous. Birch-Hirschfeld found records of six cases occurring in the first decade of life, seven in the second, eight in the third, one in the fourth, two in the fifth and one in the sixth. Of cases reported since 1935, three have occurred in the second decade of life, four in the third, five in the fourth and two in the fifth.

UNILATERALITY. In all reported cases the condition has been unilateral. Poole commented that the left eye is involved ten times as often as the right. This high ratio is not upheld by Birch-Hirschfeld's compilations, although he stated that the left eye was affected more often than the right. Kraupa and Mendl found the right eye affected in ten cases and the left eye in eight cases. In the thirteen cases described since 1935, the left eye was always affected. Excellent accounts of intermittent exophthalmos of the right eye have been given by Byers and Rumjanzewa.

It is natural that attempts have been made to explain the predominance of involvement of the left eye. Reese suggested that the jugular foramen on the left side is frequently smaller than that on the right, but this structure is remote from the lesion producing the venous changes and can have no bearing on its causation. There is no apparent reason that a congenital lesion, such as that causing this condition, should favor one side.

THE EXOPHTHALMOS ITS DIRECTION AND DEGREE. The complete syndrome of alternating exophthalmos and enophthalmos usually develops gradually and progressively. Radswitzki described a case of exophthalmos which occurred only as a result of severe coughing or vomiting up to the age of fourteen years, but thereafter a change in position of the head, holding the breath, etc., was sufficient to induce the condition, which rapidly disappeared when the head resumed the erect position. Mulder described the case of a man who until the age of twelve years exhibited intermittent exophthalmos only when he wore a tight collar but later presented the complete syndrome. Mention has already been made of Rumjanzewa's case, in which the anomaly developed during the strains of childbirth.

The eye may be protruded either directly forward or downward and outward. In a majority of reported cases mention is made only of direct protrusion. According to Birch-Hirschfeld, the superior ophthalmic vein is usually larger than the inferior ophthalmic and, consequently, the eye is usually pushed downward and outward, as well as forward. The position of the eyeball is doubtless dependent on the symmetry or asymmetry of the venous bed in the orbit.

Narrowing of the palpebral fissure during the episodes of exophthalmos was observed in Poole's and Rumjanzewa's cases and in our case. During the stage of enophthalmos the palpebral fissures on the two sides were quite, or almost, equal in width. Probably Dunphy's suggestion that during exophthalmos there may be voluntary or reflex closure of the lids as a protective measure is correct.

The amount of proptosis has been noted to vary within wide limits in different cases. Sattler and de Vincentiis observed 25 and 29 mm. respectively in their cases when the head was bent forward. In our case, 18 mm. of relative exophthalmos was observed when the patient exhaled forcibly with the nostrils compressed, but this did not represent what could have been obtained, since it was thought unwise to attain the maximum. It may be remarked that measurements of exophthalmos as usually made are only approximate; special photographic apparatus, such as that described by Birch-Hirschfeld, is necessary for accuracy.

The time required for proptosis to begin is not stated in most reported cases. Birch-Hirschfeld observed a latent period of five seconds, followed by protrusion of the eye, which reached almost its maximum in thirty seconds and its full maximum in another fifteen seconds. His patients had the head bent forward. He commented that the latent period had been stated as being from one to five minutes but that it rarely, if ever, is as long.

FACTORS INFLUENCING EXOPHTHALMOS. Often, as in our case, the condition has first been observed by a friend. Birch-Hirschfeld observed protrusion of the normal eye when the head was bent forward. This, of course, is due to gravity and is intensified when an abnormal venous bed exists.

Proptosis can be produced in most instances by pressure over the jugular vein on the side of the intermittent exophthalmos. In our case this produced about as much proptosis as did bending the head forward. Occasionally, as in Lindenmeyer's case, pressure over the contralateral vein produced proptosis when similar pressure over the homolateral jugular vein failed to do so. In such instances, either there is great congenital narrowing or absence of the homolateral jugular vein, or it has become thrombosed.

The position of the head in lateral rotation has been found to influence the position of the eye, owing to a degree of jugular constriction. Mann observed that rotation of the head to the right produced maximal venous drainage through the left jugular vein, and, conversely, rotation of the head to the left produced maximal venous drainage through the right jugular vein. In our case forcible turning of the head produced exophthalmos of the affected eye, which was more pronounced when the head was turned to the left. In Poole's photographs the effect is most striking.

Birch-Hirschfeld surmised that any obstruction to the anterior venous pathways outside the orbit resulted in additional pressure in the ophthalmic veins, and, to prove it, he devised an ingenious experiment by which the extra-orbital veins were compressed. This, however, could have no bearing on the intermittency of the exophthalmos. Krauss assumed that large congenital varicosities in the orbit might cause intermittent exophthalmos. He also assumed that an obstruction to the drainage of orbital blood, either anteriorly, as suggested by Birch-Hirschfeld, or posteriorly, could produce intermittent exophthalmos. Both these observers commented on the narrowness of the ophthalmic vein just before it enters the cavernous sinus, and Krauss remarked on there being a pronounced constriction of the superior ophthalmic vein where it lies close to the tendon of the superior oblique muscle. However, an obstruction to the veins is the one thing that cannot explain this condition; the prompt appearance of proptosis with jugular compression means that there is no obstruction in the venous channels. All textbooks are in agreement that there are no valves along the ophthalmic vein. There could not, of course, be any effective valves in intermittent exophthalmos because pressure on the juguar veins immediately produces the ocular protrusion.

ENOPHTHALMOS. Enophthalmos is not essential to the diagnosis, but it is usually present. It can only be due to absorption of orbital fat from pressure of the vascular bed (probably venous) in the orbit. Enophthalmos, when present, is apparent only when the head is in the erect position.

LIDS, TEMPORAL REGION AND FACE. It might well be expected that there would be some engorgement, or at least prominence, of the veins of the eyelids, temple and face on the side of the anomaly, since they are in communication with the orbital veins. However, this is only occasionally observed and was not present in our case. Some swelling of the lids may be observed when the eye is proptosed. The temporal region was engorged during proptosis in Marchesini's case, and the homolateral side of the face was swollen in Petrov's case. In Rumjanzewa's case there was flushing of the side of the face when the eye was protruded.

In no instance, so far as we are aware, has there been great dilatation of veins over the face and lids or over the scalp, as is so commonly observed in cases of carotid-cavernous fistula and pronounced cirsoid aneurysm.

FACIAL ASYMMETRY. In several instances retardation of growth of the homolateral side of the face has been described, but Birch-Hirschfeld concluded that this was not of particular significance because of the relative frequency of asymmetry of the face in otherwise normal persons. There can be no local reason for asymmetry of the face.

THE AFFECTED EYE. It is obvious from consideration of reported cases that the involved eye in a great majority of instances remains normal. When the eye is proptosed and remains so for a considerable time, there may be congestion of the bulbar conjunctiva. In a relatively small number of the reported cases some degree of optic nerve atrophy (14 per cent, Birch-Hirschfeld) has been present. In our case vision was slightly reduced −20/30. Birch-Hirschfeld assumed that optic nerve atrophy was due to retrobulbar hemorrhage, which is said to be, and doubtless is, an occasional complication. However, a more reasonable assumption in a majority of such cases would appear to be long-sustained direct pressure of the mass on the optic nerve.

Visual acuity may be lowered materially during the exophthalmic phase. Extreme overfilling of the retinal veins has been noted during the period of exophthalmos, and they may pulsate; but the fundus remains otherwise unchanged. Diplopia, present occasionally in our case, is not usually mentioned. Usually there is no limitation of ocular movements. The pupil remains unchanged in many cases, but pupillary dilation during exophthalmos has been described by several observers listed by Birch-Hirschfeld and was present in our case. Rumjanzewa described narrowing of the pupil during periods of exophthalmos in her case.

PULSATION OF THE EYEBALL. According to Birch-Hirschfeld, this symptom is rarely present in cases of intermittent exophthalmos. Mention of it was made in only seven of seventy-four cases included in his study and in that of Wissmann and Schulz. The symptom was present in our case and was most pronounced during maximum exophthalmos. It is entirely possible that the pulsation was overlooked in some of the reported cases in which it was not mentioned. However, in many cases special mention has been made of the absence of pulsation, and there can hardly be a doubt that it is not always present. In only one instance has a subjective murmur or objective bruit been noted. In Delord and Viallefont's case a blowing sound was heard on auscultation. Poole's patient described roaring and tinnitus. Neither was present in our case despite the known arteriovenous communication.

OTHER SYMPTOMS. In many cases the condition is asymptomatic; but pain may be the only symptom, and it may become steadily more severe. Since pain is associated with protrusion of the eye, it may be present most of the time. A sensation of fulness in the side of the face is frequently noted. In Poole's case the pain became so severe that the patient could not continue his work. Often there is complaint of dizziness and vertigo, usually not severe and occurring only during periods of exophthalmos. Birch-Hirschfeld, in a short discussion (1930), suggested that intracranial varices possibly account for these symptoms. Hippert expressed the opinion that venous anomalies influenced the vestibular apparatus in his case.

ROENTGENOGRAMS. Roentgenographic evidence has usually been reported as negative. Hippert noted a single small calcification in the sphenoid fissure, but there was a similar one on the other side. Kraupa and Mendl reported small calcifications, which they termed phleboliths, in two cases. Gastreich saw seven or eight rounded and slightly oval, smooth, pea-sized shadows. Lyding reported twelve such shadows in the orbit in his case. Such shadows are well known to occur in the defective walls of cerebral vascular beds, such as arteriovenous aneurysms in the cranial and orbital cavities, and doubtless these calcifications are of similar origin. In our case there were two calcified plaques in the outer orbit.

TREATMENT AND PATHOLOGIC FEATURES. Rychener (1942) observed improvement in a case reported by Chapman (1931) and later by Ellett (1940).

The injection of sclerosing into the orbital veins has been advocated by several authors: Hippert noted successful results in 4 cases; Ravardino reported a success, but Dunphy, a failure.

The first operative attack on the large veins of the orbit for intermittent exophthalmos was made by Schimanowsky (1907). Through an incision under the eyebrow, he clamped and twisted the large vein, perhaps the superior ophthalmic, in the back of the orbit and allowed the clamp to remain two days before being withdrawn. Cure of the exophthalmos resulted, but with ptosis and ophthalmoplegia; the state of vision was not given. Three years later he operated in another case in similar fashion except that he tied and cut the

veins. Precisely the same result was obtained. Lowenstein (1911), through a modified Kronlein approach, palpated venous tortuosities on the way to the supraorbital vein. Bleeding was severe; it was controlled by the Paquelin cautery, and the wound was packed. During the next few days the exophthalmos was extreme but gradually disappeared by the twelfth day; four days later there was an enophthalmos of 3.5 mm., and this persisted. Slight exophthalmos (1.5 mm.) persisted during jugular compression. The inferior rectus muscle was paralyzed; vision was greatly reduced immediately after operation but returned to 4/10 in four weeks and to 10/10 in nine weeks.

Germain and Weill explored the orbit of a patient who had had a retrobulbar hemorrhage and exhibited pronounced exophthalmos. A large number of dilated veins were observed within the muscle cone. In the attempt to isolate and ligate these veins there was spontaneous hemorrhage. Excision of the veins was performed. The exophthalmos was relieved. Two months later, the eye was enophthalmic, and there was external ophthalmoplegia. The state of vision was not recorded.

The only other case in which operation was done was reported by Rumjanzewa (1930), and a perfect result was obtained. The ophthalmic vein was ligated in the orbit through a supra-orbital incision; the exophthalmos was cured, without extraocular palsies. The author called it Golowin's operation—a method of attack used by him on pulsating exophthalmos.

In none of these records of operations is there any mention of pathologic observations except that the veins were large. The exposure of the orbit is doubtless too restricted to permit definition of any clearcut lesion; on the other hand, there is probably nothing in the orbit except large veins. The operation used in our case, as previously detailed, was a transcranial approach which has been evolved for orbital tumors. Since the lesion was intracranial and of a well recognized type, and since it was obliterated intracranially, there was no indication for removal of the orbital roof to inspect the orbit. This approach revealed the only extraorbital lesion that has been identified with intermittent exophthalmos. Had the orbit been explored by a Kronlein approach, the character of the underlying lesion would not have been disclosed. This arteriovenous aneurysm (not a single fistula, but coils of vessels replacing capillaries, with a larger lumen and of congenital origin) is of exactly the same character as are all arteriovenous aneurysms within the substance of the brain. Several cases of these aneurysms are cited in a paper published by one of us in 1928; one photograph of such aneurysms is included here (Fig. 1).

We do not suggest that the treatment carried out in our case is the best solution of the problem. On the contrary, the result obtained by Rumjanzewa is so much better that in another case we should probably be content to ligate the superior ophthalmic vein and leave the aneurysmal coils alone. The surgical attack is much better, and there is consequently less risk of injuring the extraocular muscles through the transcranial than through either the Kronlein or the frontal approach. The ultimate decision concerning the best type of surgical treatment will, of course, be evolved only after greater experience and after it is known whether lesions of different types may be responsible for this unusual syndrome.

However, there is a serious risk in ligating large veins ahead of an arteriovenous aneurysm. In one of our cases of cerebral aneurysm another nearby vein ruptured. It must be realized that the great venous bed emerging from the arteriovenous coils is made as an adjustment to the entering arterial blood, and reduction in the bed throws a strain on the remaining veins, all of which have relatively weak walls.

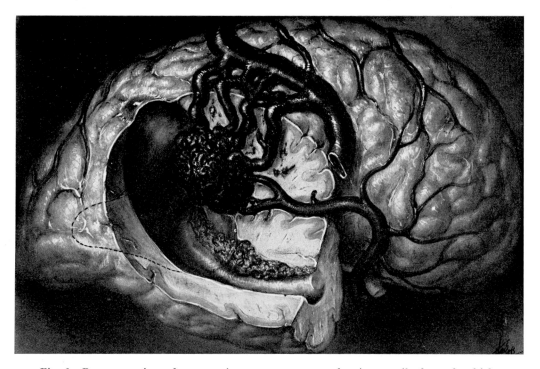

Fig. 1. Reconstruction of an arteriovenous aneurysm, showing a coil of vessels which carry arterial blood and from which the tremendously enlarged veins emerge (from Dandy, 1928, fig. 14). This drawing is shown because it is exactly like the arteriovenous aneurysm described in this paper.

Comment

In our case there could be no preoperative doubt that an arteriovenous aneurysm was causing this syndrome, i.e., in view of the pulsation of the eyeball. Nor could it be doubted that it was a "coiled" rather than a carotid-cavernous aneurysm (a fistula), which gives entirely different signs and symptoms, i.e., a murmur, constant exophthalmos and dilated, pulsating vessels in the conjunctiva and over the forehead. There are never alternating exophthalmos and enophthalmos with a fistula, nor does jugular compression affect the protrusion of the eye. The coexisting enophthalmos was new in our experience but was assumed to be due to atrophy from pressure of the dilated veins. It is noteworthy that the space-occupying mass, i.e., the vascular coils, were almost entirely in the cranial chamber, and not in the orbit. If this mass, as large as a walnut, had been in the orbit, there would have been constant exophthalmos, and never enophthalmos. Only the enlarged veins that drained the aneurysm were in the orbit, and the size of these vessels changed with the volume induced by gravity and other physiologic factors affecting venous pressure largely through the corresponding jugular vein.

A glance at Figure 1 will show the tremendous effect of arterial pressure on the size of the veins emerging from a cerebral arteriovenous aneurysm; the effect on the vein from an orbital or extraorbital aneurysm of similar type will be of precisely the same character.

It is not clear how far the pathologic changes in this case can be applied in all cases of intermittent exophthalmos. In all cases with pulsation of the eyeball there is doubtless just such a causative lesion. But in many, perhaps in the majority, of reported cases the pulsation either was not present (as determined by special mention of its absence) or was missed by the examiner. At least there must always be a large venous bed, but we know of no description of such large venous masses in the orbit. While purely venous aneurysms occur in the brain, they are uncommon, and they are not known to enlarge progressively. A true angioma would not be quickly influenced by changes in jugular pressure but would act simply as a space-occupying mass, producing a constant exophthalmos.

Until there are more pathologic confirmations of the underlying lesions in this condition, a conclusion applicable to all cases is clearly impossible.

It is possible that there are two general types of lesions causing intermittent exophthalmos, (1) arteriovenous with pulsation and (2) venous without pulsation; but speculation on this score is useless. The existence of the arteriovenous type at least is certain; that of the venous type is problematic. It is our guess that ocular pulsation has been overlooked in many cases. It is never so pronounced as in the usual pulsating exophthalmos from a carotid-cavernous fistula.

Arteriovenous aneurysm is, of course, a congenital maldevelopment, and never of traumatic origin. This accounts for its early appearance in most recorded cases. It might be asked why it is not present at birth. The answer is that the sustained arterial blood pressure causes the gradually progressive venous enlargement as the vascular coils with defective walls steadily dilate. The exact time of appearance of the syndrome, therefore, depends on the resistance of these walls, which must have wide individual variations. Doubtless many open in later life.

Conclusions

In a typical case of intermittent exophthalmos the underlyng lesion was observed at operation,—a transcranial approach—to be an intracranial arteriovenous aneurysm lying in and behind the sphenoid fissure. This case is the only one in the literature in which a cause for this rare syndrome has been disclosed. The source of the arterial part of the aneurysm is not certain; it was thought to be the middle meningeal artery.

An arteriovenous aneurysm of similar

type is probably responsible in all cases for pulsation of the eyeball. In most recorded cases pulsation was absent or missed. Whether or not there are two types of this syndrome, one with the other without pulsation, cannot be determined without subsequent pathologic studies. Doubtless, in some cases the pulsation was present but was missed by the observer.

The intermittent exophthalmos was cured by obliterating the aneurysm with the syndrome, one with and the other without electrocautery, but blindness of the affected eye ophthalmoplegia resulted.

REFERENCES

[1]Bartok, I.: Exophthalmos intermittens (case 97), abstracted. *Zentralbl. ges. Ophth.*, 25:225, 1931.

[2]Birch-Hirschfeld, A.: Der intermittirende Exophthalmus, in Graefe, A., and Saemisch, E. T.: *Handbuch der gesamten Augenheilkunde*, Ed. 2. Berlin, Julius Springer, vol. 9, pt. 1, 1917, chap. 13, pp. 105–149.

[3]Intermittierender Exophthalmus (Varix orbitae), in Schieck, F., and Bruckner, A.: *Kurzes Handbuch der Ophthalmologie*. Berlin, Julius Springer, 1930, vol. 3, pp. 16–19.

[4]Byers, W. G. M.: A Case of Intermittent Exophthalmos. *Arch. Ophth.*, 50:569–573, 1921.

[5]Chapman, T. C., cited by Rychener [case 98].

[6]Dandy, W. E.: Arteriovenous Aneurysm of the Brain. *Arch. Surg.*, 17:190–243 (Aug.) 1928.
Orbital Tumors, New York, Oskar Piest, 1941.

[7]Delord, E., and Viallefont, H.: Sur un cas d'exophtalmie intermittente. *Ann. d'ocul.*, 169:730–744, 1932.

[8]De-Petri, M.: Sugli esoftalmi intermittente e pulsante e sulla loro terapia [case 99]. *Riv. otoneurol-oftal.*, 12:306–338, 1935.

[9]de Schweinitz, G. E.: *Diseases of the Eye*. Philadelphia, W. B. Saunders Company, 1942, pp. 681–682.

[10]de Vincentiis, C.: Sull'esottalmo da neoplasia dell' orbita; da ematoma orbitario, pulsante spontaneo e traumatico; di un moncone atrofico per aneurisma dell'arteria oftalmica; su di un oc-.hio congenitamente pulsante. *Atti Accad. med.-chir. di Napoli*, 48:367–464, 1894.

[11]Dunphy, E. B., in discussion on Poole, pp. 116–117, case 109.

[12]Ellett, E. C.: Unilateral Exophthalmos. *Tr. A. M. A., Sect. Ophth.* pp. 50–91, 1940; *J.A.M.A.*, 116: 1–7 (Jan. 4) 1941.

[13]Gastreich, C.: Phlebolithen bei Orbitalvarizen mit intermittierendem Exophthalmus. *Klin. Monatsbl. Augenh.*, 88:773–777, 1932.

[14]Germain, L., and Weill, G.: Les exophthalmies

d'orgine veineuse. *Bull. Soc. d'opht. de Paris*, 9:594–597, 1927.

[15]Giqueaux, R.: Varicocele de la orbita [case 107]. *An. argent. de oftal.*, 3:25–28, 1942.

[16]Hippert, F.: Deux cas d'exophtalmie intermittente: Le varicocele de l'orbite (Exophtalmie intermittente [case 101 and 102], *Arch. d'opht.*, 53:135–146, 1936.

[17]Kraupa, E., and Mendl, K.: Ueber intermittierenden Exophthalmus. *Ztschr. Augenh.*, 89:40–50, 1936.

[18]Krauss, W.: Beitrage zur Anatomie, Physiologie und Pathologie des orbitalen Venensystems: zugleich uber orbital Plethysmographie. *Arch. Augenh.*, 66:163–204 and 285–328, 1910.

[19]Lindenmeyer, O.: Ueber Exophthalmus intermittens. *Klin. Monatsbl. Augenh.*, 68:199–203, 1922.

[20]Lipovich, N.: Abwechselnder Ex- und Enophthalmus [case 104], Sovet. vestnik oftal. 9:710–711, 1936; abstracted. *Zentralbl. ges. Ophth.*, 38: 279–280, 1937.

[21]Lowenstein, A.: Ein Fall von operative geheiltem, sogenannten intermittierenden Exophthalmus. *Klin. Monatsbl. Augenh.*, 49:183–191, 1911.

[22]Lyding, H.: Demonstration eines Falles von Phlebolithen bei intermittierendem Exophthalmus. *Klin. Monatsbl. Augenh.*, 90:245–246, 1933.

[23]Mann: Ueber den Mechanismus der Blutbewegung in der Vena jugularis interna. *Ztschr. Ohrenh.*, 40:354–359, 1901–1902.

[24]Ein neuer Beitrag zur Lehre vom Mechanismus der Blutbewegung in der Vena jugularis interna. *Verhandl. d. deutsch. otol. Gesellsch.*, 13:121–128, 1904.

[25]Marchesini, E.: Su una rara forma di esoftalmo intermittente con atrofia discendente del nervo ottico (Contributo clinico alla diagnosi defferenziale ed alla patogenesi) [case 100]. *Ann. di ottal. e. clin. ocul.*, 63:263–280, 1935.

[26]Muirhead, W. M.: Intermittent Exophthalmos [case 103]. *Tr. Ophth. Soc. U. Kingdom*, 56: 304, 1936.

[27]Mulder, M. E.: Ueber intermittierenden Exophthalmus mit Pulsation des Auges. *Klin. Monatsbl. Augenh.* 38:3–13, 1900.

[28]Petrov, A. A.: Ein Fall von einseitigem intermittierendem Exophthalmus [case 105] Vestnik oftal. 14:76–77, 1939; abstracted. *Zentralbl. ges. Ophth.*, 44:674, 1939–1940.

[29]Poole, W. A.: Intermittent Exophthalmos: Case Report [case 108]. *Tr. Am. Acad. Ophth.*, 112–118, 1942.

[30]Radswitzki, P. I.: Ein Fall von Enophthalmus mit intermittirenden Exophthalmus. *Med. obozr.*, 47:726–732, 1897; abstracted, *Centralbl. Augenh.*, 1897, p. 642.

[31]Ravardino: Guarigione di un caso di esoftalmo intermittente da varici dell'orbita. *Atti Cong. Soc. ital. di oftal.*, 1924, p. 292; cited by Birch-

Hirschfeld (1930).

[32]Reese, A. B.: Exophthalmos: Ocular Complications; Causes from Primary Lesions in the Orbit; Surgical Treatment. *Arch. Ophth., 14:* 41–52 (July) 1935.

[33]Rones, B., in discussion on Poole, p. 118 (case 110).

[34]Rumjanzewa, A. F.: Ueber den intermittierenden Exophthalmus und dessen operative Behandlung. *Ztschr. Augenh., 71:*247–253, 1930.

[35]Rychener, R. O., in discussion on Poole, pp. 117–118.

[36]Sattler, R.: A Case of One-Sided Transitory Exophthalmos with Undisturbed Function and Muscular Movements of the Eye and the Coexistence of Enophthalmos or Recession of the Globe. *Am. J. M. S.., 89:*486–489, 1885.

[37]Schimanowsky, A., cited by Rumjanzewa.

[38]Spektor, S. A.: Intermittent Exophthalmos [case 106]. *vestnik oftal.* (no. 5) *15:*73–75, 1939; abstracted, *Am. J. ophth., 23:*1070, 1940.

[39]Weisner, E.: Zwei Falle von intermittierendem Exophthalmus, *Klin. Monatsbl. Augenh., 78:* 163–165, 1927.

[40]Wissmann, R., and Schulz, A.: Ueber intermittierenden Exophthalmus. *Arch. Augenh., 91:*11–33, 1922.

LXXIV

TREATMENT OF RHINORRHEA AND OTORRHEA*

In rhinorrhea and otorrhea the cerebrospinal fluid is discharged from the nose and the ear respectively. Both conditions are due to a fistula connecting the cerebrospinal spaces—either the subarachnoid spaces or the ventricular system—with the exterior. Pneumocephalus (air in the cranial chamber) is frequently but not necessarily in association. If the fistula is large enough, air enters the cranial chamber as the fluid passes out. When there is a ball valve arrangement in the fistulous tract, coughing and sneezing may force large quantities of air into the cranial chamber, and if the frontal lobes are pierced a steadily enlarging air-filled cavity in a frontal lobe gradually erodes its way into a lateral ventricle, and the entire ventricular system together with the subarachnoid spaces is then filled with air; this is the terminal stage. The surgical attack on rhinorrhea and otorrhea, however, is precisely the same, for both are due to the same underlying cause, a fistula; closure of this cures both.

The two great causes of rhinorrhea and otorrhea are (1) fractures of the skull and (2) openings created by operative procedures. Less frequent causes are (3) erosions by tumors or infections and (4) congenital abnormalities. Fortunately many fistulas heal spontaneously. Spontaneous healing occurs particularly in otorrhea following fractures of the petrous portion of the temporal bone and is due to the relatively long course of the channel through the petrous bone and the relatively greater thickness of the soft tissue. Post-traumatic otorrhea will usually stop in less than two weeks, and frequently in a day or two. There is therefore no indication for operative intervention for otorrhea of such short duration; this is fortunate, because it would be difficult to determine the site of the fistula, i.e. whether it was in the middle or the posterior cranial fossa. Posttraumatic or postoperative fistulas into the frontal or ethmoid sinuses or fistulas created by operations on the mastoid are frequently slow to heal and may never heal, or they may close and periodically reopen. The explanation is that the drainage tract is usually larger and the soft tissues relatively thin, being only mucosal lining, usually the fistula persists too long to await nature's efforts at closure by granulation tissue.

A cerebrospinal fistula is always a potential source of meningitis or cerebral abscess, and if the draining fluid persists long enough several attacks of meningitis may occur, and eventually one will be fatal. Many years may indeed elapse before death, or it may come quickly—depending on the chance of infection within the paranasal or mastoid sinuses. Sulfonamide drugs and penicillin are helpful and may prolong life, but the danger of a fatal termination is always present nevertheless. The high percentage of recoveries from meningitis in the presence of cerebrospinal fistulas is due to the continuous drainage afforded by the opening.

It is my strong feeling that a fistula (except those following injury to the petrous bone) should never be left open longer than two weeks unless the fluid is unmistakably diminishing. Closure is now a comparatively simple, danger-free procedure and leaves nothing to chance. The only exception to this statement is closure in the presence of a known, well developed intracranial infection. In 1 of my cases (case 2) organisms were isolated from the fluid

*Reprinted from the *Archives of Surgery*, 49:75–85, August, 1944.

but there was no purulent meningitis. In case 8 a cerebral abscess became full blown three weeks after the fistula was closed, but it was certainly there before the operation; at least nothing was lost in the attempt, and had it been closed earlier the abscess would never have developed.

Plum [1] (1931) reported a fistula of eighteen years' duration; Fribourg-Blanc, Lassalle and Germain [2] (1934), one of seventeen years' duration, with intermittent closure for short periods. Wurster [3] (1937) reported one of six and a half years' duration; it finally healed spontaneously and had remained closed three years at the time of his report. Thomson reported on this condition [4] (1899) in a patient, which had persisted several years. A number of spontaneous cures are recorded in the literature, but there are many more fatalities.

LOCALIZATION OF THE BONY AND DURAL OPENINGS

When rhinorrhea follows operative procedures, the site of the fistula is along the path of the operative attack and is therefore usually not difficult to find. If the fistula follows a depressed fracture of the skull the depression may indicate its position. But if there is no depression roentgenograms of the frontal region (frontal, ethmoid and sphenoid sinuses) are all important. Even then its location may be in doubt. Drainage of fluid from one nostril predominantly is fair evidence that the fistula is on the corresponding side of the anterior fossa, but that is by no means dependable proof. Cairns [5] (1937) found the opening on the contralateral side; it was explained by a blood clot which filled the other nostril. Then, too, one of the frontal sinuses may be closed for other reasons. There are times when only an exploratory operation will determine the site of the opening. Moreover, there may be bilateral fistulas (Cairns,[5] Adson,[6] Eden,[7] Campbell, Howard and Weary [8]).

To differentiate between a fistula of the frontal and one of the ethmoid sinus may at times be difficult. It is my impression that the differential diagnosis can often be made by observing the cerebrospinal outflow, i.e., if when the head is tilted forward there is a sudden increase in the volume of fluid it is apparent that the fluid has been contained in a reservoir and is pouring over the edge and that the fistula is located in a frontal sinus. And if the flow of fluid is not altered by tilting the head, an opening in the ethmoid or in the sphenoid cells is indicated.

In 1 case (case 10) I was not able to find the opening in the bone through which fluid poured into the middle ear and thence down the eustachian tube and the pharynx and when the patient was lying down from the nose. The opening into the middle ear was found, but its closure was unsuccessful.

If there is any difference of opinion concerning the advisability of operation for cerebrospinal fistulas, it can be only in those few cases in which the site or side of the fistula cannot be determined beforehand, but even in such unusual cases bilateral exposure is preferable to the almost certain fatality that lies ahead.

METHODS OF SURGICAL CLOSURE OF THE FISTULA

The first successful treatment of rhinorrhea was reported by me in 1926.[9] Autogenous grafts of fascia lata were sutured over the dural opening behind a depressed fracture of the orbit and the frontal sinus. Before this Grant [10] (1923) had attempted to close an opening through a cranial exposure but was not successful, and Teachenor [11] (1923) debated whether to uncover a frontal fistula in order to close the dura. Cushing [12] (1927) reported successful treatment in 3 cases in which rhinorrhea followed removal of orbitoethmoid osteomas; in each a piece of fascia lata was laid over the dural defect. Prior to these cures, two patients with similar conditions had died of infection; it was these deaths that prompted the closure with fascia. Rand [13] (1930), McKinney [14] (1932), Cairns [5] (1937), Gissane and Rank [15]

(1940), Eden [7] (1942) and Campbell, Howard and Weary [8] (1942) have since reported cures by the use of fascial transplants. The fascia may be taken from the thigh or from the covering of the temporal muscle. The fascia may be sutured in place or when this is not practical laid over the defect.

To cure rhinorrhea or otorrhea, it is not necessary that both the opening in the bone and that in the dura be closed. The closure of either will cure the condition. On the whole, closure of the dura is preferable. In two of the cases in this series (cases 4 and 5) the bone was waxed (1934 and 1937). This method of closing the defect in the bone was reported by Graham [16] (1937) and later by Adson [6] (1941).

Packing the wound with iodoform gauze was advocated by Peet [17] (1928) and has been used by Gurdjian and Webster [18] (1944). However, packing of the wound is now rarely done, most wounds being closed without drainage.

TREATMENT OF FISTULAS FOLLOWING CRANIAL OPERATIONS

As previously noted, when rhinorrhea develops after a cranial operative procedure the site of the fistula is evident or nearly so. In frontal craniotomy an unusually large frontal sinus may be opened. This is such a potential risk that surgeons should always know from roentgenograms the size of the frontal sinus, and when a low frontal approach is required entry into the sinus can be avoided by correspondingly shifting the bony incision. There are times when entry cannot be avoided, as for example in attacking tumors that invade the frontal sinus. When a frontal sinus is opened a flap of dura can be reflected over the opening and tightly sutured to the overlying galea. If the opening is disclosed by rhinorrhea after the operation is completed the wound should be reopened immediately and this procedure carried out (case 3). During cerebellar operations for trigeminal neuralgia, Meniere's disease, tumor of the acoustic nerve and other conditions a mastoid cell is occasionally opened; the dura should be immediately sutured over it to prevent immediate or subsequent infection.

In another case (case 4) rhinorrhea followed a frontal craniotomy in which the frontal sinus was not opened but in which the dura had been accidentally stripped from the floor of the anterior fossa. Re-exploration revealed an opening as large as a slate pencil into an ethmoid cell, and in the opening was an old elevated fracture (of many years' duration). This was plugged with bone wax (1934); there was no corresponding dural opening. The fluid had escaped through the dural suture line, thereby gaining access to the subdural space, where it entered the defect in the bone.

In another case (case 5) an opening in the ethmoid cell was made when the orbital roof was rongeured away in preparation for the removal of an orbital tumor. This opening was waxed later in the day and the dura reflected over it and sutured in place. As a precaution against the possibility of such an accident in operations on orbital tumors, the dura covering the orbital roof is now always reflected mesially; it can then be used to cover any opening in the ethmoid cells.

Nasal operations in which the cribriform plate is punctured and operations in which hypophysial tumors are attacked by the nasal route are other sources of rhinorrhea. Neither of these was encountered in this series.

OTORRHEA FOLLOWING OPERATIONS OF THE MASTOID

There are four cases in this series in which otorrhea followed operation on the mastoid; in each case it was due to the operator's chiseling through the mastoid bone and the dura. In 3 of the cases the bony defect was in the roof of the petrous bone about 2 cm. inside the lateral wall of the skull; this is probably the most common site. According to the law of probability, therefore, this is the logical place to look for the fistula. The corresponding dural defect can be sutured and if necessary reenforced by a piece of fascia lata or more conveniently by a layer of the sheath of the temporal muscle. The latter serves just as well as fascia lata for this purpose and is immediately available in the operative area. If the dural defect is near the surface the fascia is sutured in place; if it is too deep it can be laid over the suture line and treated with 3.5 per cent solution of iodine to promote adhesions. It was possible to suture in all of these cases. In a fourth case the dural opening was just back of the mastoid bone. This opening was sutured and covered by fascia, which was merely laid over the suture line and treated with iodine solution; the dura was too thin to support additional sutures. It is evident that an attempt to find the fistula by reexploring the original wound of the mastoid would be unproductive, because nothing could be done to the dural opening unless a large area of bone were removed. The incision, therefore, is made anterior to the old incision, so that the roof of the petrous bone can be exposed and the overlying dural defect reached with adequate room for closure; the attack is entirely extradural.

In case 10 a postoperative fistula was found in an unusual site. After the removal of a tumor of the acoustic nerve (by me) that had deeply eroded the petrous bone, it was discovered that a fistula opened into the middle ear and that the fluid was discharged into the pharynx. The tumor had eroded the posterior wall of the middle ear. Since rhinorrhea was an immediate postoperative sequel, the fluid had to come from this site. The ear drum blugged almost to the point of rupture, and after two unsuccessful attempts to find the fistula it was disclosed by injecting methylthionine chloride (methylene blue) (Dr. John Baylor's idea) through the drum with a tiny needle; the walls of the fistula were then colored by the dye. But an attempt to close it with sutures and a fascial trans-

plant was unsuccessful. It would not have been possible to suture a dural graft over the large defect intracranially, but an attempt was made to wax the bed from which the tumor had been extirpated. Perhaps a more careful plastic operation with fascia would now bring results. This is the only case in the series in which there was failure to close a fistula. The patient subsequently died of meningitis; the rhinorrhea persisted one year after removal of the tumor.

RHINORRHEA AND PNEUMOCEPHALUS FOLLOWING DEPRESSED FRACTURES OF THE FRONTAL SINUS

A depressed fracture of the frontal sinus is frequently visible or palpable. In two of the cases in this series (cases 1 and 2) it was necessary only to elevate the depressed fragment and remove it temporarily to close the opening in the dura with a fascial transplant. If there is not an adequate exposed area of dura, an additional amount of the inner table of the frontal sinus must be rongeured away until the desired exposure is obtained. The elevated or removed fragment of bone can then be replaced in its proper position and will usually hold without wiring. Without the existence of a depressed fracture a lateral cranial exposure would be preferable to removing the walls of the frontal sinus.

In these cases (1 and 2) both patients had pneumocephalus, with a large frontal defect and ventricular filling. Both were unconscious at the time of admission to the hospital and both recovered. There were no other cases of pneumocephalus in the series.

RHINORRHEA FOLLOWING NONDEPRESSED FRACTURES OF THE FRONTAL AND ETHMOID SINUSES

Fractures of the frontal sinus need not of course be depressed. A linear fracture will tear the underlying dura and cause rhinorrhea. With such a lesion roentgenograms are essential to determine whether the tear is on the right, the left or at times both sides and to differentiate between a crack in the frontal and the ethmoid sinus. To locate the fracture and to disclose intracranial air are important functions of roentgenograhpy in this field.

For revealing a fistula resulting from a non-depressed fracture an intracranial exposure is almost essential and provides a much better cosmetic result. To rongeur away moth walls of a frontal sinus in order to expose and close a fistula beneath, as advocated by Teachenor [19] (1923 and 1927), could produce an unsightly deformity. A cranioplasty leaves no deformity, and the incision is entirely under the hair line. My choice of operative attack is a small bone flap, such as is used for hypophysial tumors, with a concealed incision. Whether or not the dura is opened depends on the amount of room necessary to close and reenforce the opening with fascia. With careful closure of the dura the opening in the bone need not be closed, though covering it with bone wax adds safety if the opening is small. Coleman [20] (1937) has used this method of attack. It was first tried by Grant [10] (1923) in probably the first operative attempt to cure pneumocephalus, but the operation was unsuccessful because of uncontrollable bleeding.

Adson [6] (1941) reported six cases in which rhinorrhea was cured and advocated a bilateral frontal approach with a coronal incision. Because of troublesome bleeding he routinely ligated the longitudinal sinus, at times both before and after. He reasoned that: (1) he could be sure of finding the fistula on either side (when the side was unknown) or on both sides (when bilateral); (2) better elevation of the meninges was possible because of added room, and therefore (3) better invagination of the edges of the dural fistula was possible during suturation. This is an extensive procedure, and ligation of a longitudinal sinus is a serious addition to it. Moreover, such a wide bone flap broken at the anterior border of the skull must lend itself to opening both frontal sinuses—a complic-

cation that every effort should be made to avoid. Cairns [5] (1937) made an enlarged unilateral exposure that was carried some distance across the midline, so as to include much of the other frontal lobe. I should much prefer two separate unilateral flaps (two operations) if bilateral fistulas are present (as in case 11) or even if the side of the fistula is not known (this is only occasionally uncertain). It is usually possible to get adequate exposure by an extradural unilateral approach, and if it is not possible opening the dura and evacuating the cisterna chiasmatis will provide more room than is necessary.

TREATMENT OF OPENINGS IN THE ETHMOID SINUSES

Openings in the ethmoid cells are somewhat more difficult to expose and require the small anterior bone flap just described; it may or may not be necessary to open the dura. If the dura is stripped from the anterior fossa, the opening in the bone may be waxed and a piece of temporal fascia laid over it. Treatment of the fascia with 3.5 per cent solution of iodine will promote adhesions. At this depth and with a thin, easily tearable dura, suturing is difficult or impossible. German [21] (1944) reported 5 cases in which a flap of dura was turned down from the falx cerebri and the crista galli and thrown across the dural defect. Gurdjian and Webster [18] (1944) reported a case in which this procedure was used. For this procedure the dura must of course be widely opened, as in any cranioplastic procedure.

Report of Cases

CASE 1. *Post-traumatic fistula with a ball valve arrangement into the right frontal sinus.*

T. S., a white man aged seventy, was seen on Feb. 20, 1925. There had been an intermittent discharge of watery fluid from the nose since an automobile accident forty-five days before. He was semicomatose on admission to the hospital. His pulse rate was 50 and his temperature was 99.8 F. The white cell count was 8,000. Operation for presumed subdural hematoma was done forty-five days after his injury; pneumocephalus was encountered; air spurted and the brain collapsed when the thin cortex was incised. An opening in the dura and the frontal sinus was disclosed when the frontal lobe was retracted. After the wound was closed the depressed fracture was elevated and the dural defect repaired with a transplant of fascia lata, which was sutured. Entrance of air into the cranial chamber had been by a ball valve arrangement of the fistulous tract; the dural opening was not superimposed on the break in the bone. Air, therefore, could be blown into the brain by coughing and sneezing, but the increased intracranial pressure forced the dura against an intact bony surface and prevented escape of the air. Roentgeograms taken before the cranial operation showed large ventricles and a large frontal defect completely filled with air, but because of his condition I had not waited to inspect them.

Subsequent Course.—Recovery was uneventful; the pneumocephalus immediately cleared.

This case was presented in an earlier publication and was the first in which a fistula causing rhinorrhea and pneumocephalus was cured by fascial repair of the opening.

CASE 2. *Post-traumatic fistula into the left frontal sinus with pneumocephalus and ventricular filling (Fig. 1A).*

W.F., a white man aged twenty, was seen on Nov. 23, 1928. The patient was comatose when admitted to the hospital. There was a constant drip of clear fluid from the nose. Two months previously he had been in an automobile accident, after which he was unconscious for two days and then irrational for several days. When he got out of bed rhinorrhea was observed from the left nostril and had since persisted.

On admission to the hospital his temperature was 105 F.; the spinal fluid was xanthochromic and contained 20,700 cells; the white cell count was 17,000. Streptococci were grown from the spinal fluid, but the fluid was not purulent. When his head

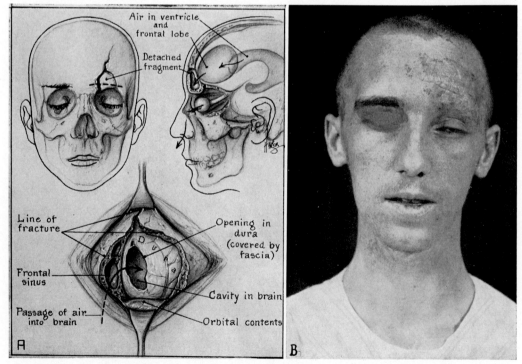

Fig. 1 (case 2).—*A*, drawings illustrating essentially the same condition as in case 1, i.e., advanced pneumocephalus with destruction of the frontal lobe and filling of the ventricular system. In this case the dural opening, which was covered with fascia, as in case 1, was also of a ball valve type, since the two openings were not superimposed. *B*, patient two weeks after operation. He was unconscious on admission to the hospital. At the present time, sixteen years after the operation, he is fighting with the United States Marines in the South Pacific.

was tipped forward a half-cup of fluid rolled out.

Roentgenograms showed the lateral ventricles filled with air and a large air-filled defect of the left frontal lobe. A depressed fracture of the left frontal bone and a crack in the right frontal sinus were disclosed. There was complete paralysis of the left oculomotor nerve.

Operation was performed on Nov. 24, 1928. The old depressed fracture of the left frontal bone was elevated. The incision was made along the supraorbital ridge. An opening 2 cm. long and 1 cm. wide was disclosed beneath it; air escaped. A piece of fascia lata was sutured over the opening and the fragment of bone replaced.

Subsequent Course.—Recovery was uneventful and the rhinorrhea did not recur (Fig. 1B). Meningitis did not develop. The patient is now serving with the marines in the South Pacific.

CASE 3. *Postoperative defect in a frontal sinus.*

T. I., a white man aged fifty-eight, was seen on Jan. 26, 1940. Immediately after removal of an enormous osteosarcoma of the skull, rhinorrhea appeared. At the time of operation the opening in the frontal sinus was not observed. On the following day the wound was reopened, and a pedicled flap of dura was reflected over the opening and snugly sutured to the galea. The rhinorrhea immediately ceased; recovery was uneventful.

CASE 4. *Post-traumatic and postoperative opening into ethmoid cells.*

E. L. a white woman aged twenty-six, was seen on Aug. 25, 1934. A glioma was removed with a section of the left frontal lobe. During the operation an assistant jerked the dura, stripping it from the anterior fossa. Rhinorrhea immediately followed the operation.

On the following day the wound was reopened, and an old elevated fracture lying in an opening in the cribriform plate was disclosed. The upturned fragment of bone left an opening as large as a slate pencil into an ethmoid cell. It was covered with wax. The dura was intact; therefore the patient had not had rhinorrhea at the time of the original cranial fracture. The fluid had now escaped through the dural suture lines into the extradural space and through this opening into the pharynx.

Subsequent Course.—There was no discharge of fluid after operation. Seven

years later (April 19, 1941) the patient died of recurrence of the tumor; there was never recurrence of the rhinorrhea.

CASE 5. *Postoperative defect in the ethmoid cells following removal of an orbital tumor by the transcranial route.*

R. H., a white woman aged thirty-five, was seen on April 7, 1937. Immediately after removal of an intracranial and intra-orbital dural meningioma, rhinorrhea appeared. It was clear that an ethmoid cell had been opened. On the following day the wound was reopened, and the open cell was found and covered with bone wax. A flap of orbital fascia was placed over the waxed opening and treated with 3.5 per cent solution of iodine to promote adhesions. Recovery was uneventful. There was no subsequent leak of cerebrospinal fluid.

CASE 6. *Postoperative defect in the left petrous bone and the dura.*

E. W., a white woman aged twenty-seven, was seen on July 3, 1934. A cerebrospinal fistula from the left ear had persisted for four years after mastoidectomy. Meningitis was said to have been present at the time of the operation on the mastoid.

At operation a circular opening (about 0.5 cm. in diameter) was exposed in the roof of the petrous bone and about 2 cm. inside the skull. There was a defect in the overlying dura, and cerebrospinal fluid was escaping. Fascia from the temporal muscle was sutured over the dural defect. Then the bony defect was covered with wax.

Subsequent Course.—The patient recovered, with no subsequent drainage of spinal fluid.

CASE 7. *Postoperative defect in the petrous bone and the dura.*

M. R., a white woman aged twenty-six, was seen on Aug. 27, 1938. Otorrhea of five years' duration following immediately after an operation on the mastoid. There was recovery from one attack of meningitis during this period.

At operation an opening (about 1 by 1 cm.) was located in the dura and in the roof of the petrous bone about 2 cm. from the lateral surface of the skull. The temporal lobe protruded through the dural opening and filled the bony defect. This fungus was cut away, the dural defect was closed with silk and a piece of fascia from the temporal muscle was sutured over the closed dura.

Subsequent Course.—The patient recovered, with no subsequent otorrhea.

CASE 8. *Postoperative defect in the petrous bone and the dura.*

F. S., a white boy aged ten years, was seen on Aug. 21, 1941. A periodic discharge of cerebrospinal fluid from the left ear was noticed after an operation on the mastoid four years before his admission to the hospital. The longest period in which the opening was closed was nine months; the patient never had meningitis.

An operation was performed on Aug. 21, 1941. Over the roof of the petrous bone, 1 cm, from the lateral surface of the skull, there was an opening as large as a lead pencil and a corresponding opening in the dura. Granulation tissue and a cerebral fungus filled the openings. The dural opening was closed with silk, treated with 3.5 per cent solution of iodine and covered with fascia from the temporal muscle. The opening in the bone was not waxed.

Subsequent Course.—No discharge of fluid was present at any time after operation.

CASE 9 *Postoperative defect in the temporal bone and the dura posterior to the right mastoid.*

S. M., a white girl aged eleven years, was seen on Jan. 7, 1944. Since an operation on a mastoid six months previous to her admission to the hospital, there had been intermittent discharge of cerebrospinal fluid from the right ear—about a quarter of a pint (118 cc.) daily. A protruding fungus filled the external auditory meatus. She had survived with complete recovery one attack of meningitis and at the time of hospitalization had a maximum temperature of 100 F. daily; the pulse rate was from 120 to 140.

At operation an opening in the temporal bone back of the petrous portion and a defect in the dura about 1 cm. square were closed with sutures and not reenforced by fascia. The fungus was removed from the external ear.

Subsequent Course.—The wound in the external ear became infected. Cerebrospinal fluid did not leak at any time after the operation, but the fever and tachycardia persisted and gradually increased. On the nineteenth day her temperature rose to 105 F. and her pulse rate increased to 170; hemiplegia and coma followed, with death twenty-six days after operation. Multiple abscesses studded the right hemisphere; Staph. aureus was isolated. Sulfadiazine had been given by mouth since her

entry into the hospital.

CASE 10. *Rhinorrhea (otorrhea?) through a postoperative defect in the mastoid following removal of a tumor of the acoustic nerve; a fistula into the middle ear.*

L. T., a white man aged 48, was seen on March 4, 1937. After removal of a large tumor of the acoustic nerve (April 27, 1937) from which there was extensive destruction of the petrous bone, rhinorrhea appeared and persisted. I was puzzled that rhinorrhea and not otorrhea developed and assumed that the fluid had in some way entered the eustachian tube mesial to the ear drum and then entered the pharynx.

After two attacks of meningitis— (1) pneumococcus type XXIX (Dec. 20, 1937) and (2) Staph. aureus (March 2, 1938) — both of which cleared promptly and miraculously with sulfanilamide, which was just then beginning to be used, the cerebellar wound was opened and the hollow in the petrous bone painstakingly waxed (March 4, 1938), but without any effect on the drainage of cerebrospinal fluid.

Dr. Baylor then found the drum bulging with fluid and injected methylthionine chloride (methylene blue) into it. A blue-stained fistula was located in the posterior wall of the middle ear. This cartilaginous opening was sutured and the adjacent mastoid waxed. The wound broke down with infection, and the sutures were extruded.

The rhinorrhea persisted. Several weeks later, on April 6, 1938, he had another attack of meningitis (Staph. aureus) and died.

CASE 11. *Spontaneous rhinorrhea.*

G. S., a white man aged thirty-nine, was seen on Sept. 15, 1943. The patient was referred by Dr. E. H. MacKinlay, of McConnellsburgh, Pa.

His complaint was "water flowing from the nose." He had had severe bilateral sinusitis ten years before I saw him; he reported drainage of pus for one year and headaches during the entire time. He has had no trouble with sinuses since then. He had had two unconscious spells: The first, a year before admission to the hospital, lasted two to three hours; the second, one week before, lasted thirty-six hours. The present illness began four months preceding hospitalization, when clear, colorless fluid began to drain from the right side of the nose. There had been no antecedent injury or infection. This drainage had been almost constant for four months. When he was standing or sitting the fluid went down the back of his throat. When he bent forward it poured out of the right nostril in a steady stream. Physical and neurologic examinations gave normal results except for the draining fluid. When he was bending forward about 2 cc. of clear colorless fluid was collected in two minutes. This came exclusively from the right nostril; however, if he turned to the left, the fluid came from the left nostril. For several years he has had occasional generalized convulsions. The blood pressure was 130 systolic and 80 diastolic; a Wassermann test of the blood gave negative results. Roentgenograms of the skull were normal, and a reexamination after the lesion was disclosed at operation did not reveal the small opening in the bone.

A diagnosis of spontaneous rhinorrhea through a frontal sinus of undetermined orgin, probably from the right sinus, was made. An exploratory operation on the small right frontal lobe was performed on Sept. 20, 1943. A slender strand of tissue slightly larger than the lead in a pencil and 1 cm. long was passed from the tip of the frontal lobe through an opening in the dura and skull—presumably the outer part of the frontal sinus—but when a probe was passed into the opening a little orbital fat protruded and was excised. It is doubtful, therefore, that this opening passed into the frontal sinus. The strand of tissue bridging the subdural space was excised for microscopic study; the tissue was of nondescript fibrous character, condensed into two circular strands; no definite nerve tissue could be identified. The dura was stripped from the anterior fossa, the bony opening plugged with wax and a piece of temporal fascia placed over the opening of the dura on its outer surface. A 3.5 per cent solution of iodine was applied to stimulate adhesions.

Subsequent Course.—The rhinorrhea continued after operation, but the patient stated that the quantity was about half as much as before. Two months later there had been no change. The frontal region was reexplored Nov. 30, 1943, but the opening was sealed over perfectly. It was then supposed that another fistula was probably on the left side. The left frontal lobe was explored on Dec. 11, 1943, and a similar strand of tissue was found at exactly the same spot as on the right. It was shorter and broader than that in the right—perhaps 0.5 cm. long and as large as a slate pencil. The arachnoid could be seen passing from the frontal lobe around the strand of tissue and was filled with cerebrospinal fluid. There were a defect in the dura and a bony opening—possibly into the outer part of the frontal sinus. The bridge of tissue was cut through, but it was too short to excise for microscopic study. The cisterna at the chiasm was opened to provide room for the operative attack on the fistula. The dura was not stripped from the floor of the skull, but a piece of temporal fascia was sutured over the opening and treated with 3.5 per cent solution of iodine to stimulate adhesions. The iodine solution was also applied to the opening in the arachnoid. It should be noted that there was evidence of congenital malformation of the left frontal lobe in that the vascular pattern was abnormal—there being two large and tortuous veins running across the outer surface of the lobe from the sylvian fissure to the longitudinal sinus. The unconscious spells were doubtless due to the congenital malformation (on the patient's first admission to the hospital ventriculography showed a normal ventricular system).

After operation the flow of cerebrospinal fluid was unchanged, and at the time of this writing (nine months later) it persists to the same degree. The findings at operation therefore did not account for the rhinorrhea. The openings in the bone could not have been into the frontal sinus.

SUMMARY AND CONCLUSIONS

Though not a common condition—11 cases in nearly twenty years—continuing rhinorrhea and otorrhea nearly always demand surgical closure of the opening in the dura or the bone, preferably both. Although spontaneous closure of the fistula does occur, it is not common, and it is not safe to delay operation in the hope that such closure may take place. The operation itself is parctically free of danger. Death following closure of a fistula is due to preexisting intracranial infection—usually one or more abscesses in the brain. The fistula may be closed in several ways: (1) suturing the dural opening; (2) suturing when possible a transplant of fascia over the dural defect; (3) suturing snugly to the overlying tissues a flap of dura or any soft tissue which has been turned over the bony opening; (4) covering the bony opening with bone wax.

Eight of the eleven patients whose cases are included in this report were permanently cured. Two (cases 9 and 10) died subsequently of intracranial infection; in 1 the infection was present at the time of operation, and in the other it appeared subsequently. One patient (case 11) remained unimproved nine months after operation; congenital openings in the dura and bone were found and closed on each side. At the time they were thought to enter the frontal sinuses, but this assumption was incorrect, because there was no benefit. The real fistula therefore was not located.

Usually the location of the fistula is readily determined by the site of a fracture or by an operation at which the opening in the bone and the dura was created. But disclosure of the fistulous tract may be exceedingly difficult, perhaps even impossible, as in case 11. In this case there has been no definite indication even of the side of the fistula. In case 10 the fistula into the middle ear as found only after injecting methylthionine chloride (methylene blue) through the bulging drum. In this case closure of the fistula in the cartilaginous wall was unsuccessful.

Pneumocephalus with a large unilateral defect in the frontal lobe and complete filling of the ventricular system was present in two cases (1 and 2) and was promptly cured after the fistula was closed.

For fistulas through the frontal sinus there are two methods of approach: (1) by elevating the depressed fracture, suturing or covering the defect with fascia and replacing the depressed fracture; (2) if there is no depressed fracture, by exposing the frontal region through a unilateral frontal bone flap with a concealed incision. This is preferable to cutting away the walls of the frontal sinus and leaving an unsightly deformity. If the side of the fistula cannot be determined, the same unilateral exposure is made on the suspected side (suggested by the side of the nose into which the cerebrospinal fluid drains), and if the opening is not found the same procedure is indicated on the other side later. Two such procedures are preferable to the single large bilateral exposure, which uncovers and usually requires ligation of the longitudinal sinus.

Drainage of cerebrospinal fluid from the nose is not pathognomonic of a fistula into the frontal or the ethmoid sinus but may occur through the mastoid bone into the middle ear and the eustachian tube, as in case 10; this, however, is exceptional.

REFERENCES

[1]Pium, F. A.: Cerebrospinal Rhinorrhea. *Arch. Otolaryng., 13:*84 (Jan.) 1931.

[2]Fribourg-Blanc, Lassalle and Germain: Deux observations de pneumatocele intracranienne. *Rev. neurol., 2:*51, 1934.

[3]Wurster, H. C.: Cerebrospinal Rhinorrhea: Report of an Unusual Case. *J. Indiana M. A., 30:* 199, 1937.

[4]Thomson, St. C.: *The Cerebrospinal Fluid: Its Spontaneous Escape from the Nose.* London, Cassell & Co., 1899.

[5]Cairns, H.: Injuries of the Frontal and Ethmoidal Sinuses with Special Reference to Cerebrospinal Rhinorrhoea and Aeroceles. *J. Laryng. & Otol., 52:*589, 1937.

[6]Adson, A. W.: Cerebrospinal Rhinorrhea. *Ann. Surg., 114:*697, 1941.

[7]Eden, K. C.: Traumatic Cerebrospinal Rhinorrhoea. *Brit. J. Surg., 29:*299, 1942.

[8]Campbell, E.; Howard, W. P., and Weary, W. B.: Gunshot Wounds of the Brain. *Arch. Surg., 44:* 789 (May) 1942.

[9]Dandy, W. E.: Pneumocephalus. *Arch. Surg., 12:* 949 (May) 1926; Pneumocephalus, in Lewis, D.: *System of Surgery.* Hagerstown, Md., W. F. Prior Company, Inc., 1943, vol. 14, pp. 311–319.

[10]Grant, F. C.: Intracranial Aerocele Following a Fracture of the Skull. *Surg., Gyne.. & Obst., 36:* 251. 1923.

[11]Teachenor, F. R.: Pneumoventricle of the Cerebrum Following Fracture of the Skull. *Ann. Surg., 78:*561, 1923.

[12]Cushing, H.: Experiences with Orbito-Ethmoidal Osteomata Having Intracranial Complications. *Surg., Gynec. & Obst., 44:*721, 1927.

[13]Rand, C. W.: Traumatic Pneumocephalus: Report of Eight Cases. *Arch. Surg., 20:*935 (June) 1930.

(April) 1944.

[19]Teachenor, F. R.: Intracranial Complications of Fracture of Skull Involving Frontal Sinus. *J.A. M.A., 88:*987 (March 26) 1927; footnote 11.

[20]Coleman, C. C.: Fracture of the Skull Involving the Paranasal Sinuses and Mastoids. *J.A.M.A., 109:*1613 (Nov. 13) 1937.

[21]German, W. J.: Cerebrospinal Rhinorrhea—Surgical Repair. *J. Neurosurg., 1:*60, 1944.

[14]McKinney, R.: Traumatic Pneumocephalon. *Ann. Otol., Rhin. & Larying., 41:*597, 1932.

[15]Gissane, W., and Rank, B. K.: Post-Traumatic Cerebrospinal Rhinorrhoea with Case Report. *Brit. J. Surg., 27:*717, 1940.

[16]Graham, T. O.: Cerebrospinal Rhinorrhoea. *J. Larying. & Otol., 52:*344, 1937.

[17]Peet, M. M.: Symptoms, Diagnosis and Treatment of Acute Cranial and Intracranial Injuries. *New York State J. Med., 28:*555, 1928.

[18]Gurdjian, E. S., and Webster, J. E.: Surgical Management of Compound Depressed Fracture of Frontal Sinus, Cerebrospinal Rhinorrhea and Pneumocephalus. *Arch. Otolaryng., 39:*287

LXXV

DIAGNOSIS AND TREATMENT OF STRICTURES OF THE AQUEDUCT OF SYLVIUS (CAUSING HYDRO-CEPHALUS)*

S trictures of the aqueduct of Sylvius (the iter) are congenital maldevelopments, characterized by a replacement of this channel with glial tissue. Histologically remnants of this epithelial-lined channel are present. At times the stricture is not complete but is so tiny that fluid can pass only intermittently, or at least incompletely.[1] Occasionally a stricture of the iter may follow a healed infection within the ventricles, but with these rare exceptions the strictures are of congenital origin.

Since the aqueduct of Sylvius is the only channel for passage of the cerebrospinal fluid that arises from the choroid plexuses of the third and both lateral ventricles, hydrocephalus involving these ventricles is a necessary and unfailing sequel when this channel is closed. There are no other collateral channels through which the fluid can be sidetracked spontaneously. When the occlusion is complete, the hydrocephalus is fulminating and produces rapid destruction of the brain. If the cranial sutures are open, the head increases in size; if they are closed, but not too tightly, when the obsturction develops, they may separate and cause moderate enlargement of the head (in childhood) ; if they are tightly closed, no enlargement can occur. The diagnosis of hydrocephalus may therefore be exceedingly simple for infants, less so but definite for children and difficult for adults. When the head cannot enlarge, hydrocephalus can be diagnosed only by convolutional atrophy shown in the roentgenograms or by ventriculography.

Hydrocephalus results from obstructions along the cerebrospinal circulatory system in four general locations: (1) the foramens of Monro, (2) the aqueduct of Sylvius, (3) the foramens of Magendie and Luschka and (4) the cisternae along the base of the brain. Of these, obstructions of the aqueduct of Sylvius account for about half of the cases of hydrocephalus in infants. Hydrocephalus arising from congenital strictures of the aqueduct of Sylvius is infrequent after infancy, though still common enough to be considered in differential diagnosis, and particularly through childhood. After infancy, tumors are responsible for hydrocephalus in perhaps 95 per cent of the cases of hydrocephalus, and in infancy congenital occlusions account for about 95 per cent of the cases. After infancy, therefore, a tumor is the presumptive cause of hydrocephalus on the law of probability. It is for this remaining group of 5 per cent, therefore, that the diagnosis of a stricture is all-important. If the diagnosis is missed, the patient is subjected to a big cerebellar operation that is unnecessary and not without danger to life. If the diagnosis is made correctly, the treatment is simple, is relatively safe and will usually cure.

DIAGNOSIS OF STRICTURE OF THE AQUEDUCT IN INFANTS

For infants the diagnosis of a stricture at the aqueduct is simple and fairly free from error. If the dye test (phenolsulfonphthalein) shows an obstruction in the ventricular system, the obstruction will be either at the aqueduct or at the foramens of Magendie and Luschka. And if the inion is low, the obstruction will be at the aqueduct; if the inion is high the obstruction will be at the foramens of Magendie

*Reprinted from the *Archives of Surgery*, 51:1–14 July–August 1945.

740

and Luschka. The height of the inion is therefore all-important. The reasons for its importance are: 1. When the foramens of Magendie and Luschka are blocked, the fourth ventricle participates in the ventricular enlargement and the resulting increased volume in the posterior cranial fossa pushes the inion upward. 2. Conversely, when the aqueduct of Sylvius is occluded, the posterior fossa does not enlarge and the inion remains low. As a matter of fact, the inion may be, and usually is lower than normal because the supratentorial pressure from the greatly enlarged lateral ventricles compresses the posterior cranial fossa and therefore lowers the inion. This is one of the most important signs in neurologic diagnosis and localization and is no less important for children than for infants. After childhood, it has but little importance.

For localization of the lesion causing hydrocephalus in infants, therefore, ventriculography is not necessary and should not be used. If the dye passes from the spinal canal into the lateral ventricles, the ventricles are not obstructed; the cerebrospinal spaces are then blocked in the cisternae (communicating hydrocephalus), and an entirely different treatment is indicated.

DIAGNOSIS OF STRICTURE OF THE AQUEDUCT IN CHILDREN AND ADULTS

Until recently, the diagnosis of stricture of the aqueduct could be made only at operation. In children the most common lesion causing intracranial pressure is a tumor, and about two thirds of these tumors are in the cerebellum. If there are cerebellar signs, the diagnosis and localization require no further diagnostic aids. But many cerebellar tumors give no signs of localization. It is from this group that strictures of the aqueduct must be differentiated, for few, if any, localizing symptoms usually result from strictures; occasionally there is a little staggering or ataxia. Ventriculography is then necessary,

and it will always accurately localize the obstruction. When this is in the anterior part of the fourth ventricle, the aqueduct and part of the fourth ventricle will be filled. A stricture can therefore be excluded. But when the air shadow shows the obstruction to be at the aqueduct, occlusion may still be due to a tumor but there may also be a stricture. Patients with this ventriculographic finding have routinely had cerebellar operations, since tumors are the probable lesions. And when tumors did not present on the surface, the exploration was carried up the fourth ventricle until the ventricular block was disclosed; at times a stricture of the aqueduct was found. When the lesion is a stricture, the conditions observed in the posterior cranial fossa are usually sufficiently normal to exclude a tumor: i.e. the cerebellar volume is not increased, the tonsils of the cerebellum are not pushed into the spinal canal (as by a tumor) and the cisterna magna is of fair size. To an experienced operator these negative findings are usually enough to make it unnecessary to carry the inspection to the aqueduct and are adequate to exclude a tumor and make the diagnosis of a stricture. With rare exceptions, when a thin diaphragm causes the block and can be opened, nothing can be done surgically to open the dense scar that usually causes the stricture. The operation therefore has done nothing but make the diagnosis and is, of course, a big and serious procedure—and certainly one to be avoided if possible.

VENTRICULOGRAPHIC DIAGNOSIS OF STRICTURE OF THE AQUEDUCT

The positive diagnosis of a stricture can now usually (not always) be made by a study of the shape of the air shadow at the obstruction as disclosed by ventriculography. The ventricular system ahead of the obstruction must be completely filled with air to insure filling of the third ventricle and of the aqueduct if it is patent. Less than complete filling leads to uncertainty and frequently to error in interpretation. The air shadow is frequently pathogonomonic of a stricture. From a somewhat dilated, or possibly normal-sized, opening of the aqueduct in the third ventricle, the air shadow tapers backward to a point in the midbrain—i.e., the shadow is funnel shaped or triangular. The shape of the shadow is determined, of course, by the character of the lesion, i.e., a scar which gradually becomes more intense as it passes backward. Usually when this lesion is present, the entire length of the open aqueduct is less than 0.5 cm. Such a shadow differs from that of an obstruction by a tumor in that the latter causes a sudden obstruction and therefore a sharp vertical line at the point of obstruction and the part of the aqueduct anterior to it is uniformly dilated, because there is no scar to constrict it. Occasionally a diaphragmatic obstruction of the aqueduct exists, and when this obtains the roentgenographic shadow is precisely like that of a tumor; such an obstruction, however, is uncommon. It will be understood, of course, that a stricture of the aqueduct always dilates the entire ventricular system ahead of the aqueduct, and it is then necessary only to concentrate the inspection of the ventricular shadows to the point of obstruction. It will also be observed that the hydrocephalus due to a stricture of the iter is frequently much greater than that caused by tumors in the posterior fossa, because in the latter the obstruction is intermittent and of ball valve character until the final stages. It is probable that for years after birth there is a tiny lumen in an aqueduct with a stricture and that eventually it closes completely. That is the only plausible explanation for the appearance of the strictures in late childhood and even beyond. However, in none of the patients who have been operated on in this hospital has any air been found beyond the aqueduct; i.e.. the strictures were then complete.

DIAGNOSIS OF STRICTURES OF THE AQUEDUCT WITHOUT VENTRICULOGRAPHY, I.E., BY THE HEIGHT OF THE INION

It is now possible to make the diagnosis of stricture of the aqueduct without operation and even without ventriculography. This had been done in 5 cases. The clue to the diagnosis is the height of the inion. Roentgenologic examination is usually a better guide to the site of the inion than palpation, because the inion may be difficult to feel with accuracy. Also, the lateral venous sinuses usually show in the roentgenogram and give additional indication of the size of the posterior cranial fossa.

The size of the posterior cranial fossa is nearly always increased in the early years of life by a tumor in this position. The inion is therefore pushed upward as an expression of the increased volume. And if the inion is not higher than normal, it usually (not always) means that there is no tumor in the posterior cranial fossa. Therefore, if the head is oversize, the sutures are separated (Macewen's sign) and there is evident hydrocephalus and, at the same time, the inion is normally placed, the diagnosis of a stricture of the aqueduct is almost assured. Exceptions to this are the following: 1. An occasional cerebral tumor will give similar signs and symptoms but can be easily differentiated by simply tapping both lateral ventricles to determine their size. A cerebral tumor may enlarge one lateral ventricle but not both. 2. A tumor of the third ventricle cannot be differentiated in this way, because the two ventricles are equally large. The latter diagnosis cannot be made without ventriculography, but it is disclosed at operation (ventriculostomy) by the absence of a large third ventricle. On the law of probability I prefer this occasional mistake to the injection of air in all cases in which a stricture of an aqueduct is the probable lesion.

ANATOMIC REASONS FOR THIRD VENTRICULOSTOMY

By a third ventriculostomy, fluid is short-circuited from the third ventricle to the cisterna interpeduncularis and the cisterna chiasmatis, which together from the central distributing station from which the cerebrospinal fluid is normally passed along to the cerebral subarachnoid spaces, where it is absorbed. It is absolutely essential that the opening in the third ventricle be made in its floor, not the roof. Nearly half a century ago the roof of the third ventricle was opened by blindly passing an instrument through the corpus callosum—the so-called *Balkenstich* procedure. An opening in the roof of the ventricle cannot cure or improve hydrocephalus, because the fluid then pours into the subdural space, where it cannot be absorbed. Moreover, the opening will not remain patient, because of subsequent cicatrization. Fluid can be absorbed only in the subarachnoid spaces. In cases of stricture of the aqueduct of Sylvius there is only one possible place—i.e., the floor of the third ventricle—from which the fluid can be sidetracked from the dilated ventricular system, where it cannot be absorbed, to the subarachnoid spaces where it is absorbed. Fortunately, the floor is membranous and thin, thereby reducing the possibility of reclosure that obtains in cases in which the walls are thicker.

TWO TYPES OF THIRD VENTRICULOSTOMY

In 1922, I [2] proposed a third ventriculostomy in the floor of the ventricle. The attack was made anteriorly through a small supraorbital approach. The third ventricle lies just behind the optic nerves, and, since these nerves in infancy are very short and there is no space between them and the olivary eminence, it was necessary to divide an optic nerve to gain access to the third ventricle. Although there were occasional successes, it was found that usually the fluid poured over the surface of the brain and an external hydrocephalus followed, i.e., the fluid poured into the subdural space, this being the path of least resistance. White (1942) [3] has continued to use this procedure, but only for adults, whose optic nerves are longer, and has reported good results. Stookey and Scarff (1936) [4] have also used this approach, but instead of cutting an optic nerve they have pushed a blunt instrument backward above the optic tracts and through the posterior wall of the floor of the ventricle—certainly a hazardous attack and one that could succeed only by luck. White also tried the Torkildsen [5] attack, by which a rubber tube is passed subcutaneously from the lateral ventricle to the cisterna magna, although he also thought it difficult to believe that such a procedure, depending on permanent patency of a rubber tube and a foreign body, could ever be successful. Sweet (1940) [6] presented a necropsy specimen of a spontaneously cured hydrocephalus. There was 4 mm. opening from the anterior part of the third ventricle into the cisterna chiasmatis. It is the only demonstration of the cause of a spontaneously cured hydrocephalus.

THE LATERAL APPROACH

An approach to the third ventricle by the temporal route was reported by me in 1932 [7] and has since been used exclusively. There are several important advantages over the frontal approach—in fact, they constitute the difference between success and failure of the third ventriculostomy in most cases. The procedure is equally applicable to infants, children and adults.

The advantages are: 1. The ventricle is opened under direct inspection—behind the infundibulum and in the cisterna interpeduncularis (not the cisterna chiasmatis), where the ventricular wall is thinnest. 2. An external hydrocephalus does not develop subsequently, because the dura lining the middle fossa of the skull ends mesially in a shelf that lies alongside the cisterna laterally.

The temporal lobe falls over this shelf and prevents fluid from pouring out. The efficacy of this sealing is evident when at operation the partially collapsed lateral ventricles are filled with fluid under pressure; the fluid does not pass into the middle fossa. 3. The optic nerves are not disturbed. 4. The approach requires a smaller operative exposure and one covered by hair.

The operative attack on the floor of the third ventricle presupposes a downward bulge of the greatly enlarged third ventricle. Occasionally this does not obtain, and the procedure cannot then be carried out unless one is willing to make a blind stab for the ventricle. Such a high, non-bulging third ventricle has been encountered twice in this series of cases, once in an infant and once in an adult. In the latter case, the anterior approach was tried subsequently, but without success. It should be noted that in children and adults the floor of the ventricle is always thicker than in infants, and, to prevent subsequent closure, a larger opening is required. In 7 cases in group I, the opening had closed after a short time, but after a second and in one case a third operation on the same or the other side the opening has persisted permanently.

A third ventriculostomy is also indicated in some cases of inoperable tumor of the cerebellum, in which there are no crippling sequelae of the tumor, such as motor paralysis or nerve palsies. It is also useful in obstructions of the foramens of Luschka and Magendie when a new foramen cannot be maintained.

THE OPERATIVE PROCEDURE

A small vertical incision is made from the zygoma upward and just in front of the ear to the edge of the temporal muscle; it then curves forward about half this distance. The incision is much like that for a temporal gasserian ganglion approach but smaller and is entirely below the origin of the temporal muscle, which is incised in a similar curve and retracted forward. A small circular area of the bone is then rongeured away and the dura opened. A flanged ventricular needle is inserted into the descending horn of the lateral ventricle and remains in place during retraction of the temporal lobe. The ventricular fluid is released through this needle by pressure of the spatula on the temporal lobe and in the exact amount necessary to expose the region about the third cranial nerve. The brain is therefore not subjected to severe pressure by retraction of the temporal lobe. The mesial shelf of the dura then comes into view, and a little more traction with the spatula exposes the third nerve and the thin wall of the cisterna interpeduncularis. The latter is incised both in front of and behind the third nerve, after which the downward bulging floor of the third ventricle is fully exposed. It is punctured with forceps and the opening enlarged by spreading the forceps or by cutting away the membrane. The flanged needle is then withdrawn and another needle connected with a funnel is inserted in its place. Isotonic solution of three chlorides is passed by gravity into the ventricle until the brain is flush with the dura (Fig. 1). The fluid emerging from the third ventricle is retained in the cisterna interpeduncularis. It is probable that external hydrocephalus will not develop so consistently following the anterior approach in the older patients because the subarachnoid spaces are open.

Infants must be placed in a head down position during the operation in order to prevent the large volume of escaping fluid from flooding the field and preventing the careful enlargement of the newly created opening. This position is not so necessary for children and adults, but some downward declination of the head is still advisable. An infant must also have the head encased in plaster of paris, to prevent collapse of the brain when the ventricle is opened.

SUMMARY OF THE RESULTS IN GROUP I (OVER 1 YEAR OLD)

There are twenty-nine patients in this group; thirteen are females and sixteen males. There were five in the first five years of life, five in the second five years, fifteen between the ages of ten and twenty, and four older than twenty; the oldest was forty-five years. On the whole, the children in this group showed few signs and symptoms except those of intracranial pressure.

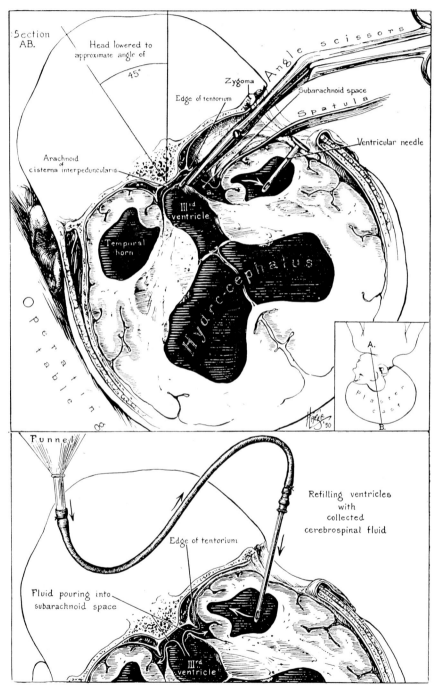

Fig. 1. The upper composit drawing indicates all the steps in the operative procedure. The lower drawing deminstrats the method of filling the ventricles with isotonic solution of three chlorides after the operation is complete. The brain then gradually fills out until it is flush with the dura.

Frequently the patients had had headaches throughout life, and usually these were periodic. The head was always oversize and usually strikingly so; the circumferences ranged from 59 to 65 cm. The cranial sutures were open, and a cracked pot sound was elicited. In many instances the sella turcica was enlarged in the anteroposterior direction owing to the pressure of the big third ventricle, and in one patient there were a partial bitemporal hemianopsia and complete destruction of the sella from the same cause. In every case extensive convolutional atrophy was seen in the roentgenograms—an almost pathognomonic indication of hydrocephalus.

Usually there was bilateral papilledema, at times with hemorrhages in the eyegrounds. One patient was blind and two others nearly so from the intracranial pressure. In only one patient was there an extraocular palsy; she had bilateral ophthalmoplegia which has persisted for thirteen and one-half years after operation; doubtless the scar at the aqueduct had included the nuclei controlling the extraocular muscles. Dizzy spells were noted in two cases.

VENTRICULOGRAPHY. In all cases a complete block has been shown at the iter; in none has air been seen beyond. However, in the period before the obstruction had become total, such a finding might well have been observed. Only in recent years have the relatively high incidence of this lesion and the number of cerebellar operations in which tumors were not found led to a more careful study of the shadow at the aqueduct. It is now believed that the funnel-shaped shadow when it occurs is characteristic of the lesion. Until this fact as disclosed, thirteen cases of stricture of the aqueduct had been found at cerebellar operations. Since then, eleven have been disclosed by ventriculography alone.

The size of the ventricles as measured by the amount of fluid required to fill them was 150, 180, 200, 205, 275, 300, 400, 525, 600, 650 and 720 cc. in 11 recorded cases. Particularly significant are the very large ventricles, i.e., over 500 cc. Cerebellar tumors may cause such large ventricles, but rarely do they cause ones as large as 500 cc.

DIAGNOSIS OF STRICTURES WITHOUT VENTRICULOGRAPHY

Even more gratifying is the further advance of making this diagnosis without ventriculography (in children). Even in adult life an unusually large head is carried over from childhood and may have the same significance; for 1 adult the diagnosis has been made in this way. The diagnosis is made when (1) the head is oversize; (2) there is a separation of the cranial sutures from intracranial pressure; (3) the x-rays show convolutional atrophy, and (4) most important, the inion is low, indicating the absence of a tumor in the posterior cranial fossa. The length of time the large head has been known to exist is also significant, strictures usually being of longer duration than tumors. In 5 cases the diagnosis has been made without ventriculography.

After childhood the lesion is still found but less frequently, and unless a large head indicates a carry-over from childhood the diagnosis would hardly be entertained before operation. With this exception, it is therefore always an operative disclosure in adults.

RESULTS OF TREATMENT

GROUP I (OVER 1 YEAR). A total of thirty-six operations (ventriculostomies) were performed in the twenty-nine cases. The reason for the seven extra operations was that the opening in the floor of the ventricle had closed before the patient left the hospital or subsequently, and a second attempt was made either on the same or on the other side. In six of these cases the subsequent operation (in one case two additional operations) was successful. The presence or absence of fulness at the site of the operation (a miniature decompression) is proof of the patency or nonpatency of the newly created opening. The decompression will be flat and soft if the hydrocephalus has been cured.

There was one operative death in the series. In one case (age seventeen) it was not possible to make an opening in the third ventricle because it did not descend far enough. An anterior approach was tried; the optic nerve was cut to reach it, but the opening was small and quickly closed over again. The patient died four months later. Three other patients died at home five weeks, three months and six months after leaving the hospital. In none of these cases was an autopsy obtained; one of these patients had made great improvement; in one there was no improvement, and no comment was made concerning the third.

From the series, twenty-four are living and cured. The time since operations is: between six months and one year, two cases; between five and ten years, 11 cases; between ten and twenty years, three cases, and in 1 case twenty-three and one-half years (Fig. 2). Four are mentally retarded in degrees; one goes to school but makes little progress; another is in high school but has difficulty keeping up with his classes; the other two are morons.

Three patients have greatly defective vision but can see. The vision is not worse than before the operation and in 1 instance has improved a little.

Aside from these defects, which are caused by the long-sustained intracranial pressure, the remaining patients are well, active and normal mentally and physically.

There are probably no groups of patients with a background of intracranial pressure that do better than those with stricture of the aqueduct and in which the procedure is so simple and safe. The earlier the diagnosis is made, the better the operative results will be.

GROUP II (UNDER 1 YEAR). The operative cures obtained in group II are far less than in the preceding one, i.e., in patients over one year of age. In the first place, the failures of the operation to sidetrack the fluid into the subarachnoid space are approximately one half, whereas for the patients over one year of age failures are very

uncommon. The reason for this difference is not too clear, and the explanation offered may or may not be correct. It is my impression that the subarachnoid spaces leading from the cisterna interpeduncularis over the cerebral hemispheres may be compressed over such a long period that they may not reopen. In several instances air has been injected intraspinally before operation, and the air has reached but not passed beyond the cisterna interpeduncularis. Since the hydrocephalus in these patients was doubtless present in intrauterine life, these spaces may never have been open and functioning. Consequently, it may be expecting too much to anticipate their reestablishment with uniformity after they have been obliterated for so long. At any rate, these spaces do open in some cases, and when this obtains the hydrocephalus is cured. For infants, therefore, assurance can never be given that a cure is attainable; it is just a chance, less than even, but the only chance, and it may be worth taking. However, even if he is cured, the chances that the child will be normal are none too good. Even with a moderate-sized head, the cerebral damage is so extensive that one wonders how a normal mentality can ever result, though is occasionally does (Fig. 2). In several of these children, there are such mental deficits and physical infirmities that they had better never been cured. For several years I have made it a rule not to operate on any hydrocephalic infant with a head that is much oversize— perhaps over 50 or 52 cm. At this size one can never be certain of the mental development, which is so varied, and for that reason the infants are probably entitled to any existing doubt; but after this stage there can scarcely be any uncertainty. Obviously the operation should be done at the very earliest time the diagnosis is made. Every week thereafter the cerebral destruction is extensive. Moreover, it is probable —though not certain—that the number of operative cures would be greater in the earlier stages. At present, a baby is rarely referred for operation before a stage has been reached when the mother can make the diagnosis as early as the physician. With a little more careful observation on the part of physicians, who must bear this responsibility, this picture could easily be changed.

Doubtless the important reasons for the difference in results from operation for hydrocephalus in infants and older children are that (1) in the latter the brain is firmer and more resistant to pressure changes than in infants and (2) the stricture is always partial for some time in children, whereas it is always total in infants. This also means that the cerebral subarachnoid spaces are open and functioning for absorption with the partial occlusions of older patients, and therefore there is every assurance that these spaces will continue to function when the fluid is short-circuited through the third ventriculostomy.

The detailed results in this group of infants—most information is obtained from correspondence—are as follows:

I. Number of patients operated on, sixty-three (twenty-six females and thirty-seven males).

2. Number of deaths in hospital, ten; number of survivals, fifty-three.

3. Latest results: Number of patients now living, twenty-one; now dead, thirty-two; no report by letter, ten.

Although there were a few deaths from intercurrent infections and other lesions, most of the patients have probably not been cured.

4. Of the thirty-two patients who are now dead, ten died in the hospital; five later died in less than a month; ten died in less than six months; six, in less than a year, and one after twelve and a half years (cause of death not known).

5. Of the twenty-one who now survive, the time since operation is: for one, less than six months; for one, less than a year; for five, less than five years; for eight, less than ten years, and for six over ten years. The three longest survivals are twelve and one-half, fourteen and one-half, and twenty-three and one-half years (Fig. 2).

6. As nearly as can be determined, the hydrocephalus in twelve has been cured. Of these, only five have a normal or nearly normal mentality. One of the twelve cured patients is deaf and blind; two have club-feet; one is unable to walk; two have convulsions, and seven are decidedly subnormal mentally.

Only once have I seen a hydrocephalic head shrink in size after the operation. In a three month old infant, the bones overlapped noticeably at the frontoparietal suture and along the midline. The circumference of the head measured 43 cm. on admission and four months later 39 cm. One could feel very prominent ridges where the bones were overlapping. Four years later the child was walking and talking and appeared to be fairly normal but the head was strikingly microcephalic; unfortunately, photographs were not obtained. The normal growth of the body was in striking contrast to the tiny head. When the child was four and one-half years old, a sudden right hemiplegia and aphasia developed and was associated with a high fever—perhaps a vascular accident but certainly not connected with the old hy-

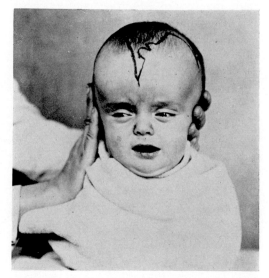

Fig. 2. At the time of operation (April 6, 1921), the patient was 5 months old and the circumference of the head was 51 cm. The anterior fontanel is outlined in ink.

drocephalus. She survived this but never regained speech or motor power on the right side. Frequent convulsions followed. Six months later she died at the age of five and one-half (five and one-fourth years after operation).

Not infrequently one sees slight overriding of the cranial bones soon after operation but, except in this one case, no appreciable reduction in the size of the head. The reason doubtless is that the bones are fairly well fixed at the base of the skull and for some distance laterally. Even when the hydrocephalus is cured, the growth of the head may continue at a subnormal rate, therefore stigmatizing the patient with an oversized head of varying degree (see photographs). For the presumably cured patients, the following increases in circumferences of the head have been recorded: (parents' measurements in most cases)

1. Head smaller than before operation after five and one-fourth years.

2. After four, six and ten years, no increase (three cases).

3. After two years, 1 cm.

4. After five and one-half years, 1 cm.

5. After nine and one-fourth years, 3.5 cm.

6. After five and one-half years, 6 cm.

7. After six years, 5 cm.

8. After twelve years, 10 cm. (measurement questionable).

SUMMARY

Strictures of the aqueduct of Sylvius are easily diagnosed in infants by (1) the dye test indicating an obstruction and (2) a low inion.

For children over 1 year old the diagnosis can now usually be made by ventriculography and without operation and frequently without ventriculography. In most of these, a partial occlusion of the aqueduct has doubtless existed for a long period before becoming complete. An oversized head, with (1) Macewen's sign (cracked pot sound) and (2) an inion normally placed or at times lower than

normal, indicates hydrocephalus without a space-occupying lesion (a tumor) in the posterior cranial fossa. By exclusion, the lesion is a stricture of the iter.

When ventriculography is used, the shape of the shadow in the aqueduct of Sylvius—funnel shaped or triangular—will frequently make the diagnosis without an unnecessary cerebellar operation for its disclosure.

A third ventriculostomy—temporal approach—is the operative choice for hydrocephalus due to a stricture of the aqueduct. It is much superior to the anterior approach because (1) external hydrocephalus does not follow; (2) it is not necessary to section a nerve (the optic nerve must be sectioned in the anterior approach), and (3) the scar is under the hair.

Cures are attained in most cases when the patient is more than a year old and in less than half the cases of infants. Excellent results are obtained in the older group. In the younger group—i.e., infants—a perfect result is obtained in very few cases. One may perhaps even question the wisdom of operating on this group, though operation is probably worth while when the head is not over 50 or 52 cm. in circumference at the time of operation.

REFERENCES

[1]Dandy, W. E., and Blackfan, K. D.: Internal Hydrocephalus. *Am. J. Dis. Child.*, *8*:406 (Dec.) 1914.

[2]Dandy, W. E.: Operative Procedure for Hydrocephalus. *Bull. Johns Hopkins Hosp.*, *33*:189, 1922.

[3]White, J. C.: Treatment of Obstructive Hydrocephalus. *Surg., Gynec. & Obst.*, *74*:99, 1942.

[4]Stookey, B., and Scarff, J.: Occlusion of the Aqueduct of Sylvius. *Bull. Neurol. Inst. New York, 5:* 348, 1936.

[5]Torkildsen, A.: A New Palliative Operation in Cases of Inoperable Occlusion of the Sylvian Aqueduct. *Acta chir. scandinav.*, *82*:117, 1931.

[6]Sweet, W. H.: Spontaneous Cerebral Ventriculostium. *Arch. Neurol. & Psychiat.*, *44*:532 (Sept.) 1940.

[7]Dandy, W. E., in Lewis, D.: *Practice of Surgery.* Hagerstown, Md., W. F. Prior Company, Inc., 1933, vol. 12, p. 247.

LXXVI

ARTERIOVENOUS ANEURYSMS OF THE SCALP AND FACE*

Arteriovenous aneurysms in the integument may occur anywhere but are more common in the head than over the remainder of the body, and most of these are in the scalp. They are not common; perhaps between 200 and 300 cases have been reported. Elkin (1924)[1] described a case from Cushing's clnic and noted that this was the only case of its kind that Cushing had seen in his entire experience up to that time in over 35,000 patients admitted to hospitals. Nine additional cases are reported; 1 of these was from Dr. Blalock's clinic and is added with his permission.

Heine (1869)[2] collected the first series of cases of arteriovenous aneurysms occurring in the head, sixty in all, but he questioned the diagnosis in fifteen. In forty-six cases the aneurysms were in the scalp (including twelve back of the ear), in 13 cases they were in the face and in one case on the tongue. The first cases in his collection were reported by Pellebon (1810), Walther (1823), Dupuytren (1828), Brodie (1829),[3] Mussey (1830),[4] Graefe (1832) and Breschat (1834). Heine ascribed the origin of most of these tumors to congenital nevi or cavernous angiomas that had been present since birth or had at least been observed soon after birth. From these, the vascular radiations gradually spread and enlarged during the years. A minority of cirsoid aneurysms had no such antecedent lesions but were known to have followed trauma and were presumably related thereto. Virchow was a dominant influence in Heine's interpretation of this lesion as being congenital. There can be no doubt that this view is correct.

Korte (1880)[5] added twenty-six cases and considered his publication a continuation of Heine's excellent report. He too concluded that most of the aneurysms were of congenital derivation but that many were due to trauma; the frequency of the latter was less than that of the former. Since these two excellent pioneer publications by Heine and Korte, many subsequent reports have shown the variations in size and distribution of the so-called cirsoid aneurysms of the scalp and face; some of them are extraordinary. The following are good examples: Muller (1891)[6] described a case in which after operative death the tremendous coils were dissected and photographed; this gave an excellent view of the naked vessels. Berger's (1898)[7] case presented one of the youngest patients (nine years), with an extremely extensive lesion, the great size of which is usually attained in later years. From Germany, large deforming aneurysms were reported by Clairmont (1908),[8] Kepler (1912)[9] and Schlochetzki (1933)[10] and from Holland by Noordenbos and Jong (1918). From England, Canada and Australia, cases have been reported by Brodie (1929),[3] Parker (1904),[11] Searby (1931),[12] Clunie (1936)[13] (aneurysms restricted to the parietal region of one side), Rundle (1938)[14] (aneurysms restricted to the forehead), Davies-Colley (1940)[15] (mass covered the forehead, nose and left eye) and Patey (1942)[16] (mass was largely in occiput); a roentgenogram of one of the enormous vessels was made after injection with iopax (uroselectan). From the United States, cases have been reported by Warren (1867),[17] Mynter (1890),[18] Meyer (1892),[19] Forbes (1895),[20] Coley (1901)[21] (unilateral involvement in the

*Reprinted from the *Archives of Surgery, 52:1–32,* January, 1946.

temporal region), Beck (1903)[22] (aneurysms in the forehead, extending over nose and cheeks), Judd (1916)[23] (one of the largest and most widespread aneurysms on record), Elkin (1924)[1] (aneurysm in the front half of the head), Matas (1933),[24] Fite (1933)[25] and Brock and Dyke (1932).[26]

From the early reports of Heine and of Korte, aneurysms back of the ear were in greatest number, but since then those of the scalp have far outstripped them. Perhaps a good index of their frequency is gained from Kepler (1912),[9] who collected thirty-two cases in the four years after Clairmont's paper (1908).[8] Forty additional cases have been collected in the past ten years, including the nine reported here. No attempt has been made to cover all the literature. In thirty-two of these forty cases, the aneurysms were in the scalp; in five cases, they were back of and including the ear, and, in one case each, they were in the eye, in the chin (Meleney, 1923)[27] and in the lip (Davies-Colley, 1940).[15] Of the aneurysms in the scalp, eight were unilateral and twenty-four bilateral. The distribution of those in the scalp was: seven largely confined to the forehead (one extending over the nose and eyes; Davies-Colley) and the remaining twenty-five in the parietal or the occipital region or both. All these aneurysms were similar, except in their anatomic expression, to the well known congenital arteriovenous aneurysms that are confined to the brain and which are certainly not less frequent.

One group of these, however, commands special attention and is a type of aneurysm not heretofore recognized; its frequency is attested by the fact that six of the nine cases reported in this paper are of this group (cases 4 to 9 inclusive). The aneurysms in these cases differ from the other aneurysms of the scalp heretofore reported in that the primary arteriovenous aneurysm is in the dura of one or both sides and the extracranial aneurysm arises from numerous perforations of the bone from branches of the dural aneurysm.

I have found in the literature only two other examples of this type of aneurysm. Both of these were reported by Brock and Dyke in a series of eight cases of arteriovenous aneurysms of the brain. One of the patients (their case 5) was the same patient that is reported on as case 9 in this series by my colleagues and me; their report was made before the patient came here for operation, and they, of course, could not know of the remarkable intracranial aneurysm that was also present. Their case 4 is identical in every respect with our cases 4, 5, 6, 7 and 8. They commented on the enlarged posterior branches (bilateral) of the middle meningeal artery, and since the patient had a left homonymous hemianopsia they assumed that the enlarged middle meningeal artery contributed the arterial component of an arteriovenous aneurysm that continued into the visual pathways in the brain. The patient also had the same bilateral pulsating aneurysms in the occipital region of the scalp. From the position of these masses in the occipital region on each side, they inferred that the aneurysms were connected with the occipital arteries. However, in the light of the demonstrations of the meningeal connections in our cases, there can hardly be a doubt that their origin was from the middle meningeal arteries and was part of the intracranial aneurysm.

Curiously, in all five cases of homonymous hemianopsia the defect of vision has been to the right, the lesion thus being placed in the left cerebral hemisphere. There would appear to be no rational anatomic explanation for this seemingly consistent localization of the aneurysm to the left side of the brain, excluding the right hemisphere. Since the hemianopsia in the case reported by Brock and Dyke was to the left, it is now clear that either hemisphere may be involved in the aneurysm. Needless to add, it would appear to be only a lucky chance that both hemispheres are not invaded, since both meningeal arteries so commonly participate in the dorsal and the extracranial aneurysms.

Report of Cases

CASE 1. *Arteriovenous aneurysm of eyelids.* A roubust man, aged thirty-seven years, entered the hospital because of a large, disfiguring growth in both upper and lower eyelids of the left side. He was positive that there had been no swelling or vascular abnormality before he had been struck over the left eye by a steel cable, five years before. The eye was then swollen shut for several days and the lids were discolored, but all the effects subsided. Two months later a small swelling was observed in the left upper eyelid on the inner side; its growth had been progressive. Two years later (three years ago) a similar swelling appeared in the left lower lid, and it too progressed. The swellings were soft and throbbing, but the patient heard no noises. Up to the time of admission, the swelling had been lacerated eight or ten times; following each there was profuse bleeding, and the blood spurted as when an artery is cut.

Examination showed large red swellings of both lids on the left. The eyeball was completely covered, and only laterally was there any indication of a palpebral orifice. The swellings pulsated strongly and synchronous with the radial pulse. The tumor could be collapsed under a compressing finger, but the pulsation had to be overcome to do it. Especially large vessels stood out at the inner side of the swelling on the left upper lid, which was at the maximum part of the tumor and doubtless was nearest the point of origin of the arteriovenous fistula. Pressure on the common carotid artery stopped the pulsations completely and made the volume of the mass shrink perceptibly. The veins over the left side of the forehead stood out fairly prominently and were tortuous; they ran vertically toward the hair line. A thrill could be felt over both swellings but not over the veins of the forehead. The conjunctiva (left) was injected, and the eyeball pulsated and protruded 6 mm. The vision in the left eye was 20/50 and in the right eye 20/20. Examination of the fundus of the eye was noncontributory; the veins were not tortuous or engorged. The visual fields were normal. The pupil reacted normally. There was no bruit audible over the head.

Impression.—Arteriovenous aneurysm.

Operation.—On April 27, 1944, the internal and external carotid arteries in the neck were ligated. We could not tell whether the arterial side of the fistula was a branch of the ophthalmic artery, a branch of the external carotid artery near the inner canthus or both through collateral circulation. There was not enough protrusion of the eyeball for an aneurysm of the entire ophthalmic artery, i. e., the great swelling was too superficial. The external and internal arteries were exposed and each compressed. Compression of the internal carotid artery reduced the pulsation slightly but definitely. Compression of the external carotid artery almost but not quite stopped it. Compression of both eliminated the pulsation. Three small plugs of muscle (sternomastoid) were inserted into the external carotid artery, and the main trunk was ligated. The internal carotid artery was then tied, and all pulsation ceased. It was noted at the time that the external carotid artery was considerably larger than the internal carotid artery. There were no untoward effects from ligation of these vessels. The reaction to the Matas test, made before operation, was negative and gave assurance that the ligation of the internal carotid artery would be tolerated. It was not expected that this operation would cure the aneurysm, because the vast collateral circulation of the external carotid artery would soon reestablish the pulsation. The ligations were necessary to reduce the circulation to a point where a later excision of the mass would be less hazardous. Without these ligations, I doubt that this vicious aneurysm could have been removed. It would certainly have been a dangerous undertaking.

There was no detectable pulsation of the masses on the following day, but three days later a faint pulsation was detected. The size of both masses was distinctly less (perhaps one fifth) than before operation, and they were softer. A definite palpebral orifice was now present, and the patient could see through the slit without pushing the masses aside.

Second Operation.—On May 6, 1944 both masses were excised. Bleeding was distinctly arterial and troublesome, but complete excision was attained without undue difficulty. Since the arterial pulsation ceased with the ligation of the internal and external carotid arteries, removal of the aneurysm immediately would have been accomplished with less bleeding than would have been obtained ten days later, when the pulsation had returned. The conjunctiva and skin of the upper lid were sufficiently good to get a fair upper lid. On the lower lid, however, the skin was so thin and the conjunctiva so reduced that the lid was largely lost. Much of the remaining lower lid subsequently sloughed from infection. On June 6 Dr. Staige Davis threw a pedicle flap from the forehead to replace the lower lid and obtained an excellent result.

CASE 2. *Arteriovenous aneurysm in mastoid region and including the ear.* A white man, aged thirty-nine, was a patient on Dr. Blalock's service and was operated on by his resident physician, Dr. Longmire. Ten years before, the patient had noticed a swelling back of the right ear. It steadily grew larger. It was not painful, but there was a roaring hum when he lay on the affected ear. It did not bleed. There was no history of trauma.

The mass measured 2.5 by 1 cm. and involved the posterior surface of the ear in its lower two thirds. It was also attached to the mastoid bone. It was not painful to touch, but a strong thrill was elicited on palpation. A loud hum was heard and was transmitted to the neck.

Operation.—At operation by Dr. Longmire on February 2, 1945, a skin flap was dissected back from the ear, carrying with it the tumor. The tumor was then excised. The superficial temporal artery was also ligated. The patient was discharged one week later; all pulsation had ceased. Fifteen months later there had been no recurrence.

CASE 3. *Arteriovenous aneurysm of scalp.* N. H., a large, healthy-looking woman aged twenty-nine, complained of headache and swelling on the head. The present illness probably dated back to birth, when it was noticed that after a normal delivery the posterior fontanel did not close and a swelling remained there. The patient did not know whether this swelling had increased in size before she was twenty, when her first baby was born, but she did know that after the childbirth the veins began to swell over her forehead and did not recede. Furthermore, with each subsequent pregnancy—and there had been seven—enlargement of the vessels developed anew. The progress of the venous enlargement was from the region of the posterior fontanel along the

midline of the head toward the front, then over the temporal and parietal regions of both sides and finally to the mesial side of both eyes. The vessels became painful and tense when venous pressure was increased by straining or coughing or stooping. She also found it more comfortable to sleep with the head elevated. The vessels had never bled. Generalized headaches had been present for four or five years, but only occasionally did they prevent sleep. Recently there had been a throbbing sensation in both ears, synchronous with heartbeats; her hearing was unaffected. She had had occasional convulsions. She was again pregnant, for the eighth time.

Examination showed a large mass of vessels in the midline of the scalp, back of the center; from this, huge, tortuous and nodular vascular trunks radiated in all directions. One large collection passed forward to the bridge of the nose and overhung the medial part of both eyes. This mass was slightly bluish. Another mass passed laterally in front of each ear, slightly covering the face. The central mass pulsated strongly; slight pulsation was present in the large vessels radiating from it, and a slight thrill could be detected on light palpation. The central mass was not tender. Compression of the superficial arteries did not influence the size of the swelling. On auscultation a slight murmur was heard; this became intensified with greater pressure of the instrument. When the finger milked the blood backward in a big vessel from the nasion to the hair line, the vessel was collapsed and a deep furrow resulted, indicating that the blood came from the central mass posteriorly. Both middle meningeal arteries were greatly enlarged in the roentgenogram and passed directly backward and upward toward the region of the extracranial angiomatous mass.

Diagnosis.—The diagnosis was congenital ateriovenous aneurysm of the scalp with a congenital coil of vessels in the midparietal region.

Operation.—On Sept. 21, 1926, the external carotid artery on both sides plus both occipital, internal maxillary and superficial temporal arteries were ligated; the external jugular veins were oversize, and they were not ligated. Temporary compression of the common carotid artery did not appear to influence the size of the mass. The large vein over the forehead was ligated at the hair line. There was essentially no change in the size of the oc- citptal mass; it may even have been a little more tense, and to the patient it seemed definitely tighter (from thrombus forma- tion). The vein over the forehead remain- ed collapsed. Six days later the pulsation in the mass had stopped (from thrombus formation) and the vessels in the mass and those radiating therefrom were firm and pulseless, with the exception of one in the right temporal region. The veins of the forehead had collapsed. The headaches and the noise in the ears were no longer pres- ent.

Second Operation.—On Jan 5., 1932 (five and one-fourth years after first operation), the patient returned because swelling in the back of her head persisted and pulsat- ed. Except for a fair-sized pulsating vessel in the occiput, there was no trace of the huge veins over the head and face that formerly were so prominent; the central mass was also much smaller. It did pul- sate, though much less than before. She wanted to get rid of it.

An elliptic incision was made around a central area of thin red skin at the top of the mass and the mass was dissected from its bed. The periosteum was thickened and was not stripped from the bone. In the layer of thickened periosteum two fair-sized arteries emerging from the pari- etal foramens were thrombosed with the electrocautery. Since there was no other source for these vessels—all the lateral chan- nels were severed—they had to come from the bone. It has been noted (in roentgen- ograms) that the middle meningeal arteries were greatly enlarged and were directed backward toward this mass. It is practi- cally certain, therefore, that the arterial supply of the tumor was ultimately from this source. Since the skin was redundant, primary closure was attained in spite of the excised central area; the wound healed without sloughing.

Subsequent Report.—On June 1, 1945, thirteen years after extirpation of the mass, the patient was perfectly well; there has been no return of the aneurysm.

Case 4. *Aneurysms of the dura, with extension extracranially.*

The patient was a normal-looking wo- man, aged thirty-eight. She complained of headache and noise in the head. She had been conscious of the noise for many years, but the headaches had began only a month ago. Both the noise and the headaches were in the left occipital region and co-

incided with a roughly circular pulsating mass 5 cm. in diameter. There was a similar mass on the right, about half as large as the one on the left. A thrill could be felt and a bruit heard over both masses. The bruit was most intense in the occipital region but could be heard over the entire head and in the neck. The veins over the frontal and the temporal regions were conspicuous.

The patient had a right homonymous hemianopsia.

Roentgenograms showed greatly en- larged middle meningeal grooves extend- ing straight back to the occipital region. In the parieto-occipital regions of both sides, the bone was extremely porous from numerous small erosions.

Operations.—On Feb. 13, 1939, an arteri- venous aneurysm in the left occipital region was removed, a flap being used. Arterial bleeding coming out of the bone was controlled by wax. The same opera- tion on the right side was performed Feb. 16, 1939. The bone was not remov- ed on either side. On April 25 the bone was rongeured away piecemeal under the previous flap (left side). The dura was extremely bloody, and coils of vessels filled the dura and projected outward to- ward the bone. They were coagulated with the electric cautery. The large middle meningeal artery was ligated. The dura was not opened.

Subsequent Note.—On May 1, 1945 (six years after the operation), the patient had had no headaches since operation. The aneurysms had disappeared.

Case 5 A man aged fifty-nine, was rather ill-looking, walked poorly and with staggering gait and was deaf to conver- sational tones. He complained of general weakness.

Since early childhood he had had inter- mittent headaches. They were now bi- frontal and occurred several times weekly; they were not associated with nausea or vomiting. For many years a subjective head noise that he could not localize had disturbed him. His hearing had been defective for over twenty-five years, and he had been totally deaf for ten years. He had a right homonoymous hemianopsia but did not know when it developed. Bilateral exophthalmos of moderate degree had also been present for years.

A year before he had begun to have general malaise and weakness and had difficulty in walking, especially in the dark (due to vestibular divisions of the auditory nerves). His wife said that he was becoming mentally sluggish, was disoriented at times and on numerous occasions had threatened suicide. There had been no convulsions.

Examination.—Examination revealed: (1) in the left occipital region an expansile, pulsating mass, 5 cm. in diameter (a systolic thrill could be heard over it); (2) in the right occipital region another mass of same kind but smaller, 3 cm. in diameter; (3) in the right vertex another similar mass (2.5 cm. in diameter); (4) over both temporal regions many tortuous pulsating vessels; (5) right homonymous hemianopsia; (6) bilateral exophthalmos; (7) bilaterally equal loss of hearing below conversational level; (8) bilateral vertical nystagmus; (9) swaying broad-based walk, with a positive Romberg sign in all directions; (10) roentgenologic evidence of enormous bilateral middle meningeal channels, directed backward to the occipital region and numerous little erosions in parietal bones, and of several small calcified areas in the left parietal and occipital lobes, and (11) stopping of the pulsation on the corresponding side by pressure on the carotid artery.

Operation.—On April 11, 1939, an occipital extracranial aneurysm on the left side was excised, a flap being used. From the bone, arterial blood spurted in dozens of places; it was controlled by waxing.

On April 19, under the cutaneous flap, the bone was rongeured away piecemeal. Dozens of little vessels were pulled out of the bone; many were thrombosed, but some still bled; they were attached to the dura and were continuous with the branches of the middle meningeal artery. This vessel was as large as a slate pencil and was ligated. The many bleeding points in the dura were coagulated with the cautery. The dura was not opened.

The patient was much improved on Dec. 12, 1939. His headaches were now only on the right side; he was much better mentally. The neurologic conditions had, of course, not changed. The middle meningeal artery was tied on the right subtemporal approach.

COMMENT. This case is very similar to the preceding one in many of the subjective and the objective findings. On July 20, 1945, six and one-fourth years after operation, the patient was free of all headaches and leading a normal life.

CASE 6 A pale, undernourished man, aged forty-six, had never been well; he had always been easily exhausted and had had numerous complaints. Generalized headaches had begun fifteen years before consultation and were intermittent until one year before he was seen, when they became constant. Since losing a good job five years before, he had been nervous, depressed and subdued and had had a definite personality change. For six weeks there had been an occasional noise in the right ear. His complaints were those characteristic of psychoneurosis. However, for the past two months he had had intermittent attacks of numbness in the left arm and leg but no actual convulsions. The examination disclosed numerous large dilated and tortuous vessels in the scalp, over which a thrill could be felt and a murmur heard. These were more pronounced in the occipital region, the vertex and both temporal regions. There was no concentrated mass of vessels as in other cases. There was a small hemangioma on the right upper eyelid and a birthmark in the midline of the upper lid, neither associated with the vascular masses.

The roentgenogram showed three small calcified areas in the leg area of the right side—doubtless the cause of his sensory seizures.

Operation.—On July 31, 1942 a bone flap was contemplated to remove the calcified areas in the right hemisphere, but the bone was covered with tiny holes from which arterial blood spurted and was controlled by wax; the sharp bleeding was from the vessels supplying the extracranial arteriovenous aneurysms. Continuation of the bone flap would have courted severe hemorrage. Instead, the bone was rongeured away by bits, and each bite of the bone was attended by brisk bleeding. The exposed dura was covered with large vessels, branches of the middle meningeal artery; these were coagulated with the electrocautery. The dura was turned back and three small bony spicules removed from the brain in the neighborhood of the longitudinal sinus; one was flat and on the surface of the pia, and each of the other two was perhaps 2 cm. in length and projected into the brain tissue. All were easily removed. In this limited exposure the suspected intracranial aneurysm was not visible.

CASE 7. A normal-looking man, aged forty-two, had had headaches for fifteen years; at first they had occurred every two or three months, lasting from a few hours to a day, and had ended with vomiting. For the past two years the headaches had been almost constant. They were mainly on the left side and affected the eyes, the face, the gums and the back of the head and neck. A visual aura had preceded the attacks; blindness lasted from thirty to forty-five minutes when headaches follow-ed, but there were many attacks of blind-ness without headaches; the blindness then lasted longer, thirty to forty-five minutes. At times there was numbness of the left hand, and at times there was difficulty in expressing himself and naming objects.

Examination.—1. There were enlarged tortuous vessels over the left parietal and occipital regions, but there was no visible or palpable localized mass of vessels. 2. A bruit was heard over the entire skull, but it was more pronounced in the left parietal and mastoid regions. 3. There was a homonymous hemianopsia to the right. 4. A roentgenogram of the skull showed a greatly enlarged left middle men-ingeal artery directed backward to the left occipital region. This involved only the posterior branch of the middle meningeal artery, the anterior branches being normal. 5. There was a small diffuse area of calci-fiication in the depths of the parietal lobe.

Operation.—On Dec. 30, 1944 both mid-dle meningeal vessels in the parietal region were ligated.

The patient returned because of con-tinued headaches and a second operation was performed, Nov. 1, 1945. The parieto-occipital region on the left side was rong-eured away piecemeal, as in the other cases, until a defect as large as the palm of one's hand was made. There was no undue bleeding from the bone except in the mastoid region, which was extremely bloody; here the bone was stripped and waxed, as in the other cases. The dura was turned back over the entire area; there was intracranial pressure of high grade, the brain bulging tremendously. A large arteriovenous aneurysm covered much of the temporal and parietal lobes; it extended from the inferior surface of the temporal lobe, covered in lesser degree the parietal lobe and emerged at the mastoid region, where the dural and ex-tracranial connections were made.

Subsequent Course.—The patient has just left the hospital. His headaches had ceased; relief of the intracranial pressure was due to the large decompression.

CASE 8. A white woman, aged thirty-one, was referred to me by Dr. Charles Wainright, of Baltimore. Her first com-plaint was dimness of vision, beginning six years before and occurring only at times, but it had been so disturbing that an ophthalmologist was consulted. At this time she was said to have had bilateral papilledema and was referred to a neuro-surgeon, who on three occasions attempted injection of air via the ventricles and the spinal canal, but without successful filling of the ventricular system. Following these procedures, headaches first appeared and were attributed by her to the punctures. The headaches had been confined to the left side. There was a sensation of fulness and a dull aching, and both were practical-ly continuous, though with variations in degree. Injections of histamine did not influence the headaches. She had had two hospital admissions to Dr. Wainwright's service, June 30, 1943 and July 18, 1945. Since her first admission she had had four convulsions; three of these were in rapid succession.

Examination.—The patient was well developed and well nourished. The only significant finding was a homonymous hemianopsia for form and color on the right side. On three occasions the Wasser-mann test of the blood elicited a positive reaction, and, on the assumption that there was a cerebral syphilitic process, she had received antisyphilitic treatment for eighteen months.

The roentgenogram showed bilaterally symmetric, large posterior branches of the middle meningeal arteries; these were di-rected backward toward the occipital region and were considered pathognomonic of an arteriovenous aneurysm of the dura. Following this interpretation, auscultation disclosed a murmur over most of the head but of greatest intensity over the parieto-occipital region and more on the left side. No mass could be felt, but after the head was shaved, preparatory to operation, a soft boggy mass was palpable mesial to the left mastoid; this pulsated strongly, and there was a thrill. There were no intra-cranial calcifications and no evidence of porosity of the bone in the roentgenogram.

The patient had been extremely emotion-al. She "cried every day" and after a "good cry the headache was always better." But a psychoneurotic headache would not have been localized to one side of the head.

Operation.—On July 26, 1945, a semicircular flap of scalp was turned back in the parieto-occipital region. Bleeding from the bone was furious; dozens of spurting vessels were waxed after the bone had been scraped. As in the preceding cases, a bone flap could not be considered, because of the excessive vascularity. This area of skull was rongeured away picemeal until dura, about 5 by 5 cm., was uncovered. The middle meningeal trunks were large, and these and numerous spurting branches in the membrane were thrombosed with the electrocautery. The bone was quickly waxed after each bite was removed. A small opening was made in the dura, and a small dural flap was begun but not completed because of bleeding. Large vessels of an arteriovenous aneurysm covered the brain. The exposure was too small to determine the arterial connections of the aneurysm.

CASE 9. A youth, aged nineteen, was referred to me by Dr. M. Douglas, of Harrisburg, Pa., Aug 29, 1933, because of a midline pulsating swelling on the forehead. (This case was reported by Brock and Dyke [1932], but before the operations.)

Present Illness.—The father had noticed a bean-sized swelling at the root of the nose when the boy was two or three years old. The tumor had grown slowly and steadily, and when the boy was six it was the size of a thumb and was then known to pulsate. Aside from a rushing noise in the head, there had been no symptoms. There was an indefinite history of a bump on the head when the boy was two, but the parents could not suggest a definite relationship to the onset of the tumor. The patient had never had convulsions.

Examination.—The tumor was in the exact midline of the forehead and extended from the hair line to the bridge of the nose; it measured 5 cm. in length and 3.5 cm. in width and was elevated about 2.5 cm. It had a bluish tinge and pulsated strongly, and a pronounced thrill was imparted to the palpating finger. At the bridge of the nose the swelling was not so high but extended to the inner canthus of the eye and gave the impression of a rather wide nose and of the eyes being farther apart than normal. There were small telangiectases over the eyelids and some on the face.

Pressure on either internal carotid artery did not eliminate the pulsation. On palpation, one had the impression of entwining vessels.

On auscultation, a murmur was heard over the mass and over the whole head and down both sides of the neck. The only positive neurologic findings were (1) general constriction of the fields of both eyes, (2) nasal hemianopsia on the left, (3) left homonymous hemianopsia for blue only and (4) reduction of visual acuity on the left to 20/50; the visual acuity on the right was 20/20.

The roentgenogram showed multiple thin, straight and curved calcified linear shadows, suggesting plaques, in walls of blood vessels. The frontal bone was extremely thin.

Impression.—The intracranial calcifications and the partial homonymous hemianopsia made an intracranial lesion certain. And since the extracranial lesion was an arteriorvenous aneurysm, it was practically certain that the intracranial lesion would be of the same character.

First Operation (Aug. 30, 1933).—A left anterior craniotomy, exposing the frontal lobe and extending close to the longitudinal sinus, was performed. The bone flap was extremely bloody; this had been anticipated because of the large middle meningeal artery shown in the roentgenogram. When the dura was turned back, an arteriovenous aneurysm so completely covered the entire exposure that little brain tissue was visible. One enormous vessel, pink from arterial blood, skirted the posterior part of the exposure and curved forward toward the tip of the frontal lobe. A second vessel, of similar size, curved backward toward the temporal lobe, where it was lost to view. These two vessels were much the largest vessels I have ever seen in the brain. They were as large as one's little finger and pulsated violently. The walls were fairly thick but not so much as those of an artery. Numerous large coiled vessels covered the frontal lobe. Three large vessels crossed to the longitudinal sinus and were thrombosed with the electrocautery and divided. A mass of vessels extended to the tip of the frontal lobe but could not be traced through the bone, i. e., to connect with the aneurysm on the forehead.

The left frontal lobe was then elevated and the internal carotid artery exposed and isolated. Perhaps half a dozen fair-sized crossing vessels of the aneurysm were thrombosed and divided before the carotid artery was reached; all were in the neighborhood of the carotid artery and completely hid it from view. The internal carotid artery was the largest I have seen before or since and was only slightly smaller than the enormous vessels on the surface of the aneurysm. The anterior cerebral artery, at least twice as large as normal, was doubly clipped and divided and the ends coagulated with the cautery; four large branches of this vessel extending to the right side were also thrombosed and divided. It was our belief that the arterial supply of the aneurysm was from the anterior cerebral artery, and it was our plan to remove the arterial component as completely as possible. This interpretation of the arterial supply may or may not have been correct. However, after these ligations the pulsation in the large trunks in the aneurysm ceased. These huge vessels on the surface were then coagulated with the cautery and were largely obliterated. This could not have been attempted during their pulsation; they would surely have ruptured. It was also noted after the operation that the pulsation in the extracranial aneurysm was absent. On the following day, however, a faint pulsation had returned, and it steadily increased. Whether this temporary cessation of pulsation resulted from the absence of pulsation in the intracranial aneurysm or from the cutting of the middle meningeal artery when the bone flap was made cannot be stated. Perhaps both may have been responsible. Certainly the middle meningeal artery supplied the aneurysm directly through the skull. No actual continuity could be established between the intracranial and the extracranial aneurysms, and it is difficult to believe that such a communication was possible with the skull intact. However, this is only an impression, which may or may not be correct.

Postoperative Course.—The patient's recovery was uneventful. He returned ten months later for removal of the extracranial aneurysm on the forehead. This was somewhat though not much smaller than before operation.

Second Operation (June 20, 1934).— The mass was exised through a midline incision. Four fair-sized vessels, with thin walls but with arterial pulsation, came through the bone into the aneurysm; these were thrombosed and the bone scraped and waxed. The aneurysm was made up of coils of small vessels.

Third Operation (June 27, 1934).—Since a fulness remained at each side of the nose and extended toward the inner canthus of the eyes, an additional extirpation of these portions was thought to be indicated to improve the appearance. On June 27 this was done on the left side, but the procedure was so bloody that the operation on the other side was not done. I am still perplexed to explain the existence of such a vascular mass after the aneurysm on the forehead had been excised.

Subsequent Course.—The patient was discharged from the hospital July 18. The extracranial aneurysm did not return.

On Jan. 2, 1937, two and one-half years later, his death was reported "cause unknown." Six months before death, convulsions had developed.

In retrospect and with a more extended experience with these lesions, I doubt that the operative attack on an intracranial aneurysm of this type is indicated. It is extremely unlikely that the entire arterial supply of such an aneurysm could ever be completely eliminated, because of the extensive circulation. In none of the other cases has the intracranial aneurysm been molested, and in only 2 has it been exposed.

COMMENT

This group of aneurysms, together with those reported on in the literature, indicates clearly that there are two sources of origin. Most of them arise congenitally, but many develop in the later years of life from trauma and without a preexisting vascular lesion. In only one of our nine cases is the aneurysm known to be traumatic in origin (case 1). In case 2 it may or may not be of traumatic origin, but it is more probably from a congenital nevus, though it was not recognized. In the remaining seven cases they are known to be congenital in origin. In the traumatic cases, it can only be said that as a result of the injury and arteriovenous connection has been established between small arteries and veins. Although there are certain sites of predilection for the congenital aneurysms, particularly the scalp and the back of the ear, they may occur almost anywhere.

In this series of seven cases of arteriovenous aneurysms of the scalp, it is clearly shown in all that the arterial component is derived from the middle meningeal artery and therefore that the arterial blood comes through the skull from the cranial chamber. This statement does not mean that all such aneurysms have intracranial connections, but it does indicate the frequency of this source of arterial supply and, I think, it also indicates that this is the usual if not the sole origin. This intracranial arterial supply explains why ligations of any and all the arteries in the scalp make no impression on the pulsation or the size of the extracranial aneurysm and also why ligation of the external carotid artery does reduce the pulsation and size to some extent. The external carotid artery cuts off blood supply from the middle meningeal artery. When both external carotid arteries are ligated—and this can be done with impunity—the pulsation of the aneurysm is completely stopped, but the effect is only transient because of the extensive collateral circulation that obtains.

There are two types of arteriovenous aneurysms of the scalp (Fig. 1): (1) that in which one, two or perhaps more preformed genuine arteries come through the skull and enter a primary congenital angiomatous mass on the exterior (in case 3 the arteries passed through the parietal foramens, one on each side) and (2) that in which numerous thin-walled vessels penetrate the skull and from an arteriovenous bed without a primary angiomatous mass in the scalp (cases 4, 5, 6, 7, 8 and 9 are of this type). In the latter group the arteriovenous bed in the scalp is smaller; at least in none of these cases has it approached the size of the beds in the first group, and in one case it was demonstrable only after the head was shaved. In five of the six cases in this group an arteriovenous component of the aneurysm was also in the cerebral

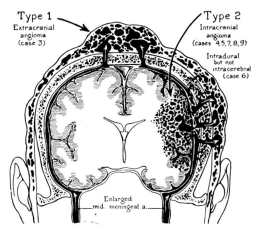

Fig. 1 Diagram showing the two types of extracranial aneurysms, both arising from the middle meningeal artery. In type 1 the extracranial aneurysm is supplied by preformed arteries coming through the skull and entering an angiomatous mass, and in type 2 there are numerous branches of the middle meningeal artery penetrating the skull over a wide area and forming the angiomatous mass, and in type 2 there are numerous branches of the middle not always extends into the cerebral hemisphere.

hemisphere. Whether or not this ever obtains in the first group cannot be stated; it has never been demonstrated, and because of the great size of the extracranial aneurysms my guess would be that there are no intracranial components. Both types are prone to have a bilateral arterial supply from the middle meningeal arteries, but in some it is unilateral and in most it is greater on one side than on the other. In the second group, the vessels penetrating the bone are so thin walled that they are not recognizable. When the galea is turned back, they rupture at the bone and are controlled by waxing. The bleeding is so furious that wax must be applied quickly and in large amount. In the first group the vessels were preformed and the firm walls permitted their isolation and control by ligatures. The diffuse vascularity of the bone in the second group is similar to that arising from the highly vascularized dura that develops over dural meningiomas.

The perforations in the skull from these

vessels frequently show in the roentgenogram, and in one case the affected region of the skull appeared moth eaten from the vascular perforations. Moreover, in these six cases the great arterial varices in the dura were seen after removal of the bone; in every case (except case 7) the bleeding was too severe to warrant turning down a bone flap; instead, the bone was removed piecemeal with rongeurs. In six of the seven cases the grooves in the oversized middle meningeal arteries were strickingly shown in the roentgenogram and were directed backward to the vascular bed in the skull. In all but two of our cases the aneurysm was in the parietooccipital region (in case 7 it was in the temporal lobe), and it is the enlargement of the posterior branch (normally inconspicuous) that is all-important in the roentgenologic diagnosis of this lesion. In 5 cases, both the right and the left meningeal arteries were about equally enlarged, although the size of the extracranial aneurysm varied on the two sides, and always the hemianoposia indicatve of the intracerebral aneurysm was unilateral.

In five of these cases there is proof that the brain as also involved in the aneurysm, for in each there was a right homonymous hemianopsia, which could be explained only by the invasion of the visual area in the occipital or temporal lobes by the aneurysm directly overlying it. In three cases (cases 5, 7 and 9) numerous calcifications in the brain indicated the extension of the aneurysm into the subjacent brain. These have been linear in two cases and diffuse in the third; the linear shadows suggest calcification of walls of blood vessels. The fact that epileptic attacks have been reported in at least 6 cases in the literature, one of Clairmont's (1908), one of Elkin's (1923) and four of ours, is suggestive but not conclusive evidence of a cerebral extension of the lesion. In one of our patients (case 6) in which the cerebral hemisphere was exposed, the seizures were not due to extension of the aneurysm into the brain but to three dense bony plaques of

congenital origin. Moreover, these plaques were at a distance from the site of the aneurysm in the dura and not subjacent, as in case 5. Since congenital lesions are not infrequently multiple and of different types, an intracranial extension of an aneurysm cannot be accepted purely on the basis of convulsions; the aneurysm may or may not be responsible. The five cases with right homonymous hemianopsia, however, could leave no doubt concerning the intracerebral extension of the aneurysm and of the convulsions when they were present. The intracranial aneurysm was demonstrated in three cases at operation. In the case of 1 patient with an enormous intracranial aneurysm, there had never been convulsions; he was nineteen years old. However, convulsions finally developed before his death, two and one half years after operation.

The large middle meningeal arteries directed toward the location of the angioma have been commented on by Clairmont (1908),[8] Elkin (1923)[1] and Rundle (1938),[14] and all considered the possibility of this source of the arterial blood. Elkin and Cushing, who operated on the patient, concluded it to be "a mistaken idea," and in a recent communication to me Elkin still maintained this view. Elkin stated that Guerin (1870) suggested the possibility that the lesion might extend intracranially. In looking at Cushing's operative sketch in the paper by Elkin it should be perfectly clear that the arterial blood does come through the bone and therefore from the middle meningeal artery, because the central mass of the aneurysm is encircled by the incision and could therefore get no possible arterial blood from the scalp; since the vessels still bled briskly, the blood had to come through the skull. Moreover, Cushing did not separate the vascular mass from the skull but was content to make numerous ties of the protruding vessels. In such circumstances, a cure, if it resulted, could have come only from extension of thrombus formation resulting from the ligatures, a not impossible outcome. In a recent letter Elkin stated that the patient was cured. A photograph of the patient after operation, however, still shows a swelling at the original site; Elkin explained this as edema of the tissues.

It is difficult to believe that such large and misdirected middle meningeal vessels do not carry pathognomonic significance concerning the arterial supply of the aneurysm, and in our direct exposure of these vessels in the seven cases this conclusion is inescapable. In one case (case 8) the diagnosis was made solely on this finding in the roentgenograms, and this led to the discovery of the murmur and the extracranial aneurysm.

It is worthy of comment that all these patients have been highly nervous, and after cure of the headaches and the head noises the nervous condition, while improved, has continued in most cases.

A review of the relative size of the extracranial component in the seven cases of arteriovenous aneurysm of the scalp leads us to believe that the size of the extracranial aneurysm is probably inversely proportional to the size of the intracranial component of the aneurysm, i.e., when the extracranial aneurysm is small, the intracranial portion is extremely large and when the extracranial part is large the intracranial part, if any, is small. This has at least been true in the cases reported here.

The Treatment

In recent years, with improvement hemostasis, most of the patients have been treated by extirpation, with little mortality. Even in the past century there were many successful extirpations, usually, but not always, in two or three stages. During the past century, however, many aneurysms were injected with corroding solutions or treated by galvanic punctures, with a surprising number of cures. The end result was attained by thrombosis of the vessels, after which the mass gradually disappeared. However, in most instances there was only improvement and frequently only for a time; one or more repetitions of the treatments brought the final disappearance of the lesion. In many cases severe infection followed the injections, and this at times induced the cure by thrombosis; but a rather large number of deaths resulted from the infections. Kummell (1883) [28] reported six deaths in fifteen collected cases in which injections had been used. The fact that severe "inflammation" helped the disappearance of the aneurysm was even recognized in the period before Lister's discovery of the cause of infection. Cures by injections are still occasionally reported. Fite (1933) [25] reported a cure by injections of boiling water. Patey (1942) [16] tied both external carotid arteries and cured the aneurysm by injections. Klass (1942), [29] using sclerosing injections, brought about the complete disappearance of a large aneurysm involving the ear; had the mass been extirpated, two thirds of the ear would have been sacrificed. Davies-Colley (1940) [15] reported a remarkable cure of a big aneurysm of the forehead and covering the bridge of the nose and an eyelid; the cosmetic result was doubtless better than by operation, since no scar remained; in another of Davies-Colley's cases, the patient died twenty-eight hours after an injection. One cannot deny the value of injections, and doubtless in experienced hands the risk is not great; moreover, there are times when the cosmetic results will be better. In safe hands, however, and certainly for aneurysms back of the hair line, surgical removal is better and safer.

During the nineteenth century, ligation of the common carotid artery, even on both sides, attained a great vogue. It is difficult to understand why the common carotid arteries should have been ligated instead of the external carotid arteries, from which the blood supply is derived and the ligation of which is harmless. The summarized results of Heine (1869) [2] and Korte (1880) [5] show this procedure to have been almost routine. The size of the aneurysm was always reduced by the ligations, but within a short time the pulsation had returned and the lesion continued to grow.

As a matter of fact, ligation of the common carotid artery can carry less effect on these aneurysms than ligation of the external carotid artery because the return flow of blood from the internal to the external carotid artery quickly overcomes the transient effect of closure of the common carotid artery. And it should again be noted that a number of hemiplegias and deaths followed ligations of the common carotid arteries. Ligation of any of the large arteries in the neck probably never cures an aneurysm and can improve it for only a short time. Thrombosis could conceivably result from such ligations and thus produce a cure, but so many failures are recorded that one is led to suspect that thrombosis occurs mainly through the venous components of the aneurysm. In our case, ligations of the external carotid arteries plus one large vein in the scalp produced widespread thrombosis that cured all the emissary vessels from the aneurysm and even reduced the angiomatous mass.

One can only marvel at the results attained by surgical treatment before Lister made open operation safe and at a time when hemostasis was far less secure. The cure of a large aneurysm of this type in 1829, by Benjamin Brodie, one of the great names in English surgery, provides most interesting reading of one of the earliest cases treated by surgery. This patient had been seen by Sir Ashley Cooper, probably the most famous surgeon in the world at that time. He had treated her with compression bandages, without result. Since the lesion was growing steadily and causing much discomfort, he yielded gracefully to Brodie's suggestion of a surgical attack that Brodie had conceived. Brodie's ingenious procedure was to pass two large curved needles at right angles through the skin and under the tumor, grazing the bone; by traction on the needles the aneurysm was elevated, and a heavy suture was then drawn around the skin beneath the needles. By drawing the suture tight, the tumor was strangulated at the base. This procedure was repeated three days later and again on the fifth day. The mass sloughed away, healed by granulation and did not recur. The accompanying copy (Fig. 2) of a drawing from Sir Charles Bell's "Surgical Observations" (1816) [30] shows the use of a tenaculum to elevate a tumor and is similar in principle to Brodie's needles.

The case reported by Warren, and Boston (1867), [17] almost forty years after Brodie's operation, is also noteworthy and the tumor was treated in much the same man-

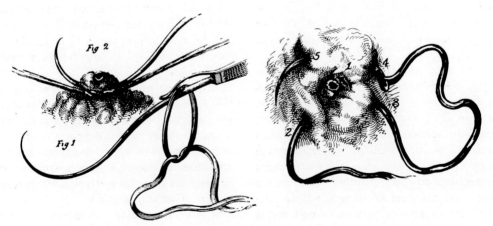

Fig. 2. Drawing taken from Sir Charles Belle, 1816, [30] showing (*a*) method of elevating vascular mass with the tenaculum and the ligature placed around it and (*b*) method of deep sutures to constrict the vascular area that is bleeding. By these two methods, Benjamin Brodie made a remarkable cure of a large arteriovenous aneurysm of the forehead in 1829. Considering the fact that this was over one hundred years ago, it is a remarkable cure.

ner. It was a case of one of the extremely large aneurysms and much like our case 1.

Included in the reports of Heine and Korte (to 1880) are records of ten cases of extirpation of the aneurysm, with cures; in six of these, both common carotid arteries were ligated after intervals of several days, and, curiously, none of the patients died, although there were two deaths following ligations of the common carotid artery. The first ligation of the external carotid artery (instead of the common carotid artery) for this purpose was probably performed by Maisoneuve (1851).

At the present time there should be little hazard in the extirpation of these aneurysms because of better hemostasis in the scalp; by the use of the electrocautery, bleeding vessels in the central mass can be coagulated. Despite the great size of the radiating, pulsating vessels, they may be compressed by the fingers on each side of the incision and the ends sealed by turning the galea over them with clamps. The central mass, which is the only part of the aneurysm that needs extirpation, is then isolated and can be quickly excised from the skull, from which the vessels enter, or the mass can be scraped off the skull with a periosteal elevator and the mouths of the bleeding vessels closed with bone wax. After removal of the central mass, the large veins that are distributed over the scalp collapse and subsequently become inconspicuous.

The type of treatment of these aneurysms depends on whether or not the arterial coil is (1) extracranial or (2) intracranial; if extracranial, removal of the mass will produce a cure; if intracranial, removal of the group of vessels emerging from the skull will cure the extracranial aneurysm, but the primary coils in the dura will continue to cause headache. For the cure of the intracranial angiomatous mass, a semicircular flap of scalp is turned down so as to expose the entire group of vessels emerging from the bone in the involved area. The bone is scraped and waxed, or as in the other group, when the ar-

terial supply to the scalp is eliminated the pulsating vessels in the scalp will collapse.

The excision of an angiomatous mass (coil of vessels) that is entirely extracranial (as case 3) is relatively simple. This can be done with (1) a semicircular flap around the angiomatous mass or (2) a straight incision over its center. In either case the mass of vessels is isolated from the scalp and dissected from the skull or scraped from the skull and the entering vessels waxed. Should the tumor invade the skin (as in case 3), a straight incision is preferable because the affected area of skin should be excised. Since the skin is redundant, the edges can be brought together without leaving a defect in the scalp. In ten of the cases collected from the literature a flap has been used and in five a straight incision, at times with a counter-incision (Parker, 1904). On the whole, the flap is easier, but if the aneurysm is over the forehead a straight incision will leave a smaller scar.

Ligation of one or both external carotid arteries is hardly advisable and is not necessary for an aneurysm in the scalp, since the bleeding is not difficult to control. Ligations of the common or the internal carotid arteries are never indicated and are strongly contraindicated. Ligation of both the external and the internal carotid arteries on one side, however, is essential for such aneurysms as those in the eyelids, as presented in case 1; both vessels contributed to its arterial supply because of the extensive collateral circulation between these vessels in the orbit. It is doubtful that this lesion could have been extirpated without these ligations. And the better time to complete the removal of an aneurysm of this type is immediately after the arteries have been ligated; delay means return of some pulsation.

If an extracranial aneurysm has been completely removed it probably will not recur. If only partially removed, it will recur unless a fortunate and hardly to be expected progressive thrombosis obliterates the aneurysmal mass.

It is not clear how far one should go in the treatment of the aneurysms with the vascular coils in the dura, from which the aneurysms of the brain and the scalp are supplied. Certainly nothing can be accomplished toward removal of the intracerebral aneurysm; extensive coagulation of the varices of the middle meningeal arteries has been done in these cases, and, I believe, with benefit. Whether or not the extracranial aneurysm would recur unless the dural vessels are also obliterated is not certain, though I should suspect that it might well do so. It seems hardly possible that the headaches would be cured without elimination of the dural vessels. It has seemed advisable to attack the dural vessels in order to increase the probabilities of success. This entails practically no risk, but it does leave a defect in the skull (which, of course, can be corrected later if desired); the skull must be removed piecemeal, since a bone flap would not be safe with such profuse bleeding. In no other condition is the skull so vascular, not even with dural meningiomas.

It might well appear that the large intracerebral aneurysm would be the source of the headache. This was true in case 7, but many similar arteriovenous aneurysms, without dural connections, have been found at operation and have not caused headache.[31] Moreover, removal of the dural and the extradural vessels does stop the headache in most instances.

It is also difficult to determine whether the aneurysms should be attacked on one or both sides when they are known to be bilateral. My judgment has been to operate on one side only when the headache or noise is unilateral and to operate on both sides when the symptoms are bilateral.

SUMMARY

Seven, and probably eight, of the nine cases of arteriovenous aneurysm of the scalp and face presented are of congenital origin; in one the aneurysm followed trauma late in life, and there was no known preexisting angiomatous lesion. This per-

centage of congenital aneurysms is approximately in accord with the incidence of such lesions from the cases in the literature. Similar aneurysms in the integument occur elsewhere over the body but less frequently than in the scalp.

In all the 7 cases of aneurysms in the scalp, the arterial supply was traced to the middle meningeal arteries and was therefore of intracranial derivation. In 1 the arterial supply was through two arteries, one on either side, and continuous with the greatly enlarged middle meningeal arteries through the parietal foramens (roentgenologically). In the other 6 there were numerous branches perforating the bone on both sides and derived from great primary plexuses of vessels in the dura (the middle meningeal arteries). In these cases, the roentgenograms disclosed greatly widened grooves of the posterior branches of the middle meningeal arteries, and these were directed to the parieto-occipital region, in hich the extracranial arteriovenous aneurysms appeared. In 1 case the anterior branch of the middle meningeal was enlarged and supplied a frontal aneurysm of the scalp.

Three of the aneurysms (all with hemianopsia) were demonstrated at operation to be in the brain: one in the frontal and temporal, one in the temporal and parietal and one in the parietal and occipital lobes. In two other cases with hemianopsia, the brain was not exposed, but intracerebral aneurysm was doubtless the cause of the hemianopsia.

In four cases, there were occasional convulsions, indicating a cerebral lesion, but in 1 of these the convulsions were not due to the aneurysm but to another congenital lesion, i.e., three closely related bony spicules in the sensory leg area. These aneurysms, therefore, may involve the dura and the brain, in addition to the scalp; the arterial supply has been from the middle meningeal artrey in all of the cases. Although in all except 1 of our cases the extracranial aneurysms were bilateral, many of the cases assembled from the literature involved only one side of the scalp.

The safest and best treatment of the aneurysms when an extracranial primary angiomatous mass exists is extirpation of the central mass; the large pulsating veins that radiate from the mass disappear when the source of the arterial blood is removed. When the primary angiomatous mass is in the dura, the vessels penetrating the bone should be waxed after the scalp has been stripped from the affected area of bone. It is probably better in these cases to expose and coagulate the dural varices and to ligate one or both (if bilateral) of the middle meningeal arteries.

Many good results have been obtained by injecting sclerosing solutions into the central mass; there may be times when this has an advantage, i.e., when the aneurysm is over the forehead and a scar would be averted or when excision of one in the ear would mean sacrificing part of the ear. Injections are probably more dangerous and are less certain than operation when the latter is performed by a good surgeon; cures from injections are due to thromboses that propagate from the venous into the arterial component of the aneurysm. In the presence of an intracranial aneurysm, sclerosing injections might well be hazardous.

Ligation of the external (not the common) carotid artery is usually not necessary as a preliminary procedure to reduce the arterial content of aneurysms of the scalp. In our case, however, the extirpation of the aneurysm in the eyelids would have been hazardous without ligations of both the internal and the external carotid arteries, both of which contributed to its pulsation because of the extensive anastomoses. Ligations of the arteries in the scalp are useless because they do not supply the aneurysm.

REFERENCES

[1]Elkin, D. C.: Cirsoid Aneurysm of the Scalp. *Ann. Surg., 80:*332, 1924.

[2]Heine, C.: Ueber Angioma arteriole racemosum aus Kopfes und dessen Behandlung. *Prag. Vrtljschr., 3:*1, 1869.

[3]Brodie, B. C.: An Account of An Aneurysm by Anastomosis of the Forehead. *Tr. Med.-Chir. Soc., 15:*177, 1829.

[4]Mussey, R. D.: Aneurysmal Tumors upon the Ear, Treated by Ligation of Both Carotids. *Am. J. M. Sc., 26:*333, 1853.

[5]Korte, W.: Beitrag zur Lehre vom Angioma arteriale racemosum. *Deutsche Ztschr. Chir., 13:* 24, 1880.

[6]Mulleh, H.: Ein Fall von arteriellem Rankenangioma des Kopfes. *Beitr. klin. Chir., 8:*79, 1891.

[7]Berger, H.: Die Extirpation des Angioma arteriale racemosum aus Kopfes. *Beitr. klin. Chir., 22:* 129, 1898.

[8]Clairmont, P.: Zur Behandlung des Angiome racemosum. *Arch. klin. Chir., 85:*549, 1908.

[9]Kepler, M.: Zur Behandlung des Aneurysma arteriole racemosum. *Beitr. klin. Chir., 78:*521, 1912.

[10]Schlochetzki, H.: Ein Beitrag zur Pathologis und Klinik der Rankenangiome der Kopfschrootte. *Beitr. klin. Chir., 157:*35, 1933.

[11]Parker, R.: Cirsoid Aneurysm of the Forehead Treated by Free Incision and Extirpation. *Brit. M. J., 1:*304, 1904.

[12]Searby, H.: Cirsoid Aneurysm of the Scalp. *Australian & New Zealand J. Surg., 1:*209, 1931.

[13]Clunie, T.: Cirsoid Aneurysm of the Scalp. *Brit. M. J., 2:*1183, 1936.

[14]Rundle, F.: A Case of Cirsoid Aneurysm of the Scalp. *Brit. J. Surg., 25:*872, 1938.

[15]Davies-Colley, R.: Cirsoid Aneurysm. *Guy's Hosp. Rep., 90:*134, 1940–1941.

[16]Patey, D. H.: A Case of Cirsoid Aneurysm of the Scalp. *Brit. J. Surg., 29:*290, 1942.

[17]Warren, J. M.: *Surgical Observations with Cases and Operations.* Boston, Ticknor & Fields, 1867, p. 451.

[18]Mynter, H.: Extensive Cirsoid Aneurysm of Scalp Obliterated by Multiple Ligatures. *Ann. Surg., 11:*93, 1890.

[19]Meyer, W.: Excision of Cirsoid Aneurysm of the Temporal Region. *New York M. J., 56:*214, 1892.

[20]Forbes, W. S.: Successful Treatment of a Large Cirsoid Aneurysm of the Scalp. *M. News, Philadelphia., 66:*663, 1895.

[21]Coley, W. B.: Cirsoid Aneurysm Successfully Treated by Excision After Ligation of the External Carotid. *Ann. Surg., 34:*414, 1901.

[22]Beck, C.: On an Aggravated Case of Aneurysma Racemosum. *Ann. Surg., 38:*496, 1903.

[23]Judd, E. S.: Cirsoid Aneurysm. *St. Paul M. J., 18:* 48, 1916.

[24]Matas, R.: Cirsoid Aneurysm of the Face and Scalp. *South. M. J., 26:*820, 1933.

[25]Fite, P.: Cirsoid Aneurysm of the Scalp. *South M. J., 26:*816, 1933.

[26]Brock, S., and Dyke, C. G.: Venous and Arteriovenous Angiomas of the Brain. *Bull. Neurol. Inst. New York, 2:*247, 1932.

[27]Meleney, F. L.: A Pathological Study of a Case of Cirsoid Aneurysm. *Surg., Gynec. & Obst., 36:* 547, 1923.

[28]Kummell, H.: Zur Behandlung des Angioma arteriole racemosum. *Arch. klin. Chir., 28:*194, 1883.

[29]Klass, A. A.: Cirsoid Aneurysm Affecting Auditory Auricle. *Canad. M.A.J., 46:*370, 1942.

[30]Bell, C.: Surgical Observations, London, Longman [and others], 1816.

[31]Dandy, W. E.: Arteriovenous Aneurysms of the Brain. *Arch. Surg., 17:*190, 1928.

LXXVII

RESULTS FOLLOWING BANDS AND LIGATURES ON THE HUMAN INTERNAL CAROTID ARTERY*

In the surgical treatment of intracranial aneurysms it is at times necessary for the safety of the cerebral circulation to partially occlude the internal carotid artery as a preliminary step before total closure of the artery. For this purpose a band of fascia lata is preferable, although a band of dura or the fascial covering of the temporal muscle is equally effective. A partial ligation is necessary when the Matas test (digital pressure on the internal carotid for ten minutes) induces signs or symptoms of cerebral anemia and, therefore, indicates an inadequate collateral circulation at the circle of Willis. Reduction in the lumen of this artery (by a band) to one-half, or more, forces the collateral channels at the circle of Willis to enlarge and carry an additional load to the brain. In a week or ten days the resulting increased blood flow through the circle of Willis is sufficient to permit total ligation of the internal carotid in the neck, or intracranially, or both. In a group of patients in whom a band has been placed for this purpose and total ligation has later been necessary, the segmant of the artery, including the band, has, at that time, been excised for gross and microscopic study, principally to learn what happens to the affected portion of the artery and to the band. Since the band is always applied just above the bifurcation of the common carotid it has been necessary to include in the resected segment of the internal carotid a small part of both the common carotid and the external carotid arteries.

The specimens for study are (1) those following partial ligation of the artery (six cases) (Fig. 1); (2) following total ligation of the internal carotid (one case), and total ligation of the common carotid (one case) (Fig. 2); and (3) a single case following ligation of the intracranial carotid by a silver clip (Fig. 2).

(1) Specimens following *partial* occlusion of the internal carotid by fascial bands (six cases):

There are six of these. In all of them the lumen of the internal carotid has remained patent, though greatly reduced in size. The intervals of time between application of the bands and removal of the specimens at operation were, sixteen, eighteen, twenty-five, twenty-seven, fifty-eight and fifty-eight days. In only one was there any indication of a thrombus within the lumen; in this case the thrombus was a tiny non-obstructing caruncle-like fibrous nodule. This patient had highly sclerosed arteries and a high grade of hypertension. Whether this condition of the arteries or the band was responsible for the thrombus is impossible to determine, though it would appear logical to assume that the band was at least a determining factor because the thrombus was directly under it. However, the intima was not infiltrated with cellular reaction.

In all cases there was an excessive bulbous mass of fibrous tissue about the bands. The size of the swelling increases with time, and at the end of 58 days was perhaps four or five times larger than the original volume of the fascial band. In the specimens of 16 and 18 days the fibrous mass is about double the size of the original band.

In all specimens the bands show marked fragmentation. Under the microscope the integrity of the bands is in large part lost in the gross and they are difficult or im-

*Reprinted from the *Annals of Surgery*, 123:3, March, 1946.

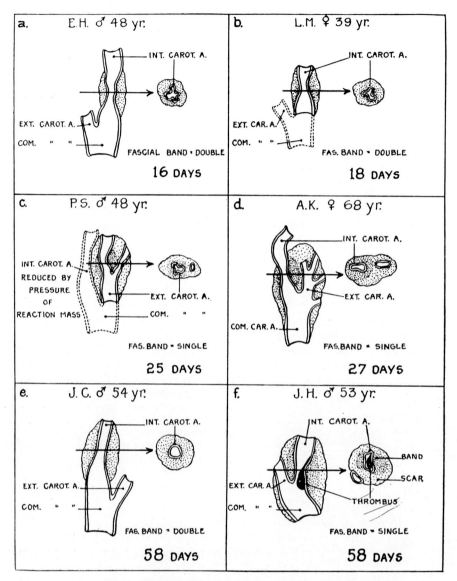

Fig.1. Showing partial ligation of the artery.

possible to delineate in the older speci-mens. There appears to be a larger mass of fibrous tissue about the single than about the double bands, and is probably due to the greater and more rapid disintegration of the single fascial layer from the arterial pulsation.

A rather surprising histologic finding is the absence of any reaction throughout the intima of the arteries, there being no tendency to vascular rupture.

In five of the six specimens the cross-section of the vessel shows marked wrink-ling of the inner lining (in the gross), but in one specimen (fifty-eight days) the lu-men was almost perfectly circular (Fig. 1).

(2) Thrombus formation within the carotids following *total* ligations (two cases) (Fig. 2):

In one case the internal carotid had been ligated two years earlier (elsewhere), and in another the common carotid had been ligated six months before (elsewhere). In each, the vessel was thrombosed for a con-

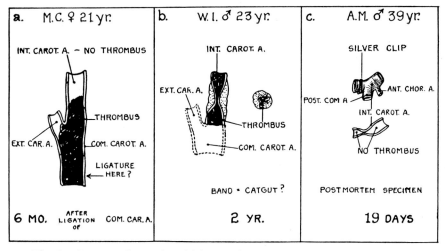

Fig. 2. Two specimens in which (a) the common carotid artery; and (b) the internal carotid artery had been ligated, elsewhere, six months and two years, respectively, before removal of the segment of the carotid arteries; and (c) the results following the application of the silver clip to the intracranial portion of the internal carotid artery 19 days after its application. It shows absence of thrombus on either side of the clip. The extent of the intra-arterial thrombus following the total ligation is shown as far as could be determined from the examination at operation.

siderable distance. The extent was determined by palpation of the arteries and by opening the internal carotid. In the case of the previously-ligated *internal* carotid, the common and the external carotid arteries pulsated freely but the internal carotid was thrombosed higher than our exposure; the upper limit of the thrombus could, therefore, not be determined (Fig 2b). In the case of total ligation of the *common* carotid six months earlier, the common carotid was totally occluded lower than our exposure and about two centimeters into the internal carotid: when the internal carotid was opened at this level there was bleeding from the cranial end but none from the cardiac end, which was full of firm thrombus; the external carotid was patent up to the bifurcation (Fig. 2a). In this case there was extensive new endotheliallined vascular spaces within the thrombus, but there is no evidence that they were continuous and the absence of bleeding proves that they were not.

It is clear from these two cases that the extent of an intra-arterial thrombus resulting from total ligation of an artery is

variable and unpredictable and is *not*, as has been frequently stated, limited by "the first sizable branch" (the external carotid).

(3) The single specimen taken nineteen days following application of a silver clip to the internal carotid is included because there was no thrombus on either side of the clip (Fig. 2c). This we have observed on at least four other occasions when the site of the clip has been subsequently exposed at a second operation; we were surprised to find the vessel patent both above and below the clip. That a thrombus is consistently absent after the application cannot, of course, be stated without many more observations. However, in a series of thirty-eight intracranial "clippings" of the internal carotid there has never been clinical evidence of cerebral thrombosis. The absence of thrombus formation within the artery in this experiment is exactly the same as the results obtained by Doctor Halsted in a large series of dogs when aluminum bands were used. The flat silver clip is doubtless comparable in its action to that of an aluminum band on the internal carotid in the neck. And

when the greatly reduced size of the intracranial portion of the internal carotid is considered, the size of the silver clip is relatively the same as the larger band in the neck.

TYPES OF BANDS

In 1905, Professor Halsted made extensive studies on the aorta and carotid with bands of different kinds. He gave up fascia lata because it disintegrated rapidly under the pulsation of the vessel. His final choice was an aluminum band for which a specially contrived roller placed the band around the vessel in a cylinder. It was then moulded with the finger until the desired degree of partial constriction or total occlusion was attained. From these studies several fundamental principles for vascular surgery were made, and have since remained unchallenged:

(1) Whether the band is partially or totally occluding there is no thrombus formation within the arterial lumen.

(2) Thrombus formation is due to injury to the intima by ligation (this was known before).

(3) Beneath an aluminum band the vascular wall becomes completely necrotic.

In his earlier experiments (1905) Doctor Halsted stated that under partially constricting bands the wall of the vessel did not become grossly necrotic after ten days. In his last published paper (1924), however, he stated that "the included portion of the wall always dies whether the occlusion is *partial* or *complete.*"

Reid (1916) carried on another series of experimental studies for Doctor Halsted, using bands of various metals, and concluded that the wall of the artery always atrophied beneath the band. This was the investigation that changed Doctor Halsted's opinion on this point. In the earlier experiments he had not made microscopic examinations of the arterial walls.

Matas (1911) used aluminum bands on the big vessels for occlusion of the carotids,

because it could be safely removed if the cerebral circulation should be inadequate. An ordinary ligature would cut through all the coats and, therefore, could not be removed without danger of rupture. He also demonstrated that necrosis of the vessel was not visible until 96 hours after the band had been applied. He has since had occasion to remove the bands from the carotid in several instances, and with return of cerebral function. An interesting case of C. H. Mayo's was referred to by Doctor Matas in this early publication: A patient upon whose carotid a thin tin band had been applied developed cerebral symptoms (loss of vision); he loosened the band but did not remove it; the vision returned and the band healed in place. Doctor Matas emphasized the fact that a ligature could not have been removed.

Since this publication the invaluable Matas test for the efficiency of collateral circulation has been introduced, and when correctly applied, the surgeon no longer guesses but can know with certainty before operation whether or not a total occlusion will be tolerated. Doctor Matas, I think, still uses the metal band on the carotid because of the reputed disintegration of fascia.

Pearse (1932) titled a publication "The Impracticability of Using Fascia for Gradual Occlusion of the Large Arteries," and concluded that at that time Halsted's aluminum band was "the best device today." In a series of experiments upon the aorta of dogs the bands of fascia were found to disintegrate and relax even when six or eight thicknesses were used. In some instances the walls of the artery ruptured beneath the bands (25 per cent). He reasoned that fascial bands were unreliable and dangerous.

Despite the above experimental evidence bands of fascia lata have been used in all of our cases, and without an untoward result of any kind. They are sewn in place at the desired constriction of the artery after the method of Kerr (1925). They have served their purpose with complete satisfaction in a series of 30 cases to date.

The danger of rupture of the internal carotid from a viable tissue is, I think, less than from a metal band. Moreover, they are just as easy to remove if that should be necessary when the constriction has been carried too far. In three of our series the bands have been removed and later replaced with less reduction of the lumen. Complete cerebral function returned in two, and partially in a third.

In the microscopic sections the intima is always viable and unchanged from the normal, *i.e.*, it does not disintegrate as under an aluminum band. There is no doubt that the fascia does disintegrate, even when doubled, but the doubling decidedly delays the fragmentation. However, this probably is not so important in the carotid because there is a greater mass of fibrous tissue about the single bands and is probably roughly proportionate to the disintegration. The volume of connective tissue produced about the band is doubtless an important factor in reinforcing the vessel. Certainly, in no instance has there been any tendency of the lumen to expand. On the contrary, I should guess that the mass of fibrous tissue probably gradually constricted the lumen farther than obtained at the time the band was applied.

Most of the experimental work has been done on the aorta—a very much more severe test for bands than the internal or common carotid. When a band is applied to the aorta there is no other sizable preformed channel by which the arterial load can be diverted to the lower part of the body. The anastomotic channels develop slowly through the dilatation of tiny communicating channels. After the carotid is tied, an increased volume of blood is immediately transferred to the other carotid and thence through the sizable trunks of the circle of Willis, which can quickly enlarge. I should not even suggest that fascial bands would be applicable to the aorta of human beings even when applied in multiple layers: but for the carotids the results are undeniable.

PROGRESSIVE OCCLUSION OF THE LARGE ARTERIES

A method by which a progressive constriction of a large artery could be induced has, until recently at least, been unsuccessful. Doctor Halsted's experimental efforts were originally begun with the hope that a partially occluding band could be still further constricted by a subsequent manipulation of the band by reopening the wound, thus making the final occlusion by steps instead of gradually. All earlier attempts to induce progressive occlusion had been through ligatures or clamps that were left extruding from the wound, and these always became infected, with disastrous results. But Doctor Halsted's bands have not been satisfactory because the wall of the vessel became necrotic.

Pearse (1940) has recently introduced, in experimental studies, a very ingenious method of gradual compression of large vessels which may or may not prove to be the answer. A layer of cellophane is wrapped around the aorta and tied: a violent and extensive cellular reaction (doubtless of chemical origin) engulfs the band and gradually constricts the vessel until it is completely closed. This fibrous mass has been strong enough to prevent rupture of the vessel. Its practicability in human cases has, I think, not been tested. Its use on the carotid artery may or may not be as good as fascia. It could hardly be better. At most, it could only make a subsequent total ligation unnecessary: and to do this would require a certainty in its efficacy which could only be acquired by an extended experience. Fortunately, in the carotid attack a progressive occlusion is not essential for success. Here, again, ligations of the carotid and of the aorta are entirely different problems: what applies to one does not apply to the other. It should also be noted that the reaction to bands of fascia lata is precisely similar to those of cellophane except in degree. The mass of fibrous tissue is, at least, an effective support for the arterial wall and it may, and probably does, cause progressive occlusion of the lumen.

INTRACAROTID THROMBOSIS FOLLOWING BANDS AND LIGATURES

It is very probable, but not certain, that a thrombus always develops in time on either side of a *ligature* on a large arterial trunk. Our two cases are examples. This is doubtless due to injury of the intima, which must always occur. And yet bands of fascia and aluminum, whether partially or totally occluding, appear not to do this. Doctor Halsted's experiments with aluminum bands and ours with fascia are proof of this.*

The development of a thrombus after ligation and its absence following application of a band, are the reasons for a better form of ligation of the internal carotid. When a clot forms in the carotid it may break off and send an embolus into the cerebral arteries, with disastrous results; or the clot may propagate from the site of the ligature and pass directly into the cerebral vessels with the same result. Either of these eventualities is the explanation for the hemiplegias and deaths that occur 12 to 96 hours after carotid ligations. I am certain that they can be avoided either by totally occluding bands of fascia or by ligating *over* a band of fascia. The ligature does not then cut the intima. The latter procedure is probably preferable and more certain. One should never trust to a ligature directly applied to a large artery.

That injury to the intima of a large artery was responsible for thrombus formation is not a new conception. The following interesting excerpts from that great English master of surgery, Sir Charles Bell (1816), show how long this has been known. "I was taught carefully to avoid drawing a ligature so tight around an artery as to cut the inner coats; and this remark was repeated both in the dissecting room and the hospital." He then made some facetious remarks about theoretic surgeons who were trying to revolutionize the surgery of blood vessels, by tying the artery and at once removing the ligature. He predicted that some bright young surgeon would put it in practice and "it was done that winter," for an aneurysm of the leg. "But as it did not cure the aneurysm, the medical world heard nothing about it." "To correct this erroneous, because partial, view of the subject, I made the following simple experiment. I put a cord around the carotid of a dog without drawing it. The ligature lay in contact with the coats of the artery but did not press upon them, nor interrupt the flow of blood through them. I was certain of the result: a clot formed where the artery was irritated by the presence of the ligature and the vessel was obstructed at that part."—"the effect of the ligature is perfect." "After this experiment I should be as fully authorized to commit the folly of using a ligature to the artery of an aneurysmal limb, thus, simply putting it around the vessel without tying it, as they who propose to effect the same purpose by cutting the coats of the vessel with the ligature and taking it off again"—and concludes that "a surgeon ought never to consider himself at liberty to deviate from a line of practice which experience has taught to be effective and safe."

One cannot be certain to whose new experimental studies Bell referred, but just at that time three important contributions were made in England on the use of ligatures on large arteries. They were by Jones (1802), Travers (1813), and Lawrence (1815), and doubtless these stimulated his sarcastic remarks. The particularly pertinent experimental studies of Travers had just appeared and very probably provoked his attack.

Jones showed that (1) a tightly drawn ligature always cut the two inner coats, only the adventitia holding fast. (Jones says this was known to Desault and was demonstrated to him [Jones] by Thomson, a surgeon in Edinburgh); and (2) a plastic exudate "lymph from the vasa vasorum" at the site of and induced by the ligature was responsible for the closure of the artery.

Travers found that after 12 hours a ligature performed no function because the reparative processes induced by injury to the vessels caused its permanent closure and, therefore, "it seemed probable" that the ligature could be removed after that time and the "dreaded inflammations" induced by the foreign body, *i.e.,* "liberation from the vessel by an ulcerative process" could be avoided. It will be recalled that at that time the long sutures were left emerging from the wound and were later (two to three weeks) sloughed out.

Lawrence then introduced silk as the ligature of choice and began the unorthodox method of cutting the ligature close to the knot, leaving it to be disposed of by nature. Many of the wounds healed by first intention, but he was at a loss to understand what eventually happened to the ligature. Shortly thereafter the absorbable suture was introduced by Physic, of Philadelphia.

The relation of thrombus formation to ligatures has long been disputed. It was long ago proposed that it was responsible for the closure of the artery. Travers decried its importance saying it was variable, "it may be present in twelve hours and may not be formed in twenty-four hours." Senn (1885) found it to occur (as did Pouteau over a century before) only at times. He quoted Porta, one of the earliest great names in experimental vascular surgery, as finding thrombi in 87 per cent of the ligations, and Schumann in 33.3 per cent. Delpine and Dent (1891) found, in a series of sheep, a distal thrombus in only one and peripheral in all. Ballance and Edwards (1891) reported a thrombus in every instance, whether the intima was injured or not.

In retrospect, it is now clear that the thrombus above and below Bell's non-constricting band was due to infection which, of course, he could not know. The same explanation doubtless holds for the results of Delpine and Dent, and of Ballance and Edwards (1891), whose experiments were performed before Lister's discovery had

taken effect.

Doctor Halsted's experiments, performed under strict surgical asepsis, gave the answer when sepsis was excluded, and our human cases are exactly the same.

The conception that a thrombus ended at the nearest sizable branch, probably dated from Jones' experiments (1802). Soon thereafter, Travers (1813) emphatically stated that the thrombus "is not bounded by collateral branches but extends into them." Ballance and Edwards also concluded that "the length of the clot, either above or below the ligature, is not dependent upon arterial branches into and beyond which the clot may not pass." Bell's plate, (Fig. 1) Bell's sketch shows a small thrombus at the site of the ligature and stopping at the mouth of an entering artery. Bell believed in this rather prevalent impression despite Travers experiments that denied it. In an earlier publication* I included a drawing of a spontaneous propagating and noninfective thrombosis that covered the entire course of the internal carotid and passed through the anterior and middle cerebral arteries and the posterior communicating arteries. One of the cases (Fig. 2a), here reported, shows that the external carotid was no barrier to its progress, and in the other case (Fig. 2b) the thrombus stopped part way up the internal carotid where there was no branch.

SUMMARY

(1) Six specimens of the human internal carotid were removed at operation for microscopic study at varying periods of time (from 16 to 58 days) after partially occluding bands of fascia lata had been placed on the vessels. Two specimens of the same vessel were studied for the extent of propagation of intra-arterial thrombosis following total occlusion of the internal carotid in one case and of the common carotid in the other. A specimen of the intracranial internal carotid was removed at necropsy nineteen days after a silver clip had totally occluded the artery.

(2) Bands of fascia lata, either single or double, were used in these and 24 additional cases, and were perfectly satisfactory in every way.

(3) Although the bands disintegrate, a dense mass of connective tissue surrounds the fascia and prevents the artery from re-expanding. Whether this mass of connective tissue produces an additional *progressive* constriction of the artery is not certain.

(4) The arterial wall does not become necrotic under the fascial band; as it does under an aluminum band. The intima is unchanged and shows no cellular reaction.

(5) Except for one tiny caruncle-like localized and nonoccluding thrombus in an elderly person with very sclerotic vessels there was no thrombus formation.

(6) In one patient whose *internal* carotid had been completely ligated (elsewhere) two years earlier, the thrombus completely filled the internal carotid higher than our incision in the neck but the common and external carotid arteries were patent. In the other patient, whose *common* carotid had been ligated (elsewhere) six months earlier, the common carotid was thrombosed lower than our exposure; the external carotid was patent and the thrombus in the internal carotid extended about two centimeters above the bifurcation, after which the artery was patent (it was divided at this level). The latter case demonstrates that the termination of a propogating thrombus is not determined "by the nearest sizable branch."

(7) The single case of a "clip" totally occluding the intracranial portion of the internal carotid, demonstrates the absence of an intra-arterial thrombus 19 days after application of the clip. In at least four other cases that have had reexploration of the intracranially-clipped carotid (in carotid cavernous arterio-venous aneurysms) the absence of a thrombus on either side of the clip has been demonstrated by palpation of the vessel. This is, therefore, a disadvantage, when thrombus formation is desired to cure the aneurysm.

REFERENCES

*It cannot be said that a thrombus will *never* occur, but in none of our cases has it been seen. However, in one case of his and one of mine there was a tiny nonpropagating, nonobstructing caruncle-like body on the lumen under the band, and presumably related to the band.
*Zentralblatt fur Neurochirurgie, 1937.

[1]Ballance C. A., and Edmunds, W.: *A Treatise on the Ligation of the Great Arteries in Continuity.* London, Macmillan & Co., 1891.

[2]Dandy, W. E.: Carotid-cavernous Aneurysms (Pulsating Exophthalmos). *Zentralbl. Neurochir.,* 2:2, 1937.

[3]Dandy, W. E.: Results Following Ligation of the Internal Carotid Artery. *Arch. Surg.,* 45:521, 1942.

[4]Dandy, W. E.: *Intracranial Arterial Aneurysms.* Comstock Publishing Company, Cornell University, 1944.

[5]Delpine, S., and Dent, C. T.: The Changes Observed in the Healthy Medium-sized Arteries and in Tendon Ligatures during the First Four Weeks after Ligation. *Med. & Chir. Trans.,* 56:367, 1891.

[6]Halsted, W. S.: The Partial Occlusion of Blood Vessels, Especially of the Abdominal Aorta. *Bull. Johns Hopkins Hosp.,* 14:346, 1905.

[7]Halsted, W. S.: Partial Progressive and Complete Occlusion of the Aorta and Other Large Arteries in the Dog by Means of the Metal Band. *J. Exper. Med.,* 15:373, 1909.

[8]Halsted, W. S.: *The Effect on the Walls of Blood Vessels of Partially and Completely Occluding Bands.* Surgical Papers. The Johns Hopkins Press, 1924, p. 585.

[9]Jones, J. F. D.: *On the Process Employed by Nature in Suppressing the Hemorrhage from Divided and Punctured Vessels.* Philadelphia, Th. Dobson, 1811.

[10]Kerr, H.: Fractional Ligation of the Common Carotid Artery in the Treatment of Pulsating Exophthalmos. *Surg., Gynec. & Obst.* 41:565, 1925.

[11]Lawrence, W.: A New Method of Tying the Arteries. *Mer. Chir. Trans.,* 6:156, 1815.

[12]Matas, R., and Allen, C. W.: Occlusion of the Large Surgical Arteries with Removable Metallic Bands. *J.A.M.A.,* 56:232, 1911.

[13]Matas, R.: Discussion on Vascular Surgery: With Special Reference to Surgery of the Carotid Tracts. *Am. J. Surg.,* 24:692, 1933.

[14]Pearse, H. E.: The Impracticability of Using Fascia for Gradual Occlusion of the Large Arteries. *Am. J. Surg.,* 16:242, 1932.

[15]Pearse, H. E.: Experimental Studies on the Gradual Occlusions of Large Arteries. *Tr. Am. Surg. A.,* 58:443, 1940.

[16]Reid, M. R.: Partial Occlusion of the Aorta with

the Metallic Band: Observations on Blood Pressure and Changes in the Arterial Wall. *J. Exper. Med.*, 24:287, 1916.

[17]Reid, M. R.: Partial Occlusion of the Aorta with Silk Sutures and Complete Occlusion with Fascial Plugs: The Effect of Ligatures on the Ar-

terial Wall. *J. Exper. Med.*, 40:293, 1924

[18]Senn, N.: Cicatrization of Blood Vessels After Ligature. *Tr. Am. S. A.*, 2:249, 1885.

[19]Travers, B.: Further Observations on the Ligatures of Arteries. *Med. Chir. Tr.*, 6:632, 1815.

LXXVIII

THE LOCATION OF THE CONSCIOUS CENTER IN THE BRAIN — THE CORPUS STRIATUM*†

In 1930 the writer reported a remarkable cerebral phenomenon that followed resection of the left frontal lobe with the remains of a bilateral frontal glioma: (the right frontal lobe and its contained tumor had been extirpated three weeks earlier with no untoward effect). Immediately after the second operation there was almost complete absence of conscious effort for a period of seventeen days when she died of pneumonia. This patient lay with her eyes open or closed, never changed position, never spoke or responded in any way. The only movement, except opening and closing the eyelids, was an occasional contraction of a hand or leg. From day to day there was no change whatever. Urination and defecation were involuntary; swallowing movements were present; there were attacks of vomiting and hiccoughing. Throughout this period there were frequent minor focal epileptic attacks involving an arm or leg and occasionally a grand mal seizure. There was no rigidity of the extremities. The reflexes were not increased: Babinski reflexes were usually negative but occasionally positive. Strong sensory stimuli would induce a mild contracture of the affected extremity; lesser stimuli had no effect. The eyelids closed when the cornea was touched.

At no time following operation was there intracranial pressure. The enormous defect created by the removal of both frontal lobes was insurance against pressure. Moreover, frequent taps of the defect revealed no pressure and finally, continuous drainage of the defect produced no change in the patient's response. Since there was never intracranial pressure to account for the loss of consciousness the explanation could only be that the conscious center of the brain had been injured directly.

At the time of the original report, it was clear that an area of the brain controlling consciousness had been affected and I assumed that the bilateral ligations of the anterior cerebral arteries were responsible. And since the right anterior cerebral artery had been sacrificed many times without effect, I assumed that the anterior cerebral arterial supply was probably responsible. A few years later Poppen (1939) encountered the same phenomenon in a patient following ligation of both anterior cerebral arteries. Poppen, too, supposed the vascular loss to be responsible but he was puzzled because he had had a series of three other cases in which both anterior cerebral arteries had been ligated without the same effect, in fact without any effect whatever. He also stated that in seven additional cases the left anterior cerebral artery had been ligated without any disturbances of consciousness. He also included a statement that in a series of ten cases the left anterior cerebral artery had been ligated at the Mayo Clinic without subsequent disturbance. Poppen concluded, after a suggestion by Fulton, that if the blood pressure was low at the time of the ligation, the loss of consciousness would follow, but if the blood pressure was not low, loss of consciousness would not result. In 1941 Poppen reported two more cases in which the low blood pressure had been elevated by transfusion before ligating the left anterior cerebral artery and nothing happened.

*Reprinted from the *Bulletin of the Johns Hopkins Hospital*, *LXXIX*: 34–58, July, 1946.

†Dr. Dandy died on April 19, 1946.

He attributed the absence of effect to the elevated blood pressure resulting from the transfusion, although the same procedure had been harmless in several earlier cases without this precaution. I know of no other clinical reports of this immediate, total and permanent abolition of consciousness following operation.

Poppen was quite correct in stating that either one or both anterior cerebral arteries can be ligated without causing loss of consciousness. I have since ligated the left anterior cerebral artery a number of times and both anterior cerebral arteries (at the genu of the corpus callosum) in at least six cases without any noticeable disturbances related thereto and with no effect on consciousness. The total abolition of consciousness cannot, therefore, be explained by the loss of circulation to the brain beyond the ligated artery or arteries. However, there is now evidence in case 6 that this vascular occlusion, whether single or bilateral, is responsible for this loss of consciousness, but in a manner entirely unsuspected by either Dr. Poppen or myself. The explanation is a retrograde thrombosis of the anterior cerebral artery from the point of coagulation of one or both torn vessels to the internal carotid artery ond including the recurrent medial striate artery (Heubner) en route. If unilateral this is the exact equivalent of ligating the anterior cerebral at the carotid and again at the anterior communicating artery, and, therefore, preventing collateral circulation to the medial striate artery which supplies part of the corpus striatum. If bilateral thrombosis occurs it is the equivalent of tying both anterior cerebral arteries at the internal carotids.

It would appear that Poppen's suggestion that a low blood pressure at the time of the ligations might lead to this loss of consciousness, may well be a very astute observation conforming to this concept, but also in a manner that he did not conceive. The low blood pressure per se could not cause this phenomenon but it is a well known fact that vascular thromboses, though always capricious, are precipitated by low blood pressure and particularly in defective vessels.

Although all of the brains in our series were inspected post mortem, still a thrombosed vessel would hardly be recognized unless one's attention was especially directed to it. Indeed in case 6 the thrombosed medial striate branch of the anterior cerebral artery was missed by myself and found by Mrs. Padget (Miss Hager) who made the drawings.

A note concerning the effect of anterior cerebral ligations should be entered here. All of the bilateral ligations of this vessel by Poppen and myself have been at the genu of the corpus callosum, the vessels being injured during resections of one or both frontal lobes; at this point these vessels lie very close together. The brain supplied by these vessels beyond this point is now known not to be important and no function is lost by their elimination. Ligation of a single anterior cerebral artery at its origin from the internal carotid would produce no ill effects because the collateral circulation from the opposite side (through the anterior communicating artery) would immediately restore the circulation. Below the anterior communicating artery it would be necessary (in man) to ligate both anterior cerebral arteries at the internal carotid artery to abolish the collateral circulation of these vessels. In one of our cases both anterior cerebral arteries were ligated alongside the internal carotid and identically the same loss of consciousness followed.

In the fifteen years since the original report, I have encountered nine additional cases in which this phenomenon— (immediate and permanent loss of consciousness) has followed operations for the removal of tumors or aneurysm (1 case). In one (Case 1) both frontal lobes were extirpated, both anterior cerebral arteries being ligated at the genu of the corpus callosum. In six (Cases 2, 3, 4, 5, 6 and 7) only the right frontal lobe was extirpated, but in each instance both anterior cerebral arteries were ligated at the genu of the corpus callosum. In two (Cases 8 and 9) tumors were dissected from the third ventricle (one recurrent) and without injury to the anterior cerebral arteries, and in one (Case 10) both anterior cerebral arteries, were ligated (clipped) alongside the internal carotid arteries in order to stop bleeding when an aneurysm ruptured during its dissection. In two of the cases, therefore, the anterior cerebral arteries were not injured and precisely the same immediate and total loss of consciousness appeared. In all of these cases intracranial pressure was known not to be the cause of loss of consciousness. Necropsies were obtained in all, but, unfortunately, all except two of the brains (Cases 9 and 10) have since been thrown away and studies of the pathological material are, therefore, not now available. In Case 7, microscopic studies were not made but the gross specimen was carefully studied before the brain was lost. Until quite recently we were content to believe that the loss of the anterior cerebral arteries explained the loss of consciousness and our attention was not directed toward the basal ganglia, where the real disturbance occurred. In Cases 9 and 10 the brains have been carefully studied. In every case the total loss of consciousness and of voluntary effort were observed immediately after the time (four-six hours) when there could be no question of any effects of anaesthesia (avertin and supplementary ether, and in Case 1, ether alone.)

CASE 1. H. M. patient, an obese woman, aged fifty-one, was admitted to the Johns Hopkins Hospital 10/31/27 (surgical history no. 15048, Path. no. 10170). She was transferred from a psychopathic hospital where she had been an inmate for six weeks because of amnesia, complete disorientation and confabulation. The first sign of organic trouble was a series of eight convulsions four years ago. These occurred soon after the death of her mother by which she was greatly overcome; she was then in the menopause. During the next year there were no convulsions but she complained of severe headaches and showed marked changes of personality; she became untidy about her person and

housework. Since then her headaches and personality changes had progressed. Her memory failed and her word was unreliable. After a stay of three weeks at the Sheppard Pratt Hospital a diagnosis of brain tumor was made.

Neurological examination revealed only bilateral papilloedema and pronounced mental changes. Ventriculography 11/1/27: left frontal tumor.

Operation 11/1/27: Excision left frontal lobe; tumor extended across the midline into the right frontal lobe. Weight of tumor and left frontal lobe was 105 grams.

It is interesting that within two weeks after the operation, her mental condition had cleared greatly.

Second Operation 11/25/27: Resection right frontal lobe with tumor. The tumor reached the surface of the frontal lobe; it therefore passed all the way through both frontal lobes. The tumor had attached itself to the falx and a segment of this was excised. The weight of the frontal lobe and tumor was 103 grams. Both anterior cerebral arteries were ligated; this was later confirmed at necropsy.

Pathological Diagnosis: Spongioblastoma multiforme (glioma).

Postoperative state: Patient l i v e d seventeen days. Throughout this time she lay motionless except for an occasional grasping movement of the hands, and an occasional movement of the feet—both in response to stimulation but never in response to command. Her eyes would open and close, but never in response to command. Only once did the eyes follow anyone in the room; on this occasion the arm was strongly flexed during a test and the eyes turned to that side. It was, in fact, the only time her eyes were seen to turn from the forward position. There was never an attempted movement to change the position of the body. There was involuntary urination at intervals and stools were involuntary. There were not infrequent tremors, and fairly frequent convulsions, involving various parts of the body singly, at times one entire side of the body, and there were a few generalized convulsions. Occasionally the jaws would grind. Hiccoughing, grunting, sighing, vomiting, moaning, moving the tongue, occurred from time to time and on at least one occasion she spat out mucus. The pulse was rapid—100 to 150 throughout, respirations varied greatly but were regular and on the whole faster than normal—20 to

40. The temperature was elevated and irregular throughout—100 to 103, until the onset of the terminal pneumonia. All extremities were flaccid throughout, never spastic. The Babinski reflex was positive bilaterally; the knee kicks were normal. The pupils reacted to light directly and consensually.

The following note was made by Dr. Frank Ford 12/1/27: Patient is in deep coma, eyes closed, makes no spontaneous movements and does not respond to stimuli. Eyes move a little but non-concomitant and do not fix. Face does not move. Jaw partly open and does not move. Arms and legs are flaccid. When arm is pricked for vena puncture there is slight flexion at elbow. Strong stimuli of feet produce minimal flexion and feeble Babinski (bilateral); no ankle clonus. Tendon reflexes are active and equal and not increased. Passive rotation of head to either side causes no change in posture of arms or legs and no demonstrable tone. There are no signs of decerebrate rigidity.

Dr. L. F. Barker 12/7/27—Twelfth day after operation—made the following note: The spontaneous movements recently have consisted of twitching of both arms and legs, yawning and coughing. On passive movements of the left arm, she opened her eyes, turned them to the right and looked at me. A little later she turned her eyes up, but when the light was turned on she turned them forward again.

The pupils are approximately equal and react promptly to light. The mouth is slightly open. On pulling the right eyelid upward she closes the left eye and on elevating the left, the right eye closes. There is marked exaggeration of the deep reflexes in the right arm, but the biceps, triceps and periostial radials are not elicited on the left. There is, however, some tonicity of the muscles on the left arm. (The reflexes on other examinations were equal, active and not increased.)

The right k.k. is active, right ankle jerk hyperactive, the left k.k. present, left ankle jerk hyperactive. Babinski positive on right, not definitely elicited on the left.

The striking features are:—

1) Bilateral total paraplegia for face and arm muscles.

2) Apparent bilateral anaesthesia.

3) Incontinent of urine and faeces.

4) I cannot be sure of vision, but I get the impression that she looked at me.

5) On clapping hands over ear, she looked at me.

6) Cannot test for aphasia, agraphia, or agnosis.

7) Some signs of motor irritation (twitching of upper motor extremities and last night a generalized convulsion).

Impression:—One gets the impression that the complete akinesis is associated with a total loss of spontaneous motor impulse. There may also be an absence of thought activity—patient lying as though in a catatonic stupor. There are no imperative expressive movements of laughing, crying or fright reactions. There is no way of testing affectivity but the patient shows no signs of affective reactions.

Remarks: Following the operation and for seventeen days thereafter there were no voluntary movements or responses, and only minimal reflex movements. At no time was there response to command. Both anterior cerebral arteries had been clipped at the genu of the corpus callosum. At that time the loss of conscious effort was attributed to these ligations, an explanation now known to be incorrect because several bilateral ligations of these vessels have been made at this point and without such effect. It should be emphasized that there was never intracranial pressure following the operation. The huge bilateral space resulting from the bilateral frontal lobectomy precluded intracranial pressure. Moreover, for several days after operation a flanged needle inserted into the frontal lobe, permitted constant drainage of the cerebrospinal fluid. Although this was unnecessary it gave further proof that there could be no intracranial pressure. Cessation of drainage produced no change in the patient's reactions and subsequent punctures of the intracranial space revealed no pressure.

CASE 2. B. Z., white male, age thirty-seven, History no. 130330; Path. no. 15698. Operation 2/5/38: Removal right frontal lobe with tumor (calcified) that extended into left frontal lobe. Much of left frontal lobe was also removed with the tumor. Weight of tumor and frontal lobes 211 grams. Both anterior cerebral arteries were thrombosed with the electro cautery.

Postoperative:. Patient lived two days, never regaining consciousness; numerous convulsions, tonic and clonic; all were mild. Swallowed, hiccoughed; slight movements of extremities; no reaction to painful stimuli. No intracranial pressure; repeated taps of the big frontal defect yielded clear fluid under no pressure.

Necropsy: Both anterior cerebral arteries occluded 2 cm. distal to the anterior communicating artery. Death from pulmonary oedema.

CASE 3. D. K., white, male, aged thirteen, Hist. no. 198213, Path. no. 16896. Operation 4/24/40: Removal large hypophyseal tumor after resection of right frontal lobe: Both anterior cerebral arteries were coagulated at the genu of the corpus callosum. Weight of tumor 15.5 grams. Weight of frontal lobe 61.5 grams.

Postoperative: Lived five days. Never regained consciousness although no intracranial pressure. Hiccoughs frequent, many light generalized convulsions. Slight movement of extremities. No effort to turn in bed. No reaction to painful stimuli. Yawned, gritted teeth, voided involuntarily.

Necropsy:—Both anterior cerebral arteries closed, 1.5 cm. distal to the anterior communicating artery. Death from pulmonary embolus. Tumor extended into posterior cranial fossa, imbedding basilar artery to middle of pons.

CASE 4. N. G. white male, age fifty-five, History no. 20791. Path. no. 16999. Operation July 18, 1940—Air injection. Removal right frontal tumor—glioma. Tumor bilateral, both anterior cerebral arteries were coagulated when an attempt was made to remove the remaining tumor on the other side. It was predicted that he would not awaken and he did not. Fifteen hours later wound was reopened and some necrotic tissue was evacuated but there was no change in his condition.

Died three days later without response. Vomited twice, twitching left hand, moaned, hiccoughed, coughed and sighed. Voided involuntarily.

Necropsy: Both anterior cerebral arteries were coagulated 2 cm. beyond the anterior communicating artery.

CASE 5. E. C. white male, age twenty-six, History no. 224686; Path. no. 17409.

Operation: 2/24/41; Ventriculography; resection right frontal lobe, and extension of tumor into left frontal lobe. Both anterior cerebral arteries were coagulated. Frontal lobe and tumor weighed 121.9 grams.

Postoperative: Patient lived fifty-one days; at no time was there any response. There were occasional slight movements

of the right arm and the leg, never purposely. The eyes opened and closed but never in response to command or stimuli. Groaned and gnashed teeth occasionally. Occasional light convulsions, both tonic and clonic. Yawned and sighed from time to time. At times his eyes appeared to follow persons moving about room but this was not certain. When a light was thrown in the eyes the eyelids closed but there was no additional movement. The knee kicks were slightly hyperactive; Babinski negative bilaterally. Slight reaction to very painful stimuli.

Necropsy: Both anterior cerebral arteries were coagulated 2 cm. distal to the anterior communicating artery.

CASE 6. H. L., white female, age forty-six: History no. 321320; Path. no. 18980.

Patient was operated upon 5/17/44 for a large dural meningioma of the olivary eminence. The intracranial pressure was so great that removal of the tumor was impossible without resection of the right frontal lobe. The tumor was so hard that its interior could not be curetted to reduce its bulk. The mass was enucleated with the finger; it weighed 17.7 grams. The frontal lobe weighed 94 grams. In removing the frontal lobe both anterior cerebral arteries were torn and coagulated over the genu of the corpus callosum.

Postoperative response: Patient did not rouse following operation and never reacted to any verbal stimuli. She hiccoughed, vomited, coughed and gagged and responded by slight movements of the hands to painful stimuli. She began menstruating on the third postoperative day. Urination and defacation were always involuntary. On the third day the wound was reopened. There was no intracranial pressure, no bleeding, and only a little necrotic tissue from the frontal resection; a large defect remained and was filled with clear fluid. The pulse constantly ranged from 110 to 130; the temperature was 101 to 103 and respirations 24 to 36 throughout the postoperative duration of life. She died of pneumonia fifteen days after operation.

Necropsy: Verified the double ligation of these vessels at the genu.

Only the gross examination of this case can be presented. It was the first to draw our attention to the corpus striatum. On the right (operated) side, there was necrosis of the *lower half* of the anterior portion of the corpus striatum, the left was intact.

This is the part of this structure supplied by the recurrent medial striate branch (Heubner) of the anterior cerebral artery. The anterior cerebral artery on this side was completely thrombosed from the point of ligation at the genu of the corpus callosum to the internal carotid artery and included the artery of Heubner. The thrombus was confirmed microscopically. On the left side there was a small thrombus at the point where the artery was torn; this ended 2 cm. above the anterior communicating artery, which was patent.

It is worthy of note that there was no trauma to the upper half of the corpus striatum on either this or the other side. The necrosis in the lower half (cross section) of the corpus striatum on the right was therefore due to occlusion of the anterior cerebral artery by a thrombus extending from the torn end of this vessel to the internal carotid artery. A similar extensive thrombus did not develop on the opposite (left side).

CASE 7. C. C., white, male, age forty. History no. 365332. Path. no. 19635.

Patient was semiconscious and unable to answer questions. There was a history of bifrontal headaches for seven years. He had been bedridden for the past three weeks. His vision was said to have been poor. There was bilateral papilloedema but no haemorrhages. The deep reflexes were slightly more active on the left. Pulse was 50 per minute.

Operation 10/10/45: Ventricular air injection; 5 cc. of air were injected into the left ventricle, 10 cc. into right: The third ventricle did not fill. The right frontal horn was depressed and dislocated to the right. Only the posterior and descending horns filled on left. Diagnosis: Bifrontal tumor, greater on left. Since the tumor was apparently bilateral, it seemed preferable to attack the right frontal lobe first.

The right frontal lobe was widely resected; the weight was 132 grams. Both anterior cerebral arteries were occluded at the genu of the corpus callosum. A tremendous encapsulated dural meningioma lay under the falx; about three-fourths or more were on the left side, the remainder bulged to the right. It shelled out very easily and with scarcely any bleeding; the weight was 116 grams. A prompt recovery was expected but patient did not rouse. The first movements were: squeezing with right hand (not left) and scratching nose

(ten hours after operation). During the next twenty-four hours there were fairly frequent movements of both hands and reflex gripping with both hands; clonic convulsions began eighteen hours after operation and were fairly frequent thereafter: some were restricted to one arm or leg, others were generalized. There were also frequent tonic spasms of either or both arms and legs; at times the whole body became rigid. Very slight movements followed strong stimuli but no spontaneous movements after twenty-four hours. At no time after the operation was there any response to commands and no attempt to turn the body. At no time was there intracranial pressure: Repeated taps of the great bilateral frontal defect insured its absence. Death occurred thirty-three hours after operation.

Necropsy: Gross examination. The injury to the corpus striatum is found at the upper anterior end of the *right* corpus striatum.

Microscopically: There were many ruptured blood vessels, much haemorrhage, areas of marked oedema and swollen degenerated fibers in the internal capsule. The lower anterior and more inferior part of the striatum, which is frequently supplied by the medial striate branch of the anterior cerebral artery was not affected by the operative procedure except for some oedema and small haemorrhages.

Both anterior cerebral arteries had been injected with India ink after death and the circulation of the striate arteries were intact on both sides.

On the left side the corpus striatum showed some old foci of perivascular round cell infiltration (syphilitic?) and a few areas of slight oedema but no haemorrhage or necrosis.

The thalamus showed no gross change.

The hypothalamus was beyond the field of operation and showed no alteration in the gross.

CASE 8. H. B., white female, age 17, history no. 44281; Path. no. 12771. Operation 9/9/32: Removal recurrent tumor third ventricle (glioma), (previous operation 7/13/32 with uneventful recovery). The tumor was adherent to the wall of the third ventricle and was removed by sharp and blunt dissection. No arteries were encountered. The approach was along the falx with retraction of the posterior part of the right hemisphere as in a pineal operation.

Postoperative: Following operation patient never made any response or conscious effort. There were slight movements of the arms and legs at times. She lay on the back and without any attempt to turn. She moaned, sighed, coughed, hiccoughed and was incontinent. There were frequent generalized convulsions, also tonic attacks with rigidity of the entire body. She lived four days without change in the state of consciousness. The lateral ventricles were large and intracranial pressure was controlled by repeated ventricular taps.

CASE 9. G. R., white, female, age twenty-five: History no. 287888; Path. no. 18351.

Operation 4/5/43: Immediately after localization by ventriculography, an ependymoma was removed from the right lateral and third ventricles. Because the tumor was rather large and deeply placed it was necessary to remove the right frontal lobe to provide the proper exposure. The anterior cerebral artery was not injured. The removal of the tumor was followed by diffuse oozing from both the third and lateral ventricles; this was controlled by packing repeatedly and with some applications of the cautery. The tumor weighed 5 grams, the excised lobe 90 grams.

Postoperative Response: There was no return of consciousness at any time before death twenty-three days later. She yawned, coughed, hiccoughed, moved both hands on a few occasions, voided and defecated involuntarily. Never was there any response to questions and only slight movements of the arms or legs to painful stimuli. From time to time there were mild focal convulsions. There was never intracranial pressure. This was shown by repeated punctures of the cerebral defect.

Necropsy: Death from pneumonia. The anterior cerebral arteries were intact.

CASE 10. J. H. M.: white male, age twenty-eight; surgical history no. 339857: Path. no. 19261.

Operation 12/22/44: Avertin and ether anaesthesia: A small arterial aneurysm of the right anterior cerebral artery was dissected until the neck of the sac was free. It ruptured when a defective clip holder cut the neck of the aneurysm. After an initial spurt of blood that quickly filled the wound, the spatula compressed the bleeding point and the wound was dry. The anterior cerebral artery on the left was seen and clipped and the neck of the aneurysm was coagulated with the electrocautery. When the spatula was removed the bleeding had entirely stopped. The only trauma was at the site of the coagulation of the neck of the aneurysm.

Postoperative Responses: The first response was ten hours after operation when he moved right hand toward face. Fourteen hours after operation he would hold your hand reflexly; eyes were wide open but blank. Pulled at dressings. Fifteen hours: moved both hands to face. Eyes open and blank. Tried to vomit; hiccoughing. Seventeen hours; twitching of whole body—started in right hand. Twenty-two hours later: Pulse 160, temperature 105.4, respiration labored. The bone flap was removed; there was slight pressure; the brain barely protruding. His condition became steadily worse; death came forty-eight hours after operation.

Remarks: In this case the lack of conscious response was essentially the same as in other cases and was due to ligation of both anterior cerebral arteries at the internal carotids. However, the element of intracranial pressure cannot be entirely subtracted from the picture; it would surely result in time from the reaction to necrotic tissue. It is my belief that signs of pressure could not have developed in the first twelve hours and during this time there were no signs of returning consciousness.

Necropsy: The brain was sketched from all aspects, sliced coronally, each section drawn and about twenty blocks made for microscopic study. The corpus striatum showed necrosis of the lower half (coronal section) in the right side and the lower third on the left. This differing quantitative distribution of necrosis conforms to the variability of the medial striate branches of the anterior cerebral artery, including the recurrent artery of Heubner.

The necrosis from the operative trauma at the base of the brain passes into the area of necrosis of the corpora striata of vascular origin and this terminates at the anterior border of the thalamus. This area of necrosis covers the anterior part of the hypothalamus but not the tuber cinereum of the corpora mamillaria. Microscopic section of this region through the hypophyseal stalk was free of oedema or necrosis.

The thalamus was not abnormal microscopically or in the gross.

ANALYSIS OF CASES WITH LOSS OF CONSCIOUSNESS

In all of the above cases, consciousness was totally lost immediately, did not return nor were there any signs of clearing, up to fifty-one days—the longest surviving period. In six of these cases death occurred within five days and in three of these within two days after operation. It cannot be said that consciousness was *permanently* lost in these cases. In four cases death occurred fifteen, seventeen, twenty-three and fifty-one days (Cases 6, 1, 9 and 5) and until the time of exitus there had been no sign of returning consciousness; in these, I have assumed the consciousness to have been permanently lost. There can be no doubt that a specific area of the brain controlling consciousness had been damaged and probably destroyed either directly or indirectly through deprivation of its blood supply. The only functions remaining were automatic.

From the results of extensive resections of the brain one can be certain that neither cerebral hemisphere above the basal ganglia plays any part in consciousness. This statement is based upon seven total *right* hemisphere removals that I have performed in man, another by Gardner and the single total removal of the *left* cerebral hemisphere by Zollinger. Moreover, while experiments in animals are not necessarily transferable to man, the famous Goltz's dogs with both cerebral hemispheres removed and with normal locomotion afterwards are at least proof that consciousness is not affected by the absence of both cerebral hemispheres in dogs. There can, therefore, be no doubt that consciousness is not related to the cerebral hemispheres; it must, therefore, be referred to the basal ganglia or the thalamus, or possibly the hypothalamus or brain stem.

From the first seven cases in this report, this phenomenon of immediate, total and permanent loss of consciousness resulted from exactly the same procedure, i.e. resection of one or both (1 case) frontal lobes; however, in the bifrontal case, loss of consciousness followed removal of the second lobe i.e. the left frontal lobe had previously been removed with no effect. It has been shown at necropsy in each of these cases that both anterior cerebral arteries were severed at the genu of the corpus callosum. But since the deprivation of the blood supply of these vessels beyond this point is now known not to cause loss of consciousness, there must be another explanation for this phenomenon. Moreover, the part of the brain that is injured and is responsible for this change must be in the immediate environs of the line of section of the frontal lobe or lobes. There is only one part of the brain that could meet this condition i.e. the corpus striatum. One might suggest a second part of the brain i.e. the anterior part of the hypothalamus but this area lies at some distance from the line of the resection and is not traumatized, (except Case 10).

From the cases in this report three have been studied carefully at necropsy (two with microscopic studies) and all of these show sharply defined necrosis of the anterior part of the corpus striatum (the head of the caudate nucleus and the lentiform nucleus (the globus pallidus and the putamen).

In two of the cases (6 and 10) this necrosis was in the lower half of the tip of the corpus striatum and was due to loss of its blood supply from occlusion of the recurrent medial striate artery (Heubner). In Case 10 the necrosis was bilateral and followed ligation of both anterior cerebral arteries at the internal carotid arteries, following which necrosis follows because the arteries can receive no collateral. It has been shown by Ayer and Aitken (1907 and 1909), Beevor (1909), and recently Alexander (1942) that all the arterial supply to the basal ganglia is by end arteries. In Case 6 the right anterior cerebral artery (and its medial striate branch) was thrombosed from the point at which the artery was occluded at the genu of the corpus callosum to the internal carotid artery and there was necrosis in the same area of the corpus striatum as in Case 10. Moreover, there was no trauma to the upper half of the corpus striatum; the necrosis was, therefore, of vascular and not traumatic derivation. It is very probable that other cases in this series have had similar extensions of the intraarterial thrombus, but without a careful study of the vessels and the basal ganglia, thromboses could easily have been overlooked.

In the remaining case (7) with postmortem study, the *upper* half of the anterior part of the corpus striatum was necrotic and had sloughed off. This was due to direct trauma that occurred in the line of the resection. This also was strictly unilateral and confined to the right (operated) side. The inferior half of the corpus striatum was oedematous but not necrotic. Whether the upper half, i.e. above the internal capsule, or the oedematous portion below was responsible for the loss of consciousness cannot be stated. The trauma was sufficiently severe to implicate the entire cross section of this structure from oedema.

Permanent loss of consciousness probably therefore results either from direct trauma to the anterior part of the corpus striatum or from deprivation of its blood supply. And since in two of these cases the necrosis of this structure was strictly unilateral, (and on the right side), one can only conclude that bilateral involvement is not necessary. Whether the same result would obtain from involvement of only the left side cannot be answered.

In none of these three postmortem examinations was there any gross change in the optic thalamus and in the two with microscopic studies there was none.

If Case 10 were alone, one could not exclude the possibility that the anterior portion of the hypothalamus might play a role as the conscious center because the traumatic necrosis includes this area (both anterior cerebral arteries were clipped at the carotids). However, in both Cases 6 and 7 the necrosis is far removed from the hypothalamus and there can be no doubt

that its exclusion cannot be questioned.

Perhaps a word of explanation is in order concerning the plane of the resected frontal lobe. The usual incision passes through the lobe transversely in a line corresponding roughly with the fronto-parietal bony suture and is well in advance of the motor area, which it roughly parallels. The incision through the lobe passes slightly forward and is usually just anterior to the genu of the corpus callosum. It should miss the anterior horn of the lateral ventricle, though not infrequently the tip of the ventricle is opened. At the base of the skull this would terminate about 2 to 3 cm. anterior to the olivary eminence. In more extensive resections of the lobe (dependent upon the posterior extent of the tumor), the incision in the cortex begins nearer the Rolandic area and in the depths the incision is curved forward in order to miss the corpus callosum and thus avoid the anterior cerebral arteries. It is in these more extensive resections that these vessels and the underlying part of the basal ganglia may be injured at the genu of the corpus callosum. Every effort is made to avoid tearing the branches of the anterior cerebral artery and thus avoid injury to the main trunks but this is not always successful; when torn the vessels are packed with wet cotton, then isolated and coagulated with the electrocautery or occasionally silver clips.

LOSS OF CONSCIOUSNESS FOLLOWING EXTIRPATION OF TUMORS OF THE THIRD VENTRICLE

In two cases (8 and 9) precisely the same loss of consciousness—total and permanent—followed removal of tumors of the third ventricle (one recurrent). In neither of these could either anterior cerebral artery be injured (post mortem verification) because the operative approach is remote from these vessels. These two cases demonstrate that the same loss of consciousness results from injury of the basal ganglia directly and without injury to the vascular supply—i.e. the anterior cerebral arteries.

These cases do not, however, indicate whether the damage that caused loss of consciousness has been done anteriorly at the corpus striatum or posteriorly at the thalamus, or both. The preceding experiments (Cases 1 to 7) are necessary for the more precise identification of the area involved.

In this connection I have reviewed a series of 5 pineal tumors operated upon with fatal result; in all of these the tumor entered the posterior part of the third ventricle and the trauma of removal affected the thalamus rather than the corpus striatum. Upon coming out of the anaesthetic there was always immediate return of consciousness with movements of all extremities. Later consciousness was lost as the postoperative oedema spread to the more anteriorly situated corpora striata. From comparison of these cases with those in which the basal ganglia are injured anteriorly, additional evidence is added that the conscious center is in the anterior part of the corpus striatum and not in the thalamus or the posterior part of the corpus striatum.

LIGATION OF THE ANTERIOR CEREBRAL ARTERIES

It has been stated that in two cases deprivation of the blood supply to the corpus striatum on one or both sides resulted in necrosis of the anterior part of the corpus striatum (of one or both sides depending upon whether one or both arteries are occluded.) [2] Although this is the general rule, in a certain percentage of cases variously estimated from one-fourth to one-third (Ayer and Aitken, Beevor, and Alexander), the anterior cerebral arteries send no branches to the corpus striatum: in these cases the blood supply is from branches of the middle cerebral arteries which (with the anterior choroidal artery) normally supply the remainder of the basal ganglia. It is evident, therefore, that elimination of the blood supply of one or

both anterior cerebral arteries will not always be followed by necrosis of the corpus striatum; but that in one-fourth or one-third of cases in which the recurrent medial striate branch (Heubner) is absent, or very small, the anterior cerebral arteries may be sacrificed without effect upon the conscious area. It should, therefore, be emphasized that when cases of bilateral ligations of the anterior cerebral arteries at the carotids are subsequently reported to be done with impunity that the anterior cerebral arteries should be carefully inspected for these branches when necropsy affords an opportunity.

It should also be emphasized that ligation of one anterior cerebral artery at the internal carotid will not normally affect the corpus striatum because of the collateral circulation through the anterior communicating artery (occasionally the anterior communicating artery is absent).

LITERATURE ON THE CONSCIOUS CENTER

I know of no instances in the literature where total and permanent loss of consciousness described above has been described from any lesion of the brain or following any experiment. A considerable literature has accumulated concerning pathological sleep, which doubtless is concerned with the center of consciousness and is a physio-pathological disturbance of it or its connections. For many years a center for sleep has been placed in the environs of the third ventricle. This conclusion has been reached through pathological material—largely tumors, from the end results of encephalitis and more recently from experiments on animals.

Sinkler (1893) reported a tumor as large as a hen's egg in the posterior part of the optic thalamus; the patient had had recurring attacks of drowsiness but the size and location of the tumor might well have induced periods of sleep from intracranial pressure. Probably in most tumor cases somnolence is due to intracranial pressure: and tumors causing ball valve obstructions of the ventricular system are particularly prone to produce recurring attacks of somnolence because of the recurring blockage of the ventricles (hydrocephalus). For this reason many tumors of the cerebellum and third ventricle, and even of the lateral ventricles produce recurring attacks of sleep. In the presence of tumors it is, therefore, always difficult to subtract the element of intracranial pressure from the local effects of the lesion.

Luksch (1924) reported a postmortem study on a twenty-seven year old patient who had had recurring attacks of stupor over a period of three weeks. She had a small metastatic abscess in the right thalamus and third ventricle; this abscess was a sequel of endocarditis. Fulton and Bailey (1929) collected a group of tumors of the third ventricle; in all their five cases there were periods of uncontrollable sleep. Their conclusion was that the region of the brain controlling sleep was in the thalamus and hypothalamus and possibly in the region of the Aqueduct of Sylvius. Globus (1940) reported two cases of intermittent, incontrollable drowsiness, both with extensive arteriosclerosis of the cerebral vessels and in each there was bilateral softening of the optic thalamus. Much the same localization was reached by Von Economo (1928) in studying brains from an epidemic of encephalitis. Penfield (1938) briefly mentioned a remarkable result in a patient from whom he had removed a tumor from the region of the pineal and with extension into the posterior part of the third ventricle. She was unconscious or nearly so for six weeks and finally recovered. It is not stated whether there were movments of the body and if so, how much. He concluded that the center for consciousness, which had been injured, was in the optic thalamus. In the light of our present experiments it would now appear more probable that oedema of the contiguous corpora striata was responsible and as the oedema cleared, consciousness belatedly returned. Had the conscious center been injured directly and so severely, the loss of consciousness would doubtless have been permanent.

If the coma was total for six weeks in Penfield's case, the period of somnolence is surpassed in only one of our patients (5), who lived fifty-one days without change. I cannot say that consciousness might not have returned in some of those with shorter survivals. One can only say that there was no indication of improvement. In one of our recent cases there was loss of consciousness for four days, then gradual return of movements and consciousness and on the fifth day there was response to command. In this patient both anterior cerebral arteries had been ligated following bilateral removal of the frontal lobes for a bilateral glioma. It was assumed that the conscious area had been traumatized but not destroyed and that as the oedema subsided the conscious area again functioned very much as in Penfield's case, but with a more rapid recovery. A similar recovery takes place in recovery from traumatic injuries of the brain and also from coma during the last stages of intracranial pressure from brain tumors, after the pressure has been relieved. In all of these examples the conscious center must be affected but not to a point beyond repair.

From experiments on animals, Hess (1932-1936) was led to place the center for sleep in the same region, i.e. the thalamus and hypothalamus. He placed electrodes in the region of the hypothalamus and the thalamus and induced sleep by stimulation. Ransom (1939) produced lesions in various parts of the thalamus and hypothalamus, running the needle through from the surface of the brain and passing a current through for brief periods. Lesions in various locations resulted. His best results in terms of sleep were in the hypothalamus (although the needle passed through the basal ganglia). Spiegel and Maba (1927) on the other hand got differing results with similar methods and obtained greater sleep from lesions in the thalamus. Stimulation experiments could hardly localize a center with accuracy for the effect of stimulation would carry beyond the point stimulated. The lesions produced in the animal experiments would appear to be near but not at the actual center for consciousness: if the center of consciousness were injured consciousness would be abolished as in our human cases.

SIGNIFICANCE OF "CONSCIOUSNESS"

There has been much discussion about the meaning of consciousness. If in its original sense consciousness implies the recognition and utilization of afferent impressions, the only way of recognizing consciousness is by the efferent manifestations of speech and motion. The definition is doubtless reversible, for if, with intact pathways of speech and movement, there is no outward expression of speech and movement, the assumption of recognition of incoming impressions could not be assumed and these functions are in all probability abolished also. In these cases practically all activities of the body (there are a few minor movements) [3] are lost except the autonomic—and that certainly means the loss of consciousness. The center for consciousness is, therefore, the "integrator" of all the voluntary activities of the brain. With the loss of this center the body becomes a vegetative organism. Doubtless it is this center of consciousness that is concerned with sleep. With its complete destruction there have been, of course, no periods of recurring sleep.

COLLATERAL FOLLOWING ARTERIAL LIGATIONS IN THE BRAIN

The collateral circulation that has maintained in very surprising degree the integrity of the frontal lobes that have been deprived of their circulation by ligation of both anterior cerebral arteries is interesting. This study is not concerned with the area of consciousness but is a secondary consideration. In Case 10 both frontal lobes looked surprisingly normal and were certainly not soft or necrotic. The microscopic study, however, did show oedema and spotty areas of necrosis throughout. In the right frontal pole near the operative site, there was fresh haemorrhage in the meninges, old and fresh heamorrhage around arterioles and many dead cells. More distally, about midway between the operative area and the Rolandic fissure, three sections showed relatively large areas of normal brain and irregular areas of necrosis. Reaching the premotor and motor cortex, there were still larger areas of normal brain and smaller foci of dead cells. In all sections little change was detected in the white matter.

The left cerebral cortex in the distribution of the anterior cerebral artery showed the same changes as the right (operated side) but to a definitely lesser degree. The section from the lower tip of the frontal pole, 4 cm. in front of the bed of the aneurysm, showed areas of necrosis and many haemorrhages, but 4 cm. more distally at the upper tip of the frontal pole there was little more than oedema. In each of two sections made 3 and 4 cm. in front of the Rolandic fissure respectively, there was found only one small focus of dead cells. Blocks taken from the motor and sensory cortex and including the gyrus cinguli on this side revealed perhaps a little oedema but no necrosis.

In Case 7 both anterior cerebral arteries were torn at the genu of the corpus callosum and death occurred thirty-three hours after operation. The following report was made on the microscopic studies of the left frontal lobe by Dr. Rich (the right frontal lobe had been removed in large part). The inferior portion of the left frontal lobe escaped infarction proximal to the ligation of the anterior cerebral artery except at the margins of the resected area where there was operative trauma. At the posterior margin of the operative site there was inflammation, haemorrhage, oedema and necrotic cells. A section 1 cm. posteriorly and 3 cm. in front of the Rolandic fissure showed a relatively large amount of well preserved brain surrounding foci of necrosis. Blocks made approximately 1.5 to 2 cm. in front of and behind the central fissure in the motor and sensory areas showed perfectly normal brain like the control sections.

In Case 6, in which only the gross specimen was examined, there was extensive necrosis of the mesial portions of both frontal lobes and of the white matter through the lobes and of the corpus callosum after fifteen days, but the greater part of the frontal lobes was surprisingly firm. Unfortunately, there is no microscopic study and a subsequent more careful review of the gross defects is not possible.

In each of the three cases there is a striking difference between the immediate and complete necrosis induced in the corpus striatum by occlusion of the medial striate arteries and the partial and delayed necrosis in the remaining distribution of the anterior cerebral arteries. The only conclusion can be that there is extensive collateral circulation between the middle and anterior cerebral arteries in the meninges over the cortex and no collateral in the vessels supplying the corpus striatum.

SUMMARY AND CONCLUSIONS

Ten cases are presented in which consciousness was immediately, almost totally and probably permanently lost after the following operative procedures: (1) resection of a frontal lobe (seven cases); (2) removal of tumors from the third ventricle (two cases); and (3) ligation of both anterior cerebral arteries at the internal carotids (one case). In four (4) of these cases the loss of consciousness lasted fifteen, seventeen, twenty-three and fifty-one days (until death) and is assumed to have been permanent.

In all of the seven frontal resections both anterior cerebral arteries wre sacrificed at the genu of the corpus callosum. In only two (Cases 6 and 7) of these brains have the basal ganglia been carefully studied (one microscopically). One of these showed direct trauma to the corpus striatum (right side) and the other showed necro-

sis of the same region (right side) from retrograde thrombosis of the anterior cerebral artery from the genu of the corpus callosum to the internal carotid artery, thus including the recurrent medial striate artery (Heubner) which supplies the anterior part of the corpus striatum. Until our attention was attracted to the basal ganglia we had been content to believe that bilateral ligations of the anterior cerebral arteries at the genu of the corpus callosum was adequate explanation for the loss of consciousness and had not carefully inspected the basal ganglia or the arterial supply. The brains have since been thrown away. We now know from other bilateral ligations of the anterior cerebral arteries at this point that deprivation of the blood supply of these vessels beyond the genu of the corpus callosum does not, per se, cause loss of consciousness.

In another case (10) both anterior cerebral arteries were ligated (clipped) at their origin from the internal carotid arteries and bilateral necrosis in the anterior portion of the corpora striata resulted and this, I think, is responsible for the loss of consciousness.

In each of the three carefully studied cases there was necrosis of the anterior part of the corpus striatum—one directly traumatic, the other two from deprivation of the blood supply. In none of the three specimens was the thalamus involved in the necrosis (two of these were microscopically studied).

In two of the ten reported cases, the same loss of consciousness followed removal of the tumors from the third ventricle and without injury of either anterior cerebral artery. These cases merely indicate that the center for consciousness is located somewhere in the basal ganglia or thalamus, but do not indicate the precise location. It is clear that in the 7 frontal lobectomies the injured part of the basal ganglia or of its blood supply must lie in the path of the resection and this could only be in the anterior part of the corpus striatum. The optic thalamus is posterior to this line of section and therefore not involved in the trauma.

The anterior part of the hypothalamus is also beyond the line of section of the frontal lobes and for that reason could not be involved.

In two of the three cases carefully examined, the lesion in the corpus striatum was strictly unilateral and on the right side; in the third it was bilateral. It is difficult to believe that a lesion of the left corpus striatum would not act similarly but our evidence does not cover this possibility.

REFERENCES

[2]Loss of consciousness does not follow ligations of both anterior cerebral arteries in dogs or monkeys (unpublished experiments).

[3]In none of the cases has there been an absolute loss of movement of the hands and feet but in all it has been within a fraction of totality. In cases 7 and 10 occasional movement of the hands to the face was a trifle more motor response than obtained in the remaining 8 cases.

[1]Alexander, L.: The vascular supply of the striopallidum. Ass. Res. Nerv. and Ment. Dis., 1942; xxi; 77.

[2]Ayer, J. B. and Aitken, H. F.: Brief on the arteries of the corpus striatum. Brit. Med. Surg. Jour., 1907; clvi; 768.

[3]Ayer, J. B. and Aitken, H. F.: A report on the circulation of the lobar ganglia. Brit. Med. Surg. Jour. (Supplement), 1909 (May), 160.

[4]Beevor, C. E.: On the distribution of the different arteries supplying the human brain. Phil. Trans. Roy. Soc. London, 1909; 200–1. Series B.

[5]Dandy, W. E.: Changes in our conceptions of localization of certain functions in the brain. Amer. Jour. of Physiol., 1930; xciii; 2.

[6]Fulton, J. F. and Bailey, P.: Tumors in the region of the third ventricle. Their diagnosis and relation to pathological sleep. J. Nerv. & Ment. Dis., 1929; lxix; 1–145–261.

[7]Gardner, W. J.: Removal of right cerebral hemisphere for infiltrating glioma: Report of Case. Journ. A.M.A., 1933; ci; 823.

[8]Globus, J. H.: Probable topographic relations of the sleep-regulating center. Arch. of Neurol. & Psychiat., 1943; xliii; 125.

[9]Hess, W.: The Autonomic Nervous System. Lancet, 1932; ii; 1199.

[10]Luksch, F.: Uber des Schlafzentrums. Zeitschr. f. d. ges. Neurol. u. psychiat., 1924; xciii; 83.

[11]Penfield, W.: Cerebral Cortex in Man: I. Cerebral Cortex and Consciousness. Archives of Neurology and Psychiatry, 1938; xl; 417.

[12]Poppen, J. L.: Ligation of the anterior cerebral artery. *Arch. Neurol. & Psychiat.*, xli; 495, 1939.

[13]Poppen J. L.: Ligation of the left anterior cerebral artery. Its Hazards and Avoidance of Complications. *Surg. Pract. Lahey Clinic*, 1941, p. 691.

[14]Ranson, S. W.: Somnolence Caused by Hypothalamic Lesions in the Monkey. *Arch. Neurol. & Psychiat.*, xli:1, 1939.

[15]Sinkler, W.: Tumor of the optic thalamus. *Tr. Am. Neurol. A.*, 1893, July 25, p. 48.

[16]Spiegel E. A. and Maba, C.: Zur zentralen Lokalisation von Storungen des Wachenzustands. *Ztschr. ges. exper. med.*, lv:164, 1927.

[17]Von Economo, C.: Theorie du Sommeil. *J. Neurol. et de Psychiat.*, xxviii: 437, 1928.

[18]Zollinger, R.: Removal of the left cerebral hemisphere. *Arch. Neurol. & Psychiat.*, xxxiv: 1055, 1935.

This Book

SELECTED WRITINGS OF WALTER E. DANDY

Compiled by

CHARLES E. TROLAND, M.D.
FRANK J. OTENASEK, M.D.

was set and printed by the Missourian Printing and Stationery Company of Cape Girardeau, Missouri. It was bound by the Becktold Company of St. Louis, Missouri. The engravings were made by the Capitol Engraving and Electrotype Company of Springfield, Illinois. The page trim size is 6¾ x 10 inches. The type page is 33 x 52 picas. The type face is Baskerville, set 10 on 12 point. The text paper is 70-lb. Hifect. The cover is Bancroft's Buckram 6470 (Maroon).

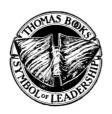

With **THOMAS BOOKS** *careful attention is given to all details of manufacturing and design. It is the Publisher's desire to present books that are satisfactory as to their physical qualities and artistic possibilities and appropriate for their particular use.* **THOMAS BOOKS** *will be true to those laws of quality that assure a good name and good will.*